MW01169996

GASTROENTEROLOGIC ENDOSCOPY

MICHAEL V. SIVAK, Jr., M.D.

Head, Section of Gastrointestinal Endoscopy
Department of Gastroenterology
Cleveland Clinic Foundation
Cleveland, Ohio

Rita Feran

Editorial Assistant

1987 W. B. SAUNDERS COMPANY
Harcourt Brace Jovanovich, Inc.
Philadelphia London Toronto
Montreal Sydney Tokyo

W. B. SAUNDERS COMPANY
Harcourt Brace Jovanovich, Inc.

West Washington Square
Philadelphia, PA 19105

Library of Congress Cataloging-in-Publication Data

Sivak, Michael V., Jr.

Gastroenterologic endoscopy.

1. Endoscope and endoscopy.   2. Gastrointestinal system—
   Diseases—Diagnosis.   I. Feran, Rita.   II. Title.
   [DNLM: 1. Endoscopy.   2. Gastrointestinal Diseases—
   diagnosis. WI 141 S624g]

RC804.E6S56 1987   616.3'307545   84–23519

ISBN 0–7216–1182–6

Editor: William Lamsback
Designer: Karen O'Keefe
Production Manager: Bob Butler
Manuscript Editors: Kate Mason and Charlotte Fierman
Illustration Coordinator: Walt Verbitski
Indexer: Linda Van Pelt

Gastroenterologic Endoscopy   ISBN   0–7216–1182–6

Last digit is the print number: 9   8   7   6   5   4   3   2

Dedicated to

Michael V. Sivak, Sr., M.D.
Benjamin H. Sullivan, Jr., M.D.

CONTRIBUTORS

JOHN I. ALLEN, M.D.
Assistant Professor of Medicine, University of Minnesota; Staff Physician, Veterans Administration Medical Center, Minneapolis, Minnesota
Endoscopy in the Postoperative Upper Gastrointestinal Tract

MILES O. AUSLANDER, M.D.
Assistant Clinical Professor of Medicine, University of California, Los Angeles, California
Endoscopic Photography

GEORGE BERCI, M.D.
Clinical Professor in Surgery, University of California, Los Angeles, School of Medicine; Associate Director, Department of Surgery, and Director, Division of Surgical Endoscopy, Cedars-Sinai Medical Center, Los Angeles, California
Emergency Laparoscopy

H. WORTH BOYCE, JR., M.D.
Professor of Medicine and Director, Division of Digestive Diseases and Nutrition, University of South Florida College of Medicine, Tampa, Florida
Hiatal Hernia and Peptic Diseases of the Esophagus; Special Varieties of Esophagitis

WILLIAM P. BOYD, JR., M.D.
Clinical Associate Professor of Medicine, Department of Internal Medicine, Division of Digestive Diseases, University of South Florida; Staff Physician, St. Joseph's Hospital, Tampa, Florida
Laparoscopy in Ascites and Peritoneal Diseases

WILLIAM D. CAREY, M.D.
Staff Physician, Department of Gastroenterology, The Cleveland Clinic Foundation, Cleveland, Ohio
Indications, Contraindications, and Complications of Upper Gastrointestinal Endoscopy

MEINHARD CLASSEN, M.D.
Professor of Medicine and Director of Medical Clinic II, Technical University, Munich, West Germany
Endoscopic Ultrasonography; Endoscopic Papillotomy

GIORGIO DAGNINI, M.D.
Head of the Laparoscopic Center, Hospital of Padua, Padua, Italy
Laparoscopy in Cirrhosis and Portal Hypertension

W. J. DODDS, M.D.
Professor of Radiology and Medicine, Medical College of Wisconsin, Milwaukee, Wisconsin
Sphincter of Oddi

D. ROY FERGUSON, M.D.
Staff Physician, Department of Gastroenterology, The Cleveland Clinic Foundation, Cleveland, Ohio
Indications, Contraindications, and Complications of ERCP

DAVID FLEISCHER, M.D.
Associate Professor of Medicine, Georgetown University School of Medicine, Washington, D.C.
Lasers and Gastrointestinal Disease

SOTARO FUJIMOTO, M.D.
Vice-Director, Department of Gastroenterology, Kyoto Second Red Cross Hospital, Kyoto, Japan
Peroral Cholangioscopy and Pancreatoscopy

J. E. GEENEN, M.D.
Clinical Professor of Medicine, Medical College of Wisconsin, Milwaukee; Director, Digestive Disease Center, St. Luke's Hospital, Racine, Wisconsin
Sphincter of Oddi

DAVID A. GILBERT, M.D.
Clinical Assistant Professor of Medicine, University of Washington School of Medicine; Chief, Division of Gastroenterology, Providence Medical Center, Seattle, Washington
Endoscopy in Gastrointestinal Bleeding

KOJI GOCHO, M.D.
Instructor of Surgery, St. Marianna University School of Medicine; Senior Staff, Second Department of Surgery, St. Marianna University Hospital, Kawasaki, Japan
Choledochofiberoscopy

DAVID Y. GRAHAM, M.D.
Professor of Medicine and Virology, Baylor College of Medicine; Chief, Digestive Disease Section, Veterans Administration Medical Center, Houston, Texas
Peptic Diseases of the Stomach and Duodenum

JAMES A. GREGG, M.D.
Assistant Clinical Professor of Medicine, Harvard Medical School; Active Staff, New England Deaconess Hospital and New England Baptist Hospital, Boston; Consulting Staff, Leonard Morse Hospital, Natwick, Massachusetts
The Intraductal Secretin Test

BERNARD H. HAND, M.S., F.R.C.S
(Deceased)
Anatomy and Embryology of the Biliary Tract and Pancreas

WILLIAM S. HAUBRICH, M.D.
Clinical Professor of Medicine, University of California, San Diego; Senior Consultant, Division of Gastroenterology, The Scripps Clinic and Research Foundation, La Jolla, California
History of Endoscopy

PROFESSOR DR. MED. HARALD HENNING
Faculty of Medicine, University of Hamburg; Clinic Foehrenkamp, Federal Institute for Salaried Employees' Insurance, Moelln, West Germany
Hepatomegaly and Inflammatory Disease of the Liver and Gallbladder

W. J. HOGAN, M.D.
Professor of Medicine, Medical College of Wisconsin; Chief, GI Diagnostic Laboratory, Froedtert Memorial Lutheran Hospital, Milwaukee, Wisconsin
Spincter of Oddi

RICHARD H. HUNT, M.B., F.R.C.P., F.R.L.P.(C)
Professor and Head, Division of Gastroenterology, McMaster University; Chief of Gastroenterology Service, McMaster University Medical Center, Hamilton, Ontario, Canada
Miscellaneous Disorders of the Colon

HIROSHI ICHIKAWA
Vice-President, Medical Instrument Division, Olympus Corporation, Lake Success, New York
Fiberoptic Instrument Technology

KAZUNORI IDA, M.D.
Professor, Ashai University; Chief of Department of Internal Medicine, Murakami Memorial Hospital, Gifu, Japan
Chromoscopy

NOBORU IIJIMA, M.D.
Emeritus Professor of Surgery, St. Marianna University School of Medicine, Kawaski, Japan
Choledochofiberoscopy

DAVID G. JAGELMAN, M.S.(Lon.), F.R.C.S.(Eng.), F.A.C.S.
Staff Surgeon, Department of Colorectal Surgery, The Cleveland Clinic Foundation, Cleveland, Ohio
Anoscopy

JARL Å. JAKOBSEN, M.D.
Staff, Department of Diagnostic Radiology, Ullevål Hospital, Oslo, Norway
The Intrahepatic Bile Ducts and Gallbladder

DENNIS M. JENSEN, M.D.
Associate Professor of Medicine, University of California, Los Angeles, School of Medicine; Gastroenterologist, University of California, Los Angeles, Center for the Health Sciences and Wadsworth Veterans Administration Medical Center, Los Angeles, California
Benign and Malignant Tumors of the Stomach

LAWRENCE F. JOHNSON, M.D.
Professor of Medicine, and Director, Digestive Disease Division, Uniformed Services University of the Health Sciences, Bethesda, Maryland; Chief, Gastroenterology Service, Walter Reed Army Medical Center, Washington, D.C.
Esophageal Motility and Miscellaneous Disorders

SHINOBU KAMEYA, M.D.
Associate Professor of Surgery, St. Marianna University School of Medicine; Associate Surgeon-in-Chief, Second Department of Surgery, St. Marianna University Hospital, Kawasaki, Japan
Choledochofiberoscopy

ICHIZO KAWAHARA
Executive Director of Endoscope Division, Olympus Optical Company, Ltd., Tokyo, Japan
Fiberoptic Instrument Technology

KEIICHI KAWAI, M.D.
Professor, Department of Preventive Medicine, Kyoto Prefectural University of Medicine, Kyoto, Japan
Peroral Cholangioscopy and Pancreatoscopy; Endoscopic Diagnosis of Cancer of the Pancreas

CHARLES J. LIGHTDALE, M.D.
Associate Professor of Clinical Medicine, Cornell University Medical College; Director, Diagnostic Gastrointestinal Unit, Memorial Sloan–Kettering Cancer Center, New York, New York
Indications, Contraindications, and Complications of Laparoscopy

BARRY J. LUMB, M.B., F.R.C.P.(C)
Assistant Professor of Medicine, Department of Gastroenterology, McMaster University; Staff, Hamilton Civic Hospitals, Hamilton, Ontario, Canada
Miscellaneous Disorders of the Colon

JAMES W. MANIER, M.D.
Clinical Professor of Medicine, University of New Mexico; Gastroenterologist, Lovelace Medical Center, Albuquerque, New Mexico.
Flexible Sigmoidoscopy

ARMANDO MARTI-VICENTE, M.D.
Chief, Laparoscopy Unit, Gastroenterology Service, Hospital Santa Crev i Sant Pau, Barcelona, Spain
Laparoscopy of Abdominal Tumors

MASATSUGU NAKAJIMA, M.D.
Guest Assistant Professor, Department of Preventive Medicine, Kyoto Prefectural University of Medicine; Director, Department of Gastroenterology, Kyoto Second Red Cross Hospital, Kyoto, Japan
Peroral Cholangioscopy and Pancreatoscopy; Endoscopic Diagnosis of Cancer of the Pancreas

H. JUERGEN NORD, M.D.
Professor of Medicine and Associate Director, Division of Digestive Diseases and Nutrition, University of South Florida College of Medicine; Chief, U.S.F. Gastroenterology Service, Tampa General Hospital; Attending Physician, H. Lee Moffitt Cancer Center and Research Institute and James A. Haley Veterans Administration Hospital, Tampa; Consulting Physician, Bay Pines Veterans Administration Hospital, St. Petersburg, Florida
Techniques of Laparoscopy

MELODY J. O'CONNOR, M.D.
Instructor of Surgery, University of Minnesota; Staff Physician, Veterans Administration Medical Center, Minneapolis, Minnesota
Endoscopy in the Postoperative Upper Gastrointestinal Tract

ROGER C. ODELL
Technical Products Manager, Surgical Products Division, Valleylab, Inc., Boulder, Colorado
Principles of Electrosurgery

MAGNE OSNES, M.D.
Professor of Medicine, University of Oslo; Staff, Department of Internal Medicine, Section for Gastroenterology, Ulleval Hospital, Oslo, Norway
The Intrahepatic Bile Ducts and Gallbladder

JOHN P. PAPP, M.D.
Associate Clinical Professor of Medicine, Michigan State University College of Human Medicine; Director, Endoscopy Unit, Blodgett Memorial Medical Center, Grand Rapids, Michigan
Endoscopic Treatment of Gastrointestinal Bleeding: Electrocoagulation

HARRISON W. PARKER, M.D.
Clinical Professor of Medicine, Medical College of Wisconsin; Director, Digestive Disease Unit, St. Joseph's Hospital, Milwaukee, Wisconsin
Congenital Anomalies of the Pancreas

JOHN L. PETRINI, JR., M.D.
Staff Physician, The Cleveland Clinic Foundation, Cleveland, Ohio
Video Endoscopy

DAVID A. PEURA, M.D.
Assistant Professor of Medicine, Uniformed Services University of the Health Sciences,

Bethesda, Maryland; Director of Clinical Services, Gastroenterology Service, Walter Reed Army Medical Center, Washington, D.C.
Esophageal Motility and Miscellaneous Disorders

JEFFREY L. PONSKY, M.D.
Associate Professor of Surgery, Case Western Reserve University School of Medicine; Director, Department of Surgery, Mt. Sinai Medical Center, Cleveland, Ohio
Percutaneous Endoscopic Gastrostomy

ASHLEY B. PRICE, B.M., F.R.C.(Path)
Consultant Histopathologist, Northwick Park Hospital, London, England
Colon Polyps and Carcinoma

GEORGE B. RANKIN, M.D.
Staff Physician, Department of Gastroenterology, The Cleveland Clinic Foundation, Cleveland, Ohio
Indications, Contraindications, and Complications of Colonoscopy

B. H. GERALD ROGERS, M.D.
Clinical Associate Professor, University of Chicago Pritzker School of Medicine; Attending Physician, Ravenswood Hospital, Consulting Physician, Augustana Hospital, Grant Hospital, and Henrotin Hospital, Chicago; Consulting Physician, Christ Hospital, Oak Lawn, Illinois
Disorders of the Large Bowel Having a Vascular Component

WOLFGANG RÖSCH, M.D.
Direktor der Medizinischen Klinik am Krankenhaus Nordwest der Stiftung Hospital zum Heiligen Geist, Frankfurt, West Germany
ERCP in Acute and Chronic Pancreatitis

YOSHIHIRO SAKAI, M.D., D.M.Sc.
Assistant Professor, Gastroenterology Department, Toho University School of Medicine; Chief of Gastroenterological Endoscopy, Ohashi Hospital, Tokyo, Japan
Technique of Colonoscopy

NOBUHIRO SAKAKI, M.D.
Lecturer, First Department of Internal Medicine, Yamaguchi University School of Medicine, Ube, Yamaguchi-prefecture; Chief, Gastrointestinal Unit, Department of Internal Medicine, Tokyo Metropolitan Komagome Hospital, Tokyo, Japan
High-Magnification Endoscopy

ROBERT A. SANOWSKI, M.D.
Clinical Professor of Medicine, University of Arizona College of Medicine, Tucson; Chief of Gastroenterology, Veterans Administration Medical Center, Phoenix, Arizona
Foreign Body Extraction in the Gastrointestinal Tract

MELVIN SCHAPIRO, M.D.
Associate Clinical Professor of Medicine, University of California, Los Angeles; Director, GI Diagnostic Laboratory, Valley Presbyterian Hospital, Van Nuys, California
Endoscopic Photography

BERNARD M. SCHUMAN, M.D.
Professor of Medicine, Medical College of Georgia; Attending Staff, Medical College of Georgia Hospital; Consultant, Augusta Veterans Administration Hospital, Augusta; Consultant, Eisenhower Hospital, Fort Gordon, Georgia
Disorders of the Duodenum

JAMES M. SENICK
Designer and Illustrator
The Endoscopy Unit

FRED E. SILVERSTEIN, M.D.
Associate Professor of Medicine, University of Washington School of Medicine; Director, Gastrointestinal Endoscopy Service, University Hospital, Seattle, Washington
Endoscopy in Gastrointestinal Bleeding

STEPHEN E. SILVIS, M.D.
Professor of Medicine, University of Minnesota; Chief, Special Diagnostic and Treatment Unit, Veterans Administration Medical Center, Minneapolis, Minnesota
Pancreatic Trauma, Ascites, Fistula, and Pseudocyst

MICHAEL V. SIVAK, JR., M.D.
Head, Section of Gastrointestinal Endoscopy, Department of Gastroenterology, The Cleveland Clinic Foundation, Cleveland, Ohio
The Endoscopy Unit; The Gastrointestinal Assistant; Introduction to Special Methods and Techniques in Gastroenterologic Endoscopy; Technique of Upper Gastrointestinal Endoscopy; Esophageal Varices; Indications, Contraindications, and Complications of ERCP; The Normal Retrograde Pancreatogram and Cholangiogram

IRENE M. SPADA, R.N.
Supervisor, Gastrointestinal Endoscopy Unit,

The Cleveland Clinic Foundation, Cleveland, Ohio
The Gastrointestinal Assistant

WOLF DIETER STROHM, M.D.
Director of Medical Clinic II, Academic Hospital of the University of Heidelberg, Heidelberg, West Germany
Endoscopic Ultrasonography

MASAHIRO TADA, M.D.
Instructor, Kyoto Prefectural University of Medicine; Director of Gastroenterology, Kyoto First Red Cross Hospital, Kyoto, Japan
Chromoscopy

TADAYOSHI TAKEMOTO, M.D.
Professor of Medicine, First Department of Internal Medicine, Yamaguchi University School of Medicine, Ubi, Yamaguchi-pref., Japan
High-Magnification Endoscopy

FRANCIS J. TEDESCO, M.D.
Professor of Medicine, Medical College of Georgia; Chief, Section of Gastroenterology, Department of Medicine, Medical College of Georgia Hospital and Clinics, Augusta, Georgia
Special Problems in Chronic Ulcerative Colitis

G. N. J. TYTGAT, M.D., Ph.D.
Professor of Gastroenterology, University of Amsterdam; Chief, Division of Gastroenterology-Hepatology, Academic Medical Center, Amsterdam, The Netherlands
Benign and Malignant Tumors of the Esophagus

JACK A. VENNES, M.D.
Professor of Medicine, University of Minnesota; Staff Physician, Section of Gastroenterology, Veterans Administration Medical Center, Minneapolis, Minnesota
Endoscopy in the Postoperative Upper Gastrointestinal Tract; Technique of ERCP

FRANCISCO VILARDELL, M.D., D.Sc.
Director, School of Gastroenterology, Universidad Autonoma; Chief, Gastroenterology Service, Hospital Santa Crev i Sant Pau, Barcelona, Spain
Laparoscopy of Abdominal Tumors

JEROME D. WAYE, M.D.
Clinical Professor of Medicine, Mount Sinai School of Medicine; Chief, Gastrointestinal Endoscopy Unit, Mount Sinai Hospital and Lenox Hill Hospital, New York, New York

Differential Diagnosis of Inflammatory and Infectious Colitis

WILFRED M. WEINSTEIN, M.D.
Professor of Medicine, Division of Gastroenterology, University of California, Los Angeles, School of Medicine; Attending Staff and Director, GI Procedures Unit, University of California, Los Angeles Medical Center, Los Angeles, California
Gastritis and Inflammatory Disorders of the Stomach

CHRISTOPHER B. WILLIAMS, B.M., F.R.C.P.
Consultant Physician, St. Mark's Hospital for Diseases of the Rectum and Colon and St. Bartholomew's Hospital, London, England
Colon Polyps and Carcinoma

DIETMER F. W. WURBS, M.D.
Dozent, Medizinische Fakultät, Universität Hamburg; Allgemeines Krankenhaus Barmbek-Gastroenterologie, Hamburg-Barmbek, West Germany
Calculus Disease of the Bile Ducts

ROBERT WYLLIE, M.D.
Staff Physician, Department of Pediatrics and Adolescent Medicine and Department of Gastroenterology, The Cleveland Clinic Foundation, Cleveland, Ohio
Esophagogastroduodenoscopy in the Pediatric Patient; Colonoscopy in the Pediatric Patient

KENJIRO YASUDA, M.D.
Staff, Department of Gastroenterology, Kyoto Second Red Cross Hospital, Kyoto, Japan
Endoscopic Diagnosis of Cancer of the Pancreas

A. ALBERT YUZPE, M.D., M.Sc., F.R.C.S.(C), F.A.C.O.G., F.A.C.S.
Professor of Obstetrics and Gynecology, The University of Western Ontario Faculty of Medicine; Chief of Gynecology, University Hospital, London, Ontario, Canada
Gynecologic Laparoscopy for the Gastroenterologist

DAVID S. ZIMMON, M.D.
Professor of Clinical Medicine, New York University School of Medicine; Co-Director, Hepatobiliary Unit, Beth Israel Hospital; Attending Physician, Medicine, Radiology and Surgery, St. Vincent's Hospital, New York, New York
Stenosis and Dilation of the Biliary and Pancreatic Ducts

PREFACE

My purpose in undertaking the editorship of this volume was to develop a standard reference that encompasses all gastrointestinal endoscopy. An additional goal was to present this knowledge in a global perspective with the recognition that there is great variability in the approach to endoscopic diagnosis, technique, and therapy throughout the world. I have taken the position that a textbook should not, perhaps cannot, define the correct and best solution to every problem. Rather, facts and information shall be presented in a judicious manner. Unfortunately, much of our knowledge must be termed empiric. This circumstance and my approach place a greater burden of discernment on the reader, although I trust that this will be a source of intellectual satisfaction as much as a challenge.

Expertise in gastrointestinal endoscopy inextricably blends the intellectual powers of observation and deduction with manual dexterity, experience, and judgment, the latter attribute being especially important in therapeutic endoscopy. True expertise, something beyond technical facility with an endoscope, is not easily achieved. It requires diligence and guidance and a strong foundation in basic endoscopic technique. The value of proper training in gastrointestinal endoscopy cannot be overstated, and the best form of instruction is that which one receives in a one to one relation with an expert endoscopist who has the innate ability and patience to train others. Apropos of teaching and expertise, I have dedicated this book in part to Dr. B. H. Sullivan, Jr. From him I have received many valuable things, the most important of which is the standard of integrity that he applied in the use of endoscopy. I also dedicate this volume to the memory of my father, Dr. Michael V. Sivak, Sr.

I am indebted to the numerous contributors to this book. For myself, and on behalf of all who will read and study this volume, I thank each of them for their efforts and for their willingness to communicate their knowledge to others. When I set out to write a first manuscript some years ago, I was aided by Ms. Rita Feran, who was at that time the medical editor for the Cleveland Clinic. She has been my assistant and a copy editor in this present work, which would not have come to fruition without her help. I offer a special thanks to my secretaries, Mrs. Jane Salamon and Mrs. Jeannie Bongorno, for their devotion and attention to detail, and also to the W. B. Saunders Company and my editors, Mr. William J. Lamsback and Mr. Carroll C. Cann, for the quality of their work and professionalism.

MICHAEL V. SIVAK, JR., M.D.

FOREWORD

This book is timely and impressive. We are all delighted that Michael Sivak has found the time, and skills, to conceive and deliver the state-of-the-art book on gastrointestinal endoscopy. He has persuaded many of the giants in the field, including several of the European and Japanese pioneers, to join with him in the enormous task of describing and assessing all of the techniques that are now available. It could not reasonably have been done before, since the subject has been developing continuously for over 20 years. Endoscopy has now come of age. The excitement and anxiety of youth have mellowed into the confidence of adulthood—with its attendant responsibilities. We can still find some new games to play, but the main task is to take stock, to provide efficient and effective services, and to provide the correct environment in which to train the next generation.

Three major issues now need to be addressed. The first is the importance of objective evaluation: real comparisons between endoscopy and related methods. Most assessments of endoscopic techniques are seriously flawed by personal bias, which is usually unconscious. All of us see what we wish to see, and indeed what we are asked to see. There are few thorough prospective or randomized studies, and long-term results of necessity cannot yet be given. Anecdotal assessments are marred by an "apples and oranges" problem; surgeons, radiologists, and medical endoscopists deal with different types of patients (as they should do if the referral system is intelligent) so that each may be correct even when they disagree.

The second issue is interrelated—to whom does the endoscope "belong"? As therapeutic applications have burgeoned and encroached upon orthodox surgery, so the limits of the gastroenterologist's training and competence are often stretched, and may be over-reached. Endoscopic therapy can be thought of simply as a new development in surgery—so it is not surprising that surgeons wish to be involved. Rather than continue this argument, which interferes with efficient clinical services, it seems better to ignore or break down the time-honored barriers and look for increasing integration between medical and surgical gastroenterology, with overlapping facilities and teaching programs. With a team approach, the endoscopist's actual label becomes less important.

The third issue concerns the relationship between endoscopy and academic gastroenterology. Much has been written on this subject, often with unhelpful vehemence. The existence of separate endoscopic and gastroenterology societies in many countries emphasizes and will continue to foster an artificial division; the endoscope is a tool, not a trade. The time spent in endoscopic training and in the performance of procedures encroaches on many other aspects of the subject, and the potential for fiberscopes to be used in basic research is virtually untapped.

Gastrointestinal endoscopy has grown from a sapling to a sturdy tree. All those interested in the field will be glad to own and study this intricate drawing of the tree as it stands in 1987. New shoots will appear and some branches will wither as alternative methods blossom. Future health and strength depend upon ensuring that the roots are well embedded in clinical and academic gastroenterology.

PETER B. COTTON, M.D., F.R.C.P.
Professor of Medicine
Chief of Endoscopy
Duke University Medical Center
Durham, North Carolina

CONTENTS

Section I

GENERAL TOPICS

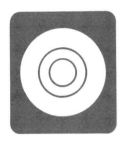

Chapter 1

HISTORY OF ENDOSCOPY

WILLIAM S. HAUBRICH, M.D.

The word *endoscopy* is derived from the Greek by combining the prefix *endo-*, "within", and the verb *skopein*, "to view or observe." The result is an apt term for the procedure of peering into the recesses of the living body. But there is more to the term than that. *Skopein* means not merely to look at something but rather to view with a purpose, to observe with intent, to monitor. The ancient Greeks had no equivalent for "endoscopy" but, being clever and wise, they would have understood its modern meaning and likely would have admired its choice.

INCEPTION OF GASTROINTESTINAL ENDOSCOPY

The original concept of using a tube to peer into the hidden cavities of the living human body is easily understood, but the technical difficulties that confronted early investigators may be difficult for modern physicians to comprehend. First was the matter of design. Few channels and cavities in the living body lend themselves to inspection by a simple, straight, rigid probe. Second was a lack of suitable materials with which to construct an endoscope. In the early 19th century metals were available, but machines to fashion metals of high tensile strength were relatively crude. Rubber was known but in short supply, and the process of vulcanization, whereby rubber is rendered strong and elastic, was not discovered until 1839. Plastics as we know them were unheard of. Third, and the greatest impediment, was a lack of adaptable light. Before the invention of the incandescent bulb, the only convenient source of artificial light was that from a burning candle, an oil or gas lamp, or an exposed, glowing platinum wire. This was the setting in which gastrointestinal endoscopy had its humble beginnings.[1]

The earliest recorded attempt at endoscopy was by Phillip Bozzini[2] of Mainz and Frankfurt who, in 1806, devised a tin tube illuminated by a wax candle fitted with a mirror. He tried to peer into the urinary tract. On hearing of this, the medical faculty at Vienna derisively dismissed the preposterous idea of "a magic lantern in the human body."

EARLY ATTEMPTS AT GASTROSCOPY

Adolf Kussmaul, a German physician who lived from 1822 to 1902 and is perhaps better remembered for his description of air-hunger as a symptom of diabetic acidosis, is generally credited with fashioning and employing what might be called the first gastroscope in 1868. In a plethora of publications related to the gastrointestinal tract, it is curious that he hardly mentioned work with a gastroscope. For an account of his work one must turn to the recollections of others.[3] Kussmaul's instrument was a straight, rigid, metal tube, passed over a previously inserted flexible obturator (Fig. 1–1A). The light source was a Desmoreaux lamp (Fig. 1–1B) that burned a mixture of alcohol and turpentine, illumination being concentrated by a reflector and a lens. The first subjects for experimentation were recruited from the ranks of sword-swallowers. Legend has it that one of the first recruits balked when he saw the prototype instrument, exclaiming, "I'll swallow a sword anytime, but I'll be damned if I'll swallow a trumpet!" Needless to say, Kussmaul's tube, while marking an epoch, was hardly practical.

The first clinician to consider seriously the special requirements of a workable gastro-

2

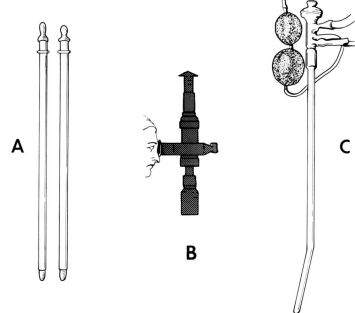

FIGURE 1–1. *A,* Kussmaul's original simple tubular endoscope with obturator in place (1868). *B,* Desmoreaux's lamp, which provided endoscopic illumination, of a sort, before the advent of the incandescent electric bulb. *C,* Mikulicz's rigid, angled gastroscope (1881); note the provision of a rubber bulb for insufflation of air. (Excerpted from Walk, L. The history of gastroscopy. Clio Medica 1965; 1:209–22.)

scope was Johann von Mikulicz-Radecki (1850–1905), a Polish surgeon more remembered for a variety of innovative operations. Mikulicz understood that the longitudinal axis of the esophagus is not the same as that of the stomach. Therefore, in 1881, he reported the design of a tube, 65 cm long and 14 mm in diameter, that was slightly angled in its distal fourth, employed an optical system, and was equipped to insufflate air (Fig. 1–1C).[4]

Illumination was originally supplied by an electrically activated, glowing, platinum wire, but this was soon replaced by a miniature incandescent globe (then called a "Mignon Lampchen" and devised by Max Nitze, developer of the first useful cystoscope). It was with this type of instrument, later refined by others, notably Rosenheim,[5] Kelling,[6] and Elsner[7] (see Fig. 1–2A), that the first informative views of the intact, living esophagus and stomach were obtained. A Cleveland surgeon, F. C. Herrick, in 1911 proposed intraoperative gastroscopy—inserting a modified cystoscope through a small gastrotomy—as a means of locating a site of bleeding in the stomach.[8] Among the early accounts of peroral gastroscopy in the United States are those by Chevalier Jackson[9] of Philadelphia and by Janeway and Green[10] of New York.

To understand the compulsion of early investigators to find a means, however crude, of diagnosing diseases of the stomach, one must remember that the earliest efforts to develop gastroscopy preceded the advent of gastrointestinal fluoroscopy and radiography. The remarkable power of x-rays was discovered by Wilhelm Roentgen in 1895.

At the juncture of the 19th and 20th centuries, the most notable accomplishments in endoscopy were by German physicians. The reason was the technical supremacy in optics and instrument manufacture by German artisans. However, these skills were soon mastered by American craftsmen, among the foremost being Reinhold Wappler of New York, who later organized American Cystoscope Makers, Incorporated, now better known by the acronym ACMI.

LAPAROSCOPY

Laparoscopy has had almost more names than early promoters. This method, by which the contents of the abdominopelvic cavity can be visualized telescopically, has also been termed *peritoneoscopy, organoscopy,* and *coelioscopy*—all meaning the same thing—to name but a few. No single name has yet gained universal usage, but "laparoscopy" has the advantage of historical precedence. It is the term commonly used in Europe and Asia and is gaining acceptance in the United States, especially by gynecologists who now utilize the procedure more often than internists or surgeons.

In 1902, Georg Kelling[11] reported at Hamburg to the 73rd meeting of a group known as German Natural Scientists and Physicians his observations of the abdominal viscera of a dog by means of a Nitze cystoscope. In the same year Dimitri Ott,[12] a Russian gynecologist, deliberately introduced a speculum into the pelvic cavity of a female patient through an incision in the posterior vaginal fornix. He referred to the procedure as "ventroscopy." Working independently in Sweden, H. D. Jacobaeus[13, 14] reported his use of the procedure in human patients and in 1912 proposed the term *laparoscopy*. Thereafter, Kelling and Jacobaeus long disputed the priority of discovery. In what may have been among the earliest efforts at medical cost containment, Kelling[15] in 1923 wrote that he used "coelioscopy" as a means of sparing his poor German patients, then in the depths of economic depression, the expense of surgical laparotomy.

Use of the procedure in the United States was first reported in 1911 by Bertram Bernheim,[16] a surgeon at the Johns Hopkins Hospital in Baltimore. He had inserted a proctoscope with a half-inch bore through the abdominal wall of a jaundiced patient and confirmed the presence of a Courvoisier gallbladder. Benjamin Orndoff[17] of Chicago used a similar device for what he called "peritoneoscopy" and published the first report of an extensive experience. Meanwhile, the procedure became widely applied in Europe, where Korbsch[18] published his *Lehrbuch und Atlas der Laparo- und Thorakoskopie* in 1927. Heinz Kalk, a renowned German proponent of laparoscopy, culminated a series of publications with his "Lehrbuch," written in collaboration with Egmont Wildhirt in 1961,[19] which emphasized the additional benefit of guided liver biopsy.

John Ruddock[20] of Los Angeles was almost a lone champion of the procedure in the United States during the 1930's. Ruddock used a modified cystoscope in hundreds of cases and proposed a number of therapeutic applications. After World War II, with the renewed importation of refined German instruments and the arrival of physicians trained in their use, laparoscopy won new adherents. Quick to perceive the value of laparoscopy were gynecologists whose specialty now comprises the largest number of laparoscopists in the United States. Prominent among endoscopically oriented gynecologists is Peter Steptoe[21] of England, who found laparoscopy essential in his development of the technique that has resulted in the current "test tube baby" boom.

CHOLEDOCHOSCOPY

Just as early clinicians were stimulated to develop gastroscopy because of dissatisfaction with palpation of the abdomen (before the era of radiographic examination), so surgeons, not content with palpating the bile ducts at operation, have sought a better means of detecting lesions within these ducts. George Berci[22] has outlined the development of endoscopy as applied to the biliary tree.

The first to attempt a view inside the living common bile duct was Bakes,[23] a German surgeon, who reported his findings in 1923. Bakes is better known as the surgeon who devised the graduated probes commonly used at operation to dilate the common duct and ampulla of Vater. A right-angled telescope specifically constructed for the common bile duct was reported by McIver[24] in 1941, and improved instruments were described 20 years later by Wildegans[25] and by Berci.[26] Predictably, fiberoptic technology was soon applied in choledochoscopy,[27] but there was then a return to the use of a rigid instrument equipped with prisms and lenses,[28] because it was more wieldy and conveyed a brighter, clearer image. This is one of the few instances in the development of endoscopy wherein the rigid lens system has prevailed over the flexible fiberoptic system.

With the demonstrated feasibility in the intact patient of cannulating the ampulla of Vater with a catheter for the purpose of radiography, it was inevitable that substitution of a small caliber fiberoptic endoscope would be proposed. Indeed, Nakajima et al.[29] reported this remarkable feat in 1978. They modified a duodenoscope (the "mother scope") by enlarging the bore of its catheter channel to 2.8 mm. They were able to pass through this channel a 2.3 mm fiberoptic endoscope (the "baby scope"), which could then be guided under direct vision into either the common bile duct or the pancreatic duct. Because the exceedingly fine caliber of the probing endoscope could contain only 3000 fibers and because the view was through a fluid medium, the image lacked the clarity associated with other endoscopic techniques. Although peroral cholangiopancreatoscopy has not gained widespread use, its accomplishment is nonetheless recognized as a tour de force.

THE REMARKABLE CAREER OF RUDOLF SCHINDLER

With the use of instruments such as those devised by Mikulicz and by Elsner,[7] Rudolf Schindler embarked on his career of lifelong dedication to the advancement of gastroscopy. Why is the career of Schindler so pivotal? Because this one man, almost single-handedly, provided an impetus for the method when the ranks of other erstwhile proponents were in disarray. Moreover, this one man sparked the promotion of gastrointestinal endoscopy throughout Europe and, later, in the United States. One can argue that there would have been others, sooner or later, who would have played the same role. Doubtless this is true, but it is also beside the point. Schindler was the man.

Rudolf Schindler was born in Berlin on May 10, 1888, the son of a banker and an artistically gifted mother who encouraged his early interests in classical music, poetry, and natural history. A fascination with marine biology and the collection of sea shells became a lifelong hobby. Young Schindler's decision to study medicine, we are told by Audrey Davis[30] (whose perceptive account of Schindler's career is recommended to the reader, along with that by Martin Gordon and Joseph Kirsner[31]), derived from his respect and admiration of his maternal uncle Richard Simon, a Berlin ophthalmologist.

On graduation from the University of Berlin, Schindler undertook a rural practice of medicine that was soon interrupted by service as a medical officer in the German army during World War I. In this setting he observed the prevalence of alimentary ailments in both the military and civilian populations, and he became convinced that much digestive debility could be attributed to morbid changes in the gastric mucosa, undetectable by conventional methods of diagnosis. The only answer, Schindler concluded, would emerge from direct observation of the internal milieu of the living stomach—in short, by gastroscopy.

On his return to practice, Schindler attended patients at the Munich-Schwabing Hospital, where, in 1920, he acquired a rigid Elsner gastroscope that had been discarded by someone whose interest had flagged. With this instrument and a later model modified according to Schindler's own suggestions (Fig. 1–2A, B), both constructed by the Munich firm of Reiniger, Gebbert, and Schall, Schindler performed hundreds of gastroscopic examinations, carefully documenting each procedure. Often gastroscopy was repeated in the same subject so as to observe the evolution of mucosal lesions. Nor did Schindler neglect to scrutinize the normal

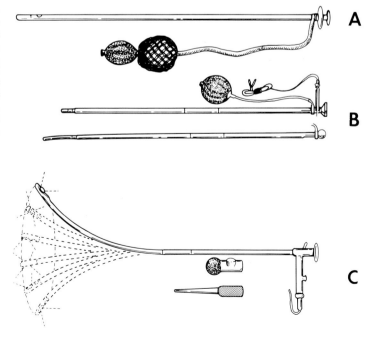

FIGURE 1–2. Early gastroscopes devised by Elsner in 1911 (A) and modified by Schindler in 1922 (B); the diameter of both was 11 mm. C, Schindler's semiflexible gastroscope, introduced in 1932. The original model had a sponge rubber ball at the tip, which Schindler later found to be a hazard; it was replaced by a tapered, finger-like rubber tip. (Excerpted from Walk L. The history of gastroscopy. Clio Med 1965; 2:209–22.)

A

B

C

stomach. He is said to have examined the stomach of his surprisingly willing housekeeper on a number of occasions. This early work, conducted with meticulous care and often in an atmosphere of hostility to the procedure, culminated in the publication in 1923 of Schindler's monumental *Lehrbuch und Atlas der Gastroskopie*.[32] This exposition, like none before it, elicited serious interest in gastroscopy by clinicians the world over. In the era before intragastric photography became feasible, gastroscopic images were vividly rendered by colored drawings or paintings, usually by professional artists who peered through the endoscope, but sometimes by the examining physicians themselves. Both Schindler's 1923 classic and the atlas compiled in 1937 by Kurt Gutzeit and Heinrich Teitge[33] can still be perused for delight and instruction, especially for their depiction of stomach lesions now seldom seen.[34]

Meanwhile, Schindler was far from satisfied with the efficacy and safety of the rigid gastroscope. He devoted himself to the design of an instrument that could be inserted with less discomfort and risk to the patient and that would provide a clearer, more extensive view of the gastric mucosa. Schindler was joined in this effort by Georg Wolf, a skilled Berlin instrument maker. The collaborative effort of Schindler and Wolf, even though marked by occasional moments of dissension, is a prime example of the alliance between clinician and engineer needed to bring to fruition new and useful ideas in the advancement of diagnostic and therapeutic instrumentation.

The idea shared by Wolf and Schindler was to construct an optical gastroscope wherein the light rays that conveyed the image could be made to follow a flexible arc. The optical principle of the articulated prisms and lenses within a bendable tube had been established by Michael Hoffmann[35] in 1911, but its incorporation in a workable endoscope proved difficult. Wolf had contrived a prototype offered for use in the inspection of condensing tubes in steam engines (today fiberscopes are used to inspect the inner mechanisms of many types of machinery). He first proposed and constructed an optical gastroscope that was flexible throughout its length, but Schindler had the better idea of combining a rigid proximal half with a flexible distal half, thus producing a more wieldy instrument that conveyed a brighter, clearer image. The result was the famous Wolf-Schindler semiflexible gastroscope, first produced in 1932 (Fig. 1–2C). In retrospect, what was considered "semiflexible" by the examiner probably was felt to be "semirigid" by the examinee.

With this instrument, Schindler[36] was able to announce to the medical world the advent of an acceptably safe, workable instrument capable of conveying informative images of the stomach's interior to the eye of the examining physician (Fig. 1–3). Schindler's achievement was readily recognized, and clinicians flocked to Munich to observe and learn the new technique. Of these, Schindler acknowledged the following workers as most influential in propagating the method: Francois Moutier of France (who published his own *Traite de gastrocopie et de pathologie endoscopique de l'estomac*[37] in 1935), Norbert Henning of Leipzig, and Kurt Gutzeit of Breslau. Among Schindler's American students were Samuel Weiss, a New York gastroenterologist, and Edward Benedict, a Boston ear-nose-and-throat surgeon. It should be mentioned that in certain prominent centers, such as the University of Pennsylvania and the Mayo Clinic, peroral endoscopy was considered in those early days to be solely in the province of what was called broncho-esophagology.

With the darkening clouds of Nazism hovering over Germany, Rudolf Schindler, whose father was Jewish, was subjected to increasing persecution by the anti-Semitic regime. He was befriended by two American colleagues, Dr. Marie Ortmayer and Dr. Walter Lincoln Palmer, who had visited Schindler's Munich clinic in the 1920's. Hearing of his plight, they invited Schindler to come to the University of Chicago as a visiting professor. In 1934 Schindler managed his escape to the United States where he found an opportunity to practice and teach his endoscopic method at the Billings Hospital. His publications, now in English, proliferated. Walter Palmer provided unstinting assistance to Schindler in publishing his textbook *Gastroscopy* in 1937. This, with subsequently revised editions[38] appearing in 1950 and 1966, was the gospel of gastroscopy for a generation of clinicians. It is worthy of note that Schindler subtitled his book, *The Endoscopic Study of Gastric Pathology*. By this, Schindler made clear his belief in the endoscopic method as an approach to an understanding of diseases and to the care of patients, not as

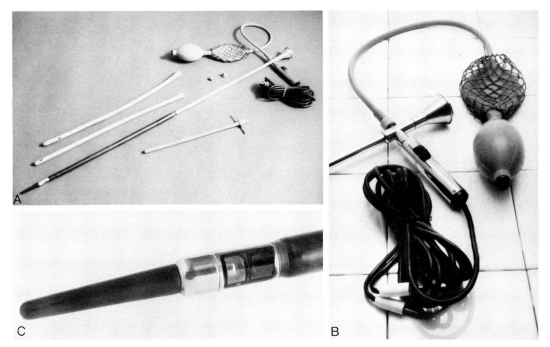

FIGURE 1–3. *A*, Schindler semiflexible gastroscope with accessories. *B*, Proximal viewing end with insufflation bulb and electrical connection. *C*, Distal end of semiflexible gastroscope. Note side-viewing optical design and tapered rubber tip. (*C*, Courtesy of Dr. Eric Lee).

an end in itself. Schindler always considered himself to be first a physician and only secondarily one who was skilled in technology.

On settling in Chicago, Schindler ever sought to improve the design and construction of the gastroscope. He allied himself with William J. Cameron, whose Cameron Surgical Company became the world's largest supplier of illuminated instruments. On Cameron's staff was a talented instrument maker, Louis Streifeneder, with whom Schindler developed a close rapport. With the supply of German equipment cut off during World War II, the Cameron Omniangle gastroscope, modeled closely after the original Wolf-Schindler design, became the standard instrument used in many clinics in the United States. Streifeneder later formed his own firm, the Eder Instrument Company, that continues a tradition of meticulous workmanship, now mainly directed to the production of laparoscopes.

In 1943, Schindler departed from Chicago to reside in Los Angeles, where he taught at the College of Medical Evangelists (now Loma Linda University) and later served as consultant at the Long Beach Veterans Administration Hospital, where his principal coworkers were Dr. Stephen Stempien and

Dr. Angelo Dagradi. At age 70 Schindler learned Portuguese and accepted an appointment to the faculty of the University of Minas Gerais at Belo Horizonte, Brazil. His wife's ill health necessitated a return to the United States in 1960.

No account of Schindler's career would be complete without mention of his wife Gabrielle (née Winkler), to whom he was wed in 1922. The use of the rigid and the semiflexible gastroscopes required an assistant who could hold and manipulate the patient's head. Moreover, it was the assistant who closely monitored the patient's reaction to examination and who sought to soothe the patient's apprehension and discomfort. Although untrained as a nurse, Gabrielle learned to perform the function of gastroscopic assistant to perfection (Fig. 1–4). It is said that on the rare occasion when Gabrielle was unavailable to assist him, Schindler declined to perform gastroscopy.

From 1960 to 1965, Schindler again served as consultant at the Long Beach Veterans Hospital. On him was bestowed the first Schindler Award by the American Society for Gastrointestinal Endoscopy in 1962. That occasion was his last attendance at an annual meeting of the group he had originally

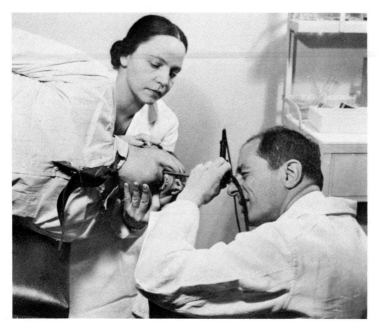

FIGURE 1–4. The Schindler team at work at the University of Chicago Clinics, about 1940. Rudolf Schindler peers through his semiflexible gastroscope as Gabrielle Schindler exhibits her art of head-holding. Note that her left index finger aids the drainage of oropharyngeal secretions. (Courtesy of Dr. Martin Gordon. From Gordon ME, Kirsner JB. Rudolf Schindler, pioneer endoscopist; glimpses of the man and his work. Gastroenterology 1979; 77: 354–61. Reproduced by permission.)

founded as the American Gastroscopy Club in 1941. His beloved Gabrielle died in 1964. Schindler then married Marie Koch, a friend of long standing from Munich, and in 1965 returned to that city where much of his early work had been accomplished. He occupied himself by preparing an atlas based on his lifetime performance of 10,300 gastroscopic examinations. Also, he found time to enjoy his music and his shell collection. Rudolf Schindler died of heart disease in Munich in 1968.[39]

Gastroscopy as it Was Performed During the Era of Rudolf Schindler

Perhaps the reader will find of interest a brief account of what it was like to perform gastroscopy in the era before the advent of fiberoptic instruments. In most centers, the procedure was considered an unusual diagnostic step to be undertaken only by an examiner rigorously trained and especially devoted to the method. The patient was carefully selected, his or her need for gastroscopy always being predicated on a previous barium meal radiographic examination. There was no talk of gastroscopy being a first-line diagnostic venture in those days, with the possible exception of the "vigorous diagnostic approach" to the bleeding patient as advocated by Dr. E. D. Palmer.[40]

Premedication usually consisted of intramuscular injection of a short-acting barbiturate. Atropine often was added to reduce gastric secretion and motility. The lens-system gastroscope was not equipped with a suction channel, this being the reason why the patient's stomach had to be emptied by an Ewald tube before the endoscope was inserted. A specially tilted table was provided for this purpose. If one followed Schindler's carefully specified method, the patient's throat was anesthetized by the injection of a numbing solution through a 25 cm rubber tube with side openings at its distally tapered end. This tube, when fully inserted, extended through the upper esophageal sphincter. This maneuver had the further advantage of slightly dilating the sphincter, thus facilitating the passage of the gastroscope.

An experienced and sturdy nurse-assistant held the head of the patient, who lay in the left lateral decubitus position. The operator's index and middle fingers guided the soft, tapered, rubber tip of the gastroscope into the proximal esophagus. The assistant then firmly and fully extended the patient's neck so as to provide a straight mouth-throat-esophageal channel, allowing smooth passage of the endoscope into the stomach. Needless to say, one hoped for an edentulous patient, whose mouth would more easily accommodate the instrument and who was without front teeth to grate on the proximal steel rod of the fully inserted gastroscope.

The semiflexible instruments employed a

side-viewing objective which provided no view of the esophagus either on insertion or on withdrawal (Fig. 1–5). Esophagoscopy required a quite different instrument and was an altogether separate procedure (Fig. 1–6). Once the gastroscope was within the stomach, air was insufflated. The distal half of the instrument, with its lenses and prisms in a rubber sheath, was partially flexible to accommodate the contours of the stomach wall, but its flexion was uncontrollable by the examiner. One could, however, precisely manipulate the torque of the instrument; the external handle, carrying electric current to the small incandescent light bulb at the distal tip, always pointed in the direction of the objective. Thus, orientation of the view in the stomach was precise. The problem was that inspection of the stomach lining was somewhat limited. The pylorus was usually seen, but never transgressed; the lesser curve of the antrum was a "blind area," as was the mucosa lying at the very tip of the endoscope.

The examiner had to be content with relatively fleeting glimpses. Discomfort to the patient, with his rigidly extended neck, hardly encouraged a leisurely look. Moreover, the gastroscopist's visual impression usually had to suffice. Photography through the instrument was managed by only a few accomplished operators.[41] There was no provision for the insertion of a biopsy forceps, except in the special "operating gastroscope" devised by E. B. Benedict,[42] an instrument found too cumbersome by most gastroscopists.

Thus it was that gastroscopy was performed in the decades from the 1930's to the 1960's. Despite the formidability of the instruments then available, complications were relatively rare, doubtless because of the caution sternly inculcated in practitioners of the art.[43] But such constraints may explain why, as late as 1966, there were only 268 members of the American Society of Gastrointestinal Endoscopy.

THE BRIEF BUT ILLUMINATING ERA OF THE GASTROCAMERA

An impediment to the appreciation of early gastroscopy was that views of the internal milieu of the stomach, and such lesions as it might bear, were limited to the visual cognizance of the examiner or to such fleeting glimpses as he might permit an observer peering over his shoulder. In a way, this was an advantage to the endoscopist; he could wax eloquent about what he saw, and none could dispute him. As might be expected,

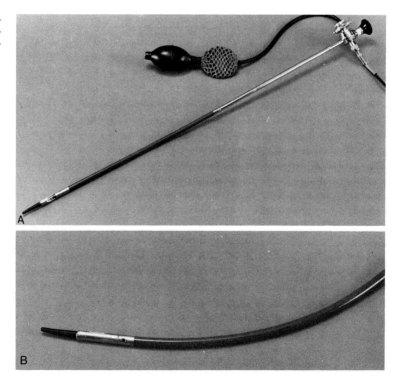

FIGURE 1–5. A, Eder-Palmer semiflexible gastroscope. Note side-viewing optics. B, Eder-Palmer instrument with tip deflected.

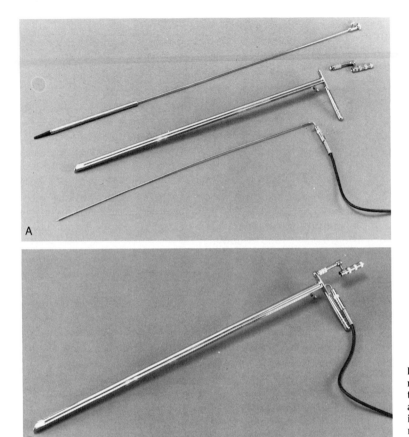

FIGURE 1–6. A, Eder-Hufford rigid esophagoscope. Note (from top to bottom) the obturator, lens assembly, examination tube, and illumination rod. B, Eder-Hufford rigid esophagoscope assembled for use.

skeptics abounded, especially when the topic was gastritis.

The first challenge to endoscopic interpretation was the use of the gastric mucosal biopsy tube devised by Ian Wood et al.[44] of Australia. The pathologist then had a section of tissue, albeit minute; the endoscopist had no documentation other than his mental image, often imperfectly recollected.

The 19th century invention of photography provided a means of recording a permanent image but, because of obvious technical inadequacies, it was long before this could be adapted to endoscopy. Lange and Meltzing[45] actually tried in 1898 to reproduce black-and-white photographic images obtained at gastroscopy, but a lack of sufficient light and the slowness of then available emulsions discouraged further use of the method.

Another idea was to construct a miniature camera, small enough to be swallowed by the patient and attached to a tube through which the camera could be controlled and retrieved by the operator (Fig. 1–7). This was a concept

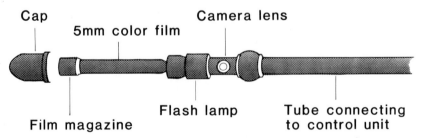

FIGURE 1–7. Diagram of disassembled distal tip of the gastrocamera apparatus. At the proximal end of the connecting tube was a control unit and rubber bulb for air insufflation of the stomach. (Adapted from Perna G, Honda T, Morrissey JF. Gastrocamera photography. Arch Intern Med 1965; 116:434–41.)

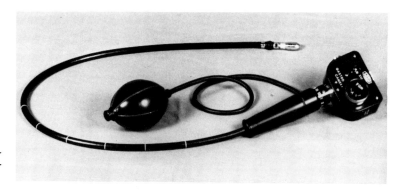

FIGURE 1–8. Early model gastro-camera manufactured by Olympus Optical Co.

ideally suited to implementation by the Japanese. Thus was developed a workable gastrocamera by Tatsuno Uji[46] in collaboration with his engineering colleagues at the Olympus Optical Company (Figs. 1–8 and 1–9).

Dr. John Morrissey[47] has related the story of how Dr. Yoshio Hara brought the first gastrocamera to the University of Wisconsin in 1962. Hara had come to the Madison campus to study cancer chemotherapy. He happened to bring along a set of vivid, full-color photographs of lesions as they appeared in the living stomach. He brought, too, the tiny camera that had captured them. Morrissey was quick to recognize the utility of the instrument and became adept in its use. Soon scores of students journeyed to Madison, eager to become gastrophotographers. Gastrocameras, gastroprojectors, and gastroscreens soon proliferated across the land (though never in the same numbers as in Japan where, according to Morrissey, in 1966 there were 10,000 gastrocameras taking pictures in half a million subjects annually).

While no finer photographs of the intact stomach have ever been obtained with any other means (the reader is invited to inspect the color plates in Morrissey's 1965 article[48]), the early gastrocamera had a major disadvantage: The operator could not see what he had photographed until the film was developed. Pictures (32 exposures on a roll of 5 mm film) were taken in rote sequence (Fig. 1–10).[49] If all went well, this produced a fairly complete survey of the stomach lining. But a gastroscope was needed to obtain a visual image. The answer: Attach the gastrocamera to a gastroscope. This was done in 1963.

FIGURE 1–9. Later gastrocamera model GTF-A manufactured by Olympus Optical Co. Note small 5 mm film cartridge placed near the distal tip of the instrument.

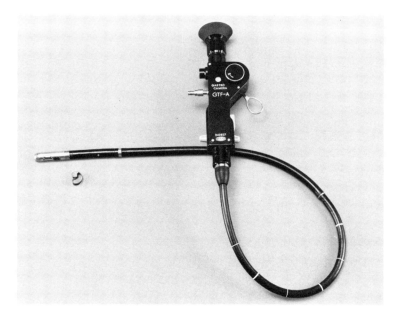

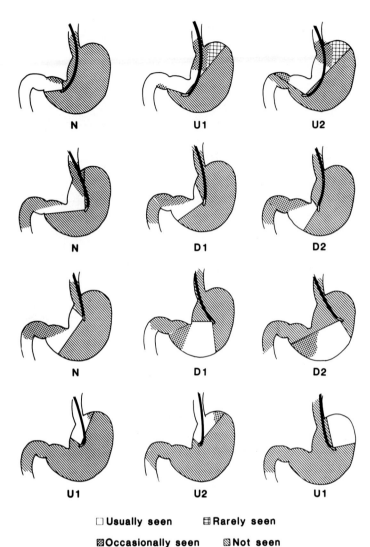

N   U1   U2

N   D1   D2

N   D1   D2

U1   U2   U1

□ Usually seen   ⊞ Rarely seen

▨ Occasionally seen   ▧ Not seen

FIGURE 1–10. Scheme of the prescribed sequence in which gastrocamera photographs were taken. The tip of the tube containing the miniature camera was first placed in the gastric antrum. N indicates the neutral position; U1, U2, D1, and D2 indicate flexion of the tip up (U) or down (D), 15 degrees or 35 degrees. The sequence was repeated as the tube was moved proximally. (Adapted from Perna G, Honda T, Morrissey JF. Gastrocamera photography. Arch Intern Med 1965; 116:434–41.)

However, as the optical system of the fiberscope was rapidly improved, it soon thereafter became much easier for most endoscopists to simply attach an external 35 mm camera to the eyepiece of the gastroscope and photograph the image conveyed by the fiber bundle. Insertion of the miniature camera into the colon was suggested,[50] but then came the colonoscope. Ease of use won over fidelity. The gastrocamera, marvelous as it was, became obsolete.

ADVENT OF FIBEROPTICS

A Transatlantic Coalition

The modern era of fiberoptic gastrointestinal endoscopy might be said to have dawned on a wintry day in Ann Arbor, Michigan, when Basil Hirschowitz picked up the January 1954 issue of *Nature*. What caught his eye were two articles on the optical properties of fine glass fibers. One of them in particular, by Hopkins and Kapany[51] of the Imperial College of Science and Technology in England, fired his imagination of how an endoscopic image might be transmitted by a bundle of fully flexible glass fibers from the alimentary tract of a patient to the eye of an examiner. The ensuing events have been described by Hirschowitz himself in a delightful account.[52]

That light would follow the curved path of a stream of water pouring from a tank was first demonstrated by John Tyndall, a British physicist, in 1870. The idea of using flexible glass fibers to propagate light was proposed in patent applications by J. L. Baird of England in 1927 and by C. W. Hansell of the United States in 1930. Schindler credited Heinrich Lamm[53] with being the first to recommend the adaptation of fiberoptics to gastroscopy. Unfortunately, Schindler gave no further thought to the matter, because he was then preoccupied with developing his system of lenses and prisms, which he knew to be feasible.

Light-carrying bundles of glass fibers are of two types: incoherent and coherent. Incoherent or random bundles intended only to transmit illumination are easily constructed. Construction of a coherent bundle intended to convey an image, wherein many thousands of fibers must be arrayed in precisely the same order at both ends of the bundle, is quite another matter. Any appreciable leakage of light from one fiber to another defeats the purpose of the coherent bundle. This principal impediment to the development of a fiberscope was overcome by Lawrence Curtiss, then an undergraduate physics student at the University of Michigan. Curtiss invented a process whereby an individual, fine fiber of optical glass could be clad in a layer of glass of lower refractive index, thus providing the fiber with an insulating coat. Hirschowitz, with whom Curtiss collaborated, credits this as the single most important innovation in the advancement of fiberoptic endoscopy.[54]

DEVELOPMENT OF THE FIBEROPTIC ENDOSCOPE

A prototype fiberscope, adapted for gastroscopy, was finally constructed at Ann Arbor in February, 1957. Hirschowitz manfully undertook to be the first to swallow this oversized worm. Unscathed, within a few days he performed the first fiberoptic gastroscopy at the University Hospital, the examinee being a young woman who harbored a duodenal ulcer. Hirschowitz demonstrated his instrument to a small, polite, but less than enthusiastic audience at the annual session of the American Gastroenterological Association later that year.[55]

I recall having been shown this prototype instrument on a visit to Hirschowitz' laboratory. It was rigged so as to convey the visage of Abraham Lincoln that adorned a 5 cent stamp. Peering into the fiberscope, I could not deny recognizing Lincoln, but the quality of the image reminded me of a picture I had seen of prototype television images displayed in the 1920's. Vivid it was not. Comparing this with the image then obtained by the lens-and-prism gastroscope, I confess I saw little future in fiberoptic endoscopy (Plate 1–1). A remarkable accomplishment, I thought, but little will come of it (Figs. 1–11 and 1–12). Now, along with thousands of other endoscopists the world over, I rejoice in my lack of prescience.

It was not until the latter 1960's that meticulous technicians, both Japanese and American, succeeded in refining construction of the first workaday fiberoptic endoscopes. Among notable improvements were those in optical clarity, in wieldiness and manipulability of the distal tip, and in provision of channels for biopsy and therapeutic maneuvers. The Japanese were especially intent on this work because of their need to precisely diagnose gastric cancer.

The first fiberoptic instrument to gain widespread use in the United States was the esophagoscope with a working length of 75 cm. This had the advantage of an end-viewing objective rather than the side-viewing objective with which Hirschowitz' early fiberscope was equipped. To those of us who previously had been obliged to attempt endoscopy of the esophagus by means of a straight, rigid, steel tube, the fiberoptic esophagoscope was a marvel. Equally pleased with this new instrument, I am sure, were our patients. Soon thereafter, the fiberoptic bundle was extended to a working length of 110 cm, and we had an easily insertable instrument with which the esophagus, stomach, and duodenum could be scrutinized, all in the same procedure. It took some of us a while to adapt our orientation in the stomach from the side-viewing to the end-viewing objective. Moreover, the earlier fiberoptic gastroscopes lacked a capacity for responsive torque, and this hampered precise control.

These and other deficiencies were promptly corrected in later models. In fact, improvements in endoscope design were so numerous and rapid during the early 1970's that one could hardly purchase a new instrument and become acquainted with its use before that instrument was rendered obsolete by a new model. Refinements will continue, no doubt, but the ungainly instrument that had its inauspicious beginning in the corner of a physics laboratory at Ann Arbor has, for a full generation, notably advanced the man-

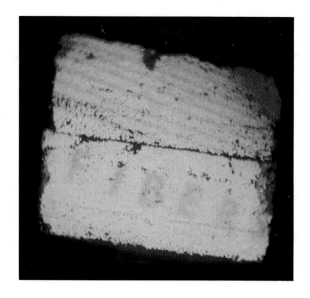

PLATE 1–1. Photograph of image with the first laboratory-made fiberscope, constructed by Basil I. Hirschowitz, Larry Curtiss, and C. Wilbur Peters at the University of Michigan in January, 1957. The fiber bundle was made in two halves, accounting for the dark line across the middle. The photograph was made with an Exacta 35 mm camera which is still used by Dr. Hirschowitz. (Courtesy of Dr. Hirschowitz.)

PLATE 1–2. Early prototype fiberoptic sigmoidoscope developed at the Illinois Institute of Technology Research. (Courtesy of Dr. Bergein Overholt.)

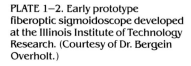
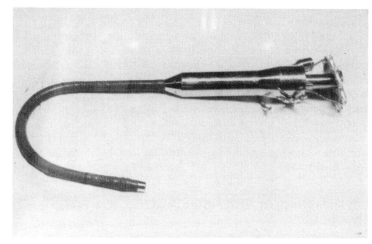

PLATE 1–3. Prototype fiberoptic sigmoidoscope made by the Eder Instrument Co. (Courtesy of Dr. Bergein Overholt.)

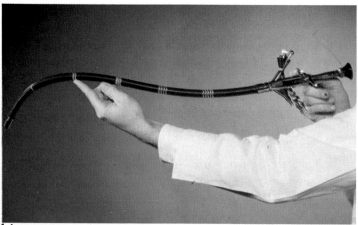

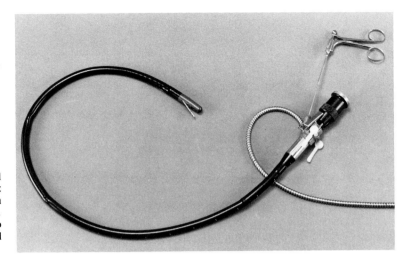

FIGURE 1–11. An early model flexible fiberoptic Hirschowitz endoscope made by American Cystoscope Makers, Inc. (ACMI). Note passage of biopsy forcep through accessory channel, and the side-viewing optics.

agement of patients with gastrointestinal disease.

COLONOSCOPY

The success of fiberoptic endoscopy perorally naturally led to its adaptation for insertion at the nether end of the alimentary tract. Specula for examination of the anus and rectum had been in wide use since well before the turn of the century. For practical purposes, the maximum length of a straight, tubular proctosigmoidoscope had been found to be 25 cm. The tortuosity of the sigmoid colon was far beyond the turning capacity of a lens-and-prism endoscope. Even

the early fiberscope could not be properly advanced in a retrograde fashion into the colon. For the development of a workable, fiberoptic colonoscope, we return to the University of Michigan at Ann Arbor.

According to Bergein F. Overholt,[56] who pioneered in the development of fiberoptic colonoscopy, the work was stimulated by an unusually disagreeable proctosigmoidoscopic examination suffered by the person of Dr. J. Howard Gowan. In 1961, Overholt was an intern at the University Hospital in Ann Arbor; as part of his application for a U.S. Public Health Service fellowship, he was interviewed by Gowan, who had just undergone a somewhat trying physical check-up at

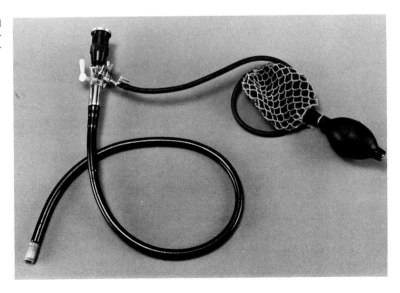

FIGURE 1–12. An early model flexible fiberoptic LoPresti endoscope made by American Cystoscope Makers, Inc. (ACMI).

the hospital. Being well-acquainted with the principles of fiberoptics, Overholt commented on the prospect of a more comfortable sigmoidoscopic procedure. Others, of course, had been tempted to set aside esthetics and insert the fiberoptic gastroscope in the anus (this procedure was later reported).[57] All manner of contrivance had been suggested to pull through the colon a fiberscope hooked onto the end of a swallowed string. But, just as the peculiar anatomy of the proximal alimentary tract had posed a problem for Kussmaul and the earliest would-be gastroscopists, so did the serpentine anatomy of the sigmoid colon present a problem to would-be colonoscopists.

Overholt, with the support of Dr. H. Marvin Pollard,[58] strived to overcome this difficulty, at first with the aid of a reverse silicone cast that reproduced the tortuous lumen of the rectosigmoid segment. There was a brief period of minor excitement in the late 1950's when silicone rubber casts of the rectosigmoid colon were conceived as a means of detecting colonic lesions. It was from such a cast that Overholt devised his life-like model. This permitted the proper adjustments in a fiberscope for torque and control that resulted in a prototype instrument that was first employed clinically in 1963 (Plates 1–2 and 1–3). Further refinement was required, and it was not until the 1967 meeting of the American Society for Gastrointestinal Endoscopy that Overholt described, to a somewhat skeptical audience, his experience in examining his first 40 patients.[59] This event took place at the same locale where Hirschowitz, also representing the University of Michigan, had first described fiberoptic gastroscopy exactly 10 years earlier. Meanwhile, Japanese workers were busily engaged in improving the colonoscope and advancing its clinical application.[60, 61]

Colonoscopy gained rapid acceptance by clinicians who had been recently introduced to the marvel of fiberoptic gastroscopy, although most operators soon found that successful colonoscopy was much more demanding than gastroscopic examination of the proximal alimentary tract. In England, Christoper Williams[62] and in the United States Hiromi Shinya[63] and Jerome Way[64] were among the early developers and most proficient teachers of colonoscopy. Thus, an additional important segment was placed within the purview of the gastrointestinal endoscopist.

ENDOSCOPIC RETROGRADE CHOLANGIOPANCREATOGRAPHY (ERCP)

The intricacies of the bile ducts and, particularly, the pancreatic duct long had intrigued physicians. The fascinating story of visualizing the biliary tree begins in 1924 with the demonstration by surgeons Evarts Graham and Warren Cole that intravenously administered iodinated phenolphthalein was selectively excreted in bile. However, even with the later use of improved agents, the radiographic image of the biliary tree was faint, and the pancreatic duct defied radiographic demonstration. In 1955 Doubilet et al.[65] described intraoperative pancreatography, but what was needed was a means of obtaining an image of the pancreatic duct without surgical intervention. In 1965 Rabinov and Simon[66] reported cannulation of the duodenal ampulla by a catheter manipulated under fluoroscopic guidance. Their painstaking procedure was successful in only one of eight patients.

Why not guide a cannula into the ampulla under endoscopic control? This was first accomplished by William S. McCune and his associates[67] at George Washington University in 1968. Again, it remained for the Japanese to perfect the technique that was described by Oi and his coworkers[68, 69] in 1970 and by Kasugai et al.[70] in 1972. Foremost among the proponents in the United States of this endoscopic technique were Jack Vennes and his colleagues[71] at the Minneapolis Veterans Administration Hospital. For his masterful teaching of the technique, Vennes received the 1978 Schindler Award of the American Society for Gastrointestinal Endoscopy.[72]

THERAPEUTIC ENDOSCOPY

Throughout much of the history of the development of endoscopy, endoscopists well understood the meaning of Mark Twain's complaint, "Everybody talks about the weather, but nobody does anything about it!" Endoscopists could regale their associates with descriptions of what they saw, but they were relatively powerless to intervene. Now the prospect has vastly changed.[73]

True, the early broncho-esophagologists, who employed rigid tubes, were fond of extracting foreign bodies that had been inadvertently or deliberately choked down by unfortunate patients. I recall well the astonishing display of trophies of incredible variety, extracted from various recesses, that lined the walls of the Chevalier Jackson Broncho-Esophagology Clinic at the Graduate Hospital in Philadelphia. Endoscopists no longer so decorate their workplaces, but the ingenious application of a variety of techniques employing fiberoptic endoscopy has expanded this mode of intervention.[74]

The therapeutic procedure most widely used by endoscopists, and probably that of greatest benefit to patients, is polypectomy. I remember having been in the audience at the meeting of the American Gastroenterological Association at Miami in 1971 when Shinya and Wolff showed motion pictures depicting the innovative technique of colonoscopic polypectomy.[63] Viewers were enthralled as they watched the improvised snare approach the polyp. A spontaneous cheer erupted when the polyp, severed, was seen to topple from its pedicle. How many patients have been since saved from carcinoma by having benign polyps removed from segments of the gastrointestinal tract accessible to fiberoptic endoscopy has yet to be proved, but surely benefit has accrued.

Control of active bleeding from lesions within the range of endoscopy, by electrocoagulation, heater probe, or laser, is the subject of ongoing investigation. No longer are strictures in the alimentary tract merely observed; they are now effectively dilated under endoscopic guidance. Even more dramatic is the endoscopic intervention in cases of calculous disease in the biliary and pancreatic ducts. Many of the pioneering and most knowledgeable investigators in these fields present the work in the following chapters.

Sometimes what looms on the horizon and may seem new turns out not to be new at all. Knowledge of what has gone before can improve one's perspective. This is illustrated by another means of endoscopic therapy. Endoscopic sclerosis of esophageal varices is not new; interest in the procedure is merely renewed. This method was first reported by Clarence Crafoord and Paul Fleckner[75] in Europe in 1939 and, a few years later, from the United States by Herman Moersch[76] and by Cecil Patterson and Milford Rouse.[77] They all announced favorable results in the short term.

What can we learn from the history of endoscopy? Two recurring themes stand out. First, almost without exception, advances in endoscopy have come about by virtue of a close collaboration between clinician and artisan; neither could have succeeded alone. Second, those clinicians who have notably contributed to endoscopy were invariably seeking an answer to a broader medical problem; none thought of himself as merely a technician pursuing technology as an end in itself.

History is looked upon as a humanistic discipline, but it has an essential role, too, in the advancement of science. To know the history of endoscopy is to pay tribute to those who have cleared the path we now tread, to understand the impediments that have been overcome, to appreciate more fully the facility we now enjoy, and to point to the prospect of still more marvelous advances to come.

References

1. Walk L. The history of gastroscopy. Clio Med 1965; 1:209–22.
2. Bozzini PH. Lichtleiter, eine Erfindung zur Anschauung innere Teile und Krankheiten. J Prakt Heilk 1806; 24:207.
3. Killian G. Zur Geschichte der Oesophago- und Gastroskopie. Dtsch Z Chir 1901; 58:499–512.
4. Mikulicz J. Ueber Gastroskopie und Oesophagoskopie. Wien Med Presse 1881; 52:1629.
5. Rosenheim T. Ueber die Beschtigung der Kardia nebst Bemerkungen über Gastroskopie. Dtsch Med Wochnschr 1895; 21:740–4.
6. Kelling G. Endoskopie fur Speiserohre und Magen. München med Wochnschr 1897; 44:934–7.
7. Elsner HD. Ein Gastroskop. Klin Wochenschr 1910; 47:593–5.
8. Herrick FC. Profuse recurrent gastric hemorrhage, with report of cases and description of an instrument for viewing the gastric interior at operation. Cleveland Med J 1911; 10:969–76.
9. Jackson C. Tracheobronchoscopy, esophagoscopy, and gastroscopy. St. Louis: Laryngoscope Co., 1907.
10. Janeway HH, Green N. Esophagoscopy and gastroscopy. Surg Gynecol Obstet 1911; 13:245–53.
11. Kelling G. Ueber Oesophagoskopie, Gastroskopie, und Kölioskopie. Münch med Wochenschr 1902; 49:21.
12. Ott DO. Die Beleuchtung der Bauchhöhle Ventroskopie als Methode bei vaginaler Koliötomie. Centralbl Gynäkol 1902; No. 31, 817–20.
13. Jacobaeus HC. Ueber die Möglichkeit die Zystoskopie bei Untersuchung seroser Hohlungen anzuwenden. Münch med Wochenschr 1910; 58:2090–2.
14. Jacobaeus HC. Ueber Laparo- und Thorakoskopie. Beitr Klin Erforsch Tuberk 1912; 25:183.
15. Kelling G. Koelioskopie und Gastroskopie. Arch Klin Chir 1923; 136:226–8.
16. Bernheim BM. Organoscopy; cystoscopy of the abdominal cavity. Ann Surg 1911; 53:764–7.
17. Orndoff BH. The peritoneoscope in diagnosis of diseases of the abdomen. J Radiology 1920; 1:307–5.
18. Korbsch R. Lehrbuch und Atlas der Laparo- und Thorakoskopie. Munich: IF Lehmann V, 1927. 58 pp.
19. Kalk H, Wildhirt E. Lehrbuch und Atlas der Lapa-

roskopie und Leberpunktion. Stuttgart: George Thieme, 1962, 247 pp.

20. Ruddock JC. Peritoneoscopy. Surg Gynecol Obstet 1937; 65:629–39.

21. Steptoe PC. Laparoscopy in gynaecology. Edinburgh: E. & S. Livingstone Ltd., 1967. 93 pp.

22. Berci G. Choledochoscopy. In: Berk JE et al., eds. Bockus's Gastroenterology, 4th ed. Philadelphia: W. B. Saunders Co., 1985.

23. Bakes J. Die Choledochlopapilloskopie nebst Bemerkungen über Hepaticusdrainage und Dilatation der Papill. Archiv Klin Chir 1923; 126:473–83.

24. McIver MA. An instrument for visualizing the interior of the common duct at operation. Surgery 1941; 9:112–4.

25. Wildegans H; Die operative Gallengangendoskopie. Munich: Urban & Schwartzenberg, 1960.

26. Berci G. Choledochoscopy: the exploration of the extrahepatic biliary system under visual control; preliminary report. Med J Australia 1961; 2:862–3.

27. Shore JM, Lippman HN. Operative endoscopy of the biliary tract. Ann Surg 1962; 156:951–5.

28. Shore JM, Berci G. The clinical importance of cholangiography. Endoscopy 1970; 2:117–20.

29. Nakajima M, Akasaka Y, Yamaguchi K, et al. Direct endoscopic visualization of the bile and pancreatic duct systems by peroral cholangiopancreatoscopy (PCPS). Gastrointest Endosc 1978; 24:141–5.

30. Davis AB. Rudolf Schindler's role in the development of gastroscopy. Bull Hist Med 1972; 46:150–70.

31. Gordon ME, Kirsner JB. Rudolf Schindler, pioneer endoscopist; glimpses of the man and his work. Gastroenterology 1979; 77:354–61.

32. Schindler R. Lehrbuch und Atlas der Gastroskopie. Munich: IF Lehmann, 1923. 132 pp.

33. Gutzeit K, Teitge H. Die Gastroskopie: Lehrbuch und Atlas. Berlin: Urban & Schwartzenberg, 1937. 342 pp.

34. Palmer ED. Gutzeit and Teitge revisited. Gastrointest Endosc 1977; 23:244.

35. Hoffmann M. Optische Instrumente mit beweglicher Achse und ihre Verwendlung fur die Gastroskopie. München med Wochenschr 1911; 58:2446–8.

36. Schindler R. Ein vollig ungefahrliches flexibles Gastroskop. München med Wochenschr 1932; 79: 1268–9.

37. Moutier F. Traite de gastroscopie et de pathologie endoscopique de l'estomac. Paris: Masson, 1935.

38. Schindler R. Gastroscopy: the endoscopic study of gastric pathology. Chicago: University of Chicago Press, 1937; revised 1950; 2nd ed., New York: Hafner Publishing Co., 1966.

39. Dagradi AE, Stempien SJ. In memoriam: Rudolf Schindler. Gastrointest Endosc 1968; 15:121.

40. Palmer ED. Clinical Gastroenterology, 2nd ed. New York: Hoeber Med Div, Harper & Row, 1963; 233–4.

41. Nelson RS. Routine gastroscopic photography. Gastroenterology 1956; 30:661–8.

42. Benedict EB. An operating gastroscope. Gastroenterology 1948; 11:281–3.

43. Schindler R. Results of the questionnaire on fatalities in gastroscopy. Am J Dig Dis 1940; 7:293–5.

44. Wood IJ, Doig RK, Motteram R, et al. Gastric biopsy. Lancet 1949; 1:18–21.

45. Lange FM, Meltzing D. Die Photographie des Ma-

genintern. München med Wochenschr 1898; 45:1585–8.

46. Uji T. The gastrocamera. Tokyo Med J 1952; 61:135–8.

47. Morrissey JF. Gastrointestinal endoscopy; 20 years of progress. Gastrointest Endosc 1983; 29:53–6.

48. Morrissey JF. The use of the gastrocamera for the diagnosis of gastric ulcer. Gastroenterology 1965; 48:711–7.

49. Perna G, Honda T, Morrissey JF. Gastrocamera photography. Arch Intern Med 1965; 116:434–41.

50. Matsunaga F, Jsushima H, Kuboto T. Photography of the colon. Gastroenterol Endosc (Japan) 1959; 1:58–63.

51. Hopkins HH, Kapany NS. A flexible fiberscope, using static scanning. Nature (London) 1954; 173:39–41.

52. Hirschowitz BI. A personal history of the fiberscope. Gastroenterology 1979; 76:864–9.

53. Lamm H. Biegsame optische Gerate. Z Instrumentenk 1930; 50:579.

54. Curtiss LE, Hirschowitz BI, Peters CW. A long fiberscope for internal medical examinations. J Am Optical Soc 1956; 46:1030.

55. Hirschowitz BI, Curtiss LE, Peters CW, et al. Demonstration of a new gastroscope, the "fiberscope." Gastroenterology 1958; 35:50–3.

56. Overholt BF. The history of colonoscopy. In: Hunt RH, Waye JD, eds. Colonoscopy: Techniques, Clinical Practice, and Colour Atlas. London: Chapman and Hall, Ltd., 1981. (Distributed in U.S. by Yearbook Medical Publishers.)

57. Lemire S, Cocco AE. Visualization of the left colon with the fiberoptic gastroduodenoscope. Gastrointest Endosc 1966; 13:29–30.

58. Pollard HM. Presentation of 1975 Schindler Award to B. F. Overholt. Gastrointest Endosc 1975; 22:62–3.

59. Overholt BF. Clinical experience with the fibersigmoidoscope. Gastrointest Endosc 1968; 15:27.

60. Oshiba S, Watanabe A. Endoscopy of the colon. Gastroenterol Endosc (Tokyo) 1965; 7:440–2.

61. Niwa H. Endoscopy of the colon. Gastroenterol Endosc (Tokyo) 1965; 7:402–8.

62. Williams CB, Muto T. Examination of the whole colon with the fibreoptic colonoscope. Br Med J 1972; 3:278–81.

63. Wolff WI, Shinya H. Colonofiberoscopy. JAMA 1971; 217:1509–12.

64. Waye JD. Colonoscopy. Surg Clin North Am 1972; 52:1013–24.

65. Doubilet H, Poppel MH, Mulholland JH. Pancreatography: technics, principles, and observations. Radiology 1955; 64:325–39.

66. Ravinov KR, Simon M. Peroral cannulation of the ampulla of Vater for direct cholangiography and pancreatography; preliminary report of a new method. Radiology 1965; 85:693–7.

67. McCune WS, Shorb PE, Moscovitz H. Endoscopic cannulation of the ampulla of Vater: a preliminary report. Ann Surg 1968; 167:752–6.

68. Oi I, Kobayashi S, Kondo T. Endoscopic pancreatocholangiography. Endoscopy 1970; 2:103.

69. Oi I. Fiberduodenoscopy and endoscopic pancreatocholangiography. Gastrointest Endosc 1970; 17:59–62.

70. Kasugai T, Kuno N, Kobayashi S, et al. Endoscopic pancreatocholangiography. I. The normal endo-

scopic pancreatocholangiogram. Gastroenterology 1972; 63:217–26.

71. Vennes JA, Silvis SE. Endoscopic visualization of bile and pancreatic ducts. Gastrointest Endosc 1972; 18:147–52.

72. Silvis SE. Presentation of 1978 Schindler Award to Jack Vennes. Gastrointest Endosc 1978; 24:263.

73. Soergel KH, Hogan WJ. Therapeutic endoscopy. Hosp Pract 1983; 18:81–92.

74. Vizcarrondo FJ, Brady PG, Nord HJ. Foreign bodies of the upper gastrointestinal tract. Gastrointest Endosc 1983; 29:208–10.

75. Crafoord C, Frenckner P. Nonsurgical treatment of varicose veins of the esophagus. Acta Otolaryngol 1939; 27:422–9.

76. Moersch HJ. Further studies on the treatment of esophageal varices by injection of a sclerosing solution. Ann Otol Rhinol Laryngol 1941; 50:1233–44.

77. Patterson CO, Rouse MO. Injection treatment of esophageal varices. JAMA 1946; 130:384–6.

Chapter 2

FIBEROPTIC INSTRUMENT TECHNOLOGY

ICHIZO KAWAHARA*
HIROSHI ICHIKAWA†

PRINCIPLES OF FIBEROPTICS

Principle of Total Internal Reflection

The heart of the flexible fiberoptic endoscope is the image-carrying fiber bundle which transmits the image through the instrument. This bundle contains tens of thousands of individual, ultra-thin glass fibers. The ability of the individual fiber to transmit efficiently the light entering the distal end of the fiber without substantial loss of brightness or change in color and without leakage of light from one fiber to adjacent fibers is basic to the development of fiberoptic instruments.

The phenomena of refraction and reflection (Fig. 2–1) explain why light can be transmitted through flexible glass fibers. Figure 2–1 shows two transparent substances. The lower substance can be assumed to be glass with a refractive index of n. The upper substance may be either air or glass of a different composition possessing a lower refractive index n'. A ray of light traveling through the lower medium and hitting the boundary surface at point P with incident angle A (Fig. 2–1a) will be refracted and travel through the upper transparent medium at angle B. The relationship between angles A and B is given by the equation

$$n \sin A = n' \sin B.$$

As the angle of incidence A is increased, the angle of the refracted ray B also increases, according to the above relationship. When A equals A_c (known as the "critical angle" of incidence), the refracted ray will travel along the boundary surface. The critical angle for any two substances is found by setting B = 90° (Sin B = 1). In this case,

$$\sin A_c = \frac{n'}{n}$$

If the angle of incidence is increased further to A_o, since A_o is greater than A_c, the ray is totally reflected at the boundary surface back into the lower medium. The angle of reflection always equals the angle of incidence. It is this condition of "total internal reflection" that enables glass fibers to transmit light. Total internal reflection can occur only when the ray is incident on a medium whose index is less than that of the medium in which the ray is traveling.

Optical Fibers

A long, cylindrical glass fiber will transmit light if its surface is clean and it is surrounded by a medium with a lower refractive index (Fig. 2–2a). However, any debris on the surface of the fiber, or any contact of the fiber

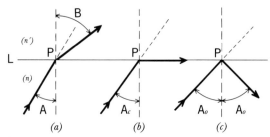

FIGURE 2–1. Phenomenon of refraction and reflection of light by a plane surface. See text for explanation.

---

*Executive Director, Olympus Optical Co., Ltd.
†Vice President, Olympus Corporation.

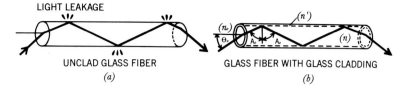

FIGURE 2–2. Path of light ray through an (A) unclad and (B) clad glass fiber.

LIGHT LEAKAGE

UNCLAD GLASS FIBER
(a)

GLASS FIBER WITH GLASS CLADDING
(b)

with adjacent fibers or other objects will disturb the boundary condition and prevent total internal reflection from occurring at that point on the surface. These conditions will result in leakage of light from the fiber, a loss in transmission, and the transfer of light from the fiber to other objects with which it comes in contact. To prevent this and to ensure a proper boundary surface, all glass fibers used for fiberoptics are clad with a very thin layer of glass (Fig. 2–2b). The cladding glass has a lower index than the core glass, a condition that guarantees total internal reflection of all rays traveling through the core glass.

A ray incident on the face of the fiber at angle θ_o (Fig. 2–3) will be refracted and travel through the core at angle A_o. At point P_1 on the boundary surface, it undergoes total internal reflection. It undergoes a second reflection at point P_2 and continues onward down the fiber, reflecting each time that it hits the boundary surface. As the angle of incidence θ_o on the face of the fiber is increased, the angle of internal reflection decreases until A_o equals A_c, the critical angle for internal reflection (see Fig. 2–3). The angle representing the maximum incidence angle for total internal reflection is referred to as the maximum acceptance angle, θ_c. A_c is a function of n and n', the index of the glass used in the core and cladding, respectively.

$$\sin A_c = \frac{n'}{n}$$

A ray incident on the boundary at an angle less than A_c will not undergo reflection but will be refracted through the cladding, out through the side of the fiber, and will be lost.

A calculation of the value of θ_c will show that it is dependent on the index of the core, cladding, and medium at the face of the fiber.

$$n_o \sin \theta_c = \sqrt{(n)^2 - (n')^2} = \text{N.A.}$$

N.A. is the numerical aperture of the fiber and equals $\sin \theta_c$ when the face of the fiber is in contact with air ($n_o = 1$ for air). The greater the difference between n and n', the greater the numerical aperture and the larger the cone of light that the fiber will accept and transmit. Because of production limitations on the glasses used for the core and cladding, the N.A. of optical fibers is generally limited to 0.52. By calculation with the above formula, θ_c (the maximum acceptance angle) is 31° for a fiber with this N.A. Light entering at angles greater than this angle will not undergo internal reflection, but will pass out through the side of the fiber.

In practice, not all light entering the face of the fiber at incident angles less than the maximum acceptance angle of incidence θ_c will be transmitted and exit at the other end of the fiber. Light transmission is also decreased by the following factors.

1. Absorption by the core glass. This loss is proportional to both the length of the fiber and the length of the path light takes within the fiber. The greater the length of the fiber and the number of internal reflections, the

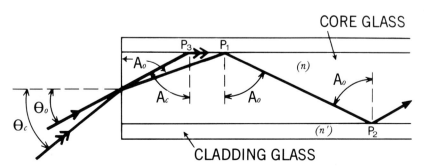

CORE GLASS

CLADDING GLASS

FIGURE 2–3. Total internal reflection and maximum acceptance angle of incidence, θ_c. See text for explanation.

greater the length of the optical path; therefore, the greater will be the absorption of the light as it passes through the fiber.

2. Although the preceding discussion indicated that at angles greater than A_c the light will be totally reflected, in practice this reflection is not 100%. The small amount of refraction or scattering that takes place is insignificant for one reflection. However, because the light may be reflected tens of thousands of times in traveling one meter, a small loss at each reflection point results in a measurable loss at the end of the fiber. Fibers of small diameter and long length have the greatest loss of this type.

3. Loss at the surface of both ends of the fiber. Some of the light falling on the surface of the fiber will be reflected by the surface instead of entering the fiber. Also, light falling on the cladding and the space between individual fibers grouped into a bundle will not be transmitted.

Fiberoptic Bundles

An individual fiber cannot transmit an image. If one observes the end of an illuminated fiber, only a spot of light of a certain color and intensity is seen. To create an image, a large number of fibers must be grouped together. The pattern formed by the color and intensity of the individual fibers is perceived by the observer as an image. For the image at one end of the bundle to duplicate the image at the other end, it is necessary that the ends of each individual fiber occupy the same relative position in both ends of the bundle. A bundle which is organized in this manner is called a "coherent" bundle (Fig. 2–4). Only coherent bundles are capable of producing an image. Therefore, they are also referred to as image guide (IG) bundles.

An important property of an IG bundle is its resolving power, i.e., the amount of image detail that the bundle can convey. A bundle's resolving power depends on the diameter of the fiber core, the thickness of the cladding, and the alignment and orderliness of the packing of the fibers within the bundle faces. The smaller the fiber and the thinner the cladding, the greater the image resolution. In practice, the thickness of the fiber cladding cannot be less than 1.5 micron for visible

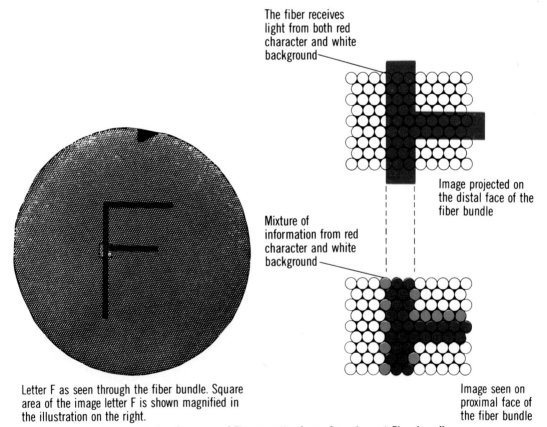

The fiber receives light from both red character and white background

Image projected on the distal face of the fiber bundle

Mixture of information from red character and white background

Letter F as seen through the fiber bundle. Square area of the image letter F is shown magnified in the illustration on the right.

Image seen on proximal face of the fiber bundle

FIGURE 2–4. Alignment of fibers on the face of a coherent fiber bundle.

light, because of production limitations as well as physical optical principles.

The ratio of the total area occupied by the individual fiber cores to the total area of the fiber bundle is referred to as the "packing fraction." Since only the cores transmit light, it is an advantage to make the packing fraction as large as possible. However, since there is a limit to the thinness of the cladding as the diameter of the core is reduced to improve resolution, a certain point is reached at which the packing fraction becomes unacceptably low. The high proportion of cladding area to core area results in a very dark image. Due to this limitation, the smallest practical fiber diameter (including cladding) is generally limited to approximately 8 μ. A typical packing fraction is 60%.

The alignment of the fibers in the faces of the bundle greatly affects the quality and resolution of the image. Imperfect alignment will result in distorted images and annoying flaws or dark areas in the image.

Individual fibers in the bundle that have been broken or damaged will produce black or gray dots in the image. The single free fiber is surprisingly strong and resistant to damage by bending or torquing. However, once the fibers are arranged in a bundle and packed into the body of an endoscope with other rigid mechanical parts, it is more susceptible to breakage. Careful design of the various components of the fiberscope, followed by carefully thought-out positioning of the fiber bundles within the endoscope, and demanding durability tests are required to ensure the safety of the fiber bundle within the instrument.

The length and number of fibers within an image guide vary greatly, depending on the type and size of the endoscope. The number of individual fibers in the image guide bundle usually ranges between 5000 and 40,000. The diameter of the bundle may vary between 0.5 mm and 3 mm. The individual fiber size also varies, a typical fiber being 8 μ to 12 μ in diameter. Due to the greater space available within the insertion tube of colonoscopes,

these instruments contain the largest image guides and, therefore, the greatest number of fibers. The image of a colonoscope is, therefore, unsurpassed by those of other types of fiberscopes. The length of the fibers used in a typical colonoscope image guide of 40,000 fibers, with each 2 meters in length, totals more than 80 km, or 50 miles.

When looking at fiberscopes, one will note two types of image guides. Early fiberscopes employed square image bundles that required much hand labor to manufacture. A totally new process (described later) allows the production of round bundles with thinner fibers. The new method is more automated and the quality of the bundles produced is more consistent.

Fiber bundles used for light transmission, as opposed to image transmission, are referred to as light guide (LG) bundles. The random packing of the fibers in an LG bundle results in an "incoherent" bundle which is incapable of producing an image. They are much less expensive to produce and are designed to maximize light carrying ability, rather than resolution. Since resolution is not a factor, the individual fibers are made much thicker (30 μ) than fibers in an IG bundle, and are therefore much more efficient at transmitting light.

Basic Optical System of a Fiberscope

A schematic of a typical optical system used in fiberscopes is shown (Fig. 2–5). The objective lens at the tip of the fiberscope forms an image of the object in view (X_o) on the distal face of the image guide (X'_o). This miniature image is limited by the size of the fiber bundle. The light representing this image is transmitted through the image guide and a duplicate image is formed on the proximal face of the bundle near the eyepiece. Since the objective lens produces an inverted image on the distal face of the bundle, the bundle must be twisted 180° to produce an upright image at the proximal face. The resulting image is a faithful reproduction of the viewed

FIGURE 2–5. A basic fiberscope optical system. I.G.—image guide.

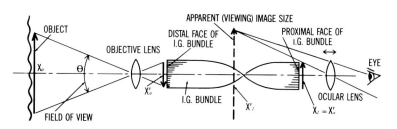

object; however, it is much too small to view with the naked eye. The diameter of the entire bundle is between 0.5 mm and 3.0 mm. The ocular lens (fiberscope eyepiece) functions as a simple magnifying glass and creates an enlarged virtual image of the image resting on the tiny tip of the bundle. This magnified image is easily observed by the endoscopist.

Magnification of the viewed object is determined by several factors. Magnification produced by the objective lens is variable and is determined by the distance between the objective lens (fiberscope tip) and the object being viewed:

$$\text{Magnification by objective lens} = M_o. = \frac{X_o'}{X_o}$$

M_o is usually much less than 1. In most fiberscopes, the distance between the objective lens and the IG bundle face is fixed. As a result, there is a limited range of distance between the object and the objective lens within which the object will still be in focus. This limited range of focus is referred to as the optical depth of field. A typical fiberscope can focus clearly on objects located approximately 3 to 100 mm from the tip of the instrument. Special high-magnification fiberscopes contain a distal focusing mechanism to vary the distance between the objective lens and the fiber bundle. With the use of this control, the fiberscope can be adjusted to focus on objects as close as 2.5 mm from the objective lens, thereby producing a greatly enlarged image of the mucosal surface. The clinical applications of this type of instrument are presented in Part 3 of Chapter 10.

Magnification of the tiny image on the proximal face of the IG bundle is determined by the focal length of the ocular lens:

$$\begin{aligned} \text{Magnification} \atop \text{of ocular lens} &= M_1 \\ &= \underline{X_1'} \text{ (apparent image size)} \\ &= X_1 \text{ (actual image size)} \end{aligned}$$

M_1 typically ranges between $15\times$ and $30\times$. It is the ocular magnification which has the greatest influence over the apparent size of the image seen by the endoscopist. It is very easy to increase the magnification of the eyepiece and create a larger image; however, this magnification will also magnify the size of the individual fibers within the image. There is, therefore, a practical limit to the

magnification of the image before the pattern of the fiber bundle becomes disturbingly exaggerated and hinders the endoscopist's interpretation of the image.

The visual magnification of the fiberscope's entire optical system M is the product of M_o and M_1:

$$M = M_o \times M_1$$

It should be noted that the field of view of the objective lens is closely related to the overall magnification of the mucosal surface. Early fiberscopes had a relatively narrow field of view (e.g., 60°). New lens designs and brighter illumination systems have allowed current fiberscopes to have fields of view up to 120°. It is important to recognize that, from the clinical viewpoint, a wide field of view may not always be desirable and appropriate. Therefore, a wide field of view is not suitable for all models.

Fiberscopes with round image guides make the most efficient use of the lens and illumination capacity of a fiberscope. Since the light output of the fiberscope illuminates a circular area, and lenses produce circular images unless masked off, a round image on a round image guide makes best use of the optical and illumination systems. If a square bundle is used, either the corners of the image will not be brightly illuminated or light must be wasted in the illumination of the unseen portion of the square field.

All fiberscopes have a diopter adjustment on the eyepiece. This allows focusing of the ocular lens to compensate for variations in the diopter of the individual endoscopist's eyesight.

Ancillary Optical Equipment— Camera

A schematic of the optical system for an endoscopic still camera is shown in Figure 2–6. The mount on the front of the camera is designed so that the camera can be placed on the fiberscope eyepiece and rotated slightly to attach it firmly to the eyepiece. A mechanical linkage built into the fiberscope eyepiece automatically changes the lens system of the ocular from one which creates a virtual image for viewing by the endoscopist to one which produces a real image which can be captured on film. When the camera is rotated for attachment, it automatically overrides the diopter setting that the physician has chosen and focuses the eyepiece properly for photography.

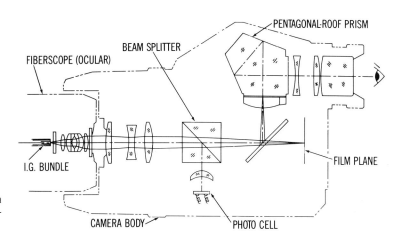

FIGURE 2–6. Optical system of an endoscopic still camera. I.G.—image guide.

A small, partially silvered prism in the camera mount diverts a small portion of the light passing into the camera to a light-sensitive transducer (photocell). This transducer electronically measures the brightness of the image and informs the endoscopic light source as to how much light has reached the film. This enables the light source to automatically produce a flash of the proper duration for a correctly exposed photograph, taking into account the size of the image on the film and the brightness of the scene.

Ancillary Optical Equipment—Teaching Attachment

An optical teaching attachment can be coupled to the eyepiece of the endoscope, allowing a second observer to view the image along with the endoscopist (Fig. 2–7). A beam splitter in the body of the teaching attachment diverts 80% of the light to a secondary IG bundle. This bundle carries the image to the secondary ocular for observation by the assistant or student. Because of the great light loss in transferring the image from one bundle to another, the brightness of the image at the secondary ocular approximately equals the brightness at the main ocular; that is, both are receiving only 20% of the original light. A camera can be attached to the main ocular if a photograph is desired while the teaching attachment is in place. A switch on the main body of the teaching attachment momentarily diverts 100% of the light to the main ocular when the photograph is being taken.

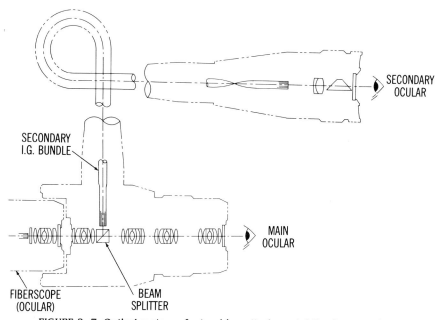

FIGURE 2–7. Optical system of a teaching attachment. I.G.—image guide.

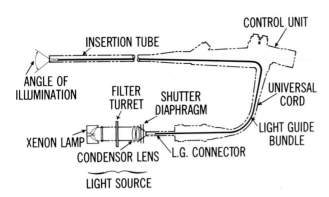

FIGURE 2–8. Fiberscope illumination system. L.G.—light guide.

Illumination System

An optical system used for endoscopic illumination is shown in Figure 2–8. An incoherent LG bundle is used to transmit light through the fiberscope. Special lens systems on both ends of the bundle are needed to capture effectively the maximum amount of light from the light source at one end of the bundle and to produce wide-angle, even illumination from the tip at the other end. Fibers used in the LG bundle are designed for a high N.A. and a high transmission ratio. To produce the highest possible packing fraction, light guide fibers are made as large as possible without compromising their flexibility and durability. At present, 30 μ fibers are commonly used.

Due to the intense heat produced by the high-intensity light sources used in endoscopy, dichroic coatings and heat-absorbing filters are employed to filter out non-visible radiation from the lamp output. In addition, heat sinks and forced air cooling systems in the light source prevent the LG bundle from overheating.

Early generation fiberscopes had a plain cover glass or a single, simple lens at the proximal end of the LG bundle to transfer light to the interior of the organ under observation. Current fiberscopes require wide-angle illumination to cover the ultra-wide visual fields of these instruments. To achieve even, wide-angle illumination, a complex lens system is required at the proximal end of the LG bundle.

PRODUCTION AND QUALITY OF IMAGE GUIDE BUNDLES

Following is a general description of an automated process that produces high-quality round bundles. This is the method used to make the IG bundles found in the majority of fiberscopes today.

Process

The individual fiber starts out as a single glass rod consisting of a core of high-quality optical glass, a cladding of glass with a lower refractive index, and a second cladding of acid leachable glass (Fig. 2–9). This original glass rod is many times larger in diameter than the final flexible glass fiber.

The necessary number of these single glass rods (usually tens of thousands) are perfectly aligned within a larger cylinder made of acid leachable glass. This large coherent bundle is called the master IG (Fig. 2–10).

The master IG is placed in an electric furnace and pulled (Fig. 2–11). The heat and tension cause the bundle to elongate and become thinner. This process is repeated many times until the individual fibers are

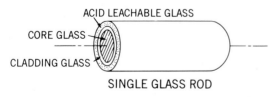

FIGURE 2–9. Composition of a glass rod which, after heating and elongation, will become an individual glass fiber.

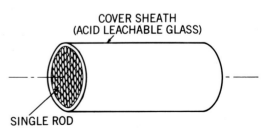

FIGURE 2–10. Master image guide (IG) bundle.

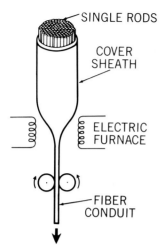

FIGURE 2–11. Process of pulling a master IG bundle to reduce its diameter.

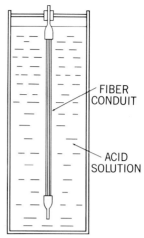

FIGURE 2–13. Rigid fiber bundle is soaked in an acid solution which dissolves the acid leachable glass and frees the individual fibers.

reduced to the desired size of approximately 10 μ. A cross section of the bundle at this stage is shown in Figure 2–12. Due to the tension of the pulling process, the acid leachable glass is forced into a hexagonal honeycomb pattern, fusing the individual glass rods into a single rigid bundle. The perfect packing and coherence of the original master IG are maintained.

Protective holders are placed over both ends of the bundle, and the bundle is soaked in an acid solution (Fig. 2–13). Only the acid leachable glass that is fusing the fibers is affected by the acid. As this glass is slowly dissolved, the fibers become free and flexible (Fig. 2–14). At this point, the individual fibers are freed from one another to convert the fragile, rigid bundle into a durable flexible bundle.

Quality

Several factors can affect the quality of the final IG bundle (Fig. 2–15), including the following: black dots caused by broken fibers, half-opaque (gray) dots caused by poor cladding or an air bubble in the fiber, and disorders in fiber alignment or dust in the fiber that is inherent in the manufacturing process.

MECHANICAL CONSTRUCTION OF THE FIBERSCOPE

The major parts and controls of a typical fiberscope are shown in Figure 2–16. At this point, various aspects of the internal construction of the fiberscope will be discussed in detail.

Distal Tip

An end view and cross section of the distal tip of a typical fiberscope are shown in Figure

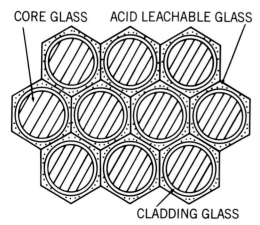

FIGURE 2–12. Cross section of the fiber bundle after the pulling process showing the fusion of the acid leachable glass.

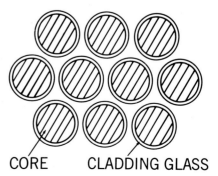

FIGURE 2–14. Cross section of the fiber bundle after the acid leaching process.

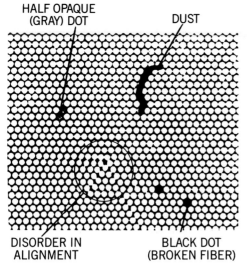

HALF OPAQUE
(GRAY) DOT　　　　　　DUST

DISORDER IN　　　　　　　BLACK DOT
ALIGNMENT　　　　　　　(BROKEN FIBER)

FIGURE 2–15. Example of various forms of fiber bundle imperfections.

2–17. On the face of the tip can be seen (1) the channel opening for suctioning and passage of accessories; (2) the complex LG lens system that distributes the light from the LG bundle into wide-angle, even illumination of the visual field; (3) the objective lens system that focuses an image of the mucosa onto the face of the IG bundle; and (4) an air/water nozzle, which supplies air for insufflation of the organ being observed and water that flows across the lens to remove substances which may obscure vision such as secretions, mucus, and blood.

Depending on the model and manufacturer, some instruments may have separate nozzles for air and water. Also available is an optional or detachable hood around the distal tip to keep the objective lens away from the mucosa and to aid, after polypectomy, in capturing and removing polyps by suction. Because of advantages in packing the various components within the distal tip, and in order to produce a more balanced illumination during close-up viewing, the LG bundle may be divided into two smaller bundles in some instrument models.

Two cross sections of the distal tip of a side-viewing fiberscope are illustrated in Figure 2–18. A roof prism is used to produce a 90° change in the direction of view. A forceps raiser is also necessary to deflect the tip of various accessories passed through the channel in order to bring them within the field of view.

Bending Section and Angulation System

The design of the bending section, which is the portion that produces controlled deflection of the distal tip, was originally developed in Japan for the gastrocamera. Four-way tip deflection was first introduced with the Olympus CF-MB/LB colonoscope in 1970. A variety of different mechanisms to control tip deflection have been developed since then.

A typical angulation system in current use is shown in Figure 2–19. Fiberscopes used

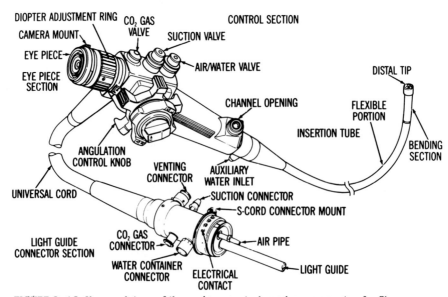

DIOPTER ADJUSTMENT RING　　CO_2 GAS VALVE　　　CONTROL SECTION
CAMERA MOUNT
SUCTION VALVE
EYE PIECE
AIR/WATER VALVE
EYE PIECE SECTION
DISTAL TIP
CHANNEL OPENING
FLEXIBLE PORTION
INSERTION TUBE
BENDING SECTION
ANGULATION CONTROL KNOB
VENTING CONNECTOR
AUXILIARY WATER INLET
UNIVERSAL CORD
SUCTION CONNECTOR
S-CORD CONNECTOR MOUNT
LIGHT GUIDE CONNECTOR SECTION
CO_2 GAS CONNECTOR
AIR PIPE
WATER CONTAINER CONNECTOR
ELECTRICAL CONTACT
LIGHT GUIDE

FIGURE 2–16. Nomenclature of the various controls and components of a fiberscope.

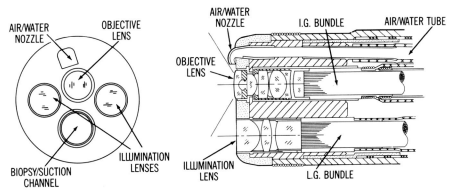

FIGURE 2–17. End view and cross section of the distal tip of a fiberscope.

for gastrointestinal purposes generally have a built-in resistance or an adjustable braking system to control the deflection of the tip, allowing the operator to remove his hand from the control knob and still maintain tip deflection. To produce tip deflection, the operator rotates the control knob, which is connected to a sprocket within the control section. This sprocket moves a chain, which in turn pulls on various wires running the length of the insertion tube. As a wire is pulled, it produces tip deflection in that direction. The bending section is constructed from interlocking metal rings. The pivot points between adjacent rings alternate by 90°, thereby giving the bending section the ability to bend in any direction. A cross-sectional view of the bending section is shown in Figure 2–20.

An important aspect of fiberscope design is determining the proper amount of free space within the fiberscope insertion tube. This free space permits the internal components to bend and move about as the fiberscope is repeatedly flexed, bent, pushed, and pulled during use. A very tight packing will place undue force on the delicate fiber bundles and result in fiber breakage. Excessively loose packing will result in wasted space. The relative position of the various components within the bending section is also very important to prevent the larger, more unyielding components from pinching the delicate fiber bundles when the fiberscope is bent.

During an endoscopic procedure, the tip of the instrument is deflected many times (Fig. 2–21). To withstand repeated, complex movements, the deflecting mechanism must be extremely durable, and should be tested extensively to guarantee that it is safe and will not fail prematurely. An example of the types of machines used to test angulation system durability during production is depicted in Figure 2–22.

Insertion Tube

Although the insertion tube, excluding the bending section, is not capable of controlled deflection, its carefully calculated flexibility

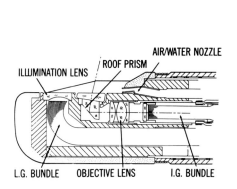

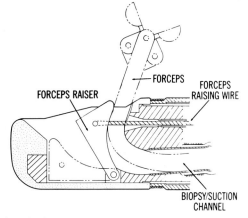

FIGURE 2–18. Cross section of the distal tip of a side-viewing fiberscope in two different planes.

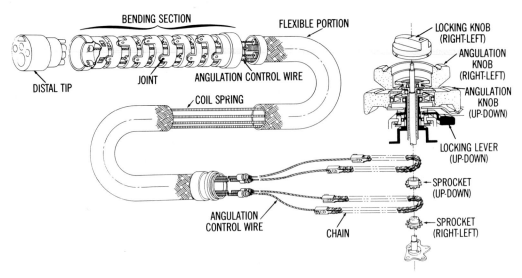

FIGURE 2–19. Bending section and angulation system of a fiberoptic endoscope.

and torque-free construction are of major importance in endoscope design. Most instruments have two-stage flexibility, i.e., the distal portion of the insertion tube is more flexible than the proximal portion. Whenever a new fiberscope is designed, the flexibility of each portion of the insertion tube requires extensive clinical testing to ensure that the fiberscope handles easily and produces minimum patient discomfort. Experience has shown that stiffer insertion tubes are more suitable for use in the relatively straight and fixed upper GI tract, whereas more flexible instruments pass more easily in the tortuous and mobile lower GI tract.

The basic construction of the insertion tube is shown in Figure 2–23. Helical steel bands form the supporting structure of the tube and give it its round shape. These bands are covered with a layer of stainless steel wire mesh. Together, these components prevent the insertion tube from twisting or stretching along its axis and also help shield the glass fiber bundles from damaging x-ray radiation.

The outer plastic sheath which covers the metal structure of the instrument also helps prevent twisting of the insertion tube as well as compression along its axis. It is important that this final covering be waterproof and able to withstand a variety of chemical agents

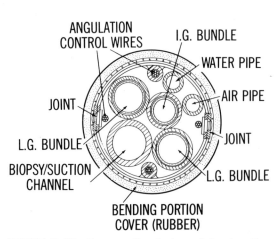

FIGURE 2–20. Cross-sectional view of the bending section of a fiberscope. L.G.—light guide; I.G.—image guide.

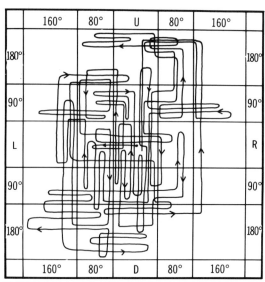

FIGURE 2–21. Data showing the degree and direction of tip deflection during typical endoscopic procedure.

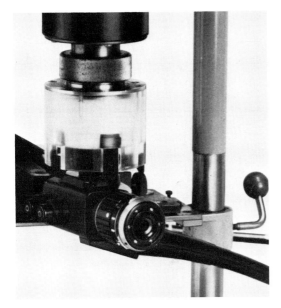

FIGURE 2–22. Instrument designed to test the durability of a fiberscope's angulation system.

including gastric acid and corrosive disinfectants. The specifications of each component of the insertion tube are carefully chosen to ensure that the completed tube has the proper flexibility and also the elasticity necessary to recover from repeated bending.

Control Section

The control section of the fiberscope is designed to be held by the left hand alone, leaving the right hand free to hold and manipulate the insertion tube. The second, third, and fourth fingers grip the instrument against the palm, leaving the left thumb free to control the up/down angulation knob and the index finger free to operate the air/water and suction valves. The right hand is used to torque and advance the insertion tube, insert

and operate accessories, control the right/left angulation knob, operate the camera, adjust the diopter of the ocular lens, and focus the objective lens as necessary. Proper technique is described in Chapter 11.

Air, Water, and Suction System

A cross section of a colonofiberscope, providing the various internal channels for air, water, and suction, is shown in Figure 2–24. This type of design, providing automatic air, water, and suction, originated in 1968 with the Olympus Model EF esophagoscope and has remained basically the same through succeeding instrument generations.

Air supplied by a pump within the light source is emitted from the nozzle on the distal tip when the opening in the air/water valve is covered. Air is used to insufflate the organ under observation and to blow water off the objective lens. When the air/water valve is depressed, water is forced from the pressurized water container through the fiberscope and out the nozzle on the distal tip.

Aspiration of either air or fluid through the fiberscope is accomplished by depressing the suction valve. An external suction pump and collection bottle are connected to the fiberscope and provide the required negative pressure. When performing electrosurgery, the endoscopist may wish to introduce CO_2 as an inert gas to reduce the risk of accidental explosion in the bowel, particularly the colon. This is done by depressing the CO_2 gas valve, which allows gas from an external regulated tank to be insufflated via the fiberscope.

Valves are provided on all of these channels to check the backward flow of material from the various openings on the distal tip into the air, water, and gas channels within the fiberscope. However, since the fiberscope is used in a pressurized environment, owing

FIGURE 2–23. Internal components and construction of the insertion tube of the fiberscope. L.G.—light guide; I.G.—image guide.

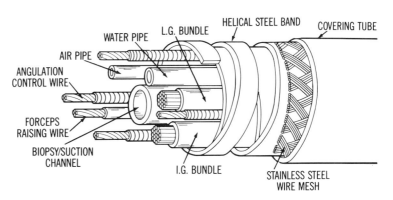

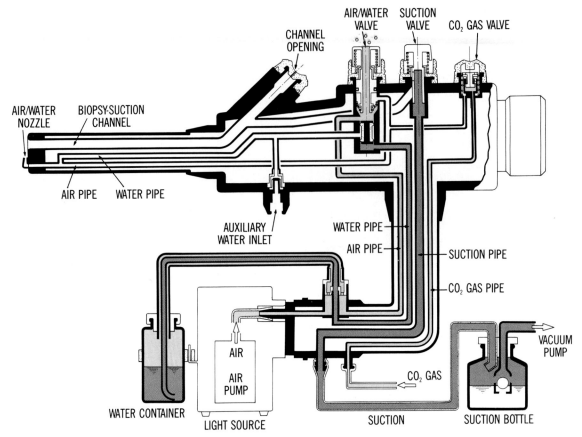

FIGURE 2–24. Air, water, suction, and CO_2 systems of a typical colonofiberscope.

to organ insufflation, and because the air within the channels of the fiberscope is compressible, it is possible for small amounts of debris to work their way slowly into the interior air, water, and gas tubing of the fiberscope. To prevent occlusion of these small tubes, and for reasons of infection control, it is important to flush and disinfect these lines thoroughly when the instrument is cleaned.

Light Guide Connector

The light guide connector (Fig. 2–25) connects to the light souce of the fiberscope and provides light and pressurized air. It also has connections for the water container, suction pump, and an S-cord (see the section on electrosurgical generators, p. 34) to safely return any electrosurgical leakage current back to the generator. A vent on the connec-

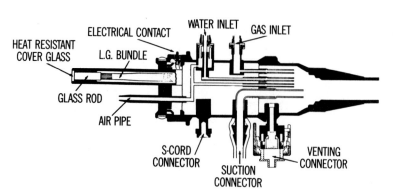

FIGURE 2–25. Cross section of the light guide connector of a fiberscope. L.G.—light guide.

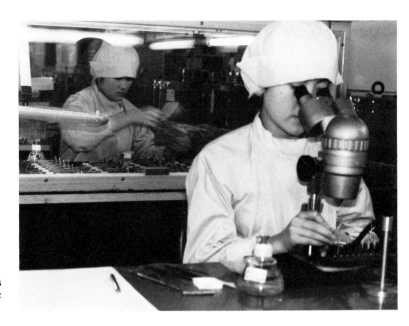

FIGURE 2–26. Optical system is assembled under a microscope in a dust-free room.

tor allows the interior of an air- and fluid-tight fiberscope to be vented before the instrument is placed in an evacuated chamber for gas sterilization.

Fiberscope Manufacturing Process

Typical modern fiberscope assembly lines are shown in Figures 2–26 and 2–27. Assembly is followed by critical adjustment and careful inspection of the entire instrument. Fiberscope manufacturers, like manufacturers of all medical devices, must meet the requirements of various regulatory agencies, such as the Food and Drug Administration. These standards influence the following areas: quality assurance programs, quality audits of critical components, production and processing controls, packaging and labeling requirements, storage and distribution, device evaluation, factory inspection, personnel training, equipment calibration, and record keeping.

ANCILLARY EQUIPMENT
Endoscopic Light Sources

A variety of endoscopic light sources are available, ranging from simple low-power halogen light sources to sophisticated high intensity xenon units. The larger, more advanced light sources generally have features

FIGURE 2–27. Final inspection of an assembled fiberscope with all pertinent data stored in a computer.

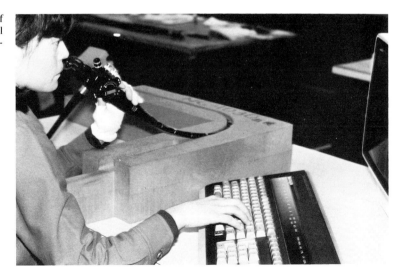

such as automatic flash photography and automatic brightness control for television and motion picture documentation. A block diagram of the function of the various components of a high-intensity xenon light source (Fig. 2–28) and the internal components (Fig. 2–29) and the front panel (Fig. 2–30) of a xenon light source are illustrated.

Electrosurgical Generators

Only solid state generators having isolated outputs should be used for endoscopic procedures. Although almost any generator that operates within the proper power range can be adapted for endoscopic use, electrosurgical units designed specifically for use with fiberscopes have several important additional safety features. One of these is a separate terminal to connect a safety return cord (S-cord) from the fiberscope (Fig. 2–31). This S-cord returns any capacitance-induced "leakage" current in the fiberscope directly to the generator, thereby avoiding potentially dangerous circuiting through the patient or physician. If proper electrical connections

have not been made, a warning system built into the generator will alert the operator and will prevent the unit from operating until these connections are correct. A second safety feature is continuous monitoring by the generator of the amount of current returning through the S-cord, as well as comparison of that amount with the total output. If a significant amount of current is detected in the S-cord, the generator automatically shuts down power output, preventing possible injury. The principles of electrosurgery are discussed in Chapter 7.

For safety, it is important that endoscopic electrosurgery only be attempted through fiberscopes specifically designed for this application. Fiberscopes with exposed metal bands on the insertion tube or noninsulated distal tips, and nongrounded fiberscopes should never be used.

Suction Pump

Either regulated wall suction or a small portable suction pump can be used for endoscopy. A more detailed explanation of the

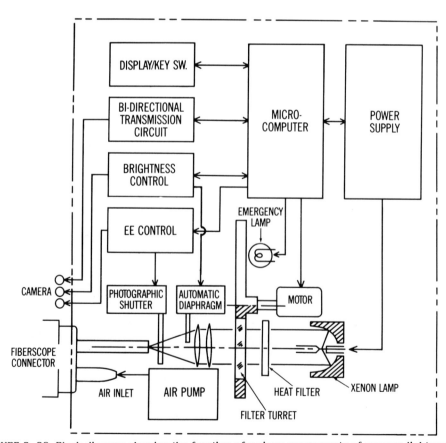

FIGURE 2–28. Block diagram showing the function of various components of a xenon light source.

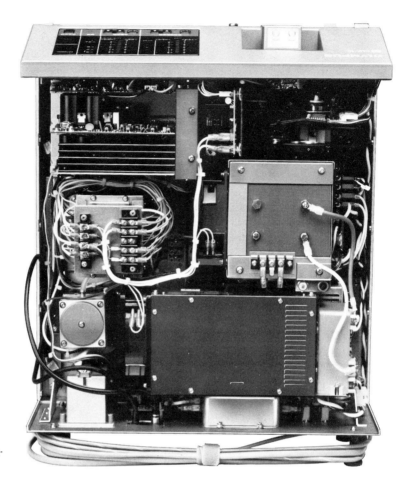

FIGURE 2–29. Internal components of a xenon light source.

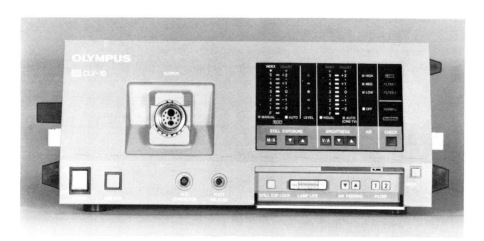

FIGURE 2–30. Front panel of a xenon light source.

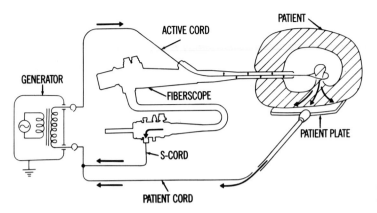

FIGURE 2–31. Schematic diagram of endoscopic electrosurgery with a safety return cord (S-cord).

automatic suction system is described on p. 31.

PHOTOGRAPHIC APPARATUS

Various technical aspects and a general overview of endoscopic photography are discussed in this section. A detailed consideration of gastrointestinal photography is given in Chapter 4.

Still Cameras

The function of the internal components of a still camera specifically designed for endoscopic use is shown diagrammatically in Figure 2–32. The layout of the actual components within the camera is shown in Figure 2–33.

Endoscopic cameras are designed to operate in conjunction with the fiberscope's light source to produce properly exposed photographs automatically. To do this, various electrical signals are sent through the fiberscope, allowing communication of the camera and light source concerning the timing of the shutter sync, brightness of the image, duration of the flash, and any data that are to be imprinted on the film.

When the camera release button is depressed, the following sequence of events occurs automatically (Fig. 2–34). The light source shutter closes, cutting off all light

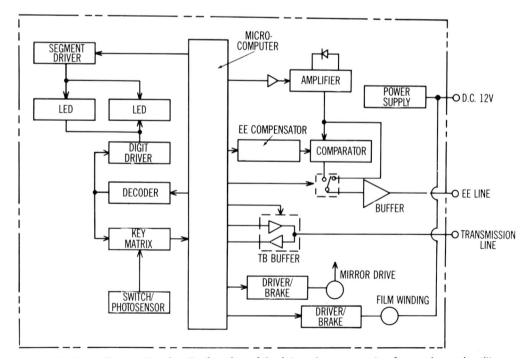

FIGURE 2–32. Block diagram showing the function of the internal components of an endoscopic still camera.

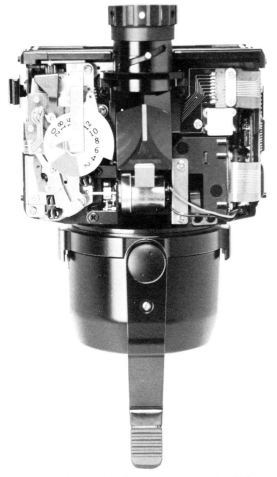

FIGURE 2–33. Layout of actual components within an endoscopic camera.

source to be processed by an automatic exposure circuit. When this circuit has determined the film has received proper exposure, the flash is terminated and the light source shutter closes. After a brief interval, the camera shutter timer reaches the end of its preset cycle (0.25 second) and the camera shutter also closes. The light source then returns to the normal light intensity for observation.

Because of the photocell and the electronic exposure circuit, the photographic system automatically compensates for variations in subject-to-fiberscope distance, magnification, and subject coloration, which influence the amount of exposure required. An adjustment on the light source allows the system to accept several different types of color slide and color print films.

An example of the type of information presented in the viewfinder of the endoscopic camera is shown in Figure 2–35. In addition to the endoscopic image, there are also exposure indicators that warn the physician, before the photograph is taken, whether the image is so dark or so bright that it is beyond the capability of the system to expose the film properly. In this case, the physician can either move closer to the subject to brighten the image, move farther away, or insert a filter to darken the image, as the case may require.

There is also an indicator light in the viewfinder, which shows when the light source flash is completely charged and ready to be used again. In addition, the date can be displayed at the bottom of the image by a clock built into the light source. The date can be imprinted on the film along with the image, if desired. If an optional data setting unit is used, any combination of alphanumeric characters can be imprinted on the film as well.

from the light source. The camera shutter opens. The light source shutter opens and the flash is triggered. At this moment, the photocell located in the camera begins measuring the intensity of the light entering the camera and feeds this information to the light

FIGURE 2–34. Sequence of camera and light source shutter operation controlling exposure during endoscopic photography.

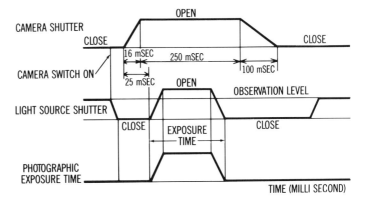

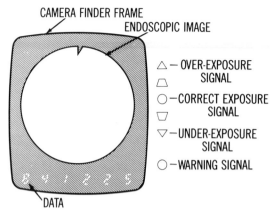

FIGURE 2–35. Information displayed in the viewfinder of an endoscopic camera.

Instant, Cine, and TV Cameras

In addition to the still camera, there are other types of photographic equipment that can be connected to the fiberscope. Instant print cameras are available which will produce an endoscopic photograph in 90 seconds. Motion picture cameras provide high-quality documentation for teaching purposes. With the advent of compact, lightweight TV cameras, the use of motion pictures has declined. An endoscopic TV system allows assistants, radiologists, and others in the room to observe the procedure, which can also be recorded on video tape.

TOTAL ENDOSCOPIC SYSTEM

A large variety of accessories and ancillary equipment are required for modern endoscopy. A total endoscopic system is depicted schematically in Figure 2–36.

CLEANING, STERILIZATION, AND MAINTENANCE OF FIBERSCOPE AND ACCESSORIES

Meticulous cleaning of the fiberscope immediately after use is important to keep the instrument free of accumulated organic debris and in good mechanical working order. An improperly cleaned instrument will also render any subsequent disinfection or sterilization procedure completely ineffective, since the surface layer of debris will shield underlying microorganisms from the biocidal action of the disinfectant.

Many recent fiberscope models are completely watertight and can be placed under an open faucet or totally immersed without installing caps or making other modifications.

The entire exterior surface can be easily washed with a sponge or soft brush. It is also possible to completely disinfect or "cold" sterilize all exterior surfaces and internal channels of these watertight instruments by immersing them in an appropriate disinfectant solution. All detachable parts, such as distal hoods, forceps valves, air/water and suction valves, water containers, and tubes, should be removed from the instrument and cleaned and sterilized separately. It is important to note that many instruments, particularly earlier models, are not watertight. Therefore, immersion in water or other solutions or contact of certain parts (the control section, for example) of these instruments with fluids will result in serious damage. The manufacturer's instructions for cleaning and disinfection should always be studied carefully before putting a fiberscope to use.

Two common types of disinfectant solutions are safe and effective for use with fiberscopes. These are glutaraldehydes and iodophors. Many brands are available. It is suggested that the user consult the endoscope manufacturer concerning the suitability of particular disinfecting agents before using them to disinfect the instrument. Instrument manufacturers can suggest products that they have tested and that did not damage their instruments after long-term use.

It is important that the instrument be thoroughly rinsed after using a cold disinfectant solution and that all interior channels be flushed with clean water and air dried. Many disinfectants are toxic or irritating to body tissue and must be completely rinsed from the instrument before further patient use. It is important that the instrument be properly dried before storage. Moisture in the interior channels of the fiberscope will promote the growth of microorganisms, and water drops that are allowed to dry will leave a film or stain on electrical contacts and lens surfaces.

Ethylene oxide gas (ETO) sterilization is suitable for sterilizing the entire instrument. The fiberscope must be completely dry before ETO sterilization. The venting valve on new air- and fluid-tight instruments must be opened before placing them in a gas sterilizer. This allows the pressure inside the instrument to equilibrate with the chamber pressure. If the instrument is not vented, as the vacuum is being drawn in the sterilization chamber, the atmospheric pressure inside the fiberscope will cause expansion and bursting of the rubber sheath covering the bending section of the instrument.

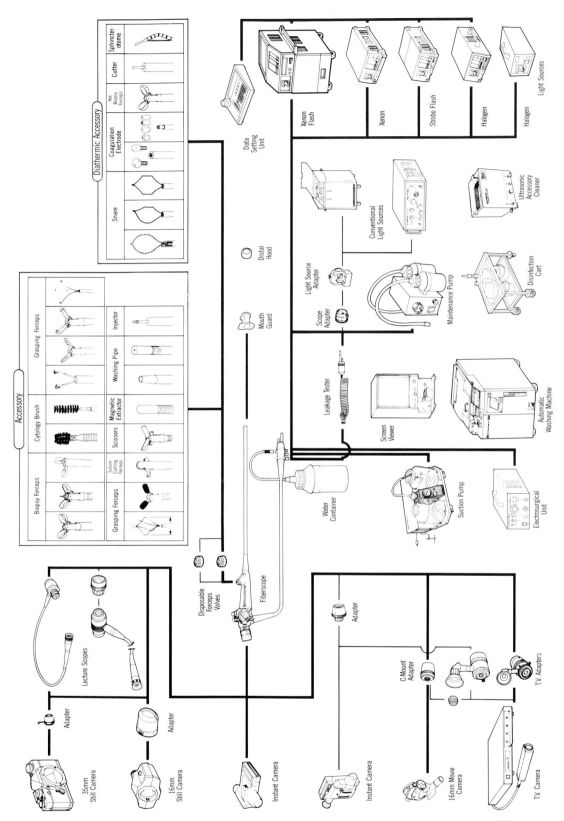

FIGURE 2–36. Endoscopic System Chart. A complete endoscopic system includes not only a variety of fiberscopes but also a complete line of accessories and ancillary equipment.

After exposure to ETO, the fiberscope must be aerated to remove any residual ETO that has been absorbed by the plastic and rubber parts of the instrument. Seven days are required if aeration is performed at room temperature. The use of an aeration chamber can shorten aeration time to approximately 10 hours. The fiberscope manufacturer should be consulted concerning the maximum temperature, pressure, and humidity that the instrument can withstand during sterilization and aeration cycles.

Although the fiberscope cannot be placed in an autoclave, many accessories such as biopsy forceps, polypectomy snares, cytology brushes, water containers, and mouthpieces can be sterilized by this method, which makes use of high pressure steam. Because of the shorter cycle of steam sterilization, this method may be more convenient in some situations.

The use of an ultrasonic cleaner is recommended to remove particulate matter from the delicate hinges of biopsy forceps and other hard-to-clean areas of endoscopic accessories. An automatic washing and disinfecting machine (Fig. 2–37) may be desirable in a busy endoscopy suite, since it saves time in cleaning and will clean and disinfect the fiberscope automatically.

SAFETY

Mechanical Safety

As with any medical instrument, fiberscopes must be manufactured according to the Good Manufacturing Practice (GMP) standards of the United States Bureau of Medical Devices. However, for the greatest safety, an endoscope manufacturer must consider all possible types of malfunction, and his instruments should be designed so that a malfunction, if it should occur, will not cause harm to the patient. An example of this type of design philosophy is an angulation system that cannot jam or malfunction with resultant locking of the instrument's tip in a deflected position, thereby preventing removal of the instrument from the patient. Another example is an insufflation system that cannot malfunction in a manner which would produce potentially dangerous continuous insufflation. A final example is the use of a braided wire consisting of numerous strands of extremely fine wire (as many as 49) in the instrument's angulation system. Although a braided wire with only a few, thicker wires could be used, if one of the strands became frayed or cut, a thick wire would be strong enough to puncture the outer sheath of the

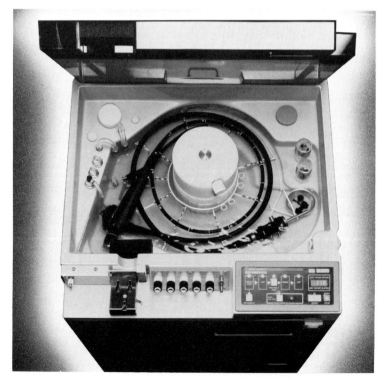

FIGURE 2–37. A machine designed to automatically wash and disinfect watertight fiberscopes.

insertion tube and injure the patient; the thinner wire would not.

With many mechanical devices, it is easy to increase durability by simply increasing the size and weight of critical components, thereby strengthening them and preventing future failure. It is possible to substantially increase the durability of a fiberscope by strengthening or redesigning certain components; however, this may severely compromise the safety and effectiveness of the instrument. For example, using larger, thicker wires in the angulation system would reduce the amount of stretching that might occur but would compromise safety, as explained in the preceding paragraph.

Other changes to improve durability might be adding a thicker protective covering over delicate fiber bundles to prevent fiber breakage, using a heavier supporting structure in the insertion tube to prevent damage due to patient bites, reducing the amount of tip deflection to reduce stress on the internal components, and increasing the thickness of the rubber sheath to eliminate water leakage due to pin holes. These and many more changes could be made to produce an instrument which would require little or no repair during its lifetime. However, the results of these changes would be a fiberscope with a large, stiff insertion tube, limited tip deflection, reduced accessory channel size, and a larger, heavier control section. Since these changes are unacceptable, modern fiberscope design represents a delicate balance between the various features the physician requires and the best design in terms of ultimate durability.

Another important design factor is the necessity for the fiberscope to "yield" before the patient does. The flexibility of the instrument and the tactile feedback of the control knobs allow the physician to gauge the force the instrument is exerting on the patient. This required "feel" of the instrument also puts important limitations on the type of materials used in the fiberscope and the manner in which the instrument is constructed.

Electrical Safety

UL (Underwriter Laboratories) and IEC (International Electrotechnical Commission) standards apply to the ancillary electrical equipment used with fiberscopes. The basic concerns of these standards are (1) to prevent patient or operator shock due to leakage of line voltage and (2) to maintain the electrical safety of the equipment should some internal component fail or malfunction.

Fiberscopes are now designed so that they are electrically isolated from ground. This prevents current from flowing through the fiberscope and patient should a fault occur in attached ancillary equipment. This also prevents the fiberscope from acting as the return electrode if the return electrode should become dislodged or disconnected when electrosurgery is performed with a ground-referenced electrosurgical generator.

Due to the nature of high frequency current, it is impossible to eliminate capacitive coupling of the fiberscope and an electrosurgical accessory passed through it. Therefore, it is essential that there are no unnecessary exposed metal parts on the insertion tube, which could possibly result in an electrosurgical burn to the patient. The use of a safety bypass cord (S-cord) and a protective eyeshield for metal, electrically nonisolated eyepieces is also recommended. Despite all the safety features incorporated into modern instruments and because of the potential hazards of electrosurgery, the therapeutic endoscopist should be thoroughly trained in electrosurgical procedures and aware of all possible complications.

Chapter 3

THE ENDOSCOPY UNIT

MICHAEL V. SIVAK, JR., M.D.
JAMES M. SENICK

The concept of devoting a specific area of a hospital, outpatient clinic, or even a private office to gastrointestinal endoscopy is relatively recent. Not many years ago, endoscopic procedures were usually performed in converted consultation/examination rooms or a surgical suite. Although many factors have made allocation of dedicated space for gastrointestinal endoscopy inevitable, the uniform characteristic, operative in virtually every health care facility that offers endoscopic services, is growth.

Gastrointestinal endoscopes have undergone remarkable changes over the past 20 years (see Chapter 1). As a result, certain diagnostic procedures such as upper gastrointestinal endoscopy have become technically less difficult and are thus performed by greater numbers of physicians. The ready availability of such procedures, combined with their diagnostic superiority, has naturally led to greater utilization.

Gastrointestinal diseases themselves have added impetus to this evolution, so that gastrointestinal endoscopy developed rapidly in a country such as Japan where gastric carcinoma is a significant problem. Colon cancer and the recognition of its relation to the colon polyp have clearly promoted the development of colonoscopy and flexible sigmoidoscopy in the United States. Factors such as these have thus contributed to the steady growth year by year in the number of endoscopic procedures performed.

There have also been profound changes in the complexity of endoscopic procedures. For example, development of a side-viewing endoscope in the early 1970's provided an important new approach to investigation of diseases of the duodenal papilla, bile duct, and pancreas. Although diagnostic endo-

scopic retrograde cholangiopancreatography (ERCP) has been supplanted to some degree by other methods such as ultrasonography and computed tomography (CT), the addition of an electrosurgical wire to the standard cannula provided endoscopic access to the biliary system and pancreas that became the basis for a variety of more complicated therapeutic maneuvers. There are numerous examples of endoscopic treatment methods, all of which have added complexity that requires sophisticated instruments, a multitude of specific accessories, and specially trained personnel.

Whether considering a large tertiary care center or a small community hospital, the two attributes of growth in numbers of procedures and expanding complexity of methods are common to every endoscopy unit. There are, however, other common characteristics.

This chapter will not attempt to define an ideal endoscopy unit. The operational characteristics of a given unit are determined by unique factors, so that no single design can be suitable in every case. Rather, the purpose will be to define principles of design and function that can be applied in most instances. By considering the endoscopy unit as a concept rather than a place, certain general rules and guidelines can be evolved that are applicable in many situations.

MEGATRENDS

Other forces molding the form of the endoscopy unit (not medical in the sense of individual patient care) might be termed sociologic and economic. They differ greatly from country to country, so that generalization creates difficulties. Nonetheless, it cannot be denied that gastrointestinal endoscopy, and hence the gastrointestinal endos-copy unit, is and will be influenced to some degree by external factors.

Outpatient Procedures

The shift toward outpatient endoscopy is a universal trend. Although morbidity and mortality are associated with some therapeutic procedures, many such procedures, as well as diagnostic endoscopy in general, can be performed safely on an outpatient basis. In the United States the trend toward outpatient services is in part motivated by cost containment, although outpatient procedures also simplify administrative matters and are more convenient for patients. Emphasis on outpatient procedures influences the design and operation of an endoscopy unit; more space must be available for dressing, preprocedure holding, and postprocedure recovery, and additional personnel are required

Primary Diagnostic Endoscopy

Another emerging trend is that of providing endoscopic services on request. In the future, a substantial portion of relatively simple diagnostic procedures such as esophago-gastroduodenoscopy (EGD) will be performed at the request of a referring physician without prior consultation, much the same as a radiologist performs an upper gastrointestinal x-ray series. This type of endoscopic procedure is referred to by a variety of names, such as primary diagnostic endoscopy or primary panendoscopy. Such a system presently works best in a closed staff environment in which there is an established referral pattern of patients for endoscopy and in which the endoscopist has an existing professional relationship as well as direct communication with the physicians who request endoscopy.

Expertise in Gastrointestinal Endoscopy

Because of the increasing complexity of endoscopy, it is a foregone conclusion that every gastroenterologist or surgeon cannot perform every procedure. Many more complex therapeutic procedures will be developed that will require a high level of expertise, something that can be developed and maintained only by performing such procedures on a regular basis. The ever increasing

skill required for proficiency in new endoscopic procedures will make it more and more difficult to become competent in all endoscopic procedures within presently constituted training programs. It is unlikely, therefore, that large numbers of physicians will be competent in all endoscopic procedures in the future. This has important implications for the endoscopy unit because of the changing and variable qualifications of the physicians who perform procedures. Within any professional staff, most members will execute the more conventional procedures such as EGD and colonoscopy, whereas complex, usually therapeutic procedures will become restricted to fewer individuals. The opposite approach, that each physician performs every indicated procedure on his or her patient, almost certainly leads to a decrease in the quality of services performed within an endoscopy unit. In any community, finite limits on the number of patients who require a particular endoscopic skill plus the necessity of constant practice in order to maintain proficiency virtually assure a lower standard of practice within an endoscopy unit if every endoscopist attempts all procedures. In some, but not all, places the practice of endoscopy is organized on the basis of these realities.

Socioeconomic Factors

Developmental advances in the field of endoscopy over the past 10 to 15 years have evolved at relatively low cost. However, future technologic gains that require computers, videosystems, lasers, and specialized endoscopes and other instruments will have a higher monetary cost. It is doubtful that every hospital will be able to afford a "state of the art" endoscopy unit in the future.

It would be inappropriate to comment on the sociologic consequences of systems of health care delivery, except that there can be no doubt that these influence the practice of endoscopy and the structure of endoscopy units.

When systems of health care delivery are centrally planned by government agencies, it is common that complex procedures requiring high levels of skill and expensive equipment are performed by a relatively small number of individuals in a few centers. Economic issues are a major driving force in such a system, so that the allocation of funds for staff and equipment determines the pattern of medical practice.

Economic forces are becoming increasingly important in health care delivery in the United States, although these forces operate differently. In this country the trend is toward a competitive, "market-place" strategy in which health care delivery systems must vie for fixed or even reduced "health care dollars." To an ever increasing extent, the "health care dollar" is spent by organizations, the so-called "third party payers," rather than by individuals. The third party has traditionally been an insurance company or government agency, but increasingly other third parties such as corporations will negotiate for health care benefits. Economic factors such as these favor larger, efficient, flexible, and responsive institutions that have an economy of scale. The large "for profit" health care company is a derivative of these changes. Another result is the consolidation of smaller health care institutions to achieve an economy of scale. Thus, there are hospital mergers and acquisitions, as well as affiliations and amalgamations as "networks" to provide total health care systems. The essence of competition is that over the course of time there are fewer competitors.

It is impossible to know the long-range consequences of these forces with regard to an endoscopy unit. One net result may be that within any health care system (a "network" of hospitals, for example) endoscopic services may also be consolidated. It is logical to expect that specialized endoscopic procedures will be concentrated at one or a few locations within an organization. The end result may be a system that more closely resembles those in which governmental agencies are responsible for centralized planning of health care; i.e., complex procedures that require high levels of skill and expensive equipment will be performed by a relatively small number of individuals in a few centers.

Acting as a Unit

The short-range, narrow view of endoscopic expertise is that the endoscopy unit must be only a place where individual physicians independently perform their work; i.e., it provides a service not only to patients but to their physicians. A different view is that the endoscopy unit is made up collectively of physicians who perform endoscopy, gastrointestinal assistants, equipment, and rooms and that the unit as a whole performs services for patients and referring physicians within a specific setting such as a hospital, city, or any geographic area. Complex procedures that require high levels of skill and much expensive equipment are performed by a relatively small number of designated individuals. This usually results in endoscopic services that are not only efficient and productive but of the highest quality.

An organized endoscopy unit in which the resources of staff and equipment are deployed to attain the highest levels of patient services comes about in a variety of ways. Perhaps the most common mode over the past decade has been the presence of an "acknowledged expert." This person characteristically has a natural aptitude for endoscopy, has an interest in developing new procedures, and is the first to acquire a specific endoscopic skill, frequently by working with the actual person who developed a technique, and is therefore the first to introduce procedures into a specific hospital or clinic or city or geographic area. Expertise is thus established and an adequate referral base of patients is assured. The expert eventually attracts one or more colleagues, the endoscopy unit being essentially built around these individuals, and the expert is customarily designated the director of a unit. It should not be misconstrued that this has always taken place according to a deliberate plan. In many cases it would be more accurate to say that the endoscopy units of high quality have evolved around one or more experts. Such serendipity will probably not promote the development of a unit in the future.

The "acknowledged expert" method of building an organized endoscopy unit has been practical for the goal of productive, efficient, high quality endoscopic services. However, this course may be incommensurate with future requirements. Obviously, the quality of endoscopic services becomes dependent on the presence of one or more individuals, and loss of the expert(s) for whatever reason means an immediate decrease in quality. However, a more subtle difficulty lies in the fact that expertise in endoscopy is not all that is required of a unit director. Because of the growth in numbers and complexity of procedures, the unit director must (some would say unfortunately) become a manager with responsibility in many areas in which expertise in endoscopy is irrelevant.

ENDOSCOPY UNIT FUNCTION

A large endoscopy unit (25 to 35 or more procedures per day) is a complicated place in which a great number of different procedures are performed. It is no small task to organize the use of available space, numerous pieces of equipment, and various staff members to accomplish a heavy schedule of procedures with a minimum of confusion. By the same token, the operation of such a unit becomes difficult to comprehend as the numbers and complexity of procedures increase. Planning for future needs and growth becomes even more perplexing. In view of the seeming complexity of the endoscopy unit, problem solving as well as establishing and achieving goals can be an arduous process that sometimes amounts to a series of educated guesses. From the standpoint of daily operations, problem solving, and future goals, it is essential that one clearly understands the way in which a unit functions. To this end there are certain management tools that can be used. These are actually abstract concepts, but they provide insight into function as well as a workable apparatus for analysis and problem solving. These devices are the procedure unit, the weighted scale, and the endoscopy room.

The Procedure Unit

Most endoscopists regard an endoscopic procedure only in terms of actual use of an endoscope in a patient. From an operational standpoint a procedure is more complicated. However, any endoscopic procedure, whatever the type, can be reduced to a series of basic steps (Table 3–1). These can be subgrouped into preprocedural, procedural, and postprocedural categories. The basic procedure components taken together are termed a "procedure unit." From a manufacturing viewpoint the business of an endoscopy unit is to produce endoscopy procedure units.

The actual endoscopic component of the procedure unit is but one part of a relatively complex process. The length of time required for each component varies according to the type of endoscopic procedure, although the endoscopy itself may require a short length of time relative to the time needed for the other steps. Diagnostic EGD, for example, requires only 5 to 10 minutes.

TABLE 3–1. **The Procedure Unit**

Preprocedure
Scheduling
Patient check-in
Patient instruction, interview
Patient preparation
Premedication
Room/equipment preparation

Procedure
Examination/procedure
   (handling of biopsy and other specimens)

Postprocedure
Patient recovery
    Monitoring
    Postprocedure instructions/scheduling
    Discharge
Room/equipment cleaning, turn-around
Charting/report generation
    Written chart notation
    Report dictation
    Typing report
    Review/signature of typed report
    Processing of report to chart
    File copy of report
(Data processing)*
(Billing)*

*Variable activity. May not be performed in some endoscopy units.

But the components of scheduling, preparing the patient for the procedure, preparation of the procedure room and equipment, administration of sedative drugs, cleaning, and report generation require the same amounts of time as colonoscopy, even though the colon examination may be three to four times as long as the EGD.

The Weighted Scale

Although all procedure units are identical, actual endoscopic procedures differ in many respects. From the managerial point of view the fundamental variables are the time required and the number of personnel and items of equipment. The procedure unit concept is useless unless it is adjusted for these factors. One method of doing this is to employ a weighted scale for procedures.

It is no longer possible to assess the amount of work performed in an endoscopy unit simply by counting the number of procedures performed. A "raw count" does not take into consideration complicated procedures that require more time, equipment, and personnel. One way to deal with this is to develop a weighted scale for procedures.

The weighted scale is an equivalent value system that adjusts a total procedure count for degree of complexity. The number as signed in the scale to any procedure relates the complexity of the procedure to an arbitrary reference procedure. The reference base of our scale is the diagnostic EGD (without biopsy or other ancillary procedures), since this procedure should be the fastest and least complex in terms of personnel and equipment required. Diagnostic EGD is assigned a value of 1.0 on our scale. A value of 1.0 in our system is equivalent to approximately 30 minutes. A part of the equivalent value table presently used in our endoscopy unit is shown in Table 3–2.

The procedure unit may be arbitrarily assigned any weighted value in the scale. Since the basis of our scale is the simple EGD, which is also the procedure most commonly performed, it is practical to assign its value (1.0) in the weighted scale as the value of one procedure unit also. Giving the procedure unit an arbitrary reference value in the weighted scale facilitates manipulation and analysis. In our unit, therefore, when we speak of procedure units, we mean something that is equivalent to a simple diagnostic EGD.

Our weighted scale was developed in relation to the time and effort required of the gastrointestinal assistant (GIA) in accomplishing a procedure unit. The GIA calculates and records the weighted value of each procedure according to the guidelines in Table 3–2. Adjustments are permitted for especially lengthy and difficult procedures or for those that require an unusual number of items of equipment.

To be most effective, each endoscopy unit must develop its own weighted scale for procedures, because there are unique aspects in the way each unit functions that cannot be accounted for in a universal scale. For example, until recently ERCP procedures in our unit have been performed off floor in a radiology suite. Thus, transport time and additional time to place necessary equipment on carts are calculated into the procedure equivalent value for ERCP. Our equivalent values also reflect the fact that endoscopy procedures are taught in our unit. Teaching is almost always inefficient. As a rule, supervised instruction increases the time required for a procedure by a factor of about one-third. This added time must also be factored into the scale. In a non-teaching institution the time equivalent for a weighted scale value of 1.0 might be reduced to 25 or 20 minutes.

When endoscopic photodocumentation is a routine practice, it must be calculated into the weighted scale. Although only 1 or 2 minutes are needed to snap a few pictures, additional minutes are consumed by procurement of film, handling, record keeping, processing, and filing the film. It may seem trifling

TABLE 3–2. **Cleveland Clinic Weighted Scale of Endoscopic Procedures**

Procedure		Value
EGD		1.00
EGD with heat probe or Bicap probe		2.00
Other procedures with EGD		1.50*
Sclerotherapy		1.75
Esophageal dilation (bougie)		0.50
Colonoscopy		2.00
Limited colonoscopy		1.50
Polypectomy	(add)	0.25
Multiple polypectomies (7 to 10 polyps)		3.00
Colonoscopy with sequential biopsy for dysplasia (CUC)		2.50
Colonoscopy with heat probe or Bicap probe		3.00
Peritoneoscopy		3.00
ERCP		3.00
Sphincterotomy		4.00
ERCP, sphincterotomy, stent placement		4.50
Sphincter of Oddi manometry		1.50
Laser, all types		2.75
Percutaneous endoscopic gastrostomy		2.00
Any major complication, any procedure (e.g., respiratory arrest, hemorrhage)	(add)	3.00
Any procedure done on hospital floor (except laser and ERCP)	(add)	0.50

*Polypectomy, dilation over guide wire, insertion of endoprosthesis, for example.

to view photographic documentation as important with respect to the efficiency of a unit. However, if 5000 procedures are performed per year, with some abnormality being found in about half of the examinations, and if 2 minutes are used in obtaining photographs in these 2500 cases (actual photography plus all other aspects of photodocumentation—certainly an underestimate), the policy of photodocumentation consumes 5000 minutes per year. If one procedure unit is equal to 30 minutes, photodocumentation requires 167 procedure units per year. Although there is a certain monetary cost for film, cameras, and adapters, the real cost to the overall function of a unit is the time required for photodocumentation. This is neither an argument for or against photodocumentation. However, if photodocumentation is the policy of a unit, it must be calculated into the weighted scale.

The procedure unit/weighted scale methodology has many invaluable uses with respect to analysis, planning, and problem solving. It can be a measuring device to gauge the work output and performance of a unit more accurately. For example, in our unit in 1984 the average weighted value of all procedures was 1.4. Multiplying the total number of procedures performed in 1984 by 1.4 converts the total count to an equivalent number of simple diagnostic EGD procedures, i.e., converts it to procedure units. The average weighted value for all procedures in 1985 increased to 1.53, which indicates that further growth in complexity of procedures during 1985 was not reflected in a simple count of procedures.

The weighted scale method of analysis of procedure activity can be used in planning for acquisition of more space, equipment, and staff. The theoretic maximum capacity of a given unit can be assessed in terms of procedure units once the average weighted value and the time value for one procedure unit are established. This calculation would be as follows: the number of available rooms multiplied by the number of working hours per day multiplied by the number of working days per year multiplied by the time value for 1.0 procedure unit (or a weighted scale value of 1.0) divided by the average procedure equivalent value multiplied by the efficiency expected of the unit. The last value, expected efficiency, is somewhat arbitrary, but if not included, the calculation assumes that every room in the unit operates at 100%

efficiency, something that is not attainable. A more reasonable efficiency factor would be about 70%. It is also a simple matter to calculate the actual efficiency of a unit by comparing the weighted procedure count with the theoretic maximum at 100% efficiency.

Our weighted scale was developed to justify an increase in the number of GIAs. Although a steady increase in the number of procedures performed could be easily demonstrated, this "raw count" alone did not seem to justify the additional personnel. However, in addition to increasing numbers of procedures, there was also a corresponding increase in procedure complexity that was not reflected in the count. In essence, the workload of the GIAs had increased to a much greater extent than the procedure count suggested. This became clear when the weighted scale was applied to the procedure count. Our subjective impression of a more substantial workload was converted to an actual measurement that everyone could understand—and that justified an increase in staff, I might add. Needless to say, our GIAs are among the strongest supporters of this method of performance assessment.

The Procedure Room

At least two persons are required for every endoscopic procedure (in addition to a patient): the endoscopist and a GIA. The procedure table should be considered the focus of the room. It so happens that for most procedures the assistant and the endoscopist perform their respective roles at opposite sides of the procedure table. Although in some cases the assistant may stand at the head of the table, the basic rule of specific places within the room is established by the way in which endoscopic procedures are performed. It is necessary to have access to the table from at least three (and preferably four) sides, so that the table is almost always placed at or near the center of the room. The next logical step conceptually is to divide the room in half, with one side for the assistant and the other for the endoscopist.

A well-designed procedure room takes greatest advantage of this simple but valuable principle of dividing the room in half according to the activities of assistant and endoscopist. The first variables to consider are size and shape of the room. Based on experience, an endoscopy room should never be smaller than 300 square feet (approximately 35 square meters). This is the floor space required for a basic procedure room and does not take into account special procedures that require larger items of equipment such as a fluoroscope or laser. It is also my personal experience that a room of this size becomes inadequate when used for more than one special purpose procedure or for the development of new and highly specialized procedures.

The shape of the room is another consideration. Unfortunately, this is sometimes dictated by the overall dimensions of the building, placement of stairwells and elevators, plumbing, and a host of other factors. When possible, however, a somewhat rectangular room with the procedure table oriented along the longer dimension is more suitable. A room with this configuration might have dimensions of about 15 by 20 feet. In a room of this size the work surfaces, cupboards, and storage facilities are within easier reach of the endoscopist and assistant.

An endoscopy room in our unit with approximately the dimensions described above is shown as an example (Fig. 3–1). Drawing a diagonal line from the lower left to the upper right corner of the figure illustrates the approximate division of this procedure room into endoscopist and GIA areas. Within a procedure room are many and varied other items of equipment, some of which are discussed in Chapter 5.

THE ENDOSCOPY UNIT

Acquisition of Space

Few endoscopy units have been designed specifically for gastrointestinal endoscopy. Rather, portions of a hospital or clinic have

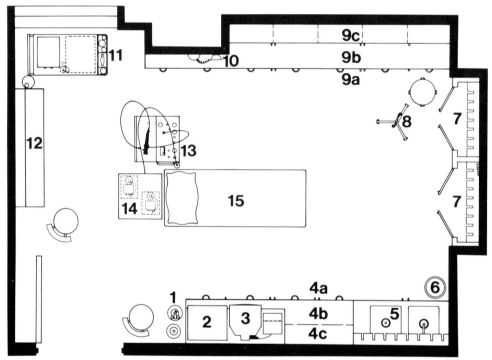

FIGURE 3–1. Typical endoscopy procedure room. A diagonal line drawn from the left lower to the right upper corner divides the room into a right triangular half for the GIA and a left triangular half for the endoscopist. Beginning at the right and proceeding clockwise around the room are the areas for storage (7), cleaning (5), and assistant work surfaces (4a–c). Proceeding clockwise from the left side of the room there is space for charting (12) and space for the usual position of the endoscopist (13). In back of the endoscopist there is also work space (9a–c) that may also be used for items such as lecturescopes and cameras. The rectangular arrangement of the room places the respective countertop work surfaces for the assistant and endoscopist within easy reach even during a procedure (1—oxygen tanks, 2—videotape deck, 3—television monitor, 4a—storage below, 4b—countertop, 4c—cupboard, 5—double sink with rack above for hanging endoscopes, 6—waste basket, 7—storage closets with hanging racks, 8—IV pole, 9a—storage below, 9b—countertop, 9c—cupboards, 10—sphygmomanometer, 11—cart for emergency endoscopy, 12—shelf with x-ray view boxes above, 13—light source, 14—accessory table for GIA, 15—procedure table).

usually been converted for this purpose. To a certain extent, this means that function must fit form; i.e., the design of the unit must conform to the space allotted. Fitting the basic components of the unit into available space frequently leads to a less than ideal design with respect to the flow of activities within the unit. Seifert and Weismüller[1] have recently stated that a completely satisfactory gastrointestinal endoscopy unit probably does not exist in the Federal Republic of Germany, a remarkable statement from a country with high standards of endoscopic practice.

Another liability inherent in the renovation of existing space is a lack of flexibility. The space available is usually subdivided according to specific functions, and rooms are constructed for designated purposes. However, it often becomes necessary to change the function of a specific room or rooms as the demand for endoscopic services increases and new procedures and newly developed equipment are added. Such shifts in emphasis will be possible to the degree that foresight is exercised in designing adaptability into the unit.

An endoscopy unit is usually developed in response to problems that have arisen in meeting the demand for services. The unswerving desire of administrators to economize wherever possible often leads to construction of a unit that is adequate for current needs, but poorly positioned for future growth. Existing problems are solved, but there is little anticipation of future difficulties. This leads to an obsolescence cycle in which a series of units will have been constructed that meet the needs of the moment or at best the immediate future. The capacity for growth in numbers and complexity of procedures is a distinct luxury, and built-in provisions for growth are seldom encountered. Rather, it is more usual that growth is compromised in a fashion that is, based on past performance, almost predictable.

Principles of Design

In many respects, all endoscopic procedures are alike in that the same basic steps are required to complete one procedure unit (see Table 3–1). From this standpoint, endoscopic procedures can be considered uniform and interchangeable when designing an endoscopy unit. From another perspective, they are also dissimilar. In relation to the

design and function of the unit, the differences in procedures relate to requirements for diverse items of equipment and variation in procedure room size.

Division of Floor Space

The physical design of an endoscopy unit must accommodate the basic steps in the general procedure unit (see Table 3–1). Space must be allotted to each of these components whether the endoscopy unit consists of a single procedure room or has several rooms. Thus, any floor plan for a unit must subdivide available space according to the fundamental functions listed in Table 3–3.

In assigning available space(s) to specific function(s) (Table 3–3), some areas may serve a dual purpose. Areas can be set aside in the procedure room for cleaning, storage, and charting (see Fig. 3–1); patients may be interviewed in the procedure room; scheduling and secretarial functions can be located in a single area.

With maximum consolidation, the simplest possible endoscopy unit must consist of four rooms or areas designated as follows: (1) patient reception, (2) scheduling/secretarial, (3) procedure room (with cleaning, storage, charting areas), and (4) patient dressing/recovery room or area. At the opposite extreme is the referral center unit that is substantially larger than the simplest model, there being much greater floor space and many more rooms. However, the available space, albeit greater, is nevertheless allocated according to the same basic functional plan no matter what the size of the unit (Table 3–3). In the simplest unit, space for storage, cleaning, and charting is provided within the procedure room itself, whereas separate larger areas, even actual rooms, might be provided for these functions in a sizable referral center unit. Scheduling, secretarial, and patient reception might be served by a single area in the simplest unit model, whereas individual

TABLE 3–3. **Allocation of Space in the Endoscopy Unit**

Scheduling
Patient reception
Patient interview room(s)
Patient dressing/recovery room(s)
Procedure room(s)
Cleaning
Storage
Charting/dictation
Secretarial

areas are often allocated to these functions in the large unit.

Independent and Interdependent Procedure Rooms

The degree to which the procedure rooms of a large unit function independently of one another is an important design decision.

In the simplest unit model the single procedure room serves many functions; the elements of the procedure unit (see Table 3–1) are substantially contained and accomplished within this room. A larger unit design can preserve this approach by placing as many elements of the procedure unit as possible in the procedure room.

The opposite approach is to accomplish as many procedure unit elements (see Table 3–1) away from the procedure room as are feasible, so that the only activity performed in this room would be the endoscopy per se. Other areas and rooms in the unit are then provided and designated for other components of the procedure unit. Single rooms for cleaning and for storage could serve all procedure rooms. A centralized pattern for cleaning/storage versus a more dispersed scheme with facilities for cleaning/storage perhaps in each procedure room, or divided between two procedure rooms, is one of the main differences in design among units. Centralized storage/cleaning provides flexibility in the use of procedure rooms, since the same equipment can be used in more than one room. However, it also increases scheduling intricacy, since care must be taken to avoid simultaneous procedures that require the same item of equipment. Administration of sedative drugs can also be accomplished outside the procedure room with the use of a cart exchange system, so that the sole purpose of the procedure room becomes the procedure itself.

The arrangement of the physical counterparts of the various procedure unit elements also has a bearing on staffing. For example, with a central cleaning/storage room it may be efficient to assign a GIA to this responsibility alone, perhaps on a daily rotating basis.

Multifunctional versus Dedicated Procedure Rooms

In the simplest model (one procedure room), all procedures in the repertoire are necessarily performed in one room. As the number of procedure rooms increases, an independent room philosophy can be maintained, except that if carried to its logical conclusion, this results in a group of extraor-

dinarily well equipped, functionally independent procedure rooms, any one of which could serve alone as a respectable endoscopy unit. This is, of course, facetious, and in practice such a unit would be highly unusual. In fact, as procedure rooms become more numerous, they are diversified according to various functions, each room being designed, equipped, and arranged with an emphasis on one or a few types of procedures.

The way in which different procedures are diversified among available procedure rooms is one of the major differences among endoscopy units. To a large extent this reflects the pattern of procedures performed in the unit, which in turn depends on referral patterns, the demand for particular procedures, and the interests and expertise of the professional staff. Thus, in one unit an emphasis on laparoscopy might require a room designated for this purpose. A center with a large referral base for ERCP would logically require a separate room for this purpose. None of the factors that influence the pattern of the types of procedures performed in a unit is static. Rather, the pattern always changes over the course of time, especially as new techniques are developed. It is probably safe to predict, for example, that the demand for colonoscopy procedures will continue to accelerate in coming years.

A tradeoff necessarily occurs when a room is designated for a precise function. Altered for a specific purpose by the way it is scheduled and equipped, perhaps even with respect to physical changes in the floor plan, it becomes less suitable for other procedures. Essentially, the unit as a whole becomes less flexible and less adaptable to changes in the pattern of procedures. A unit in which rules for room utilization are relatively inflexible tends to be inefficient. Certain functions, such as scheduling, are simplified, but procedure rooms may stand idle. If demand for endoscopic services is high, this translates to limitations of access, delays in scheduling procedures, and dissatisfied patients and referring physicians. At the other extreme is the concept of the capability to perform virtually any procedure in any room. The tradeoff here is more complex scheduling and a greater tendency toward disorganization in the management of the daily activities unless each room is so well equipped that procedures can be scheduled ad lib in any room without concern for availability of assistants and equipment. The price for the latter approach is the high cost for duplicate staff and equipment. Endoscopy units become unique as they attempt to balance these two extremes.

Special and Routine Procedures. One method of establishing a balance in a unit between dedicated and multifunctional procedure rooms is to divide procedures into "routine" and "special" types. Routine procedures have the following characteristics: (1) are usually, but not always, high volume; (2) can be performed by numerous endoscopists; (3) are usually diagnostic; (4) require fairly standard, relatively unsophisticated equipment that is readily available in the unit; and (5) have significant variation day to day (even hour to hour) in demand. Special procedures tend to have the following attributes: (1) are performed by fewer endoscopists; (2) often require special, perhaps expensive, equipment and therefore are available only as a one-of-a-kind item within the unit; (3) have lower volume relative to that for routine procedures; (4) frequently are more time consuming; and (5) may require more than one GIA. It is frequently useful to divide routine procedures into high and low volume. The definition of a "high-volume" procedure is arbitrary, but generally applies to any procedure that constitutes 20% or more of the volume of all procedures.

The process of dividing procedures into routine and special categories is unique in each unit. Although EGD and colonoscopy would be typically categorized as routine in most units, other large units might include ERCP and laparoscopy. This depends on two factors: the pattern and numbers of procedures performed and the availability of equipment. It is unusual to find the capability to perform ERCP in more than one room in any given unit, so that by default ERCP becomes a special procedure with a designated room. In our unit, ERCP, laparoscopy, laser endoscopy, percutaneous endoscopic gastrostomy tube placement, certain dilation procedures, and esophageal prosthesis placement are "special," whereas all other procedures are "routine" and can be performed in any room. EGD, colonoscopy, polypectomy, some types of dilation, and most methods for control of bleeding, including sclerotherapy, can be performed in any of our rooms. Certain provisions are made in scheduling. For example, it is best not to alternate or mix EGD and colonoscopy procedures in a given room. Therefore, EGD procedures are usually scheduled first. However, colonoscopy procedures may nevertheless begin at any time in a given room during the working day, and, in fact, a room might be scheduled entirely for colonoscopy on any given day.

Achieving Balance. As a general rule, specific rooms should be designated for special procedures. Usually this follows without much deliberation, since the availability of special equipment is limited. However, as far as possible, routine procedures should not be restricted to specific procedure rooms. For maximum efficiency, it should be feasible to conduct routine procedures in any room, even rooms designated for special procedures. A large referral center unit should have adequate equipment to carry out routine, high-volume procedures simultaneously in most or all procedure rooms, including those designated for special purposes.

Since by definition certain routine procedures are high volume, it might seem logical to assign specific rooms for such procedures while excluding other activities from these rooms. Depending on circumstances this may be efficient or restrictive. If the number of routine procedures of one type, EGD for example, is sufficient to reasonably expect that a room will be fully utilized in the performance of this one procedure, then it may be efficient to designate one or more procedure rooms for this purpose. However, another characteristic of the routine procedure is that the demand for this type of service varies a great deal on a day to day basis (even hour to hour in a highly active unit). Over longer periods of time there will be changes in the numbers and patterns of procedures performed.

In deciding the mix of multifunctional and dedicated rooms within a unit, it is important to analyze efficiency and the effect that limiting room usage has on the scheduling process.

A retrospective approach to assessing efficiency is to determine the average number of hours per day that a unifunctional, designated room is not in use in relation to the desired overall efficiency of room utilization in the unit. If, for example, this is significantly greater than about 30%, the use of the room for a single specific function may be inefficient, i.e., the procedure activity in question does not justify restriction of a room. Conversely, utilization of the room at greater than targeted efficiency may mean that demand exceeds capacity. If at the same time other rooms designated specifically for other procedures are not in use more than about 30% of the time, the overall unit is not functioning at maximum efficiency.

There is a further element in balancing dedicated versus multifunctional room usage that is potentially more damaging to the orderly function of the endoscopy unit. Rigid adherence to specific room designations may restrict patient access. One way to determine this is to track overall scheduling activity of the unit with special attention to schedule lag. This is the length of time required to complete a procedure unit beginning with the moment of contact between the endoscopy unit and the patient and/or referring physician. It is important to consider all types of procedures performed in the unit, since the time required for completion of one type may be within objectives, whereas that for another may be unsatisfactory. The many possible reasons for such an imbalance include limited staff availability. However, in some cases it may be due entirely to or at least compounded by an inflexible adherence to a policy of dedicated room usage.

The uncontemplative "trigger" reaction to apparently excessive demand for a routine procedure is to acquire another designated room. A more discerning approach is first to determine whether or not the way in which the unit functions is the problem. This emphasizes the basic importance of trying to think about the endoscopy unit from an abstract conceptual point of view rather than as a physical cluster of rooms.

The blend of unifunctional special procedure rooms and multifunctional routine procedure rooms should never become absolute and unchangable. If past experience is any guide, it can be assumed that the pattern, numbers, complexity, and general mix of procedures will continue to change. Therefore it is important that a unit be constructed so that the function of any room can be altered when necessary. A "few small rooms" for EGD, for example, is very imprudent. A unit cannot be set up today that will serve all the foreseeable and unforeseeable needs of the next decade. The only answer to this problem is flexibility in design.

Ultra High Volume Procedures. Certain procedures may be performed in such numbers that the sheer volume is overwhelming and the function and efficiency of the unit are compromised. It usually becomes necessary to consider such ultra-high-volume procedures as separate categories in relation to other endoscopic procedures. The only procedure that in general qualifies in this respect at present is screening flexible sigmoidoscopy. Flexible sigmoidoscopy does not fit the procedure unit concept, i.e., it differs significantly from other endoscopic procedures with respect to scheduling, patient preparation and recovery, and time required. These differences in relation to other procedures would not be so important were it not for the high volume of these procedures. In great numbers the special characteristics of an ultra-high-volume procedure tend to dominate the function of the unit. It would seem to be not only efficient but also responsive to patient needs to design a specific room or rooms in the endoscopy unit for this purpose. However, it makes more sense to divorce the truly ultra-high-volume procedure physically and functionally from the rest of the endoscopy unit.

The dissociation of flexible sigmoidoscopy from the rest of the endoscopy unit need not be absolute. For example, scheduling might be done in the same place and by the same personnel for both procedures. Staff can rotate from one unit to the other. However, at any point in time, the function of the flexible sigmoidoscopy unit should be independent of the endoscopy unit. Patient flow patterns should not intersect nor should patients use the same dressing facilities. To some degree toilet facilities might be shared in a well-designed unit, but in this case care must be taken that the requirements for flexible sigmoidoscopy preparation do not overwhelm the capacity to prepare patients for colonoscopy.

Ultra high volume could become problematic with respect to EGD in relation to the growing utilization of this examination as a primary diagnostic procedure in place of the upper gastrointestinal x-ray series. From a conceptual and operational point of view it may be reasonable to separate facilities for primary upper gastrointestinal diagnostic endoscopy from the other procedure activities. Such a separation can be physical and/or functional to greater or lesser degrees. Another possible concept is to separate special (frequently therapeutic) procedures from routine high volume diagnostic procedures.

Thus, laser, ERCP (with a high volume of therapeutic endoscopy), endoscopic methods of hemostasis, and other therapeutic procedures might be done in one area of the unit, while EGD and colonoscopy might be performed in another. Operationally these two areas would work at different paces, and require different methods of scheduling, different types of equipment, and different levels of staffing.

The Multidisciplinary Unit

It is possible to dispense with specific gastrointestinal endoscopy scheduling/secretarial, reception, and patient dressing/recovery areas in a multifunctional unit in which a variety of other non-gastrointestinal diagnostic and therapeutic procedures are performed. This is not germane here, since a gastrointestinal endoscopy unit as an entity does not exist in this type of unit. However, this plan has the advantage of cost containment in that some equipment, staff, and spaces are shared among disciplines, but it is extremely restrictive in terms of growth, both in numbers and complexity of procedures. Furthermore, the similarity among different types of endoscopic procedures is superficial with regard to the instruments required and to actual procedures, so that cross training of assistants for more than one discipline has its limits. Shared units frequently lead to scheduling conflicts and apportionment of time and room availability to the various specialties that use the unit, a practice that in effect means that each specialty has its own unit but that it is operated at something less than full-time.

Certain expensive pieces of equipment, e.g., a C-arm fluoroscope or Nd:YAG laser, might be shared between two or more specialties if the volume of cases for all users is small and the demand for use of a machine is expected to remain static. However, when two or more departments must combine their patient activity to justify the acquisition of an expensive device, a laser for example, there is reason to wonder whether or not this represents an improvement in patient care, since the number of procedures in any category of usage is by definition small. Nevertheless, cost is a significant factor in the function of a unit. Except where the volume of procedures is very high, ERCP is usually performed away from the endoscopy unit in a radiology suite because of the cost of x-ray equipment. In general, however, the efficiency of an endoscopy unit decreases in proportion to the number of procedures performed away from the unit.

Location

Location of an endoscopy unit in the hospital setting is not an inconsequential question. Although options as to site are often not available (see Aquisition of Space), placement of the unit in relation to other hospital departments has a direct bearing on efficiency. In the 1983 report of the British Society of Gastroenterology, the second most common problem encountered in endoscopy units, after limited size, was excessive distance from other hospital departments.[2] The endoscopy unit has a natural relationship with many other areas of the hospital, including the emergency room, radiology department, and intensive care units, since it is frequently necessary to perform endoscopic procedures in these areas. At the same time the unit must be convenient to hospital wards. When certain beds are reserved for specific types of disease or for specific hospital departments, placement of the endoscopy unit near those wards set aside for patients with gastrointestinal diseases is advantageous.

Since more and more endoscopic procedures are being performed on an outpatient basis, convenient outpatient access becomes a necessity. For hospital units built at a time when there was less emphasis on outpatient procedures, patients must endure a series of signs, maps, and conflicting directions that begin at the hospital front door, a symbolic portal that is not necessarily "patient friendly."

A location for a unit that is desirable in every way is an impossibility, as this would require that the hospital be built around the unit. Fortunately, close physical relationships within the hospital have relative degrees of importance. To some degree these priorities are determined by practice methods. As a general rule, however, proximity to the radiology suite and easy outpatient access should be given precedence in determining unit location. In addition to the fact that ERCP and related procedures may be performed in the radiology suite, many radiologic and endoscopic procedures are complementary. This facilitates patient evaluation in that patients may undergo a series of procedures in each of the two units without returning to their hospital beds between diagnostic studies. Proximity also facilitates a cooperative professional relationship between radiologist and endoscopist that enhances patient care.

Number of Procedure Rooms

The number of procedure rooms required is a very basic consideration in planning an endoscopy unit. It is a simple matter to calculate the needs of the moment, but the future, be it further growth in numbers and complexity (or contraction of growth), is more difficult to predict. Past experience helps to some extent, and in this respect records of past unit activity are extremely helpful. But there are no formulas for future activity, and forecasts are at best educated guesses. Some variables in this calculation are common to all units, such as the socioeconomic factors and other trends described above. However, each unit faces unique questions peculiar to its environment. Such an analysis can be far reaching and can include such diverse factors as the level and quality of competing organizations and the demographic characteristics of the population that the unit serves. In the final analysis, however, growth is strongly related to the quality of the unit. Is it innovative in a critical way? Is it responsive to the needs of patients and referring physicians? Is the proficiency of its staff high? Does it function efficiently?

The theoretic maximum capacity of an endoscopy room can be calculated in procedure units using the weighted scale. It is first necessary to calculate the number of working days per year (approximately 256 days based on a 5-day work week and 5 or 6 holidays per year) and the working hours of the unit (usually 7 hours). The time corresponding to a 1.0 procedural equivalent is a relative value that must be estimated for each individual unit (1.0 equals about 30 minutes in our unit). Thus, the theoretic maximum number of procedure units (diagnostic EGD equivalents) that can be performed in one room during one year is 3584 ($256 \times 2.0 \times 7$). However, this is a theoretic value that assumes that all procedures performed are diagnostic EGD. To arrive at a more realistic number it is necessary to allow for the average degree of difficulty of the procedures performed. In our unit in 1985 the average weighted value

of all procedures was 1.53. Thus, the theoretic maximum number of procedures that a single room can accommodate in our unit is 2342 (3584 divided by 1.53). This, however, assumes 100% efficiency in the use of the room, a level that is not possible. A more attainable efficiency for use of a room would be about 60% to 70%. Thus, the capacity of one of our endoscopy rooms is about 1500 procedure units per year.

Support Rooms

Although the procedure room(s) is the nucleus of every endoscopy unit, many other kinds of rooms or designated areas are also necessary. A relatively complete list of possibilities is given in Table 3–4. It is doubtful that actual facilities in the majority of units are so complete. However, such a complement of rooms is not an unreasonable goal for a large referral unit.

Dressing Room

The term dressing room is preferred for the preprocedure holding and postprocedure recovery area for patients, although in some units this is termed the recovery room. In most units a single dressing room serves all procedure rooms. This arrangement is most common because it allows for the most efficient use of space and staff. However, other plans are possible, such as a dressing/recovery area for each procedure room, although this is usually impractical. There are other potentially useful modifications of the basic arrangement, provided adequate space and equipment are available. One would be

TABLE 3–4. **Endoscopy Unit Rooms (Full Complement)**

Reception
Procedure room(s)
Appointment desk
Dressing room
Toilet facilities (women/men)
Interview room(s)
    Offices
    Director of unit
    Medical staff
    Head nurse
    Secretaries
    Word processing
    Computer facilities
    Records
Staff changing, toilet facilities, locker room
Nurse base area, utility room
Conference room—staff, students
Library
Storage room(s)

separate areas for inpatients and outpatients. Hospitalized patients do not require extensive dressing facilities, although they often require closer postprocedure monitoring while awaiting transport to their hospital beds. Conversely, outpatients who are presumably in better condition require more elaborate dressing facilities, but perhaps less close observation after the procedure. The hospital patient recovers from the procedure on a hospital guerney, whereas the outpatient requires a bed. Furthermore, it is somewhat inconsiderate to mix relatively healthy patients with those who are seriously ill or dying. Separation of inpatients and outpatients in the dressing room does require some duplication of space, since the ratio of inpatient to outpatient procedures will fluctuate from day to day (in our unit this may change by as much as 30% to 40% from one day to the next).

The major concern with respect to the dressing room is its size, i.e., what is the required ratio of dressing room bed spaces to procedure rooms. There are various formulas but these can be deceptive, since an ideal ratio depends greatly on methods of practice. For example, the types and dosages of sedative drugs used may necessitate more prolonged observation. Another major factor is the number of outpatient therapeutic procedures that require protracted postprocedure observation. Just as there is a trend toward performance of routine diagnostic procedures on an outpatient basis, there is also a trend toward use of outpatient therapeutic procedures.[3, 4] Thus, any formula for dressing room bed space must be modified according to individual circumstances.

One basis for determining the number of beds needed is the average time a patient spends in the dressing room. This depends in part on how the room is used. Usually patients are brought to the dressing room and assigned a space to be utilized throughout the procedure. Because outpatients require a place for personal belongings and to gown for the procedure, assignment of a dressing room space upon arrival is most satisfactory. Clothes and other personal belongings can be placed in a lockable cabinet, the key to which the patient retains throughout the procedure (e.g., on a bracelet). The result of this method, however, is that a certain number of bed spaces are reserved but unoccupied while patients are in the procedure room. It is possible to circumvent this by simply not assigning a space until after the procedure. Theoretically, this would be more efficient and allow a reduction in the ratio of dressing room bed spaces to procedure rooms. However, in a large unit the flow of patients to and from multiple procedure rooms is always so unpredictable that this method allows for only a slight reduction at best in the ratio of recovery beds to procedure rooms. Furthermore, it makes changing clothes and handling personal belongings more difficult, and it usually deprives the patient of some privacy.

The average time required for recovery after a procedure can be determined by actual observation (e.g., a dressing room log). For many routine procedures, however, the recovery time is about equal to the length of the procedure. For routine diagnostic EGD, for example, this is usually about 30 to 45 minutes.

For maximum efficiency at least two dressing room spaces should be available for each procedure room; a patient should be ready and waiting in one bed while the second bed awaits the patient undergoing the procedure. One procedure room at 100% efficiency can sustain 14.0 procedure units per day. At 70% efficiency this is reduced to 9.8 procedure units per day. This would mean that about 19.6 hours of dressing room time would be required for one procedure room per day. Based on an 8-hour working day, this means that about 2.45 beds would be required to support one procedure room. However, the average weighted value for procedures performed in a unit is never 1.0, since all procedures other than basic EGD are by definition longer and/or more complex and therefore given a higher value in the weighted scale. If the average weighted value for procedures in a unit is 1.5, the actual number of procedures performed in one room in one day could be as low as 6.5. Theoretically, only 1.6 dressing room spaces would be needed for this level of activity, although this does not take into account the length and difficulty of the procedure nor the fact that more extended periods of recovery are required for some procedures. Thus, the ideal ratio of beds for a unit operating rooms at 70% efficiency with an average weighted scale value of 1.5 would be between 1.6 and 2.45 beds per procedure room. A unit with four procedure rooms would therefore require about ten recovery beds.

Lavatory Facilities

The number of toilets required depends in part on methods of preparation for colonoscopy. In my opinion the best method is that of colon lavage and that this is best accomplished within the endoscopy unit itself under the supervision of a GIA. However, this requires the maximum lavatory facilities of all possible methods. It takes about 3 to 4 hours to complete this type of preparation. It is mandatory that one toilet be available during this period of time for each patient undergoing colon lavage. There must be duplicate facilities for men and women.

Interview Rooms

The requirements for preprocedure and postprocedure interview rooms relate for the most part to the level of outpatient activity in the unit. When this is high (e.g., 70% of procedures), more rooms will be needed. In a unit with this level of outpatient procedure activity, a ratio of about one interview room to every two procedure rooms is usually satisfactory.

Other Rooms

Requirements for other types of rooms shown in Table 3–4 depend on the size and functions of the unit.

The reception area or reception room generally serves as a waiting room for family and friends. It may also serve as a step-down recovery unit following certain procedures when extended close monitoring is not necessary, but it is still desirable that a patient remain in the unit for several hours.

As the endoscopy unit increases in size, it usually becomes necessary to separate the appointment desk from other functions such as reception. In a large unit, scheduling can be so complex that a separate area with specific appointment secretaries becomes necessary.

With increasing size comes increasing administrative complexity and a more complicated administrative structure that requires a director, who should be a physician, and a chief GIA, who should be a nurse. These individuals constitute the nucleus of a management team, and their offices should be nearby, if not within, the endoscopy unit. It may be prudent to allocate office space for other physicians within the unit, depending on the amount of time they spend in endoscopic activities. Consultation/examination rooms must also be provided in this case.

A conference room, although not absolutely essential, is of great value, especially in teaching units. Many different meetings may be scheduled in an endoscopy unit, such as in-service demonstrations of new equipment, management conferences, teaching conferences for both trainees and GIAs, and problem-solving discussions. A pleasantly appointed conference room not only provides a convenient, time-saving meeting place but also helps to promote "esprit de corps" simply by virtue of the fact that there is a common ground.

A library is essential in units where endoscopy is taught. This is not a library in the ordinary sense, although some books on endoscopy should be provided. Rather it should contain audiovisual materials such as television tapes that demonstrate and illustrate endoscopic procedures and findings.

When photography is important, as for photodocumentation, scientific publications, and teaching, it is prudent to set aside a small area in the unit for handling, storing, and labeling photographs.

A large unit (25 to 35 procedures per day) will require at least one secretary who will be occupied entirely with report generation, including typing and filing of copies. With a standardized format for endoscopy reports plus word processing capability, one experienced secretary should be able to generate about 20 to 25 reports per day.

Computerized record-keeping systems (see below) become more necessary as the volume of procedures increases. Computers can be expensive, and because valuable data can be lost as a result of unauthorized use or tampering, it is advisable to set aside a restricted area for data storage.

Unusable Space

In designing an endoscopy unit it is important to realize that all the floor space allocated for the unit cannot be used for the various rooms that one wishes to construct. About 30% of the available space will be taken up by corridors, walls, building supports, stairwells, etc.

Floor Plan

The last step in designing an endoscopy unit is the arrangement of the desired rooms in a floor plan. Often an ideal room arrangement is prevented by the configuration of a building. Even when floor space is adequate, the shape of the building may not accommodate a desired design. The compromises made at this stage determine what is good and bad about the layout of a unit, and every unit has a little of each.

Any arrangement of rooms should be made with traffic flow patterns in mind. The major flow is from reception to dressing room to procedure room and back again to dressing room and then reception. Thus, the dressing room should be relatively near the procedure rooms. If at all possible, there should be separate routes to and from the procedure room. If a separate room (or rooms) for cleaning and storage of equipment is used, it must obviously be near the endoscopy rooms. In all cases it is highly desirable that heavy traffic flow patterns do not intersect.

Procedure rooms are often grouped in one area of the unit. This is not absolutely necessary, and arranging the procedure rooms around the dressing room or at opposite sides of a central dressing room can have advantages. However, this usually eliminates central cleaning and storage of endoscopes.

Support rooms, other than the dressing room and cleaning and storage rooms, can usually be located away from the more active areas of the unit. However, personnel, equipment, and rooms for report generation should be clustered if at all possible. Appointment and reception areas should also be close together, since some communication between these areas is often needed.

Floor plans for three hypothetical units are shown in Figures 3–2 to 3–4. The plan shown in Figure 3–2 was designed for a unit that performs about 1000 procedure units per year. Figure 3–3 depicts a floor plan for a medium-sized unit that performs about 3000 procedure units per year. A design to accommodate a large referral center unit performing 6000 or more procedure units per year is shown in Figure 3–4.

EQUIPMENT

Many of the various items of equipment needed in an endoscopy unit are discussed in Chapter 5, which also considers deployment of equipment to achieve maximum efficiency. Some general ideas concerning management of capital equipment will be discussed.

Information on the life expectancy of a gastrointestinal endoscope in terms of number of procedures would be of great value. Unfortunately there is no such information. The number of times an endoscope can be used depends entirely on the manner in which it is used. In units where there are numerous endoscopists with varying levels of skill and where endoscopic procedures are taught, an endoscope may not last very long. If an endoscopy unit has an efficient record-keeping system that tracks the usage of an instrument as well as its repair record, it is not too difficult to determine the average lifespan of an endoscope.

The number of endoscopes necessary for routine procedures depends on how the unit functions. It has been suggested that at least three upper gastrointestinal endoscopes should be available for each room in which EGD is performed (one being cleaned, one as backup, and one in use).[5] This ratio is too high, and one backup instrument for every room is unnecessary unless a simultaneous malfunction of every instrument is expected. Two upper gastrointestinal endoscopes for each multifunctional procedure room in which EGD is performed should be adequate.

In a large unit (5000 or more procedures per year) repair costs are a significant budget item. The actual cost of repairs will again depend on the skill and care exercised in using the instruments. With careful record keeping it is possible to cost account major repairs.

SYSTEMS

One of the objectives of this chapter is to emphasize a conceptual approach to the endoscopy unit, i.e., to think in terms of its functions and insofar as is possible to make the physical form of the unit fit these functions. Systematic methods for directing daily activities are crucial to orderly function. Such systems are also based on management concepts. Two of the most important systems are scheduling and record keeping.

Scheduling

If the procedure room is the heart of the endoscopy unit, the daily schedule is its nervous system. When 25 or more procedures requiring numerous different pieces of equipment and procedural skills are being performed daily by several physicians, there is obviously an enormous potential for disorder and confusion. The extent to which this potential remains latent and unrealized is a direct indication of managerial skill in designing a scheduling system.

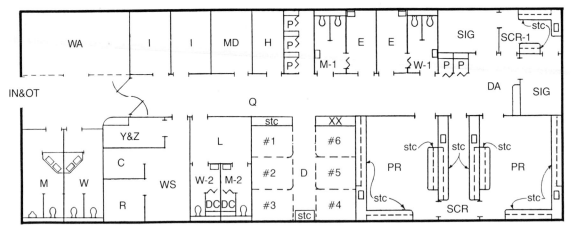

4,250 net. sq. ft.

FIGURE 3–2. Architect's drawing of hypothetical endoscopy unit in which approximately 1000 procedure units would be performed per year.

C	Computer Room	6′ × 8′	Q	Corridor	8′ W
D	Dressing Room*	18′ × 21′	R	Medical Records Room	8′ × 20 ′
DA	Dictation Area	2′ × 6′	SCR	Cleaning and Storage	8′ × 20′
DC	Dressing Cubicle	3′ × 4′	SCR-1	Cleaning and Storage	8′ × 12′
E	Enema Room	6′ × 12′	SIG	Sigmoidoscopy Room	8′ × 12′
H	Head Nurse	6′ × 12′	stc	Storage Cabinets†	
I	Interview and Consultation Room	8′ × 12′	WA	Waiting Area‡	11′ × 21′
			WS	Word Processing/Secretarial Area	9′ × 17′
IN	Inpatient Entrance/Exit				
L	Staff Lounge	9′ × 12′	W	Women's Restroom	8′ × 18′
M	Men's Restroom	8′ × 12′	W-1	Women's Toilet/Patient	6′ × 11′
M-1	Men's Toilet/Patient	6′ × 12′	W-2	Women's Toilet and Dressing Area/Staff	6′ × 11′
M-2	Men's Toilet and Dressing Area/Staff	6′ × 11′	XX	Linen Storage	2′ × 8′
MD	Medical Staff	8′ × 12′	Y&Z	Receptionist/Appointments Room	6′ × 12′
OT	Outpatient Entrance/Exit				
P	Preparation Cubicle	3′ × 4′	▭	Sink	6′ × 12′
PR	Procedure Room	16′ × 20′			

*Broken line indicates bed space.
†Broken line indicates above counter wall-mounted cabinets.
‡Approximate seating for 18 people. Broken line indicates 5′ high temporary partition.

The primary task in devising a method of scheduling is to determine which procedure component will be most restrictive. There may be an abundance of procedure rooms but limited numbers of endoscopists, assistants, and/or instruments. Some deficiencies and imbalances are easier to correct than others. When there are adequate numbers of staff, the overriding factors that control the schedule are the availability of procedure rooms and to a lesser extent the availability of equipment for special procedures. These two factors necessarily govern the schedule.

The endoscopy schedule also reflects the basic philosophy for procedure room utilization. The efficiency and capacity of the unit increase in proportion to the number of procedure rooms that are considered multifunctional, although greater numbers of multifunctional rooms increase the complexity of the schedule. When there is dogmatic restriction of procedure types to specific rooms, the schedule is uncomplicated, but there is a loss of flexibility in responding to day by day fluctuations in the demand for procedures.

The first step in devising a schedule is to set up a timetable for each available procedure room. This timetable should be divided into units of time that equal one procedure unit (e.g., 1.0 procedure unit = 30 minutes).

Special procedures (see definition above) should then be restricted to specific rooms to the degree that necessary items of equipment are limited or unique in the unit. Thus, one room might be designated for ERCP (more desirable would be the simple designation "fluoroscopy"), another for laser endoscopy, and perhaps another for laparoscopy. These designated rooms, however, should not stand idle in the absence of special procedure activity. If properly designed and equipped, a laser room or laparoscopy room will serve nicely for EGD and colonoscopy and any number of other procedures. Even an ERCP room can be used for other procedures when necessary.

A multifunctional room scheduling scheme requires careful thought and judgment by the appointment secretary, who must have insight into the function of a unit. Such an individual must be a tactician with the ability to effectively deploy and coordinate staff, equipment, and rooms. In a highly multi-functional room system, close cooperation

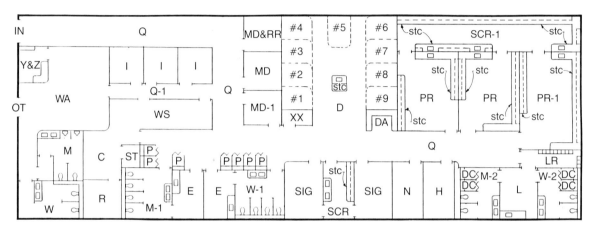

7700 net. sq. ft.

FIGURE 3–3. Architect's drawing of hypothetical endoscopy unit in which approximately 3000 procedure units would be performed per year.

C	Computer Room	10′ × 12′	PR	Procedure Room	16′ × 20′
D	Dressing Room*	24′ × 30′	Q	Corridor	8′ W
DA	Dictation Room	5′ × 8′	Q-1	Corridor	4′ W
DC	Dressing Cubicle	3′ × 4′	R	Medical Records	10′ × 10′
E	Enema Room	8′ × 12′	SCR	Cleaning/Storage	8′ × 14′
H	Head Nurse	8′ × 14′	SCR-1	Cleaning/Storage	9′ × 48′
I	Interview and Consultation Room	9′ × 9′	SIG	Sigmoidoscopy Room	10′ × 14′
			ST	Storage Room	5′ × 6′
IN	Inpatient Entrance/Exit		stc	Storage Cabinets†	
L	Staff Lounge	10′ × 13′	W	Women's Restroom	10′ × 17′
LR	Staff Locker Room	5′ × 16′	W-1	Women's Toilet/Patient	13′ × 13′
M	Men's Restroom	12′ × 13′	W-2	Women's Toilet and Dressing Area/Staff	12′ × 13′
M-1	Men's Toilet/Patient	12′ × 14′			
M-2	Men's Toilet and Dressing Area/Staff	12′ × 13′	WA	Waiting Area‡	16′ × 22′
			WS	Word Processing and Secretarial Area	8′ × 27′
MD	Medical Staff	10′ × 10′			
MD-1	Medical Staff	9′ × 10′	XX	Linen Storage	4′ × 8′
MD&RR	Medical Staff and Residents' Room	9′ × 10′	Y&Z	Receptionist and Appointments	8′ × 10′
N	Nurse Utility Station	8′ × 14′	▭	Sink	
OT	Outpatient Entrance/Exit		▢	Locker	
P	Preparation Cubicle	3′ × 4′			

*Broken line indicates bed space.
†Broken line indicates above counter wall mounted cabinets.
‡Approximate seating for 30 people.

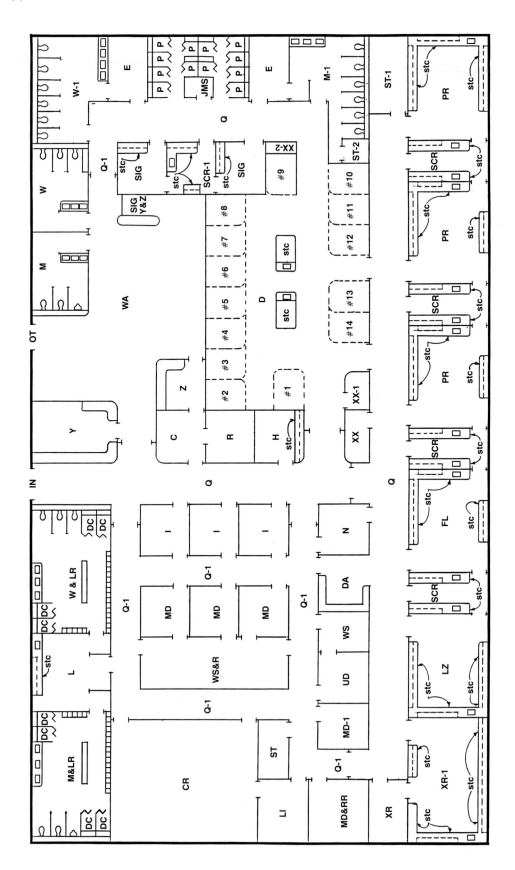

14,540 net sq. ft.

FIGURE 3–4. Architect's drawing of hypothetical endoscopy unit in which 6000 procedure units would be performed per year.

C	Computer Room	10' × 10'
CR	Conference Room*	24' × 30'
D	Dressing Room*	33' × 49'
DA	Dictation Area	10' × 11'
DC	Dressing Cubicle	3' × 4'
E	Enema Room	8' × 13'
FL	Fluoroscopy	16' × 20'
H	Head Nurse	10' × 10'
I	Interview and Consultation Room	10' × 10'
IN	Inpatient Entrance/Exit	
JMS	Janitorial/Maint. and Storage	4' × 6'
L	Staff Lounge	15' × 16'
LI	Library	10' × 12'
LZ	Laser Room	16' × 20'
M	Men's Restroom	11' × 16'
M-1	Men's Toilet/Patient	264 sq. ft.
M&LR	Men's Toilet and Locker Room/Staff	16' × 24'
MD	Medical Staff	10' × 10'
MD-1	Medical Staff	9' × 10'
MD&RR	Medical Staff or Residents' Room	12' × 12'
N	Nurse Utility Base	10' × 10'
OT	Outpatient Entrance/Exit	
P	Preparation Cubicle	3' × 4'
Q	Corridor	8' W
Q-1	Corridor	6' W
R	Medical Records	10' × 10'

SCR	Cleaning/Storage	8' × 16'
SCR-1	Cleaning/Storage	10' × 10'
SIG	Sigmoidoscopy Room	10' × 10'
SIG/Y&Z	Sigmoidoscopy Rec./Appointment Desk	6' × 8'
ST	Storage Room	6' × 12'
ST-1	Storage Room	8' × 15'
ST-2	Storage Room	5' × 5'
stc	Storage Cabinets†	
UD	Unit Director	10' × 10'
W	Women's Restroom	11' × 16'
W-1	Women's Toilet/Patient	283 sq. ft.
W&LR	Women's Toilet and Locker Room	16' × 24'
WA	Waiting Area‡	24' × 32'
WS	Word Processing/Secretarial Area	8' × 10'
WS&R	Word Processing Secretarial and Records Area	10' × 30'
XZ	X-Ray Equip. Room	8' × 12'
XR-1	X-Ray Room	16' × 24'
XX	Linen Storage	5' × 10'
XX-1	Linen Storage	5' × 8'
XX-2	Linen Storage	2' × 6'
Y	Receptionist Area	12' × 17'
Z	Appointments	10' × 10'
▯	Sink	
▯	Locker	

*Broken line indicates bed space
†Broken line indicates above counter wall-mounted cabinets.
‡Approximate seating for 56 people.

between the appointment secretary and the head nurse is essential for success. With such cooperation it is entirely possible to shift and adjust staff, rooms, and equipment on an hour to hour basis to achieve a highly flexible system that adapts quickly to delays in one or more procedure rooms, urgent requests for examinations, equipment breakdown, and a variety of other foreseen and unforeseen circumstances. Our endoscopy schedule, based on room availability, is illustrated in Figure 3–5. The schedule is a sheet of paper about 3 feet long. Each of the four columns represents one procedure room. If properly folded, each of the columns on the schedule can be photocopied separately. These copies can then be distributed to the GIAs, one for each procedure room.

The work habits of physicians can be one of the more difficult problems in scheduling. Although most physicians consider themselves not only hard working but also productive, their schedules and work habits may be at odds with those of the unit as a whole. Teamwork is less ingrained as a work ethic. Therefore, an important stratagem is to induce the endoscopists to think in terms of overall productivity and goals of the endoscopy unit. One step in this direction is to persuade them to accept assigned, regularly scheduled work periods in the unit. In medical communities where primary diagnostic endoscopy is accepted, certain procedures can be scheduled with whatever endoscopist is working within the unit at the time requested by the patient and/or referring physician.

Records, Statistics, and Computers

The administration and hence the operation of an endoscopy unit are facilitated by reliable and readily available statistical data. Certain types of information, such as complication rates and types of complications, are relevant to high standards of patient care. When the volume of cases is high and a number of endoscopists and GIAs perform procedures, a recurring complication of a particular procedure may become evident as a pattern indicating a breakdown in technique only by reference to data on complications over an extended period. Accurate methods of endoscopy record keeping support and promote scientific inquiry.

A record-keeping system is also a management tool. Data and statistics may seem mundane and irrelevant in a small unit where standards of care are readily assessed, scientific inquiry has a low priority, and management is a relatively simple part-time business. However, recall and subjective assessment are crude administrative techniques that are poorly suited not only for recognizing and dealing with problems but also for guiding the unit toward its goals. When problems arise (such as low staff morale, confusion and delays in scheduling, poor condition of instruments, high cost, low productivity, out of date equipment, inadequate numbers of or poorly trained GIAs, excessive delays between procedures, problems with supplies, declining referrals, dissatisfied referring physicians, dissatisfied patients, an insufficient number of procedure rooms, crowded working conditions, and incompetent personnel), the first query is whether the fault lies in the system of management or perhaps even the lack of a system. When problems are numerous and interrelated, there may be a basic inability to define and understand the difficulty, which is often due to a lack of information.

The computerized data base has revolutionized almost every human activity except the endoscopy unit. A glance at Table 3–1 and a rudimentary knowledge of the capabilities of computers lead to the inevitable conclusion that the procedure unit could be streamlined by combining and delegating as many "secretarial" tasks as possible to the computer. Thus, scheduling, sending written instructions and appointment confirmations to patients, and report generation are functions that can be performed by a computer. With proper software and a relatively inexpensive computer, it is entirely possible to dispense with handwritten chart notes, report dictation and typing, and all file copies. Rather, the endoscopist interacts with the computer by responding to a series of questions. Based on these responses, the computer can produce an accurate, "hard copy" English language (or any language) report that can be placed in the patient's chart within minutes. Best of all, the patient's record then becomes part of a computerized endoscopy data base (eliminating the file copy) that can be manipulated to provide information that has a bearing on the management of the endoscopy unit.

There are relatively inexpensive computers that can perform these mundane tasks. What is lacking is the appropriate software. One

GASTROINTESTINAL ENDOSCOPY APPOINTMENTS

ROOM #1 (438) **M T W T F** **DATE:**

DR/RM APPT	PATIENT'S NAME	CHART NO	PROCEDURE	REMARKS	REF DR
7:30					
8:00					
8:30					
9:00					
9:30					
10:00					
10:30					
11:00					
11:30					
12:00					
12:30					
1:00					
1:30					
2:00					
2:30					
3:00					
3:30					
4:00					

COMMENTS________________

ROOM # OR (LASER)

DR/RM APPT	PATIENT'S NAME	CHART NO	PROCEDURE	REMARKS	REF DR
PM 1:00					
1:30					
2:00					
2:30					
3:00					

COMMENTS________________

GASTROINTESTINAL ENDOSCOPY APPOINTMENTS

ROOM #2 (434) **M T W T F** **DATE:**

DR/RM APPT	PATIENT'S NAME	CHART NO	PROCEDURE	REMARKS	REF DR
8:00					
8:30					
9:00					
9:30					
10:00					
10:30					
11:00					
11:30					
12:00					
12:30					
1:00					
1:30					
2:00					
2:30					
3:00					
3:30					
4:00					

COMMENTS________________

ROOM # DESK 20 ERCP

DR/RM APPT	PATIENT'S NAME	CHART NO	PROCEDURE	REMARKS	REF DR
8:00					
8:30					
9:00					
9:30					
10:00					
1:30					
2:00					
2:30					
3:00					

COMMENTS________________

GASTROINTESTINAL ENDOSCOPY APPOINTMENTS

ROOM #3 (433) **M T W T F** **DATE:**

DR/RM APPT	PATIENT'S NAME	CHART NO	PROCEDURE	REMARKS	REF DR
8:00					
8:30					
9:00					
9:30					
10:00					
10:30					
11:00					
11:30					
12:00					
12:30					
1:00					
1:30					
2:00					
2:30					
3:00					
3:30					
4:00					

COMMENTS________________

OUT DATES

DOCTOR'S NAME	DATES	TIME	COMMENT

GASTROINTESTINAL ENDOSCOPY APPOINTMENTS

ROOM #4 (436) **M T W T F** **DATE:**

DR/RM APPT	PATIENT'S NAME	CHART NO	PROCEDURE	REMARKS	REF DR
8:00					
8:30					
9:00					
9:30					
10:00					
10:30					
11:00					
11:30					
12:00					
12:30					
1:00					
1:30					
2:00					
2:30					
3:00					
3:30					
4:00					

ON CALL PATIENTS

M T W T F **DATE:**

DR/RM APPT	PATIENT'S NAME	CHART NO	PROCEDURE	REMARKS	REF DR

COMMENTS________________

FIGURE 3–5. Cleveland Clinic endoscopy schedule based on 4 procedure rooms. (M T W T F = Monday, Tuesday, etc.; DR/RM APPT = space for endoscopist's initials near specified appointment time; REF DR = referring physician.) Note space provided to list unavailable endoscopists ("OUT DATES"). A space is also provided for "on call" hospitalized patients should a time slot become available as a result of a cancellation or "no show."

problem is that endoscopy units are very different. Also, a great variety of disorders and varying circumstances are encountered during any endoscopic procedure, not to mention the variety of procedures themselves. The Computer Committee of the American Society for Gastrointestinal Endoscopy has developed a computer program that performs many report generation functions. The purpose of this program, now in a field testing stage, is to permit large numbers of endoscopists to pool endoscopic information by virtue of use of the same data base program. This might also be considered an experiment to determine whether or not this approach is readily accepted by endoscopists.

The endoscopy data base of the Cleveland Clinic was developed in the early 1970's. Our system utilizes a VAX–11/780 computer (Digital Equipment Corp) and a Professional 350 microprocessor (Digital Equipment Corp). The VAX–11/780 is a high-performance computer that is shared (time share, i.e., each on-line user is permitted 0.1 second in turn) with other departments and which is located in the information services center of the Foundation. The Professional 350 within the endoscopy unit interfaces with the VAX–11/780 via a modem. The data base itself, which now contains the records of approximately 65,000 endoscopic procedures, resides with the VAX–11/780. Records are added to the data base using the Professional 350 microprocessor. Each record is based on a "code sheet," which is simply a sheet of paper with various check-off items, each of which has a computer code. A "code sheet" is completed by the endoscopist at the conclusion of each procedure.

Some information in each procedure record ("code sheet") pertains to diagnosis and therapy and has no bearing on management of the unit. However, certain data can be used to track unit activity. For example, it is possible to review any category of procedure activity by any day, month, or year. Since our unit is involved in teaching, a record of the types and numbers of procedures performed by any trainee in the last 15 years is available within minutes. Each instrument in the unit also has a code, so that it is possible to determine how many times an instrument has been used. Some types of information (purchase orders, instrument repair records) are kept in the endoscopy unit on the microprocessor. Generally, the amount of data in these records is small compared with the

endoscopy data base proper, and therefore the small memory (10 megabytes) of the microprocessor is more than adequate.

STAFFING

Endoscopists

From a managerial viewpoint it is necessary to know how many endoscopists are in a unit. This is not the same as how many physicians perform procedures, since the majority will not be full-time endoscopists. However, it is useful to calculate the equivalent number of full-time endoscopists using the part-time contributions of each of the staff members.

It is easy to estimate the number of procedures (using the weighted scale method to allow for more complex procedures) that one full-time endoscopist can perform in one year based on 256 working days per year and a 7-hour day. This number should then be modified by taking into account scheduled staff meetings, conferences, vacation and meeting time, and perhaps a day or two for illness. An estimate of the efficiency of the unit should be added, since the endoscopist cannot be more efficient than the least efficient component of the system. This works out to about 1800 procedure units. This computation should not be used out of context, since it is based on a hypothetical institution that has three or four conferences per week; 30 days of vacation and meeting days per year for a tired, middle-aged endoscopist; an expected endoscopy unit efficiency of 70%, and other assumptions. The actual maximum output of a full-time endoscopist in terms procedure units can, however, be calculated for any institution. The actual number of procedures will also be less because the endoscopist usually performs a variety of procedures that are more complex, i.e., have a higher weighted scale value, than a simple EGD.

It is important to note that 1800 procedures per year exceeds the maximum theoretic capacity of one procedure room by about 300 procedures.

The purpose of these computations is to determine whether or not there are sufficient numbers of procedure rooms, items of equipment, and GIAs in relation to the number of endoscopists. Obviously, the staff of few, if any, units is made up of full-time endoscopists. However, the part-time contributions of the actual members of the staff can be converted to the number of full-time endoscopist equivalents. The easiest method is to determine how much time each endoscopist spends in the unit during an average week. Since there are 10 half days in a week, a full-time individual would have a score of 10. Often, an endoscopist will perform procedures on a half-day basis. A physician who performs procedures three mornings per week would have a score of 3; someone working three mornings and two afternoons would score 5. Totaling the scores for all endoscopists and dividing by 10 yields the number of full-time endoscopist equivalents performing endoscopy. This analysis assumes that the unit is fully operational and that procedures are performed throughout the day (idle rooms and GIAs are very expensive). There are other ways to use this method of analysis. For example, when it appears that limited space is restricting procedural activity and acquisition of additional rooms or even construction of a new unit is contemplated, a similar calculation can be made based on the amount of time that each endoscopist thinks he or she needs to perform procedures.

Gastrointestinal Assistants

The number of GIAs required in a unit is a very important determination. Of all the types of personnel who contribute to one procedure unit, the GIA has the most functions and duties. The maximum ability of a GIA in terms of procedure units per year will be lower than that of the endoscopist or the procedure room itself. Applying the methods of analysis used throughout this chapter results in a figure of about 1000 procedure units per year. This therefore translates to a ratio of about 1.5 GIAs per procedure room or 1.8 GIAs per equivalent full-time endoscopist.

The role of the GIA in the endoscopy unit is discussed in Chapter 5. In terms of management of the unit there are many ways to deploy assistants. These methods are also considered in Chapter 5.

Other Personnel

Many other important personnel are part of a well-organized endoscopy unit. There is a necessary process for redelegating responsibilities in relation to the procedure unit as the volume and complexity of procedures performed increase. The easiest way to conceptualize this is to think in terms of one procedure unit (see Table 3–1) and the various types of personnel needed to accomplish one unit of work. Early in the development of the unit one employee may be responsible for more than one component. With growth, more employees will be required and each will be responsible for a smaller number of components in the procedure unit. For example, in a small unit (not more than 1000 procedure units per year) one secretary might handle appointments, report generation, statistics, and filing. However, as volume increases, the number of employees required to accomplish each of the steps in the procedure unit increases, and each employee must focus on a smaller number of components.

After the head nurse and director of the unit, one of the most important members of the team is the appointment secretary, especially in a unit that has a flexible method of scheduling, as described above. At a level of about 2500 to 3000 procedure units per year, a unit should have one person assigned to this job.

A suggested staff for a unit that performs between 6000 and 8000 procedure units per year is shown in Table 3–5.

There is a fascinating, exciting quality to the day to day activity in a large endoscopy unit. The truly well-organized, efficient, highly productive unit requires the support of many individuals with a remarkable variety of skills and knowledge. In addition to the usual team members who generate procedure units there are many other necessary support personnel. One of the most valuable is a highly qualified biomedical engineer. Some others are computer specialists, audiovisual personnel, photographers, administrative assistants, and specialists in human engineering.

TABLE 3–5. **Suggested Staff Levels for a Large Endoscopy Unit**

Unit director (1)
Full-time endoscopist equivalents (4.5)*
Administrative assistant (1)
Head nurse—GIA (1)
GIAs (7)†
Appointment secretary (1)
Receptionists (2)
Secretaries (2)

*Includes Unit director.
†Includes head nurse.

EFFICIENCY

As a rule it is not possible to eliminate any of the basic elements in the procedure unit (see Table 3–1). To assess the efficiency of an endoscopy unit it is only necessary to study the way in which each of the basic steps in the procedure unit is accomplished. There are numerous definitions of efficiency, all of which depend upon overall objectives.

Standards of Patient Care

A high standard of patient care should be an obvious goal. Generally this pertains to certain aspects of the endoscopy procedure itself that can be assessed by reviewing factors such as complication rates and numbers of unsuccessful procedures. For example: How often are colonoscopy procedures cancelled because of poor preparation? Is there a high incidence of sepsis in association with ERCP? What percentage of colonoscopy procedures are not accomplished to the cecum? Additional, less tangible but no less consequential considerations are the qualifications, training, and morale of the staff, including the GIA.

From the administrative standpoint, however, there are other important factors with respect to efficiency. Generally these pertain to time and cost.

Cost Effectiveness

What does it cost to generate one procedure unit? Such a question is often considered secondary in importance to patient care. The issue of cost effectiveness often engenders a defensive posture behind the argument that attempts at improved cost effectiveness automatically decrease standards of care. Although there are always critical cost levels at which further reductions adversely affect patient care and staff morale, it is also true that excessive costs in an era of fixed and, in some cases, limited financial resources are also a threat to the quality of patient care.

Many components of the procedure unit are labor intensive, i.e., they require people. A quick method of assessing the total cost of operating an endoscopy unit is to add up the number of staff.

Equipping an endoscopy unit is expensive. However, capital equipment, maintenance, and supplies are less important than the payroll. From a long-range accounting point of view, the financial commitment to a staff member in terms of salary and benefits far exceeds that of almost any piece of equipment. Even the most expensive laser or fluoroscope represents a one-time cost that can be amortized over several years, even with allowances for periodic repair. With proper care many endoscopes can be used for 1000 or more procedures before a major overhaul is necessary. A member of the endoscopy unit staff, however, represents a repeated cost year to year that will only increase with periodic salary increases and seniority.

Time Effectiveness

How much time is required to accomplish one procedure unit? This also has a direct bearing on patient care. If the time required is excessive, delays in scheduling are the usual result. This can be extremely costly for hospitalized patients. Delays in scheduling are a major restricting factor in the growth of an endoscopy unit. In some cases growth is restricted by limitations on space and/or staff. But in others it may seem that space and staffing of a particular unit should be more than adequate for continued growth. When such growth is not apparent, there are many possible reasons, including a declining referral base and poor-quality patient services. However, another factor, often more difficult to define, is inefficient use of existing resources.

References

1. Seifert E, Weismüller J. How to run an endoscopy unit? Experience in the Federal Republic of Germany. Results of a survey of 31 centers. Endoscopy 1986; 18:20–4.
2. The British Society of Gastroenterology. Report 1983. Design of Gastrointestinal Endoscopy Units. 1984; 1–28.
3. Korula J. Outpatient esophageal variceal sclerotherapy: safe and cost-effective. Gastrointest Endosc 1986; 32:1–3.
4. Drell E, Prindiville T, Trudeau W. Outpatient endoscopic injection sclerosis of esophageal varices. Gastrointest Endosc 1986; 32:4–6.
5. Larson DE, Ott BJ. The structure and function of the outpatient endoscopy unit. Gastrointest Endosc 1986; 32:10–4.

Chapter 4

ENDOSCOPIC PHOTOGRAPHY

MILES O. AUSLANDER, M.D.
MELVIN SCHAPIRO, M.D.

Endoscopic photography is used to document findings that are visualized at endoscopy. Such documentation may be of benefit and interest to physicians who refer patients for endoscopic procedures, and it may also be of use to endoscopists at the time of follow-up examinations as a reference to prior procedures. However, the greatest current use of endoscopic photography is in teaching and education. It is the means by which an endoscopist illustrates and compares his or her observations with those of colleagues and it is a major technique for instructing new students in gastrointestinal endoscopy. High quality endoscopic photography is in a sense a universal method of communication among those who practice this art (Plate 4–1).

Photographs may be obtained from the viewing eyepiece of an endoscope using still, motion picture, or television cameras. A television image may also be produced in direct fashion by means of a charge-couple sensor device at the end of an endoscope. Such an image may be recorded on video tape or photographed. An image can be recorded on negative film to produce a photographic print, directly on "instant film" for a print, or on reversal film in order to make photographic slides.

Obtaining a high quality endoscopic image requires careful preparation of the patient and endoscopic technique. Requirements for additional light, selection of film, and camera type will also be discussed.

HISTORY OF ENDOSCOPIC PHOTOGRAPHY

During the early years of the endoscopic era, documentation of findings was limited to a "word-picture." These descriptions, often influenced by the examiner's personal bias, served as the primary medical and legal forms of endoscopic documentation until the present. The technical advances in endoscopic photography give promise of an era when quality photographic documentation of both normal and abnormal findings will be the standard of practice.

The results of early attempts to obtain quality photographs through the lens endoscope were inconsistent. The portions of the upper gastrointestinal tract which could be photographed were limited to areas that were especially well lighted, and the requisite equipment was not only cumbersome but required special expertise in photography. Thus a series of artists' drawings of normal and pathologic endoscopic findings supplied the best illustrations for teaching in the early days of gastrointestinal endoscopy.

The quality of early photographs taken through the semi-rigid lens endoscope improved with the availability of color film, but the techniques of photography were still very difficult to acquire,[1–5] and it was not until the inception of the fiberoptic era in endoscopy that the situation improved significantly.[6] The fiberoptic bundle not only provided a marked increase in illumination of the object to be photographed, but also improved the quality of the visualized image. This advance in light transmission capability, coupled with single lens reflex (SLR) camera technology, led to high quality still photography (Plate 4–2). Furthermore, both 8 mm and 16 mm motion picture photography also became possible.[7]

The miniaturization of photographic equipment by Japanese manufacturers led to development of the gastrocamera,[8] the history of which is discussed in Chapter 1. This

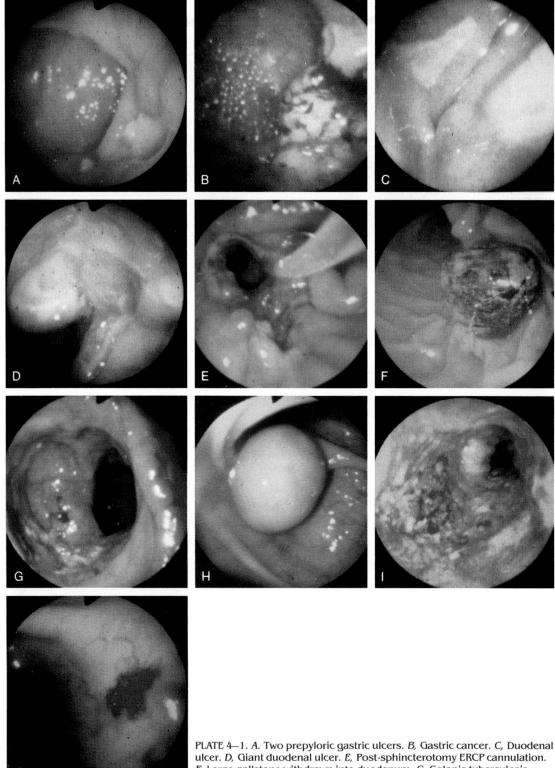

PLATE 4–1. *A.* Two prepyloric gastric ulcers. *B,* Gastric cancer. *C,* Duodenal ulcer. *D,* Giant duodenal ulcer. *E,* Post-sphincterotomy ERCP cannulation. *F,* Large gallstone withdrawn into duodenum. *G,* Colonic tuberculosis. *H,* Colonic polyp. *I,* Ulcerative colitis. *J,* Colonic vasculae ectasia.

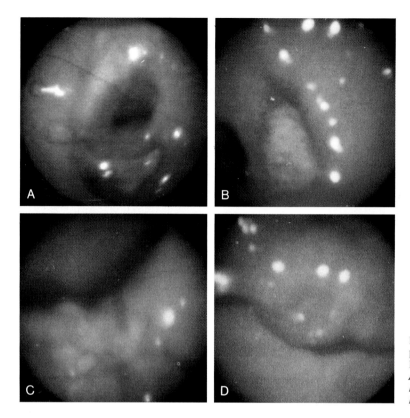

PLATE 4–2. Endoscopic photographs made with the early Hirschowitz flexible endoscope. A, Two prepyloric gastric ulcers. B, Gastric ulcer. C, Gastric cancer. D, Giant gastric rugal fold.

blind examination utilized a camera at the distal end of an insertion tube. High-quality photographs of the stomach were made in rote fashion by inserting the tube to varying depths and with the patient in a variety of positions. Subsequently the film strip was processed, and the image projected onto a screen for interpretation of the findings.[9] Gastrocamera technology was later combined with fiberoptic technology, which permitted direct visual examination and allowed an examiner to obtain high quality photographs of the endoscopic findings as they were observed (Plate 4–3).[10]

Photographs made with gastrocamera instruments are, in the opinion of many experts in endoscopic photography, the best quality still photographs that can be obtained with an endoscope. However, technical advances incorporated target biopsy and therapeutic capabilities into endoscopes, and use of the miniature camera system in the distal tip of the endoscope was abandoned. The approach to photography returned to methods of recording the image produced by a lens attached to the optical fiber bundle. Some of the technical aspects of coupling a camera to an endoscope are discussed in Chapter 2.

Improvements in fiber bundle technology, the availability of highly sensitive film with reduced grain as a characteristic, the provision of high intensity light delivery systems, and the development of automatic camera systems have allowed routine production of photographic slides and/or prints wherever and whenever the examiner elects. These photographs, however, require time for processing and are therefore not immediately available as part of the endoscopic record.

Early attempts at endoscopic "instant" photography were the natural outgrowth of technology developed by the Polaroid Corporation. However, the instant film which was initially available, especially when used with standard cameras adapted to the endoscope, did not provide satisfactory results (Fig. 4–1). Although this situation has improved with higher speed instant film and automatic endoscopic cameras designed for instant photography, light transmission through thin diameter endoscopes is often less than that necessary for this type of film, and this reduces the quality of the photographs to a considerable degree.[11]

One of the drawbacks of still photography is that it is not a record of the total endoscopic

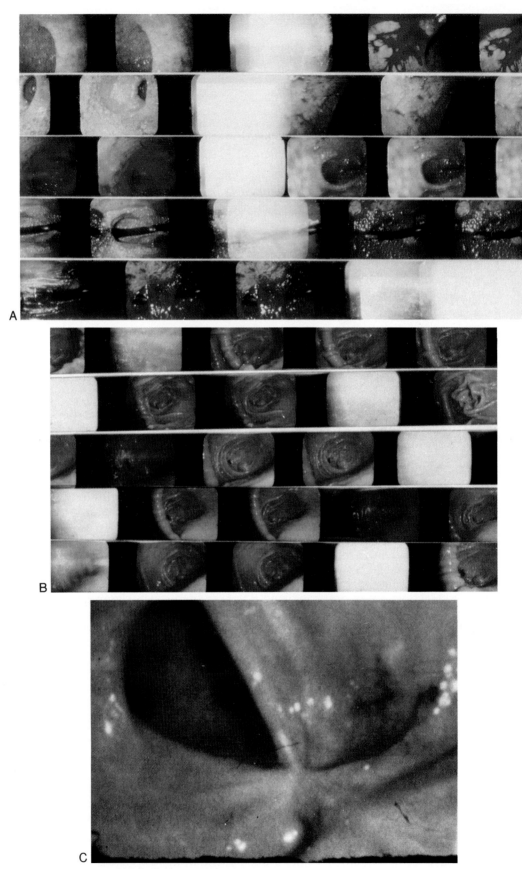

PLATE 4–3. *See legend on opposite page.*

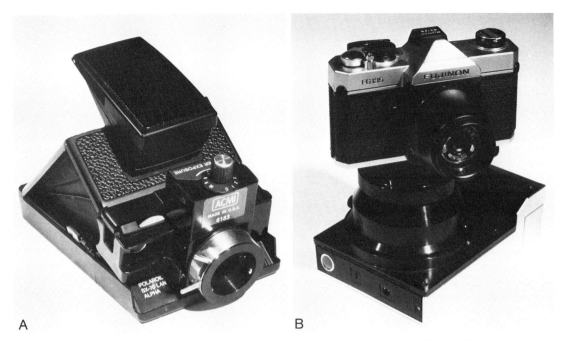

A   B

FIGURE 4–1. Instant photographic system modifications. A, ACMI adaptor for Polaroid SX-70. B, Polaroid adaptor for 35 mm endoscopic camera.

examination. In addition the quality of such photographs as an accurate record of an examination or a specific lesion is influenced by the examiner's ability to obtain good pictures as well as his or her bias for or against the concept of documentation. Motion picture films and television videotapes obtained through the viewing bundle are much more accurate in terms of documentation, but they require additional equipment and are expensive; therefore, they are rarely used routinely for documentation even by endoscopists who favor their use.

Recent improvements in camera technology offer a promise of more routine utilization.[12] The VideoEndoscope system introduced by Welch Allyn, Inc.[13–15] allows the endoscopist to videotape an entire examination or only its pertinent parts. Essentially, anything observed by an endoscopist using a VideoEndoscope may be retained permanently, and total documentation is possible with very little additional effort. The VideoEndoscope is discussed in Part 6 of Chapter 10.

BASIC PHOTOGRAPHY

Recording an image on film follows the same basic principles whether it is an endoscopic photograph or a vacation snapshot. The human eye is a magnificent optical device. It adjusts to light levels rapidly and automatically and retains its sensitivity even with low intensity levels. Its resolution (defined as the ability to separately distinguish lines placed close together) is extremely fine. This high resolution is maintained even when very bright and very dark objects are viewed together (high contrast). The brain further enhances our ability to obtain information from the image. A stereoscopic image is obtained when both eyes view an object, and this provides a perception of depth. The brain also adds color balance to vision to make the color of an object that which we always associate with the object. For example, a white cloud looks white at midday, when the ambient light is actually somewhat blue (color temperature about 5600 degrees Kelvin); it still looks white in the later afternoon,

PLATE 4–3. Photographic film strips made with the Olympus Gastrocamera, Model GTF-A. A, Gastric bleeding. B, Normal stomach. C, Healing gastric ulcer (enlargement).

when the sunlight has turned quite yellow (about 3600 degrees Kelvin). Proper photographic technique requires that certain corrections be performed in order to obtain an image that the eye regards as "normal."

The first requirement for a good photograph is a good subject. The object should be clear, well lighted, and positioned so that the image fills the viewfinder without extraneous background. Frequently an inexperienced photographer will mentally subtract extraneous factors from his view. These may be unwanted highlights, dark areas, or debris. Often the photographer will in reality be attempting to capture on film a mental conception of an object, which is actually a composite of many different views of the object; the camera does not have this capability. When the pictures are studied later, they seemingly do not do justice to the exciting endoscopic views.

Lighting requirements depend on the ability of the camera lens system to transmit light and on the sensitivity of the film. In general the more light available, the more control the photographer has over the photographic image. The illumination should be fairly even. Contrast range is defined as the ratio of the brightest segment or highlight to the darkest segment or shadow. The contrast range of a gray poodle against a medium gray background is only 1.5 to 1. A skier in a navy blue jacket against a snowy background may create a contrast of 1000 to 1. A high contrast range in an image may limit the film's ability to capture detail at the extremes of the lighting range.

Transmission and focusing of the image of the object onto the film is performed by the lens. The amount of light which the lens is capable of transmitting is measured as the f-stop, which is the ratio of the focal length of the lens to the diameter of the aperture in millimeters. F-stop markings are logarithmic—2.0, 2.8, 3.5, 5.6, 8.0, etc. The amount of light transmitted is doubled with each stepwise decrease in the f-stop setting.

The camera provides a totally darkened container for transportation of the film. The camera shutter opens for a precisely defined period of time to allow light to strike the film. Shutter speeds (in seconds or fractions of a second) are marked in doubling intervals such as 1/125, 1/250, 1/500. Many cameras have a light meter which measures the light entering the lens and can automatically set the lens aperture, shutter speed, or both to provide a correct exposure. Light meters may measure a selected central spot in the viewfinder or, more commonly, a broader central area with more weight placed on the central section.

Photographic film consists of a light-sensitive emulsion of silver halide particles layered onto a supporting medium. Color film has three emulsion layers with colored dyes. Color negative film produces a reversed image (e.g., white for black, yellow for blue), with an overall orange tint or mask. When this negative is printed, the image is reversed back to the original. During the printing process, color filtration can correct overall color imbalances. Specific negative films for daylight or tungsten lighting are unnecessary since the printing process corrects the color differences. The quality of the finished print is directly dependent on the quality of the negative. A larger negative size, higher resolution, and high tolerance of contrasting light conditions result in a better print.

Color reversal or slide film also creates a negative image, but during processing a true positive results within the emulsions. The slide can be viewed with a hand viewer or projected onto a screen. The image can be transferred to a print, using instant film and a slide printer or by a photoprocessor. Color slide film cannot be color corrected for projection. The emulsion is less tolerant of incorrect exposure or color balance. For this reason, slide films are made for daylight conditions (including electronic flash) as well as tungsten (incandescent) lighting.

Instant film also produces a true positive image within the finished print. The complex layering of emulsions and developing chemicals may be separated as in peel-apart type film such as Polaroid 668, or it may be self-contained as in Polaroid 600 film. Because the finished print is produced within the light sensitive emulsion, color correction is not possible and print size is limited. Instant slide film is also available, with processing chemicals stored in a separate cartridge. This film can be processed to finished slides within five minutes.

Films vary in their sensitivity to light, measured as the ISO number (formerly ASA). Doubling this number indicates that the film's sensitivity is twice as great, and that it can therefore capture an image with half the available light needed by a film with an ISO number one half as large. Color slide film used by professionals for magazine covers has an ISO of 25. The fastest negative film presently available has an ISO of 1000, i.e., it is more than five times faster. Films vary in their tolerance to over- or underexposure. In general, negative color film can be overexposed by two f-stops or underexposed by one f-stop and still provide adequate prints. Slide film can tolerate overexposure by only one half f-stop or underexposure by one f-stop.

The ability of film to resolve fine detail is inversely related to its sensitivity. Slow film (indicated by a low ISO number) is coated with silver particles of very fine size (grain), and therefore it is able to resolve over 100 lines per millimeter. Faster films are not capable of this degree of resolution. This also means that the ability to preserve fine detail is compromised when pictures made with faster films are enlarged or projected. The sensitivity of a film to light is often referred to as its "speed."

To review, good photography demands a good, well-illuminated subject. The lens must transmit the image with minimal distortion and with a clear focus. The camera controls the amount of light striking the film and transports the film for sequential exposures. Photographic films vary in ability to record different light levels with fine resolution. Table 4–1 lists the presently available types of color film used for endoscopic photography.

TECHNIQUE OF ENDOSCOPIC PHOTOGRAPHY

Basic Principles

Obtaining photographs of the body's interior using fiberoptic light transmission adds another dimension to an already difficult task. The object or area to be photographed must be free of debris and not covered by water or other fluid. The subject should be centered in the field, and close enough to fill the viewing field. To ensure even lighting, a perpendicular view is desirable but may be difficult to obtain. The light available for viewing depends on the output of the light source, the capacity of the light transmitting fibers, the distance and reflectance of the object, and the quality and capabilities of the optical fiber bundle (except for Video-Endoscopes) and lenses. (Refer to Chapter 2 for a consideration of the construction of fiberoptic endoscopes.)

Light sources vary tremendously with respect to light output. Smaller and older units employ a halogen bulb of about 150 watts. This gives a yellow balanced light which requires tungsten balanced slide film. The very best light sources employ a 300 watt xenon bulb that provides daylight balanced illumination. The light is transmitted via fiberoptic bundles to the endoscope tip. The light transmission of a fiberoptic bundle decreases over the course of time and is affected by exposure to radiation and iodophor cleaners. The object reflects light to the viewing lens. A dark (low reflectance) object such as a blood clot in an ulcer requires more illumination than normal mucosa. A distant subject, such as the gastroesophageal junction viewed in retroflexion from the distal body or antrum of stomach, also requires more light. The reflected light must then pass through the distal lens, the coherent, or image guide (IG), fiberoptic bundle, and the objective lens. These are affected by the same factors as the light guide (LG) bundles. In different endoscopes, the IG bundle also varies in diameter and in the number of fibers it contains. A pediatric bronchoscope used for neonatal upper endoscopy, for example, transmits only a fraction of the light of a flexible sigmoidoscope, owing to differences in the number of light transmitting fibers. In addition, broken fibers will decrease light transmission and may distort the image (Plate 4–4). Video-Endoscopes, whose image is formed electronically, still depend on a light source and fiberoptic bundles for illumination of the object. In general the television medium is more sensitive to light than conventional photographic film.

Film Format

After achieving the best possible endoscopic photographic technique and maximizing available light, a film format must be selected. By far the most popular is the 35 mm format. The 35 mm camera uses film that is 35 mm wide and is available in lengths with a capacity for 24 to 36 exposures, each measuring 24 by 35 mm. For many years cameras that used only half of the frame of the 35 mm format were employed in most gastrointestinal laboratories (Fig. 4–2). These were very economical in terms of film, but they are no longer available (Plate 4–5). Although there are hundreds of 35 mm camera models, only a few are commonly used for endoscopic photography, since lens mounting rings are not interchangeable and only

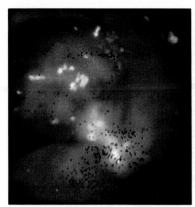
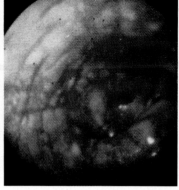
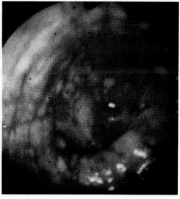

PLATE 4—4. Broken optical fiber bundles obscuring gastric ulcer.

PLATE 4—5. Half-frame images demonstrating esophagitis.

those cameras with adaptors for endoscopes can be used.

Most major endoscope manufacturers produce high quality cameras (Tables 4–2 and 4–3; Fig. 4–3). Brand selection depends on the types of endoscope and light source used. The 35 mm single lens reflex camera transports film from a cylinder-shaped cassette across the shutter aperture and onto a take-up spool. The shutter is the focal plane type, which means that a thin slit in a fabric or metal sheet travels across the film. The speed at which this slit travels determines the exposure. The focal plane shutter is covered by a front curtain until exposure. The lens mounting ring opens into the mirror box. This contains a rapid return mirror which directs the image into the viewfinder until the moment of exposure. The hinged mirror flips upward out of the way when an exposure is made and then returns to its original position after the picture has been taken. Cameras for general photography have a viewfinder screen usually featuring a split image range finder and microprism-focusing

collar. Since endoscopic systems have a fixed focus, this screen should be replaced with a plain screen if possible (Fig. 4–4). If, however, this screen is in place, its focusing aids should be ignored, since endoscopic systems do not require focusing.

Ancillary Features

The basic camera body is embellished with a variety of features, only some of which are applicable to endoscopic photography. Automatic exposure, an important feature in many cameras, utilizes a light-sensitive cell, either a silicon or gallium photodiode, in the mirror box to determine the light level. This cell may be directed at the mirror, thereby measuring the light just prior to exposure, or it may be placed at the base of the box to measure the light reflected from the front curtain and film during the exposure. Cameras also may be automated to set the aperture of the lens, the shutter speed, or both. Since endoscopic lenses have a fixed aperture, only cameras that have automated shutter speed are used.

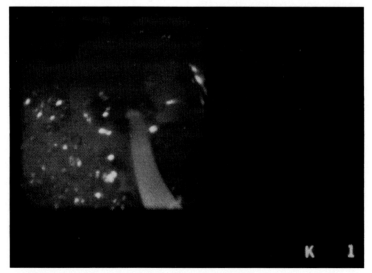

PLATE 4—6. Data back imprints code "K 1" on edge of the ERCP slide.

TABLE 4–1. **Types of Color Film Available for Endoscopy**

Type of Film	Manufacturer	Name	ISO
35 mm Color negative	Agfa	AgfaPan	100, 400
	Fujinon	Fujicolor	100, 200, 400
	Kodak	VR	100, 200, 400, 1000
35 mm Color slide	Agfa	Agfachrome	64, 100, 200
	Fujinon	Fujichrome	50, 100, 400
	Kodak	Kodachrome.	25, 64
		Ektachrome Tungsten	160
		Ektachrome	64, 200, 400
	Polaroid	Polachrome	40
	3M	Tungsten	640
		Daylight	400, 1000
Instant color	Polaroid	668	
		SX-70	
		779	
		Sun 600	
110 Size color negative	Fujinon	Fujicolor	100
		Fujicolor	400
	Kodak	Kodacolor	100
		Kodacolor	400
110 Size color slide	Fujinon	Fujichrome	100
		Fujichrome	400
	Kodak	Ektachrome	200
		Ektachrome	400
Filmstrip	Olympus	SCA-3	
		SCA-4	

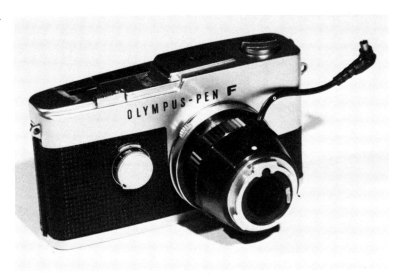

FIGURE 4–2. Olympus Pen-F half-frame camera.

TABLE 4–2. **Endoscopic Cameras**

Manufacturer	Format	Model	Comments
Fujinon	35 mm	FG-135	
	110 mm	FG-110	Auto advance
Olympus	35 mm	OM-1N	
	35 mm	OM-2N	Auto exposure
	35 mm	OM-4	Spot meter, auto
	Filmstrip	SCA-3, 4	Auto advance
Pentax	35 mm		
Polaroid	Instant	Endocamera	

Certain endoscopes and light sources, such as those manufactured by Olympus, determine the light necessary for correct exposure by means of a meter within the endoscope head, and set a shutter in the light source to provide this level of illumination. Camera metering is therefore unnecessary. Other light sources and endoscopes benefit from camera metering. Most cameras, such as the Olympus OM-2N, are light sensitive to an area that is larger than that of the actual endoscopic image. These cameras will average the dark borders when calculating the exposure. A correction must be made for this type of metering by setting the ISO level on the camera about two to four times higher than the actual film rating. For example, one would set the camera at ISO 1600 when using Ektachrome ISO 400 film. Other cameras, such as the Olympus OM-4, measure a small central spot; in this case such correction may not be necessary.

Certain options available for most 35 mm cameras can be helpful in endoscopic photography. For example, the normal hinged camera back can be replaced with a data back (Fig. 4–5). This will imprint letters and numbers onto the edge of the film during exposure, such as patient identification numbers, dates, and other codes, that can be used to identify the film (Plate 4–6). A motorized film winder is also helpful for rapid sequence photography and allows the endoscopist to keep a finger at the shutter release. This can be of assistance when the subject is moving or is difficult to view satisfactorily (Fig. 4–6).

Camera Adaptors

The camera is attached to the endoscope using an adaptor (Table 4–3; Fig. 4–7). This firmly connects the camera and allows image transmission to the film (Fig. 4–8). Adaptors frequently have electrical contacts for transmitting information to the light source, since some light sources control the exposure time or light intensity and some provide a flash. In such cases the moment of exposure and the light level measured by a meter in the control section of some endoscopes must be communicated to the light source via these contacts.

Some adaptors have no lenses, and merely orient the camera properly to the endoscope viewing lens. Others have lenses, some of which magnify the image. Magnifying the image on the film does not increase resolution, but only its size. Endoscopic photography systems do not have to be focused. Endoscope lens systems have a fixed focus with a depth of field (the range within which objects are in focus at the film plane) of about 3 to 100 mm from the tip. Endoscopes have a diopter adjustment in the viewing lens by means of which the instrument may be ad-

TABLE 4–3. **Endoscopic Adaptors**

Manufacturer	Camera Mount	(to) Endoscope	Model
ACMI	Olympus	ACMI	WI 1010
Fujinon	Olympus	Fujinon	POL-01
Olympus	Olympus	Olympus	SM-26
	Olympus	Olympus OES	A10-M2
Pentax	Olympus	Pentax	

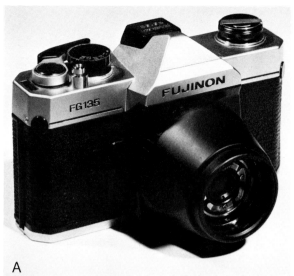

A

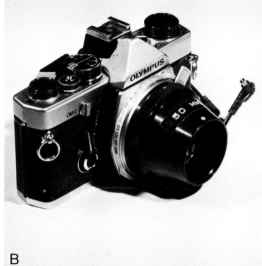

B

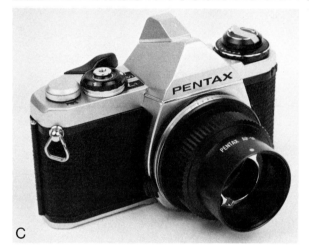

C

FIGURE 4–3. 35 mm cameras for endoscopic photographs. A, Fujinon 135. B, Olympus OM-2. C, Pentax.

FIGURE 4–4. Installing focusing screen of Olympus OM-2 camera.

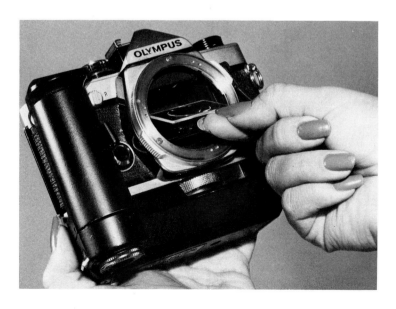

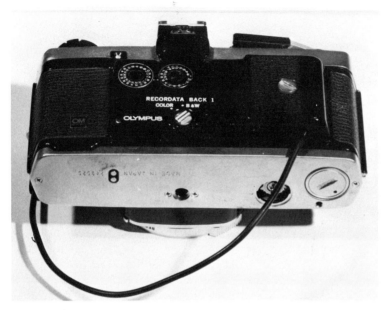

FIGURE 4–5. Data back for Olympus OM-2.

FIGURE 4–6. Motor drive for Olympus OM-2.

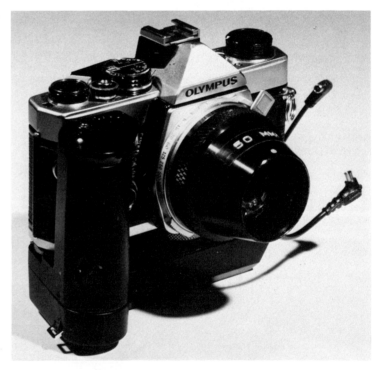

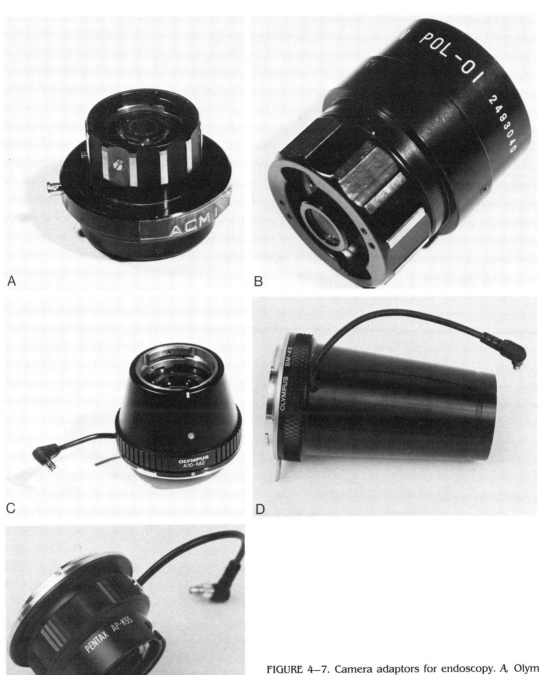

FIGURE 4–7. Camera adaptors for endoscopy. *A,* Olympus adaptor to ACMI endoscope. *B,* Olympus adaptor to Fujinon endoscope. *C,* Olympus camera to Olympus OES-endoscope. *D,* Olympus camera to Olympus endoscope (enlarged 4). *E,* Olympus camera to Pentax endoscope.

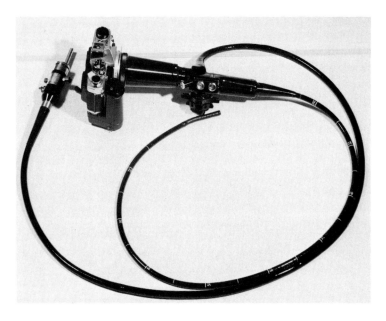

FIGURE 4–8. Olympus OM-2 with SM-45 enlarging adaptor on Olympus GIF-XQ endoscope.

justed to the endoscopist's eyesight. For photography this should be at the zero correction or infinity setting (Fig. 4–9). Some camera adaptors automatically make this adjustment when the camera is attached to the endoscope. If an endoscopist normally wears glasses, they should be worn for endoscopic photography. The eyepiece can be easily set by sharpening any black dots (broken fiber bundles) in the viewscreen.

Film Selection

If an interval of several days between film exposure and the finished print is acceptable,

then color negative film should be used. Kodak produces a high resolution VR line of color negative film in ISO speeds of 100, 200, 400, and 1000. Fujinon Fujicolor is available in 100, 200, and 400 speeds. Because the grain size increases and resolution decreases with increased film speed, a 400 speed film is a good compromise. Color balance is corrected during printing; therefore, there is no need for a special film for halogen versus xenon lighting. High quality photographic lenses can resolve over 50 lines per millimeter, but this level of resolution cannot be matched by endoscopic optics. VR 400 film can resolve over 50 lines per millimeter while

FIGURE 4–9. Olympus endoscope diopter adjustment at zero.

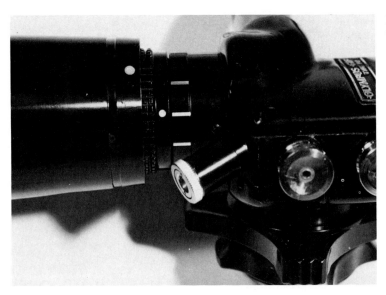

providing the sensitivity needed for low light conditions.

Slide film is available from Kodak in the Ektachrome series with ISO speeds of 64, 200, and 400 in daylight balance for use with xenon bulb light sources, and 160 in tungsten balance for halogen bulb sources. Fujichrome is available in 50, 100, and 400 speeds. 3M Corporation produces an ISO 640 tungsten and 400 and 1000 speed daylight slide film.

Although the resolution of slower films is superior, the 400 speed daylight film is more acceptable, since satisfactory photographs can be produced in spite of variations in available light, a condition that commonly occurs during endoscopic photography. Tungsten balanced 160 speed film may not be fast enough for certain conditions encountered in endoscopic photography. It can be exposed with an EI (exposure index; correlates with ISO number) of 320 by setting this on the camera. If this is done, the manufacturer or photofinisher must be required to use a one stop "push" during processing. This push processing results in a longer developing time, so that the film's sensitivity is increased, although with some compromise in quality. A new professional slide film, Ektachrome P-800/1600 (available from Kodak), can be push processed for acceptable slides at an EI of up to 3200. This may have application under unusual low light conditions.

In summary, camera and film are chosen according to the type of photograph desired and the endoscopic equipment available. Two examples are as follows.

To obtain slides using an Olympus CLV light source and a GIF XQ10 upper endoscope, an Olympus OM-1N camera (no automatic exposure) is loaded with Ektachrome 400 film. The camera light meter is turned off. The manual shutter speed is set at ¼ second. The endoscope eyepiece diopter adjustment is set on infinity. The Olympus A10-M2 adaptor connects the camera to the endoscope. The CLV light source exposure index is adjusted by trial and error for the specific conditions, but generally placed on 5. Photographs are now taken with automatic exposure control provided by the light source.

To use the Fujinon FUL-300 light source and Fujinon UGI FP endoscope with an Olympus OM-2 camera to produce a photographic print, the camera is loaded with Kodak VR 400 film. The camera ISO dial is set to 1600 (Fig. 4–10). The camera is set to automatic (Fig. 4–11) and attached with the Fujinon POL-01 and Olympus SM-25 adaptors. The light source is set to "exposure" and level 8. Exposures are controlled automatically by the camera.

Other popular formats for endoscopic photography employ smaller film. Specialized cameras using either 110 size film, which renders 13 by 17 mm exposures, or 16 mm film strips are available. These small cameras may have intrinsic automatic film advance, and many also have auto exposure. The Olympus SCA-3 camera can be used on older Olympus endoscopes, whereas the SCA-4 is used with the OES line of Olympus instruments. The SCA cameras utilize the light

FIGURE 4–10. Olympus OM-2 camera with ISO set to 1600.

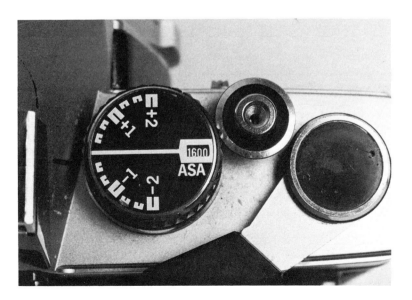

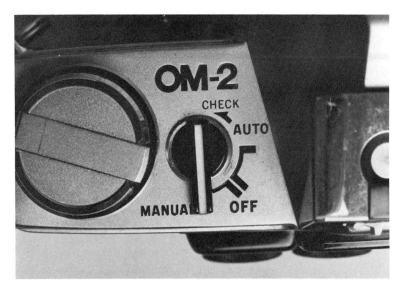

FIGURE 4–11. Olympus OM-2 camera meter setting dial.

source exposure control system. The Fujinon FG-110 camera uses 110 film size with automatic exposure (Fig. 4–12). The camera can be triggered by a button on the newer line of Fujinon instruments. These cameras are easy to use and provide quality images. The final picture is about one third the size of those obtained with 35 mm cameras. This is adequate for snapshot-size prints, but limited with respect to slide projection.

INSTANT PHOTOGRAPHY

Instant photographic film is available from Polaroid in peel-apart and self-contained forms for black and white and a variety of color applications. The instant photography camera most commonly used for endoscopy is the Endocamera manufactured by Polaroid and marketed by several endoscope manu-facturers along with specific mounting adaptors (Fig. 4–13). This camera uses Polaroid 779 self-developing film packs with an ISO speed of 600. The film is similar to Polaroid Sun Camera 600 film except that the color balance curve is modified to take into account a relatively short shelf storage time. The camera automatically expels the exposed print, electrical power for this being supplied by a battery in the film pack itself. Proper exposure with this system is determined by trial and error. Shutter speed will vary between 1/30 second and 1/2 second, depending on the light source and endoscope. Fuji-

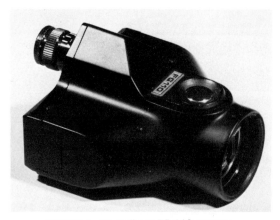

FIGURE 4–12. Fujinon FG-110 camera.

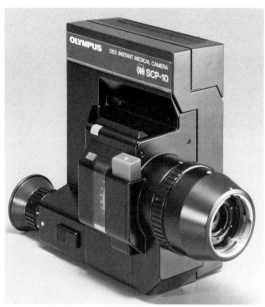

FIGURE 4–13. Polaroid endocamera EC-3 with Olympus mount.

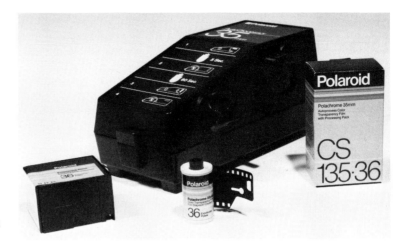

FIGURE 4–14. Polachrome 35 mm slide system.

non FUL-300 and ACMI 1012 light sources have a special flash setting which can be employed to improve the quality of the print by increasing available light.

Instant photographs were initially obtained with an SX-70 single lens reflex camera made by Polaroid and a special adaptor made by ACMI (see Fig. 4–1*A*). The faster 600 speed film could be used with the SX-70, but this required that plastic tabs be shaved from the edges of the film packs. This system produced excellent prints but was cumbersome. Special camera backs are now available so that Polaroid film packs can be used with standard 35 mm cameras (see Fig. 4–1*B*).[16] The disadvantage is a substantial loss of light in the lens magnifying system.

Instant film is also available in the Polaroid Polachrome slide film system. This 35 mm transparency film is available in standard cassettes which have 12 or 36 exposure lengths. After exposure of the roll, the film can be processed in less than five minutes in the available processing machine using chemicals supplied with the film (Fig. 4–14). A slow ISO number of 40 markedly limits the film's application to endoscopic photography.

Another film system that has applications for endoscopy is the slide printer. Sold by a variety of manufacturers, this type of device can print a standard slide onto Polaroid instant color film (Fig. 4–15). The print is finished within minutes of exposing the slide. This capability can be used to broaden the use of endoscopic photography. For example, standard slides can be made for instructional purposes and documentation while at the same time a print can be made available for the patient's permanent record.

ENDOSCOPIC TELEVISION PHOTOGRAPHY

Endoscopic television photography is the most convenient form of dynamic photodocumentation. Video cameras have almost completely replaced endoscopic motion pictures, and in many centers television is used routinely for all endoscopic procedures. Cameras, monitors, and videotape recorders are available from several manufacturers. Video endoscopy is performed by one of two techniques.

1. In the first method, using standard endoscopes and light sources, the image at the eyepiece may be diverted to several types of special video cameras, all of which are characteristically small and lightweight (Fig.

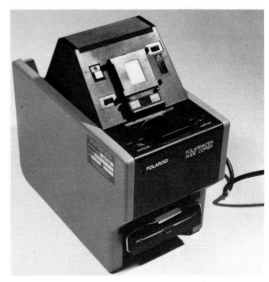

FIGURE 4–15. Polaroid Polaprinter slide copier.

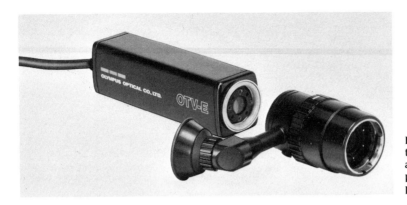

FIGURE 4–16. Small lightweight television camera (Model OTV-E) and beam splitter made by Olympus for endoscopic television photography.

4–16). The gastrointestinal tract is generally viewed through the videocamera eyepiece with a supplemental monitor as optional equipment. The availability of a monitor greatly increases the endoscopist's capacity for teaching, especially when large groups of students are being instructed. The procedure may be recorded on magnetic tape, employing the usual home video casette records in Beta or VHS format. The higher quality ¾ inch U-Matic format tape may also be used. Image-splitting adaptors are available for all major endoscopes (Fig. 4–17). These divert an endoscopic image to the endoscopist at the expense of a small decrease in the light available to the camera.

2. A more direct method of video endoscopy has recently been introduced. This type of imaging system utilizes a charge-couple sensor placed at the distal tip of the insertion tube, by means of which an image is formed electronically for viewing on a television monitor.[13] The television image has been found to be of very high quality.

It is a relatively simple matter to add an auxiliary videocamera to a standard endoscope. The excellent image obtained by endoscopes produced by major manufacturers reproduces well in television format. The use of a light source with automatic light level control such as the Olympus CLV or Fujinon FUL-300 is desirable. This feature, when used with compatible endoscopes, senses the level of the light returning to the endoscope head and signals the light source to adjust the light output to maintain the viewing level. Thus, light level is always constant regardless of viewing conditions. The image splitter (beam splitter) is placed onto the endoscope eyepiece. The camera is attached to the image splitter. The image can then be viewed by means of the image splitter eyepiece or the television monitor, and it can be preserved for future reference by videotape recording.

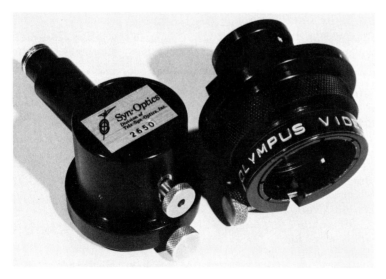

FIGURE 4–17. Syn-Optics video image splitter for Olympus endoscopes.

Television cameras are very sensitive to light, and therefore good recording conditions are almost always encountered. Basically, if it can be seen, it can be captured on videotape.

A log of the subject matter including reference to tape recorder counter numbers should be maintained. Actual inclusion of patient identification information and perhaps other data on the same videotape as the endoscopic subject material is also desirable.

References

1. Segal HL, Watson JS Jr. Color photography through the flexible gastroscope. Gastroenterology 1948; 10:575–85.
2. Nelson RS. Routine gastroscopic photography. Gastroenterology 1956; 30:661–8.
3. Nelson RS. Gastroscopic photography. Gastroenterology 1958; 35:74–8.
4. Keever IC, Barborka CJ. Electronic flash gastroscopic color photography. Gastroenterology 1959; 36:743–8.
5. Barrett B. Gastroscopic color photography with incandescent light. Bull Gastrointest Endosc 1961; 8(2):13–4.
6. Hirschowitz B. Photography through the fiber gastroscope. Am J Dig Dis 1963; 8:389–95.
7. Berci G, Merei F, Kont LA. A new approach to clinical film recording with special reference to endoscopy. Med Biol Illus 1966; 16:37–43.
8. Uji T. The gastrocamera. Tokyo Med J 1952; 61:135–8.
9. Morrissey JF, Thorsen WB Jr. The usefulness of the gastrocamera. Gastroenterology 1968; 54:321–2.
10. Morrissey JF, Tanaka Y, Thorsen WB. The relative value of the Olympus model GT-5 gastrocamera and Olympus model GTF gastrocamera fiberscope. Gastrointest Endosc 1968; 14:197–200.
11. Schapiro M, Auslander MO. A comparison of endoscopic photography systems. (Abstr) Gastrointest Endosc 1982; 28:144.
12. Nelson RS, Korinek JK. Routine color television recording in gastrointestinal endoscopy. (Abstr) Gastrointest Endosc 1984; 30:158.
13. Sivak MV, Jr, Fleischer DE. Colonoscopy with a VideoEndoscope: preliminary experience. Gastrointest Endosc 1984; 30:1–5.
14. Schapiro M, Auslander MO. A comparison of the video endoscopic system to fiberoptic endoscopy in the community hospital. (Abstr) Gastrointest Endosc 1984; 30:160.
15. Classen M, Phillip J. Electronic endoscopy of the gastrointestinal tract. Endoscopy 1984; 16:16–9.
16. Greene LS. Instant endoscopic photography. (Abstr) Gastrointest Endosc 1982; 28:151.

Chapter 5

THE GASTROINTESTINAL ASSISTANT

IRENE M. SPADA, R.N.
MICHAEL V. SIVAK, JR., M.D.

THE ROLE OF THE GASTROINTESTINAL ASSISTANT (GIA)

The evolution of gastroenterology over the past several decades encompasses ever increasing knowledge and steadily improved methods of diagnosis and therapy. The diversity and greater use of endoscopic procedures have resulted in even more profound changes. What could not be anticipated at the inception of fiberoptic endoscopy is the extent of its development so that the field now embraces and supplants many aspects of diagnosis and therapy that historically have belonged to surgery and radiology.

Changes in gastroenterology and endoscopy have significantly affected the field of nursing. The comfort and safety of a patient undergoing gastrointestinal endoscopy, vis-a-vis rigid endoscopy, formerly depended largely on the skill and attention of the endoscopy assistant. Just as rigid endoscopy is an art no longer practiced by most endoscopists, so also few gastrointestinal assistants are cognizant of the role of the "head holder." In one respect this is unfortunate since the modern-day gastrointestinal assistant has little awareness of the background and early development of this form of nursing. Although not essential, an appreciation of the role of the assistant from an historical perspective adds greatly to the sense of profession and of participation in the development of an important field.

Although much has changed for the endoscopist and assistant, the fundamental relationship remains the same. During the early days of endoscopy the assistant had two basic functions that have remained essentially unaltered: custody and preparation of endoscopic instruments and a role in maintaining the comfort and safety of the patient. The specific ways in which these functions are carried out, however, have changed substantially. Responsibility for the endoscopic instruments now extends to a large endoscopy unit that includes numerous items of equipment. Patients now undergo many different procedures that require the use of many items of equipment, each procedure having unique potential complications and special difficulties for patients.

In the past there was a more personal relationship between the assistant, the endoscopist, and the patient since there were fewer of each of these participants. Now, many patients require the services of the assistant during the course of a day. Furthermore, an assistant may work with many endoscopists in a given unit, making it more difficult to recognize and adapt to the methods and even idiosyncrasies of each physician.

The remarkable increase in the number of procedures performed presents new problems for the assistant with respect to patient comfort and safety. Heretofore, the assistant might have been responsible for the postprocedure recovery of one or a few patients, whereas he or she now has responsibility for an entire room full of patients with various disorders who have undergone any number of different procedures. Safety in rigid endoscopy once depended on holding the patient's head properly and monitoring his or her respiration and cardiac function. Although the exact position of the patient is perhaps less important now, attention to the patient's vital functions is no less essential. When large numbers of procedures are performed, they become "routine," and this, plus the inherent low complication rate for most endoscopic procedures, can lead to a false sense of security. In a busy unit the many tasks to be performed can distract the attention of the assistant from the most critical function of patient monitoring.

The assistant's custody of the instruments also has a direct bearing on patient safety. The endoscopist and patient both expect that all instruments will be in working order and that the success and safety of the procedure will not be compromised by poor condition of the equipment. This has ramifications that range from instrument malfunction during a critical stage of a procedure to disease transmission by inadequately cleaned instruments. A high volume of procedures presents special problems with respect to proper cleaning and maintenance of equipment.

The avoidance of pain, discomfort, and patient injury as a direct result of an endoscopic procedure is essentially the responsibility of the endoscopist. However, in many respects the assistant shares this responsibility. For example, every patient approaches any procedure with trepidation. The size and intense activity of a large endoscopy unit can compound this anxiety by virtue of a seeming lack of individual attention and consideration. Because of these factors the role of the endoscopy assistant with respect to the emotional preparation of the patient for a procedure becomes even more vital, while at the same time requiring more well-developed skills and experience.

THE GIA

Evolution of the GIA Concept

The relationship of nursing to gastrointestinal endoscopy in the past was usually that of a part-time assistant, since the volume and variety of procedures performed did not fully occupy a nurse in most institutions. The growth and evolution of gastrointestinal endoscopy have necessitated a change in this relationship to such an extent that the role of the endoscopy assistant has become a highly specialized area of expertise within the field of nursing. It is appropriate that this full-time profession with its special requirements and qualifications be given its own designation, hence the term gastrointestinal assistant (GIA).

Qualifications

Certain fundamental qualifications are required for an individual to become a GIA. The GIA should be trained in the basic aspects of patient care; prior experience that involves contact with patients is desirable. The GIA must be familiar with the essential aspects of cardiovascular and respiratory physiology and must be able to assess quickly and accurately the cardiopulmonary status of any patient. Certification in cardiopulmonary resuscitation (CPR) should be required, including a thorough knowledge of all drugs and equipment used in CPR.

Medications are administered in most endoscopic procedures, so that the GIA must be knowledgeable about dosages, methods of administration, side effects, and interactions of the various drugs used. Since the medications used in endoscopy are often controlled substances, the GIA must be licensed and qualified to handle these agents.

The special personality or character traits that are desirable in a GIA are relatively few, but the most important of these are conscientiousness and attention to detail. From an intellectual viewpoint the GIA's job is not difficult to master. The difference between an adequate and an excellent GIA is the quality of thoroughness and punctilious attention to the numerous small aspects of patient care, procedures, and the equipment. By virtue of their training, experience, and temperament, nurses are uniquely qualified for the role of GIA.

FUNCTIONS OF THE GIA

The Procedure Unit

The endoscopy "procedure unit" was discussed in Chapter 3. The essential elements in this concept are that in many respects all endoscopic procedures are alike since they all have certain steps in common and that the actual endoscopic component of the procedure unit is only part of a more complex process (Table 5–1). The GIA has responsibility for more steps and more tasks to accomplish in the endoscopy procedure unit than any of the other personnel, including the endoscopist.

The length of time required for the endoscopic component of the procedure unit is highly variable and depends on the type of procedure, whether or not any abnormalities are encountered, and the skill of the endoscopist. Thus, a routine diagnostic upper gas-

TABLE 5–1. **Functions of the GIA in the Procedure Unit**

Preprocedure
Scheduling
Patient check-in*
Patient instruction, interview*
Patient preparation*
Premedication*
Room/equipment preparation*

Procedure
Examination/procedure* (handling of biopsy and other specimens)*

Postprocedure
Patient recovery
Patient monitoring*
Patient postprocedure instructions/scheduling*
Patient discharge*

Room/equipment cleaning, turn-around*

Charting/report generation
Written chart notation
Report dictation
Typing report
Review/signature of typed report
Processing of report to chart
File copy of report

(Data processing)

(Billing)

*Functions normally performed by GIA.

trointestinal endoscopy can be accomplished in 5 to 10 minutes, although a complex colonoscopic polypectomy may require a significantly longer period of time. As a general rule, there is less variation in the time required for the steps in the procedure unit that are accomplished by the GIA. The time required for preparation of the instruments and procedure room, cleaning, and postprocedure monitoring of the patient is relatively fixed regardless of the type of procedure performed.

Preprocedure Functions

The main preprocedure duties of the GIA include preparation of the patient, proper arrangement of the procedure room, and preparation of the endoscopic equipment. In some units the GIA may also have a partial role in scheduling the procedures, a function that is usually the responsibility of the GIA supervisor. This role is discussed below.

Preparing the patient for endoscopy has several facets that may differ according to the type of procedure to be performed.

First Contact

Some time after the patient arrives at the endoscopy unit he or she must be brought to the dressing room and shown the place he or she will occupy before and after the procedure. The GIA can explain what must be done in preparation for the procedure, such as disrobing and gowning. Some patients may require assistance. Although these details are seemingly mundane and unimportant, they offer the GIA an ideal opportunity to meet with the patient and to establish rapport.

It should be verified that the patient has accomplished all necessary steps in the preparation process prior to coming to the endoscopy unit. For example, when preparation for colonoscopy has been carried out by the patient, it is nevertheless useful to review the process with the patient to confirm that cleansing of the colon will be adequate for the examination. It is not unusual to discover that the patient has encountered difficulty with some aspect such as self-administration of enemas. An alert GIA can sometimes salvage this situation with additional enemas and so avoid loss of valuable time.

Medical History

It is of value to inquire about any recent change in the patient's overall medical status. As a general rule this line of questioning can be based on chart notes and should focus on the patient's cardiovascular and pulmonary status, any change in gastrointestinal symptoms, and the use of medication. Recent changes in gastrointestinal symptoms such as the onset of protracted vomiting, worsening and/or prolonged abdominal pain, and the appearance of bloody diarrhea sometimes necessitate changes in an investigative plan.

Medications

The use of medications prior to a procedure is a common area of confusion for patients. Essential drugs may have been discontinued in the mistaken belief that this was a necessary part of fasting. Conversely, the patient may have continued the use of an agent that he or she did not consider to be a medication, for example, a liquid antacid. Some patients continue to take iron preparations orally during the standard preparation for colonoscopy, which often precludes adequate preparation of the colon.

The GIA should be particularly careful with insulin-dependent diabetics. In our unit we usually ask the diabetic patients to administer one-half the morning dose of insulin at the usual time. Procedures are scheduled early in the day for these patients, and the second half of the usual insulin dose is given along with a morning meal after the patient recovers from the procedure. However, errors nevertheless occur with this simple plan, especially in patients on a stable dosage who have a consistent routine for insulin administration.

The GIA should also ask about the use of sedative and hypnotic drugs that have a bearing on the selection of medications and dosages for the procedure. The anxiety prone patient may find it necessary to take such a drug before coming to the endoscopy unit. Chronic users of this type of medication may also have a tolerance to some agents. Finally, it is essential to ask about any drug allergies, especially if antibiotic prophylaxis will be used for the procedure.

Description of the Endoscopic Procedure

In our unit all patients receive a written description of the procedure they are to undergo. Ideally they receive this far enough in advance of the procedure that they are able to express any concerns or questions that may arise after studying the written outline. The printed material contains information on the goal of the study, steps the patient must take to prepare for the procedure, a general description of the way in which the endoscopy will be performed, and some basic facts concerning complications, including signs and symptoms along with specific instructions in the event that the patient encounters evidence of a complication after discharge from the unit. This type of instruction serves as a point of reference for the patient and often fills in gaps in the patient's memory regarding the physician's instructions. Although the printed description is necessary and valuable, it is impersonal and may strike some patients as legalistic. It seldom offers the patient a sense of confidence or reassurance. Regardless of how well it is written, it is unrealistic to believe that all the information it contains will be correctly interpreted by every patient. Therefore, it can never substitute totally for an informed consent or be the sole vehicle for conveying instructions and information to the patient.

The responsibility for the formal explanation of the endoscopic procedure is delegated to the GIA in some units. However, it remains the primary responsibility of the endoscopist to advise the patient of the indication(s), methodology, and possible complications of the endoscopic procedure; the GIA may, nevertheless, play an important role in this process. Questions often arise in the patient's mind some time after contact with the physician. A patient may sometimes be reluctant to discuss concerns and questions that may be considered trivial or unimportant to the physician. It is necessary to repeat important points in the description for some patients, especially when the information has become distorted by anxiety. The GIA is usually the first person with a medical background whom a patient encounters immediately before a procedure. At this time, when the sense of uneasiness is greatest, patients are most likely to ask questions. Furthermore, patients often recognize the GIA as not only someone with knowledge of the endoscopy procedure, but also as a person to whom they can relate to in a more personal and direct way than may occur in the traditional "doctor-patient" relationship.

Most of the common questions that patients ask are predictable and can be anticipated by the experienced GIA: "will it hurt," "is it dangerous," "will I gag," "will I be able to breathe," "I don't like needles," "how long will it take." The GIA should answer these questions forthrightly and directly. There is, however, a natural human tendency to offer support to a person in emotional distress so that the GIA must be careful not to offer excessive reassurance and should never attempt to completely dismiss from the patient's mind any of the potentially unpleasant parts or hazardous prospects of a procedure. It is equally important not to overly stress these aspects.

Psychologic Preparation

Almost all patients are apprehensive to some degree. Many patients control this well, but in others there is overt fear and aversion. The way that this is dealt with can influence the course and outcome of the procedure. If the patient is at ease, the procedure will be better tolerated, the endoscopist will have adequate time to complete the procedure, and smaller amounts of sedative drugs will be required. Although the value of this psychologic preparation in addition to the pharmacologic preparation is easily recognized, the emotional needs of patients may be difficult to resolve. Success is in some measure dependent on the natural attributes and personality of the GIA. Under normal circumstances the physician endoscopist is regarded as a benefactor; otherwise the patient would not permit the procedure. However, this is not to say that the patient is always at ease and comfortable with the physician, who is often perceived as an "authority figure." In contrast the GIA is in a less formal and more personal position to offer the type of reassurance that lends to the emotional confidence that all of the participants place the patient's welfare first and foremost. The simple phrase, "I am . . . and I will be with you through the procedure" can be as effective as any drug, the key words being I, with, and you.

Premedication

Sedative drugs are usually administered before endoscopic procedures, the two most widespread classes in use being narcotics and benzodiazepine agents. These may be given in a variety of ways, although intravenous administration is probably preferred. Anticholinergic drugs are rarely used for most routine endoscopic procedures with the exception of laparoscopy. In almost all cases the dosage of medication is varied according to the patient's age, weight, and general medical condition, and it is administered slowly while observing the patient's response. Endoscopists also differ with respect to methods of intravenous administration. For a relatively short diagnostic procedure in a motivated patient, some endoscopists administer a small dose(s) by direct intravenous injection. For a more prolonged procedure in which some discomfort is expected, the endoscopist may prefer to maintain intravenous access so that additional amounts of sedative drugs may be given. Generally, a "heparin-lock" is adequate for this purpose, although a slowly running intravenous infusion is sometimes requested for procedures that involve some risk, such as bleeding. In our unit direct intravenous injection of drugs is performed only by a physician or by a GIA under the direct supervision and observation of a physician.

In some units sedatives and other drugs are administered prior to bringing the patient to the endoscopy room. Generally, this requires a cart-exchange system between the dressing room and the procedure room. In most units intravenous sedation is given in the procedure room immediately before a procedure.

The GIA has primary responsibility for the drugs used in the endoscopy unit. This includes the maintenance of a proper inventory of agents commonly used and the handling of controlled substances as prescribed by law. In addition, the GIA is also responsible for preparing correct dosages of drugs for use during procedures.

Preparation of the Procedure Room and Equipment

An important duty of the GIA is to prepare the procedure room for each endoscopy. The bed linen for the examination table should be changed completely between cases. The room itself should be clean and kept in good order. The need for various items of equipment should be anticipated. Our scheduling system is based on room availability. The master schedule sheet can be easily separated into individual sections that cover the activity for each individual room on a daily basis. A copy of this is placed in each procedure room and the dressing room station and a master schedule is kept by the GIA supervisor. Using this schedule the GIA working in each room can plan ahead with respect to the equipment needed for each procedure and can also anticipate the special preferences of each endoscopist since the physician's name is also listed on the schedule. When appropriate, marginal notes and remarks are included on the schedule to indicate special requirements, especially with respect to therapeutic endoscopy.

It would be impossible to list all the various items of equipment needed for the many different diagnostic and therapeutic endoscopic procedures. There are also differences among institutions in the way procedures are performed, and these modifications often necessitate additional accessories and pieces of equipment. The ability to organize all equipment and to keep the procedure room and unit functioning smoothly is a skill based on a thorough understanding of endoscopic procedures, and one that can only be learned by actual practice.

Functions During Endoscopy

Some general remarks on the assistant's role in the main types of endoscopic procedures will be discussed. It is impossible to include every variation in the activities of the GIA during every type of procedure.

Esophagogastroduodenoscopy

Usually it is only necessary for a patient to partially disrobe for esophagogastroduodenoscopy (EGD) on an out-patient basis. It is ordinarily sufficient to remove outer garments above the waist, but not undergarments, and then put on a hospital gown. Eye glasses and dentures should be removed.

Some, but not all, endoscopists prefer topical pharyngeal anesthesia. There are several methods of doing this, such as an anesthetic spray administered by the GIA or a gargle with a viscous anesthetic agent. It is well to inquire again about any drug allergies before any medication is administered in the procedure room.

The patient is then positioned on the examination table. One or two pillows should be provided. If sedative drugs are to be given, the patient usually first assumes a supine position, although he or she may be placed directly in the left decubitus position for endoscopy if there is convenient intravenous access. Once the medication is given, the GIA adjusts the patient to the proper position for the procedure. For upper gastrointestinal endoscopy the patient is generally on his or her left side, knees flexed, left arm under pillow, right arm on the right side, with head and chin tilted slightly downward toward the chest.

Except in the case of edentulous patients a mouthguard is placed between the patient's teeth to protect both the instrument and the patient's teeth during the examination. One of the GIA's main responsibilities is to insure that the mouthguard remains in the proper position during the procedure. There is a tendency for the mouthguard to fall out or to be pushed out by the patient during the procedure. Some endoscopists prefer to lubricate the insertion tube of the endoscope for upper gastrointestinal endoscopy and therefore a supply of lubricant should be at hand. Because the insertion tube also becomes coated with secretions, gastric juice, and mucus during the procedure, it may become slippery and difficult to handle. We therefore keep a washcloth and a few sponges on the pillow near the patient's head for the endoscopist to use in grasping the instrument.

All endoscopists in our unit pass the endoscope under direct observation without inserting a finger into the patient's mouth (see Chapter 11). During direct vision passage of the endoscope through the pharynx and cricopharyngeus, it is necessary that the GIA maintain the patient's head in the proper position. There is a natural tendency for patients to extend the neck and to move away from the instrument. Gentle words of reassurance and encouragement offered by the GIA are frequently helpful as the instrument is being passed. Just as the instrument enters the esophagus we place a disposable oral suction catheter in the left side of the patient's mouth next to the mouthguard. This can be bent to fit comfortably in the mouth and has a blunt tip (Fig. 5–1). The purpose of this is to remove any fluid that the patient regurgitates as well as oral secretions during the passage of the instrument.

During the endoscopic procedure the GIA must keep the patient in the proper position on the examination table and monitor the cardiopulmonary status, especially respiration. Some endoscopists prefer that the lights be dimmed in the room; others do not. The room should never be so dark, however, that it becomes difficult to monitor the patient. The GIA must also insure that the mouthguard and suction device remain in proper position and must be alert for unexpected vomiting, as aspiration is one of the major complications of upper gastrointestinal endoscopy.

Several types of specimens, including tissue, cells, and secretions, may be collected at endoscopy. In these various procedures the

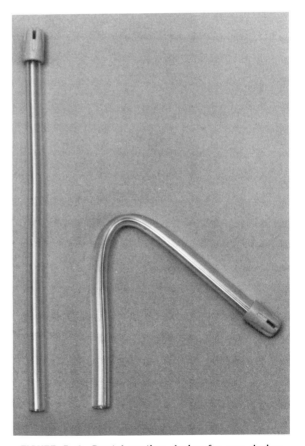

FIGURE 5–1. Dental suction device for use during esophagogastroduodenoscopy (left). The device may be bent at any angle to fit comfortably in a patient's mouth alongside the mouthguard and the endoscope.

GIA has several functions: preparing the necessary accessories and equipment; assisting in actual collection of specimens; handling specimens, including proper labeling of containers and preparing the necessary forms used for submitting the specimens to the laboratory; and cleaning certain accessories.

Although all endoscopic biopsy forceps are basically similar in design, there are differences. The most important is the variation in diameter necessitated by the differences in accessory channel diameter according to the type and manufacture of an endoscope. This variation is a minor problem in a large unit that has many endoscopes. It should never be necessary to interrupt a procedure to search for the correct forceps; this can be avoided by storing each endoscope and its related accessories (including cleaning brush) in the same place (see Storage of Instruments below). When the endoscope is set out for use (or replaced in storage), its set of accessories should always be included. Biopsy forceps may differ slightly in some other respects; they may have open or closed forceps cups, or there may be a bayonet spike enclosed within the cups. The GIA must determine the type of forceps preferred by the endoscopist.

Probably the second most commonly used accessory is the sheathed cytology brush. In some cases this may be used to obtain specimens such as exudate from the esophageal surface to determine the presence of *Candida albicans*. However, this accessory is most commonly used to obtain cells from the surface of a lesion for cytologic study. A new cytology brush should be used for each procedure and then discarded, since this type of accessory is very difficult to clean adequately. Otherwise it may be possible to transfer malignant cells from one patient to the cytologic sample from another patient. Commercially available disposable cytology brushes are relatively inexpensive.

Most often the endoscopist directs the GIA to open and close the biopsy forceps. It is important that the GIA and endoscopist agree on the specific and simple directions such as "open" and "close." The forceps should always be checked to be certain that it works properly before it is given to the endoscopist. The forceps can be broken if opened or closed too forcefully. The endoscope may be damaged as well as the forceps if the latter is opened while within the acces-

sory channel or if it is withdrawn into the channel while open. An alert and experienced GIA can recognize that the forceps is partially or completely within the channel if an unusual opposing force is encountered when opening of the device is attempted. This may save the unit expensive repair and replacement costs and is particularly important when trainees are obtaining biopsies. Even an experienced endoscopist may attempt to open the forceps while it is partially within the channel when he or she encounters difficulty in obtaining a specimen and for whatever reason must approach the lesion closely. Closure of the forceps should not be abrupt or forceful. Brusque closure will sometimes cause the forceps cups to shear off a firm lesion without obtaining a specimen. An experienced GIA can sometimes appreciate that a lesion is unusually firm or hard as the forceps closes; this tactile perception is often associated with malignancy. As the forceps is removed from the accessory channel of the instrument, simultaneously wiping it with a gauze pad will prevent dripping of fluid on the patient. This also cleans and dries the coil somewhat and makes for easier handling.

The GIA is also responsible for the proper handling of tissue and cytologic specimens. The methods of doing this should be coordinated with the special requirements of the pathology and cytology laboratories. These will vary from hospital to hospital. In our unit biopsy specimens are gently teased out of the forceps cup and onto a small disc of filter paper (one paper disc per biopsy) using a toothpick. The paper and specimen are then placed in a bottle containing Hollandes' fixative solution. We do not attempt to orient the specimen in any way since our pathologists do not require this. Most endoscopic biopsy specimens are small, and attempts to rearrange the specimen on the paper damage the tissue. Cytologic specimens obtained by brushing are placed on a frosted microscope slide by simply brushing the specimen onto the glass. With a good specimen there is usually material for two slides. The slide is then placed in Carnoy's solution.

The GIA is usually responsible for proper identification of the biopsy specimens and completion of the pathology request forms. This obligation should never be taken lightly since confusing the specimens from one patient with those from another or mislabeling may have serious consequences. Therefore, the methodology for handling specimens should be rigidly established and adhered to in every unit.

When the endoscopist indicates that biopsy or other specimens will be obtained, the first step in our unit is to complete the necessary forms and label the containers. The forms and labels with each patient's name and identification number are prepared in advance of the procedure. Although it would seem obvious, it is nonetheless necessary to state that the most important aspect of this is that the patient's name and identification number are correct. The GIA then asks the endoscopist for the specific information that is to appear on the request form, starting with the location of the biopsy and then the endoscopic diagnosis and finally any information that the endoscopist wishes to communicate to the pathologist. When the pathology laboratory permits submission of multiple specimen containers from different locations with a single request form, it is mandatory that each container be labeled in some way with a corresponding indication of this label on the request form. In our unit each frosted glass slide used for a cytologic specimen is also labeled in pencil at one edge with the patient's surname.

Sclerotherapy of esophageal varices is a commonly performed therapeutic procedure in conjunction with EGD. Injection of the sclerosant solution is almost always performed by the GIA and requires precise communication between the assistant and the endoscopist. The directions given by the endoscopist should be unambiguous, and a simple set of terms should be used. In our method the GIA reports the volume of sclerosant injected in increments of one-half milliliter to allow the endoscopist to slow or increase the rate of injection. Intravariceal injections are used predominantly in our technique (see Chapter 16). It is often possible for an experienced GIA to recognize that the needle is not within a vessel or that a vessel is thrombosed according to the degree of resistance encountered while injecting. For each procedure we prepare 50 ml of sclerosant solution, 10 ml for each of five 10-ml syringes. The 10-ml syringe is the easiest for the GIA to handle. Since most sclerosants are injurious to the eyes, care must be taken that the syringe not be abruptly disconnected from the injector. If this should occur, the sclerosant may be sprayed in the eyes of the physician, patient, or GIA. To prevent this

we always wrap a gauze sponge around the connection while injecting. The total volume used and number of injections are recorded by the GIA.

Certain complications are possible with sclerotherapy. Those that may occur suddenly during the procedure include vomiting and aspiration of blood and gastric contents during injections for acute variceal hemorrhage and the onset of active bleeding during the procedure. In a few instances in our experience balloon tamponade has been necessary for control of acute bleeding. Therefore we keep the necessary equipment at hand and are also prepared to administer vasopressin.

Colonoscopy

The functions of the GIA during colonoscopy differ somewhat from those attendant to upper endoscopy. Assistance is usually required with changing the patient's position during the procedure. It is usually necessary to apply additional lubricant to the insertion tube near the patient's anus at times during the procedure (we place a small amount of lubricant on a gauze pad; however, several other methods may be used). In addition to the usual monitoring of the patient it is essential in this procedure to observe the patient for signs of excess discomfort or pain and evidence of abdominal distention.

There are substantial variations in colonoscopy technique among endoscopists (see Chapter 40). The endoscopist may request that the GIA hold the instrument at the anus as he shifts his hand from the insertion tube to the lateral deflection knob. In our unit, however, the GIA is never permitted to advance or withdraw the colonoscope. Some endoscopists use external counterpressure on the patient's abdominal wall during the procedure. Generally, pressure is applied to the mobile segments of the colon that are on a mesentery (see Chapter 40). There are many individual variations for this part of the procedure. If external counterpressure is requested, the GIA should ask the endoscopist to indicate the place and direction to apply pressure on the abdominal wall, especially if the GIA is not familiar with the endoscopist's methods. The patient should be forewarned of this maneuver and should be observed for evidence of pain or excessive discomfort. The suction-accessory channel of the colonoscope sometimes becomes clogged during colonoscopy. This can often be cleared by forcing water and/or air back through the channel

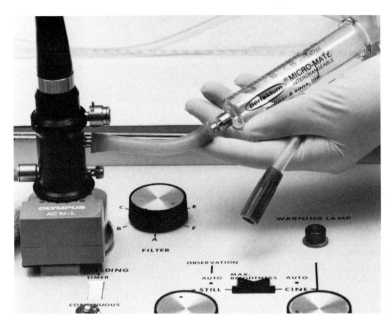

FIGURE 5–2. Method of clearing accessory channel during colonoscopy by disconnecting the suction tubing and flushing air and/or water through the channel.

(Fig. 5–2). During this maneuver it is necessary that the endoscopist depress the suction valve.

The GIA usually has several important functions in the process of polypectomy. Modern electrically isolated electrosurgical generators provide a margin of safety for endoscopic polypectomy (see Chapter 7). In addition, the patient is almost always awake, albeit sedated, during the procedure so that it is unlikely that an inadvertent burn will lead to tissue necrosis. But these factors do not in any way reduce the responsibility of the GIA for the safety of this procedure.

All connections between the active electrode snare and the generator, as well as those for the indifferent plate electrode, must be made correctly. This equipment must be inspected periodically to be sure that the wires and connections are not worn or broken. In addition, the GIA must be certain at all times that there is a good contact between the plate and the patient, especially if the patient's position has been changed between successive polypectomies. Braided polypectomy snare wires should be checked carefully for any small broken wires in the braid. A broken strand can result in stray electrosurgical currents. These are usually difficult to see but can be found by gently running a gauze sponge over the open snare loupe.

The generator output is usually set by the GIA; the settings should always be verified before proceeding with polypectomy and

never assumed to be correct, especially if the generator is used for a variety of procedures by different endoscopists. Even if the GIA is thoroughly familiar with an endoscopist's particular technique, it is always wise to announce the settings before proceeding. It is best also that the GIA have an understanding with every endoscopist that polypectomy must not begin until the GIA announces that everything is ready. A certain amount of the active snare wire may be exposed within the control handle of the polypectomy device. Well-designed devices limit the degree of exposure of the active elements, but a burn will still result if such a component is touched during activation of the generator.

Closure of the snare loupe is a critical phase of endoscopic polypectomy. Since the GIA and the endoscopist must cooperate closely in this maneuver, it is essential that the directions the endoscopist will use be established and clearly understood by the GIA in advance. As with biopsy technique, simple directions work best, e.g., "close" (to close the loupe), "open," "open slightly," "open full," "open half," etc. (to open the loupe). In the method that we use, the endoscopist repeats the direction to "close" until the loupe is against the stalk of the polyp. Electrosurgical polypectomy encompasses several variations in technique (see Chapters 7 and 45) that determine how tightly the snare loupe must be closed. Excessive force may guillotine the polyp and result in bleeding, or it may inhibit the sparking necessary to produce electrosurgical cutting. Inadequate closure may also prevent adequate coagulation and/or cutting. It is virtually impossible to describe the correct amount of tension to be applied to the snare wire; the GIA can learn this through experience, and this learning process is based entirely on close cooperation and communication with the endoscopist. As the snare is closed, the GIA can often appreciate that viable tissue is still present within the loupe since the effort to close meets with a certain resistance. It is also possible to sense the point that the snare cuts through tissue. The degree of closure of the loupe can also be gauged by observing the control handle.

Endoscopic Retrograde Cholangiopancreatography (ERCP)

The tasks associated with ERCP are similar to those for EGD with some additions such as the injection of contrast medium. ERCP may also require a greater variety of accessories than most other procedures. Certain ERCP procedures have a higher risk of complications, depending on the nature of the disease. In some clinical situations there is a higher risk of sepsis.

As with biopsy, polypectomy, sclerotherapy, and any cooperative therapeutic procedure, injection of contrast medium requires precise communication between endoscopist and assistant. Excessive force with an increased rate and volume of injection usually causes discomfort and in the pancreatic duct may contribute to postprocedure pancreatitis. Generally, the endoscopist controls the rate of injection by reference to the fluoroscopic image. The GIA should also watch the filling of the ductal systems fluoroscopically, although instructions from the endoscopist should primarily direct the filling procedure. Some special types of ERCP catheters may be used, such as ones with a tapered tip and those with a small metal tip for cannulation of a stenotic papilla or the minor papilla (ERCP technique is discussed in Chapter 25).

Aseptic technique is mandatory in ERCP, since in some clinical situations contrast medium may be injected into a closed space such as a pancreatic pseudocyst or beyond a tight stricture in the bile duct. The introduction of bacteria into a closed space without proper drainage can lead to septicemia and abscess formation. One of the major sources of contamination is the light source water bottle. Because of this danger, our water bottles are gas sterilized and changed daily. All catheters and other accessories are also sterilized in a similar manner. Although it is not possible to make ERCP a sterile procedure, measures such as these are known to reduce the incidence of serious infection.

Endoscopic sphincterotomy (ES), along with its ancillary therapeutic maneuvers in the bile and pancreatic ducts, is one of the most demanding of all therapeutic procedures for both the endoscopist and the GIA. The papillotome is usually operated by the GIA in response to established instructions. It is necessary that the GIA be thoroughly familiar with the technique of sphincterotomy. There are also a number of variations of ES, most of which require special papillotomy devices (see Chapter 29). Extraction of bile duct stones may require different devices during a procedure, including various baskets, mechanical lithotriptors, and balloons. Breakage of certain accessories commonly occurs so that back-up equipment must always be available. Biliary stenting requires that a number of different types of stents be available in different sizes. Insertion of a large-diameter prosthesis requires not only an endoscope with a large accessory channel, but also several types of catheters and guide wires (see Chapter 31). Many other pieces of equipment may be needed during any given procedure. The GIA must know the names and understand the use of each of these items. As virtually any accessory may be called for quickly and unexpectedly, the entire complement of devices and accessories must be well organized and within easy reach. In our unit every device and accessory is placed in its own package. Each of these packages is labeled; one side of the envelope is also clear plastic so that the contents can be seen without opening the envelope (Fig. 5–3). The envelopes and their contents are gas sterilized.

Pediatric Endoscopy

There are some important differences in the role of the GIA in pediatric endoscopy and endoscopy in adults (see Chapter 13). For example, in most children endoscopy requires two assistants. One performs those functions normally associated with adult procedures while the other holds and comforts the child. Generally, the endoscopes used are the same as those for adults except that in small children smaller diameter instruments must be used. Dosages of medications differ in some cases.

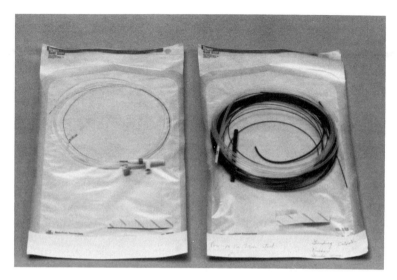

FIGURE 5–3. Package used for ERCP accessories. The contents of the package may be gas sterilized after the package is sealed. The transparent side of the envelope plus labeling allows the GIA to identify quickly which accessories are contained in the package.

Certain additional supplies are required when pediatric endoscopy is performed in an endoscopy unit. These include diapers, small gowns, bottles, toys, and candy. CPR also differs slightly in infants and children. For example, certain items of equipment must be available in smaller sizes.

Charting

In our unit the GIA has a limited role with regard to entry of notations in the patient's chart, except that all medications given must be noted, including the dosage, route, and time of administration.

Postprocedure Functions

The GIA has two main tasks after endoscopy: (1) monitoring the patient's recovery and (2) cleaning the instruments.

Patient Monitoring

The length of time that a patient must remain under observation varies and depends on type and dosage of the sedative drugs given and the nature of the procedure. Even after a patient recovers from the medication it may be necessary to continue observation in the case of therapeutic procedures that carry a risk of complications. Generally, proper postprocedure monitoring requires determination of vital signs and observation of the patient for any signs of pain or discomfort. In our unit the GIA is permitted to discharge patients from the dressing room. The assistant also enters postprocedure notations in the chart using a standard format. Discharge instructions are given by the GIA; this includes a printed sheet that provides information on possible delayed complications and instructions for the patient should a complication develop.

Cleaning

In addition to cleaning and preparing the room for the next procedure the GIA must clean the endoscope and other equipment used during the procedure.

Water and then air should be flushed through the air-water channel of the endoscope immediately after the procedure. This is done by disconnecting the water bottle and then blocking the air-water inlet on the universal cord of the endoscope with a finger while the endoscopist depresses the air-water valve. By doing this the light source will pump out all the water remaining in the channel; air is pumped through the channel once it is emptied of water.

Clean water should also be drawn through the suction channel, followed by room air. We use transparent suction tubing so that the color and the contents of the suctioned water can be seen. The cleaning brush is then passed through the accessory suction channel(s) of the endoscope.

Proper cleaning requires the use of a sink with a fairly large basin. In addition, a rack on the wall above the sink on which the instrument may be hung is extremely useful. This allows the insertion tube of the instrument to hang down into the basin (see below under Procedure Room Organization). The main supplies we use in cleaning an endoscope are listed in Table 5–2. The GIA should always wear gloves during the cleaning procedure.

TABLE 5–2. **Supplies Required for Cleaning Endoscopes**

1. Large plastic or metal basin
2. Plastic bottles (3)
   a. Soap
   b. Disinfectant solution
   c. 70% alcohol
3. Cotton-tipped applicators
4. Plastic cups (3)
   a. Clean rinse water
   b. Disinfectant
   c. Alcohol for soaking accessory channel valve and distal insertion tube hood (where applicable)
5. Gauze pads (4″ × 4″)
6. Channel cleaning adapter
7. Syringe (20 or 50 ml)
8. Pick-up forceps
9. Hydrogen peroxide

Debris and secretions should be removed from the opening of the accessory channel valve with the cotton-tipped applicator. The control section of the endoscope should then be cleaned, especially around the controls, the suction and air-water valves, deflection locks, and deflection knobs. This must be done carefully with older non-immersible instruments, since the instrument will be damaged by water or other fluids that enter the control section. A gauze sponge moistened with 70% alcohol is usually adequate for this purpose. Any disinfecting or sterilization process will be ineffective if mechanical cleaning of the instrument has not been thorough.

About 50 ml of disinfectant solution should be flushed through the accessory channel. Glutaraldehydes and iodophors are two commonly used disinfectant solutions. The fiberscope manufacturer should always be consulted to determine that the solution to be used will not damage the endoscope. The next step is to flush about 200 ml of clean water through the channel to wash out the disinfectant. This is a very important step since disinfectants are usually toxic.

The insertion tube is first washed with soapy water, then rinsed with clear water using a gauze sponge. The insertion tube is then washed again, this time with the disinfectant solution, and rinsed again with clear water and a gauze sponge. All of the disinfectant solution must be removed. The insertion tube is finally wiped down with a gauze sponge soaked in 70% alcohol.

It is possible to disinfect newer air- and water-tight fiberscopes more completely, as well as some electronic endoscopes, by completely immersing them for a period of time,

after removing all detachable parts, in a disinfectant solution. We prefer Cidex for a period of 10 to 20 minutes.

Air should be flushed through the accessory channel to remove water droplets. Stagnant water within the channel promotes the growth of microbes. Hanging the instrument when not in use allows the accessory channel to drain and helps to avoid this problem. The accessory channel valve should be cleaned separately and replaced in the instrument.

Thorough mechanical cleaning and the use of a disinfecting agent are generally satisfactory after most endoscopic procedures. Automatic washing and disinfecting machines are available commercially that carry out essentially the same process as described. Whether or not these machines are a worthwhile investment in time saving is a personal decision.

Despite the adequacy of mechanical cleaning and disinfection, certain clinical situations remain that cause some concern for possible transmission of infectious agents. Although the risk of this is low, we do keep a separate set of older, infrequently used instruments for the examination of patients who may harbor transmissible agents and for patients at exceptionally high risk for infection. These instruments are cleaned in the usual way, but they are also subjected to ethylene oxide gas sterilization.

Sterilization with ethylene oxide gas is discussed in Chapter 2. Certain essential points merit repeating. A fiberscope must be completely dry, the venting valve on fluid/air-tight instruments must be opened to avoid damage to the instrument, and the instrument must be aerated to remove all residual gas before it can be used again. Aeration requires up to 7 days at room temperature, but this can be shortened to 24 hours or less with the use of an aeration chamber. The fiberscope manufacturer should always be consulted for each type of instrument that will be sterilized with ethylene oxide. Autoclave sterilization destroys fiberscopes, but certain accessories may be sterilized by this method.

Adequate mechanical cleaning of a biopsy forceps after a procedure is difficult because of the numerous crevices and small places in this accessory. The forceps can be soaked in hydrogen peroxide before cleaning in soapy water and then rinsed in clear water or be gas sterilized whenever necessary to insure proper disinfection. Ultrasonic cleaning devices are used for this purpose in some units. Because it is possible that small amounts of blood may adhere to the forceps, some units sterilize the biopsy forceps after each use.

GIA Productivity and Staffing Level

Weighted Scale

Although the procedure unit concept considers endoscopic procedures in terms of their similarities, in fact endoscopic procedures also differ significantly for the GIA. From a systems management viewpoint, the major differences among procedures relate to the number of personnel required, the time required for the endoscopic portion of the procedure, and the number of items of equipment needed.

The concept of a weighted scale rating system for procedures is presented in Chapter 3. The essential features of this concept are as follows: Because of differing degrees of complexity of procedures it is not possible to assess the activity and productivity of an endoscopy unit by a simple procedure count. Every procedure performed in a unit is given a number value that relates the complexity and difficulty of the procedure to an arbitrary reference procedure that is given a value of 1.0 on the scale. The reference base procedure in our unit is the diagnostic EGD without biopsy or other ancillary procedure (see Table 3–2, Chapter 3). It is important to establish a time equivalent for this procedure (in our unit 1.0 is equal to 30 minutes). The total of the weighted scale values for any given period of time relates procedural activity to the reference procedure, in this case EGD. The total of weighted scale numbers therefore states procedure activity in terms of the diagnostic EGD. A procedure unit in our system therefore becomes equivalent to a simple diagnostic EGD.

Although the procedure unit/weighted scale methodology has many applications with regard to analysis, planning, and problem solving, we developed it mainly to assist in gauging GIA productivity. It became apparent that the work output of the unit as an entity (including all personnel and resources) seemed to be substantial, but that this was not totally reflected in the procedure count. A steady increase in the complexity of procedures had taken place so that productivity was actually at a much higher level than suggested by the count total. The workload of the GIA had increased to a greater degree than could be determined from existing data. Although the subjective impression of the unit staff of an increasing workload was correct, it was difficult to substantiate this for those without direct knowledge of the function of an endoscopy unit or of the fact that endoscopy procedures are not the same. Based on the count, for example, requests for additional personnel were not entirely justified. The procedure unit/weighted scale system of analysis, however, more accurately reflects the actual performance and productivity of a unit.

The GIA has a central position in the procedure unit/weighted scale methodology. As noted, the assistant has responsibility for more steps in the procedure unit than any other participant, including the endoscopist. In developing the weighted procedure scale, the time and effort of the GIA were primary considerations. At the conclusion of every procedure a weighted scale value is calculated by the GIA using a set of guidelines (see Table 3–2, Chapter 3). The assistant can also adjust the value within certain limits for especially long and difficult procedures or those that utilize an unusual amount of equipment. Our scale is already adjusted to account for those procedures that require transport of equipment to and from other areas of the medical center and to reflect the participation of trainees.

Staffing

From the standpoint of productivity, and especially cost effectiveness, it is of great importance to know the actual number of GIAs that an endoscopy unit requires. Although equipment can be very expensive, the greatest cost factor is usually the payroll. The basic problem in determining the number of GIAs required is that there are imbalances in the amount of time required of the GIA, the endoscopist, and the procedure room to accomplish one procedure unit. In terms of procedure units, one GIA is not equivalent to one endoscopist or to one procedure room.

The maximum number of procedure units that a GIA can produce in a given time can be calculated using the procedure units/weighted scale method (see Chapter 3). This will always be less than the maximum capability of one endoscopist, and it is always less than the maximum capacity of one procedure room, the latter being due principally to the need to monitor patients postprocedure. A

GIA who assists with the endoscopic portion of a procedure may not actually be the one who performs postprocedure functions such as cleaning and patient monitoring, but these functions nevertheless require GIA time and this must be considered. Other adjustments must be included in calculating maximum productivity such as vacation days, conferences, and the expected efficiency for the unit as a whole. Expected efficiency is difficult to analyze. Individuals almost always assume that they function at a level approaching 100%, but it is difficult to exceed the maximum possible efficiency of the endoscopy unit as a whole. No unit functions at 100% efficiency since this requires that every procedure be performed with virtually no delay and that all equipment and personnel be fully occupied at all times. A more reasonable prospect would be 70% of the theoretical maximum capacity. This would also, therefore, be a reasonable expectation for GIA productivity.

Using these various methods of analysis, a reasonable expectation for the productivity of one GIA is 1000 procedure units per year. To determine the necessary level of GIA staffing for a unit, however, it is also necessary to know the maximum capacity (in terms of procedure units) of the available procedure rooms. It is also necessary to know the number of full time equivalent endoscopists working in the unit along with the maximum number of procedure units that each full-time equivalent can produce.

The capacity of a procedure room will differ from unit to unit. It will depend on a variety of factors, including the expected efficiency of the unit. Once these determinations are made, it is a simple matter to calculate the actual and theoretical maximum efficiency of an endoscopy unit as a whole (see Chapter 3). Based on certain assumptions, the capacity of one procedure room is about 1500 procedure units per year.

It is not difficult to estimate the number of procedures that one endoscopist working full-time can accomplish in a given time (see Chapter 3). Certain corrections can be included to account for time away from the unit for various reasons. The expected efficiency can also be included as a factor, although this must be based on the maximum efficiency possible for the unit itself. Using these various assumptions, the maximum productivity of a single full-time endoscopist is about 1800 procedure units per year. Since most endoscopists perform a variety of different procedures rather than simple diagnostic EGDs alone (the base reference procedure in the weighted scale), the actual count of procedures will almost always be less than 1800. The theoretical maximum productivity in terms of procedure units of one full-time endoscopist exceeds that of a single procedure room by about 300 procedure units.

With reference to the ratio of GIAs to endoscopists it is also necessary to know how many full-time endoscopists work in a unit. This is not equivalent to the number of physicians that perform endoscopy, since most physicians are not full-time endoscopists and only perform procedures during a portion of a working day. Nevertheless, it is possible to calculate the equivalent number of full-time endoscopists based on estimates of part-time (or in a few cases the full-time) contributions of each staff member (see Chapter 3).

These calculations indicate that there should be a ratio of about 1.5 GIAs per procedure room or 1.8 GIAs per equivalent full-time endoscopist. The final step in calculating the level of GIA staffing required in a unit is to determine whether the number of endoscopists or number of procedure rooms will be the limiting factor on productivity. If the number of full-time endoscopist equivalents exceeds the capacity of all of the unit's procedure rooms, then GIA staffing should be based on the number of rooms available. Conversely, if the limiting factor is the number of full-time equivalent endoscopists, GIA staffing should be calculated based on a ratio of 1.8 GIAs per each equivalent full-time endoscopist. In practice, other factors must also be considered such as the demand for procedures. In recent years this has been steadily increasing, but it should not be assumed that this will continue.

Many small, seemingly unimportant tasks must be performed in an endoscopy unit. Many of these tasks pertain to supply and logistics (see below). Time and effort are required to keep a unit clean and orderly. The morale of the GIA staff requires that time be set aside for discussions, in-service meetings pertaining to new equipment, and education. Rigid calculations of the required staffing level often ignore these less tangible, less noticeable, but not less important activities of the GIA. In the long run, the efficiency and the quality of the work produced by a unit will be greater if some estimate of the time and manpower needed for these tasks is included when determining the level of staffing appropriate for a unit.

In almost any endoscopy unit it is necessary that some procedures be performed away from the unit. The reasons for this are varied: the type of practice (e.g., a large number of procedures for acute hemorrhage), the need to share expensive equipment such as a laser with other departments, the need to have the services of a radiologist and an x-ray suite for certain procedures such as ERCP, and a variety of other factors. The types and numbers of procedures performed away from the endoscopy unit have a bearing on the number of assistants needed. Transport of equipment to and from the endoscopy unit is always time consuming. For complex procedures such as therapeutic biliary endoscopy the variety and amount of equipment would prohibit transport were it not for the fact that x-ray equipment is usually available only in a radiology department. Although a complete complement of equipment could be maintained in the radiology suite, this is only a partial solution. In addition to the fact that certain useful pieces of equipment, such as a light source, would not be used for significant periods of time, the GIA still has the problems of cleaning, storing, restocking supplies as they are consumed, and refurbishing worn equipment. From a managerial viewpoint, this approach means in essence that an additional part-time procedure room requires GIA staffing. In a large medical center complex, travel time to and from the endoscopy unit and an off-unit procedure site may be significant. When two or more off-unit sites are used routinely, travel time during a day can be equivalent to two or three procedure units. For these reasons having a large number of procedures performed away from the unit requires additional GIA staff.

THE GIA SUPERVISOR

Just as the growth and evolution of gastrointestinal endoscopy have fostered the position of the GIA, so the growth of the endoscopy unit has engendered the position of GIA supervisor. Sustained increases in the numbers and complexity of procedures have also brought about a substantial increase in the staff of most units. During the early development of endoscopy a single individual usually accomplished most of the GIA tasks entailed in a single procedure unit. In the modern unit, however, there is often a substantial division of labor because of the greater number of procedures. Thus, one GIA may only assist with the endoscopic portion of a procedure, another is responsible for instrument cleaning and preparation, and still another is concerned only with post-procedure patient monitoring. Various assignments are usually rotated among the GIA staff. Because of the intricacy of new therapeutic techniques, more than one GIA may be needed for some procedures. Such an intricate operation has a high potential for disorder and confusion, a point strongly in favor of the need for a specific supervisor of GIA personnel.

Extensive experience in gastrointestinal endoscopy, including a thorough knowledge of all procedures, is a major qualification for the position of GIA supervisor. However, a comprehensive background in endoscopy is not the only quality required. Such an individual occupies a pivotal position in the organizational structure of the unit. In this role the GIA supervisor is directly and most immediately involved in the allocation of the resources of personnel, equipment, and procedure rooms. This central role obligates the supervisor to participate in the day to day scheduling of procedures. The GIA supervisor also shares responsibility in meeting the endoscopy unit's standards of quality, for the maintenance of plant and equipment, for GIA training, for the development and evaluation of new procedures and equipment, and for the logistics of consumable supplies. The GIA supervisor directs the activities of the GIA staff throughout the working day and also interacts with many people who support the operation of the unit but who are not staff members, such as manufacturer's representatives, the biomedical engineer, radiation safety officer, pharmacist, and many others. Thus, it is highly desirable that the GIA supervisor have managerial and organizational skills in addition to a total grasp of the field of gastrointestinal endoscopy.

It is mandatory that the importance of the GIA supervisor's many functions be clearly recognized and that these functions be considered apart from the activities of other GIA personnel. The GIA supervisor and the physician head of the unit form the nucleus of the unit's management team. It is unrealistic to expect that a single individual can accomplish these managerial tasks and still perform the more usual duties of a GIA. Paradoxically, therefore, the GIA supervisor must become less involved with the actual steps of the procedure unit.

Scheduling

Endoscopy unit efficiency requires a systematic approach to the scheduling of procedures. Certain aspects of this are discussed in Chapter 3. As a guiding principle, the design of any system should be based on the most restrictive factor. This may be any one or more of the following: procedure rooms, endoscopists, assistants, or instruments. In our unit the schedule is based on the procedure rooms (see Chapter 3). The scheduling system will also reflect a basic philosophy of room utilization, e.g., to what extent a room can accommodate various procedures. The complexity of a scheduling process increases in proportion to the degree to which procedure rooms are multifunctional in a unit. Multifunctional rooms increase efficiency and flexibility, but they also demand more sophisticated scheduling methods. There is usually a mixture of multipurpose and dedicated or semidedicated rooms in every unit.

Virtually no scheduling system can anticipate the minute to minute changes in the daily activity of a large endoscopy unit unless a superficial orderliness is achieved at the expense of productivity. There are unforeseen delays in patient preparation, last minute cancellations, mistakes in scheduling, procedures prolonged beyond the allotted time, complications, equipment breakdown, urgent and emergency requests for service, absence of staff members due to illness, delays in starting procedures for any number of reasons, and many other foreseeable and unforeseeable ways in which the daily activities can be disrupted. When there is a close working relationship and communication between an appointment secretary and the GIA supervisor, the resources of the unit can be quickly redeployed to adjust the schedule to changing circumstances on an hour to hour basis. The result of this relationship is a flexible, efficient, and productive system.

Logistics

An incredible amount and variety of equipment are required for the efficient functioning of an endoscopy unit. The capital equip-

ment, i.e., endoscopes, light sources, lasers, x-ray machines, etc., is the most obvious. However, a less evident but no less ubiquitous or important category of equipment is that of consumable supplies. The list is seemingly endless: antibiotics, arm boards, aspirin, batteries, Band-Aids, biliary stents, biopsy channel valves, cytology brushes, cleaning solutions of all types, colon lavage solutions, diapers, dental suction devices, enemas, emesis basins, facial tissue, gauze sponges, glass slides, hospital gowns, intravenous tubing and solutions, light source lamps, lubricants, laboratory requisitions, nasobiliary tubes, needles, paper towels, photographic film (various types), sheets, silicon lubricant, specimen bottles, sedative drugs, suction tubing, syringes, tape, tongue depressors, toothpicks, toys, videotape cassettes, washcloths, x-ray monitoring badges, etc. In addition, endoscopic accessories are another category of equipment that must be replaced periodically. This includes items such as snare wires, papillotomes, biopsy forceps, Bicap and heat probes, and stone extraction balloons. Although much of this seems mundane, it must not be taken for granted. Every endoscopy unit, if it is to function smoothly, must have an inventory supply system, and this should also be the responsibility of the GIA supervisor.

Deployment of GIA Staff

The physical design of an endoscopy unit must accommodate the basic steps of the procedure unit. Since space must be allocated for each fundamental component of the procedure unit, the floor plan of the unit also locates the work stations of the GIAs.

It is highly inefficient for a GIA who assists at the endoscopic segment of the procedure unit to also perform postprocedure patient monitoring, since this results in a significant lapse of time between procedures. Furthermore, the simplest possible endoscopy unit must be divided into four rooms or areas: (1) patient reception, (2) scheduling/secretarial, (3) procedure room (with cleaning, storage, and charting areas), and (4) patient dressing/recovery area. These factors dictate that at a minimum all but the smallest units with a single procedure room will require at least two GIAs.

As the size of an endoscopy unit increases, there are many more questions of design that must be answered. The degree to which procedure rooms function independently of one another must be resolved. Even in a unit with many procedure rooms and a large amount of floor space, individual procedure rooms can remain semiautonomous by retaining many of the procedure unit steps. In practical terms this means that the procedure room must contain facilities for cleaning and storage as well as for all drugs, accessories, and other paraphernalia required for a variety of procedures. This endoscopy unit "philosophy" also demands some duplication of equipment. In essence, however, each procedure room in such a scheme will have its own daily schedule of cases. In general, this system requires one GIA for each active procedure room. When procedure room utilization approaches 75%, at least one GIA will be required for each procedure room in the unit.

A design that utilizes an interdependent room concept is another option. In such a system, as many elements of the procedure unit as possible are removed from the procedure room and performed in other areas and rooms provided for these purposes. A unit design might use a single space for cleaning and storage of instruments that is central to all of the procedure rooms. To utilize such a plan to maximum advantage it is necessary to assign at least one GIA to cleaning and preparation of endoscopes. Consolidation of the cleaning and storage functions for groups of two or more procedure rooms within the unit is another possibility. The advantages of this are space saving and simplified interchange of equipment between the associated rooms. Since cleaning and storage for the unit as a whole are not truly centralized in such a plan, however, it is usually impractical to assign an individual exclusively to these duties unless the unit is exceptionally large and a GIA can be fully occupied at each of the cleaning-storage substations.

Preparation, cleaning, and storage of endoscopes and accessories are relatively uncomplicated tasks. It is possible, therefore, to hire a less highly trained individual to perform only these functions. In such cases this activity is usually regarded as a separate job description that is not filled by a GIA. This has certain advantages and disadvantages. One view is that it is desirable that a GIA be familiar with all aspects of endoscopy, that expensive equipment is better cared for by individuals who understand and respect its

purposes, and that these tasks will be performed with greater care by someone more directly involved with the patients for whom the equipment is intended. Although it is essential that this type of work be performed in a careful and expeditious manner, it is nevertheless relatively routine and perhaps unexciting. If the activity of a fully qualified GIA is to be limited to this work, then it is best to rotate this assignment among the GIA staff. The opposite view is that hiring a person with lesser qualifications for this position is economical and also frees GIAs for activities that are more concerned with direct patient contact.

The basic task elements of the procedure unit can be subdivided in other ways. Patient preparation for procedures can also be accomplished outside the procedure room. This method usually requires a cart exchange system between the procedure rooms and dressing room. Since sedative drugs are administered before the patient reaches the procedure room, using such a system requires that the patient be attended by a GIA. It can be efficient in a large unit that uses such a system to assign a GIA exclusively to the patient exchange function. This function could also include an assisting role in postprocedure observation in the dressing room in conjunction with another GIA assigned only to monitoring. The patient exchange GIA could also be responsible for preparation of the procedure room between cases except for instruments and equipment.

The number of GIAs required in the dressing room depends on the number of patients who can be accommodated, which in turn should relate to the number of procedure rooms (see Chapter 3). The number of GIAs will also depend on the types of procedures being performed. The length and intensity of postprocedure monitoring are less if a high percentage of procedures are simple diagnostic EGDs. If, however, there are many outpatient therapeutic procedures that require closer observation for more extended periods of time, then the workload of the GIA will be greater. During 1985 in our unit the average weighted scale value for all procedures was 1.53, at which level of activity one experienced GIA managed 8 bed spaces.

Various types of procedures are performed in most endoscopy units. Many of these procedures will be considered routine, whereas others might be termed special procedures. Those in the special category tend to be therapeutic and are usually performed less frequently relative to the numbers of routine examinations. This mix will be reflected in the design of the unit, specifically with respect to the ratio of dedicated rooms for specific procedures to multifunctional rooms. From a managerial viewpoint it is important that individual GIAs not become identified with certain procedures. Although it can be argued that the result of restricting certain procedures to one or a few GIAs improves the quality of the procedure, this tends to segregate the GIAs into groups. The implication of this is a hierarchy within the GIA staff, that some members have greater importance than others. This managerial stance, that only certain individuals are capable of performing particular procedures, can be inefficient and may be a source of friction within the GIA staff. In this same context, it is essential that GIA assignments be rotated among the endoscopists who work in a unit. Allowing an endoscopist to identify those GIAs he or she will work with, or permitting GIAs to select endoscopists to work with according to their preferences, makes it impossible to develop and maintain a team approach. Such a predicament may be inadvertent and its consequences may only become evident as it impedes growth of the unit. It must always be the primary goal of the GIA supervisor that the GIA staff functions as a unit.

The various endoscopy procedures performed in a given unit may be broadly classified into "routine" and "special." The attributes of each of these are discussed in Chapter 3. Special-type procedures are usually therapeutic and often require distinctive, expensive, one-of-a-kind equipment within the unit. Some special procedures require relatively large numbers of equipment. These factors increase the magnitude of preparation for the procedure as well as the postprocedure work of the GIA. Depending on the skill of the endoscopist, special procedures can be more time consuming. In addition, they are intrinsically more complex for both the endoscopist and the GIA. The assistant must often perform a number of tasks, including patient monitoring, at the same time. Although one GIA is the minimum requirement for a special procedure, in some cases the difficulty of the procedure, patient safety requirements, and the need to perform a number of tasks simultaneously justify the presence of a second GIA. Endoscopic sphincterotomy, especially with additional therapeutic maneuvers such as insertion of a biliary stent, is an example of such a procedure.

GIA Training

In-service Conferences

Associated with the increase in the scope and complexity of endoscopic procedures is a corresponding increase in the complexity and number of items of endoscopic equipment. New procedures are constantly being developed. Another aspect of this change and growth is that the GIA must also acquire new knowledge and skill concurrently. There is considerable value, therefore, in regularly scheduled in-service conferences.

Training

Much of the present knowledge and skills that the GIA requires are based on practical experience. Since little instructive information has been published, this knowledge resides mostly with individual nurses who have themselves participated in the growth and development of gastrointestinal endoscopy and the endoscopy unit. This knowledge and skill are therefore not part of any formal training curriculum and can only be learned at present through practical instruction from an experienced GIA.

The fact that the art and skills that qualify a nurse as a GIA reside with relatively few individuals is inauspicious for the future development of gastrointestinal endoscopy. The method of training GIAs is essentially that of passing information and experience from one individual to another. Even the methods and techniques used in training new GIAs, as well as the actual experience of teaching those who undertake this activity, are known to relatively few nurses. Thus, in many large units the training and supervision of a number of GIAs are the responsibility of one nurse with a number of years of service and experience. The loss of this individual, through retirement, for example, is equivalent to a substantial loss of ability to train new GIAs.

The training of GIAs is a stepwise process. It is first necessary to provide an overview of the way in which endoscopy is performed through observation. The student GIA must learn the primary parts of a gastrointestinal endoscope along with the correct methods of handling this type of instrument, especially with respect to proper techniques for cleaning and storage.

In our experience, GIA training is best conducted by learning one procedure at a time, upper gastrointestinal endoscopy serving as the initial basic training procedure. This method of instruction is similar to our system for training gastrointestinal endoscopists. The use of one fundamental procedure as a prototype in instruction simplifies the learning process. Rather than confronting the trainee with many different endoscopes, accessories, and procedures, the subject matter is broken down into smaller parts that fit into a natural progression in which the information and knowledge acquired in earlier stages of training can be built upon and modified as the GIA is introduced to colonoscopy and later ERCP. In this respect it is also best to introduce therapeutic procedures only after the assistant is thoroughly familiar with basic diagnostic endoscopy.

In order to properly assist at endoscopy it is essential that a GIA have a basic understanding of the way in which endoscopic procedures are performed by the endoscopist. This knowledge of the procedure itself should include the indications and contraindications, and should in particular include its major complications and the signs and symptoms of untoward events. Familiarity with the procedure allows the GIA to be alert to possible patient discomfort and to recognize potential hazards and difficulties for the endoscopist. Furthermore, it also allows the GIA to anticipate the need for accessories, other items of equipment, and medication.

A well-designed procedure room supports the performance of endoscopic procedures in a number of ways. For example, items of equipment, the examination table, work surfaces, storage spaces, sink, etc. are located according to the role they play in the procedure unit (see Chapter 3). The organization of the procedure room should be presented early in the course of training at a time when the new GIA is learning about the endoscopy procedure itself. With an understanding of the objectives and actual performance of an endoscopic procedure, it is relatively easy to comprehend the seemingly complex organization of a procedure room; as the relation between form and function of the procedure room becomes more apparent, the new GIA is also better able to understand and recognize his or her role in the procedure unit.

Equipment

The GIA supervisor plays an essential role in maintaining the endoscopy unit equipment. The quality of the procedures performed in the unit, the safety of patients, and the overall efficiency of the unit depend substantially on the cleanliness and good condition of the equipment. The growth of endoscopy has also fostered growth in the commercial sector so that many manufacturers now sell endoscopic equipment. Although competition is desirable in many respects, it also leads to differences in price, quality, durability, design, safety, and availability. Consideration must also be given to provisions for service and compatibility with existing equipment. The choice of equipment can therefore be difficult; proper selection requires a thorough familiarity with available items. Manufacturers also make improvements in their products so that equipment must be reevaluated continuously. The GIA supervisor plays an essential role in this process and collects and synthesizes the opinions and experience of the unit's staff.

New endoscopic procedures are being developed constantly. Each new technique requires further skills and knowledge on the part of the GIA. In a large unit, one GIA, often the GIA supervisor but not necessarily the same individual in each case, can be assigned to assist in the development of new procedures and to evaluate new equipment. The knowledge and information derived in this process must then be disseminated to other GIA staff members.

METHODS

The methods of experienced GIAs differ in many ways. This applies not only to the specific process of assisting at procedures, but also to the general activities within the endoscopy unit. There are different systems for cleaning and storage of instruments, for preparation of patients for procedures, for moving patients to and from the procedure room, for handling emergency situations, and for a great variety of other functions. It is uncertain whether these differences are important and whether the approach of one individual to a given procedure is more satisfactory than that of another. Most likely there are unique aspects of each experienced GIA's methods that would be useful to others. Although there have been recent efforts to better disseminate this type of knowledge, these have been rudimentary in relation to the number of endoscopy units and the remarkable growth of this field.

Although there are no standardized techniques for GIAs, an attempt to develop a standardized methodology would have merit. The purpose of this would not be to define recommended or approved methods, either arbitrarily or by consensus, or even to impose uniformity. Rather the value of a more standardized approach lies in the establishment of a frame of reference and guiding principles for future GIAs.

Although it is impossible to discuss the many methods and techniques used by the GIA, several will be considered here.

Procedure Room Organization

The arrangement of the contents of the procedure room follows naturally from the general manner in which endoscopic procedures are performed. A simple but useful plan of organization for the room, as discussed in Chapter 3, is one that provides specific work areas for the GIA and the endoscopist with the examination table placed centrally. Ideally, the GIA's area should have a large countertop work surface as well as adequate storage areas, all within easy reach during a procedure.

Some features of a procedure room that pertain to the GIA's functions can be illustrated by reference to a procedure room in our unit (Fig. 5–4). This diagram is also used in Chapter 3 to point out the general features of a procedure room. During a procedure the GIA works in the section of the room between the examination table (number 15 in Fig. 5–4) and the bottom of the figure. During a procedure there is a countertop work surface with cupboards above and below (number 4a–c in Fig. 5–4) (Fig. 5–5A,B) behind the GIA. Cleaning and storage facilities are provided in one area within the room. Instrument storage cupboards are to the right in the diagram (number 7 in Fig. 5–4) (Fig. 5–6). We prefer to hang our en-

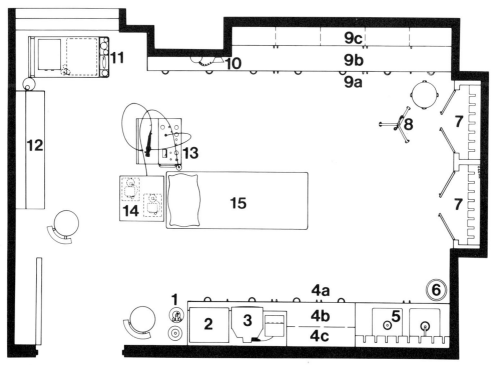

FIGURE 5–4. Typical endoscopy procedure room. 1—oxygen tanks, 2—videotape deck, 3—television monitor, 4a—storage below, 4b—countertop, 4c—cupboard, 5—double sink with rack above for hanging endoscopes, 6—waste basket, 7—storage closets with hanging racks, 8—IV pole, 9a—storage below, 9b—countertop, 9c—cupboards, 10—sphygmomanometer, 11—cart for emergency endoscopy, 12—shelf with x-ray view boxes above, 13—light source, 14—accessory table for GIA, 15—procedure table. The GIAs' work areas are at the bottom of the figure during a procedure and at the right for cleaning and storage.

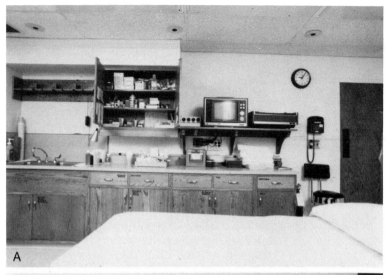

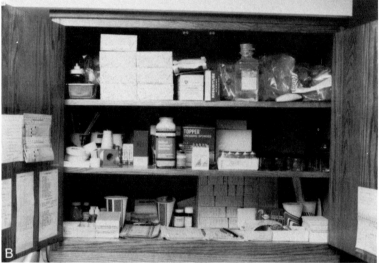

FIGURE 5–5. *A*, View of the GIAs' work area during a procedure from the endoscopist's side of the table (looking from the top toward the bottom of the diagram in Figure 5–4). Note countertop work area (4b in Fig. 5–4), with cupboards for storage below (4a in Fig. 5–4) and above (4c in Fig. 5–4). A phone extension is also provided for the GIA. (A separate extension is also provided on the endoscopist's side of the examination table.) *B*, Closer view of over counter cupboard (4c in Fig. 5–4) containing various paraphernalia used in procedures.

doscopes for storage as in Figure 5–6. Near the instrument cupboards in the right corner of the diagram is a double sink with a rack for hanging instruments while they are being cleaned (number 5 in Fig. 5–4) (Fig. 5–7). A small work table is placed at the head of the examination table for the GIA (number 14 in Fig. 5–4) (Fig. 5–8). This table has wheels so that it can be moved away from the head of the examination table. It provides an additional work surface and also holds various items of equipment, e.g., the electrosurgical generator that will be needed during the procedure. The position of this table allows the GIA to perform certain tasks, working with specimens for example, without turning his or her back to the patient or endoscopist.

Some Special Equipment

Carts

Regardless of how well an endoscopy unit and a hospital are equipped, certain endoscopic procedures must be performed away from the unit. This means that virtually every item of equipment needed for the procedure must be transported. The best method of transferring the equipment for a procedure to another site is by use of a cart. The type and amount of equipment needed will vary according to the nature of the procedure. The procedures include emergency endoscopy for gastrointestinal bleeding with endoscopic methods of hemostasis, ERCP with

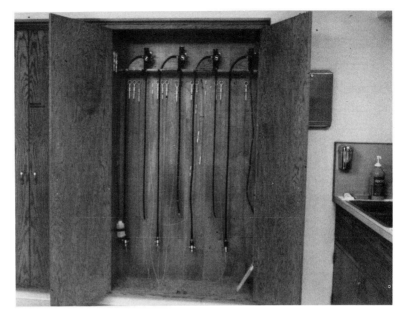

FIGURE 5–6. Instrument storage cupboards (number 7 in Fig. 5–4). Sets of accessories are also hung in these cupboards with the endoscopes they are used with.

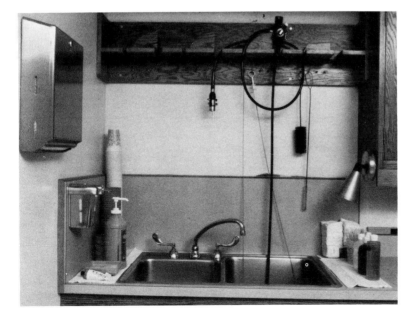

FIGURE 5–7. Double sink with instrument rack above for cleaning endoscopes (number 5 in Fig. 5–4).

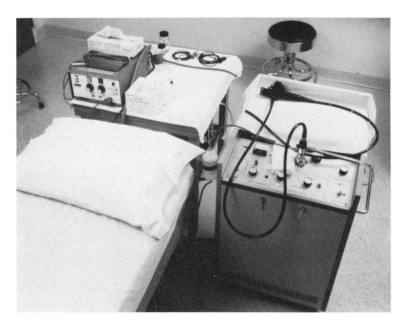

FIGURE 5–8. View of a portion of the procedure room depicted in Figure 5–4 showing small work table at the head of the examination table. There are electrical outlets on the floor below this table. The table may be rolled about if necessary. In the illustration the table holds an electrosurgical generator, gloves, facial tissues, specimen bottles, connecting wires for electrosurgical devices, and sponges. On the lower shelf of the table (not seen) there is space for Gomco suction machines.

FIGURE 5–9. Emergency cart. The items carried by this cart are listed in Table 5–3.

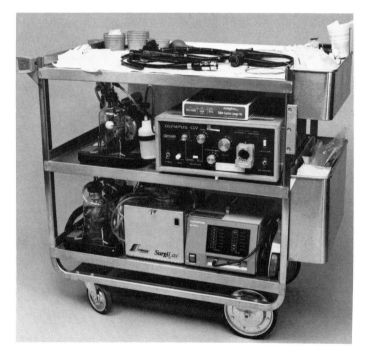

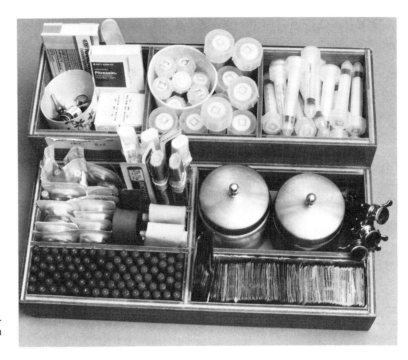

FIGURE 5–10. Small box containing paraphernalia used in administering drugs.

endoscopic sphincterotomy, laser endoscopy, and bedside sigmoidoscopy. It is difficult to set up a general purpose cart that would be suitable for all of these procedures.

For procedures that are frequently performed away from the unit a single cart may be equipped and maintained for this purpose. The usual example is the "emergency cart" for EGD for acute upper gastrointestinal bleeding (Fig. 5–9). The equipment on the emergency cart that we use routinely in our unit is listed in Table 5–3. We prefer a relatively simple cart with open shelves and large wheels. This allows for the interchange of various items of equipment so that the cart can be used for various purposes. Certain items commonly used in the endoscopy unit can also be placed on small carts with wheels so that they can be moved from one procedure room to another. It is often useful to place an electrosurgical generator on such a cart.

TABLE 5–3. **Emergency Cart Equipment**

Basin for water
Plastic cups
Mouthguard
Gauze sponges (4″ × 4″)
Gloves
Lubricant
Cytology brush
Cleaning brush
Biopsy forceps
Hugginson pump
Light source
Fiberoptic panendoscope
Lecturescope ("teaching attachment")
Heater probe (with large and small probes)
Gomco suction (2)
Forms
Viscous lidocaine (Xylocaine) spray
50-ml syringe with blunt needle
Gastric lavage kit
Sclerosing needles (2)
Introducer (for accessory channel valve)

Items kept in plastic bag:
   3% Sotradecol (one 2-ml ampule)
   Sterile 95% alcohol
   12-ml syringes (6)
   Normal saline (two 10-ml vials for injection)

Boxes

Certain small and frequently disposable items of equipment are required for specific parts of the procedure unit. Such items are often used at the same time. An example would be the needles, tourniquets, Band-Aids, alcohol prep sponges, and syringes for premedicating patients. One method of organizing items of equipment that are used together is to put them in small boxes or baskets (Fig. 5–10).

Chapter 6

ENDOSCOPY IN GASTROINTESTINAL BLEEDING

DAVID A. GILBERT, M.D.
FRED E. SILVERSTEIN, M.D.

The purpose of this chapter is to review the role of endoscopic diagnosis in upper and lower gastrointestinal bleeding. Several excellent reviews of this subject have been published.[1-3]

ENDOSCOPY IN UPPER GASTROINTESTINAL BLEEDING

Upper gastrointestinal bleeding is commonly encountered in clinical medicine. It is estimated that annually between 50 and 150 patients per 100,000 population are hospitalized for bleeding.[4, 5] Therefore, in the United States, with a population of approximately 200 million, about 200,000 patients present with upper gastrointestinal bleeding yearly. Despite major advances in monitoring and intensive care, there has been little change since 1940 in the mortality rate of approximately 10% for such patients.[6] One possible explanation, reflecting advances in other aspects of medical care, is that patients in recent studies are older (the majority being over age 60) than patients studied three to four decades ago, and therefore they often have a variety of other serious illnesses.

We will discuss the usefulness of endoscopy for the bleeding patient, specifically the information gained by endoscopy that may aid in management and influence the ultimate outcome of the bleeding episode. This issue was the subject of a recent National Institutes of Health consensus workshop in the United States.[7]

Approach to the Patient

When a patient presents with upper gastrointestinal bleeding, an initial brief assessment is appropriate. Often this requires the judicious and expeditious use of the entire range of the physician's skills. The assessment may be carried out during or immediately after institution of resuscitative measures. It should include inquiry concerning prior incidents of upper gastrointestinal bleeding, known peptic ulcer disease or gastrointestinal malignancy, and ingestion of drugs that cause gastrointestinal inflammation or ulceration. Symptoms of recent bleeding, such as melena, passage of red blood per rectum, and hematemesis, should be elucidated. Historical or physical evidence of other intercurrent illnesses must not be overlooked, because certain conditions such as diabetes, various forms of heart disease, and hypertension have a bearing on management. During the brief but thorough physical examination, some estimate must be made of the acuteness and severity of the bleeding. Accurate determinations of the heart rate and blood pressure, including orthostatic changes in blood pressure, are essential. A careful inspection for signs of liver disease, including spider telangiectasia, jaundice, and ascites, is also essential. Emesis and stool specimens should be examined if possible.

As the assessment proceeds, resuscitative measures should be instituted, starting with placement of one or more large-bore intravenous catheters. According to the estimated severity of blood loss, appropriate fluids should be given for volume replacement and hemodynamic stabilization. Based on an estimate of the volume of blood loss and the severity of bleeding, an appropriate number of units of whole blood or packed cells should be typed and crossmatched. In some situations, it may be necessary to use rapid methods for crossmatching, in consultation with blood bank personnel, especially when there is a danger of exsanguination.

Appropriate consultations should be sought as the patient is being admitted rather than as urgent measures when the patient's condition suddenly deteriorates. These consultations are based on the overall assessment of the patient's status; however, as a general rule it is best that a gastroenterologist and a surgeon be involved to some degree in the majority of cases. The level of such consultation can range from active participation by both members of this team in the management of gravely ill patients to a request that consultants remain available for assistance should the need arise.

Laboratory tests appropriate at initial presentation include hematocrit, hemoglobin, and white cell count. Coagulation studies, such as a bleeding time to assess platelet function, platelet count, prothrombin time, and partial thromboplastin time, may also be of importance. Serum electrolyte values and simple tests of renal function should be obtained. If there is any question of liver disease, basic liver function tests should be included, because underlying liver disease has been identified as a significant risk factor in the outcome of a bleeding episode.[8, 9]

Diagnostic and Management Considerations Following Initial Assessment and Resuscitation

The diagnostic and management issues that arise subsequent to the initial assessment and resuscitation, will be examined in detail. These are:

1. Determination of the level of the bleeding.
2. Assessment of the severity of active bleeding.
3. Diagnosis of the cause of the bleeding.
4. Prognostic value of endoscopy.
5. Timing of endoscopy.
6. Effect of the endoscopy on patient outcome.
7. A rational approach to endoscopy in the patient with upper gastrointestinal bleeding.

Determination of the Level of Bleeding

The level of bleeding should be determined as soon as possible after the patient's condition is stabilized. Although in many cases it is obvious that bleeding is upper gastrointestinal in origin, in some cases the level of bleeding is uncertain. Immediate management may not be altered by this information, but knowledge of the bleeding level will have a profound impact on the sequence and extent of the patient's workup. If the patient reports hematemesis and can be considered a reliable observer, it may be assumed that the source of bleeding is proximal to the ligament of Treitz. However, the patient may be obtunded, the reliability of the patient may be questionable, or in some cases hematemesis may not have occurred. In such instances it is essential that a tube be passed into the stomach to sample the gastric contents for blood. An 18 French sump tube is recommended.

In a retrospective series of 353 patients with gastrointestinal bleeding, Luk et al.[10] reported a less than 1% chance of bleeding proximal to the ligament of Treitz if the gastric aspirate did not contain blood. However, in the prospective national survey by the American Society for Gastrointestinal Endoscopy (ASGE),[11] which included data on 2225 patients who were evaluated for upper gastrointestinal bleeding, an active source of bleeding was found by endoscopy in 15.9% of patients whose gastric aspirates were clear. The differing conclusions of these two studies may be explained by the retrospective nature of the report of Luk et al. and by the fact that only 209 of 353 patients had endoscopy in this study. The endoscopic diagnoses in the patients with clear nasogastric aspirates in the National ASGE Survey are listed in Table 6–1. Duodenal ulcer was the most common finding, although gastric and esophageal lesions are represented. It can be concluded that a gastric aspirate positive for blood confirms that bleeding is from the upper gastrointestinal tract, although a negative aspirate does not eliminate this possibility.

There are several reasons for a clear gastric aspirate in the presence of upper gastrointestinal bleeding. The nasogastric tube may curl in the distal esophagus, thereby preventing sampling of the stomach contents; the stomach may have emptied itself of blood and bleeding may have stopped; or the bleed-

TABLE 6–1. **ASGE Bleeding Survey:**
Endoscopic Findings in 214 Patients with Clear
Nasogastric Aspirates*

Finding	No. Patients	Incidence (%)
Duodenal ulcer	64	29.8
Gastric erosions	57	26.5
Gastric ulcer	47	21.9
Esophagitis	23	10.7
Duodenitis	21	9.8
Varices	11	5.1
Mallory-Weiss tear	10	4.7
Neoplasm	8	3.7
Stomal ulcer	7	3.3
Esophageal ulcer	2	0.9
Telangiectasia	0	
Other	18	8.4
None	24	11.2

*From: Gilbert DA, Silverstein FE, Tedesco FJ, et al.: The national ASGE survey on upper gastrointestinal bleeding. III. Endoscopy in upper gastrointestinal bleeding. Gastrointest Endosc 1981; 27:94–102. Reprinted with permission.

ing lesion may be distal to the pylorus with no reflux of blood into the stomach, which may occur with an ulcer in the descending duodenum or an aortoduodenal fistula. On occasion, especially with difficult bleeding problems, endoscopy may be necessary to determine if bleeding is, in fact, emanating from an upper gastrointestinal source.

Assessment of the Severity of Active Bleeding

Patients with upper gastrointestinal bleeding are a heterogeneous group. They vary in general medical status from relatively healthy to very ill with concomitant systemic illnesses. Similarly, there is great variation in the severity of blood loss. Patients may present in shock or in stable condition with a history of having black stools several days earlier. The initial assessment of bleeding activity is important from the standpoint of prognosis as well as immediate management. In the ASGE survey, bleeding activity in patients with up-

per gastrointestinal hemorrhage, judged by color of gastric aspirate (Table 6–2) or color of stool (Table 6–3), significantly correlated with outcome in terms of mortality, need for more than five-unit transfusions, need for surgery, and occurrence of a complication during the bleeding episode.[8] Combining data on the color of the nasogastric aspirate and stool color provides additional insight into prognosis (Table 6–4). Patients with brown stools and clear nasogastric aspirates had a relatively low mortality, whereas those with red nasogastric aspirates and red stools had a mortality rate approaching 30%.[8]

Stomach lavage may provide an additional assessment of the severity of bleeding. Prior to diagnostic endoscopy, a large-bore (32–36 French) soft rubber tube should be passed via the mouth to the stomach to gently lavage the stomach. The purposes of this are to determine the activity and rate of bleeding, to clear the stomach of clots and fluid, to facilitate endoscopy, and to reduce the possibility of aspiration during endoscopy. This tube should have extra holes cut at its tip to assure adequate drainage of the irrigation fluid. The patient is placed in a left decubitus position with his head in a slightly dependent, downward position. About 150 to 200 ml of irrigation fluid may be introduced at one time. Whenever possible, fluid should be allowed to flow out of the stomach without using suction. This decreases the risk of traumatic injury to the gastric wall that results in submucosal lesions that may be confused at endoscopy with gastric erosions or mucosal hemorrhages. The tube should be allowed to drain passively by gravity into a container at the bedside. If the tube does not drain, squeezing it with a milking motion often dislodges a clot from the intragastric tip and allows it to drain properly. Also, changing the position of the tube by moving it in and out slightly will frequently restore proper drainage.

The purpose of lavage is not to stop bleed-

TABLE 6–2. **ASGE Bleeding Survey: Nasogastric Aspirate Color and Patient Outcome***

Nasogastric Aspirate Color	No. Patients	Mortality (%)	Complications (%)	>5 Units of Blood (%)	Surgery (%)
Clear	234	6.0	8.6	12.0	9.8
Coffee-grounds	650	9.2	10.6	26.0	12.9
Red (blood)	734	17.9	18.9	41.3	22.9

*From: Silverstein FE, Gilbert DA, Tedesco FJ, et al.: The national ASGE survey on upper gastrointestinal bleeding. II. Clinical prognostic factors. Gastrointest Endosc 1981; 27:80–93. Reprinted with permission.

TABLE 6–3. **ASGE Bleeding Survey: Stool Color and Patient Outcome***

Stool Color	No. Patients	Mortality (%)	Complications (%)	≥5 Units of Blood (%)	Surgery (%)
Brown	465	11.0	9.9	16.3	12.3
Black	1312	8.1	10.8	24.8	13.5
Red	373	20.1	16.4	45.3	26.3

*From: Silverstein FE, Gilbert DA, Tedesco FJ, et al.: The national ASGE survey on upper gastrointestinal bleeding. II. Clinical prognostic factors. Gastrointest Endosc 1981; 27:80–93. Reprinted with permission.

ing. There are no controlled studies that support the notion that lavage with cold or warm saline or water, with or without vasoconstrictors, will stop acute gastrointestinal hemorrhage. One study in an animal model of iced lavage solutions with and without vasopressin failed to demonstrate the efficacy of this procedure for the control of acute upper gastrointestinal hemorrhage.[12]

Endoscopy can effectively establish the level or degree of gastrointestinal bleeding. If seen endoscopically early in the course of the bleeding episode, bright red blood emanating from a lesion establishes the presence of active, ongoing bleeding. In fact, there are situations in which, although bleeding appears to have stopped based on clinical assessment, an actively bleeding lesion, including a spurting artery, may be found at endoscopy. This finding alerts the medical/surgical team to the serious nature of the patient's condition. Endoscopy can also identify risk factors associated with an increased likelihood that bleeding will recur (to be discussed). Techniques such as the use of

TABLE 6–4. **ASGE Bleeding Survey: Nasogastric Aspirate and Stool Color Versus Mortality***

Nasogastric Aspirate Color	Stool Color	No. Patients	Mortality (%)
Clear	Brown	38	7.9
	Black	149	4.7
	Red	41	7.3
Coffee-grounds	Brown	128	7.8
	Black	412	8.3
	Red	84	19.1
Red (blood)	Brown	160	19.4
	Black	382	12.3
	Red	171	28.7

*From: Silverstein FE, Gilbert DA, Tedesco FJ, et al.: The national ASGE survey on upper gastrointestinal bleeding. II. Clinical prognostic factors. Gastrointest Endosc 1981; 27:80–93. Reprinted with permission.

technetium-labeled red blood cells with gamma camera scanning to determine activity and location of bleeding[13] and visceral angiography[14, 15] are needed only rarely to assess the degree of upper gastrointestinal bleeding. (They are discussed in detail in the following section on lower gastrointestinal bleeding.)

Diagnosis of the Cause of Bleeding

Several approaches can be used in determining the cause of bleeding. The first is clinical acumen. Using the history of the patient's bleeding episodes, one can venture a guess as to the current cause of bleeding. However, several studies suggest that the accuracy of this is as low as 40%.[16, 17] In the ASGE survey, an ulcer was found to be the cause of gastrointestinal bleeding in less than 50% of patients with a history of gastric or duodenal ulcer; a similarly poor correlation was observed with a history of reflux esophagitis.[11] In patients with portal hypertension and known varices who presented with upper gastrointestinal bleeding, it has been reported that 30% to 50% were bleeding from sources other than varices.[18–20] The actual bleeding sources in patients with known varices that were not bleeding, as reported in the ASGE survey, are listed in Table 6–5.

Upper gastrointestinal barium x-ray studies have been reported as useful in determining the cause of upper gastrointestinal bleeding. Single contrast x-rays have demonstrated lesions such as varices, carcinoma of the stomach and esophagus, and deep gastric and duodenal ulcers.[21] The results of some studies have even suggested that a vortex of blood can be seen spurting into the gastrointestinal lumen which has been filled with barium, thereby making possible a diagnosis of active bleeding.[22] This is, however, a rarely observed phenomenon. The results of other investigations indicate that with the enhanced resolution of air contrast x-rays, subtle mu-

TABLE 6–5. **ASGE Bleeding Survey:**
Final Diagnosis in 109 Patients
with Varices at Endoscopy
that Were Not the Cause of Bleeding*

Diagnosis	No. Patients	Incidence (%)
Gastric erosions	62	56.8
Mallory-Weiss tear	16	14.6
Gastric ulcer	15	13.8
Duodenal ulcer	15	13.8
Esophagitis	12	11.0
Duodenitis	7	6.4
Esophageal ulcer	3	2.7
Neoplasm	3	2.7
Stomal ulcer	1	0.9
Telangiectasia	1	0.9
Other	3	2.7

*From: Gilbert DA, Silverstein FE, Tedesco FJ, et al.: The national ASGE survey on upper gastrointestinal bleeding. III. Endoscopy in upper gastrointestinal bleeding. Gastrointest Endosc 1981; 27:94–102. Reprinted with permission.

TABLE 6–7. **ASGE Bleeding Survey:**
Endoscopic Diagnoses in Upper
Gastrointestinal Bleeding
(2097 Patients)*

Diagnosis	No. Patients	Incidence (%)
Gastric erosions	620	29.6
Duodenal ulcer	477	22.8
Gastric ulcer	457	21.9
Varices	323	15.2
Esophagitis	269	12.8
Duodenitis	191	9.1
Mallory-Weiss tear	168	8.0
Neoplasm	78	3.7
Esophageal ulcer	46	2.2
Stomal ulcer	39	1.9
Telangiectasia	10	0.5
Other	152	7.3

*From: Gilbert DA, Silverstein FE, Tedesco FJ, et al.: The national ASGE survey on upper gastrointestinal bleeding. III. Endoscopy in upper gastrointestinal bleeding. Gastrointest Endosc 1981; 27:94–102. Reprinted with permission.

cosal lesions such as varioliform gastritis or erosive esophagitis can be diagnosed.[23]

Many studies have compared the accuracy of endoscopy with that of upper gastrointestinal barium x-ray in the diagnosis of gastrointestinal bleeding.[24–26] Three representative prospective studies are compared in Table 6–6. These demonstrate that accuracy with respect to determination of the site of bleeding is approximately 25% to 50% with single contrast x-rays, with 70% to 95% for fiberoptic panendoscopy. Although the air contrast upper gastrointestinal technique is more sensitive than single contrast studies, it is not as accurate as endoscopy.[27] Endoscopy can detect superficial mucosal abnormalities such as esophagitis, gastritis, and Mallory-Weiss tears. Ulcers are identified with greater accuracy by endoscopy than by x-ray.[24]

There are other drawbacks to the use of upper gastrointestinal barium x-ray studies in the evaluation of the bleeding patient. Barium obscures the gastrointestinal mucosa and makes subsequent endoscopy impossible for at least 6 to 12 hours. Similarly, diagnostic and therapeutic visceral angiography cannot be undertaken for several hours. Thus, it is generally accepted that endoscopy is superior to roentgenography in determining the cause of bleeding. In a small percentage of stable patients (5% to 10%) in whom endoscopy fails to disclose the bleeding source, an upper gastrointestinal series may be helpful.

Visceral angiography is less available than endoscopy and does not give a precise diagnosis of the bleeding lesion. Complications may occur from the arterial puncture and injection of the contrast agent. Angiography is generally reserved for the patient with problematic recurrent bleeding in whom angiographic therapy is a consideration. Technetium-labeled red blood cell studies are rarely helpful for diagnosis of the cause of upper gastrointestinal bleeding.

The incidence of the various causes of upper gastrointestinal bleeding has been accurately determined using endoscopy (Table 6–7).[11] It is reported that multiple lesions are found in approximately one third of patients.[11, 28–30]

Prognostic Value of Endoscopy

Several investigators have suggested that certain endoscopic findings predict a poor clinical outcome. Such findings may, therefore, identify patients who may benefit from earlier and, in some cases, more aggressive therapeutic intervention. Findings that pre-

TABLE 6–6. **Endoscopy Versus x-ray in**
Diagnosis of Upper Gastrointestinal Bleeding*

Author	No. Patients	Identification of Site By Endoscopy (%)	By X-ray (%)
Katon and Smith[24]	90	93	30
Morris et al.[25]	54	69	22
McGinn et al.[26]	134	88	53

dict hemorrhage will be considered here in terms of nonvariceal and variceal bleeding.

In a study, principally of nonvariceal bleeding, by Morgan et al.,[31] 6 factors (5 clinical and 1 endoscopic) were found that predicted the likelihood of recurrent bleeding and mortality. In 66 patients, no single factor was significantly associated with a poor outcome, but the presence of 3 or more factors was highly predictive. The specific endoscopic findings examined were upper gastrointestinal ulcer and cancer.

Stigmata of recent hemorrhage have been described endoscopically in patients with upper gastrointestinal bleeding as a clot or black spot adherent to the lesion, or a visible vessel in the base of the lesion. Foster et al.[32] observed such changes in 47% of 233 patients with presenting symptoms of hematemesis or melena. In 89 patients with peptic ulcer, they observed that those patients whose ulcers had stigmata of recent hemorrhage had a significant increase in recurrent bleeding and that they required surgery significantly more often than patients who did not have these findings. These workers concluded that the endoscopic stigmata of recent hemorrhage were better predictors of these less favorable outcomes than age, shock, or serious underlying disease.

The degree of active bleeding at endoscopy has also been shown to correlate with an unfavorable outcome. In the ASGE survey, patients with either oozing or pumping blood from a lesion at endoscopy had a more than twofold increase in mortality and need for surgical treatment during the bleeding episode than did patients without these findings.[11] In addition, there was an association between active bleeding at endoscopy and a requirement for more than 5 units of transfused blood. These correlations with poor outcome were especially strong in patients with actively bleeding duodenal ulcers.

Recently, attention has been focused on the significance of a visible vessel seen at endoscopy in the base or rim of an ulcer. In a retrospective study, Griffiths et al.[33] noted that, in a group of 157 ulcer patients, 28 (18.5%) had a visible vessel associated with an ulcer. These 28 patients subsequently experienced either uncontrollable bleeding or recurrent bleeding. In the other 129 patients, without visible vessels, only 26% had uncontrollable or recurrent hemorrhage (p <.001).

In 3 subsequent, prospective trials of endoscopic hemostatic therapy, the frequency of a visible vessel in an ulcer base was 10%, 20%, and 48%.[34-36] The 48% figure derives from a study in which the ulcer crater was washed at endoscopy by a water jet with the catheter tip placed 1.0 cm from the ulcer. This removed overlying blood, mucus, clots, and other debris, and probably revealed ulcer vessels that would not have been visible otherwise. In practice, such vigorous methods are not routine and are probably best avoided unless endoscopic hemostatic therapy is planned. In all 3 of these studies, patients with visible vessels experienced further bleeding or required surgery more frequently than patients without a visible vessel in an ulcer base. An incidence rate for recurrent bleeding approaching 50% has been reported in patients with visible vessels.[36] Other stigmata of recent hemorrhage (central spot in an ulcer base) are associated with recurrent bleeding in 10% of patients. It should be noted that vigorous preparation of the lesions, as previously described, may alter the natural history and increase the chance of recurrent bleeding. Nevertheless, it appears that the observation of a visible vessel in an ulcer crater indicates a propensity for recurrent bleeding that may require endoscopic or surgical intervention.

In an effort to reduce mortality and the need for surgery, some investigators have adopted an aggressive interventional approach in patients with stigmata of recent hemorrhage. This hypothesis has been tested in 4 controlled trials of endoscopic therapy. Papp[37] reported a controlled trial of prophylactic monopolar electrocoagulation in a group of 32 patients with visible vessel ulcers. Bleeding recurred in 1 of 16 treated patients, in contrast with 13 of 16 untreated patients. Using the high-power argon laser, Swain et al.[38] demonstrated a significant reduction in recurrent bleeding in treated vs. untreated patients with visible vessels. Another trial using the same laser at similar power levels demonstrated no such benefit.[35] Neither of these laser trials demonstrated any benefit from laser treatment of ulcers that had only a central spot in their bases. The neodymium-YAG (Nd:YAG) laser has been used in two trials. That by Rutgeerts et al.[39] did not show any benefit in terms of a decrease in recurrent bleeding or surgical intervention in 43 patients with visible vessels or fresh clots in ulcer bases. In a small, controlled trial in patients with visible ulcer vessels, the incidence of resumed bleeding and the need for emergency surgery decreased with Nd:YAG laser treatment.[34] It has been reported in both argon and Nd:YAG laser trials that laser therapy initiated bleeding that was not controlled by further therapy.[38, 39] Although no perforations have been reported in these studies, the risk of full-thickness bowel wall injury is underscored by histologic studies showing that visible ulcer vessels are often located in the serosal layer of extremely deep ulcers.[40] Controlled studies of endoscopic therapy in patients with visible vessels or other stigmata of recent hemorrhage have provided conflicting results, and further data on the efficacy of these or other endoscopic therapeutic modalities are required. Careful clinical judgment must be exercised when considering the application of these techniques in the prophylactic therapy of visible ulcer vessels in patients who present with upper gastrointestinal bleeding. (Endoscopic electrocoagulation and laser photocoagulation are discussed in Chapters 8 and 9, respectively.)

The observation that large varices are more prone to bleeding than small varices was first made in esophagoscopic studies nearly three decades ago.[41, 42] Both the diameter and linear extent of the varices correlated with bleeding risk in these early investigations. Dagradi[43] pointed out the increased risk of hemorrhage from varices that have "cherry red" spots on their surface. In a retrospective study of 172 patients with a history of variceal bleeding, Beppu et al.[44] expanded these observations to include a variety of "red color signs" on the surface of varices. When present, these connoted a six- to sevenfold increased incidence of bleeding.

A study of considerable interest is that of Lebrec et al.,[45] who evaluated variceal size in 100 patients with their first manifestation of cirrhosis. There was a highly significant correlation between large variceal size and the prevalence of a recent episode of bleeding caused by varices or acute gastric erosions. Furthermore, there was a significant increase in recurrent bleeding during a subsequent 1-year follow-up in patients who had large varices at the first admission.

Based on these observations, it has been suggested that a vigorous therapeutic approach be taken in patients with large varices. Lebrec et al.[45] suggested variceal size as an important consideration in the selection of patients for portacaval shunt surgery. An alternative therapeutic approach is endoscopic variceal sclerotherapy. To evaluate whether aggressive endoscopic intervention is justified in patients with large varices at endoscopy but no prior bleeding, Paquet[46] performed a prospective 2-year controlled clinical trial of sclerotherapy in such patients. Although the follow-up intervals are not clearly stated, of 32 patients who received sclerotherapy, only 2 had suffered further bleeding (9.1%), in comparison with 22 of 33 patients (67%) managed without prophylactic sclerotherapy (p <.02). Fourteen patients died in the control group; 2 died in the sclerotherapy group.

Thus, in both retrospective and prospective studies, large variceal size appears to indicate a higher risk of bleeding from varices. Whether prophylactic sclerotherapy with its attendant risks is warranted in patients with large varices that have not bled remains to be confirmed in other large, controlled clinical trials. Esophageal varices and sclerotherapy are discussed in greater detail in Chapter 16.

Timing of Endoscopy

Once diagnostic endoscopy has been decided upon, several factors will influence the timing of the procedure. Optimally, endoscopy should be performed in a hemodynamically stable patient. Expert assistance from support medical and technical personnel is mandatory. Although not advocated by all authors,[20] gastric lavage to remove intragastric blood and clots usually improves endoscopic visualization.[47]

The goal of diagnostic endoscopy in upper gastrointestinal bleeding is to identify the most likely source of hemorrhage. Active hemorrhage at endoscopy, the presence of a clot, or a visible vessel in a lesion have been interpreted as evidence that the lesion in question is the actual source of bleeding. Several investigators have evaluated the timing of endoscopy in relation to the yield for these signs of active or recent bleeding. In a group of 109 patients with hematemesis or melena, Forrest et al.[47] observed a significantly higher number of actively bleeding lesions at endoscopy when the procedure was performed within the first 24 hours after admission in comparison to endoscopy at 24 to 48 hours. Leinicke et al.[48] compared the results of endoscopy in 276 bleeding patients in whom most endoscopies were performed within 12 hours of admission or at onset of in-hospital bleeding with the results of endoscopy in 103 patients in whom endoscopy was delayed for 24 hours. Active bleeding or a clot on the lesion was seen in 62% of the group undergoing early endoscopy and in 14% of the late endoscopy group. Foster et al.[32] found a similarly high incidence of signs of recent hemorrhage or active bleeding when endoscopy was performed within 12 hours of initial hematemesis or melena. In patients who underwent endoscopy within 12 hours, 34 of 49 (69%) had these endoscopic signs, compared with 75 of 181 (42%) who had endoscopy after 12 hours.

In the ASGE survey, the frequency of finding an oozing or pumping lesion at endoscopy decreased significantly as the interval between admission to endoscopy increased from 24 to 96 hours (Table 6–8).[11] As in earlier reports, endoscopy during the first 12-hour period following admission yielded the highest frequency of actively bleeding lesions. However, the yield of actively bleeding lesions was not significantly higher if endoscopy was performed during the first 3 to 6 hours following admission.

From these data, it may be concluded that the best chance to observe signs of active or recent upper gastrointestinal bleeding at endoscopy occurs within the first 12 hours after admission or after onset of bleeding in-hospital. The presence of these signs may be especially useful in ascribing the cause of bleeding to a particular lesion when other lesions without such stigmata are present at endoscopy. From a practical standpoint, the data support the use of immediate endoscopy for patients who are admitted and stabilized during daytime and early evening hours. Conversely, examination of patients during nighttime hours may be deferred until early the next morning. This policy assures the availability of medical and technical personnel during the procedure. However, nighttime endoscopy cannot be deferred if important and urgent management decisions will be based upon endoscopic findings. This is the situation in patients with torrential hemorrhage, continued bleeding, or recurrent bleeding.

Effect of Endoscopy on Patient Outcome

The issue of whether endoscopy affects the outcome in patients with gastrointestinal bleeding has been debated at considerable length.[49] The results of studies on this question are conflicting, but most demonstrate little or no benefit from endoscopic diagnosis of upper gastrointestinal bleeding in terms of a decrease in mortality, in number of blood transfusions, or in duration of hospitalization.[25, 28, 50–55]

Hoare[56] reported the results of a retrospective study supporting the thesis that endoscopy may benefit patients. In this study, 156 patients with acute upper gastrointestinal bleeding were divided into 2 groups. The endoscopy group of 51 patients was managed by a physician whose policy was to perform endoscopy within 48 hours of admission. The 105 control patients had an upper gastrointestinal x-ray within this same time period after admission. Mortality was 5.7% in the endoscopy group and 15.2% in the x-ray group. Surgery, when indicated, was performed in both groups by the same surgeons and with the same frequency. However, surgery was performed significantly earlier and mortality from surgery was less in the patients who underwent endoscopy.

One study frequently cited as evidence against the beneficial effect of early endoscopy on patient outcome was reported by Peterson et al.[57] In this prospective study, 206 bleeding patients who were stabilized within 6 hours of admission were randomly assigned to a routine endoscopy or nonendoscopy group. All patients were treated with antacids. No significant differences were noted with regard to hospital deaths, recurrence of bleeding, transfusion requirements

TABLE 6–8. **ASGE Bleeding Survey: Interval From Admission to Endoscopy Versus Active Bleeding at Endoscopy**

| Interval (hr) | No. Patients | Active Bleeding | |
		No. Patients	Incidence (%)
0–12	663	275	41.5
13–24	340	100	29.4
25–36	115	37	32.3
37–48	135	30	22.2
49–60	36	9	25.0
61–72	68	7	10.3
73–84	31	5	16.1
85–96	29	5	17.2
>96	180	36	20.0

*From: Gilbert DA, Silverstein FE, Tedesco FJ, et al.: The national ASGE survey on upper gastrointestinal bleeding. III. Endoscopy in upper gastrointestinal bleeding. Gastrointest Endosc 1981; 27:94–102. Reprinted with permission.

for recurrent bleeding, or duration of hospital stay. Long-term follow-up revealed one gastric lymphoma in the non-endoscopy group that was overlooked during the initial examination.

Unfortunately, most of the available studies and data on the benefits of endoscopy and upper gastrointestinal bleeding are limited. Many are retrospective or have included groups of patients managed by different physicians; in some studies, patient entry was not consecutive; in others, cohorts managed several years apart are compared. In some series, patients in both groups underwent both endoscopy and x-ray; in others, there is a high proportion of incomplete endoscopies. Often, as in the study by Peterson et al.,[57] patients were not stratified according to underlying illnesses or causes of bleeding and, in addition, therapy was not modified by the information gained at endoscopy.

To investigate adequately the question of benefit from endoscopy in upper gastrointestinal hemorrhage, a study must be designed to balance the endoscopy and non-endoscopy groups of patients in terms of underlying risks for adverse outcome. As noted earlier, the presence of underlying illness significantly modifies the outcome in patients with upper gastrointestinal bleeding.[8] If death was nearly inevitable in 5% of patients studied, and these patients were not evenly allocated to the endoscopy versus the non-endoscopy group, an outcome bias could occur that would overshadow any potential beneficial effect of diagnostic endoscopy. It is therefore essential that studies of the question of benefit take into account the importance of risk factors in the bleeding patients, such as underlying illness and the source of bleeding. Only when the groups are comparable with respect to these features will it be possible to assess critically a possible difference in outcome resulting from the improved diagnostic accuracy provided by endoscopy.

Another major factor that confounds analysis of the current data pertaining to endoscopy and upper gastrointestinal bleeding relates to therapy. Few treatments of the various causes of upper gastrointestinal bleeding are of proven effectiveness.[1] If the accurate information obtained at endoscopy cannot be used to direct specific effective therapy, an improved outcome from diagnosis alone is unlikely. In the study by Peterson et al.,[57] all patients were treated with an antacid regimen whether or not they were assigned to endoscopy or control groups. It is not surprising that the outcomes for the two groups were similar.

In the future, endoscopic therapy may allow the physician to take advantage of the knowledge of the cause of bleeding obtained at endoscopy by treating the patient at the time of endoscopy. Therapy with the Nd:YAG laser,[31, 39] argon laser,[35, 36] BICAP electrocoagulation probe,[58] heater probe,[59] or monopolar electrocoagulation devices[37] may effectively stop bleeding in certain clinical circumstances. With effective endoscopic therapy it may be possible to show that a precise endoscopic diagnosis results in therapeutic benefit to the patient with upper gastrointestinal bleeding.

A Rational Approach to Endoscopy in Upper Gastrointestinal Bleeding

There are many unresolved issues with respect to the role of endoscopy in upper gastrointestinal bleeding. Although it has not been definitively shown that endoscopy is of benefit with regard to mortality, most gastroenterologists, endoscopists, and surgeons believe that endoscopy should be performed in patients with bleeding from the proximal gastrointestinal tract. In most cases, endoscopy provides an accurate diagnosis. It establishes the level and site of the bleeding, provides an assessment of the degree of active bleeding, and is of predictive value in terms of risk for further bleeding when hemorrhage has stopped. This information may be critical for immediate or long-term management decisions. Shunt surgery, for example, would be disastrous in a patient with portal hypertension if, in fact, the patient was bleeding from a duodenal ulcer. Referral of a patient with variceal bleeding for ulcer surgery is equally unacceptable. Endoscopy can affect the decision to operate, the timing of surgery, and the type of surgery to be performed.[60] Finally, in a patient who has bled from a peptic ulcer, an accurate endoscopic diagnosis will affect plans for short- or long-term medical therapy or surgery if recurrent bleeding becomes a problem. Endoscopic therapy may be appropriate in certain clinical circumstances.

Although most patients with upper gastrointestinal bleeding should undergo endoscopy,[27] under certain circumstances it may be appropriate to omit endoscopy. Endoscopy may not be necessary, for example, in the postoperative patient with a miniscule amount of coffee-grounds material in the nasogastric aspirate or in the young individual with minimal hematemesis during an acute viral illness.

Our current approach may be summarized as follows. When the patient is first examined, an orogastric tube is passed into the stomach during or following resuscitation to determine if there is ongoing bleeding. If the bleeding has stopped, the patient is stabilized, appropriate laboratory tests are performed, and blood is replaced to raise the hematocrit to the 25% to 30% range. Appropriate consultations are obtained. Endoscopy is performed 6 to 12 hours after admission. If bleeding does not stop, as manifested by continued red drainage from the orogastric tube during lavage, unstable vital signs, or persistent bloody stools, immediate endoscopy is performed as soon as the patient is reasonably stable. At this point a diagnosis is usually confirmed and decisions concerning therapy can be made. Another situation in which immediate endoscopy may be performed arises when a patient has been stabilized but then has a recurrence of significant bleeding. When balloon tamponade is contemplated or an aortoduodenal fistula is suspected, a patient is a candidate for immediate endoscopy.

The patient with torrential hemorrhage presents a special situation. Immediate exsanguination is a direct threat. Bleeding of this magnitude may occur in hemorrhage from esophageal varices, a posterior duodenal ulcer that has eroded the gastroduodenal artery, a gastric ulcer that has eroded the left gastric artery, or an aortoduodenal fistula. Often the correct therapy is immediate operative intervention. Endoscopy prior to operation may delay surgery and increase the risk to the patient.[60] Furthermore, with this type of excessive bleeding it may be impossible to perform an endoscopy adequate for diagnosis of the bleeding lesion. For these reasons, immediate surgical consultation is essential. The patient may then be taken to the operating room, and while under general anesthesia with an endotracheal tube in place, upper gastrointestinal lavage and endoscopy may be performed. This can be done as preparations are being made for surgery. With this approach, all the essential elements for diagnosis and management are brought together quickly, and the surgeon and endoscopist can plan therapy based on the endoscopic observations.

Preparation for Endoscopy

Endoscopy in the patient with upper gastrointestinal bleeding is one of the most difficult endoscopic examinations and optimally should be performed by an experienced endoscopist. Several aspects of the procedure merit further discussion.

Premedication

The frequency with which various drugs are used as endoscopic premedication in patients with upper gastrointestinal bleeding, as reported in the ASGE survey, is shown in Table 6–9.[11] Although diazepam is commonly administered, in the unstable bleeding patient it may be hazardous to use heavy sedation.[20] Meperidine may cause a fall in blood pressure that can distort clinical interpretation of the vital signs and estimation of intravascular volume. Patients with underlying liver disease may tolerate sedative drugs poorly. However, in some patients a small dose (2 to 5 mg of diazepam or 25 to 50 mg of meperidine) can make the procedure easier for the patient.

The majority of patients in the ASGE survey received a topical pharyngeal anesthetic prior to endoscopy.[11] However, the use of this type of premedication in bleeding patients is debatable. Although they may help the patient tolerate the procedure, topical anesthetic agents have cardiovascular and central nervous system effects and may increase the risk of aspiration during endoscopy.[61] This is especially true if a sedative has also been administered. In most patients, our current practice is to use a topical pharyngeal anesthetic and small intravenous doses of diazepam prior to the procedure.

TABLE 6–9. **ASGE Bleeding Survey: Endoscopic Premedication (2097 Patients)***

Drug	No. Patients (%)	Mean Dose†	Range (mg)
Diazepam	1474 (70.2)	10 ± 6.9	0.5–90
Merperidine	821 (39.2)	57 ± 22.0	5–150
Topical anesthetic	1186 (56.6)		
Atropine	317 (15.1)	0.6 ± 0.4	0.02–0.6
Glucagon	40 (1.9)	1.0 ± 0.2	0.2–1.0
Other	171 (8.2)		

*From: Gilbert DA, Silverstein FE, Tedesco FJ, et al.: The national ASGE survey on upper gastrointestinal bleeding. III. Endoscopy in upper gastrointestinal bleeding. Gastrointest Endosc 1981; 27:94–102. Reprinted with permission.

† ± 1 standard deviation

Endoscope Components and Accessories

The endoscope selected for use in the bleeding patient must function properly. Excellent light and visual resolution are essential, as is mechanical capability for such maneuvers as retroflexion. The function of the water wash to clean the lens should be checked. Leaks in the air insufflation system can produce a frustrating and potentially hazardous situation for the patient if it is impossible to adequately inflate the esophagus and stomach for examination. Similarly, suction is essential to remove gas and secretions. The accessory channel must be patent so that endoscopic therapeutic devices may be passed. These functions should be carefully checked prior to the procedure.

There is a trend in endoscopy toward use of instruments with the smallest possible diameter for all types of procedures. These instruments are easy to pass and highly maneuverable. However, for upper gastrointestinal bleeding, larger-diameter instruments may be preferable because these have larger accessory channels, and their increased channel diameter is necessary for passage of certain therapeutic devices and for the removal of blood and clots. These instruments typically have an insertion tube diameter of approximately 1.2 cm with accessory (suction) channels as large as 3.7 mm in diameter. Additional advantages are excellent visual resolution and the incorporation of an excellent light delivery bundle. These factors enhance the quality of diagnostic and therapeutic endoscopy in the bleeding patient.

Complications of Upper Gastrointestinal Endoscopy

The risks of upper gastrointestinal endoscopy in bleeding patients are, as expected, higher than those encountered in routine diagnostic endoscopy. The most recent comprehensive data are contained in a prospective ASGE survey.[62] In this study 274 physicians reported complications from 2320 endoscopies in bleeding patients (Table 6–10). Endoscopic complications occurred in 21 patients, or 0.9% of all examinations. In 3 patients, 3 complications occurred during repeat endoscopy.

Twelve complications were considered major; 9 of these occurred during emergency endoscopy. The major complications were perforation in 5 patients, aspiration pneu-

TABLE 6–10. **ASGE Bleeding Survey: Complications of Endoscopy (2320 Endoscopies)***

Major Complication	No.	Minor Complication	No.
Perforation	5†	Mucosal tear	3
Aspiration	4†	Medication reaction	3
Hemorrhage	3†	Hypotension	1
		Atrial fibrillation	1
		Anoxic episode	1

*From: Gilbert DA, Silverstein FE, Tedesco FJ, et al.: National ASGE survey on upper gastrointestinal bleeding: Complications of endoscopy. Dig Dis Sci 1981; 26:55s–9s. Reprinted with permission.
†One death in each of these groups.

monia in 4, and hemorrhage in 3. One death attributable to the endoscopic complication occurred in each of these 3 subgroups (0.1%).

This ASGE survey[62] is the third of the ASGE membership concerning complications of upper endoscopy. Both earlier reports were retrospective. In 1967, the experience of 128 ASGE members was surveyed[63]; in 35,448 examinations, there were 31 complications (0.09%) and 6 deaths (0.02%). A minority of the ASGE members in the survey used flexible fibergastroscopes for these examinations; most used semiflexible instruments. In 1974, an ASGE survey indicated a complication rate of 0.13% in 211,410 endoscopic examinations of the upper gastrointestinal tract. Cardiopulmonary events were the most common type of complication, followed by perforation and bleeding.[64, 65]

The complication rate in the third ASGE survey[62] (0.9%) is higher than that in either of the two previous studies. In 2320 procedures, a major complication occurred in 1 per 193 examinations and a minor complication in 1 per 257 procedures. The mortality rate associated with endoscopy was approximately 1 per 700 patients. The prospective nature of this most recent survey, and the fact that the patient population was composed of seriously ill and bleeding patients explains to some extent the higher incidence of complications. In other endoscopic series of patients with upper gastrointestinal bleeding, the complication rate ranges from 0.7% to 8.0%.[6, 16, 20, 66, 67] The latter figure was reported in a study by Paul and Huchzermeyer[67] that included a group of 98 patients who had upper gastrointestinal bleeding while in intensive care units. Cotton et al.[20] reported 1 perforation in a series of 196 patients undergoing diagnostic endoscopy for upper gastrointestinal bleeding, and Allan and Dykes[6] reported 1 fatal case of aspiration pneumonia in a series of 100 bleeding patients who underwent endoscopy. In a survey of French endoscopists, emergency endoscopy for upper gastrointestinal bleeding was the most hazardous type of endoscopy.[68] Thus, the complication rate as determined in the ASGE survey appears consistent with other observations on the risks of endoscopy in this patient population.

COLONOSCOPY IN LOWER GASTROINTESTINAL BLEEDING

Bleeding from the lower gastrointestinal tract may manifest as bright red blood per rectum, melena, or simply occult blood in the stools. The clinical approach to these different types of bleeding varies, as may the role and yield of colonoscopy.

Active Bleeding with Bright Red Blood per Rectum

Initial Approach

The initial approach to the patient who is passing bright red blood per rectum is similar to that for acute upper gastrointestinal bleeding. Immediate attention should be given to resuscitation and establishment of reliable venous access. The assessment should include inquiries about prior bleeding episodes, prior diarrhea, recent change in bowel habits, recent weight loss, and known diverticular disease. Special attention should be given to the digital rectal examination and examination of the abdomen. As noted, it is critical in any patient with digestive tract hemorrhage to establish the level of bleeding as upper or lower gastrointestinal. This is best accomplished by first passing a tube into the stomach. If the gastric aspirate is positive for blood, the source of bleeding is proximal to the ligament of Treitz, and the presence of red rectal bleeding usually indicates a rapid rate of upper gastrointestinal blood loss. When the gastric aspirate is negative for blood in the setting of passage of bright red blood per rectum, an upper gastrointestinal source is still a possibility depending on the patient's symptoms, other relevant history, and physical signs.[10, 11] A brief upper gastrointestinal endoscopy may be warranted in this situation.[3, 69] If this is negative, attention may be turned to evaluation of the lower gastrointestinal tract.

The initial area of interest is the perianal region, which should be evaluated for the presence of a fissure, fistula, and hemorrhoids and evidence of Crohn's disease. Hemorrhoidal bleeding can be significant in quantity and result in a confusing clinical picture. A useful way to identify bleeding hemorrhoids is to have the patient sit on a toilet and bear down gently. After 15 to 30 seconds the perianal area may be examined with the aid of a mirror and flashlight. The flashlight beam is reflected by the mirror for illumination, and the mirror provides convenient observation of the perianal area. Prolapse of actively bleeding internal hemorrhoids may be noted in this way, whereas simply having the patient bear down in the knee-chest or left lateral position usually fails to reveal this common cause of bleeding.

Following the perianal and digital rectal examinations, sigmoidoscopy should be performed with a rigid sigmoidoscope to look for evidence of inflammatory bowel disease, infectious colitis involving the rectosigmoid or a bleeding neoplasm. The large lumen of a rigid sigmoidoscope permits removal of blood and stool, but visibility in the acutely bleeding patient is often limited. The presence of guaiac-positive stool from within the rectum or sigmoid does not preclude a hemorrhoidal source. Blood from hemorrhoidal bleeding may ascend in a retrograde fashion to the descending colon and pass later into the rectum.[69]

The fiberoptic sigmoidoscope is being increasingly used by many physicians. The diagnostic yield for fiberoptic sigmoidoscopy in the well-prepared patient is superior to that for rigid sigmoidoscopy.[70, 71] However, with acute lower gastrointestinal bleeding, visualization may be limited as with rigid sigmoidoscopy, and passage of the fiberoptic instrument may be difficult. Nevertheless, in many patients flexible sigmoidoscopy, after brief preparation with an enema, may be an efficient screening examination. In addition to the more proximal extent of the mucosal examination possible with this instrument, an evaluation of the mucosa immediately above the anus may be obtained by gentle retroflexion of the sigmoidoscope tip within the rectum.

Further Diagnostic Studies

If an actively bleeding source is found during this preliminary evaluation, further diagnostic studies may be unnecessary. If no diagnosis is made, the choices of subsequent tests include barium enema x-ray studies, colonoscopy, angiography, and radionuclide scanning.

Barium Enema X-ray Studies. Barium enema with or without air contrast is not advised for the patient with acute lower gastrointestinal bleeding.[3, 69] Although it may disclose a possible explanation for the bleeding, the barium enema has several disadvantages. The quality of the examination is compromised in the unprepared or poorly prepared bleeding patient and the yield is low. Diagnosis of either of the two main causes of lower gastrointestinal bleeding, diverticula and angiodysplasia,[3] is not possible. Although the presence of diverticula may be indicated, these occur in over a third of patients older than age 60,[72] and the x-ray study cannot determine whether the source of bleeding is diverticular or which diverticulum is bleeding. Similarly, angiodysplastic lesions are flat and not detectable by barium x-ray studies.[73] Other disadvantages include retention of barium in the colon, which makes subsequent preparation for colonoscopy difficult and visceral angiography impossible. Claims that barium may have some hemostatic role in patients with colonic bleeding have not been confirmed.[74]

Colonoscopy. The role of colonoscopy in diagnosis of acute lower gastrointestinal bleeding has received considerable attention. Although initial experience suggested that technical difficulties precluded adequate endoscopic examination,[75, 76] recent investigators reported that definite diagnosis is possible in 70% to 80% of patients.[77, 78] A representative distribution of findings in 40 patients in a study by Jensen et al.[79] is given in Table 6–11.

In most cases management decisions are directly influenced by the information obtained at colonoscopy. These include the need for angiography, angiographic therapy, or endoscopic hemostatic therapy as well as the need for surgery, type of operation, and the timing of surgical intervention.

Several practical points with regard to the performance of colonoscopy in patients with colonic bleeding should be emphasized. In the patient with massive hemorrhage, preparation of the colon, except with one or more enemas, may be impossible. However, the cathartic effect of blood may clear the lumen of fecal residue to a significant extent.[77] When hemorrhage is less than massive, an

TABLE 6–11. Results of Emergency Colonoscopy in 40 Patients with Massive Hematochezia*

Finding	No. Patients
Angioma	14
Polyps or cancer	6
Active diverticular bleeding	4
Focal colitis	2
Suspected small bowel source	2
Bleeding polyp stalk	1
Endometriosis	1
Negative colon, ulcer at upper endoscopy	5
No bleeding site identified	5

*From: Jensen DM, Machicado GA, Tapia JI.: Emergent colonoscopy in patients with severe hematochezia. (Abstr) Gastrointest Endosc 1983; 29:177. Reprinted with permission.

oral purge with an electrolyte or Golytely solution is possible and desirable.[80] Adequate preparation by this method may require that the patient drink 4 to 8 liters of the purge solution to clean the colon.[79]

Colonoscopes with large accessory (suction) channels (>3.5 mm in diameter) facilitate removal of fecal material, blood, and residual fluid from the purge preparation. Some investigators prefer a double-channel colonoscope. With this type of instrument various irrigating devices can be connected to a washing catheter passed via one of the channels. Such a system provides a relatively forceful but atraumatic stream of water that can be directed to fragment clots of blood and wash the mucosal surface.

The technique for emergency colonoscopy requires cautious insertion, with a constant view of the bowel lumen. It has been suggested that overinsufflation and excess distention of the colon may aggravate hemorrhage.[79] According to some investigators, total colonoscopy may not be necessary if a bleeding lesion is identified before the cecum is reached,[79] but, in general, pancolonoscopy is most advantageous.

As with endoscopy in upper gastrointestinal bleeding, excessive sedation for colonoscopy should be avoided in patients with lower gastrointestinal bleeding, so as not to confound the evaluation of hemodynamic and mental status.[79] Some colonoscopists use glucagon to slow motility.

In summary, the role for colonoscopy in patients with active lower gastrointestinal bleeding is expanding. With rapid colonic purge using electrolyte or Golytely solutions and colonoscopes with large suction channel diameters, the feasibility of colonoscopic evaluation has improved. The examination may be performed at the bedside, obviating the need for transferring the patient to a special diagnostic facility. Furthermore, with the availability of hemostatic techniques that can be applied through the colonoscope, early colonoscopic evaluation, diagnosis, and treatment of patients with active lower gastrointestinal bleeding will become increasingly attractive.[81–83]

Angiography. Visceral angiography can be an important tool in the evaluation and therapy of certain bleeding patients. Nusbaum and Baum[14] found that angiography can determine the presence of ongoing bleeding with loss of as little as 0.5 to 1.0 cc of blood per minute into the intestinal lumen. The location of the bleeding can be identified, and in some cases a specific source is indicated. Available data indicate that the specific bleeding site can be identified by angiography in more than 75% of patients.[15] In addition to the diagnostic capability of angiography, infusion of vasoconstrictors or embolization techniques may be employed to control bleeding in some situations.[15] As with any angiographic procedure, complications may be associated with arterial catheterization as well as injection of contrast material.

Radionuclide Scanning. Technetium-labeled red blood cell scanning has simplified the determination of obscure gastrointestinal bleeding and localization of its level in the gastrointestinal tract. Bleeding rates as low as 0.1 cc per minute may be detected by this method.[13] Because of its diagnostic sensitivity, simplicity, low cost and low risk, the technetium-labeled red blood cell scan is an attractive procedure for certain patients with suspected active hemorrhage.

Recent Rectal Bleeding

Lower gastrointestinal bleeding stops spontaneously in most patients.[3] Although the clinical situation is less urgent in patients with recent bright red blood per rectum than in those with massive colonic hemorrhage, a similar evaluation of hemodynamic status and transfusion requirements is necessary. However, many of these patients are stable and may be evaluated in the outpatient department.

The approach to this problem should include a thorough history and physical examination, including digital rectal examination, hemoccult testing, and flexible or rigid sigmoidoscopic examination. In contrast to patients with massive bleeding, a barium enema x-ray study may often be the next appropriate diagnostic investigation. This should be an air contrast study, which has greater diagnostic accuracy than a single contrast study.[84]

The role of colonoscopy in patients with recent rectal bleeding has been evaluated by several investigators.[85–88] When a barium enema x-ray study discloses a polyp or mass lesion, subsequent colonoscopy may be necessary to better define the nature of the abnormality and, in the case of a polyp, to remove it. Colonoscopy is usually necessary in patients with recent rectal bleeding when sigmoidoscopy and barium enema findings are normal or disclose only diverticula. Diverticula are common in patients in whom lower gastrointestinal tract bleeding is most likely to develop; the presence of diverticula does not mean that they are the cause of bleeding. Several studies have been undertaken to assess the role of colonoscopy in patients with rectal bleeding and negative or equivocal barium enema studies except for diverticulosis. These investigations demonstrate a 30% to 40% yield of significant lesions found by colonoscopy that were overlooked by sigmoidoscopy and barium enema studies (Table 6–12).[85–88] Although many of the reported x-ray procedures were single contrast and there is no certainty that the lesions found at colonoscopy were the cause of bleeding, these reports emphasize the improved diagnostic sensitivity of colonoscopy over barium enema in this group of patients.

In view of the data from these studies, it may be appropriate to omit the barium enema study in many patients with recent rectal bleeding in favor of colonoscopy as the initial method of evaluation. In others a barium enema study may complement or confirm the colonoscopic findings, especially if colonoscopy reveals no abnormalities or the examination is not completed to the cecum. If both colonoscopy and barium x-ray studies reveal no abnormalities in the colon, an upper gastrointestinal tract source should be considered.

Melena

Melenic stool results from oxidation of hematin or other hemoglobin breakdown

TABLE 6–12. **Colonoscopic Abnormalities in Patients with Recent Rectal Bleeding***

Author	No. Patients	Cancer (%)	Polyps (%)	IBD† (%)	TEL‡ (%)	Other (%)
Tedesco et al.[85]	258	(11.2)	(22.1)	(7.4)	(6.6)	(1.6)
Teague et al.[86]	215	(12.5)	(13.4)	(7.4)	(1.0)	(7.0)
Swarbrick et al.[87]	239	(9.6)	(16.3)	(10.0)	(1.7)	(2.1)
Brand et al.[88]	306	(8.2)	(23.6)	(3.6)	(3.6)	(0.7)

*Normal sigmoidoscopy/barium enema studies or presence of diverticulosis.
†IBD—inflammatory bowel disease.
‡TEL—telangiectasia.

products. Experimentally, in patients who were undergoing surgery for appendicitis, as little as 300 cc of blood instilled into the cecum caused melena.[89] A patient with a colonic lesion may have black stools if the bleeding is slow, hematochezia does not occur, and colonic motility is sufficiently slow to allow time for oxidation of hemoglobin and its breakdown products. Although melena usually indicates an upper gastrointestinal bleeding source, occasionally it may be the presenting manifestation of a colonic lesion. These lesions are usually found in the proximal colon.

Investigation of the colon is generally recommended in patients with melena and a negative upper gastrointestinal examination. The role of colonoscopy was evaluated in 53 patients with unexplained melena in a retrospective review.[90] All patients had had negative or nondiagnostic upper and lower gastrointestinal barium x-ray examinations and negative upper gastrointestinal endoscopic examinations. Of the 53 patients, 42 had single contrast and 11 had double contrast barium enemas. Melena had been present from 1 week to longer than 12 months. Abnormalities were found at colonoscopy in 16 of the 53 patients (30%). Four patients had neoplastic polyps 5.0 mm or greater in diameter, 5 had invasive carcinoma, 6 had vascular ectasias, and 1 had Crohn's disease. Most of the lesions were located in the right side of the colon.

Occult Lower Gastrointestinal Bleeding

Testing for occult blood in the stool has become an important screening procedure for colorectal disease.[91] A discussion of the sequential evaluation of patients with stools positive for occult blood is beyond the scope of this chapter, but interesting data are available regarding the yield of colonoscopy in such patients. When sigmoidoscopy is normal and the barium enema is either normal or discloses only diverticulosis, the incidence of significant abnormalities at colonoscopy is approximately 20%.[85, 86, 88] Benign and malignant neoplasms are the most common abnormalities, followed by angiodysplasia. In many patients with occult gastrointestinal bleeding, colonoscopy may appropriately precede barium enema, and the results may preclude the need for x-ray studies.

Complications of Colonoscopy

Available data from series of patients with acute lower gastrointestinal bleeding who have undergone colonoscopy do not indicate any increase in complications.[78, 79] The overall complication rate for diagnostic colonoscopy is estimated at less than 1%, and that for colonoscopic polypectomy at approximately 2%.[92, 93] Although preliminary data from the recent prospective ASGE colonoscopy survey indicate a somewhat higher incidence of complications (2.8%), the majority of these were minor.[94]

Visualization is likely to be poor during colonoscopy in patients with active lower gastrointestinal bleeding, and the instrument must be inserted with caution. Electrosurgery is hazardous in the unprepared colon because of the risk of explosion.[95] Carbon dioxide insufflation during such procedures is advisable if electrosurgery is contemplated.

Summary

The use of colonoscopy in patients with lower gastrointestinal bleeding will likely increase. In the recent ASGE colonoscopy survey, gastrointestinal bleeding was cited as the indication for colonoscopy in 42.3% of 6614 patients, and was the most common indication for the examination.[96] The recognized diagnostic superiority of colonoscopy over barium enema studies, the ability to bring about hemostasis by endoscopic methods, the capability for removal of polyps, and the ability to rapidly prepare the colon for examination account for this development. Further advances in colonoscopic hemostatic treatment methods may augment the value of colonoscopy in patients with lower gastrointestinal bleeding.

References

1. Gilbert DA, Silverstein FE, Auth DC, Rubin CE. Nonsurgical management of acute nonvariceal upper gastrointestinal bleeding. Prog Hemost Thromb 1978; 4:349–95.
2. Larson DE, Farnell MB. Upper gastrointestinal hemorrhage. Mayo Clin Proc 1983; 58:371-87.
3. Peterson WL. Gastrointestinal bleeding. In. Sleisenger MH, Fordtran JS, eds. Gastrointestinal Disease: Pathophysiology, Diagnosis, Management. Philadelphia: WB Saunders Company, 1983; 177.
4. Cutler JA, Mendeloff AI. Upper gastrointestinal bleeding. Nature and magnitude of the problem in the US. Dig Dis Sci 1981; 26:90s–6s.
5. Schiller KFR, Truelove SC, Williams DG. Haematemesis and melaena with special reference to factors influencing the outcome. Br Med J 1970; 2:7–14.
6. Allan R, Dykes P. A study of the factors influencing mortality rates from gastrointestinal haemorrhage. QJ Med 1976; 45:533–50.
7. Roth HP, coordinator. Endoscopy. What is its role in upper GI bleeding? Dig Dis Sci 1981; 26:1s–5s.
8. Silverstein FE, Gilbert DA, Tedesco FJ, et al. The national ASGE survey on upper gastrointestinal bleeding. II. Clinical prognostic factors. Gastrointest Endosc 1981; 27:80–93.
9. Koff RS. Benefit of endoscopy in upper gastrointestinal bleeding in patients with liver disease. Dig Dis Sci 1981; 26:12s–6s.
10. Luk GD, Bynum TE, Hendrix TR. Gastric aspiration in localization of gastrointestinal hemorrhage. JAMA 1979; 241:576–8.
11. Gilbert DA, Silverstein FE, Tedesco FJ, et al. The national ASGE survey on upper gastrointestinal bleeding. III. Endoscopy in upper gastrointestinal bleeding. Gastrointest Endosc 1981; 27:94–102.
12. Gilbert DA, Saunders DR. Iced saline lavage does not slow bleeding from experimental canine gastric ulcers. Dig Dis Sci 1981; 26:1065–8.
13. Winzelberg GG, McKusick KA, Strauss HW, et al. Evaluation of gastrointestinal bleeding by red blood cells labeled in vivo with technetium-99m. J Nucl Med 1979; 20:1080–6.
14. Nusbaum M, Baum S. Radiographic demonstration of unknown sites of gastrointestinal bleeding. Surg Forum 1963; 14:374–5.
15. Athanasoulis CA, Waltman AC, Novelline RA, et al. Angiography—its contribution to the emergency management of gastrointestinal hemorrhage. Radiol Clin North Am 1976; 14:265-80.
16. Palmer ED. The vigorous diagnostic approach to upper-gastrointestinal tract hemorrhage. A 23-year study. JAMA 1969; 207:1477–80.
17. Allen HM, Block MA, Schuman BM. Gastroduodenal endoscopy. Management of acute upper gastrointestinal hemorrhage. Arch Surg 1973; 106:450–5.
18. McCray RS, Martin F, Amir-Ahmadi H, et al. Erroneous diagnosis of hemorrhage from esophageal varices. Am J Dig Dis 1969; 14:755–60.
19. DaGradi AE, Mehler R, Tan DTD, Stempien SJ. Sources of upper gastrointestinal bleeding in patients with liver cirrhosis and large esophagogastric varices. Am J Gastroenterol 1970; 54:458–63.
20. Cotton PB, Rosenberg MT, Waldram RLP, Axon ATR. Early endoscopy of oesophagus, stomach, and duodenal bulb in patients with haematemesis and melaena. Br Med J 1973; 2:505–9.
21. Allan RN, Dykes PW, Toye DKM. Diagnostic accuracy of early radiology in acute gastrointestinal haemorrhage. Br Med J 1972; 4:281–4.
22. Herlinger H. Other diagnostic approaches to upper gastrointestinal bleeding: Utility of contrast radiology. Dig Dis Sci 1981; 26:76s–7s.
23. Stevenson GW, Cox RR, Roberts CJC. Prospective comparison of double-contrast barium meal examination and fibreoptic endoscopy in acute upper gastrointestinal haemorrhage. Br Med J 1976; 2:723–4.
24. Katon RM, Smith FW. Panendoscopy in the early diagnosis of acute upper gastrointestinal bleeding. Gastroenterology 1973; 65:728–34.
25. Morris DW, Levine GM, Soloway RD, et al. Prospective, randomized study of diagnosis and outcome of acute upper-gastrointestinal bleeding: endoscopy versus conventional radiography. Am J Dis Dis 1975; 20:1103–9.
26. McGinn FP, Guyer PB, Wilken BJ, Steer HW. A prospective comparative trial between early endoscopy and radiology in acute upper gastrointestinal haemorrhage. Gut 1975; 16:707–13.
27. Morrissey JF. Clinical approach to diagnostic endoscopy in patients with upper gastrointestinal bleeding. Dig Dis Sci 1981; 26:6s–11s.
28. Hellers G, Ihre T. Impact of change to early diagnosis and surgery in major upper gastrointestinal bleeding. Lancet 1975; 2:1250–1.
29. Paul F, Seifert E, Otto P. Urgent Endoscopy of Digestive and Abdominal Diseases. Basel: Karger, 1972; 64.
30. Sugawa C, Werner MH, Hayes DF, et al. Early endoscopy. A guide to therapy for acute hemorrhage in the upper gastrointestinal tract. Arch Surg 1973; 107:133–7.
31. Morgan AG, McAdam WAF, Walmsley GL, et al. Clinical findings, early endoscopy, and multivariate analysis in patients bleeding from the upper gastrointestinal tract. Br Med J 1977; 2:237–40.
32. Foster DN, Miloszewski KJA, Losowsky MS. Stigmata of recent haemorrhage in diagnosis and prognosis of upper gastrointestinal bleeding. Br Med J 1978; 1:1173–7.
33. Griffiths WJ, Neumann DA, Welsh JD. The visible vessel as an indicator of uncontrolled or current gastrointestinal hemorrhage. N Engl J Med 1979; 300:1411–3.
34. MacLeod IA, Mills PR, MacKenzie JF, et al. Neodymium yttrium aluminium garnet laser photocoagulation for major haemorrhage from peptic ulcers and single vessels: a single blind controlled study. Br Med J 1983; 286:345–8.
35. Vallon AG, Cotton PB, Laurence BH, et al. Randomised trial of endoscopic argon laser photocoagulation in bleeding peptic ulcers. Gut 1981; 33:228–33.

36. Storey DW, Bown SG, Swain CP, et al. Endoscopic prediction of recurrent bleeding in peptic ulcers. N Engl J Med 1981; 305:915–6.

37. Papp JP. Electrocoagulation in upper gastrointestinal bleeding. Dig Dis Sci 1981; 26:41s–3s.

38. Swain CP, Bown SG, Storey DW, et al. Controlled trial of argon laser photocoagulation in bleeding peptic ulcers. Lancet 1981; 2:1313–6.

39. Rutgeerts P, Vantrappen G, Broeckaert L, et al. Controlled trial of YAG laser treatment of upper digestive hemorrhage. Gastroenterology 1982; 83:410–6.

40. Swain CP, Bown SG, Salmon PR, et al. Nature of the bleeding point in massively bleeding gastric ulcers. (Abstr) Gut 1982; 23:A888.

41. Palmer ED, Brick IB. Correlation between the severity of esophageal varices in portal cirrhosis and their propensity toward hemorrhage. Gastroenterology 1956; 30:85–90.

42. Baker LA, Smith C, Lieberman G. The natural history of esophageal varices; a study of 115 cirrhotic patients in whom varices were diagnosed prior to bleeding. Am J Med 1959; 26:228–37.

43. Dagradi AE. The natural history of esophageal varices in patients with alcoholic liver cirrhosis. An endoscopic and clinical study. Am J Gastroenterol 1972; 57:520–40.

44. Beppu K, Inokuchi K, Koyanagi N, et al. Prediction of variceal hemorrhage by esophageal endoscopy. Gastrointest Endosc 1981; 27:213–8.

45. Lebrec D, DeFleury P, Rueff B, et al. Portal hypertension, size of esophageal varices, and risk of gastrointestinal bleeding in alcoholic cirrhosis. Gastroenterology 1980; 79:1139–44.

46. Paquet KJ. Prophylactic endoscopic sclerosing treatment of the esophageal wall in varices—a prospective controlled randomized trial. Endoscopy 1982; 14:4–5.

47. Forrest JAH, Finlayson NDC, Shearman DJC. Endoscopy in gastrointestinal bleeding. Lancet 1974; 2:394–7.

48. Leinicke JA, Shaffer RD, Hogan WJ, Geenen JE. Emergency endoscopy in active upper GI bleeding (UGB): Does timing affect the significance of diagnostic yield? (Abstr) Gastrointest Endosc 1976; 22:228–9.

49. Eastwood GE. Does the patient with upper gastrointestinal bleeding benefit from endoscopy? Dig Dis Sci 1981; 26:22s–6s.

50. Winans CS. Emergency upper gastrointestinal endoscopy: Does haste make waste? Am J Dig Dis 1977; 22:536–40.

51. Keller RT, Logan GM Jr. Comparison of emergent endoscopy and upper gastrointestinal series radiography in acute upper gastrointestinal haemorrhage. Gut 1976; 17:180–4.

52. Dronfield MW, McIllmurray MB, Ferguson R, et al. A prospective randomized study of endoscopy and radiology in acute upper-gastrointestinal-tract bleeding. Lancet 1977; 1:1167–9.

53. Sandlow LJ, Becker GH, Spellberg MA, et al. A prospective randomized study of the management of upper gastrointestinal hemorrhage. Am J Gastroenterol 1974; 61:282–9.

54. Allan R, Dykes P. A comparison of routine and selective endoscopy in the management of acute gastrointestinal hemorrhage. Gastrointest Endosc 1974; 20:154–5.

55. Graham DY. Limited value of early endoscopy in the management of acute upper gastrointestinal bleeding. Am J Surg 1980; 140:284–90.

56. Hoare AM. Comparative study between endoscopy and radiology in acute upper gastrointestinal haemorrhage. Br Med J 1975; 1:27–30.

57. Peterson WL, Barnett CC, Smith HJ, et al. Routine early endoscopy in upper-gastrointestinal-tract bleeding. N Engl J Med 1981; 304:925–9.

58. Auth DC, Gilbert DA, Opie EA, Silverstein FE. The multipolar probe—a new endoscopic technique to control gastrointestinal bleeding. (Abstr) Gastrointest Endosc 1980; 26:63.

59. Protell RL, Rubin CE, Auth DC, et al. The heater probe: a new endoscopic method for stopping massive gastrointestinal bleeding. Gastroenterology 1978; 74:257–62.

60. Schrock TR. Does endoscopy affect the surgical approach to the patient with upper gastrointestinal bleeding? Dig Dis Sci 1981; 26:27s–30s.

61. Katon RM. Complications of upper gastrointestinal endoscopy in the gastrointestinal bleeder. Dig Dis Sci 1981; 26:47s–54s.

62. Gilbert DA, Silverstein FE, Tedesco FJ, et al. National ASGE survey on upper gastrointestinal bleeding: Complications of endoscopy. Dig Dis Sci 1981; 26:55s–9s.

63. Katz D. Morbidity and mortality in standard and flexible gastrointestinal endoscopy. Gastrointest Endosc 1969; 15:134–41.

64. Silvis SE, Nebel O, Rogers G, et al. Endoscopic complications. Results of the 1974 American Society for Gastrointestinal Endoscopy Survey. JAMA 1976; 235:928–30.

65. Mandelstam P, Sugawa C, Silvis SE, et al. Complications associated with esophagogastroduodenoscopy and with esophageal dilation. Gastrointest Endosc 1976; 23:16–9.

66. Noel D, Delage Y, Liguory C, et al. Hémorrhagies digestives d'origine haute chez les sujets de plus de 65 ans. Apport de l'Endoscopie. Nouv Presse Med 1979; 8:589–91.

67. Paul F, Huchzermeyer H. Results and complications of emergency endoscopy for acute gastrointestinal bleeding in patients on intensive care units. In: Abstracts of the IV European Congress of Gastrointestinal Endoscopy. Stuttgart: Georg Thieme Verlag, Stuttgart, 1980.

68. Hancy A, Condat M, Cougard A, et al. Les accidents de la fiberoscopieoeso-gastro-duodenale. Enquete nationale portant sur 150,000 fibroscopies oesogastroduodenales. Ann Gastroenterol Hepatol 1977; 13:101.

69. Waye JD. Lower gastrointestinal bleeding. In: Bayless TM, ed. Current Therapy in Gastroenterology and Liver Disease, 1984–1985. Philadelphia: B. C. Decker, Inc., 1984; 359.

70. Bohlman TW, Katon RM, Lipshutz GR, et al. Fiberoptic pansigmoidoscopy. An evaluation and comparison with rigid sigmoidoscopy. Gastroenterology 1977; 72:644–9.

71. Winnan G, Berci G, Panish J, et al. Superiority of the flexible to the rigid sigmoidoscope in routine proctosigmoidoscopy. N Engl J Med 1980; 302:1011–4.

72. Painter NS, Burkitt DP. Diverticular disease of the colon, a 20th century problem. Clin Gastroenterol 1975; 4:3.

73. Boley SJ, Brandt LJ, Mitsudo SM. Vascular lesions of the colon. Adv Intern Med 1984; 29:301–26.

74. Adams JT. Therapeutic barium enema for massive diverticular bleeding. Arch Surg 1970; 101:457–60.

75. Hedberg SE. Endoscopy in gastrointestinal bleeding: a systematic approach to diagnosis. Surg Clin North Am 1974; 54:549–59.

76. Sivak MV Jr, Sullivan BH Jr, Rankin GB. Colonoscopy; a report of 644 cases and review of the literature. Am J Surg 1974; 128:351–7.

77. Rossini FP, Ferrari A. Emergency colonoscopy. In: Hunt RH, Waye JD, eds. Colonoscopy: Techniques, Clinical Practice, and Colour Atlas. London: Chapman and Hall, 1981; 289–99.

78. Forde KA. Colonoscopy in acute rectal bleeding. Gastrointest Endosc 1981; 27:219–20.

79. Jensen DM, Machicado GA, Tapia JI. Emergent colonoscopy in patients with severe hematochezia. (Abstr) Gastrointest Endosc 1983; 29:177.

80. Caos A, Manier J, Benner K, et al. "Golytely" preparation for colonoscopy in acute lower gastrointestinal hemorrhage: preliminary findings. (Abstr) Gastrointest Endosc 1983; 29:157.

81. Frühmorgen P, Bodem F, Reidenbach HD, et al. Endoscopic laser coagulation of bleeding gastrointestinal lesions with report of the first therapeutic application in man. Gastrointest Endosc 1976; 23:73–5.

82. Kiefhaber P, Nath G, Moritz K. Endoscopical control of massive gastrointestinal hemorrhage by irradiation with a high-power neodymium-Yag laser. Prog Surg 1977; 15:140–55.

83. Jensen DM, Machicado GA, Silpa ML. Treatment of GI angioma with argon laser, heater probe, or bipolar electrocoagulation. Gastrointest Endosc (Abstr) 1984; 30:134.

84. Thoeni RF, Menuck L. Comparison of barium enema and colonoscopy in the detection of small colonic polyps. Radiology 1977; 124:631–5.

85. Tedesco FJ, Waye JD, Raskin JB, et al. Colonoscopic evaluation of rectal bleeding: a study of 304 patients. Ann Intern Med 1978; 89:907–9.

86. Teague RH, Thornton JR, Manning AP, et al. Colonoscopy for investigation of unexplained rectal bleeding. Lancet 1978; 1:1350–2.

87. Swarbrick ET, Fevre DI, Hunt RH, et al. Colonoscopy for unexplained rectal bleeding. Br Med J 1978; 2:1685–7.

88. Brand EJ, Sullivan BH Jr, Sivak MV Jr, Rankin GB. Colonoscopy in the diagnosis of unexplained rectal bleeding. Ann Surg 1980; 192:111–3.

89. Luke RG, Lees W, Rudick J. Appearance of the stools after the introduction of blood into the caecum. Gut 1964; 5:77–9.

90. Tedesco FJ, Pickens CA, Griffin JW Jr, et al. Role of colonoscopy in patients with unexplained melena: analysis of 53 patients. Gastrointest Endosc 1981; 27:221–3.

91. Winawer SJ, Sherlock P, Schottenfeld D, Muller DG. Screening for colon cancer. Gastroenterology 1976; 70:783–9.

92. Rogers BHG, Silvis SE, Nebel OT, et al. Complications of flexible fiberoptic colonoscopy and polypectomy. Gastrointest Endosc 1975; 22:73–7.

93. Frühmorgen P, Demling P. Complications of diagnostic and therapeutic colonoscopy in the Federal Republic of Germany. Results of an inquiry. Endoscopy 1979; 11:146–50.

94. Gilbert DA, Hallstrom AP, Shanyfelt SL, et al. The national ASGE colonoscopy survey—Complications of colonoscopy. (Abstr) Gastrointest Endosc 1984; 30:156.

95. Rogers BHG. Complications and hazards of colonoscopy. In: Hunt RH, Waye JD, eds. Colonoscopy: Techniques, Clinical Practice, and Colour Atlas. London: Chapman and Hall 1981; 237–64.

96. Gilbert DA, Shaneyfelt SL, Silverstein FE, et al. The national ASGE colonoscopy survey—analysis of colonoscopic practices and yield. (Abstr) Gastrointest Endosc 1984; 30:143.

Chapter 7

PRINCIPLES OF ELECTROSURGERY

ROGER C. ODELL

INTERACTION OF ANIMAL TISSUE AND ELECTROSURGICAL CURRENT

Effect of High-Frequency Current on Tissue

Tissue cells act as electrical conductors because of their electrolyte composition. A direct current causes cellular membrane depolarization in a tissue. If depolarization occurs in neuromuscular tissue, the result is excitation, and the subject experiences a shock. In the body, alternating current below a frequency of 100,000 cycles per second (cps) causes tissue ions to be pulled alternately to and fro because of the rapid reversal of current flow. Depolarization occurs but is rapidly counteracted owing to reversal of the current. The subject therefore experiences tetanic neuromuscular activity.

If a very-high-frequency alternating current is applied (i.e., greater than 100,000 cps), cellular ions change position to a small degree because of the rapidity of reversal in the direction of the current. Depolarization does not occur, and there is no neuromuscular excitation or shock. However, such a current imparts a degree of kinetic energy to the cells, and ions become excited and collide with other cellular particles. This kinetic energy raises the temperature of the cell, so that the effect of very-high-frequency alternating current on tissue is not electrical but thermal.

Electrosurgical effects are possible with any frequency between 100,000 cps (100 kHz) and 4,000,000 cps (4 MHz). However, at the upper end of this range the current is much more difficult to contain (vide infra). Below 100 kHz there is a potential for electrical shock. Therefore, most generators produce radio-frequency currents of about 500 kHz. (Since the high frequency needed to produce electrosurgical effects is in the same range as the electromagnetic radiation of radio waves, it is often called radio frequency).

Factors That Influence Tissue Heating

Total heat attained in a tissue by this process varies with certain factors. It will increase directly with the resistance (ohms) offered by the tissue to current flow, the measure of current flow itself (amps), and the duration of the time that the current is flowing.

Tissue Resistance

The total heat attained in a tissue is equal to the resistance in ohms multiplied by the square of the current amps. (total heat = resistance × amps².) High tissue resistance to a current generates more heat than the same current in a tissue of low resistance. A good conductor with low resistance will not undergo much heating.

Tissue resistance varies with the type of tissue and its water content. Skin, for example, forms a high-resistance (100,000 ohms) protective barrier for the body. Water is a pure conductor and therefore decreases the resistance to a current (and heating effect). Conversely, dry desiccated tissue has a high resistance.

Current Density

One of the most important principles of electrosurgery that has a direct bearing on clinical effect is current density. The heating effect in a circuit will vary inversely with the cross-sectional area of the tissue through which the current is flowing at any given point. The effect of cross-sectional area of a conductor on heating is expressed in the concept of current density, which is defined as amps/cm^2. Temperature is directly related to the square of the current density, that is, $T = (amps/cm^2)^2$. Current density (and heating effect) are increased by increasing the current or decreasing the cross-sectional area of the conductor through which the current flows. Decreased current and/or increased cross-sectional area will decrease current density and heating.[1]

This cross-sectional area can be changed by varying the surface area of an electrode. The smaller the diameter of the snare wire (electrode), the greater the current density and the greater the temperature rise in adjacent tissue. Current density is diminished as the current encounters larger surface areas of the body. A metal plate of large surface area is used as an indifferent dispersing electrode, and by the principle of current density the heat generated by current at this electrode is dissipated over a large area. If the surface area of contact is sufficient, the patient does not sense that the plate is "hot." (The indifferent plate electrode is often incorrectly referred to as the "ground plate.")

The patient plate should be placed as close to the operative site as possible so that the current will encounter the smallest tissue volume and least resistance. This enables one to use the lowest possible power setting to obtain the desired result. Hairy skin, scars, bony prominences, and bent or twisted plates will decrease the area contact of the skin with the plate, and increase the risk of a thermal burn. In order to decrease the high resistance offered by the skin, the indifferent electrode should be coated with a good conductive gel. Proper placement of the plate must be maintained during changes in patient position.

Electrosurgical Generator Power Output

The current in amps that is caused to flow in tissue is directly related to the power output in watts of the electrosurgical machine (watts = volts × amps). A power increase therefore results in an increase in current density (CD = amps/cm^2). Tissue in contact with a large surface area electrode can be brought to the same temperatures obtained with a smaller surface area electrode by increases in the power and current.

The electrosurgical current output of the generator can be used in one of two modes.

In the monopolar mode the active electrode is usually small. By virtue of small size the current density is high and heat energy is concentrated close to the electrode. The second electrode, by means of which the circuit is completed through the patient to the generator, is large (vide supra). However, two small electrodes can be used, one of which replaces the indifferent electrode plate. The electrosurgical current completes its circuit through any tissue that is between the two active electrodes, and electrosurgical effects occur in the vicinity of both electrodes. The best example of the bipolar output in present use is the bipolar or multipolar coagulating probes in which two or more sets of active electrodes are combined in a single device. For practical purposes, the clinical effect of the bipolar output is limited to tissue desiccation (vide infra). The clinical use of the two types of generator output for control of gastrointestinal bleeding is discussed in Chapter 8.

The bipolar output has been used in other ways. For example, two active electrodes are employed in the technique of bipolar polypectomy.[2] This technique requires a twin accessory channel endoscope and two separate electrode devices, one inserted via each instrument channel. Once the tissue—a polyp stalk, for example—is grasped with both electrodes, current will flow only through the tissue between the two electrodes. In practice, this technique is difficult to control and it is not used often or widely.

If the bipolar output is to be used, the output of the electrosurgical generator must be greatly reduced. Since the current will flow through a small volume of tissue, the resistance it encounters will be significantly less than that offered to the flow of current by the large volume of body tissues in the monopolar circuit. If the usual settings for monopolar electrosurgery are used in a bipolar technique, current density will be extremely high, cutting will be immediate, and there will be virtually no hemostasis. The commercially available generators specifically designed for multipolar coagulation of bleeding sites take this into account. They are usually limited to a bipolar output that can only be used with their companion multipolar probes.

There are many electrosurgical generators available commercially. Typically, a generator will be provided with two knobs that regulate power output, one for the coagulation waveform and one for the cutting. These are calibrated with arbitrary numbers. A given number setting on one machine usually has no relation whatsoever to the same number setting on a machine of different manufacture. Furthermore, the increase in power output from one setting to the next in ascending order is not precisely linear. For example, if the dials are provided with settings from 1 to 10, advancement to the next higher setting does not necessarily provide a 10% increase in power. In practical terms, the endoscopist must be thoroughly familiar with the characteristics of the electrosurgical generator in use. It is also advisable to eliminate variability when performing electrosurgery by using only a single type of machine. Some manufacturers have replaced the dials on recent models of electrosurgical generators with digital wattage indicators. These improve the ability to adjust power output and permit greater reproducibility in the performance of each successive procedure. Self-adjusting output power circuitry has also been introduced (Valleylab, Inc). This innovation regulates generator output so that a preset energy level is delivered through the widely ranging tissue impedances encountered during an electrosurgical procedure. Constancy in the power output allows for a more consistent and reproducible electrosurgical tissue effect.

Time

The longer the period of time a current is flowing, the more heat will be generated. If, for example, a given power setting is applied for a given length of time, a certain temperature will be attained. If the power setting is decreased, the same temperature can be attained with a longer duration of current flow. But this will also allow more heat to be conducted away from the high-current density area. The distribution of heating will be different. Generally speaking, the longer the power is applied, the greater the depth of heating.

Clinical Effects of Electrosurgery

The manner in which electrosurgical current is applied to tissue determines the clinical effect. There are three possible effects: desiccation, cutting, and fulguration.

Electrosurgical desiccation produces tissue coagulation at low power and without an electrical spark discharge ("sparking") between the electrode and the tissue. Electrosurgical cutting involves an electrical spark discharge between electrode and tissue that produces a cutting effect. Electrosurgical fulguration also involves sparking to tissue but without a significant cutting effect. Fulguration can coagulate large bleeding vessels and char (carbonize) tissue.

When radio-frequency current jumps across an air gap to tissue, the bright light in the gap is technically known as a "spark." An "arc" is a similar phenomenon that requires longer intervals to become established and probably does not play a significant role in electrosurgery.

Electrical Waveforms

There are two basic electrosurgical waveforms; these are referred to as coagulation (COAG) and cutting (CUT). With most types of electrosurgical generators used by gastrointestinal endoscopists, the selection of waveform is performed by activation of one of two pedals of a foot switch. It is often erroneously assumed that activation of one of these waveforms during electrosurgery will produce the tissue effect indicated by its name—that is, COAG will produce hemostasis, and use of CUT will result in an incision. This is not entirely correct. Depending on other circumstances, the name of the waveform used may have no relation to the clinical effect produced. This misconception can lead to serious flaws in electrosurgical technique.

The COAG and CUT waveforms can also be mixed. The type of current produced is usually referred to as blended current, or BLEND. Usually, a switch on the electrosurgical generator is provided to change the output to a BLEND waveform. Then activation of the CUT pedal results in BLEND. Selection of higher blend modes, i.e., BLEND 1, 2, or 3, results in greater hemostasis. An increase in the blend setting produces an increase in crest factor (vide infra); the net therapeutic effect produced by increasing the settings (e.g., 1, 2, 3) in a BLEND mode is greater coagulation and dragging of the active electrode when a cutting effect is desired. An increase in power output may be required to obtain a cutting effect.

Since other variables, such as the size of the electrode, have a bearing on the clinical effect of electrosurgery, there is no "right" or correct generator setting for any particular type of endoscopic electrosurgical procedure. If the proper setting for a particular procedure is not known from prior experience, then it must be determined by trial and error. This must be redetermined if another variable factor in the technique is changed—a change in the diameter of the snare wire, for example. The trial-and-error process should begin at a low power output setting. The setting may then be increased in steps until the desired clinical effect is observed.

The selection of either the CUT or COAG waveforms only has relevance to the clinical electrosurgical effects of cutting and fulguration. The selection of waveform has no importance in electrosurgical desiccation; this can be accomplished with either CUT/BLEND waveform or even with COAG.

Electrocutting Current (CUT Waveform)

The essential characteristic of the CUT waveform is that it is a continuous sine wave. If the voltage output of the generator is plotted over time, a pure cutting (CUT) waveform is a continuous sine wave alternating from positive to negative at the operating frequency of the generator, typically 500 kHz (Fig. 7–1).

Electrocoagulating Current (COAG Waveform)

The waveform of COAG is pulsed—that is, it is switched on and off for small fractions of a second. The number of pulses (and also the number of pauses) per second is on the order of 20,000. Therefore, the COAG waveform consists of short bursts of a radiofrequency sine wave (Fig. 7–2). The frequency of the sine wave is 450 kHz.

The on-off characteristic of COAG waveforms must also be described by means of a quantity called the crest factor. This is defined as the ratio of peak voltage to average (root mean square, RMS) voltage. Crest factor = peak voltage/RMS (effective average) voltage. The crest factor of a pure CUT sine wave is 1.6. The crest factor of typical COAG waveform is 7.0 to 8.0 and is essentially constant over the entire control range. This difference in crest factor means that the peak voltage with COAG is higher than that with

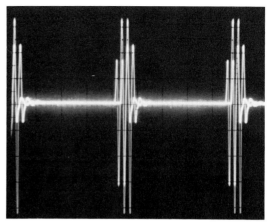

FIGURE 7–2. Oscilloscope picture of COAG waveform. Note interrupted voltage peaks.

CUT; the average (RMS) voltage may or may not be the same, depending on other circumstances. For BLEND modes 1, 2, and 3, typical crest factors are 2.3, 3.0, and 4.0.

The most important feature of the COAG waveform is the pause between each burst.

Blended Current (BLEND)

High-frequency current can be pulsed for shorter periods of time, or can be interrupted for progressively longer intervals. This produces a "blended" type of waveform with characteristics of both primary types.

Electrosurgical Desiccation

Of the three electrosurgical effects, desiccation is technically the simplest because any electrical waveform (CUT, COAG, or BLEND) can be used and only low power output levels are required from the electrosurgical generator. In desiccation, a current is passed through the tissue; the tissue offers a resistance to current flow, and an increase in heat energy results (Fig. 7–3). This is exactly the same phenomenon as the resistance wire in a toaster or stove that becomes hot when the current passes through it. When the tissue becomes hot, the water is slowly driven out of the tissue, hence the name "desiccation." The observable effect is that the tissue first turns light brown and then it will bubble and steam as tissue water is driven off.

Tissue desiccation can be accomplished with either the monopolar or the bipolar output. However, the bipolar output is optimal for desiccation in that cutting and fulguration will not occur. Even at very high power settings there is almost no tendency for cutting or fulguration to occur. Mono-

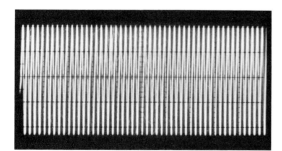

FIGURE 7–1. Oscilloscope picture of CUT electrosurgical waveform.

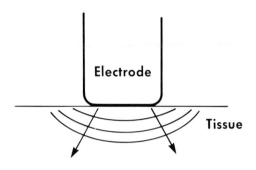

TYPICAL CURRENT=0.5 AMP RMS

FIGURE 7–3. Diagrammatic representation of electro-surgical desiccation. The electrode is in good contact with tissue. Deep coagulation spreads radially. Relatively soft, light brown eschar will result. RMS = root mean square (effective average).

polar output is designed primarily for cutting and fulguration. Low generator settings must be used in order to confine the effect to desiccation when the monopolar output is used.

The exact generator setting (i.e., the power output of the machine) needed for tissue desiccation depends on the surface area of the active electrode in contact with the tissue. The larger the electrode contact area, the more current is required to produce the same current density. Also, with higher control settings more current will be delivered, and therefore desiccation will proceed at a faster rate.

Electrosurgical Cutting

The objective with electrosurgical cutting is to heat tissue so rapidly that tissue water is quickly converted to steam. The sudden increase in water vapor pressure in the cell literally causes it to explode, thus leaving a cavity in the cell matrix. The heat generated is dissipated in the steam and therefore it is not conducted through the tissue to dry out adjacent cells. If the electrode is moved and fresh tissue is contacted, additional cells are exploded, and if the process is continued an incision will be made. Electrosurgical cutting involves sparking to tissue (vide supra) (Fig. 7–4). A hot cautery wire—that is, a heated wire with no electric current passing into the tissue—can also cut tissue, and the tissue events are the same as those described above. However, there are additional effects of electrosurgical cutting. To better understand this, it will be useful to consider an example.

Suppose one begins by desiccating tissue with a small wire electrode using the mono-

polar output, CUT waveform, and a generator setting that produces a relatively high power output. Because the power level (which corresponds to the heat delivered per second) is high, the tissue becomes desiccated quickly. As water leaves the tissue, its electrical resistance increases. Voltage, the force that drives current through a resistance, is also the force that drives electrical sparks across an air gap. If the voltage is high enough (a condition established by setting the generator for high power output) a spark will jump to the nearest moist tissue, since air, once it is ionized, is a better conductor than desiccated tissue.

Once spark to the tissue is established, tissue heating is the result of two phenomena. The first is the tissue heating produced by the current passing through the resistance of the tissue at the point where the spark strikes the flesh. The remainder of the heating comes from energy dissipated in the spark itself. Electrons collide with the tissue as does the radiant heat from the spark itself. The heat (energy) originating in the spark is actually greater than that arising in the tissue as a result of the current flow. The total heat energy of these two phenomena taken together is extremely concentrated and is thus capable of exploding cells. In contrast, cutting is practically impossible with the desiccation phenomenon alone.

One of the essential features to produce the clinical effect of electrosurgical cutting is the spark to tissue. If this does not occur, no incision will result.

Electrosurgical Fulguration

To produce the clinical effect of tissue fulguration, the active electrode must not be in contact with the tissue. Sparking is essential

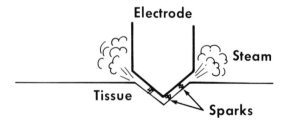

TYPICAL CURRENT=0.1 AMP RMS

FIGURE 7–4. Diagrammatic representation of electrosurgical cutting. The electrode is separated from tissue by a thin layer of steam. Short, intense sparks flash cells into steam. Hemostasis can be minimal and the process mimics the scalpel.

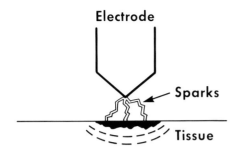

TYPICAL CURRENT= 0.1 AMP RMS

FIGURE 7–5. Diagrammatic representation of electrosurgical fulguration. The electrode is free from tissue. Long sparks to tissue result in superficial coagulation first, then deeper necrosis as fulguration continues. Eschar is hard and black.

in this process. Long sparks jump from the electrode to the tissue (Fig. 7–5). The first effect of this is superficial coagulation, but this is followed by deeper necrosis as the process is continued. Eventually a hard, black eschar will develop. The distance that sparks travel during fulguration is greater than that in the clinical effect of electrosurgical cutting.

Suppose that a COAG waveform has the same peak voltage as the CUT waveform described in the above example. Because the voltage is the same, the sparks can jump the same distance as with the CUT waveform, but the average power delivered (the amount of heat per second) is less because the COAG current is turned off most of the time (Fig. 7–6). The fulguration process may fail as the eschar develops because desiccated tissue has a much higher resistance. The voltage is now inadequate to produce a spark. This may be overcome by moving the electrode somewhat closer to the tissue, although as the gap is narrowed the clinical effect may change to

desiccation. If, however, the COAG waveform is given the same average (RMS) voltage as the CUT waveform and thus could deliver the same quantity of heat per second, fulguration would continue. Since the COAG waveform is turned off most of the time, it can only achieve the same average (RMS) voltage as the CUT waveform by having very large peak voltages during the periods when the generator is on (Fig. 7–7).

A good COAG waveform, that is, one with high peak voltage, can spark to tissue without significant cutting effect because the heat is more widely dispersed by the long sparks and because the heating effect is intermittent. The temperature of the water in the cells is not raised high enough to cause it to flash into steam. The cells are dehydrated slowly but are not torn apart to form an incision. Because of the high peak voltage of a quality COAG waveform, it can drive a current through very high resistances. This makes it possible to fulgurate long after the water is driven out of the tissue and to actually char it to carbon.

Tissue "coagulation" is a general term that includes both desiccation and fulguration. To reiterate an important point, selection of the COAG waveform output of the electrosurgical generator does not necessarily mean that tissue "coagulation" will result.

Fulguration can be contrasted with desiccation in several ways. Sparking to tissue with any practical fulguration generator always produces necrosis anywhere the spark lands. This is because each cycle of voltage produces a new spark and each spark has an extremely high current density at the point where the spark enters the tissue. In desiccation, the current is no more concentrated than the area of contact between the electrode and the tissue. As a result, desiccation may or

FIGURE 7–6. In this diagram peak voltages of CUT (top) and COAG (bottom) waveforms are the same, but power is about one third less in the COAG waveform.

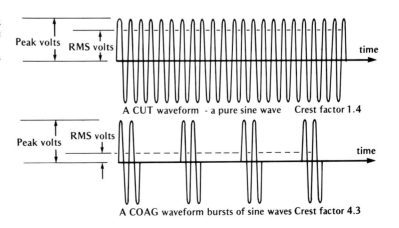

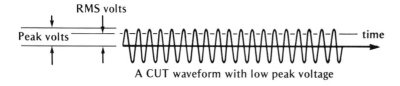

A CUT waveform with low peak voltage

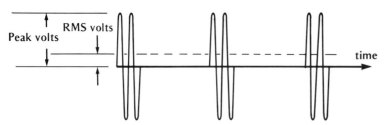

FIGURE 7–7. The COAG waveform (*bottom*) with equal power (energy per second) to that of the CUT waveform (*top*). COAG peak voltage is about three times higher in this example than in in Figure 7–6. Note that RMS (average) voltages are equal in both waveforms.

may not produce necrosis, depending on the current density. For a given level of current flow, fulguration is always more efficient at producing necrosis. In general, fulguration requires only one fifth the average current flow of desiccation.

If a ball electrode is pressed against moist tissue, the electrode will begin in the desiccation mode, regardless of the waveform. The initial tissue resistance is quite low and the resulting current will be high. But as the tissue dries out, its resistance rises until the electrical contact is broken. Although the electrode is now in contact with dry tissue, sparks will jump to the nearest moist tissue in the fulguration mode if the voltage is high enough.

Blended Cut

Blended current (BLEND) is a cutting waveform with moderate hemostatic effect. That is, the walls of the incision made with the BLEND current will be well fulgurated, depending on the fineness of the electrode. The finer the electrode, the cleaner the cut and the lesser the hemostatic effect.

POLYPECTOMY

Technique of Polypectomy

Polypectomy can be performed through virtually any type of endoscope with an accessory channel. The procedure is performed with a wire snare that is looped around the polyp and closed like a noose. There are several possible methods of severing the polyp. One is to apply electrosurgical current first to desiccate the polyp, then to cut through the peduncle electrosurgically. It is also possible to make the cut mechanically by tightening the thin snare wire around the

polyp stalk after the polyp blood supply has been coagulated and the tissue softened by electrosurgical desiccation. Polypectomy can also be accomplished in one maneuver by cutting with a blended current. Each approach has its advantages and limitations. A detailed presentation of colonoscopic polypectomy from the clinical standpoint is given in Chapter 45.

Initial Desiccation to Provide Hemostasis

If desiccation is to be performed first, separately from cutting, it can be accomplished with either COAG or BLEND waveforms at relatively low generator settings (e.g., on a Valleylab unit from 1 to 3 or a digital display of 20 to 40 watts).[3, 4] The degree of desiccation must be judged by the tissue blanching that begins within the tissue in contact with the snare wire and then spreads downward (Fig. 7–8). The desiccation must be just the right amount, regardless of whether the actual cut is to be made mechanically or electrosurgically. If it is too little, the stalk may bleed; if it is excessive, the stalk may become too hard and dry to cut either mechanically or electrically.[5] Water in the tissue is an

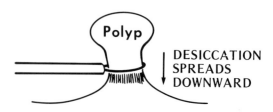

DESICCATION
SPREADS
DOWNWARD

DESICCATION FIRST FOR HEMOSTASIS

FIGURE 7–8. Diagrammatic representation of initial desiccation of polyp stalk prior to mechanical or electrosurgical cutting of stalk.

Current required is proportional to the square of the polyp diameter since current density should be the same.

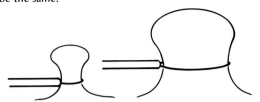

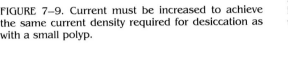

FIGURE 7–9. Current must be increased to achieve the same current density required for desiccation as with a small polyp.

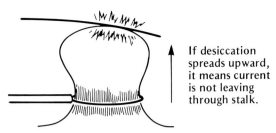

If desiccation spreads upward, it means current is not leaving through stalk.

FIGURE 7–10. Clinical effect of electrosurgical current is altered by contact of the polyp with opposite wall of the bowel.

essential factor for electrosurgical cutting. If it is not present, the snare wire may become stuck half-way through the peduncle.

Fortunately, polypectomy-related accidents are rare with relatively small (1 to 2 cm in diameter) polyps. However, with a large or sessile polyp, the technical problems and difficulty of polypectomy are compounded and the possibilities for a complication increase.

When desiccating a large polyp the generator output must be set higher if the degree of desiccation is to be the same as that used for a small polyp (Fig. 7–9). This is because the snare loop encompasses a larger volume of tissue, and thus the current density will be lower if the power output is not increased as the desiccation process is begun. However, as the snare wire is tightened, and the effective diameter of the loop decreases, the current density in the tissue increases. When the snare becomes very tight and the diameter becomes very small, the current density will rise as the inverse of the square of the diameter of the snare loop.

During electrosurgical polypectomy, current is always trying to complete a circuit by returning to the patient plate (indifferent electrode). Once the stalk is well desiccated and resistance in this area of tissue increases, current can also seek other routes of lesser resistance to complete the circuit. If, for example, the polyp is in contact with the opposite wall of the colon, the current will continue to flow off the polyp through this point of contact (Fig. 7–10). If the point of contact is small enough—that is, if the current density is high enough—a mucosal burn will result. This can be minimized by moving the polyp about in the colon, usually by moving the snare forward and backward, so that the polyp does not remain in contact with a specific point on the opposite wall for any appreciable length of time. Current flowing by an aberrant path such as this influ-

ences the electrosurgical effect within the stalk of the polyp.

Mechanical Cutting After Desiccation

After desiccation, a polyp may be severed from its stalk by mechanically closing the snare loop (Fig. 7–11). There is again an optimum amount of desiccation that will soften the tissue without drying it excessively. Some endoscopists recommend that a BLEND current be applied while tightening the snare to pull it through the polyp stalk. The advantage of this is that any undesiccated tissue at the center of the stalk will be desiccated as the maneuver is performed. Furthermore, if sparking to tissue and electrosurgical cutting should occur, the cutting will have a hemostatic component sufficient to avoid bleeding. Mechanical cutting is likely to become electrosurgical cutting when BLEND current is used in this manner because the electrode area touching the tissue becomes smaller and smaller as the cut proceeds, that is, as the current density increases.

Electrosurgical Cutting After Desiccation

Transection of the polyp after desiccation can be done electrosurgically using either CUT or BLEND. The generator setting will depend on the size of the polyp stalk, the degree of desiccation, and the diameter of the snare wire.

The most common misunderstanding about polypectomy technique concerns the fact that clinical electrosurgical cutting can

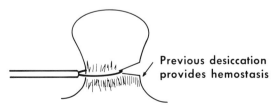

Previous desiccation provides hemostasis

FIGURE 7–11. Diagrammatic representation of mechanical transection of a polyp stalk after electrosurgical desiccation.

only occur when sparks are free to jump to the tissue. The tighter the snare is held, the less likely that this will happen and that cutting will begin. The snare must have a poor electrical contact with the tissue. A good technique to use after desiccation, therefore, is to loosen the snare wire slightly before applying the CUT waveform current.

The snare wire thickness is also critically important because it directly affects the area of metal in contact with the tissue; that is, current density is directly related to the diameter of the wire. For a given power output of the generator, a relatively thin wire produces a higher current density than a thick wire. Currently available snare wires range from 0.3 to 0.8 mm (0.012 to 0.040 inch) in diameter. Snare wires with a thickness greater than about 0.45 mm (0.025 inch) are not recommended because the thicker wires result in difficulty in starting a mechanical or electrosurgical cut. Whenever the snare wire diameter is changed, the generator setting must be changed accordingly.

The snare wire diameter also affects the degree of hemostasis. The thicker the wire the greater the degree of coagulation. Increasing the snare wire diameter, for example, could have the same effect as changing the current from pure CUT to BLEND. But, as explained above, it is harder to initiate clinical cutting with a thick wire.

Electrosurgical Cutting in One Maneuver

In this technique the polyp is severed with a BLEND current without desiccating first. Blended current is used to insure that the tissue along the course of the incision is well fulgurated. Pure CUT does not provide sufficient hemostasis. The generator output is usually set at its mid-range, but lower settings are advisable for removal of small polyps using a small diameter snare wire. When cutting with the blended mode, the speed at which the electrode moves through the tissue affects the hemostasis. The faster the electrode travels, the less hemostasis. Consequently, the snare should be closed slowly to provide maximum hemostasis.

It is also possible to cut tissue electrosurgically using the COAG as a blended current, and also to cut with the COAG only. This occurs if the snare wire is extremely fine (0.3 to 0.4 mm) and a high generator setting is used. The higher the crest factor (i.e., the more hemostasis), and the thicker the snare wire, the greater the skill required to cut electrosurgically. With a relatively thick wire (0.45 mm) the grasp on the polyp must be extremely light to allow the electrosurgical cutting to start promptly. In practice this is difficult to accomplish.

An advantage of grasping the polyp stalk lightly is that there is less tendency for normal bowel wall to be pulled into the snare where it will be harmed. Some endoscopists use "home-made" snares to achieve this delicate "feel." These snares consist of a 0.4 mm diameter wire that is formed into a loop and passed through a plastic tube. The bare wire ends are clamped with a forceps and manipulated by an assistant who must apply an exact degree of closure on the snare. The forceps are modified by wiring them to a cable that goes to the monopolar output of the generator. After the assistant has adjusted the tension, the foot switch is activated.

With conventional commercial snares, the control of tension is not as precise. Nevertheless, there is a definite sensation or feel that can be appreciated as the snare loop closes on the stalk of the polyp. This is one of the most important functions of the gastrointestinal assistant in endoscopy. An inexperienced assistant is not aware of this and may close the snare completely and amputate the polyp. This is more likely to occur with a thin stalk that resists closure to a lesser degree and so offers a more subtle sensation of tension on the closing snare loop. Once aware of the danger of bleeding as a result of mechanical amputation of a polyp, the newly initiated assistant may act in the opposite extreme and close the snare too loosely. The endoscopist must pay careful attention to the instruction of gastrointestinal assistants in this procedure.

When prompt onset of electrosurgical cutting is desirable, as is the case with electrosurgical severing of the polyp in one maneuver, it can also be facilitated by using a very thin snare wire and blend current.

Another useful modification that enables prompt electrosurgical cutting is the "rapid start" option that is built into some electrosurgical generators. This modification helps to initiate sparking and therefore cutting when an electrode is in relatively close and firm contact with the tissue.

Occasionally the electrosurgical cutting may not start promptly with large polyps, even though the snare is held loosely. Instead of cutting, the endoscopist will see the tell-tale color changes of desiccation creeping down the polyp toward the stalk. If the desiccation has coagulated the tissue enough to provide hemostasis, the endoscopist can confidently switch to a pure CUT current at an appropriate generator setting. This will usually get the cut started. A pure CUT current will "start" better than any other mode, but it provides little hemostasis.

The Art of Endoscopic Polypectomy

In the final analysis, endoscopic polypectomy is actually an art that is based on a knowledge of electrosurgical principles. There is no objective measure of the "right" amount of desiccation, for example. Rather, polypectomy is a subjective procedure based on observation, experience, and judgment, all of which must be applied in the assessment of and approach to the removal of any polyp.

All the described polypectomy techniques can be made to work successfully, but each is an art that should be learned from an endoscopist instructor who uses these techniques successfully. It is advisable for beginners to use exactly the same equipment, snare, settings, and technique used by the instructor. The use of one instructor's mode and power settings with another instructor's snare and technique can result in disaster.

ENDOSCOPIC PAPILLOTOMY (SPHINCTEROTOMY)

Endoscopic papillotomy is an endoscopic electrosurgical procedure. The technique and other aspects of the procedure are discussed in Chapter 29. Briefly, a special catheter equipped with an external wire at its distal end is introduced beyond the papilla of Vater and into the common bile duct under direct vision and with the aid of fluoroscopy. A wire linkage in the catheter control handle flexes the tip of the catheter by bowing a length of electrode wire along one side of the tip. The electrosurgical generator is activated using a blended CUT current, and the sphincter is incised by the wire electrode. The electrosurgical generator must have an appropriate wattage range, generally 55 to 65 watts when using BLEND 1 current.

Injury to the pancreas is one of the potential complications of this procedure. To avoid this it is essential that the electrosurgical cutting be well controlled with no starting delay during the incision. Delay in starting the cut will desiccate surrounding tissue including the pancreas. Technique is important in making the output controllable.

Cutting will not occur until sparks can jump freely from the electrode to the tissue. If the electrode wire is pulled firmly against the tissue, sparking will not occur until the tissue has been sufficiently desiccated and sparks are forced to jump across the dried tissue. Therefore, if there is a delay in the onset of cutting less force should be applied with the electrode wire, not more force. This is done by decreasing the tension on the wire, another important function of the assistant. An increase in tension on the wire (the natural tendency) will increase the delay, and when the electrode finally does begin to spark, the process may be more difficult to control, so that the incision is carried too far and in some cases results in perforation of the duodenum. The "rapid start" option available with some electrosurgical generators is also helpful in avoiding a delay in the onset of cutting.

As with endoscopic polypectomy, the beginning endoscopist is advised to obtain first-hand training in papillotomy from an endoscopist with experience in this procedure. He should then proceed by duplicating his instructor's equipment, generator settings, and technique as closely as possible.

HAZARDS OF ELECTROSURGERY

The potential hazards of endoscopic electrosurgery include high-frequency current burns, low-frequency shock and ventricular fibrillation, explosion of colonic hydrogen and methane, and pacemaker hazards.

Thermal Burns

If high-frequency current flows through a small area of contact in an unexpected and mistakenly created circuit, a high local current density and thermal burn can result. Visitors to the endoscopy unit or assistants can be part of such a circuit. Current may also follow unexpected paths if they are of less resistance than the intended circuit through the plate. Anything that breaks the high ohmic barrier of the skin increases this risk. Fortunately, in the majority of endoscopic electrosurgical procedures the patient is awake, albeit sedated. An electrosurgical thermal burn hurts. On the other hand, an unconscious patient can be severely burned.

A grounded electrosurgical unit is one in which the return circuit for current from the patient plate is connected to ground (Fig. 7–12A). The operational capacity of such a machine is not greatly impaired by a malfunction of the patient plate or wire, as current will always seek to complete a circuit. If a break occurs in the patient plate–return electrode component in the circuit, the current flow is from the active electrode through the patient, through a new path to ground, and hence back to the generator via its ground (Fig. 7–12B). Various points in a new circuit may be of high resistance. However, it will only be necessary to increase the power in order to continue electrosurgery. If a higher than usual setting is suddenly required to produce clinical effect with this type of machine, the power lines should be checked immediately, as this may indicate a break in the return to generator circuit. Most grounded units have a sentry circuit that monitors the integrity of the return connections. When there is a break an alarm sounds with some systems, although the better designed ones disable the output of the generator. Safety, therefore, depends largely on the sentry system. Sentry systems usually require a second connection to the patient plate, and should this connection be broken the sentry system becomes inoperative. Also, such a system does not monitor proper patient-to-plate contact.

The power output of many modern, solid state electrosurgical generators is electrically isolated. With this type of unit, in contrast to a grounded unit, the return circuit is not grounded (Fig. 7–13A). Therefore, no circuit through the patient to ground and back to the machine can exist. If there is a break in the dispersing plate (indifferent electrode) or cable, or even in patient-to-plate contact, the machine will automatically decrease its power output and cease to function (Fig. 7–13B). The chance of inadvertently causing a thermal burn in the patient is greatly decreased with this type of machine. Isolation of the patient plate and return wires also means that 60 cps fault currents cannot travel to ground by using the components of the electrosurgical system.

The isolated electrosurgical generator does have two inherent disadvantages that are not characteristic of a grounded unit. The first of these is that the problem of capacitance (vide infra) and induction of radio-frequency leakage current is compounded.

Secondly, if the active electrode of an isolated system is sparked to ground external to the patient, current can flow from ground through the patient and return to the generator via the plate and return cable. A thermal burn can result at the point of patient grounding if the current density is high. If the dispersing electrode of an isolated unit is inadvertently grounded, the system takes on the characteristics of a grounded electrosurgical unit.

Perfect isolation of an electrosurgical machine is not possible. If a machine is poorly isolated, current leakage can be large. A poorly isolated machine is inferior to a grounded one.

It should be obvious that one of the most

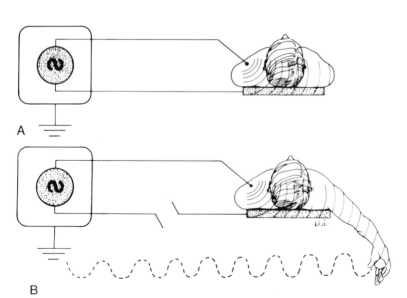

A

B

FIGURE 7–12. A, Schematic diagram of electrosurgical circuit through patient when the generator is grounded type. Current returns to the generator via the indifferent plate and return cord. B, A break in the return circuit is illustrated. High-frequency current follows a new path from the patient's hand to ground and then returns to the generator via ground. A thermal burn to the patient's right hand may occur.

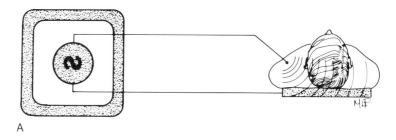

FIGURE 7–13. *A*, Schematic diagram of electrosurgical circuit when the generator is an isolated type. *B*, If a break occurs in the return circuit, the power output of the machine is shut down.

important safety features for use of electrosurgery is careful inspection of all equipment prior to use. The gastrointestinal assistant should be trained to follow a mental check list when electrosurgery is about to be performed to be absolutely certain that all components are in correct working order. The endoscopist should be alert to anything out of the ordinary in performing the procedure, such as an unusual demand for an increased power output from the generator or conversely a lack of power output and substandard clinical performance of the equipment. In circumstances such as these, the equipment and all connections should be checked immediately rather than persisting in the attempt to produce the desired effect.

Leakage Bypass Cables for Endoscopes

Some of the longer colonoscopes have over 150 pf of capacitive coupling between the snare wire and the metal supporting structure of the insertion tube and other metal parts of the endoscope. Capacitance and its effects can result in induction of high-frequency fault currents and thermal burns. Very-high-frequency currents can become capacitively connected to other conductors by virtue of proximity and in spite of insulating material. Generally, the degree of capacitance is related to the frequency of the current. The higher the frequency, the more

difficult it is to contain these fault currents. This is why electrosurgical generators operate near the lower end of the frequency range of electrosurgical currents.

Since the supporting structure of an endoscope consists of interconnecting helical steel bands covered by a layer of stainless steel wire mesh, the instrument may act as one component of a capacitor. (Refer to Chapter 2 for details of instrument construction). By means of this capacitive coupling, energy can be transferred from the active snare wire to the body of the colonoscope. This energy is a potential threat to the endoscopist and patient because the voltage that appears on the metal components of the colonoscope will try to drive a current from the exposed metal parts to the patient return electrode. The current may travel unexpected paths through the endoscopist's or patient's body to make this journey.

Because of their shorter length, some gastroscopes have only 25 pf capacitance between the active electrode wire and the metal structure of the endoscope. Therefore, some of the precautions discussed in the following paragraphs may not be necessary during endoscopic electrosurgery with these instruments.

Fortunately, the problem is not as severe as one would expect from 150 pf of coupling. This is because most of the metal framework of the colonoscope is just under the black plastic covering over the flexible portion. As a result, the metal components have much greater capacitance coupling to the patient's body than to the active electrode. This second capacitance couples most of the leakage current safely back to the patient's body and then to the patient return electrode.

Prior to 1977, many colonoscopes were manufactured with the metal frame connected to ground through the light source. It would seem that this should drain off any possible leakage current and therefore increase electrical safety, but this is not the case. Because the generator-to-patient circuit is isolated from ground, leakage current only returns to the generator via the patient return (indifferent) electrode. This can be accomplished by attaining the return electrode directly, or by reentering the patient's body and then the return electrode. Theoretically, the leakage current could cause injury if it entered the patient's body at some small point (high current density) of contact to ground.

Because of the theoretical threat posed by leakage current, at least two endoscope manufacturers recommend the use of leakage bypass cables. This may be referred to as an "S-cord" or a "bypass wire." In either case, the cables are designed to connect the metal frame of the endoscope to the patient return electrode (Fig. 7–14).

Bypass cables solve one safety problem but introduce a new one. If the indifferent plate electrode loses contact with the patient's skin, then the metal frame of the endoscope will become a substitute patient electrode, and all the electrosurgical currents will travel to it by all paths available. The circuit would then be from the active electrode through the patient to the endoscope, and finally from the endoscope to the generator via the patient re-

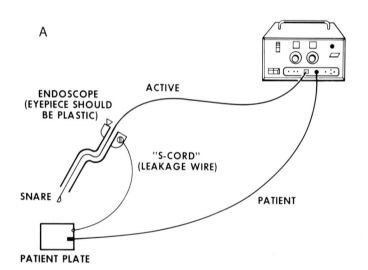

FIGURE 7–14. A, B: Diagrams showing connection of S-cord or leakage bypass wire.

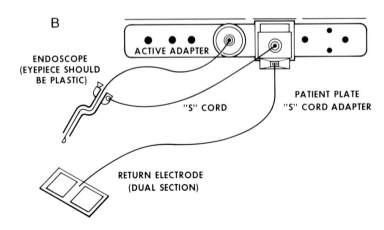

turn electrode, the latter now being merely a connection in the circuit. This is potentially worse than the original problem.

There are three ways to deal with the problem of capacitive coupling and leakage currents within the colonoscope.

In 1980, two manufacturers incorporated safety circuits into their electrosurgical generators. One type monitors the return currents from both the S-cord and the patient plate, insuring that the patient return electrode is collecting the majority of the current. Therefore, patient plate contact is assured. The other utilizes a "return electrode monitor" (REM) that has an interrogation circuit that measures the impedance at the pad-to-patient interface (patient return electrode) sites. This system serves two purposes. The first is to ensure that the patient is in contact with the indifferent (return) electrode. The second function is to ensure that the area of contact is sufficient to protect against a burn—that is, to ensure that partial contact with the plate does not result in a high current density in which the plate becomes an active electrode.

If an electrosurgical generator does not have an incorporated safety circuit, the bypass cable (S-cord) can be used if scrupulous care is taken to keep the patient return electrode in proper contact with the patient's skin.

The third alternative is to use the colonoscope without a bypass cable. If this is not used, the endoscopist must be aware that there will always be a small voltage on the metal parts of the colonoscope that theoretically could be a threat to him and his patient. The minimum precautions if this practice is adopted should be a plastic eyepiece to protect the endoscopist's eye and surrounding tissues from leakage current, and a thorough examination of the colonoscope insulation before each procedure.

Explosion Hazard During Colonoscopic Polypectomy

Because of hydrogen gas accumulations in the bowel, some authors recommend clearing the bowel with carbon dioxide gas before using electrosurgical current during colonoscopy. Since this gas is absorbed rapidly from the colon and eliminated by the lungs, its use may be contraindicated in patients with carbon dioxide retention due to chronic pulmonary disease. Rogers[6] demonstrated

that this technique was safe in normal patients and those with mild to moderate pulmonary disease, but he did not investigate its safety in patients with severe pulmonary disease and significant carbon dioxide retention.

Explosions are possible only when there is a mixture of a flammable gas and oxygen. To totally eliminate the possibility of an explosion one must either flush the bowel with an inert gas prior to beginning electrosurgery, or oxygen must not be introduced during the procedure. Most authors agree that there is no need for carbon dioxide.[7, 8] However, if carbon dioxide is not used, the risk of explosion is directly related to the adequacy of the preparation of the colon. If mechanical cleansing is unsatisfactory and the colon has not been evacuated properly, the risk of explosion increases. The use of mannitol for bowel preparation has been shown to produce dangerous concentrations of explosive gas in the colon.[9] If the preparation process includes mannitol, carbon dioxide must be employed for insufflation during colonoscopy if electrosurgery is to be used.

Pacemaker Hazards

Electrosurgery presents several special hazards to a patient with a pacemaker. Deactivation of certain demand pacemakers by electrosurgical frequency currents has been reported.[10] The bipolar electrodes of certain pacemakers are sensitive to radio-frequency electromagnetic radiation, which can be generated by an electrosurgery machine. No direct physical contact with the generating apparatus is required, and ventricular fibrillation has been produced experimentally with machines placed three feet from the subject.

A myocardial burn and ventricular fibrillation produced by the tip of an external pacemaker catheter has been reported.[11] The electrosurgical unit was a simple grounded type and a break occurred in the patient plate connection. In effect, the pacemaker catheter became the return electrode in the circuit. This would not occur with an isolated machine, since the output of this type of generator would shut down if current were not returning to the generator by the designated circuit.

For patients with pacemakers it is recommended that the indifferent electrode be placed in contact with the body at a point as far removed from the heart as possible. Radio-frequency current will follow the shortest path to the indifferent electrode, and if possible the heart should not be included in this path. Use of the bipolar output mode of the generator automatically fulfills this objective.

Early models of fixed-rate pacemakers were prone to increase their firing rate when subjected to radio-frequency interference. However, manufacturers of later models have incorporated various features into pacemaker design that block or control the effects of radio-frequency interference. Caution is required and consultation with pacemaker manufacturers is urged for patients with pacemakers for whom electrosurgery is being contemplated.

References

1. Curtiss LE. High frequency currents in endoscopy: A review of principles and precautions. Gastrointest Endosc 1973; 20:9–12.

2. Williams CB, de Peyer RC. Bipolar snare polypectomy—a safer technique for electrocoagulation of large polyp stalks. Endoscopy 1979; 1:47–50.

3. Gaisford WD. Gastrointestinal fiberendoscopy. Am J Surg 1972; 124:744–9.

4. Gaisford WD. Gastrointestinal polypectomy via the fiberendoscope. Arch Surg 1973; 106:458–62.

5. Dagradi AE, Riff DS, Norum TM, et al. A complication of colonoscopic (cecal) polypectomy. Am J Gastroenterol 1976; 65:449–53.

6. Rogers BHG. The safety of carbon dioxide insufflation during colonoscopic electrosurgical polypectomy. Gastrointest Endosc 1974; 20:115–7.

7. Ragins H, Shinya H, Wolff WI. The explosive potential of colonic gas during colonoscopic electrosurgical polypectomy. Surg Gynecol Obstet 1974; 138:554–6.

8. Bond JH Jr, Levitt MD. Factors affecting the concentration of combustible gases in the colon during colonoscopy. Gastroenterology 1975; 68:1445–8.

9. Taylor EW, Bentley S, Youngs D, et al. Bowel preparation and the safety of colonoscopic polypectomy. Gastroenterology 1981; 81:1–4.

10. Wajszczuk WJ, Mowry F, Dugan NL. Deactivation of a demand pacemaker by transurethral electrocautery. N Engl J Med 1969; 280:34–5.

11. Geddes LA, et al. New electrical hazard associated with electrocautery. Med Instrum 1975; 9:112–3.

Chapter 8

ENDOSCOPIC TREATMENT OF GASTROINTESTINAL BLEEDING: ELECTROCOAGULATION

JOHN P. PAPP, M.D.

An endoscopic approach to the treatment of upper gastrointestinal bleeding became possible with the development of flexible fiberoptic endoscopy. For four decades, only the esophagus and stomach could be viewed with rigid instruments. Simultaneous with the refinement of fiberoptic endoscopy was the development of better power sources that enabled the endoscopist to use a coagulation mode in addition to the cutting mode. This chapter discusses the experimental work and clinical applications of various methods of electrocoagulation in the treatment of gastrointestinal bleeding. A discussion of one promising new approach, the heater probe, is also included. The use of lasers for gastrointestinal hemostasis is presented in Chapter 9, and the principles of electrosurgery may be found in Chapter 7.

BIPOLAR ELECTROCOAGULATION

In order to reduce tissue injury and yet produce effective hemostasis, an effort was made to develop bipolar electrocoagulation probes. In effect, this type of instrument combines two active electrodes in a single device that can be passed through the accessory channel of an endoscope. The large surface area return electrode is eliminated from the electrosurgical generator system.

Open laparotomy canine experiments have demonstrated a reduced depth of tissue injury with bipolar, compared with monopolar, electrocoagulation.[1, 2] However, about twice the number of applications and joules* of energy were required to stop bleeding of experimentally produced standard-sized acute ulcers using a bipolar probe in conjunction with a Valleylab SSE2-K (Valley Lab, Boulder, CO) electrosurgical generator, when compared with the use of a 3 mm diameter monopolar electrode.[2] Machicado et al.[3] studied the effect of bipolar electrocoagulation on standard-sized esophageal and duodenal ulcers, using the Valleylab SSE2-K unit and prototype electrode (MediTech Corp., Watertown, MA). Bleeding was stopped in all 20 esophageal ulcers after $21(\pm 1)$ applications; transmural injury occurred in 15%. Hemostasis was achieved in 21 bleeding duodenal ulcers, but $30(\pm 4)$ applications were required, with associated transmural injury in 20%.

Johnston et al.[4] compared endoscopically applied monopolar and bipolar electrocoagulation in the treatment of bleeding gastric ulcers in dogs. A monopolar probe (Model CD-3L, Olympus Corp., New Hyde Park, NY) was used with the infusion of saline and compared with a Medi-Tech bipolar probe. The monopolar probe produced hemostasis in all 30 bleeding ulcers with a mean of 16 applications of 0.5 second duration. Transmural injury occurred with treatment of 16 of the 30 ulcers. Bleeding from 29 of the 30 ulcers was stopped with the bipolar

---

*A joule is the energy expended in 1 second by a current of 1 ampere at a potential of 1 volt.

143

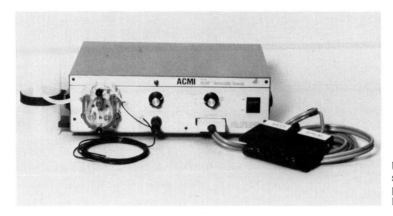

FIGURE 8–1. BICAP hemostatic system (American-ACMI). Note foot pedals for irrigation via probe and bipolar probe'at left.

probe after a mean of 25 applications, and in 5 instances transmural injury was noted. These findings were similar to those of Protell et al.[2] Johnston and coworkers[4] concluded that the bipolar electrode produced less mucosal injury, that it was technically more difficult to use than the monopolar probe, and that both were effective in producing hemostasis.

A new type of bipolar electrode was developed in 1979 by Drs. David Auth and Fred Silverstein in Seattle, Washington and subsequently marketed as the BICAP hemostatic system (American-ACMI, Stamford, CT) (Fig. 8–1). The bipoles include 3 equally spaced longitudinal electrodes along the side and 3 over the rounded tip of a cylindrical probe, making a total of 6 circum-active electrode points in a single device (Fig. 8–2) Two probe sizes, 2.4 mm and 3.2 mm diameter,

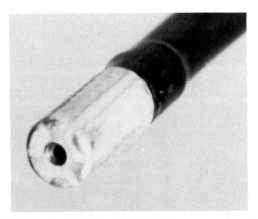

FIGURE 8–2. Distal tip of BICAP electrode probe. Note arrangement of six electrode points. Three (representing one electrode pole) arise from center of probe, and three (representing the other pole) are arranged in between. This allows the endoscopist to apply the probe from several angles with contact of at least two opposite electrode poles to tissue.

are available. A central opening in the probe allows constant or intermittent fluid infusion. Auth and colleagues[5] reported effective hemostasis in experimental canine gastric ulcers with limited depth of injury with this device (set at output 7 for 1 second).

The technique of application of the BICAP is very important. The electrode is placed within 2 to 3 mm of a bleeding vessel, and firm pressure is applied. Subsequently, the BICAP hemostatic source is activated at a setting of 9 for 2 seconds. This sequence is repeated, working around the circumference of the bleeding vessel until coagulation has occurred. The probe is then placed firmly on the vessel itself, and several applications are made until complete hemostasis occurs.

In a preliminary study by Verhoeven and coworkers[6] using the BICAP probe in patients, hemostasis was achieved in 10 of 10 bleeding gastric ulcers (bleeding resumed in one), 4 of 5 bleeding duodenal ulcers (one recurrent hemorrhage), and 2 of 2 marginal ulcers. Subsequently, Tytgat's group (personal communication, 1983) used this probe in 40 patients, with initial success in 35 and failure in 5. The 5 failed treatments included 4 duodenal ulcers and 1 gastric ulcer. In 9 of the 35 successfully treated patients, bleeding resumed after several hours to several days. Nine patients required surgery and 6 died (4 postoperative). The lesions treated included 30 gastric and duodenal ulcers, 2 Mallory-Weiss lacerations, 5 telangiectasias, 2 bleeding sites postpolypectomy, and 1 instance of suture line bleeding after surgery.

A multicenter clinical trial reported by Gilbert et al.[7] assessed the efficacy and safety of the BICAP, using the 2.4 mm probe. Bleeding was stopped in 15 of 16 gastric ulcers and in 11 of 14 duodenal ulcers, but hemorrhage recurred in 7 gastric and 3 duodenal ulcers. Hemorrhage was controlled in 3 of 4 stomal ulcers and 3 of 4 Mallory-Weiss lacerations. Last, 6 telangiectatic lesions were treated and bleeding resumed in 1 of these. In summary, electrocoagulation using the BICAP probe stopped active bleeding from 38 lesions. However, when the failure to control bleeding is combined with episodes of resumed bleeding, 50% of gastric ulcers and 43% of duodenal ulcers were considered as treated unsuccessfully.

Risa and colleagues[8] reported similar results using the 2.3 mm BICAP probe. Of 12 patients with actively bleeding duodenal ulcers, bleeding was stopped in 5, could not be stopped in 4, and recurred in 3 patients. Hemostasis was achieved in 3 of 8 patients with actively bleeding gastric ulcers, 2 ulcers continued to bleed and 3 resumed bleeding after hemostasis. Bleeding from 2 marginal ulcers, 1 Mallory-Weiss laceration, and 1 telangiectasia was successfully treated. The success rate for BICAP treatment in this series, including absence of recurrent bleeding, was 41.6% and 37.5% in bleeding duodenal and gastric ulcers, respectively.

Winkler et al.[9] reported complete success with use of the BICAP in 13 patients. The bleeding lesions treated included esophagitis, an ulcer in a hiatal hernia, Mallory-Weiss lacerations, gastritis, duodenitis, duodenal ulcers, vascular malformations of the duodenum, and hemorrhagic adenocarcinoma of the stomach. No recurrent bleeding was reported.

Jensen and coworkers[10] tested either the heater probe or BICAP in the treatment of 11 bleeding episodes from ulcers. Two patients resumed bleeding and 2 continued to bleed and required surgery. Based on a 63% success rate, they felt that further study and evaluation of the BICAP in the treatment of gastrointestinal bleeding would be worthwhile.

Yamamoto et al.[11] reported on the use of a modified bipolar probe in experimentally produced bleeding in dogs. The electrodes of this 3.4 mm bipolar electrocoagulation device, which were spaced 0.5 mm apart in a square pattern, were 2.4 mm long and 1 mm in diameter. Distilled water was constantly perfused at 20 ml/min through the electrode. An Olympus UES power source at a coagulation dial setting of 1- and 2-second pulses was used. The bipolar probe was applied directly to bleeding vessels. A mean of 3 applications produced hemostasis in the case of bleeding mesenteric and gastric serosal vessels. Since the probe was effective in animal experiments, it was used to treat 35 episodes of gastrointestinal bleeding in 32 patients (16 gastric ulcers, 8 duodenal ulcers, 3 stomal ulcers, bleeding gastric erosions in 4 patients, 2 gastric carcinomas, 1 Mallory-Weiss laceration, and 1 episode of post-biopsy bleeding). Bleeding was arrested in all patients after a mean of 6.8 applications. Five individuals resumed bleeding from 2 hours to 15 days after treatment, and 2 of them underwent successful repeat bipolar electrocoagulation.

The advantages of this type of bipolar electrocoagulation technique were summarized by Yamamoto and coworkers[11] as follows: no adherence to tissue because of constant profusion of distilled water; effective application of the probe both tangentially and vertically; and limited depth of tissue injury.

A new bipolar technique, the "hot squeeze," was recently described by Mills et al.[12] They designed a bipolar electrode that could be used for grasping a bleeding vessel to occlude its lumen and for applying bipolar electrocoagulation to produce hemostasis. These workers compared their "hot squeeze" technique for hemostasis with the BICAP, liquid and dry monopolar electrocoagulation, and the heater probe; they concluded that bond strength (mean bursting pressure of a vessel) was significantly better with their technique. They believed the major advantage of their technique to be better sealing of larger bleeding vessels in comparison with other endoscopic thermal methods, but they recognized that the use of this technique is difficult. It remains to be seen whether endoscopists will be able not only to identify an actively hemorrhaging vessel but also to grasp and hold it long enough to apply several pulses of thermal energy.

HEATER PROBE

The development of a heater probe for endoscopic use was reported by Protell et al,[13] in 1978. In essence, they refined a centuries-old method to stop bleeding by using a "hot iron." The heater probe is a hollow aluminum cylinder with an inner coil. Its outer surface is coated with Teflon (Fig. 8–3). The aluminum cylinder effectively transfers heat to tissue from either its ends or sides. Two probe sizes are available (3.2 mm and 2.4 mm in diameter). Both have a coaxial channel for washing blood and debris from

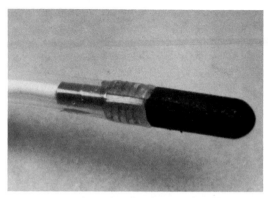

FIGURE 8–3. Distal tip of heater probe. Note outer
Teflon-coated surface and inner cylinder that can be
seen through the transparent outer tubing proximal
to Teflon-coated tip.

the target area. They can be inserted through
the accessory channel of most endoscopes.
Both probes reach operating temperature,
which is preset at 140 to 150 degrees centi-
grade, in less than 5 seconds. The amount of
energy in joules is also preset, prior to using
the probe, at 1 to 29 joules. Heat is produced
by dissipation of electrical energy from within
the probe tip to the aluminum cylinder and
then conveyed to the target tissue.

The technique of application is important.
The probe is applied to a vessel with firm
pressure in order to join its walls. Several
applications of energy at 1-second durations
may be necessary to produce hemostasis. The
usual amount of energy used per application
is 15 joules.

In endoscopic canine experiments, the 3.2
mm diameter heater probe stopped bleeding
in 18 of 19 unoperated heparinized dogs.[13]
A mean of 15 applications was required for
complete hemostasis. Although there were
no perforations, 6 dogs had histologic damage to all layers of the gastric wall. This
finding caused some concern over predictability of tissue injury depth.

Jensen and colleagues[14] reported less injury using a 3.2 mm probe on standardized
canine gastric ulcers in an open-closed heparinized model. In their study, bleeding was
stopped in 14 of 15 ulcers, using 15 joules
per 12 applications, but 13% had full-thickness injury. When 20 joules per 10 applications were used, 14 of 15 ulcers stopped
bleeding and no full-thickness injury was
noted. Similarly, the 2.4 mm probe at 15 and
20 joules, using approximately the same
number of applications, produced no full-
thickness injury.

Swain et al.[15] compared the effectiveness
of dry monopolar, liquid monopolar (i.e.,
simultaneous water perfusion and electrocoagulation), bipolar (BICAP), and heater
probe instruments for controlling active
bleeding. All were equally effective at optimal
pulse settings of 20 joules, 70 joules, 17
joules, and 15 joules, respectively. However,
liquid and dry monopolar electrocoagulation
produced full-thickness injury in 58% and
69% of experimental canine ulcers, respectively. These workers concluded that the
heater probe was almost as effective as monopolar electrocoagulation (dry or liquid), but
that the heater probe's modest tissue damage
made it the most promising technique.

Jensen and coworkers[10] reported use of
the heater probe and BICAP in patients with
bleeding ulcers and hemangiomata, but did
not indicate which modality was used or how
many applications were necessary to produce
hemostasis. However, it was concluded that
the two techniques were safe and effective,
and that controlled randomized trials should
be initiated.

The advantages of the heater probe are as
follows: it is portable; it is without electrical
hazard, because electrical currents are completely contained within the catheter and
controller; it has a coaxial channel for water
irrigation; the rate of energy delivered is
controlled and preset; the tip of the probe is
Teflon-coated to lessen adherence to tissue;
it can be applied at different angles in addition to directly vertical; it is effective (Plate
8–1); and it is relatively inexpensive. Further
clinical studies with a controlled randomized
format are eagerly awaited.

MONOPOLAR ELECTROCOAGULATION

There are 3 basic electrosurgical modes:
cut, fulgurate, and desiccate. The word coagulation can mean either fulguration or
desiccation. Fulguration is defined as sparking to tissue to produce necrosis without a
cutting effect. Electrosurgical desiccation is
defined as tissue necrosis caused by the application of an electrosurgical electrode to
tissue so that there is no sparking or cutting
effect.

When an active electrosurgical electrode is
pressed firmly against moist tissue such as
gastrointestinal mucosa, no sparking occurs.
This mode is called electrocoagulation (desiccation). When the power source is activated,
current flows from the active electrode

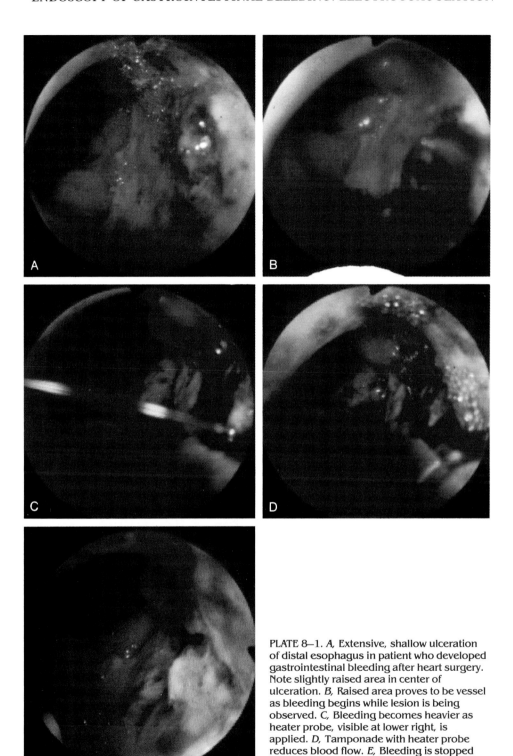

PLATE 8–1. *A*, Extensive, shallow ulceration of distal esophagus in patient who developed gastrointestinal bleeding after heart surgery. Note slightly raised area in center of ulceration. *B*, Raised area proves to be vessel as bleeding begins while lesion is being observed. *C*, Bleeding becomes heavier as heater probe, visible at lower right, is applied. *D*, Tamponade with heater probe reduces blood flow. *E*, Bleeding is stopped after three applications. (Photographs courtesy M.V. Sivak, Jr., M.D.)

through the target tissue, through the patient, and returns through an indifferent electrode of large surface area on the patient's skin to the generator. Tissue necrosis is controlled by current density. The heating effect of electrosurgical current is always proportional to the current density, which varies inversely with the area of the electrode.

These principles are considered in detail in Chapter 7. Although there are many variables in the mode of electrocoagulation, experience over the last several years has led to the conclusion that the most important parameter is the amount of energy delivered to the target tissue per application. This parameter is measured in joules.

Early efforts to study the effects of electrocoagulation focused on the size and depth of tissue injury, duration of current application, and amount of current used. Blackwood and Silvis[16] were first to report attempts to quantitate the effects of electrocoagulation on the canine stomach. They used a monopolar electrode with a Bovie electrosurgical unit, which is classified as a spark-gap generator, at settings 25, 50, 75, and 100 for 3 seconds. The animals were gastroscoped and lesions were produced in the body of the stomach at various Bovie settings with the monopolar electrode "held lightly" against the mucosa. They concluded that a setting of 50 or less on the Bovie produced optimal coagulation; lesions of known diameter could be produced accurately; depth of injury correlated with the diameter of the mucosal defect; and the technique could have important therapeutic and research applications.

Blackwood and Silvis,[17] continuing their interest in endoscopic monopolar electrocoagulation, studied the effect of amperage and duration of current application on the depth of tissue necrosis in the gastric wall of anesthetized dogs. In these experiments the Cameron-Miller electrosurgical unit (Model 26-265G) was used rather than the Bovie unit. Numerous lesions were produced at varying durations of current flow and varying settings. Single applications of 400 to 425 milliamperes (mA) for 1.0 to 1.5 seconds resulted in mucosal necrosis and minimal muscle necrosis. When the time of application was prolonged to 2 seconds or the current increased to 500 mA, there was a significant increase in the extent of muscle necrosis. Repeated applications to the same area increased the depth of necrosis by 70% to 80%. Electrode contact with mucosa was difficult to standardize, resulting in variable application of thermal energy, resistance, and current flow. These workers concluded that standardization of the technique of electrocoagulation presented difficulties.

Using a Cameron-Miller monopolar coagulator electrode (Model 80-7051) and coagulator unit (Model 80-7910), the author and coworkers[18] produced canine gastric mucosal lesions endoscopically via gastrotomy at varying durations of current flow and generator output settings. Contrary to the findings of Blackwood and Silvis,[17] the size of the ulcer produced did not correlate with depth of injury at the higher settings of 6.5 and 7.0. At settings 5 through 6, the mucosa could be electrocoagulated for 1 to 7 seconds with depth of injury limited to the submucosa. When submucosal coagulation necrosis occurred, large vessels were found to be thrombosed, with no effect on deeper vessels. Variable degrees of injury occurred at higher settings and at longer application times because of the formation of coagulum around the monopolar electrode and the impossibility of applying the same electrode pressure for each lesion produced.

The author and coworkers[19] produced duodenal and esophageal lesions using the same canine model and the same probe and coagulator unit described above at variable durations of current flow and generator settings. Coagulation necrosis of the mucosa and the internal muscle layer occurred in the duodenum at settings 4.5, 5.0, and 5.5 at 1- and 3-second coagulation intervals. Higher settings resulted in transmural injury. Whereas 600 mA at setting 5.0 for 1 second produced mucosal injury in the duodenum, 600 mA at setting 6.0 for 1 second resulted in transmural injury. Therefore, one cannot depend on amperage alone to gauge depth of injury. Hyperamylasemia was noted after duodenal electrocoagulation but did not correlate with the extent of coagulation necrosis. Mucosal injury was produced in the canine esophagus at settings 4.5 to 5.0 for 1 second, but higher settings for 1 and 3 seconds resulted in transmural injury. It was concluded that electrocoagulation in the duodenal bulb was safe at settings of 4.5 to 5.5 for 1 to 3 seconds, but was safe only at settings of 4.5 to 5 for 1 second in the esophagus.

Amperage used in a given application of current was again an unreliable predictor of depth of injury.[19] Application of 600 mA at setting 5.5 for 1 second resulted in muscularis injury in the esophagus; at setting 5.0 for 3 seconds, transmural injury occurred. Sugawa et al.[20] reported very different findings using the Cameron-Miller electrode and coagulator unit in the esophagus; at output dial settings of 5.0 and 7.0 for 5 to 7 seconds, no transmural injury was noted. Mann and Mann,[21] using the Cameron-Miller electrode (Model

80-7960), found no transmural injury in the esophagus or duodenum at settings 5, 6, and 7 for 1, 3, and 5 seconds. However, transmural injury was found with applications at dial settings 5 to 7 for 5 seconds. These discrepancies may be explained by the model and technique selected. Mann and Mann[21] used the open canine model in which the stomach, duodenum, and esophagus were opened surgically and lesions made by monopolar electrocoagulation. The author and coworkers[18, 19] made lesions via the endoscope through a gastrotomy, and all dogs in their studies were sacrificed at 7 days for histologic evaluation. Another variable that was dissimilar in the studies of Mann and Mann,[21] Sugawa et al.[20] and the author et al.[18, 19] was the pressure of the monopolar electrode on the mucosa. These variables may explain why Sugawa et al.[20] reported that settings of 3.0 and 5.0 for 3, 5, 7, and 10 seconds resulted in only muscular layer necrosis and no serosal injury in the dog stomach.

Piercey and coworkers[22] have systematically evaluated the efficacy and safety of monopolar electrocoagulation using an analogue computer inserted between an electrosurgical generator and the active electrode. The analogue computer measured actual energy delivered to the target tissue and could be adjusted to deliver a predetermined amount of energy. By using a force gauge with a predetermined energy of 20 joules, the effect of electrode pressure on the depth of injury was measured. When electrocoagulation was applied as might be done clinically, or predetermined by power leveling, all bleeding from ulcers in an open-stomach canine model stopped, but full-thickness injury to the gastric wall occurred with equal frequency with each method. It was concluded that despite analogue computer assistance in controlling energy delivered during monopolar electrocoagulation of experimental canine gastric ulcers, the depth of injury was unpredictable and excessively deep.

Techniques

Therapeutic endoscopy is impossible unless the stomach is clear of blood clots. Once the patient has been hemodynamically stabilized, an Edlich gastric lavage tube should be passed per os into the stomach and lavage with 2 or more liters of iced saline instituted. Thereafter, the patient is sedated as required. Intravenous diazepam is recommended. After passing the endoscope with the patient in the left lateral decubitus position, a careful inspection of the esophagus should be made for varices, esophagitis, ulceration, tumor, and Mallory-Weiss laceration. Once in the stomach, the endoscope is passed along the lesser curvature to the antrum, avoiding the gastric pool. After inspection of the antrum and pylorus, the endoscope is advanced into the duodenal bulb and the second portion of duodenum. If no lesion is seen and the bile is yellow, the endoscope can be withdrawn into the stomach for delineation of the source of bleeding. Care must be taken not to occlude the suction channel while aspirating blood and fluid from the gastric pool, because vision may be partially or totally obscured. If this does occur, it can usually be cleared by forcing a jet of water or air through the accessory channel. This can be done with a modified large-bore needle with attached syringe, which is inserted through the accessory channel valve. The needle should be modified by blunting the tip.

If an ulcer is found that is without stigmata of recent bleeding, no endoscopic therapy is needed, because it is unlikely that the ulcer will rebleed. If active bleeding from a visible vessel, a visible vessel without bleeding, a clot in an ulcer base with blood oozing from its base, or a "red spot" is seen in the crater, then therapeutic endoscopy should be considered, because of the high risk of continued bleeding or resumption of bleeding with these types of endoscopic findings (Plate 8–2).[23] Electrocoagulation should not be attempted if torrential bleeding is present or in esophageal varices.

The endoscopist must make a judgment when bleeding is very heavy. If the patient is in a precarious state, even a brief unsuccessful attempt at electrocoagulation may result in valuable time lost before surgery. The endoscopist must consider the nature of the bleeding, the status of the patient, and his or her own capabilities. Occasionally, a clinical situation arises in which bleeding is torrential but surgery cannot be considered for other reasons. The techniques of Gaisford,[24] Matek et al.,[25] and the author[26] may be used in applying monopolar electrocoagulation.

According to the method of Gaisford,[24] once a bleeding source is identified, a jet of saline via an irrigator electrode cannula is directed at the lesion to identify precisely the bleeding vessel. If the vessel is 1 mm or less

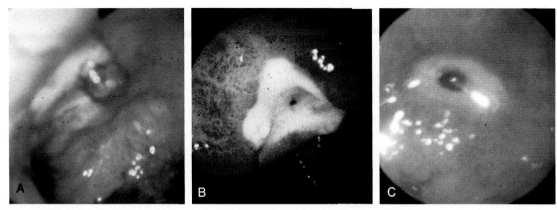

PLATE 8–2. Endoscopic view of ulcers. A, Duodenal ulcer with visible vessel in center of crater. B, Gastric ulcer with "red spot" in center of crater. C, Duodenal ulcer with "red spot" in center of crater.

in diameter, an ACMI prototype monopolar electrode approximately 2.4 mm in diameter is placed directly on the vessel, and pressure is applied to coapt the vessel. Simultaneously, coagulating current is applied in short durations of about 1 second (range 0.56 to 2 seconds). If a larger vessel is found, applications of coagulating current are made around the circumference of the lesion until bleeding stops. Subsequent to this, current may be applied directly to the vessel. The number of applications around and on the vessel depend upon the specific lesion but usually range from 4 to 10. Gaisford has used several different power sources, most commonly the Valley Lab SSE-2 generator at coagulation dial settings from 5 to 7.

Matek et al.[25] modified the technique of the author[26] by simultaneously instilling distilled water via a special electrode known as the EHT electrode (electro-hydro-thermo-electrode) during monopolar electrode application. A high-frequency Electrotom 170 RF machine (Martin, Tuttlingen) was used as the power source. Five holes were placed in the tip of the monopolar electrode and distilled water was perfused at a rate of 20 to 40 ml per minute. Insufflation of CO_2 as well as instillation of saline and hydrogen peroxide through the probe were also studied, using standard canine gastric ulcers; however, distilled water proved to be the most satisfactory. At a generator output level of 6, the electrode was activated against the bleeding lesion while simultaneously perfusing distilled water. Current was continuously applied, in a few cases up to 180 seconds.

Matek and colleagues[25] described the following advantages of their technique: (1)

lower levels of energy were used; (2) coagulation time could be lengthened in a therapeutic range with reduced penetration of tissue; (3) charring at the bleeding site was almost completely avoided; and (4) visibility was improved.

These workers[27] further modified their technique by adding a spring mechanism that guaranteed that the EHT electrode was pressed against tissue with a virtually constant force. Experimentally, 50 standardized gastric bleeding lesions were successfully arrested in dogs using this technique at power settings 6 through 8.

The author[26] described a third technique in 1976. Once a lesion is identified endoscopically as the site of bleeding, the Cameron-Miller monopolar electrocoagulation electrode is passed through the accessory channel and placed within 2 to 3 mm of the vessel. The electrode is activated for 2 to 3 seconds per application. Several applications may be necessary to stop bleeding, as the electrode is moved circumferentially around the vessel. The Cameron-Miller electrocoagulation unit (Model 80-7910) is usually set on 5. If coagulum accumulates around the electrode, the probe must be withdrawn from the endoscope and cleaned.

If blood is found oozing from beneath a clot, the clot can be either washed away by a jet of water (rarely successful) or removed by the electrode. The electrode can be used to dislodge the clot from the ulcer or can be embedded into the clot and, at a power setting of 4, coagulated onto the probe. The clot is then lifted off the ulcer and the electrode withdrawn into the accessory channel, causing the clot to fall off. (Charred tissue and clot on the surface of the electrode act as an insulating layer that increases electrical resistance and impedes the output of the generator.) The ulcer base is then viewed and therapy directed at a specific bleeding point. An arterial vessel should never be directly electrocoagulated, because it will virtually explode from the vaporizing heat, resulting in active bleeding from a retracted vessel, which is a difficult therapeutic problem for the endoscopist.

If active bleeding is present, visibility will often be poor, and therefore the patient and endoscope must be positioned in such a way that the stream of blood is directed away from the endoscope. This sometimes means that the patient must be turned to a supine or, in some techniques (e.g., Gaisford), to a right lateral decubitus position. The supine position should be avoided because of the hazards of vomiting and aspiration of blood and clots when bleeding is active. The electrode should not be activated while going through blood. It should be activated when firmly on mucosa. Steady, firm pressure must be applied which nevertheless permits some give and elastic response of the wall at the treatment site. Once bleeding stops, one must resist the temptation to coagulate the vessel directly.

The amount of energy required to stop bleeding will vary with the size of the vessel, the amount of impedance, the milieu of tissue and fluids around the vessel, and how often the electrode is cleaned. In an attempt to quantitate the amount of energy in joules needed to produce hemostasis, the author and colleagues[28] used an analogue computer in conjunction with an electrosurgical generator. An average of 103 joules per 4 applications was necessary to stop a bleeding duodenal rim vessel 1 mm in diameter, at a setting of 5 for 2.5 seconds duration per application. Nonbleeding visible vessels 2 and 3 mm in diameter required 5 applications for a duration of 2 seconds each at a setting of 5. The range of joules used was 63 to 105. Three arteriovenous malformations were electrocoagulated at setting 5 for approximately 2 seconds per each of 5 applications, using 30 to 56 joules.

The principle in the author's technique is that coagulation of a bleeding vessel occurs in the submucosa. By applying heat energy around the vessel, the tissue surrounding it shrinks thus narrowing the vessel. Simultaneously, the application pressure exerted with the electrode coapts the vessel. These two events result in coagulation of the vessel and cessation of bleeding.

Clinical Experience

Early experience using monopolar electrocoagulation in Europe was reported by Koch et al.[29] They described successful coagulation procedures in 15 bleeding patients; however, 3 perforations and 1 death occurred. This report dampened enthusiasm for further evaluation of monopolar electrocoagulation in Europe during the early 1970's. In 1970 Youmans and coworkers[30] reported the use of monopolar coagulation with a cystoscope via a gastrostomy to produce hemostasis of a bleeding vessel in a malignant ulcer in one patient and in multiple stress ulcerations in another patient. This successful use of monopolar electrocoagulation stimulated several research groups in the United States to search intensively for ways of using monopolar electrocoagulation to control bleeding in the gastrointestinal tract. While experimentation proceeded, marked advances in the development of fiberoptic endoscopes and power units also occurred. These allowed for better visualization, for better aspiration of blood via larger suction channels, and the ability to visualize not only the esophagus and stomach, but also the duodenum.

Since 1971, at the Blodgett Memorial Medical Center, the author has performed diagnostic endoscopy in 681 patients to evaluate the cause of their acute upper gastrointestinal bleeding. Of this group of patients, 353 had ulcer disease as follows: 205 duodenal, 176 gastric (including 26 marginal ulcers), and 10 esophageal. Of the 205 duodenal ulcers, 52 were actively bleeding; 51 of the 176 gastric ulcers, or 28.9%, were actively bleeding (44 of 150 gastric ulcers and 7 of 26 marginal ulcers). Arterial bleeding was present in 2 of 10 esophageal ulcers. This experience is similar to the American Society for Gastrointestinal Endoscopy (ASGE) national study on upper gastrointestinal bleeding that is discussed in Chapter 6.

In an uncontrolled but consecutive series from 1971 to 1983, all patients with upper gastrointestinal bleeding were endoscoped within 12 hours after admission (Blodgett Memorial Medical Center) or, if in-hospital, within 6 hours after bleeding occurred. No patient was excluded from consideration for endoscopic hemostasis because of severity of hemorrhage. About 20% of these patients bled while being treated in-hospital for other problems. Early experience in this series has been reported.[31-34] A total of 119 patients have undergone endoscopic electrocoagulation on 123 occasions. In addition to the patients with bleeding duodenal (52), gastric (51), and esophageal (2) ulcers (mentioned in the previous paragraph, 16 of 48 patients had Mallory-Weiss lacerations with active arterial bleeding. Fourteen of the Mallory-Weiss lacerations were successfully electrocoagulated. This experience was reported in part in 1980.[35] In addition to the above lesions, treatment was successful in a miscellaneous group of patients with the following lesions: 2 gastric fundal varices, 2 esophageal ulcers, and 8 gastric and duodenal arteriovenous malformations.

Of the 119 patients, electrocoagulation was unsuccessful in 8 (6 duodenal ulcers and 2 Mallory-Weiss lacerations) for two reasons: (1) torrential bleeding obscuring vision and (2) inability to place the probe near the bleeding vessel due to the positioning angle of the probe and vessel. These patients were treated surgically after endoscopic identification of the site of bleeding. Of the remaining 111 patients, 12 resumed bleeding from 4 hours to several days later (6 gastric and 6 duodenal ulcers). Four patients were retreated with complete cessation of bleeding. Seven underwent surgery; 1 death was due to persistent bleeding from an ulcer. One patient had a cardiac arrest while awaiting surgery.

Many of the patients in this study were elderly. The average age of those with gastric and duodenal ulcers was 63 and 69, respectively. Multiplicity of medical problems requiring intensive care was common in this group. Despite the severity of their illnesses, only 10 of 119 patients died during a 1-year follow-up. Six died while hospitalized, but only 1 from persistent bleeding despite surgery. This mortality of 5% (6 of 119) is significantly better than that in other reports, where mortality is 20% to 50% in patients older than 60.[36] Four patients died several months later from carcinomatosis. It is important to point out that those patients in this study with active bleeding from ulcer disease or Mallory-Weiss lacerations would have required surgery had electrocoagulation not been done. The risk of surgery was considered to be high in more than one third of the patients, and over 20% were not considered to be surgical candidates under any circumstances. No morbidity or mortality occurred as a result of electrocoagulation. In addition, the number of hospital days and cost of hospitalization were substantially reduced, based on retrospective analysis.[33, 34]

Other physicians have reported their experience with monopolar electrocoagulation. In 1975 Sugawa et al.[37] treated 6 patients and achieved initial hemostasis in all. The bleeding lesions were as follows: 1 Mallory-Weiss laceration, 1 gastric ulcer, gastric erosions in 3 patients, and 1 gastric polyp. Two patients resumed bleeding and required surgery (1 gastric erosion and 1 gastric ulcer). In 1978, Volpicelli and colleagues[38] reported complete initial success with monopolar coagulation in 12 patients with ulcers (6 duodenal, 5 gastric, and 1 esophageal). There was no further bleeding from 1 gastric ulcer that had resumed bleeding and was retreated.

Gaisford[39] reported a large series in 1979. His success rate was 92% in treatment of 71 patients with endoscopic electrocoagulation. Hemorrhage recurred in 6 patients. Gastric ulcers were responsible in 4 of these patients, who were successfully re-electrocoagulated. Of the remaining 2 patients with recurrent hemorrhages, 1 had a Mallory-Weiss laceration, and 1 a gastric leiomyosarcoma; both underwent surgery. The total series of lesions treated by Gaisford in the 71 patients were as follows: 4 esophageal ulcers, 6 Mallory-Weiss lacerations, 2 gastric varices, 29 gastric ulcers (8 with erosive gastritis), 2 gastric polyps, 2 gastric leiomyomas, 3 pyloric channel ulcers, 13 duodenal ulcers, and 8 jejunal ulcers. No complications were reported.

In 1980, Hojsgaard and Wara[40] reported an 89% success rate for cessation of bleeding (41 of 46 patients). Of the 52 patients in their study, treatment could not be attempted in 6 because of massive bleeding. Five patients who were unsuccessfully electrocoagulated underwent surgery with no further bleeding. Seven patients had recurrent hemorrhages between the first and sixth day after electrocoagulation (4 gastric and 3 duodenal ulcers). If the 5 unsuccessfully treated patients and the 6 untreated cases are considered together, then the success rate was 80% in this series. The following lesions were electrocoagulated: 15 gastric ulcers, 10 prepyloric ulcers, 12 duodenal ulcers, and 9 anastomotic ulcers. One fourth of the patients were 78 years of age or older. Similar results were obtained when Wara et al.[41] combined electrocoagulation with cimetidine treatment.

When their series became larger, Wara et al.[42] again reported their experience. Over a period of 1 year, 69 consecutive patients with active bleeding verified by endoscopy were entered into their study. Electrocoagulation failed to control bleeding in 5 patients and could not be applied in 6 because of massive bleeding in 4 and technical difficulty in the treatment of 2. Electrocoagulation was repeated successfully in 6 of 9 patients with recurrent bleeding. Retreatment was not considered in the remaining 3. These workers used a specially designed Olympus monopolar cannula that allowed simultaneous irrigation and coagulation. The electrosurgical unit employed was an Erbotom F2, using 40% to 60% of its maximum 170 watt power output. No morbidity or mortality resulted from the electrocoagulation procedure. Wara and coworkers concluded that endoscopic electrocoagulation can be successful, especially if applied during quiescent phases of massive hemorrhage.

Fischer[43] reported successful electrocoagulation in 33 of 34 bleeding lesions using the Cameron-Miller suction-coagulator (Model 80-7051) and Valley Lab SSE-2 and Neo-Med cautery units. Several short applications, lasting 0.5 to 2 seconds, of coagulation current were applied at a setting of 5, with irrigation between applications. Endoscopy was performed in all patients on an emergency basis to evaluate upper gastrointestinal bleeding. The following lesions were treated: 16 duodenal ulcers, 11 gastric ulcers, gastric erosions in 3 patients, 1 marginal ulcer, 2 Mallory-Weiss lacerations, and duodenitis in 1 patient. Bleeding from 1 Mallory-Weiss laceration could not be stopped and the patient was treated surgically. Fischer reduced his operative mortality from approximately 20% to zero in patients with active upper gastrointestinal bleeding who required surgery, because the use of monopolar electrocoagulation changed an emergent operation to a more elective type in many patients.

When the total number of patients studied in these various reports are combined, electrocoagulation was successful in achieving hemostasis in 258 of 284 patients (91%). Endoscopic electrocoagulation was unsuccessful in 9% of patients, who then under-

went surgery. About 10% had recurrent hemorrhages (28 of 284), but 11 of the 28 underwent repeat electrocoagulation which resulted in no further bleeding.

Arteriovenous Malformations

The technique of monopolar electrocoagulation of arteriovenous malformations is the same whether the lesion is in the stomach or duodenum. The electrode is pressed firmly, but allowing for some "give" in the wall and mucosa, at the periphery of the lesion and moved in a circular direction until the lesion is completely encircled. Only one application of energy is given per area. If an arteriovenous malformation is greater than 1 cm in diameter, repeat electrocoagulation working toward the center may be necessary at another time. The center of the lesion should never be electrocoagulated initially since significant bleeding may result.

The author and coworkers[28] successfully treated 3 patients with arteriovenous malformations (1 stomach and 2 duodenum) while studying the effects of electrocoagulation with an analogue computer. Time of coagulation varied from 0.9 to 2.2 seconds. Thirty to 56 joules per application were used with the Cameron-Miller coagulator unit on setting 5.

Farup et al.[44] used monopolar electrocoagulation successfully in the treatment of 5 patients with arteriovenous malformations (2 gastric and 3 duodenal). Sassaris et al.[45] treated 2 patients with gastric vascular ectasias with a hot biopsy forcep; in only 1 patient was the treatment successful. However, other investigators have had complete success in preventing further bleeding with use of the hot biopsy forcep.[46, 47]

Because of the possibility of using monopolar electrocoagulation in the treatment of vascular ectasias in the colon, the author and coworkers[48] studied the effect of the Cameron-Miller electrode and Olympus hot biopsy forcep on dog colon mucosa, using electrocoagulation and fulguration at varying durations of current flow and generator output settings. Applications of more than 1 second at settings of 4.5 to 6.0 on the Cameron-Miller unit and of 3 to 6 on the Valley Lab SSE3 unit produced transmural tissue injury.

Rogers[34] used the hot biopsy forcep to treat 35 patients with arteriovenous malformations in the colon, with no morbidity or mortality. This technique is considered in detail in Chapter 44. Other investigators have had success with this method.[34, 49, 50]

The Visible Vessel

It is interesting that only a few authors have pointed out the significance of the visible vessel in an ulcer crater, despite the increasingly aggressive use of endoscopy as a diagnostic and therapeutic modality in the 1970's in patients with upper gastrointestinal bleeding.[51, 52] Until recently, the early observations of these few authors were largely ignored. Now questions have been raised such as: "Why do patients rebleed?" and "Are there stigmata which indicate that surgical, endoscopic, or medical therapy is appropriate?"

Foster et al.[23] defined stigmata of recent bleeding for ulcers as follows: (1) fresh bleeding from a lesion, (2) fresh or altered blood clot or black slough adherent to the ulcer, and (3) a vessel protruding from the base or margin of an ulcer.

Storey and colleagues[53] prospectively studied 47 patients with ulcers and stigmata of bleeding. Nineteen of 34 patients (56%) with a visible vessel sustained recurrent bleeding compared with 1 of 13 patients (8%) with other stigmata of bleeding. In 40 patients with ulceration and no stigmata, no further bleeding occurred. Vallon et al.[54] studied the significance of the presence of stigmata in the ulcer base of untreated patients in a randomized trial. Of 13 actively bleeding ulcer vessels, 11 (83%) continued to bleed. Hemorrhage resumed in 8 of 16 visible vessels that were not bleeding initially. In some cases, spots were noted in the ulcer crater, and in 4 of 39 such instances (10%) there was recurrent bleeding. Of 39 patients with no stigmata of hemorrhage, only 1 patient had recurrent bleeding. However, repeat endoscopic evaluation showed that the actual lesion causing the bleeding was missed at the initial endoscopy.

Similar findings have been reported by Domschke et al.[55] In their study, 56 ulcers with visible vessels resumed bleeding; recurrent hemorrhage occurred in 8% of ulcers with blood oozing from the ulcer or around a clot, a black spot in the crater, or blood clot adherent to the crater. No bleeding occurred in those patients with ulcer disease but no stigmata of hemorrhage.

Swain and coworkers[56] reported recurrent hemorrhage in 42 of 72 patients (58%) with visible-vessel–associated ulcer disease compared with 2 of 28 patients (7%) with other stigmata of hemorrhage. Several authors have reported that actively bleeding vessels continue to bleed or resume bleeding in 78% to 100% of cases.[54, 57–59]

In a randomized prospective study of 32 patients with recent upper gastrointestinal bleeding from ulcers that had visible vessels at endoscopy, 16 patients were randomized to a control group and treated medically.[60] The other 16 patients had immediate electrocoagulation using the Cameron-Miller monopolar probe. In this study by the author,[60] the control group comprised 7 patients with gastric and 7 with duodenal ulcers. Six of the visible gastric ulcer vessels and 7 of the duodenal ulcer visible vessels resumed bleeding (a total of 81%). Of the 15 patients treated immediately with electrocoagulation, 10 had visible gastric ulcer vessels and 6 had duodenal ulcer vessels. Repeat hemorrhage occurred from a visible vessel in a gastric fundal ulcer after 3 days; the remaining 15 patients (93%) had no further bleeding. The length of hospitalization for those successfully treated by immediate electrocoagulation was 8.3 days, similar to that for the 3 patients in the control group who stopped bleeding spontaneously, and 52% better than the mean of 15.9 days for those with recurrent bleeding. Cost of hospitalization was reduced an average of $1900 (1979 dollars) in those treated immediately by electrocoagulation, compared with those with recurrent hemorrhage.[60] There is no question that the endoscopic findings of a visible vessel and other stigmata of recent hemorrhage associated with an ulcer identify patients at high risk for further bleeding. It is logical that endoscopic therapy should be applied in these cases to control bleeding and prevent further episodes as well as to eliminate the need for surgery.

CONCLUSION

Appropriate measures to resuscitate the patient with gastrointestinal bleeding must be undertaken prior to diagnostic or therapeutic endoscopy. In order to have adequate endoscopic visualization, gastric lavage must be performed to remove clots. The only appropriate initial diagnostic modality is upper gastrointestinal endoscopy. Once a source of bleeding is found, the endoscopist must study the lesion for evidence (stigmata) of recent bleeding. If, in the case of an ulcer, a vessel is seen in the crater or at its margin, or if other stigmata are present, the endoscopist must decide whether an endoscopic treatment modality should be applied.

Bipolar electrocoagulation has been only recently introduced for widespread clinical use. Although it was effective according to one report, success was limited in other studies, and the rate of recurrent hemorrhage was high. Further comparison studies with monopolar electrocoagulation in upper gastrointestinal bleeding are required if this modality is to gain acceptance as a treatment option.

Initial data relating to the heater probe suggest that it is safe and effective. However, much of this information is drawn from studies in experimental models, and although this method is promising, clinical trials are necessary to prove its effectiveness and safety in bleeding patients.

Monopolar electrocoagulation has been studied to a much greater extent and is reported to be effective in stopping active bleeding in over 80% of instances in which it has been employed. However, clinical data are derived almost entirely from uncontrolled series.

There are several possible techniques for using monopolar electrocoagulation. Meticulous attention to detail is required in using any of the three described in this chapter. Skill and experience are also without doubt important elements in the effectiveness of this procedure. The amount of energy (which can be measured in joules) per unit of time is important and will vary for different lesions and patients. Monopolar electrocoagulation is not only effective in stopping active bleeding from ulcers and Mallory-Weiss lacerations but it also prevents recurrent bleeding from vascular malformations and from visible vessels found in association with ulcer craters.

Monopolar electrocoagulation appears to be safe and effective. It is also relatively inexpensive and readily available. It has been shown to reduce the need for emergency surgery as well as the length and cost of hospitalization.

Editor's note: Some recent data support the effectiveness of bipolar electrocoagulation in the endoscopic control of bleeding from peptic ulcers. See reference 61.

References

1. Moore JP, Silvis SE, Vennes JA. Evaluation of bipolar electrocoagulation in canine stomachs. Gastrointest Endosc 1978; 24:148–51.
2. Protell RL, Gilbert DA, Silverstein FE, et al. Computer-assisted electrocoagulation: bipolar vs. monopolar in the treatment of experimental gastric ulcer bleeding. Gastroenterology 1981; 80:451–5.
3. Machicado GA, Jensen DM, Tapia JI, Mautner W. Treatment of bleeding canine duodenal and esophageal ulcers with argon laser and bipolar electrocoagulation. Gastroenterology 1981; 81:859–65.
4. Johnston JH, Jensen DM, Mautner W. Comparison of endoscopic electrocoagulation and laser photocoagulation of bleeding canine gastric ulcers. Gastroenterology 1982; 82:904–10.
5. Auth DC, Gilbert DA, Opie EA, Silverstein FE. The multipolar probe—a new endoscopic technique to control gastrointestinal bleeding. (Abstr) Gastrointest Endosc 1980; 26:63.
6. Verhoeven AGM, Bartelsman JFWM, Huibregtse K, Tytgat GNJ. A new multipolar coagulation electrode for endoscopic hemostasis. In: Stomach Diseases. Current Status. Proceedings of the 13th International Congress on Stomach Diseases. Amsterdam-Oxford, Princeton: Excerpta Medica, 1981; 216–21.
7. Gilbert DA, Verhoeven T, Jessen K, et al. A multicenter clinical trial of the BICAP probe for upper gastrointestinal bleeding. (Abstr) Gastrointest Endosc 1982; 28:150.
8. Risa L, Miscusi G, Caruso C. L'elettrocoagulatore multipolare BICAP net trattament delle emmoragie digestive. Advan Dig Surg Endosc (Rome) 1983; 117–23.
9. Winkler WP, Comer G, McCray RS. Initial experience with BICAP multipolar electrocautery in the control of upper gastrointestinal hemorrhage. (Abstr) Gastrointest Endosc 1983; 29:169.
10. Jensen DM, Machicado GA, Tapia JI, Beilin DB. Clinical hemostasis with heater probe or bipolar electrocoagulation for severe gastrointestinal bleeding. (Abstr) Gastrointest Endosc 1983; 29:162.
11. Yamamoto H, Hajiro K, Matsui H, et al. Endoscopic bipolar electrocoagulation: development of a new bipolar coagulator for stopping gastrointestinal bleeding. Gastroenterol (Jpn) 1982; 17:75–9.
12. Mills TN, Swain CP, Dark JM, et al. The "hot squeeze" bipolar forceps. A more effective endoscopic method for stopping bleeding from large vessels in the gastrointestinal tract. (Abstr) Gastrointest Endosc 1983; 29:184–5.
13. Protell RL, Rubin CE, Auth DC, et al. The heater probe: A new endoscopic method for stopping massive gastrointestinal bleeding. Gastroenterology 1978; 74:257–62.
14. Jensen DM, Tapia JI, Machicado GA, et al. Endoscopic heater and multipolar probes for treatment of bleeding canine gastric ulcers. (Abstr) Gastrointest Endosc 1982; 29:151.
15. Swain CP, Mills TN, Shemesh E, et al. Which electrode? A consumer's guide to endoscopic electrocoagulation of upper gastrointestinal bleeding. (Abstr) Gastrointest Endosc 1983; 29:187–8.
16. Blackwood WD, Silvis SE. Gastroscopic electrosurgery. Gastroenterology 1971; 61:305–14.
17. Blackwood WD, Silvis SE. Standardization of electrosurgical lesions. Gastrointest Endosc 1974; 21:22–4.

18. Papp JP, Fox JM, Wilks HS. Experimental electro-coagulation of dog gastric mucosa. Gastrointest Endosc 1975 22:27–8.

19. Papp JP, Fox JM, Nalbandian RM. Experimental electrocoagulation of dog esophageal and duodenal mucosa. Gastrointest Endosc 1976; 23:27–8.

20. Sugawa C, Shier M, Lucas CE, Walt AJ. Electrocoagulation of bleeding in the upper part of the gastrointestinal tract. A preliminary experimental clinical report. Arch Surg 1975; 110:975–9.

21. Mann SK, Mann NS. Effect of monopolar electrocoagulation on esophagus, stomach, and duodenum in dogs. Am J Gastroenterol 1979; 71:568–71.

22. Piercey JR, Auth DC, Silverstein FE, et al. Electro-surgical treatment of experimental bleeding canine gastric ulcers: development and testing of a computer control and a better electrode. Gastroenterology 1978; 74:527–34.

23. Foster DN, Miloszewski KJ, Losowsky MS. Stigmata of recent haemorrhage in diagnosis and prognosis of upper gastrointestinal bleeding. Br Med J 1978; 1:1173–7.

24. Gaisford WD. Endoscopic electrohemostasis of active upper gastrointestinal bleeding. Am J Surg 1979; 137:47–53.

25. Matek W, Fruhmorgen P, Kaduk B, et al. Modified electrocoagulation and its possibilities in the control of gastrointestinal bleeding. Endoscopy 1979; 11:253–8.

26. Papp JP. Endoscopic electrocoagulation of upper gastrointestinal hemorrhage. JAMA 1976; 236:2076–9.

27. Matek W, Fruhmorgen P, Kaduk B, et al. The healing process of experimentally produced bleeding lesions after hemostatic electrocoagulation with simultaneous instillation of water. Endoscopy 1980; 12:231–6.

28. Papp JP, Auth DC, Silverstein FE. Analogue computer evaluation of monopolar electrocoagulation in patients having had UGI bleeding. (Abstr) Gastrointest Endosc 1980; 26:73.

29. Koch H, Pesch HJ, Bauerle H, et al. Experimentelle Untersuchungen und Klinische Erfahrungen zur Electrokoagulation Blutende Lasionen im oberen Gastrointestinaltrakt. Fortschr Endoskop 1972; 10:67–71.

30. Youmans CR Jr, Patterson M, McDonald DF, Derrick JR. Cystoscopic control of gastric hemorrhage. Arch Surg 1970; 100:721–3.

31. Papp JP. Endoscopic electrocoagulation in upper gastrointestinal hemorrhage. A preliminary report. JAMA 1974; 230:1172–3.

32. Papp JP. Endoscopic electrocoagulation of upper gastrointestinal hemorrhage. A preliminary report. JAMA 1974; 230:1172–3.

33. Papp JP. Endoscopic electrocoagulation of actively bleeding arterial upper gastrointestinal lesions. Am J Gastroenterol 1979; 71:516–21.

34. Papp JP: Electrocoagulation. In: Papp JP, ed. Endoscopic Control of Gastrointestinal Hemorrhage. Boca Raton: CRC Press, 1981; 31–42.

35. Papp JP. Electrocoagulation of actively bleeding Mallory-Weiss tears. Gastrointest Endosc 1980; 26:128–9.

36. Himal HS; Watson WW, Jones CW et al. The management of upper gastrointestinal hemorrhage: a multiparametric computer analysis. Ann Surg 1972; 179:489–93.

37. Sugawa C, Shier M, Lucas CE, Walt AJ. Electrocoagulation of bleeding in the upper part of the gastrointestinal tract. A preliminary experimental clinical report. Arch Surg 1975; 110:975–9.

38. Volpicelli NA, McCarthy JD, Bartlett JD, Badger WE. Endoscopic electrocoagulation: an alternative to operative therapy in bleeding peptic ulcer disease. Arch Surg 1978; 113:483–6.

39. Gaisford WD. Endoscopic electrohemostasis of active upper gastrointestinal bleeding. Am J Surg 1979; 137:47–53.

40. Højsgaard A, Wara P. Gastroduodenal haemorrhage treated by endoscopic electrocoagulation. Ugeskr Laeg 1980; 142:501–10.

41. Wara P, Højsgaard A, Amdrup E. Endoscopic electrocoagulation combined with cimetidine: a pilot study of the applicability in active bleeding from gastroduodenal ulcer. Acta Chir Scand 1980; 146:431-4.

42. Wara P, Højsgaard A, Amdrup E. Endoscopic electrocoagulation—an alternative to operative hemostasis in active gastroduodenal bleeding? Endoscopy 1980; 12:237–40.

43. Fischer MJ. Endoscopic electrocoagulation of bleeding upper gastrointestinal lesions. Mil Med 1981; 146:407–9.

44. Farup PG, Rosseland AR, Stray N, et al. Localized telangiopathy of the stomach and duodenum diagnosed and treated endoscopically. Endoscopy 1981; 13:1–6.

45. Sassaris M, Pang G, Hunter F. Telangiectasia of the upper gastrointestinal tract: Report of six cases and reviews. Endoscopy 1983; 15:85–88.

46. Weaver GA, Alpern HD, Davis JS, et al. Gastrointestinal angiodysplasia associated with aortic valve disease: Part of a spectrum of angiodysplasia of the gut. Gastroenterology 1979; 77:1–11.

47. Weingart J, Lux G, Elster K, Ottenjann R. Recurrent gastrointestinal bleeding in Osler's disease successfully treated by endoscopic electrocoagulation in the stomach. Endoscopy 1975;7:160–4.

48. Papp JP, Nalbandian RM, Wilcox RM, Ludwig EE. Experimental evaluation of electrocoagulation and fulguration of dog colon mucosa. Gastrointest Endosc 1979; 25:140–6.

49. Nüesch HJ, Kobler E, Bühler H, et al. Angiodysplasien des Kolons—Diagnose und Therapie. Schweiz Med Wochenschr 1979; 109:607–8.

50. Tedesco FJ, Griffin JW Jr, Khan AQ. Vascular ectasia of the colon: clinical, colonoscopic, and radiographic features. J Clin Gastroenterol 1980; 2:233–8.

51. Cotton PB, Rosenberg MT, Waldron RP, Axon AT. Early endoscopy of oesophagus, stomach and duodenal bulb in patients with haematemesis and melena. Br Med J 1973; 2:505–9.

52. Allen HM, Block MA, Schuman BM. Gastroduodenal endoscopy: management of acute gastrointestinal hemorrhage. Arch Surg 1973; 106:450–5.

53. Storey DW, Bown SG, Swain CP, et al. Endoscopic prediction of recurrent bleeding in peptic ulcers. N Engl J Med 1981; 305:915–6.

54. Vallon AG, Cotton PB, Laurence BH, et al. Randomized trial of endoscopic argon laser photocoagulation in bleeding peptic ulcers. Gut 1981; 22:228–33.

55. Domschke W, Lederer P, Lux G. The value of emergency endoscopy in upper gastrointestinal

bleeding: Review and analysis of 2014 cases. Endoscopy 1983; 15:126–31.

56. Swain CP, Bown SG, Salmon PR, et al. Nature of the bleeding point in massively bleeding gastric ulcers. (Abstr) Gastroenterology 1983; 84:1327.

57. MacLeod IA, Mills PR, MacKenzie JF, et al. Neodymium yttrium aluminum garnet laser photocoagulation for major haemorrhage from peptic ulcers and single vessels: a single blind controlled study. Br J Med 1983; 286:345–8.

58. Rutgeerts P, Vantrappen G, Broeckaert L, et al. Controlled trial of Yag laser treatment of upper digestive hemorrhage. Gastroenterology 1982; 83:410–16.

59. Griffiths WJ, Neumann DA, Welsh JD. The visible vessel as an indicator of uncontrolled or recurrent gastrointestinal hemorrhage. N Eng J Med 1979; 300:1411–3.

60. Papp JP. Endoscopic electrocoagulation in the management of upper gastrointestinal tract bleeding. Surg Clin North Am 1982; 62:797–806.

61. O'Brien JD, Day SJ, Burnham WR. Controlled trial of small bipolar probe in bleeding peptic ulcers. Lancet 1986; 1:464–7.

Chapter 9

LASERS AND GASTROINTESTINAL DISEASE

DAVID FLEISCHER, M.D.

The therapeutic extension of fiberoptic endoscopy is a natural consequence of its diagnostic use. Of the numerous modalities available, laser therapy is one of the most fascinating and appealing because it is a powerful means of treatment delivered with pinpoint precision and without actual tissue contact. The laser–tissue interaction is predictable, and the range of application for this single modality is very wide. It should be emphasized that laser technology is in its infancy; therefore, it is difficult to estimate its future impact on gastrointestinal endoscopy. This chapter focuses on the development of lasers for use in gastroenterology and on their current applications, limitations, and exciting prospective for potential new roles in the treatment of gastrointestinal disease.

HISTORICAL BACKGROUND

Although Einstein is credited with conceptualizing the laser in 1917, it was four decades later when the first laser was actually built. In 1960, Maiman[1] unveiled the ruby laser. During the 1960's there was some experimentation with laboratory lasers of different wavelengths for treatment of a variety of tumors, some gastrointestinal. The first attempt to transfer the photocoagulative application in use in ophthalmology to the digestive tract was by Goodale et al.[2] in 1970. Citing the work of Ketcham and coworkers,[3] who had demonstrated that laser radiation could produce small vessel thrombosis, they reported control of bleeding gastric erosions using a carbon dioxide laser with a rigid gastroscope. A flexible waveguide that would allow carbon dioxide laser use with flexible

158

fiberoptic endoscopes had not yet been developed.

Nath and coworkers,[4, 5] working with the Kiefhaber group, were the first to describe transmission of a laser beam through a flexible endoscope. This set the stage for endoscopic laser therapy of gastrointestinal disease in humans. About the same time in the mid-1970's, Dwyer et al.[6] in the United States and Kiefhaber[5] and Frühmorgen and colleagues[7] in Germany were successful in using endoscopic laser therapy to produce hemostasis in patients with upper gastrointestinal bleeding. This remained the major focus of laser therapy for several years. In 1979, Kiefhaber,[8] in a review of the use of lasers for gastrointestinal bleeding, reported that there were 37 centers (3 in the United States) using lasers for this purpose.

Early in the 1980's it became apparent that the laser could be applied to problems other than gastrointestinal bleeding; interest in the therapy of neoplastic disease burgeoned. In concert with the generally encouraging reports of laser therapy for bleeding and of expanding applications to other digestive disorders, enthusiasm for lasers grew until, by 1984, more than 400 centers (200 in the United States) were equipped with lasers.

PHYSICAL PRINCIPLES OF LASER THERAPY

The word LASER is an acronym for *l*ight *a*mplification by *s*timulated *e*mission of *r*adiation. This phenomenon occurs when a substance is excited to a higher energy state and stimulated to emit light as it returns to a lower energy state. The process can be amplified when the photons produced interact

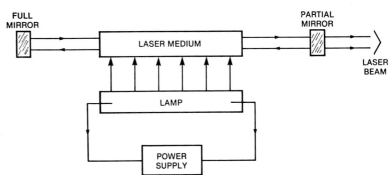

FIGURE 9–1. Schematic of solid laser medium excited by an optical source. (From: Enderby C. Medical laser fundamentals. *In*: Fleischer D, Jensen D, Bright-Asare P, eds. Therapeutic Laser Endoscopy in Gastrointestinal Disease. Boston: Martinus Nijhoff, 1983.)

between two mirrors. If one of the mirrors is 100% reflective and the other only partially reflective, the beam can escape from the mirrored chamber. The laser light is intense, monochromatic, and easily focused. These characteristics allow lasers to be utilized for endoscopic therapy.

The heart of any laser is the medium that is used to generate the beam. The type of medium determines the wavelength that is produced, and this in turn gives each type of laser its specific properties. If the lasing medium is a gas (e.g., argon), it can be excited by an electrical discharge; if it is a solid (e.g., neodymium:yttrium aluminum garnet; Nd:YAG) a different energy source must be used—in most cases an intense lamp light. The lamp is energized by an electrical power supply (Fig. 9–1).

Three main types of laser have been used therapeutically in medicine (Table 9–1). These are the argon, carbon dioxide, and Nd:YAG lasers. As mentioned, wavelengths differ among these three lasers and this affects the visibility of the beam and depth of penetration. Only the argon and Nd:YAG lasers are being used with flexible waveguides; therefore, only these two have been used with fiberoptic instruments. Technologic advances may allow use of the carbon dioxide laser with flexible instruments in the near future.

Laser–Tissue Interaction

Cummins[9] emphasized that the fundamental events that occur with laser–tissue interaction are absorption and scattering. The differences in laser-tissue interactions among the three lasers are mainly due to the presence of water and hemoglobin in biologic tissues. In each, energy absorption varies according to wavelength (Fig. 9–2). Hemoglobin is highly absorptive of light at short wavelengths, but its light-absorptive capacity is low within and beyond red wavelengths. Water is highly absorptive with long wavelengths, but its absorption is low in the visible range. The energy produced by the argon laser, therefore, is highly absorbed by hemoglobin, but energy absorption is low for water. Both hemoglobin and water absorb to some extent the energy produced at the wavelength of the Nd:YAG laser.

Scattering is the second important factor.[10] Some energy is scattered as a laser beam enters tissue. This occurs initially as the beam strikes a given surface; some further scattering occurs within the tissue substance. Upon entering tissue, scattering may occur in many directions, and as a result energy is either absorbed or rescattered. Tissue interaction is therefore more complex than simple, straight-line penetration of the beam (Fig. 9–3). Penetration is defined and measured as the depth at which the energy level is only

TABLE 9–1. **Characteristics of Medical Lasers Currently in Use***

Type	Wavelength (μm)	Penetration Depth	Visible	Adaptable to Flexible Endoscope
Nd:YAG	1.06	Least superficial	No	Yes
Argon	0.05	Intermediate	Yes	Yes
Carbon dioxide	10.6	Most superficial	No	No

*From: Fleischer D. Lasers in gastroenterology. Am J Gastroenterol 1984; 79:406–15.

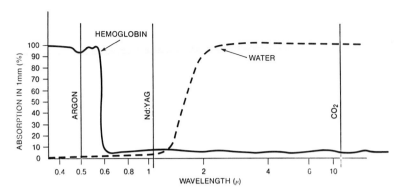

FIGURE 9–2. Wavelength range and absorption of argon, Nd:YAG, and carbon dioxide lasers. Argon has high absorption in hemoglobin, and carbon dioxide has high absorption in water. (From: Enderby C. Medical laser fundamentals. *In:* Fleischer D, Jensen D, Bright-Asare P, eds. Therapeutic Laser Endoscopy in Gastrointestinal Disease. Boston: Martinus Nijhoff, 1983.)

10% of the initial energy level. The tissue penetration of the Nd:YAG laser is about 4 mm; that is, at a tissue depth of 4 mm, the amount of energy remaining is about 10% of the incident energy. Argon laser penetration is approximately 1 mm, and that for the carbon dioxide laser is about 0.1 mm.

The phenomena of absorption and scattering are interdependent and determine the pattern of light intensities at all points within the tissue. Wavelength, tissue constituents, and therapeutic spot size are the major determinants of the intensity pattern. Spot size is the area of the tissue surface that is struck by the laser energy. Spot size for a given fiber diameter with a fixed angle of beam divergence is proportionate to the physical distance between the fiber and tissue (Fig. 9–4). The actual effect on tissue is further dependent on the power output at which the machine is set and on the pulse duration (length of time that the laser beam is applied

to tissue). As tissue is heated, critical temperature levels for endothelial damage, cell death, protein coagulation, blood vessel constriction, and tissue vaporization are attained. These translate into endoscopic manifestations and histologic events that determine the anatomic outcome (Table 9–2).

Mechanism of Clinical Effects

From a clinical point of view the tissue events can be classified into two categories: coagulation and vaporization. It is the coagulative effect that achieves hemostasis in acute gastrointestinal bleeding and eliminates lesions that have a potential to bleed, such as vascular ectasias and visible vessels in ulcer craters. It is the vaporizing effect by which tissue is ablated in endoscopic laser photodestruction of neoplastic tissue and by which normal tissue is incised for therapeutic purposes (e.g., infundibulotomy, drainage of cys-

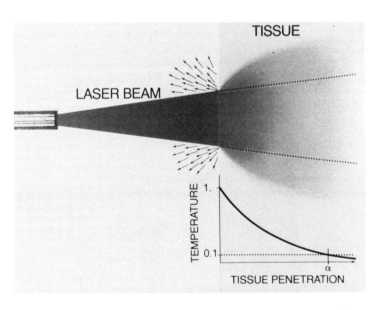

FIGURE 9–3. Tissue penetration. Laser beam penetration is not uniform and depends on the interrelationship of absorption and scattering. (From: Enderby C. Medical laser fundamentals. *In:* Fleischer D, Jensen D, Bright-Asare P, eds. Therapeutic Laser Endoscopy in Gastrointestinal Disease. Boston: Martinus Nijhoff, 1983.)

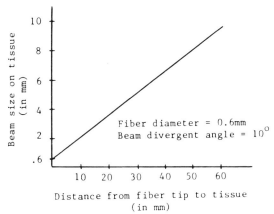

FIGURE 9–4. Relationship of beam size on tissue and distance from tip of fiber to tissue. With a divergent beam, spot size will be related to distance. (From: Enderby C. Medical laser fundamentals. *In:* Fleischer D, Jensen D, Bright-Asare P, eds. Therapeutic Laser Endoscopy in Gastrointestinal Disease. Boston: Martinus Nijhoff, 1983.)

tic lesions). These applications are cataloged in Table 9–3.

COAGULATIVE LASER THERAPY

Animal Experiments

Although the initial experimental assessment of laser therapy for gastrointestinal hemorrhage was performed with a carbon dioxide laser,[2] most of the important work in animals was performed with argon and

TABLE 9–2. Relationship Between Temperatures and Tissue Event*

Critical Temp. (°C)	Histologic Event	Endoscopic Manifestation
45	Cell death, edema, endothelial damage, vasodilation	Erythema, edema cuff
60	Protein coagulates	Tissue turns gray-brown, blood turns black
80	Denatured collagen contracts, blood vessels constrict	Tissue "puckers"
100	Tissue water boils	Vaporization causes divot
210+	Dehydrated tissue burns	Blackened tissue disappears, ± glowing embers

*From: Fleischer D.: Lasers in gastroenterology. Am J Gastroenterol 1984; 79:406–15.

TABLE 9–3. Gastrointestinal Application of Lasers*

Coagulation
    Active hemorrhage
        Active bleeding
        Recent bleeding (e.g., visible vessel)
    Recent hemorrhage—not currently bleeding
        Angiodysplasia
        Varices
        Hemorrhoids
Vaporization
    Neoplastic disease
        Palliation
        Curative treatment
        Ancillary (e.g., placement of esophageal prosthesis)
    Benign stricture or web
    Biliary disease
        Infundibulotomy
        Strictures
        Fracture "gallstones"
    Cyst drainage

*From: Fleischer D.: Lasers in gastroenterology. Am J Gastroenterol 1984; 79:406–15.

Nd:YAG lasers. In 1974, Frühmorgen et al.[7] described the acute effect of the argon laser on the gastrointestinal viscera of human autopsy specimens and cats. The first report from the United States of laser-induced hemostasis in an animal model was by Dwyer et al.[11] in 1975.

Extensive animal experiments with lasers in the control of bleeding have been done by Silverstein and coworkers.[12–14] They evaluated laser-induced hemostasis in ulcers created by the instillation of 0.1 N hydrochloric acid and by a mechanical "ulcer maker" in both endoscopic and laparotomy models. These investigators also carefully examined the histologic effect of photocoagulation. The majority of these studies were done with the argon laser and power outputs varying from 1 to 10 watts. The development by these workers of a gas-jet–assisted waveguide provided a means of blowing blood away from a bleeding site, "thereby exposing the underlying vessel to the argon beam, rather than having the energy of the blue-green beam absorbed by the overlying red blood."[12]

Others amplified the results of these initial investigations. Butler and Morris[15] used the argon laser to treat endoscopically induced bleeding lesions in the duodenum of rhesus monkeys. Bown and coworkers[16] evaluated the efficacy and safety of the argon laser. Jensen et al.[17] compared argon laser photocoagulation and bipolar electrocoagulation in the treatment of bleeding duodenal and esophageal ulcers. In 1979, both Silverstein[18] and Waitman[19] and their colleagues compared the argon laser with the Nd:YAG laser in the treatment of experimentally induced bleeding canine gastric ulcers. Each group concluded that both types of lasers achieved hemostasis, but that the argon laser produced less tissue damage and was therefore safer.

Dixon et al.[20] studied the safety of the Nd:YAG laser with regard to penetration and risk of perforation, and determined that an energy density (watts/cm²) 3 times that required to control bleeding was necessary to cause perforation. All of 9 dogs with experimentally induced perforations survived a 2-week observation period.

Similar studies with the Nd:YAG laser were performed by Rutgeerts[21] and Johnston and their coworkers.[22] After extensive investigation, they determined optimal Nd:YAG laser treatment parameters that maximize hemostatic efficacy while minimizing tissue injury. Longer pulse duration, larger spot size, and increased total energy were associated with the greatest degree of tissue injury. Geboes et al.[23] demonstrated by means of transmission electron microscopy that laser phototherapy produces endothelial damage followed by formation of a platelet thrombus in the damaged vessel. In further experiments with bleeding canine gastric ulcers, Johnston and coworkers[24] discussed the limitations and set guidelines for endoscopic use of the argon laser.

Dennis et al.,[25] using an experimental model having a single bleeding artery at the base of a gastric ulcer, observed that treatment of this type of single bleeding arterial lesion with the Nd:YAG laser resulted in much less tissue damage than that encountered in experiments that utilized the mechanical "ulcer maker." This was an important paper because this study approximated more nearly the situation with bleeding gastric ulcers in humans. With the "ulcer maker," an elliptical-shaped tissue is cut from the mucosa, and bleeding arises from several incised vessels in the margin and base rather than from a single artery. Although experimental models employing the "ulcer-maker" have been extremely useful in gathering data, the development of the single-vessel model underscores the fact that data gathered in animal experiments are not always fully translatable as events in humans.

The aforementioned experimental investigations were concerned with photocoagula-tion of bleeding ulcers and erosions. The unique work of Jensen et al.[26] assessed endoscopic laser therapy for bleeding esophageal varices in a canine model. The Nd:YAG and argon lasers were compared with a variety of other hemostatic modalities (injection sclerotherapy, heater probe, ferromagnetic tamponade, bipolar electrocautery, and monopolar electrocautery). Only the Nd:YAG laser and injection sclerotherapy proved useful in stopping acute variceal hemorrhage in this model.

Human Studies

Acute Hemorrhage

The first reports of endoscopic laser therapy in humans were published in the mid-1970's. At about the same time, Dwyer,[6] Kiefhaber,[5] and Frühmorgen[7] and their colleagues achieved hemostasis in humans. Although the initial reports were composed of uncontrolled series, they are noteworthy. In 1979, Kiefhaber[8] summarized the worldwide experience with endoscopic laser therapy of upper gastrointestinal bleeding (Fig. 9–5). A total of 1729 patients had been treated. Initial control of bleeding was achieved in 84% (range 70%–100%) of 196 patients treated with argon laser in 7 centers. In 90% (range 74%–100%) of 1533 patients treated with the Nd:YAG laser in 31 centers, initial hemostasis was accomplished. This survey did not consider the incidence of recurrent bleeding or follow-up of patients.

The largest experience with laser therapy for gastrointestinal bleeding is that of Kiefhaber.[27] From 1975 to 1982, he treated 994 episodes of acute bleeding in 625 patients. Bleeding lesions included esophageal varices, Mallory-Weiss lacerations, ulcers, erosions, vascular anomalies, and tumors. His overall success rate for achieving initial hemostasis was 94%. He reported a reduced mortality for acute and chronic bleeding from ulcers with laser treatment compared with other methods of management used prior to its introduction.

Although the above-mentioned information is compelling, it must be stressed that there are little data available from controlled studies, and therefore a critical sense and caution must be maintained. These reports must be interpreted in light of the fact that approximately 70% to 80% of all episodes of upper gastrointestinal bleeding are self-limiting and abate without specific therapy.[28]

ARGON LASER					Nd:YAG LASER				
Investigator	Country	Bleeding Lesion	Patients	Initial HS %	Investigator	Country	Bleeding Lesion	Patients	Initial HS %
Brunetaud	France	87	80	87	Kiefhaber	Germ.	587	459	94
Waitman	USA	58	20	94	Schonekas	Germ.	334	298	93
Frühmorgen	Germ.	43	41	83	Dwyer	USA	106	71	87
Dwyer	USA	34	21	70	Posi/Sander	Germ.	83	61	97
Le Bodic	France	18	14	82	Rhode	Germ.	83	61	92
Laurence	England	12	10	70	Ramirez	Mex.		80	
Manegold	Germ.	10	10	100	Weinzieri	Germ.	77	70	74
					Ghezzi	Italy	75	65	87
		254	196		Vantrappen	Belg.	53	50	96
					Wotzka/Kaes	Germ.	48	35	81
					Ultsch/Bader	Germ.	37	27	88
					Stauber	Austria	30	28	80
					Fielder/Waldm.	Germ.	30	25	90
					Kreutzer	Austria	29	25	90
					Richter	Germ.	25	20	92
					Escourrou	France	22	20	75
					Immig	Germ.	22	14	82
					Knop/Hausamen	Germ.	22	20	82
					Marcon	Canada	20	18	75
					Ihre	Sweden	15	15	93
					Dixon	USA	15	12	100
					Troidl	Germ.	12	10	85
					Viets	Germ.	11	11	100
					Beckly	England	11	9	82
					Classen/Wurbs	Germ.	10	10	100
					Zimmermann	Germ.	5	5	100
					Soehendra	Germ.	3	3	100
					Stadelmann	Germ.	3	3	100
					Tijtgat	Neth.	3	3	75
					Deyhle	Switz.	3	3	100
					Mockel	Germ.	2	2	100
							1776	1533	

Initial HS = Initial Hemostasis.

FIGURE 9–5. Worldwide summary (as of September, 1979) of series using gastrointestinal laser therapy. (From: Kiefhaber P. Laser endoscopic experience. Brussels 5th International Symposium on Digestive Endoscopy, Brussels, 1982.

Although laser therapy effectively halts bleeding, the incidence of recurrent bleeding, morbidity, transfusion requirements and complications as well as days of hospitalization required and ultimate outcome for patients must be considered. Controlled, randomized studies are essential to establishment of the overall value of laser therapy for upper gastrointestinal bleeding.

There is information available from 9 controlled studies of the efficacy of lasers in the setting of acute upper gastrointestinal bleeding (Table 9–4).[10–18] The Nd:YAG laser was used in 6 of these studies and the argon laser in 3. There are some differences in design of these trials, and considerable differences in respect to interpretation of the results. The six Nd:YAG laser studies will be discussed first.

Five of the 6 Nd:YAG studies include for the most part patients with bleeding ulcers. The exception is the study by Fleischer,[29] which focused on acutely bleeding esophageal varices. Laser therapy effectively stopped hemorrhage in 7 of 10 patients, while all control patients continued to bleed from varices. However, recurrent bleeding remained problematic, and it was concluded that laser treatment in this study did not affect overall outcome. However, laser photocoagulation may have a place as a temporary measure in stabilizing patients with esophageal variceal bleeding, prior to more definitive treatment.

Rutgeerts, et al.[30] divided 152 patients with hemorrhage in the upper digestive tract into three groups: in Group I, 23 patients had acute, spurting arterial bleeding; 86 patients in Group II had active oozing-type bleeding, but not spurting hemorrhage; and 43 patients in Group III had recent bleeding, a finding based on the presence of stigmata of recent hemorrhage (SRH), but no active bleeding. The authors did not use a corresponding control population for Group I because they felt that this would be unethical. Initial hemostasis was achieved in 20 of the 23 patients, and in 9 of the 20 this was

TABLE 9–4. **Controlled Trials of Laser Therapy for Upper Gastrointestinal Bleeding**

Investigator	Laser type	No. of Patients	Lesion	Category	Laser benefit	Reported Complications	Endoscopic Exclusions
Rutgeerts et al.[30]	Nd:YAG	152	All UGI sites except varices, gastritis	i. Spurting artery ii. Active ooze iii. SRH	Yes Yes No	None	Lesion not visualized —
Ihre et al.[31]	Nd:YAG	135	All UGI sites	i. Acute bleeding ii. Inactive	No No	None	—
Escourrou et al.[32]	Nd:YAG	83	Ulcers	Acute bleeding	No	NR	TI
Swain et al.[34]	Nd:YAG	123	Ulcers	i. Acute bleeding ii. SRH	Yes Yes	Laser-induced bleeding	TI
Fleischer[29]	Nd:YAG	20	Varices	Acute bleeding	+/−	Laser-induced bleeding Gas distention Aspiration	—
MacLeod et al.[33]	Nd:YAG	12	Ulcers	Active + Inactive VV	Yes	NR	TI
Vallon et al.[35]	Argon	136	Ulcers	i. Spurting ii. VV iii. SRH	+/− No No		—
Swain et al.[36]	Argon	76	Ulcers	i. VV ii. SRH iii. Clot	Yes No No	Laser-induced bleeding	TI
Jensen et al.[37]	Argon	12	Ulcers	Active bleeding	Yes	Laser-induced bleeding	TI

UGI = upper gastrointestinal; SRH = stigmata of recent hemorrhage; VV = visible vessel; NR = not reported; TI = technically impossible; +/− = uncertain, perhaps beneficial.

permanent. In 11 patients there was recurrent bleeding. Fourteen of the 23 patients (62%) in Group I had to undergo surgery. The overall mortality rate for this group was 30% with 3 of 7 deaths (2 postoperative) being due to hemorrhage or shock. Of the 86 patients in Group II with active, oozing lesions, 46 were treated by laser and 40 were assigned to a control group. There were significantly more patients who continued to bleed in the control group than in the laser-treated group, and there was a numerical reduction in recurrent bleeding after initial hemostasis as well as a reduction in the number of operations in laser-treated patients. The overall mortality was similar in both groups. For the 43 patients in Group III with inactive bleeding but with SRH, the incidence of recurrent bleeding and of operation was reduced, although not to a significant extent, and there was no reduction in mortality.

Ihre and coworkers[31] evaluated 135 patients with upper gastrointestinal bleeding. All types of bleeding lesions, active and inactive, were included. The laser group included 23 patients with acute bleeding, the control group 19. Eight of the 23 patients randomized to laser therapy were not treated because of technical problems. Fourteen of the 15 patients who were treated stopped

bleeding, but 7 had repeated hemorrhage. Overall, those with acute bleeding treated by laser fared no better than the control group with respect to continued or recurrent bleeding, the need for emergency surgery, and mortality. There was no difference in these parameters for 43 laser-treated patients and 50 control patients who were not actively bleeding at endoscopy.

A study of Nd:YAG therapy in acute upper gastrointestinal bleeding by Escourrou et al.[32] enlisted 83 patients, 41 of whom were assigned to a control group; the remaining 42 patients were randomized to laser therapy, although 8 of these were later excluded because endoscopic therapy was not possible. The groups did not differ with regard to permanence of hemostasis, need for surgery, or mortality.

The fifth of the 6 controlled Nd:YAG laser studies is a small series reported by MacLeod and colleagues.[33] Permanent hemostasis was found to be more frequent in a group of laser-treated patients with ulcers with visible vessels (includes active and inactive bleeding) than in a control group.

A high quality study by Swain et al.[34] deserves emphasis. In this study of 464 patients presenting with upper gastrointestinal bleeding to two London hospitals, 232 had peptic ulcers; of these 232 patients, 147 had either active bleeding or SRH. Twenty-four of the 147 patients were excluded from the study; of the remaining 123, 62 were treated with Nd:YAG laser and 61 served as controls. Control of bleeding was more effective in the laser-treated group (p <.02) and mortality was less (p <.05).

The results of 3 argon studies by Vallon,[35] Swain,[36] and Jensen[37] are mixed. In the trial reported by Vallon et al.[35] in 1981, 136 patients with bleeding peptic ulcers were divided into 3 groups and randomized to laser therapy or control. Group I included 28 patients with actively bleeding ulcers; Group II included 35 patients with nonbleeding visible vessels, and Group III included 73 patients with nonbleeding ulcers without visible vessels but with a "central spot." In the category of patients with spurting-type arterial hemorrhage (Group I), initial hemostasis was obtained in 10 of the 15 laser-treated patients; the remaining 5 required surgery. Four of the 13 control patients in Group I also stopped bleeding. Two laser-treated patients in this group had recurrent bleeding, making a total of 7 laser-treated patients in Group I that required surgery. Although fewer laser-treated than control patients in Group I required emergency operations, the difference was not significant. In both groups (II and III) of patients with SRH but no active bleeding, laser therapy did not appear to confer benefit with regard to prevention of recurrent bleeding or need for surgery.

The study by Swain and coworkers[36] culled 76 patients with actively bleeding peptic ulcers or SRH accessible to laser therapy from a group of 330 patients with acute upper gastrointestinal hemorrhage. They divided these patients into 3 groups. Group I was comprised of patients with visible vessels; Group II patients had other SRH, and Group III patients had clots overlying the crater. All 3 groups included patients with both active and inactive bleeding. Laser therapy in the patients with visible vessels (Group I) induced hemostasis, reduced the recurrence of bleeding, and decreased mortality. There were no differences between laser-treated and control patients in Groups II and III.

The last of the 3 controlled trials of argon laser treatment is a small series reported by Jensen et al.[37] Permanent hemostasis was greatest and the need for emergency surgery diminished in a group of patients with peptic ulcers treated by laser.

Information concerning complications is available for 7 of the 9 trials. No perforations were reported with either Nd:YAG or argon laser. (The reported incidence from uncontrolled series is about 1% to 2%.) There is general agreement that laser therapy can paradoxically increase the severity of bleeding. If the laser beam causes vaporization of a vessel, an increase in hemorrhage may result. In one patient with variceal bleeding, aspiration and death occurred, perhaps related to prolongation of the procedure. There was one case of severe gaseous overdistention leading to respiratory compromise. The coaxial gas flow that is used with most laser fibers is still problematic for many investigators. The risk of complications from endoscopic laser therapy increases with the amount of energy delivered and the length of the procedure.

What can be concluded from the controlled trials of laser therapy for acute upper gastrointestinal bleeding? First, only very limited amounts of data exist. About 800 patients have been included in these 9 controlled studies, in which the patient population is heterogeneous; some were actively bleeding; some were not. The best data relate to bleeding ulcers. There is a trend apparent in those studies that focus upon specific lesions with either active bleeding or visible vessels that suggests clinical benefit from laser therapy. Recurrence of bleeding is a continuing concern. Uncontrolled series focused mainly on success of initial hemostasis. Resumption of bleeding occurred in 10% to 30% of patients in the controlled trials. Finally, complications in these studies of endoscopic therapy were few with both Nd:YAG and argon lasers. This is particularly noteworthy, since the patient population with acute upper gastrointestinal bleeding is generally at high risk.

Recurrent Recent Hemorrhage

Angiodysplasia

The use of fiberoptic endoscopy routinely in gastrointestinal bleeding has demonstrated that angiodysplastic lesions in the proximal digestive tract may be responsible for the hemorrhage. Generally, bleeding is self-limited but may be recurrent. If vascular ectasias are within range of the endoscope, they are amenable to endoscopic therapy. One of several treatment modalities that has been employed is laser photocoagulation (Plate 9–1).

Several reports describe endoscopic obliteration and clinical benefit with both argon

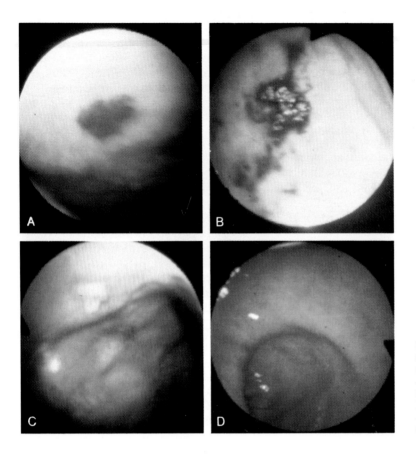

PLATE 9–1. Gastric angiodysplasia. *A,* 8-mm lesion on angulus before therapy. *B,* Immediately after laser treatment. *C,* At treatment site 2 days later; note small ulcer. *D,* One week later, site shows complete healing.

and Nd:YAG laser therapy for angiodysplastic lesions.[38–42] Waitman et al.[38] treated 50 patients with argon laser. Thirty-three patients had complete cessation of bleeding during a follow-up of 6 months to 4 years. The other 17 had markedly reduced blood loss. Bowers and Dixon[39] and Jensen et al.[40] similarly reported benefit with argon laser therapy in patients with angiodysplasia and in a group with classic hereditary, hemorrhagic telangiectasia (Osler-Weber-Rendu syndrome). These workers demonstrated a decrease in episodes of bleeding as well as reduced transfusion requirements. Benefit was also reported by Fleischer[41] and Etienne and coworkers[42] with use of the Nd:YAG laser. No perforations were reported in any of these studies. All investigators found that when the laser beam strikes a large abnormal vessel it may initially cause a dormant lesion to bleed; however, further treatment generally brings the hemorrhage under control.

These encouraging clinical responses are especially noteworthy because many patients with vascular ectasias within endoscopic range also have the same lesions in the more distal small intestine. This suggests that although angiodysplastic lesions may occur in the stomach and small intestine, those in the stomach and duodenum are more apt to be responsible for most of the blood lost. Since there is no evidence that these lesions are pathologically dissimilar it is probable that the gastric environment accounts for the greater tendency for the proximal lesions to bleed. Whether this is related to acidity, digestive enzymes, trauma from undigested food, or variations in motility or other factors is unknown.

Angiodysplasia of the colon, particularly the cecum, has been treated with both argon and Nd:YAG lasers. The principles of treatment are similar. Results are best when it has been clearly established that the colonic lesion has bled and that it is not just an incidental finding. The risk of perforation is greater in the right colon because its wall is thinner than that in other areas of the gastrointestinal tract.

Varices

Although there is no consensus as to the best treatment for nonbleeding esophageal varices that have recently bled, there is increasing interest in nonsurgical approaches. Propranolol, which lowers portal pressure, was shown in one study to reduce further bleeding.[43] Percutaneous transhepatic obliteration of varices has had some support among interventional radiologists. There has been renewed interest in endoscopic sclerotherapy, a technique first used in the 1930's[44] (described in detail in Chapter 16). A variety of new surgical procedures are also under evaluation. Thus, laser therapy has not assumed a prominent role in the treatment of variceal bleeding, although obliteration of varices has been carried out using a lateral aiming fiber as first reported by Hashimoto et al.[45]

Hemorrhoids

The use of the Nd:YAG laser and concurrent cryotherapy to treat hemorrhoids has been described in one report[46] that suggested that this offers an advantage over conventional therapy because it is effective and safe, causing the least possible damage to adjacent tissues.

ABLATIVE LASER THERAPY

Animal Experiments

The ablation of neoplastic tissue with lasers antedates their experimental use for treatment of gastrointestinal bleeding. The first animal experiments with ablative laser therapy were done in the 1960's[47–57] with a variety of lasers. In 1963, McGuff et al.[47–49] demonstrated that ruby laser energy could destroy solid metastatic nodules in the liver; they also treated methylcholanthrene-induced fibrosarcomas and malignant melanomas in hamsters. These workers speculated that the effect of the laser on tumor tissue differed from that of heat generated by electrosurgical cautery and also that the laser effect was different for different tumors. They believed that the effect was related to wavelength, power density, cumulative energy, pigmentations of tissue, vascularity of tissue, and the ratio of dose and target area to tumor size.

In 1964, Minton and colleagues[50, 51] described the use of the Nd:YAG laser to destroy melanomas, sarcomas, and mammary adenocarcinoma in animals. A helium-neon and a nitrogen laser were used by Klein and coworkers[52] to treat melanomas, osteogenic sarcomas, and bladder carcinoma in mice. Minton et al.[53] described in 1965 treatment of multiple intra-abdominal tumor implants

in rabbits, using a neodymium laser, and treatment of melanomas and sarcomas in mice.[54] In a study by Mullins and coworkers[55] chemically induced primate hepatomas were destroyed using the neodymium laser. Ketcham and Minton[56] reported further studies in 1965 with laser radiation as chemotherapy. In a review of the role of lasers in cancer, Ketcham et al.[3] predicted that lasers would become an integral part of many biomedical laboratories because of their ability to destroy selected components of the living cell.

The basis for destruction of tumors in the experiments described is, for the most part, the thermal effect of the laser energy; that is, the laser provides a mechanism for producing tissue damage with heat.

Some exciting work using lasers to produce tumor-destructive effects by different mechanisms is ongoing in two other areas. One of these is the use of selective tumor photosensitizing agents. Much work has been done in this area with hematoporphyrin or one of its congeners.[58–63] Hematoporphyrin was reported to accumulate in malignant tissue by Auler and Banzer[58] and Figge et al.,[59] who noted that the red fluorescence could be used for tumor localization. In 1960, Lipson and Baldes[60] reported on a method of preparing an acetic acid derivative of hematoporphyrin—hematoporphyrin derivative (HpD)—that had greater affinity for malignant tissue than hematoporphyrin. They stated that with a suitable light source, sufficient fluorescence for localization was obtained with low dose HpD, thereby opening the prospect for development of HpD in the clinical diagnosis and localization of malignant disease.

Since it is a dye, HpD absorbs light, with maximum absorption occurring at a wavelength of approximately 405 nm. However, it also absorbs light of 630 nm wavelength. This wavelength penetrates tissue to a deeper extent than the lower violet wavelength. The biologic effects with red light (the higher wavelength) occur in the tumor at a depth of approximately 5 to 15 mm. Absorption of the light by HpD produces a photochemical reaction that may cause tissue death by releasing singlet oxygen. The intensity of this reaction is less severe or absent in adjacent nonmalignant tissue because this contains less HpD. Dye and light must be used in combination, since neither alone causes a reaction.[64] Thus, HpD photoradiation has the potential to aid both diagnosis and therapy of malignant disease.

The second area of exciting new research in laser treatment of neoplastic disease involves the use of very small doses of laser energy designed to selectively destroy malignant cells in tissue culture systems.[65–66] Only a small fraction of the energy necessary to cause thermal destruction may damage cellular organelles. It is hoped that selected wavelengths can be found that preferentially injure neoplastic cells without damaging normal ones.

Human Studies

Neoplasms of the esophagus, stomach, duodenum, ampulla of Vater, colon, and rectum have been treated with endoscopic laser. For the most part, the objective of this has been palliation, but on some occasions curative treatment has been intended and achieved.

Endoscopic management of gastrointestinal cancer has several appealing aspects: (1) it averts surgery and general anesthesia with their attendant morbidity; (2) it diminishes considerably the likelihood of systemic side effects; (3) it can be performed under direct vision; and (4), unlike radiotherapy, there is no maximum dose, so that if the tumor recurs in the same area, treatment can be repeated. It is limited in that it does not affect pathologic tissue outside the gastrointestinal lumen, and it is this which makes it generally palliative.

The goal of palliative treatment is usually to relieve obstruction or to reduce blood loss. Generally, attempts to eliminate pain have been ineffective, presumably because pain is related to neoplastic spread outside the gastrointestinal lumen. Therapy for bleeding may be either by coagulating bleeding sites on the tumor surface or by destruction of the tumor and thereby of its vasculature. Treatment for bleeding is usually ineffective in the case of excessively large tumors (e.g., greater than 8 cm in any dimension). The author and his colleagues have successfully reduced or eliminated bleeding from primary esophageal, gastric, and colorectal neoplasms. In addition, bleeding lesions metastatic to the gastrointestinal tract (e.g., renal cell carcinoma metastatic to stomach) have also been treated successfully.

Technique of Ablative Laser Therapy

Endoscopic laser therapy for ablation of neoplastic tissue is performed by the follow-

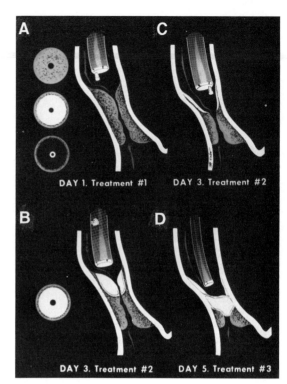

FIGURE 9–6. Treatment technique using endoscopic Nd:YAG laser with quartz waveguide delivery system. A, Endoscope advanced to superior margin of tumor, with waveguide protruding out of biopsy channel. Treatment (Day 1) begins centrally around residual lumen proceeding toward but not to wall. *Cross sections at left*: Initial changes are coagulative: with continued thermal damage, vaporization occurs. B, On Day 3 (48 hours later) the laser-treated tissue is necrotic. C, After necrotic tissue is removed, laser-treatment is performed at same endoscopic session, this time a few centimeters distal to orginal site on Day 1. D, The same process is repeated on Day 5. Treatment progresses until lumen is opened through entire length of neoplastic tissue. (From: Fleischer D. Lasers in gastroenterology. Am J Gastroenterol 1984; 79:406–15.)

ing technique (Fig. 9–6). The endoscope is advanced to either the proximal or the distal margin of the tumor. In some instances luminal narrowing is so marked that even the smallest endoscopes cannot traverse the tumor to its distal margin. The quartz waveguide that carries the laser beam is passed out of the accessory channel of a conventional endoscope (Fig. 9–7). Often a two-channel endoscope is used. The laser energy is preselected so that when the beam hits the tissue, vaporization will occur.

With the technique used by Fleischer and Kessler,[67] the Nd:YAG laser is usually set at an output of 90 to 100 watts for pulses of 2 seconds or greater, using a 1.0 cm distance

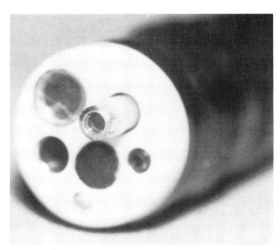

FIGURE 9–7. Quartz waveguide extending from endoscopic accessory channel. (From: Fleischer D. Lasers in gastroenterology. Am J Gastroenterol 1984; 79:406–15.)

to the tumor. The beam is aimed at the neoplastic tissue closest to the lumen, and treatment progresses in increasingly larger concentric circles toward but not to the wall of the organ (Plate 9–2). If the lumen is wide enough to allow passage of the endoscope, treatment may be carried out at various levels; if it is not, then treatment for a given session is completed when the cross section of tumor has been vaporized. Subsequent treatments are then given approximately every other day until the goals of laser therapy are achieved. Maximal tissue necrosis usually occurs during the 48 hours between treatments and is well tolerated by patients.

At the beginning of each repeat laser session, the previously treated neoplastic tissue that plugs the lumen must be removed to allow progressive "coring-out" of the new alimentary canal (Fig. 9–8). This may be done by pushing the necrotic tissue distally with the endoscope if the obstruction is not complete, aspirating it with a large bore nasogastric tube (e.g., 34 French), or by withdrawing the tissue with endoscopic accessories passed through the endoscopic channel (e.g., biopsy forceps). An ultrasonic aspirator would seem ideal, but current technology does not allow endoscopic adaptation of this instrument.

The largest area of experience with laser therapy of gastrointestinal neoplasms in the United States is with esophageal cancer. Of the potentially curative treatments for this disorder, surgery and radiotherapy are most commonly employed. Unfortunately, pallia-

tive treatment of esophageal cancer is far more common than is curative treatment.

Currently, methods of palliation for esophageal cancer include surgery, radiotherapy, bougienage, esophageal endoprosthesis insertion, and gastrostomy or pharyngostomy. More recently, chemotherapy has been used. Endoscopic methods of palliation are discussed in Chapter 17. The goal of palliation is the relief of dysphagia, odynophagia, chest pain, or bleeding. Each palliative modality may be of benefit in selected cases, but each carries specific limitations. These must be weighed by the physician as he chooses the best course of action for the individual patient.

In one series (Fleischer and Sivak)[68] we treated 40 patients with esophageal carcinoma with endoscopic Nd:YAG laser therapy. These patients were not considered to be curable by any conventional treatment. In all patients, the goal of therapy was palliation. About one half had had recurrence after previous therapy. In most, dilation was no longer effective. All had been rejected as operative candidates even for palliation because of the location of the tumor or because of the patient's overall clinical status. The major reason for therapy was dysphagia. Most could eat only liquids or a few solids. Tumors ranged in length from 5 to 11 cm, and luminal occlusion was greater than 90% in the majority. Symptomatic improvement occurred in 37 of 40 patients, and over 90% of these 37 were able to eat either most solids or all foods after laser treatment. Endoscopic luminal diameter at the narrowest point increased from a mean of 2.8 mm to 11.5 mm. Radiographic improvement was usually readily apparent (Fig. 9–9). Clinical improvement generally lasted from 3 to 6 months. Laser therapy was repeated in some patients.

The benefit of this treatment must be evaluated in the light of potential and actual complications. No episodes of sepsis or major bleeding were encountered. Of the 40 patients in this series, 5% experienced a marked degree of pain during laser therapy. Fever and leukocytosis generally occurred following laser therapy within 12 to 24 hours, but resolved without treatment or evidence of culture-proven infection. Perforations or tracheo-esophageal fistulas developed in 5 patients. Perforation occurred from 1 day to 6 months after the last laser treatment. In 2 of the 5 patients, it was relatively clear that the perforation was laser-related. In the other 3 it was difficult to determine the cause

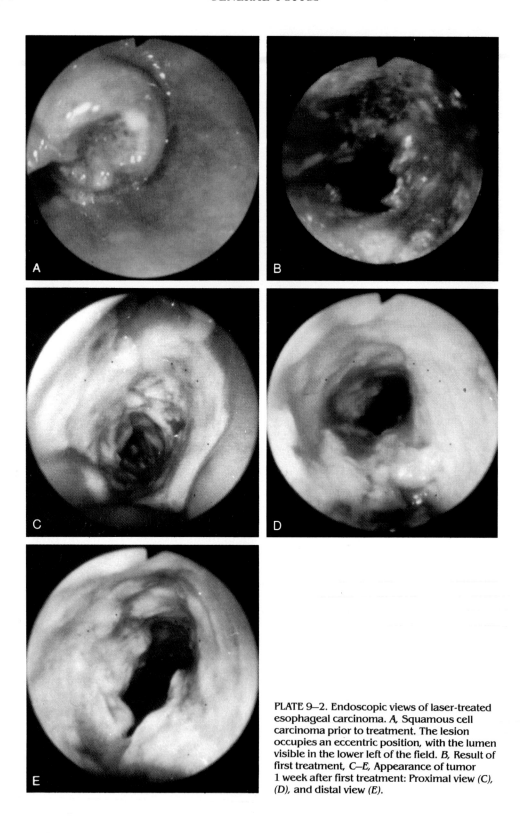

PLATE 9–2. Endoscopic views of laser-treated esophageal carcinoma. *A,* Squamous cell carcinoma prior to treatment. The lesion occupies an eccentric position, with the lumen visible in the lower left of the field. *B,* Result of first treatment, *C–E,* Appearance of tumor 1 week after first treatment: Proximal view *(C),* *(D),* and distal view *(E).*

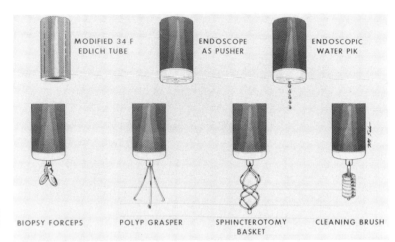

FIGURE 9–8. Modalities available for removing laser-treated (now necrotic), malignant tissue.

BIOPSY FORCEPS   POLYP GRASPER   SPHINCTEROTOMY BASKET   CLEANING BRUSH

because perforation is a recognized complication of the primary disease, radiation therapy, and esophageal dilatation, and all these factors existed in the 3 patients. We concluded that there was little question that quality of life improved for most patients treated.

Mellow et al.[69] reported similar results using endoscopic laser therapy in a group of patients with esophageal cancer. They also demonstrated a longer dysphagia-free duration of time and prolonged survival when the laser-treated group was compared with similar patients treated by radiotherapy.

As experience with endoscopic laser therapy for esophageal malignancy has increased, it has become possible to separate patients into those most likely to benefit and those

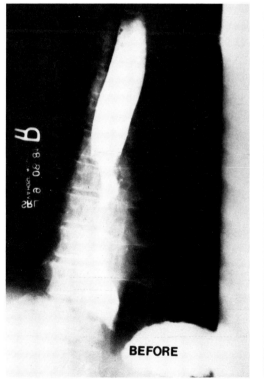

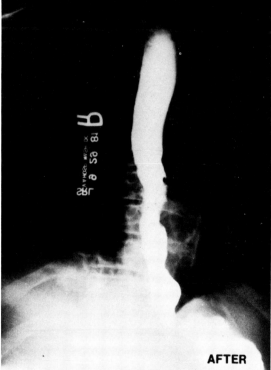

FIGURE 9–9. Barium swallow demonstrating appearance of obstructing squamous cell carcinoma before (*left*) and after (*right*) endoscopic Nd:YAG laser therapy. (From: Fleischer D. Lasers in gastroenterology. Am J Gastroenterol 1984; 79:406–15.)

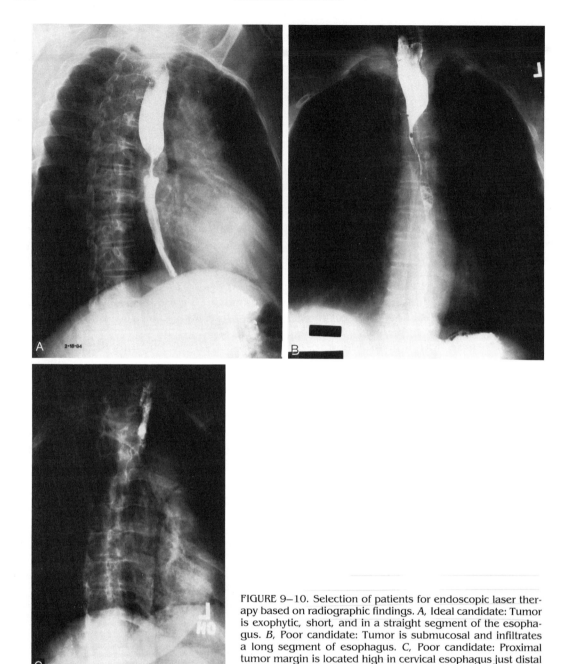

FIGURE 9–10. Selection of patients for endoscopic laser therapy based on radiographic findings. A, Ideal candidate: Tumor is exophytic, short, and in a straight segment of the esophagus. B, Poor candidate: Tumor is submucosal and infiltrates a long segment of esophagus. C, Poor candidate: Proximal tumor margin is located high in cervical esophagus just distal to cricopharyngeus.

who are less than ideal candidates. The histopathologic characteristics of the tumor are not important determinants. This is not surprising, since luminal opening is achieved by thermal destruction. Tumors of ideal candidates are endoscopically exophytic rather than predominantly submucosal, are located in straight segments of the esophagus, and are relatively short (less than 6 cm) rather than long (greater than 10 cm). Patients with tumors just distal to the cricopharyngeus do less well because the treatment of such tumors is technically difficult and occasionally dysphagia may persist even after the lumen is opened, presumably because of neuromuscular dysfunction. Radiographic examples demonstrating these points are shown in Figure 9–10.

Some exciting work using photoradiation therapy for palliation of esophageal malignancies has been done by McCaughan et al.[70] Seven patients with severe or complete malignant obstruction of the esophagus were treated with photoradiation after presensitization with HpD. For therapy, light (625 to 635 nm) was delivered from a tunable dye argon laser system. All tumors treated (adenocarcinoma, squamous cell carcinoma, and melanoma) responded, and swallowing improved. This method, however, is also photosensitizing, and patients must avoid exposure to sunlight for extended periods.

There are several reports of laser therapy for gastric cancers. Fleischer and Sivak[71] described seven patients with recurrent adenocarcinoma at the cardia treated by Nd:YAG laser therapy. Relief of symptoms was obtained in all patients after 1 to 3 treatment sessions (mean 2.2). No complications were encountered. If the patient had had an esophagogastrectomy, laser therapy was technically easy since the area of tumor recurrence was short in length (Fig. 9–11). Swain et al.[72] described palliative relief of gastric outlet obstruction with argon laser treatment. The patient returned home able to swallow minced solid food.

Several Japanese investigators have described endoscopic Nd:YAG laser therapy for gastric cancers. In a report by Imaoka and coworkers[73] on treatment of 15 gastric neoplasms, curative therapy was described in some patients with early gastric cancer. Treatment was effective in approximately 50% of the patients with stenosing gastric adenocarcinoma. These workers reported effective treatment of gastric adenomas and leiomyomas in addition to adenocarcinoma. Iwasaki et al.[74] claimed clinical benefit in 80% of patients treated for malignant stenosis at the gastric cardia. Ichikawa and coworkers[75] reported variable effects when gastric cancers were treated by Nd:YAG laser. Their studies suggested that histologic tumor type influenced results, and that undifferentiated adenocarcinoma, signet ring cell carcinoma, and mucinous adenocarcinoma were less responsive than other gastric neoplasms. Mizushima et al.[76] reported beneficial results with Nd:YAG laser therapy for gastric polyps. In a report on the treatment of 18 "borderline" neoplasms and 16 early gastric cancers, Ito and colleagues[77] concluded that laser therapy may be beneficial in such cases. In France, Brunetaud et al.[78] have used both argon and Nd:YAG lasers for palliative treatment of gastric carcinomas. Richey and Dixon[79] used both argon and Nd:YAG laser treatment to ablate premalignant gastric polyps in one patient. In none of the above studies are complications of laser therapy reported.

Tumors of the duodenum and ampulla of Vater are rare, but there are instances of laser treatment of such tumors that were causing symptoms of obstruction or blood loss. Both Bowers and Sivak (personal communications) treated such patients. The patient treated by Sivak had recurrent bouts of

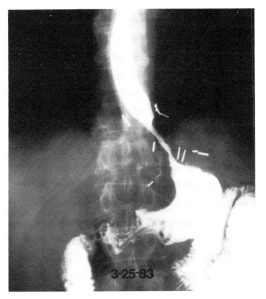
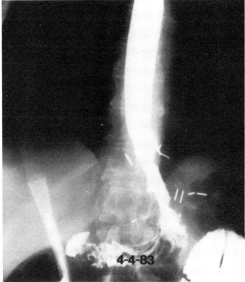

FIGURE 9–11. Barium swallow demonstrating appearance of adenocarcinoma of the stomach recurrent at site of previous esophagogastrectomy before (left) and after (right) endoscopic Nd:YAG laser therapy.

pancreatitis secondary to a tubulovillous tumor of the ampulla of Vater. The tumor remained after local surgical resection was attempted, and duodenoscopic laser therapy was undertaken with the prospect of decreasing episodes of pancreatitis and destroying premalignant tissue. The patient responded over the short term (6 months); however, bouts of pancreatitis returned, and a benign lesion was extirpated by means of a modified Whipple procedure.

There is growing experience with proctoscopic and colonoscopic laser therapy for colorectal neoplasms. These neoplasms can be categorized as follows:

1. Malignancies in which there is widespread disease and no chance for surgical cure; in such cases treatment is palliative.
2. Large premalignant polyps not amenable to electrosurgical snaring.
3. Resectable malignancies and large polyps for which the patient has refused surgery.
4. Familial polyposis in which a rectal stump with polyps remains after subtotal colectomy and ileorectal anastomosis.

Lambert and Sabhen[80] treated 209 colorectal lesions in 200 patients; 131 of these lesions were carcinomas, and the remaining 78 were adenomas too large to be removed by polypectomy. All but 9 lesions were in the rectum or sigmoid. These workers reported successful endoscopic treatment and clinical benefit in most cases, with few complications.

Bowers[81] has used both argon and Nd:YAG lasers to photocoagulate rectal polyps in patients with Gardner's syndrome who had undergone subtotal colectomy. More than 500 polyps were removed in 8 patients who were followed at regular intervals. Treatments on an outpatient basis have been well tolerated, and no significant complications occurred. Bowers[81] in conjunction with John Dixon had favorable results with treatment of a small number of incurable colorectal cancers with a Nd:YAG laser.

Summary

At the present time, laser therapy can be considered among the treatment options under certain circumstances for palliation of esophageal carcinoma. Most authorities emphasize that this measure should be considered when other measures have failed or cannot be considered.

Although laser photodestruction is effective, it has not been compared in controlled studies with other methods of management of obstructing carcinoma. Therefore, it is difficult to list these methods in any order of preference; the physician must consider the known success rate, potential benefits and risks of the various procedures when making decisions about management of individual cases. As data accumulate and technology and methodology improve, it is likely that the role and place of these modalities will shift to a considerable extent.

The available data concerning laser treatment of gastric and duodenal malignancies are limited. It appears that in some circumstances—obstruction in particular and perhaps gastric bleeding—laser therapy is effective. However, this approach is still largely investigational, and is therefore not as yet generally recommended as a treatment modality for neoplasms. As with therapy of esophageal carcinoma, data continue to accumulate, and it is reasonable to expect laser therapy to have an increasing role in treatment of gastric and duodenal malignancies.

Only preliminary data are available concerning the various endoscopic applications of laser energy in colon and rectal tumors; therefore, these must also be considered investigational although they hold considerable promise.

LASER THERAPY FOR TREATMENT OF OTHER GASTROINTESTINAL DISORDERS

The laser has been employed endoscopically to vaporize tissues other than neoplasms. Benign esophageal webs and anastomotic strictures occurring after end-to-end anastomatic stapling procedures have been treated to improve luminal patency.[82] Gertsch and Mossman[83] have removed obstructing duodenal webs by endoscopic Nd:YAG laser treatment. The laser has also been used to drain pseudocysts contiguous to the gastrointestinal tract.[84]

Laser applications in biliary tract diseases are under ongoing investigation. The distal bile duct infundibulum has been incised in patients with obstructive biliary disease, in whom endoscopic sphincterotomy was not technically feasible.[84] Intrahepatic and extrahepatic biliary obstruction have been treated using laser fibers passed via a choledochoscope.[85] Experiments are in progress by Mills et al.[86] to assess the feasibility of using lasers to fracture gallstones.

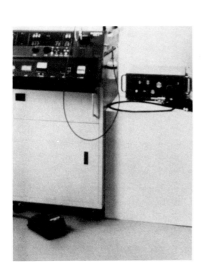
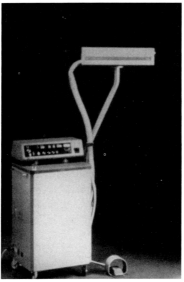
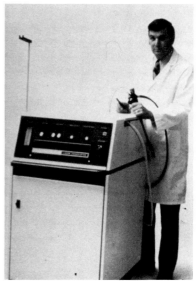

FIGURE 9–12. Commercially available Nd:YAG lasers. *From left to right*: Molectron (Cooper), Medilas (Endolase), and Olympus. (From: Fleischer D. Lasers in gastroenterology. Am J Gastroenterol 1984; 79:406–15.)

COMPONENTS AND SETTING OF ENDOSCOPIC LASER UNITS

Components

A functional endoscopic laser unit consists of the laser itself, endoscopic equipment, and the setting in which the laser is to be used.[87] Several Nd:YAG laser systems and at least one argon system are commercially available (Fig. 9–12). These systems may cost from $70,000 to $100,000. The actual laser that generates the light energy makes up only a small portion physically of the machine, most of the space being dedicated to electrical, cooling, and gas circulating systems. The beam is transmitted via a quartz fiber that is usually housed in a circular "plastic" catheter (Figs. 9–13 and 9–14). Between the actual fiber and the catheter is a free space through which a gas can flow. The purpose of this coaxial gas flow is to keep the fiber clean and to blow away blood and other debris from the surface of the treatment site. The fiber emits the beam at a certain angle of divergence (usually between 4 and 10 degrees). Because of this divergence, the tissue surface area struck by the beam (spot size) will vary according to the distance from the tissue. The greater the distance, the larger the spot size. Therefore, if power output and pulse duration are kept constant as the laser is fired, the concentration of energy (energy density) at the treatment site will vary according to this distance.

Laser systems can be used with commercially available endoscopes, but slight modifications are usually required. The distal tip of the endoscope may be damaged by heat and reflected energy. Endoscope manufacturers can convert the black "plastic" tip to a

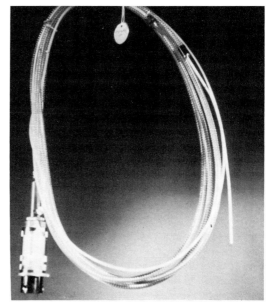

FIGURE 9–13. Typical quartz waveguide. At one end is adaptor for connecting to laser unit; the beam will be emitted at the other end. Flexible waveguide permits use with fiberoptic instruments. (From: Fleischer D. Lasers in gastroenterology. Am J Gastroenterol 1984; 79:406–15.)

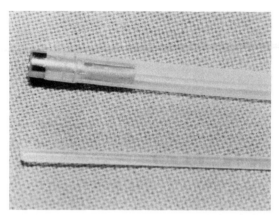

FIGURE 9–14. Standard appearance of laser delivery apparatus. *Top:* Complete unit with outer catheter surrounding quartz waveguide; *bottom:* naked waveguide. (From: Fleischer D. Lasers in gastroenterology. Am J Gastroenterol 1984; 79:406–15.)

white equivalent that is less readily damaged (Fig. 9–15). Many laser endoscopists prefer two-channel endoscopes because use of a coaxial gas type fiber can lead to overdistention of the bowel unless the gas can be exhausted. A T-adapter is available to facilitate this (Fig. 9–16). As alternatives, a suction tube can be attached onto the insertion tube of the endoscope as an extra channel, or an endoscope with a single large accessory channel can be used.

Ophthalmic Safety Accessories

Ophthalmic safety is important. A laser beam striking the eye may cause considerable damage, depending upon its intensity. The carbon dioxide laser can damage the corneal surface by absorption of water. Exposure of the retina to the argon or YAG lasers can cause damage, with resultant blind spots in vision. Therefore, safety glasses or filters are mandatory. These are made of a material that absorbs the particular wavelength of laser light being used. For carbon dioxide lasers, ordinary glass can be used. In the case of an argon laser, the filter material is orange, a color that blocks the blue-green light of the argon laser. Since this filter will color-distort the endoscopic view, it is put in place mechanically during actual firing of the laser. In the case of the YAG laser, the filter material is transparent in the visible spectrum and can be left in place during the entire procedure since it does not impair vision.

Ophthalmic safety levels for laser exposure have been determined by the American National Standards Institute. For typical endoscopic treatment, levels of Nd:YAG laser reflected light from the mucosa through the endoscope can be as much as 100 to 200 mW/cm^2, thereby necessitating a filter over the ocular of the endoscope. The filters typically have attenuations of about 1000, which reduces the reflective energy reaching the eye well below the hazardous level. If a laser is used in an open system (as opposed, for example, to the "closed system" of the digestive tract, which is the site of most gastrointestinal endoscopic procedures), the eye could be accidentally exposed to the entire energy of the laser beam; therefore, safety glasses are an absolute requirement.[10]

Location

Although laser machines are usually mounted on wheels and can be moved, from a practical point of view they are not readily portable. In most instances, therefore, they are located in the routine endoscopic area, a dedicated endoscopic suite, the operating room, or in intensive care areas. The choice of setting will vary with circumstances. Key factors in this choice are availability of space (a room size of at least 300 to 400 square feet is recommended), the component medical and surgical physician specialties that will make use of the laser, availability of support personnel, ready access to the area, and local politics. The ideal suite is a multipurpose one with adequate space and ancillary equipment

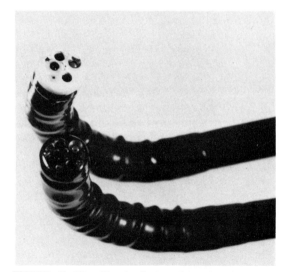

FIGURE 9–15. Standard two-channel endoscope (Olympus GIF-2T): one endoscope with regular tip and one with modified white tip. (From: Fleischer D. Lasers in gastroenterology. Am J Gastroenterol 1984; 79:406–15.)

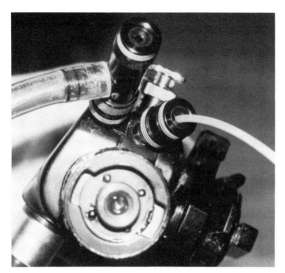

FIGURE 9–16. Endoscopic modifications for laser therapy waveguide passing into right channel of endoscope. Left channel has been modified with T-adapter to allow for tubing attachment for exhaust of recirculating gas. Note protective filter placed over viewing ocular. (From: Fleischer D. Lasers in gastroenterology. Am J Gastroenterol 1984; 79:406–15.)

for all contingencies that patients may present with, plus the flexibility to accommodate other procedures. Because lasers require special electrical power and an adequate water supply and drain capacity, these needs must be anticipated in advance of installation. Electrical codes may differ from city to city and from one area of the hospital to another. These factors may significantly increase the overall cost of acquiring laser capability.

Multidisciplinary Centers

As the use of lasers has expanded, both for the treatment of gastrointestinal diseases and for other medical-surgical diseases, the concept of a multidisciplinary laser center has emerged. A multidisciplinary unit is both logical and economical; since resources are centralized, the physician has access to several types of lasers, and costs are shared. Prototypes of multidisciplinary laser centers may be found at Sinai Hospital in Detroit, the University of Utah at Salt Lake City, and Lille University in France,[88] and this concept is flourishing in Japan.

LASERS IN HUMAN DISEASE: A PERSPECTIVE

There are many reasons for the increasingly widespread use of lasers for therapy of gastrointestinal disease. Initial results have been reasonably encouraging; the spectrum of application has broadened considerably; laser endoscopy is not difficult technically; the complication rate has been acceptably low; and injury to health-care personnel has not been reported. Furthermore, endoscopic laser therapy can often approach lesions for which existing treatment options are not ideal. The great versatility of this powerful tool is demonstrated by its investigative use in a variety of gastrointestinal disorders other than tumors. The same laser used to treat gastrointestinal disorders can be used in other subspeciality areas such as bronchoscopy and urology.

It should be pointed out that laser endoscopy has its drawbacks. Commercially available lasers are expensive. Lasers are not portable in practice and, unlike other devices used to treat gastrointestinal bleeding, cannot be taken to the bedside. Rather, the patient, often critically ill, must be brought to the laser. Comparative data are lacking to determine if endoscopic laser therapy is superior to the less expensive, more portable modalities. Technologic problems remain with both laser and endoscopic systems that make therapy difficult in some circumstances. As with all modalities, endoscopic access to a lesion is not always ideal. Efforts must be made to resolve these problems.

At present, only a few laser energy wavelengths are available for use. Conceivably, many more wavelengths can be utilized; these may have an element of specificity that makes their use safer and more effective than currently available wavelengths. In the future, tunable (selectable) lasers should be available which allow specific wavelength selection. A role in diagnostic evaluation is probable, either in association with fluorescent dyes (e.g., earlier diagnosis of premalignant conditions such as dysplasia in inflammatory bowel disease) or using totally new methods. Computer adaptations should assist precise delivery of dosage. Tissue-sensitizing agents may render abnormal tissue more susceptible to laser destruction. Advances can be expected in the development of waveguides and endoscopic delivery systems that will facilitate access to pathologic processes. Videoendoscopes already in use (see Chapter 10, Part 6) may provide new diagnostic and therapeutic capabilities when incorporated with laser technology.[89]

In conclusion, it should be stressed that application of laser technology in medicine in general, and in gastrointestinal disease in particular, is in its infancy. However, all indicators predict an ever-increasing role for lasers in gastrointestinal endoscopy.

Editor's note: The use of lasers in gastrointestinal endoscopy, as noted in this chapter, continues to evolve. References 90 to 98 are several recent reports of interest.

References

1. Maiman TH. Stimulated optic radiation ruby. Nature (London) 1960; 187:493–4.
2. Goodale RL, Okada A, Gonzales R, et al. Rapid endoscopic control of bleeding gastric erosions by laser radiation. Arch Surg 1970; 101:211–4.
3. Ketcham AS, Hoye RC, Riggle GC. A surgeon's appraisal of the laser. Surg Clin North Am 1967; 47:1249–63.
4. Nath G, Gorisch W, Kiefhaber P. First laser endoscopy via a fiberoptic transmission system. Endoscopy 1973; 5:208.
5. Nath G, Gorisch W, Kreitmair A, Kiefhaber P. Transmission of a powerful argon laser beam through a fiberoptic flexible gastroscope for operative gastroscopy. Endoscopy 1973; 5:213.
6. Dwyer RM, Yellin AE, Craig J, et al. Gastric hemostasis by laser phototherapy in man. A preliminary report. JAMA 1976; 236:1383–4.
7. Frühmorgen P, Reidenbach J, Bodem R, et al. Experimental examinations on laser endoscopy. Endoscopy 1974; 6:116.
8. Kiefhaber P. International experience with lasers for gastrointestinal bleeding. Proc III International Laser Congress, Detroit, 1979.
9. Cummins L. Laser tissue interaction. *In:* Fleischer D, Jensen D, Bright-Asare P, eds. Therapeutic Laser Endoscopy in Gastrointestinal Disease. Boston: Martinus Nijhoff, 1983; 9–38.
10. Enderby CE. Medical laser fundamentals. *In:* Therapeutic Laser Endoscopy in Gastrointestinal Disease. Fleischer D, Jensen D, Bright-Asare P, eds. Boston: Martinus Nijhoff, 1983; 1–8.
11. Dwyer RM, Haverback BJ, Bass M, Cherlow J: Laser-induced hemostasis in the canine stomach. JAMA 1975; 231:486–9.
12. Silverstein FE, Auth DC, Rubin CE, Protell RL. High power argon laser treatment via standard endoscopes. I. A preliminary study of efficacy in control of experimental erosive bleeding. Gastroenterology 1976; 71:558–63.
13. Silverstein FE, Protell RL, Piercey J, et al. Endoscopic laser treatment. II. Comparison of the efficacy of high and low power photocoagulation in the control of severely bleeding experimental ulcers in dogs. Gastroenterology 1977; 73:481–6.
14. Silverstein FE, Protell RL, Gulacsik C, et al. Endoscopic laser treatment. III. Development and testing of gas-jet–assisted argon laser waveguide in control of bleeding experimental ulcers. Gastroenterology 1978; 74:232–9.
15. Butler ML, Morris W. Use of argon laser in the treatment of experimentally induced upper gastrointestinal bleeding in primates. Gastrointest Endosc 1978; 24:117–8.
16. Bown SG, Salmon PR, Kelly DF, et al. Argon laser photocoagulation in the dog stomach. Gut 1979; 20:680–7.
17. Jensen DM, Machicado GA, Tapia JI, et al. Bipolar electrocoagulation and argon laser photocoagulation of colonic lesions. (Abstr) Gastrointest Endosc 1980; 26:69.
18. Silverstein FE, Protell RL, Gilbert DA, et al. Argon vs. neodymium YAG laser photocoagulation of experimental canine gastric ulcers. Gastroenterology 1979; 77:491–6.
19. Waitman AM, Grant DZ, DeBeer R, Chryssanthou C. Endoscopic laser photocoagulation: Comparison of argon and neodymium-YAG. (Abstr) Gastrointest Endosc 1979; 25:52.
20. Dixon JA, Berenson MM, McCloskey DW. Neodymium-YAG laser treatment of experimental canine gastric bleeding. Gastroenterology 1979; 77:647–51.
21. Rutgeerts P, VanTrappen G, Geboes K, Broeckaert L. Safety and efficacy of neodymium-YAG laser photocoagulation: An experimental study in dogs. Gut 1981; 22:38–44.
22. Johnston JH, Jensen DM, Mautner W, Elashoff J. YAG laser treatment of experimental bleeding canine gastric ulcers. Gastroenterology 1980; 79:1252–61.
23. Geboes K, Rutgeerts P, Vantrappen G, et al. A microscopic and ultrastructural study of hemostasis after laser photocoagulation. Gastrointest Endosc 1980; 26:131–3.
24. Johnston JH, Jensen DM, Mautner W, Elashoff J. Argon laser treatment of bleeding canine gastric ulcers: Limitations and guidelines for endoscopic use. Gastroenterology 1981; 80:708–16.
25. Dennis MB, Silverstein FE, Gilbert DA, Peoples JE. Evaluation of Nd:YAG photocoagulation using a new experimental ulcer model with a single bleeding artery. Gastroenterology 1981; 80:1522–7.
26. Jensen DM, Silpa ML, Tapia JI, et al. Comparison of different methods for endoscopic hemostasis of bleeding canine esophageal varices. Gastroenterology 1983; 84:1455–61.
27. Kiefhaber P. Laser endoscopic experience. Brussels 5th International Symposium on Digestive Endoscopy, Brussels, 1982.
28. Fleischer D. Etiology and prevalence of severe persistent upper gastrointestinal bleeding. Gastroenterology 1983; 84:538–43.
29. Fleischer DE. Nd:YAG Endoscopic laser therapy for active esophageal variceal bleeding. (Abstr) Gastrointest Endosc 1985; 31:4–9.
30. Rutgeerts P, VanTrappen G, Broeckaert L, et al. Controlled trial of YAG laser treatment of upper digestive hemorrhage. Gastroenterology 1982; 83:410–6.
31. Ihre T, Johansson C, Seligsson U, Torngren S. Endoscopic YAG-laser treatment in massive upper gastrointestinal bleeding. Report of a controlled randomized study. Scand J Gastroenterol 1981; 16:633–40.
32. Escourrou J, Frexinos J, Bommelaer G, et al. Prospective randomized study of YAG photocoagulation in gastrointestinal bleeding. *In:* Atsumi K, Nimsakul N, eds. Laser—Tokyo '81. Tokyo: Inter Group Corp., 1981; S–30.
33. MacLeod IA, Mills PR, MacKenzie JF. Neodymium YAG laser photocoagulation for major acute upper gastrointestinal haemorrhage. (Abstr) Gut 1982; 23:A905.
34. Swain CP, Bown SG, Salmon P, et al. Controlled trial of Nd:YAG laser photocoagulation in bleeding peptic ulcers. Lasers Surg Med 1983; 3:111.
35. Vallon AG, Cotton PB, Laurence BH, et al. Ran-

domised trial of argon laser photocoagulation in bleeding peptic ulcers. Gut 1981; 22:228–33.

36. Swain CP, Storey DW, Northfield TC, et al. Controlled trial of argon laser photocoagulation in bleeding peptic ulcers. Lancet 1981; 2:1313–6.

37. Jensen DM, Machicado GA, Tapia JI, et al. Endoscopic argon laser photocoagulation of patients with severe upper gastrointestinal bleeding. (Abstr) Gastrointest Endosc 1982; 28:151.

38. Waitman AM, Grand DZ, Chateau F. Argon laser photocoagulation treatment of patients with acute and chronic bleeding secondary to telangiectasia. (Abstr) Gastrointest Endosc 1982; 28:153.

39. Bowers JH, Dixon JA. Argon laser photocoagulation of vascular malformations in the GI tract. Short term results. (Abstr) Gastrointest Endosc 1982; 28:126.

40. Jensen DM, Machicado GA, Tapia JI, et al. Endoscopic treatment of hemangiomata with argon laser in patients with gastrointestinal bleeding. In: Atsumi K, Nimsakul N, eds. Laser—Tokyo '81. Tokyo: Inter Group Corp., 1981; 20–5.

41. Fleischer DE. Nd:YAG laser photocoagulation for upper gastrointestinal angiodysplasia. (Abstr) Gastrointest Endosc 1981; 26:122.

42. Etienne J, Raimbert P, Dorme N. Successful Nd:YAG laser photocoagulation in Rendu Osler's and Willebrand's diseases. In: Atsumi K, Nimsakul N, eds. Laser—Tokyo '81. Tokyo: Inter Group Corp., 1981; S-26–7.

43. Le Brec D, Poynard T, Hillon P, Benhamou JP, Propranolol for prevention of recurrent gastrointestinal bleeding in patients with cirrhosis. A controlled study. N Engl J Med 1981; 305:1371–4.

44. Crafoord C, Frenckner P. New surgical treatment of varicose veins of the oesophagus. Acta Otolaryngol (Stockholm) 1939; 27:422–9.

45. Hashimoto D, Miyahara T, Yoshimura R. Prophylactic treatment of esophageal varices. 5th International Congress for Lasers in Medicine and Surgery, Detroit, 1983.

46. Eddy HJ. Treatment of hemorrhoids with the Nd:YAG laser: A preliminary report. (Abstr) Lasers Surg Med 1983; 3:155.

47. McGuff PE, Bushnell D, Soroff HS, et al. Studies of the surgical applications of laser (light amplification by stimulated emission of radiation). Surg Forum 1983; 14:143–5.

48. McGuff PE, Deterling RA Jr, Bushnell D, et al. Laser radiation of malignancies. Ann NY Acad Sci 1965; 122:747–57.

49. McGuff PE, Deterling RA Jr, Gottlieb LS, et al. Effects of laser radiation on tumor transplants. Fed Proc (Balt) 1965; 24:S-150–4.

50. Minton J, Ketcham A, Dearman JR. Tumoricidal factor in laser radiation. Surg Forum 1964; 15:335–6.

51. Minton JP Ketcham AS. The laser, a unique oncolytic entity. Am J Surg 1964; 108:845–8.

52. Klein E, Fine S, Laor Y, et al. Interaction of laser radiation with biologic systems. II. Experimental tumors. Fed Proc (Balt) 1965; 24:S-143–9.

53. Minton JP, Ketcham AS, Dearman JR, et al. The application of pulsed, high-energy laser radiation to multiple intraabdominal tumor implants in experimental animals. Surgery 1965; 58:12–21.

54. Minton JP, Ketcham AS, Dearman JR, et al. The effect of neodymium laser radiation on two experimental malignant tumor systems. Surg Gynecol Obstet 1965; 120:481–7.

55. Mullins F, Hoye R, Ketcham AS, et al. Studies in laser destruction of chemically induced primate hepatomas. Am Surg 1967; 33:298–303.

56. Ketcham AS, Minton JP. Laser radiation as a chemical tool in cancer therapy. Fed Proc (Balt) 1965; 24:S-159–60.

57. Minton JP, Zelen M, Ketcham AS. Some factors affecting tumor response after laser radiation. Fed Proc (Balt) 1965; 24:155–8.

58. Auler H, Banzer G. Untersuchungen über die Rolle der Porphyrine bei geschwulstkranken Menschen und Tieren. Z. Krebforsch 1942; 53:65–8.

59. Figge FH, Weiland GS, Manganiello LO. Cancer detection and therapy: affinity of neoplastic, embryonic, and traumatized tissues for porphyrins. Proc Soc Exp Biol Med 1948; 68:640–1.

60. Lipson RL, Baldes EJ. The photodynamic properties of a particular hematoporphyrin derivative. Arch Dermatol 1960; 82:508–16.

61. Diamond I, McDonagh AF, Wilson CB, et al. Photodynamic therapy of malignant tumours. Lancet 1972; 2:1175–7.

62. Dougherty JJ. Activated dyes as anti-tumor agents. J Natl Cancer Inst 1974; 52:1333–6.

63. Tomson SH, Emmett EA, Fox SM. Photodestruction of mouse epithelial tumors after oral acridine orange and argon laser. Cancer Res 1974; 34:3124–7.

64. McCaughan JS Jr, Guy JT, Hawley P, et al. Hematoporphyrin-derivative and photoradiation therapy of malignant tumors. (Abstr) Lasers Surg Med 1983; 3:199.

65. Fu-Shou Y. The effect of laser irradiation on human liver carcinoma cells (BEL-7404 line). In: Atsumi K, Nimsakul N, eds. Laser—Tokyo '81. Tokyo: Inter Group Corp., 1981; 7–38.

66. Nakata M, Ohnishi T, Kamikawa K. Anti-tumor effects of near ultraviolet irradiation. In: Atsumi K, Nimsakul N, eds. Laser—Tokyo '81. Tokyo: Inter Group Corp., 1981; 22–4.

67. Fleischer D, Kessler F. Endoscopic Nd:YAG laser therapy for carcinoma of the esophagus: A new form of palliative treatment. Gastroenterology 1983; 85:600–6.

68. Fleischer D, Sivak M. Endoscopic Nd:YAG laser palliation for obstructing esophagogastric carcinoma. (Abstr) Lasers Surg Med 1983; 3:172.

69. Mellow MH, Pinkas H, Frank J, et al. Endoscopic therapy for esophageal carcinoma with Nd:YAG laser: prospective evaluation of efficacy, complications, and survival. (Abstr) Gastrointest Endosc 1983; 29:165.

70. McCaughan JS, Micks W, Laufman L, et al. Palliation of esophageal malignancy with photoradiation therapy. Cancer (in press).

71. Fleischer DE, Sivak MV. Recurrent gastric adenocarcinoma treated by endoscopic Nd:YAG laser therapy. (Abstr) Gastrointest Endosc 1983; 29:161.

72. Swain CP, Bown SG, Edwards D, Salmon PR. Neoplastic gastric outflow tract obstruction relieved by argon laser at endoscopy. Gastrointest Endosc 1984; 30:31–2.

73. Imaoka W, Okuda J, Ida K, Kawai K. Treatment of digestive tract tumor with laser endoscopy—experimental and clinical studies. In: Atsumi K, Nimsakul N, eds. Laser—Tokyo '81. Tokyo: Inter Group Corp., 1981; S-7–10.

74. Iwasaki M, Sasako M, Konishi T, et al. Clinical application of Nd:YAG laser endoscopy. In: Atsumi K, Nimsakul N, eds. Laser—Tokyo '81. Tokyo: Inter Group Corp., 1981; S-14–7.

75. Ichikawa T, Nakosawa S, Ema Y. Effects of Nd:YAG laser irradiation on gastric cancers, including histology. *In:* Atsumi K, Nimsakul N, eds. Laser—Tokyo '81. Tokyo: Inter Group Corp., 1981; S-18–21.

76. Mizushima K, Harada K, Namiki M, et al. Endoscopic therapy of the YAG laser in early gastric cancer and gastric polyp. *In:* Atsumi K, Nimsakul N, eds. Laser—Tokyo '81. Tokyo: Inter Group Corp., 1981; S-31.

77. Ito Y, Sugiura H, Kano T, et al. Endoscopic laser treatment of borderline lesions and early gastric carcinomas. *In:* Atsumi K, Nimsakul N, eds. Laser—Tokyo '81. Tokyo: Inter Group Corp., 1981; 10–2.

78. Brunetaud JM, Houcke P, Delmotte JS, et al. Laser in digestive endoscopy. *In:* Atsumi K, Nimsakul N, eds. Laser—Tokyo '81. Tokyo: Inter Group Corp., 1981; 20–31.

79. Richey GD, Dixon JA. Ablation of atypical gastric mucosa and recurrent polyps by endoscopic application of laser. Gastrointest Endosc 1981; 27:224–7.

80. Lambert R, Sabhen G. Laser therapy for colorectal neoplasms. 5th International Congress of Laser Medicine and Surgery, Detroit, 1983.

81. Bowers J: Laser therapy of colonic neoplasms. In: Fleischer D, Jensen D, Bright-Asare P, eds. Therapeutic Laser Endoscopy in Gastrointestinal Disease, Boston: Martinus Nijhoff, 1983; 139–50.

82. Chen P, Wu C, Chi-Sin C, et al. YAG laser endoscopic treatment of an esophageal and sigmoid stricture after EEA stapling. Gastrointest Endosc 1984; 30:258–60.

83. Gertsch P, Mossman R. Endoscopic treatments of a congenital duodenal diaphragm. Gastrointest Endosc 1984; 30:254–5.

84. Brunetaud JM, Mosquet L, Bourez J. Laser applications in nonbleeding digestive lesions. (Abstr) Lasers Surg Med 1983; 3:137.

85. Kouzou Y. Cholangiographic surgery with Nd:YAG laser. Proc 5th International Congress of Laser Medicine and Surgery, Detroit, 1983.

86. Mills TN, Watson GN, Swain P, et al. Thermal vs. photo-acoustic fragmentation of biliary calculi using continuous wave and giant pulse lasers. (Abstr) Lasers Surg Med 1983; 3:156.

87. Overholt B. Use of lasers in community hospitals in the United States. *In:* Fleischer D, Jensen D, Bright-Asare P, eds. Therapeutic Laser Endoscopy in Gastrointestinal Disease, Boston: Martinus Nijhoff, 1983; 187–92.

88. Brunetaud JM, Mosquet L, Bourez J, Wierez AM. Organization of a multidisciplinary laser center. *In:* Fleischer D, Jensen D, Bright-Asare P, eds. Therapeutic Laser Endoscopy in Gastrointestinal Disease, Boston: Martinus Nijhoff, 1983; 167–72.

89. Sivak MV Jr, Fleischer DE. Colonoscopy with a videoendoscope™: Preliminary experience. Gastrointest Endosc 1984; 30:1–5.

90. Mathus-Vliegen EM. Complications and pitfalls of laser therapy. Endoscopy 1986; 18(Suppl 1):69–72.

91. Mathus-Vliegen EM, Tytgat GN. Nd:YAG laster photocoagulation in colorectal adenoma. Evaluation of its safety, usefulness, and efficacy. Gastroenterology 1986; 90:1865–73.

92. Mathus-Vliegen EM, Tytgat GN. Laser photocoagulation in the palliation of colorectal malignancies. Cancer 1986; 57:2212–6.

93. Cello JP, Grendell JH. Endoscopic laser treatment for gastrointestinal vascular ectasias. Ann Intern Med 1986; 104:352–4.

94. Bown SG, Swain CP, Storey DW, et al. Endoscopic laser treatment of vascular anomalies of the upper gastrointestinal tract. Gut 1985; 26:1338–48.

95. Rutgeerts P, Van Gompel F, Geboes K, et al. Long-term results of treatment of vascular malformations of the gastrointestinal tract by neodymium Yag laser photocoagulation. Gut 1985; 26:586–93.

96. Swain CP, Kirkham JS, Salmon P, et al. Controlled trial of Nd-YAG laser photocoagulation in bleeding peptic ulcers. Lancet 1986; 1:1113–7.

97. Brunetaud JM, Mosquet L, Houcke M, et al. Villous adenomas of the rectum. Results of endoscopic treatment with argon and Nd:YAG lasers. Gastroenterology 1985; 89:832–7.

98. MacLeod IA, Mills PR, MacKenzie JF, et al. Neodymium yttrium aluminium garnet laser photocoagulation for major haemorrhage from peptic ulcers and single vessels: a single blind controlled study. Br Med J 1983; 286:345–8.

Chapter 10

SPECIAL METHODS AND TECHNIQUES IN GASTROENTEROLOGIC ENDOSCOPY

INTRODUCTION

MICHAEL V. SIVAK, JR., M.D.

This chapter, the largest in this volume, has several special purposes: to present new endoscopic techniques that are generally considered investigational at present and to present established but special endoscopic methods of diagnosis that are not in widespread use. However, all of the methods presented offer at least the prospect of enhanced endoscopic diagnosis or therapy. Certain special endoscopic skills are required of those who would utilize these techniques, although they are not beyond the capability of experienced endoscopists. The information in the various chapter sections can serve as a foundation for those who have an interest in any of these procedures. However, in certain instances these techniques and methods utilize endoscopic instruments that have special characteristics. Many are prototype instruments that are only available on a limited basis throughout the world. An exception is the videoendoscope, which is now available in most countries. However, the place of this instrument in gastrointestinal endoscopy remains uncertain; although a satisfactory endoscope, the videoendoscope offers some potential and as yet unrealized advantages over standard fiberscopes. Another exception is percutaneous endoscopic gastroscopy, which is becoming an established and accepted technique.

Part 1

ENDOSCOPIC ULTRASONOGRAPHY

WOLF DIETER STROHM, M.D.
MEINHARD CLASSEN, M.D.

It is now possible to produce small ultrasound probes that can be mounted on the distal insertion tube of a fiberoptic endoscope.[1-4] The combination of endoscopy of the upper gastrointestinal tract with ultrasonography increases diagnostic range; the endoscopic evaluation of the mucosal surface is supplemented by ultrasonographic analysis of the histologic layers of the gastrointestinal wall. Sonographic imaging of contiguous organs is also possible. Endoscopic access to sonographic target organs overcomes certain barriers to ultrasound imaging such as intestinal gas and bony structures, and permits the use of higher ultrasound frequencies by virtue of the proximity of the probe and target organs which reduces the necessary penetration depth of the ultrasonic beam.[5, 6]

Endosonographic studies were first undertaken in urology and gynecology. Transrectal, transurethral, and transvaginal access provided a simple ultrasonographic route to the pelvic organs,[7-12] by means of which probes were introduced into the body without endoscopic observation. For ultrasonographic endoscopy of the upper gastrointestinal tract, however, endoscopic visualization is necessary to orient the probe in the required positions. The first ultrasound gastroscopes were described in 1980.[1, 3] In contrast to these prototypes, ultrasound gastrointestinal fiberscopes now permit high-resolution ultrasonographic investigation of the upper gastrointestinal tract and immediate surrounding organs and structures in small sections. This allows sonographic analysis of the walls of the esophagus and stomach and, by transesophageal, transgastric and transduodenal ultrasonographic endoscopy, the organs of the mediastinum, especially the heart, and those surrounding the stomach, i.e., liver, bile duct, pancreas, hepatic-renal angle and splenic-renal angle.

TECHNOLOGY OF ENDOSCOPIC ULTRASONOGRAPHY

At present, ultrasound endoscopes can be classified according to the orientation of the ultrasonographic "section" relative to the axis of the insertion tube of the endoscope. There are two general categories: those which provide a sector scan perpendicular to the insertion tube and those which give a parallel or linear scan. A linear array device employs a series of individual transducers which are arranged lengthwise along the insertion tube. The transducer elements are electronically triggered in sequence to provide a rectilinear scan. Sector scanning instruments may be classified as mechanical and electronic. The electronic or phased array scanner operates on the same principle as the linear array device, except that the transducer components are oriented to produce a perpendicular scan. Mechanical devices provide a sector scan by mechanically rotating a transducer in the distal end of the endoscope, or by rotating an acoustical mirror which reflects the scanning beam into a perpendicular orientation. There are technical problems and advantages with each type. Only the mechanical sector scanning instrument will be discussed in this section.

The ultrasound endoscopic system made by Olympus/Aloka GF-EU1/EU-M1 has an optical component that orients the endoscopic view in an oblique direction relative to the insertion tube, and an ultrasound probe at its distal end (Fig. 10–1A). The diameter of the instrument tip is 13 mm. The distal end of the instrument is rigid over a length of 45 mm from the tip. The ultrasound probe is surrounded by a plastic capsule (Fig. 10–1B) within which a small reflector rotates at an angle of 45 degrees. This rotation is accomplished by a small motor and cable which

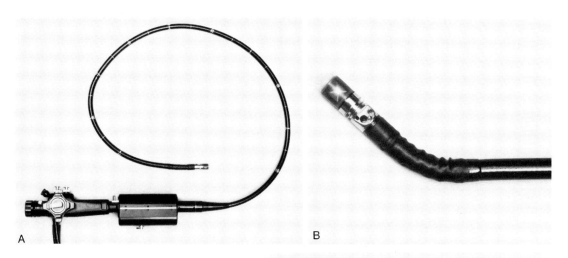

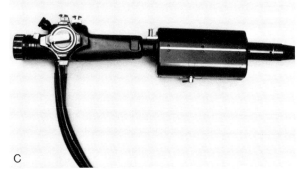

FIGURE 10–1. *A,* Ultrasound gastrointestinal fiberscope unit (Olympus GF-EU1). *B,* Distal end of ultrasound gastrointestinal fiberscope. *C,* Proximal control section of ultrasound gastrointestinal fiberscope with deflection knobs and housing for motor that rotates mirror by means of a cable.

runs through the insertion tube of the endoscope, the motor being housed below the deflection controls of the instrument (Fig. 10–1*C*). The ultrasonic impulses are produced by a crystal in the tip of the instrument. The reflector sends these into the body perpendicular to the insertion tube. The rotating reflector encompasses a semicircular field. The reflected ultrasound echoes reach the transducer via the rotating mirror, and are transmitted to a display monitor (Fig. 10–2).[2] A linear dot series marker is also incorporated into the monitor. This is calibrated so that the dots are 1 cm apart.

The ultrasound frequency is 7.5 MHz. This frequency is somewhat higher than that possible with extracorporeal systems. In general there is an inverse relation between frequency and depth of penetration: the higher the frequency, the less the depth of penetration and vice versa. However, higher frequencies result in better resolution. Since a lesser depth of penetration is required when the ultrasound probe is near the target organ, greater resolution is possible. This is one of the theoretical advantages of endoscopic ultrasonography. The system presented here provides a display of 16 × 10 cm. The best

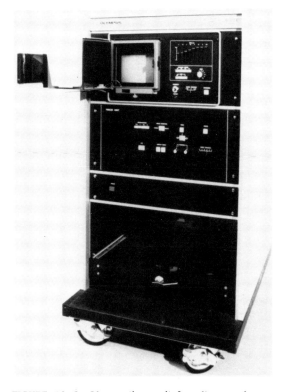

FIGURE 10–2. Observation unit for ultrasound gastrointestinal fiberscope (Olympus/Aloka (EU-M1).

quality image occurs in a section of 9 × 6 cm. Within this small section there is high quality resolution in all planes, with the resolution in the near range being particularly good.

With the Olympus/Aloka GF-EU1/EU-M1 system, endosonographic evaluation as well as some degree of endoscopic investigation are possible at the same time. However, the axis of view of the sonographic system diverges from the optical system axis by 90 degrees. It is not possible to obtain endoscopic biopsies with this system.

THE ENDOSCOPIC ULTRASONOGRAPHIC PROCEDURE

Instruments

Endoscopic ultrasonography should be performed on a table which can be tilted. Fluoroscopy should be readily available. Elements of the ultrasound investigation may be recorded by instant photography, or large segments may be preserved on video tape. An assistant is required to control the ultrasound endoscope during the scanning and documentation phases of the examination. Ideally the investigator should be highly proficient in endoscopy and ultrasonography. Since the ultrasound probe is oriented mainly by reference to the ultrasound images in addition to the approximate positioning by endoscopy, the sonographic portion of the procedure should not be delegated to an endoscopist inexperienced in ultrasonography. This dual capability is rare in a single individual in many places. In Europe, for example, a single individual is more likely to be competent in ultrasonography and endoscopy. Conversely, in the United States, ultrasonography is usually the province of the radiologist, and therefore the procedure requires two individuals with different areas of expertise. However, to perform this type of procedure satisfactorily, it is necessary that the endoscopist acquire a working knowledge of ultrasonographic anatomy.

Preparation

The pharmacologic preparation for the procedure is the same as for the more routine endoscopic procedures. Although the procedure lasts somewhat longer than diagnostic esophagogastroduodenoscopy, it is well tolerated by patients.

Position

The patient lies on the left side during introduction of the instrument. For the endosonographic investigation he or she lies prone since the topographical relations of the organs become distorted and unfamiliar with the patient in the left decubitus position. However, for scanning the pancreatic tail the left side position is recommended, and for the region of the pancreatic head a right side position.[13] When the patient's position is changed during the investigation, the instrument is drawn back to the fundus of the stomach. For scanning in the distal parts of the stomach, a semi-upright position is recommended, especially if the procedure is being performed when the stomach is filled with water.

Technique

After performing esophagogastroduodenoscopy for orientation, the tip of the instrument is placed in the desired position. Some endoscopists find this particular instrument difficult to use as an endoscope and may prefer to perform an examination of the upper gastrointestinal tract with a standard instrument first. Seven endosonographic scanning positions in the upper gastrointestinal tract are described[14]: deep duodenal intubation; at the level of the papilla of Vater; and in the duodenal bulb, the antrum, body of stomach, fundus, and the esophagus (Fig. 10–3). In the first three duodenal positions,

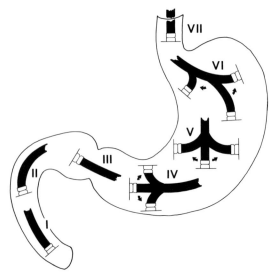

FIGURE 10–3. Seven positions of ultrasound endoscope in upper gastrointestinal tract.[14]

the examination is somewhat restricted because the narrow duodenum limits instrument maneuverability and because it is difficult to orient the probe in this location. However, these disadvantages are balanced by the extended range of scanning which brings the right kidney, the lateral parts of the right lobe of the liver, and the caudal portion of the pancreatic head into view. The positions in the antrum and body of the stomach afford more maneuverability.

Ultrasonographic endoscopy provides new dimensions for study of the intra-abdominal organs. In contrast to conventional extracorporal ultrasonography, the probe is surrounded by organs. Therefore an entirely different type of three-dimensional orientation is necessary. Since scanning may be performed in almost any direction and an almost unlimited variety of sections from the gastrointestinal tract are possible, standardization of section planes and positions facilitates orientation. The main goal is to find stable ultrasound windows which will permit adequate observation of the surrounding organs.[15]

During the investigation the probe (instrument tip) may be maneuvered by three different methods:[16] (1) flexion of the tip using the instrument's deflection controls, (2) rotation of the insertion tube on its long axis, and (3) parallel shifting by advancing the insertion tube or drawing it back (Fig. 10–4).

Deflection permits scanning in practically any section plane. Horizontal sections of the body appear to be the most useful in ultrasonographic endoscopy. They are supplemented by longitudinal and oblique sections. By convention, horizontal sections are oriented from the vantage point of the patient's feet. The right side of the image is always the patient's right side looking from the feet upward. For longitudinal and sagittal sections, cephalad is to the left and caudad to the right. In the antrum, horizontal sections are achieved by inversion of the instrument (Fig. 10–4A). As a result of this maneuver, the ultrasound display is reversed (left for right). This may be corrected by reversing the image electronically on the monitor. Scanning in longitudinal and sagittal planes causes similar problems. Sagittal sections are easily achieved from the antrum with the instrument tip in a straight configuration. In the body, tip deflection is necessary. Bending the instrument tip to the left reverses the display screen (Fig. 10–4B). Rotational movements are necessary to orient the display. If the instrument tip is surrounded by and in contact with gastric mucosa on all sides, which can be achieved by suctioning all the air from the stomach in most cases, then rotation will provide a 360-degree scan. With the patient in the prone position and without deflection of the instrument tip, a dorsally directed scan is obtained. The insertion tube must be rotated to a ventral scanning position if organs ventral to the gastrointestinal tract (the heart

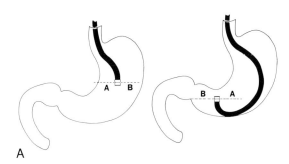

A

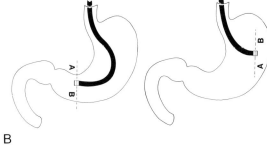

B

FIGURE 10–4. Moving the probe in ultrasonographic endoscopy. *A,* Horizontal sections; *B,* longitudinal sections; *C,* rotation; *D,* parallel shifting.

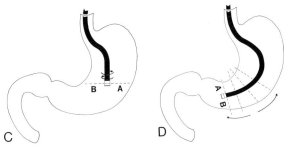

C   D

or liver, for example) are to be scanned. However, rotation to a ventral scanning position again reverses the display (left for right) (Fig. 10–4C), which can be corrected electronically with the Olympus/Aloka equipment.

The third method of moving the probe, parallel shifting, produces a series of parallel sections (Fig. 10–4D). This is advantageous for scanning larger organs. Unfortunately, present techniques allow only a short series of parallel section scans.

Common Bile Duct

Imaging the common bile duct is usually possible from the antrum. There are two recommended techniques:

1. An oblique position may be developed from the longitudinal plane with a straight instrument tip.

2. Sharp inversion and compression of the instrument's tip into the prepyloric antrum thus approaching the choledochal region (Fig. 10–5A). From this position, the splenic vein may be found and followed by flexion of the tip into a horizontal plane or by drawing the instrument backward slightly.

Pancreas

The pancreas is best imaged in horizontal sections. The proper positions for the probe are reached with a straight instrument tip as well as by inversion (Fig. 10–5B). To adequately scan the different parts of the pancreas it may be useful to change the patient's position as previously described. It is also advantageous to fill the stomach with 100 to 200 ml of water, and to scan the pancreas through intragastric liquid.[13]

Splenic-Renal Angle

Endosonographic imaging of the splenic-renal angle is relatively easy technically because of the close anatomic relation of the body of the stomach to the spleen and left kidney. The instrument is placed on the greater curvature of the stomach with the tip straight. Rotatory movements of a slight degree allow scanning of large parts of the spleen and the upper pole of the left kidney

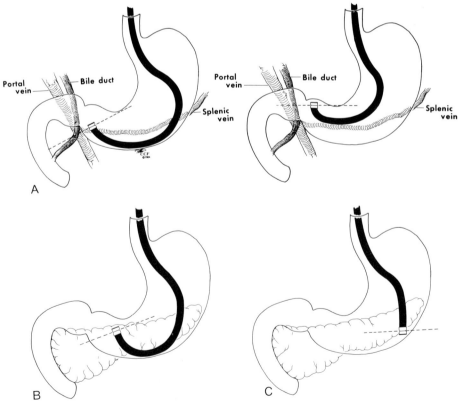

FIGURE 10–5. Investigation technique in sonographic endoscopy. A, Imaging of common bile duct; B, imaging of pancreas; C, imaging of splenic-renal angle.

(Fig. 10–5C). The left adrenal region can also be imaged in this position.

Stomach

Sonographic imaging of the gastric wall is possible only after introducing 100 to 200 ml of water into the stomach. To prevent the formation of bubbles, a liquid antifoaming agent can be added. The patient must be positioned so that the area to be investigated is covered by liquid. The probe is positioned within the fluid and the stomach wall is scanned from a distance of 1 to 3 cm. According to Caletti et al.,[17] there are four recommended positions:

1. Prepyloric with scanning of the antrum and pyloric region.

2. Middle antrum for scanning the lesser curvature or the region of the angulus (in this position the antrum and body are scanned simultaneously, the antrum being nearer to the probe).

3. Deeply positioned in body with imaging of the lesser curvature (antrum and body again may be scanned at the same time, but now the body is nearer the probe).

4. Body (body and fundus are imaged, but not the antrum).

Esophagus

To insure that the ultrasound probe is positioned at the required distance from the esophageal wall, a latex balloon is placed over the tip of the instrument before it is introduced. The balloon is filled with water as scanning is begun in the esophagus. With this method, satisfactory imaging of the esophageal wall to define mucosal or submucosal processes is possible.[17]

ANATOMIC ASPECTS

Position I: Distal Duodenum

Endoscopic ultrasonography is usually begun in the descending duodenum. Sonographic orientation is by reference to the inferior vena cava and aorta (Fig. 10–6). The inferior vena cava may be recognized as it collapses during the respiratory cycle (Fig. 10–7). By careful rightward rotation of the instrument, the hepatic-renal angle is visualized, and the right kidney and adrenal region are imaged (Fig. 10–8).

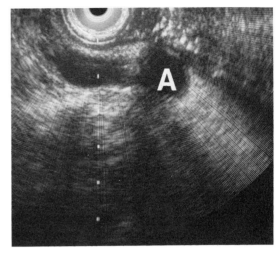

FIGURE 10–6. Position I. Vena cava and aorta (A) in horizontal section. Semicircle of the instrument lies in the vicinity of great vessels. White marks = 1 cm.

Position II: Papilla of Vater

From this position it is possible to image the pancreatic head by clockwise rotation of the instrument. Portions of the portal system such as the superior mesenteric and splenic veins can be visualized. The common bile duct may be scanned, along with the head of the pancreas and its ducts (Fig. 10–9).

Position III: Duodenal Bulb

By withdrawing the instrument to the duodenal bulb, sagittal sections are obtained. But this instrument position is difficult to maintain, and in most cases contact with the intes-

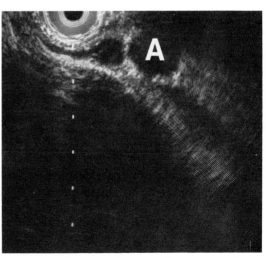

FIGURE 10–7. Collapse of vena cava.

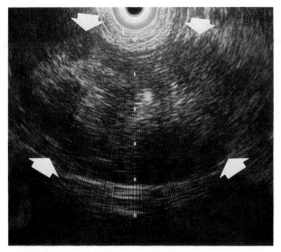

FIGURE 10–8. Position I. Longitudinal section of right kidney (*outlined by arrows*).

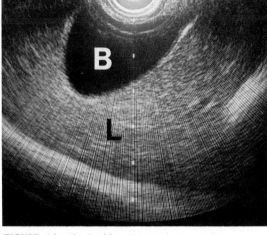

FIGURE 10–10. Position III. Oblique section of gallbladder and surrounding liver (L).

tinal wall is unsatisfactory. However, the gallbladder (Fig. 10–10), parts of the right lobe of the liver, the porta hepatis and segments of the portal vein may be imaged.

Position IV: Gastric Antrum

If the instrument tip is deflected and inverted within the prepyloric antrum, important horizontal scans of the region of the pancreatic head are obtained. From this position practically all of the head of the pancreas may be scanned (Fig. 10–11). The instrument's high resolution provides good visualization of small vessels, the main pancreatic duct (duct of Wirsung), the accessory pancreatic duct (duct of Santorini), and the

common bile duct. The common bile duct lies close to the probe and must be distinguished from the portal vein and inferior vena cava (Fig. 10–12). The gallbladder can be scanned from this position, and its recognition facilitates orientation. The liver is imaged by rotating the instrument into a ventral scanning position.

Position V: Body of the Stomach

The body of the stomach is an important scanning position in endoscopic ultrasonography. From this location the entire pancreas may be scanned in most cases. By rotating clockwise and withdrawing at the same time, the splenic vein may be followed in its course

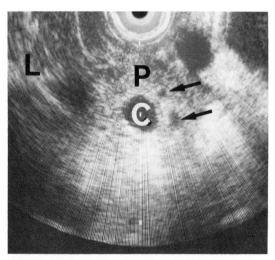

FIGURE 10–9. Position II. Head of pancreas (P). C = Vena cava; arrows = pancreatic ducts; L = liver.

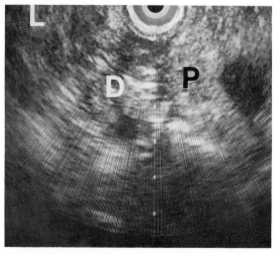

FIGURE 10–11. Position IV. Pancreatic head (P) is seen from antrum. D = Duodenum; L = liver.

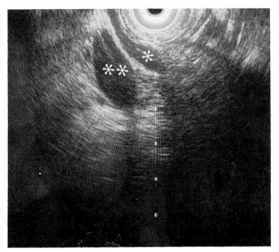

FIGURE 10–12. Position IV. Longitudinal section of normal common bile duct (*) ventral to the portal vein (**).

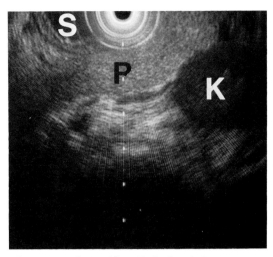

FIGURE 10–14. Position V. Body of the pancreas. Same patient as in Figure 10–13. By rotating and withdrawing from this position the scan moves from the pancreatic head to the body and to the tail of the pancreas. K = kidney.

(Figs. 10–13 through 10–15), and in so doing an image of the splenic-renal angle is achieved (Figs. 10–16 and 10–17). The probe may be brought into virtually direct contact with the left kidney and spleen (Fig. 10–18). Visualization of the left renal vein provides an additional guide for imaging the tail of the pancreas, this position being ideal for scanning this structure (Fig. 10–19).

Position VI: Fundus of the Stomach

In this position the left lobe of the liver and the spleen and diaphragm are visualized. Hepatic veins flowing toward the caval vein may be followed by parallel shifting. The

aorta is defined especially well in this position. By carefully advancing the instrument, the celiac region with hepatic and splenic arteries are scanned (Fig. 10–20).

Position VII: Esophagus

Transesophageal sonographic endoscopy allows systematic investigation of the heart. The instrument is rotated to a ventral scanning direction to obtain a four-chamber view of the heart. The mitral and tricuspid valves may be well visualized, and the atria and atrial septum as well as the semilunar valves and the great vessels can be clearly seen.

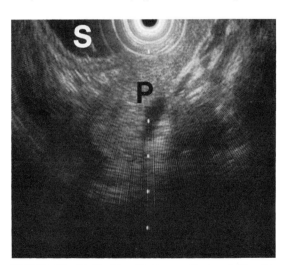

FIGURE 10–13. Position V. Pancreatic head (P) with splenic vein. Instrument lies in liquid-filled stomach (S).

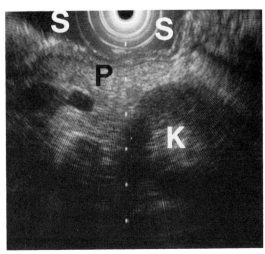

FIGURE 10–15. Position V. Tail of the pancreas (P) with splenic vein and kidney (K). S = Stomach.

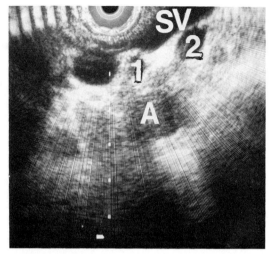

FIGURE 10–16. Position V. Splenic vein and celiac region with celiac trunk. 1 = Hepatic artery; 2 = splenic artery; SV = splenic vein; A = aorta.

DISCUSSION

Knowledge of sonographic anatomy is of great importance in orienting the ultrasound probe. The most important guides are the gallbladder, the liver, and vessels such as the splenic vein, inferior vena cava, and aorta. However, there are important individual variations in the relation of the stomach to its adjacent organs. In every patient these various organs must be located in optimal sonographic windows. For example, the stomach, because of variations in size and shape, does not always provide an ideal ultrasonographic position in relation to the liver and pancreas. In some cases the pancreas may be difficult to find. Access to the splenic-renal

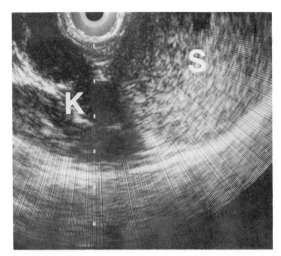

FIGURE 10–18. Position V. Kidney (K) and spleen (S) are well-accessed by endosonography.

angle containing the tail of the pancreas, however, is usually not difficult.

Organ structure can be imaged using this system with a hitherto unknown quality of resolution. This high resolution is conspicuous in visualization of the contours of vessels and hollow organs. The different layers of the wall of the gallbladder may be discerned. The normal pancreatic duct may be visualized in most cases. The structure of parenchymatous organs, such as the liver, pancreas, and kidney is similar with conventional ultrasonography. With endoscopic ultrasonography, however, there is greater differentiation of the parenchyma of these organs because of the high resolution. To illustrate, the liver parenchyma is relatively homogeneous, but a minute granulated pattern is

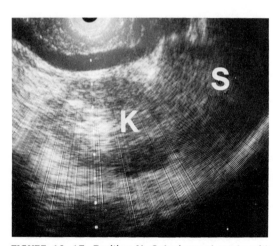

FIGURE 10–17. Position V. Splenic-renal angle with right kidney (K), spleen (S) and splenic vein.

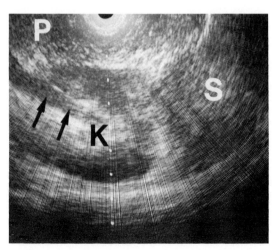

FIGURE 10–19. Position V. Splenic-renal angle. K = Kidney; S = spleen; arrows = renal vein; P = pancreas.

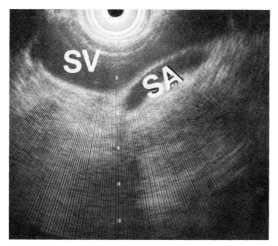

FIGURE 10–20. Position VI. Splenic vein (SV) and splenic artery (SA).

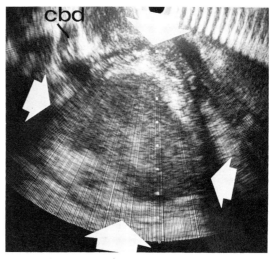

FIGURE 10–22. Hemorrhagic pancreatic pseudocyst (*arrows*) compromising the common bile duct (cbd).

discernible in endosonographic scans of the pancreas. Dark papillary areas are found in images of the renal parenchyma.

DIAGNOSTIC SPECTRUM

Early experiences with endoscopic ultrasonography suggest that this new technique may improve the diagnosis of some disorders;[18–24] the possibilities will be described for individual organs in the following section.

Pancreas

Since the pancreas may be incompletely examined by conventional sonography because of its hidden position in the abdomen,

ultrasonographic endoscopy may prove to be an important advance in diagnosis. The improved and detailed image of the pancreas should permit the addition of new differential points and criteria for diagnosis of pancreatic disease.

It has been suggested that endoscopic ultrasonography will improve the differentiation of carcinoma from pancreatitis.[25–27] In chronic pancreatitis very small cysts and minute calcifications are often discernible. The wall of a pseudocyst may be studied by endoscopic ultrasonography, especially that of cysts arising in the tail of the pancreas (Fig. 10–21). The demarcation of pseudocysts in

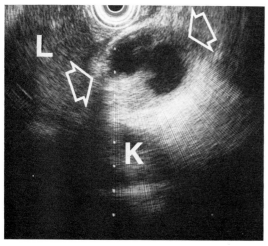

FIGURE 10–21. Position V. Pseudocyst (*arrows*) of the tail of the pancreas. L = Liver; K = kidney.

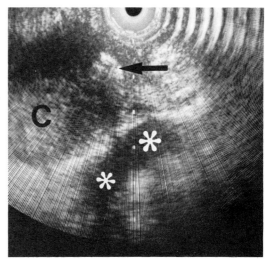

FIGURE 10–23. Pancreatic pseudocyst (C) with calcifications (*arrow*). ** = Caval vein in longitudinal section.

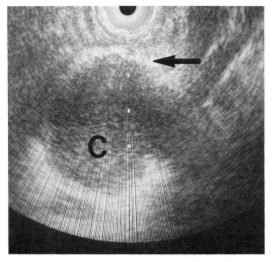

FIGURE 10–24. Pancreatic pseudocyst (C) (same patient as in Figure 10–23). Horizontal section. Calcifications are visible (arrow).

Lesions that produce stenosis of the ampulla of Vater can be demonstrated clearly, and it is possible to find minute tumors of the ampulla which may be undetectable by conventional sonography (Fig. 10–28). It is possible to detect dilation of the main pancreatic duct, which often occurs with such lesions (Fig. 10–29). The widened duct has a sharply defined wall and follows a regular course through the pancreas in contrast to the changes that occur with chronic pancreatitis, in which the dilated main duct is irregular and often focally widened to cystic proportions. This would correspond to the "chain of lakes" appearance of severe chronic pancreatitis demonstrated by retrograde pancreatography. The wall of the dilated main pancreatic duct in chronic pancreatitis displays bright ultrasonic echoes, and stones may be found within the duct (Fig. 10–30).

Bile Ducts

It is not difficult to demonstrate the bile ducts, especially the distal common duct, by sonographic endoscopy (Fig. 10–31). The detection of papillary and bile duct tumors is an important goal for endosonography. Our early experience in patients with common bile duct stones suggests that endoscopic ultrasonography may be superior to conventional ultrasonography in the detection of common bile duct stones.[28] Biliary calculi have a typical pattern of echogenic reflection and shadow (Figs. 10–32 and 10–33). Endoscopy has an advantage over conventional ultrasonography in this respect because imaging is not impaired by the presence of air in the duodenal bulb.

Since the gallbladder is easily demon-

relation to surrounding structures is improved by this technique (Figs. 10–22 through 10–24). Pancreatic carcinoma is characterized by a "flame-like" border or by plug-like or pin-like infiltrations of the tumor into the surrounding tissue (Figs. 10–25 through 10–27). Carcinoma is further characterized by a speckled or piebald pattern clearly discernible from the finely granulated appearance of the normal pancreas. A dark border at the outer margins of the tumor appears to be characteristic. However, the structural pattern of carcinoma may vary considerably in different patients. This may explain why it is not possible in all patients to differentiate between chronic pancreatitis and carcinoma based on changes in the ultrasonographic tissue structure pattern.

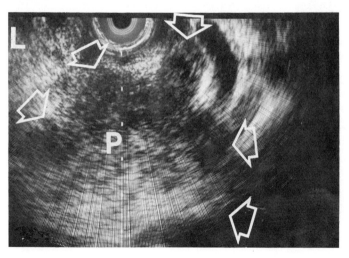

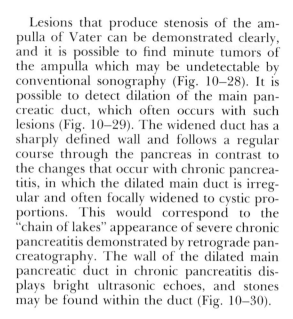

FIGURE 10–25. Carcinoma of head of pancreas (between arrows). Dilated common bile duct in front of portal vein on right side of sonogram. Position of common bile duct on sonogram is due to side inversion of the image as a result of inversion of the instrument. L = Liver; P = pancreas.

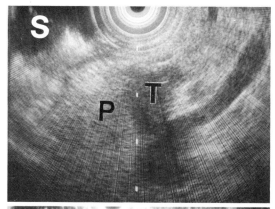

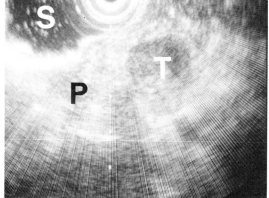

FIGURE 10–26. Pancreatic tumors. *A,* Pancreatic carcinoma (T). P = Head of pancreas, S = waterfilled stomach. *B,* Insulinoma of the pancreas (T) with sharp contours, which characterize the benign process.

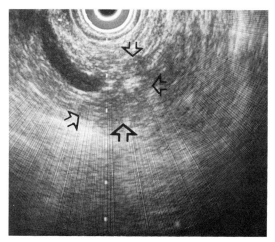

FIGURE 10–28. Carcinoma of papilla of Vater (*between arrows*) with dilation of the main pancreatic duct.

gallbladder can be imaged to demonstrate small polyps or other processes. A malignant disorder is characterized not only by thickening of the wall, but also by destruction of the normal layer structure (Fig. 10–34). Since extracorporeal ultrasonography allows optimal imaging and detection of gallbladder stones, cholelithiasis is probably important in endoscopic ultrasonography only as an incidental finding (Fig. 10–35).

Liver

Endoscopic ultrasonography does not permit scanning of all portions of the liver. The excellent resolution of the procedure may be used to advantage in those areas of the liver which can be imaged from the vantage point

strated by endosonography (see Fig. 10–10), information may be obtained that is additive to that from other investigative techniques, when an inflammatory process must be differentiated from a tumor. The wall of the

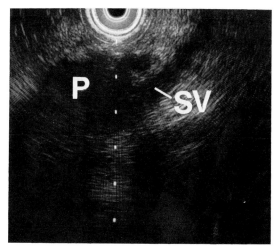

FIGURE 10–27. Carcinoma of body of pancreas (P). SV = Splenic vein.

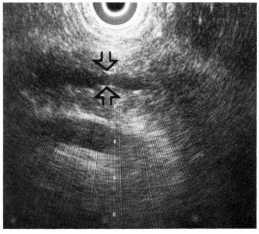

FIGURE 10–29. Dilated main pancreatic duct (*arrows*) in the body of pancreas (same patient as in Figure 10–28).

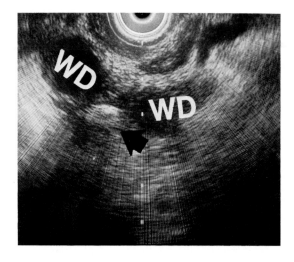

FIGURE 10–30. Dilated main pancreatic duct (WD) with stones (*arrow*).

FIGURE 10–31. Common bile duct (CBD). Prepapillary stone is defined by the asterisks on the right and a small stone is present between the two asterisks on the left.

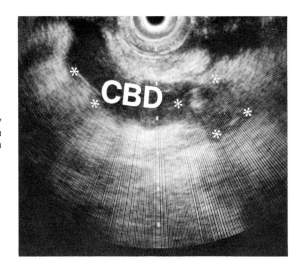

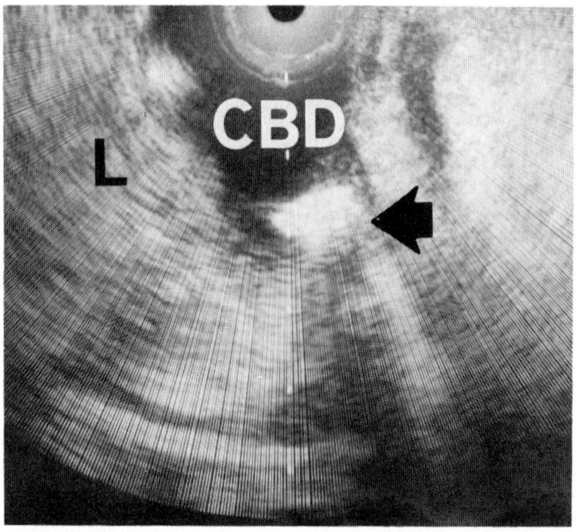

FIGURE 10–32. Prepapillary stone (*arrow*) in widely dilated common bile duct (CBD). L = liver.

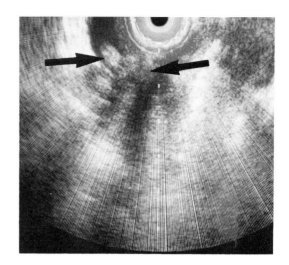

FIGURE 10–33. Three small prepapillary stones in a slightly dilated common bile duct (*arrows*).

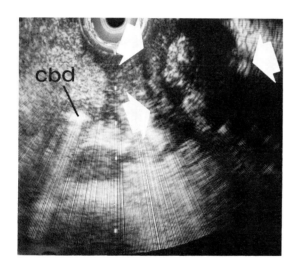

FIGURE 10–34. Carcinoma of gallbladder (*arrows*). Some large stones are present in the gallbladder. In the common bile duct (cbd), presence of a biliary prosthesis results in a bright echo.

FIGURE 10–35. Gallstone (*arrow*) in a normal gallbladder (B).

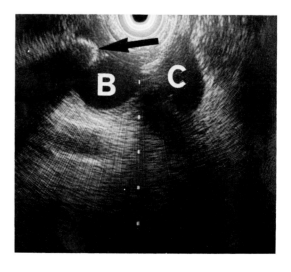

of the stomach. The procedure might prove to be useful if conventional ultrasonography is negative when focal lesions are suspected. The demonstration of very small lesions that might be overlooked normally or of "micro-metastases" is feasible (Fig. 10–36). A clinical situation may arise with a cystic process involving the liver when it is important to differentiate between a malignant and benign etiology. In the case of an echinococcus cyst, for example, analysis of the wall structure can be important. In one case in our experience, endosonography demonstrated a multilayered structure in a calcified echinococcus cyst that was not found by conventional sonography (Fig. 10–37).

Stomach

The wall of the stomach may be studied by endoscopic ultrasonography in any area, but scanning is only possible if carried out through a liquid interface. With this technique, the wall is differentiated into a characteristic pattern with several layers.[29] The wall is about 3.7 ± 0.6 mm (mean ± S.D.) thick. In the body of the stomach the gastric rugae present an undulating pattern, while in the antrum the mucosal side of the image is flat (Figs. 10–38 and 10–39). In the body as well as the antrum, five layers are clearly discernible by their differing densities. On the basis of our studies, the following five layers are discriminated: (1) inner echo-dense layer, (2) inner echo-poor layer, (3) middle echo-dense layer, (4) outer echo-poor layer, and (5) outer echo-dense layer. We assume,

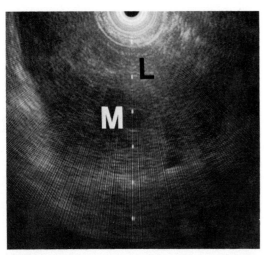

FIGURE 10–36. Liver metastasis (M). L = Normal liver tissue.

in agreement with Fukuda et al.,[13] that the two inner layers relate to the mucosa and the muscularis mucosae. The middle layer probably corresponds to the submucosa while the outer echo-poor layer represents the muscularis propria. This layer is usually not included in the mucosal folds, or if present it is only to a small degree. The outer echo-dense layer is very thin and not always demonstrable. It probably represents the serosa.

An increase in the thickness of the stomach wall may be gauged endosonographically. In our experience it has been possible to demonstrate which gastric wall layer is responsible for the increased wall thickness in every case (Fig. 10–40). In gastric ulcer a funnel-like crater in the layers of the wall with interruption of the usual structure is seen endosonographically. Alterations are also noted in the surrounding tissue with thickening of the serosa (Fig. 10–41) and submucosa. There are no reliable ultrasonographic criteria, as yet, for differentiation of benign from malignant gastric ulcers. Such differentiation of benign from malignant tumor masses, however, appears to be possible. A benign mass is sharply demarcated against its surrounding tissue (Fig. 10–42). A malignant process is more irregular, and infiltration and destruction of the gastric wall can be demonstrated. Malignant tissue is echo-poor and is easily differentiated from its surroundings, which are rich with ultrasonographic echoes. Tumor infiltration produces a clefted pattern. Destruction of the normal multilayered wall structure appears to be a sign of malignancy (Figs. 10–43 through 10–45). An endosonographic diagnosis of a malignant tumor must, at the present time, be supported by biopsy and tissue diagnosis.

Esophagus

The published experience with respect to determination of the extent of carcinoma or ulcerative processes in the esophageal wall is limited. However, the malignant process is discernible (Fig. 10–46). There is destruction of the normal layering of the esophageal wall, and the extent of a carcinoma can be assessed in both longitudinal and horizontal directions. Tumor masses infiltrating the mediastinum may also be depicted, and lymph node metastases are detectable. Preliminary investigations have shown[17] that esophageal var-

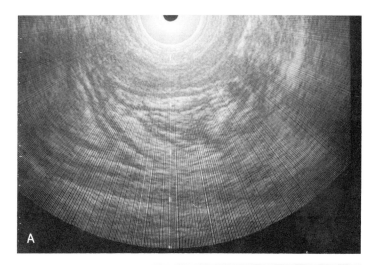

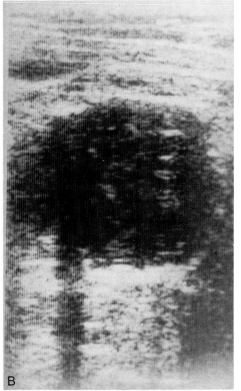

FIGURE 10–37. Membranous structure of an echinococcus cyst of the liver. *A*, Sonographic endoscopy. *B*, Conventional sonography, linear array scan, 2.2 MHz.

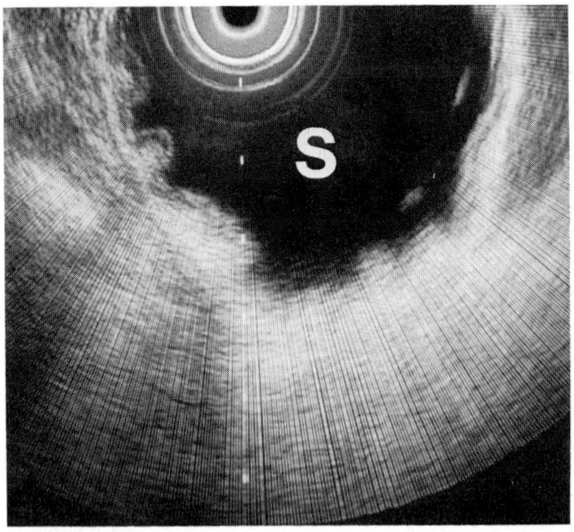

FIGURE 10–38. Gastric endosonography showing body of stomach and undulating five-layer gastric wall. S = Gastric lumen.

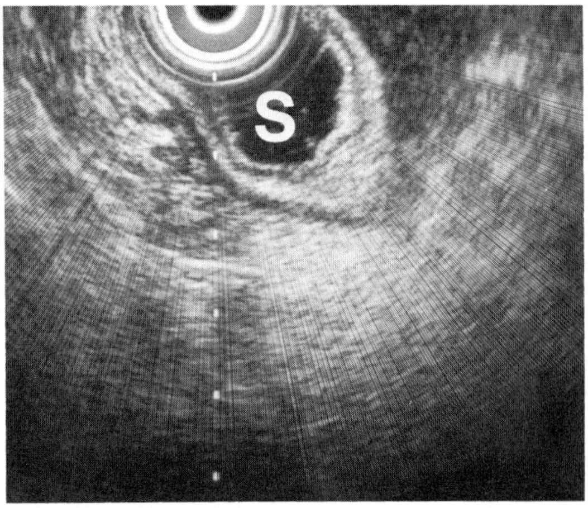

FIGURE 10–39. Endosonography of antrum of stomach showing circumscribed thickening of middle, echo-rich layer (submucosa). S = Gastric lumen.

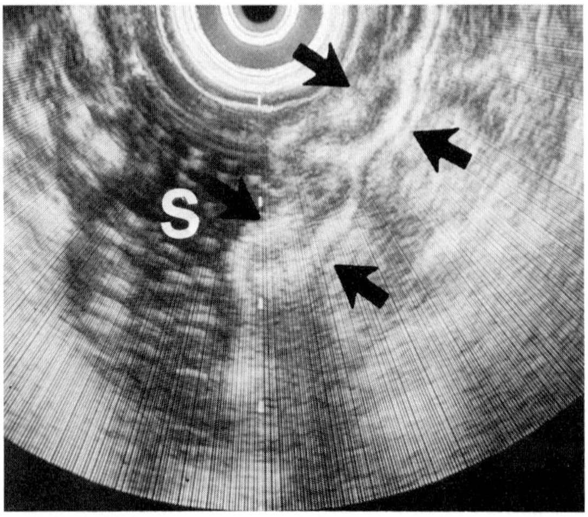

FIGURE 10–40. Gastric wall thickening in foveolar hyperplasia (*arrows*). S = Gastric lumen.

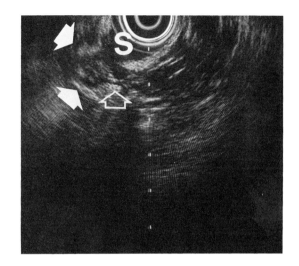

FIGURE 10–41. Benign ulcer of gastric antrum (*arrows*). S = Gastric lumen.

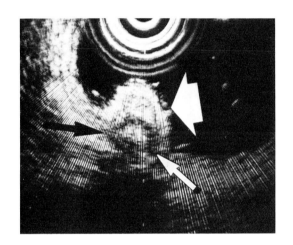

FIGURE 10–42. Benign gastric tumor (confirmed histologically neurofibroma).

FIGURE 10–43. Malignant polyp (T) of body of stomach with infiltration of mucosa (*arrows*). S = Gastric lumen.

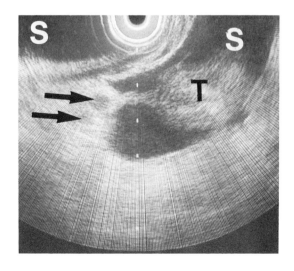

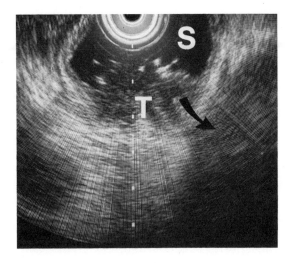

FIGURE 10–44. Ulcerating carcinoma (T) of body of stomach with infiltration (arrow). S = Gastric lumen.

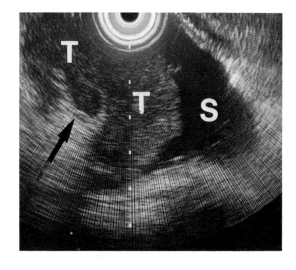

FIGURE 10–45. Adenocarcinoma of stomach. Dark tumor tissue (T) in echo-rich surrounding tissue shows signs of infiltration (*arrows*). S = Gastric lumen.

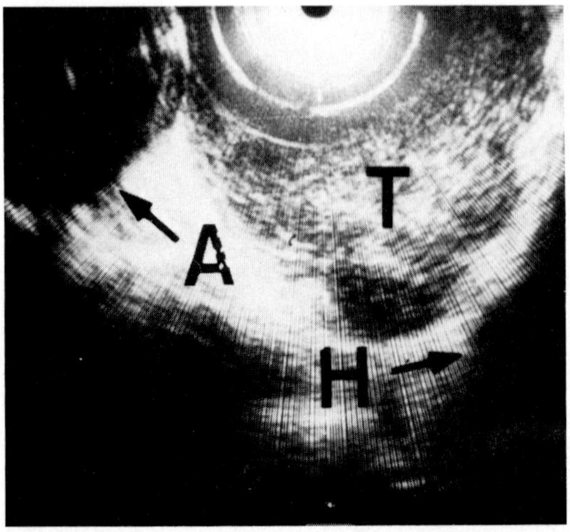

FIGURE 10–46. Esophageal carcinoma (T) between aorta (A) and heart (H). The instrument tip is covered by a water-filled balloon.

ices can be demonstrated by endosonography.

Heart

The advantage of sonographic endoscopy for imaging the heart is based on the close anatomic relationship between the esophagus and atria. Endosonographic detection of atrial septal defect was successful in 95% of patients, whereas detection by conventional echocardiography was successful in only 30% of cases.[30] Intravenous injection of cold saline into a cubital vein produces an echo-dense cloud that may be seen to cross the septum. There are certain advantages of endoechocardiography in the estimation of end diastolic and end systolic heart volume and in the diagnosis of aortic stenosis.[30–32]

SUMMARY

Endoscopic ultrasonography is an investigational procedure that is still in the stage of development and testing. The list of possible indications is incomplete and must be refined. The special advantages of the procedure must be stressed and developed to the point that the procedure is clinically useful and justified in certain patients. For example, it may provide unique information in all disorders that result in thickening of the gastric wall. However, for disorders of the liver and gallbladder, it seems unlikely that the procedure will add significant information in the majority of cases over and above that obtained with existing methods of investigation. Conversely, it may prove to be useful in pancreatic carcinoma and malignant disorders of bile ducts as wall as in tumors found within the hepatic-renal and splenic-renal angles, including those originating in the adrenal glands.

Endoscopic ultrasonography may be useful in any case in which conventional ultrasonography leaves diagnostic questions unresolved because of technical problems or insufficient sonographic resolution.

Although endoscopic ultrasonography can potentially be considered a secondary diagnostic method, it is interesting to speculate on the possibility of detecting small pancreatic carcinomas or adrenal tumors. At the present time, the technique is too involved to be considered as a screening investigation. However, refinement in technique and better instruments may permit some form of screening or perhaps incorporation of the method into the routine upper gastrointestinal examination, although such applications are purely speculative. It has been shown that endosonography is very useful in a variety of individual cases,[13, 16, 19, 20, 22, 23] but a great deal of further study and evaluation is required to define the sensitivity and specificity of the technique in a wide variety of disorders along with a critical comparison of its potential advantages with those of conventional methods of investigation.

Differentiation of benign from malignant disorders in a variety of organs is an important consideration. Whether endosonography is superior to conventional ultrasonography in this respect is unanswered. It is attractive to believe that it will be more sensitive and specific in the diagnosis of pancreatic carcinoma. Relatively small lesions have been detected.[21] In addition, the malignant character of pancreatic lesions is thought to be more demonstrable by endosonography than by conventional ultrasonography.[25] The endoscopic approach may be of value in assessment of the extent of certain lesions prior to surgery, as for example, gastric carcinoma. Regional metastasis may be detected by endosonography.[17]

As with any new method, endosonography has important problems,[33] and the procedure is not yet sufficiently developed to recommend general clinical use. The relatively long, rigid distal instrument tip makes maneuvering difficult. Inversion of the mechanical sector scanner with its rotating reflector creates difficulties with interpretation of the images. However, electronic linear array devices produce images that are small, and orientation may be especially difficult.[4, 20, 22]

The technique of endoscopic ultrasonography must be refined. With present methods it is not possible to image all intra-abdominal organs and regions in all patients. The pancreas can be visualized in about 70% to 80% of cases; the gallbladder and the spleen in 50% to 60% of cases.[34] However, it is possible to improve technique to the point that all parts of the upper gastrointestinal tract and its surrounding organs can be imaged.[13]

Editor's note: There have been technical changes in the instruments for sector scanning endoscopic ultrasonography. The most important is the image display of the Olympus system that now provides a 360 degree scan. This obviates some rotatory movements required in the technique described in this section. References 35, 36, and 37 are recommended.

References

1. DiMagno EP, Buxton JL, Regan PT, et al. Ultrasonic endoscope. Lancet 1980; I:629–31.
2. Strohm WD, Jessen K, Phillip J, Classen M. Endoskopische Ultraschalltomographie desoberen Verdauungstraktes. Dtsch med Wochenschr 1980; 106:714–7.
3. Strohm WD, Phillip J, Hagenmüller F, Classen M. Ultrasonic tomography by means of an ultrasonic fiberendoscope. Endoscopy 1980; 12:241–4.
4. Yamanaka T, Sakai H, Yoshida Y, et al. Ultrasonic endoscopy for the diagnosis of abdominal lesions. Gastroenterol Endosc 1982; 24:598–607.
5. Lutz H, Rösch W. Transgastroscopic ultrasonography. Endoscopy 1976; 8:203–5.
6. Strohm WD. Limits of ultrasound tomography and features of endoscopic ultrasonography. Scand J Gastroenterol 1984; 19(Suppl 94):7–12.
7. Frentzel-Beyme B, Aurich B. Erste Ergebnisse der transrektalen Prostatasosnographie (TPS). In: Kratochwil A, Reinold E, eds. Ultraschalldiagnostik 81. Stuttgart–New York: Thieme, 1982; 308–9.
8. Gammelgaard J, Holm HH. Transurethral and transrectal ultrasonic scanning in urology. J Urol 1980; 124:863–8.
9. Hanrath P, Kremer P, Langenstein BA, et al. Transosophageale Echokardiographie. Dtsch med Wochenschr 1981; 106:523.
10. Nakamura S, Niijima T. Staging of bladder cancer by ultrasonography: a new technique by transurethral intravesical scanning. J Urol 1980; 124:341–4.
11. Popp LW, Leuken RP, Müller–Holve W, Lindemann HJ. Gynaekologische Endosonographie. Ultraschall 1983; 4:92–7.
12. Rageth JC, Vontobel HP. Der Beitrag der Sonographie zur urologischen Diagnostik. Ultraschall 1982; 3:62–8.
13. Fukuda M, Nakano Y, Saito K, et al. Endoscopic ultrasonography in the diagnosis of pancreatic carcinoma. The use of a liquid-filled stomach method. Scand J Gastroenterol 1984; 19(Suppl 94):64–76.
14. Strohm WD, Classen M. Endoskopische Ultraschalltomographie im oberen Gastrointestinaltrakt. Internist 1982; 23:556–64.
15. Strohm WD, Classen M. Endoskopische Ultraschalltomographie (EUT). Technik, normale und pathologische Befunde. In: Ultraschalldiagnostik 82. Stuttgart–New York: Thieme, 1983; 426–8.
16. Strohm WD, Classen M. Endoskopische Ultraschalltomographie. Z Gastroenterol 1983; 21: 104–15.
17. Caletti G, Bolondi L, Labò G. Ultrasonic endoscopy—the gastrointestinal wall. Scand J Gastroenterol 1984; 19(Suppl 102):5–8.
18. Classen M, Strohm WD, Reifart N. Development in endoscopic ultrasound tomography. In: Kawai K, ed. Frontiers of GI Endoscopy. Japan: Olympus Optical Co., 1982; 3–8.
19. Gandolfi L, Rossi A, Solmi L, Leo P. L'ultrasonografia endoscopica addominale. Esperienze preliminari. Giorn Ital Endoscop Dig 1982; 5:71–8.
20. Heyder N, Lutz H, Lux G. Ultraschalldiagnostik via Gastroskop. Ultraschall 1983; 4:85–91.
21. Yasuda K, Tanaka Y, Fujimoto S, et al. Use of endoscopic ultrasonography in small pancreatic cancer. Scand J Gastroenterol 1984; 19(Suppl 102):9–17.
22. DiMagno EP, Regan PT, Clain JE, et al. Human endoscopic ultrasonography. Gastroenterology 1982; 83:824–9.
23. Lux G, Heyder N, Lutz H. Ultraschallendoskopie—Moeglichkeiten einer kombinierten Untersuchungsmethode. In: Henning H, ed. Fortschritte der gastroenterologischen Endoskopie 1983; 12:152–8.
24. Strohm WD, Classen M. Neues über Ultraschallendoskopie. In Henning H, ed. Fortschritte der gastroenterologischen Endoskopie, 1983; 12:147–51.
25. Classen M, Strohm WD, Kurtz W. Pancreatic pseudocyst and tumors in endosonography. Scand J Gastroenterol 1984; 19(Suppl 94):77–84.
26. Strohm WD. Endoskopische Sonographie bei Pankreaserkrankungen. In: Henning H, ed. Fortschritte der gastroenterologischen Endoskopie 1983; 12:159–62.
27. Strohm WD, Kurtz W, Hagenmüller F, Classen M. Diagnostic efficacy of endoscopic ultrasound tomography in pancreatic cancer and cholestasis. Scand J Gastroenterol 1984; 19(Suppl 102):18–23.
28. Strohm WD, Kurtz W, Classen M. Detection of biliary stones by means of endosonography. Scand J Gastroenterol 1984; 19(Suppl 94):60–4.
29. Strohm WD, Classen M. Endoskopisch-sonographische diagnostik der magenwand. Dtsch med Wochenschr 1983; 108:1425–7.
30. Reifart N, Strohm WD. Detection of atrial septum defects by transoesophageal two-dimensional echocardiography with a mechanical sector scanner. In: Hanrath P, Bleifeld W, Souquet JS, eds. Cardiovascular Diagnosis by Ultrasound. Transoesophageal, Computerized, Contrast, Doppler Echocardiography. The Hague, Boston, London: M. Nijhoff, 1982; 247–50.
31. Jaeger N, Radeke HW, Adolphs AD. Die pathologische Harnblase im sonographiscen Bild. Ultraschall 1983; 4:98–105.
32. Reifart N, Strohm WD, Classen M. Erfahrungen mit der endoskopischen Echokardiographie. Herz Gefaesse, 1983; 3:688–94.
33. Silverstein E, Giuliani D, Daigle R. Endoscopic ultrasound. Acta Endoscopica 1983; 13:1–5.
34. Sivak MV Jr, George C. Endoscopic ultrasonography: preliminary experience. Scand J Gastroenterol 1984; 19(Suppl 94):51–9.
35. Endoscopic ultrasonography. Proceedings of the 4th International Symposium on Endoscopic Ultrasonography. Tytgat GNJ, Tio TL, eds. Scan J Gastroenterol 1986; 21(Suppl 123):1–169.
36. Tio TL, den Hartog Jager FCA, Tytgat GNJ. Endoscopic ultrasonography of non-Hodgkin lymphoma of the stomach. Gastroenterology 1986; 91:401–8.
37. Gordon SJ, Rifkin MD, Goldberg BP. Endosonographic evaluation of mural abnormalities of the upper gastrointestinal tract. Gastrointest Endosc 1986; 32:193–8.

Part 2
CHROMOSCOPY

KAZUNORI IDA, M.D.
MASAHIRO TADA, M.D.

ESOPHAGUS, STOMACH, AND DUODENUM

The fine detail of the structure of the gastrointestinal mucosa is not delineated during conventional endoscopy. Yamakawa et al.[1] reported in 1966 that spraying a blue dye solution over gastric mucosa was useful in revealing such structures as the area gastrica. However, the results with this method were not always satisfactory because gastric mucus was also colored by the dye. In 1972 we reported a new procedure to eliminate gastric mucus.[2] With this method, the results of dye-spraying are consistently effective. Various dyes have now been applied in gastrointestinal chromoscopy on the basis of this initial success. Chromoscopy provides a unique approach to accurate diagnosis of many gastrointestinal disorders, a variety of new findings, and information which cannot be obtained by standard endoscopy.

Premedication

No special premedication is necessary for chromoscopy except for the examination of the stomach. Gastric mucosa is covered with large quantities of mucus which inhibits observation. Therefore, procedures for the elimination of mucus are always necessary for chromoscopy of the stomach.

An anticholinergic agent is given intramuscularly to suppress evacuation of the mucus-clearing solution from the stomach. The gastric mucus-clearing solution consists of dimethylpolysiloxan, Pronase (a proteinase enzyme) (Kaken Pharmaceutical Co., Ltd.), and sodium bicarbonate (Fig. 10–47). The temperature of the solution should be about 40° C, which promotes the activity of the enzyme. Sodium bicarbonate maintains the Pronase solution at optimal pH value. The mucus-clearing solution must wash over all gastric mucosal surfaces. This may be accomplished by asking the recumbent patient to roll over once every minute for about 15 or 20 minutes.

Dyes Used in Chromoscopy

Blue dyes such as indigo carmine and methylene blue are the most suitable for observation of gastrointestinal morphology and staining phenomena, because the blue color contrasts sharply with the reddish mucosa. Lugol's solution and Congo red are also useful for certain purposes. Although no side effects from the dyes used in chromoscopy have occurred, only the smallest amount of dye solution required for the examination should be used. At the conclusion of the procedure any remaining pools of dye should be aspirated.

Methods for Spraying the Dye Solution

There are two spraying methods: direct and indirect. With the direct method, which can be used throughout the gastrointestinal tract, a dye solution is sprayed over the mucosa during endoscopic observation by means of a syringe and a Teflon catheter inserted through the accessory channel of the endo-

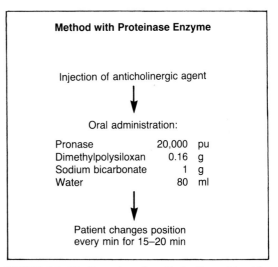

FIGURE 10–47. Procedure for elimination of gastric mucus, using a proteinase enzyme.

scope. The indirect method is used only in the stomach. After premedication and gastric mucus-clearing procedures have been completed, the patient takes the dye orally and repeats the process of repeatedly changing position by rolling over, so that the dye reaches all gastric mucosal surfaces.

Technique and Application

Three basic types of chromoscopy are employed in gastrointestinal endoscopy at the present time: these are the contrast, staining, and reaction methods (Table 10–1).

Contrast Method

The contrast method highlights irregularities in the mucosal architecture by pooling of a blue dye solution in mucosal grooves and other interstices. This improves the precision of endoscopic diagnosis by defining minute and inconspicuous lesions that might otherwise be overlooked with conventional endoscopic methods. Some of the applications of this method are as follows:

1. Observation of the minute structure of the gastrointestinal tract, e.g., the area gastrica, duodenal villi, and colonic area.

2. Confirmation of the existence of a very small lesion, e.g., a gastric erosion or a small colonic polyp.

3. Differentiation of certain lesions as either benign or malignant.

4. Determination of the extent of infiltration of a malignant lesion.

5. Certain applications in conjunction with magnifying endoscopy.

Dye spraying may be either direct or indirect with the contrast method (Fig. ·10–48). In the direct method, 0.2% indigo carmine solution is sprayed after the standard endoscopic evaluation has been completed. If the stomach is to be examined, the mucus-clearing procedure must be completed before the endoscopy. In the indirect method, which is applied only in the stomach, 10 ml of a 3% indigo carmine solution are given orally at the same time that the patient takes the mucus-clearing solution. We prefer this simple indirect method. An indigo carmine solution of greater than 0.3% should not be used in the direct method because areas of abnormal redness or whitish color will be obscured. When the contrast method is used, observation and photography must be carried out quickly because the dye solution, applied either directly or indirectly in the case of the stomach, flows away after a while.

Staining Method

The staining method is based on absorption of dye by epithelial cells, or permeation of the dye into necrotic tissue.[3] Thus, this is a more specific method of chromoscopy, since an absorptive function, with reference to a dye, of the mucosa or of certain lesions is being evaluated at endoscopy.

The staining method can be used to diagnose certain diseases, pathologic conditions, and states of the mucosa that are difficult to recognize with certainty by conventional endoscopic observation. Some examples are gastric intestinal metaplasia and the state of the colonic mucosa in ulcerative colitis, that is, whether the inflammatory process is active or healed.

It is again necessary to eliminate mucus from the stomach if the staining method is to be used in this organ. Direct and indirect methods of dye application may be used in the stomach as outlined in Table 10–2, but the indirect method is preferable because directly sprayed dye promptly flows away and is not fully absorbed. In the duodenum, small

TABLE 10–1. **Chromoscopy**

Method	Mechanism	Application	Dye
Contrast	Dye collects in mucosal depressions	More precise diagnosis	Indigo carmine
Staining	Absorption or permeation of dye	Intestinal metaplasia; intestinal and colonic diseases	Methylene blue
Reaction	Reaction with cell constituent or secretion		
Lugol		Esophagitis; esophageal CA	Lugol's solution
Congo red		Defines acid-secreting mucosa	Congo red or Congo red–Evans blue

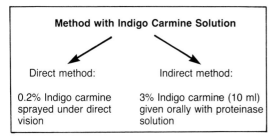

FIGURE 10–48. Contrast method, using indigo carmine solution.

intestine, and colon, however, a 0.1% to 0.5% dye solution is sprayed directly over the mucosa. After 1 to 2 minutes, the mucosa must be washed with water to observe the stained surface.

Reaction Method

In the reaction method, a dye applied to a mucosal surface reacts with a constituent of the epithelial cell or with some mucosal secretion. There are two types, the Lugol method and the Congo red method.

Lugol Method

Non-keratinized squamous epithelial cells contain abundant glycogen, which reacts with Lugol's solution.[4] This reaction has been used in the diagnosis of esophageal diseases such as esophagitis and carcinoma.[5]

After standard endoscopic evaluation, 1.5% to 3.0% Lugol's solution is sprayed directly over the entire esophageal mucosal surface. Normally, the mucosa turns brown within 1 to 2 seconds, and this discoloration then fades within a few minutes. If the reaction is abnormal, the spraying can be repeated.

Congo Red Method

The Congo red method is based on the reaction that occurs between this dye and

secreted hydrochloric acid.[6] It is therefore useful in defining the extent of the acid-secreting normal fundic mucosa. In this method the color of the normal fundic mucosa changes from red to dark blue; the antral mucosal surface does not change color.

The original technique for the Congo red method is as follows. After conventional endoscopic observation, a mixture of 0.3% Congo red and 5% sodium bicarbonate solution is sprayed over the gastric mucosa. Tetragastrin, 5 μg/kg, is then injected intramuscularly. The mucosa is then observed for 15 to 30 minutes until there is no further extension of discolored areas.

This method is not suitable for morphologic observation. We have attempted to modify the original method so that the microstructure of the mucosal surface can be observed at the same time (Fig. 10–49). This modified method, using Congo red and Evans blue dye is applicable in clinical practice and allows simultaneous observation of the acid-secreting mucosa and the microstructure of normal or abnormal gastric mucosa.

Endoscopic Appearance

Esophagus

Reaction Method

After direct spraying with Lugol's solution, the normal esophageal mucosa is stained brown or dark brown and has a fine mucosal pattern suggesting a wrinkled texture. Areas

TABLE 10–2. **Methylene Blue Staining Method**

Direct Method
1. Procedure for elimination of gastric mucus
2. Conventional endoscopic evaluation
3. Spray 0.1% to 0.5% methylene blue solution on mucosa
4. Wash mucosa with water 1 to 2 minutes later
5. Endoscopic chromoscopic observation

Indirect Method
1. Procedure for elimination of gastric mucus
2. Oral administration of 20 ml of 0.5% to 0.7% methylene blue solution in conjunction with the gastric mucus–eliminating solution
3. Patient rolls over once every minute for 15 to 20 minutes
4. Endoscopic chromoscopic observation

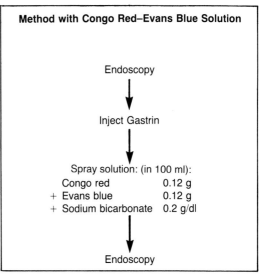

FIGURE 10–49. Modified Congo red method, using Congo red–Evans blue solution.

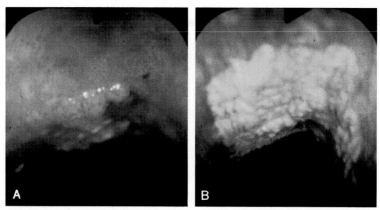

PLATE 10–1. Superficial cancer of the esophagus. *A,* Conventional endoscopy. *B,* After being sprayed with Lugol's solution, the cancer is more clearly delineated.

of leukoplakia stain a striking dark brown. Esophagitis with or without erosions and esophageal cancer are not stained by Lugol's solution. This method is useful for detecting early cancer and for defining the boundaries of invasive cancer. A superficial esophageal carcinoma, shown in Plate 10–1*A,* is well delineated as a whitish lesion after spraying with Lugol's solution (Plate 10–1*B*). In another example, esophagitis is not clearly evident by standard endoscopic observation (Plate 10–2*A*), although irregularly shaped and linear erosions are obvious after dye spraying (Plate 10–2*B*).

Stomach and Duodenum

Contrast Method

Using the contrast method, the normal, that is, acid-secreting fundic mucosa of the proximal stomach is thick and reddish, whereas the pyloric (antral) mucosa and non–acid-secreting fundic mucosa that is affected by fundal gastritis are thin and yellowish (Table 10–3).[7] The appearance of both non-secreting mucosae, when observed in the proximal stomach, corresponds to atrophic gastritis. The term area gastrica, it will be recalled, refers to small areas superimposed upon the gastric mucosa by a system of furrows. These grooves subdivide the mucosa into areas (area gastrica) 1 to 5 mm in diameter. In the normal fundic mucosa (proximal stomach) the gastric pits (foveolae) open within these areas. Between 3 and 7 gastric glands open into each gastric pit. The area gastrica of the normal fundic mucosa are usually regular in size and arrangement; those of the other non–acid-secreting mucosa are generally irregular. The former are called type F and the latter type P. Each type is divided, based on appearance, into 4 subtypes (Fig. 10–50 and Plates 10–3 and 10–4). At the higher end of the scale, i.e., F3 or P3, the mucosa is atrophic.

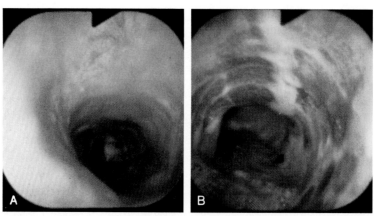

PLATE 10–2. Esophagitis. *A,* Conventional endoscopy. *B,* After spraying Lugol's solution. It is clear that the erosive process is not healed completely.

TABLE 10–3. **Chromoscopic Features of Fundic and Pyloric (Antral) Mucosa**

Mucosa	Fundic Mucosa	Pyloric (Antral) Mucosa
Thickness	Thick	Thin
Color	Reddish	Yellow
Luster	Glossy	Dull
Area gastrica		
Size	Regular	Regular—irregular
Shape	Uniform	Uniform—multiform
Contour	Well-defined	Poorly defined
Arrangement	Close, regular	Regular—irregular

The distal border of the normal fundic types of mucosa in the stomach can be easily recognized because of the differences in mucosal characteristics and the pattern of the area gastrica. This border is not uniform in position in the stomach from individual to individual, especially along the lesser curvature. Two general types are recognized. In the open type, the lesser curvature of the gastric body is covered with non–acid-secreting fundic mucosa; in the closed type, the lesser curvature mucosa is acid-secreting normal fundic (Fig. 10–51). The open and closed types are subdivided into three subtypes according to the extent of the normal fundic mucosa; that is, in the order of Type Co to O_3 the extent of the normal fundic mucosa progressively decreases, and there is a corresponding decrease in acid secretion. An example of a patient with a Type C_2 pattern is shown in Plate 10–5.

The contrast method is very effective in detection of early gastric cancer, especially minute and Type IIb carcinomas (Japanese classification of early gastric cancer), and in recognition of the extent of cancer infiltration in the mucosa.[8] An example of early gastric cancer in the body of the stomach (Type IIc, similar to IIb) is shown in Plate 10–6.

The contrast method is useful in differentiating benign from malignant ulcers and may aid in determining whether or not an ulcer is recurrent.

A small erosion which produces a very shallow depression without elevation of the surrounding mucosa is very difficult to detect endoscopically. However, with the contrast method it is not difficult to recognize such lesions and to define their size, shape, number and distribution (Plate 10–7).

Minute gastric cancers, those less than 5 mm in diameter, often have the shape and appearance of an erosion. They are not only difficult to detect endoscopically, but when discovered their true nature may not be recognized. An example of a minute cancer located on the posterior wall of the antrum is shown in Plate 10–8. In this case only a slight mucosal abnormality was suspected endoscopically, but this suspicion led to spraying with indigo carmine dye, which revealed one erosion with irregular margin located in atrophic mucosa. This malignancy was 3 mm in diameter (Fig. 10–52).

Although superficial gastritis receives little attention as a disorder or disease entity, it can accompany gastric erosions that are thought by some investigators to produce a variety of symptoms including epigastric dis-

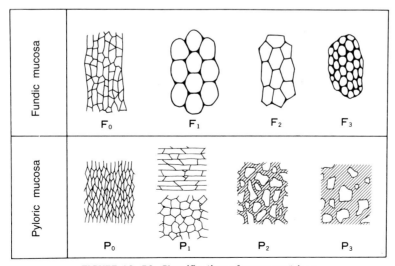

FIGURE 10–50. Classification of areae gastricae.

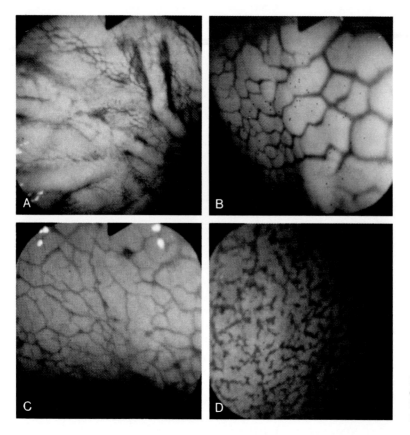

PLATE 10–3. Examples of each classification of areae gastricae in the fundic mucosa. A, F O; B, F 1; C, F 2; D, F 3.

PLATE 10–4. Examples of each classification of areae gastricae in the pyloric (antral) mucosa. A, P O; B, P 1; C, P 2; D, P 3.

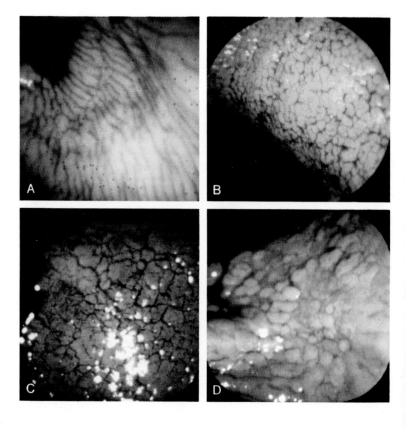

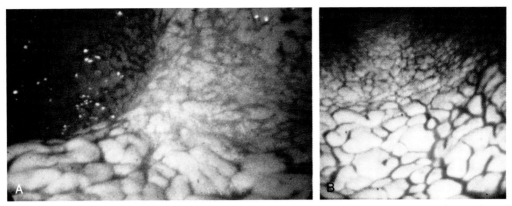

PLATE 10–5. Fundopyloric mucosal border. *A,* Region of the stomach proximal to the angulus in a patient with closed type distribution. *B,* Mucosal border on greatercurvature of antrum.

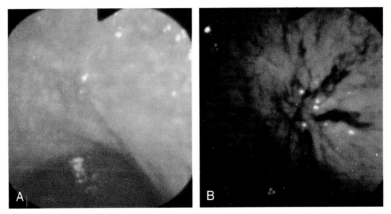

PLATE 10–6. Early gastric cancer (type IIc, similar to type IIb). *A,* Conventional endoscopy. *B,* Direct contrast method demonstrates irregular erosion, greater involvement and spread into the surrounding mucosa, and abnormal red granulation and tapered folds. All findings indicate malignancy.

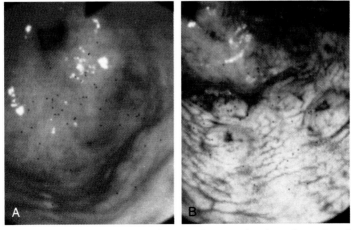

PLATE 10–7. Erosive gastritis, antrum. *A,* Conventional endoscopy showing a few red spots. *B,* Multiple small erosions demonstrated by contrast chromoscopy with indigo carmine solution.

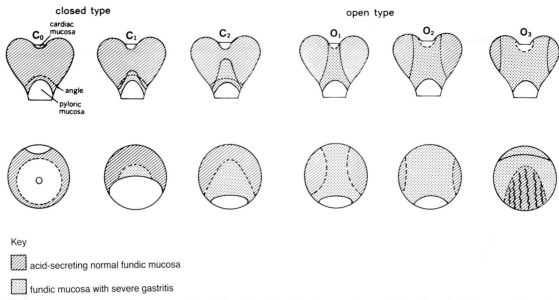

Key

▨ acid-secreting normal fundic mucosa

▦ fundic mucosa with severe gastritis

FIGURE 10–51. Schematic diagram illustrating the closed and open types of (*fundic-pyloric*) *mucosal* border pattern in the stomach as well as the subclassifications of each type. The top row of figures represents the entire stomach opened as a gross specimen along the greater curvature. The bottom row of figures illustrate endoscopic views of the stomach corresponding to the figures in the top row.

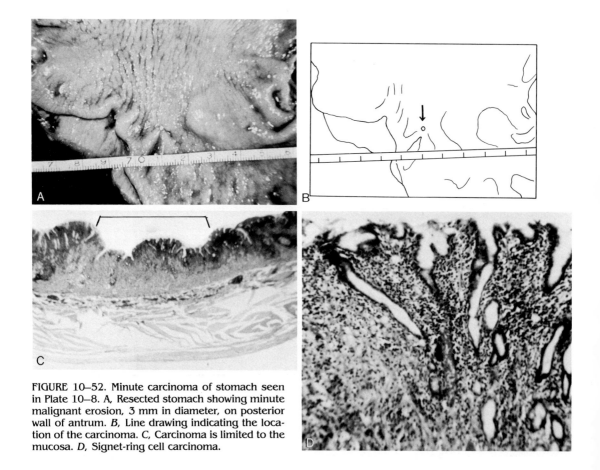

FIGURE 10–52. Minute carcinoma of stomach seen in Plate 10–8. A, Resected stomach showing minute malignant erosion, 3 mm in diameter, on posterior wall of antrum. B, Line drawing indicating the location of the carcinoma. C, Carcinoma is limited to the mucosa. D, Signet-ring cell carcinoma.

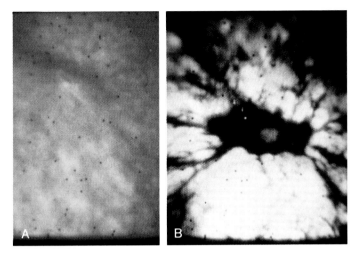

PLATE 10–8. Minute carcinoma of stomach. A, Conventional endoscopy. B, Malignant erosion revealed by indigo carmik contrast method.

PLATE 10–9. Comb-like redness and linear erosions, gastric body. A, Comb-like redness by conventional endoscopy. B, Linear erosion on a reddened fold, revealed by contrast method.

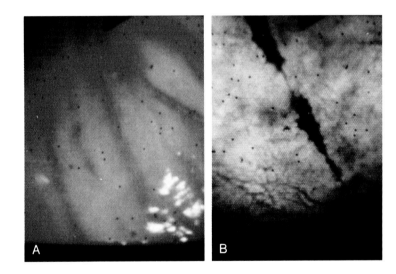

PLATE 10–10. A, Subtle comb-like redness with linear distribution in antrum. B, Multiple small erosions in antrum demonstrated by contrast chromoscopy.

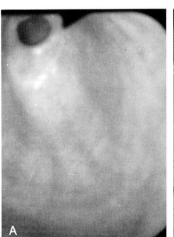

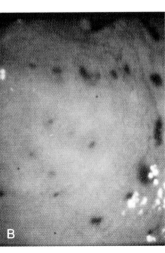

comfort. Superficial gastritis may be manifest as redness of the mucosa. There may be a comb-like pattern, that is, multiple, long, frequently narrow red lines in the mucosa, which are arranged in a parallel fashion. Comb-like redness, such as redness on the surface of ridge-like folds as shown in Plate 10–9, is considered to be a sign of superficial gastritis. This linear distribution pattern is frequently found in the antrum and may be accompanied by erosions in the same distribution pattern (Plate 10–10). The clinical significance of mucosal abnormalities such as superficial gastritis is debatable. This subject is developed fully in Chapter 21. It is our view that symptoms may result from superficial gastritis, and that the use of contrast chromoscopy will reveal associated erosions in many patients with comb-like redness and unexplained epigastric discomfort or pain.

The villous pattern of the duodenum and individual villi are clearly defined by the contrast method. In Plate 10–11, two micro-erosions are shown in a duodenal bulb, in which the mucosal pattern has otherwise a normal villous appearance. Such erosions are found frequently. The contrast method is also helpful in determining whether a duodenal ulcer has healed completely. In the example shown, standard endoscopic observation appears to demonstrate a small duodenal ulcer, but contrast chromoscopy reveals that the mucosa over the lesion has a finely granular surface and is not open (Plate 10–12).

Staining Method

Two groups of stomach lesions are defined by in vivo staining chromoscopy. Group 1 comprises the lesions that have absorptive cells and regular papillae; like villi, they are stainable by spraying methylene blue on their surface. The papillae thus stained can be seen when the tip of the endoscope is close to the mucosal surface or by high-magnification endoscopy (Plate 10–13). The lesions in Group 2 do not have the stainable, regular papillae. The staining method in this group is based on permeation of methylene blue into tumor tissue. The lesions in Group 1 include intestinal metaplasia, elevated, atypical epithelium, and polyps consisting of intestinalized mucosal tissue. Group 2 comprises protruded gastric cancers that are covered by necrotic tissue and debris.

Gastric intestinal metaplasia is accurately diagnosed using the staining method. The appearance of intestinal metaplasia in the antrum is illustrated in Plate 10–14A. The darkly stained lesion in the middle of the stained area is an elevated early gastric cancer. A magnified view of its surface is also shown in Plate 10–14B. The observation that this polypoid lesion in an area of metaplasia does not have regular stainable papillae indicates a Group 2 classification, and this differentiates it as a malignant polypoid growth. By discriminating the staining pattern of Group 1 from Group 2, benign and malignant polypoid lesions can be differentiated.[9]

The villi of normal duodenal mucosa are well stained with methylene blue. (Abnormal staining and magnification of villi stained with methylene blue are discussed below.) Relatively inconspicuous duodenal ulcers can be easily recognized with this staining method (Plate 10–15). This method will reveal complete or incomplete healing of an ulcer and will demonstrate complete versus incomplete re-epithelialization. An ulcer scar takes the same stain as surrounding mucosa, and this indicates complete re-epithelialization and therefore complete healing with a likelihood that a particular ulcer will not recur.

Reaction Method—Congo Red

Although the original Congo red method demonstrates only the extent of acid-secreting mucosa (Plate 10–16), the modified method delineates minute gastric mucosal structures, such as area gastrica, before discoloration by the Congo red dye occurs (Plate 10–17A). Once discoloration takes place, the junction of the acid- and non–acid-secreting mucosal areas is sharply defined (Plate 10–17B).

Muscosal Border and Gastroduodenal Disease

As noted above, the distribution pattern for acid-secreting normal fundic mucosa and the other non–acid-secreting one in the stomach, and hence the border between these two areas, differs from individual to individual. In general the demarcation between the two mucosal-type areas moves in an orad direction with increasing age, that is, in a group of patients the predominant classification changes from Co toward O_3 as age increases (Fig. 10–53). Gastric cancer and polyp formation, within this classification, will be found with the highest frequency in patients with the greatest proximal extent of the pyloric (antral) type mucosa, that is, those in Type O_3. Furthermore, there is a gradual increase in the frequency of these disorders

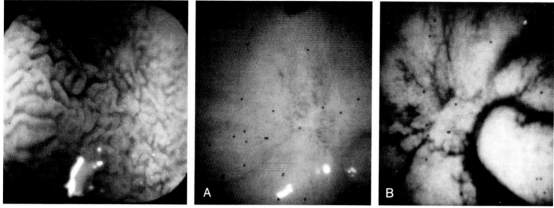

PLATE 10–11.   PLATE 10–12.

PLATE 10–11. Normal villi and two small erosions in the duodenal bulb (contrast method).
PLATE 10–12. Duodenal ulcer scar. *A,* Conventional endoscopy suggests that crater is still open. *B,* Contrast chromoscopy demonstrates fine granular pattern, indicating that the crater is closed.

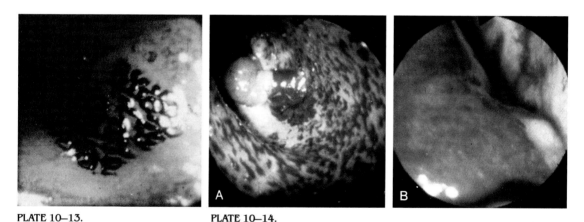

PLATE 10–13.   PLATE 10–14.

PLATE 10–13. Close-up view of intestinal metaplasia stained with methylene blue.
PLATE 10–14. *A,* Appearance of intestinal metaplasia (staining method) and elevated early carcinoma in antrum. *B,* Close-up view of the carcinomatous portion of the lesion which has no regular papillae.

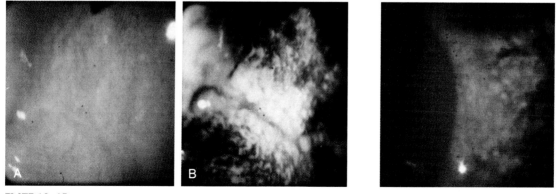

PLATE 10–15.   PLATE 10–16.

PLATE 10–15. Short linear ulcer, duodenal bulb. *A,* Conventional endoscopy. *B,* Staining method reveals a linear ulcer surrounded by non-stained mucosa.
PLATE 10–16. Endoscopic appearance after original Congo red method. Very dark purple color develops in acid-secreting mucosa.

Age
(cases)

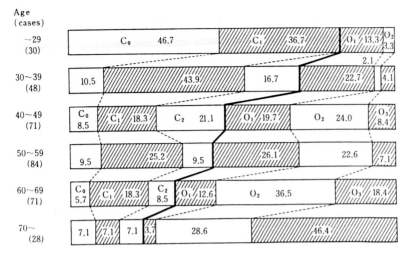

FIGURE 10–53. Types of mucosal border by age group.

as the classification changes from Co toward O_3. Conversely, the frequency of duodenal ulcer, gastric erosions, and superficial gastritis decreases as the border moves in an orad direction; that is, the highest incidence will be found with the Co classification.

The more proximal the location of a peptic ulcer, the more proximal the demarcation between the two types of mucosa. In other words, an ulcer in a proximal position will be found in fundic mucosa, which occupies a relatively small percentage of the total gastric mucosal surface area, and generally the acid output of the stomach will be low. It is interesting that more than 90% of patients with active duodenal ulcers have a closed-type mucosal pattern, and that open Types O_2 and O_3 are not found. The comb-like redness characteristic of superficial gastritis, as expected, is more often found when the mucosal pattern is a closed type.

SMALL INTESTINE AND COLON

Chromoscopy of the Small Intestine

Applications of chromoscopy in the small intestine mainly focus on observation of the villi; high-magnification fiberscopes are frequently used in conjunction with chromoscopy of the small bowel. High-magnification endoscopy is presented in greater detail in Part 3 of this chapter.

Technique

Two of the various magnifying endoscopes suitable for close observation of the villi are the type SIF-M magnifying enteroscope (Olympus Corp.) and the type CF-HM mag-

nifying colonoscope (Olympus Corp.). The latter is available commercially. The specifications of several types that are useful in conjunction with chromoscopy are outlined in Table 10–4. Use of the SIF-M and CF-HM for close observation permits photography at magnifications of 10 to 35 times.

The magnifying enteroscope or colonoscope is introduced into the small intestine via the anus or mouth. The CF-HM can only be used for observations in the ileum, but the SIF-M can be used for examination of all segments of the small intestine. With the instrument in place, and after the standard inspection, 10 ml of a 0.1% methylene blue solution are sprayed on the mucosa. Staining of the villi occurs rapidly.

Magnified View of Villi

The villi may have any of several different shapes or forms that can be described as finger-like, leaf-like, and ridged-convoluted, along with a variety of other shapes.[10] The villi of the duodenal bulb are ridge-shaped, but those in the distal duodenum are finger-like (Plate 10–18). A few villi with a wider form (tongue-like) may be found among the finger-shaped villi, but these are thought to be a variation of normal (Plate 10–19). Villi near the ileocecal valve have a ridged-convoluted form similiar to that of those in the duodenal bulb. In inflammatory bowel diseases, the villi are irregular in shape or their form is lost completely. In an area of tuberculous scarring of the intestine the villi are finger- or leaf-shaped but vary in size, and their arrangement is irregular and sporadic (Plate 10–20); also, the absorption of meth-

TABLE 10–4. **Specifications of Magnifying Colonoscopes**

Specification	CF-MB-M Type I	CF-MB-M Type II	CF-HM	CF-UHM	SIF-M
Length (mm)	1270	1270	1670	1270	2101
Working length (mm)	1110	1105	1420	1035	1860
Insertion tube outer diameter (mm)	14	13	14.4	14	10
Bending angle (degrees)					
Up/down	120	180	180	120	150/120
R/L	120	140	160	110	90
Biopsy channel diameter (mm)	2.8	2.8	2.8	2.8	2.8
Optics—angle of view (degrees)	75	50	70	100* 0.213†	65
Observation range (mm)	5–∞	2–∞	2.3–∞	3–100* 0.095–0.105†	2.4–45
Magnification	10×	25×	35×	170×	10×

*Conventional optical system.
†Magnifying optical system.

ylene blue in the area of the scar is inferior to that occurring with normal villi. In Crohn's disease, the villous pattern is irregular with leaf or ridge-convolution forms (Plate 10–21). It is interesting that in Crohn's disease the villi that are distant from an obvious inflammatory focus, and that seem to be intact by unaided endoscopic observation, actually have an atrophic appearance when studied by high-magnification chromoscopy.

When a villus becomes abnormal, there is a striking reduction in the total number of epithelial cells constituting it. Thus a leaf-shaped villus has only one eighth the cells found in a normal structure. Such morphologic abnormalities can be found, for example, in the intestinal villi of post-gastrectomy patients. It is thought that these and similar abnormalities correspond to a malabsorptive condition in the mucosa, and that they reflect the pathophysiologic state of the small intestine.

Chromoscopy of the Colon

Technique

The colonic mucosal surface, on close observation, is granular in appearance and demarcated into small areas by nonspecific grooves (Fig. 10–54). When a blue dye such as indigo carmine or methylene blue is

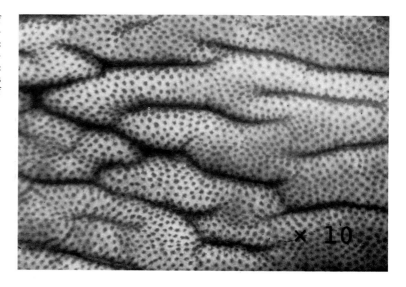

FIGURE 10–54. Close-up view of normal colon mucosa, using dissecting microscope. The surface shows granularity and demarcation by nonspecific grooves. The granules are actually minute pits that correspond to the crypts of Lieberkühn.

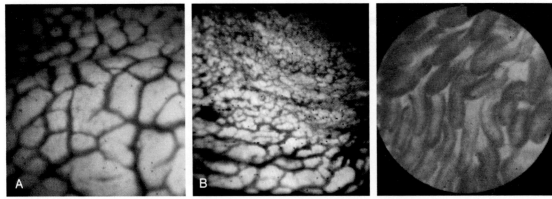

PLATE 10–17.   PLATE 10–18.

PLATE 10–17. Endoscopic appearance after Congo red–Evans blue method. A, Areae gastricae after spraying Congo red–Evans blue solution. B, Blue area corresponds to fundic mucosa.
PLATE 10–18. Normal villi (finger-shaped).

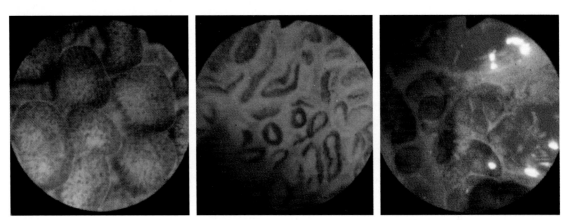

PLATE 10–19.   PLATE 10–20.   PLATE 10–21.

PLATE 10–19. Tongue-shaped villi.
PLATE 10–20. Atrophic villi of intestinal tuberculosis.
PLATE 10–21. Irregular villi of Crohn's disease.

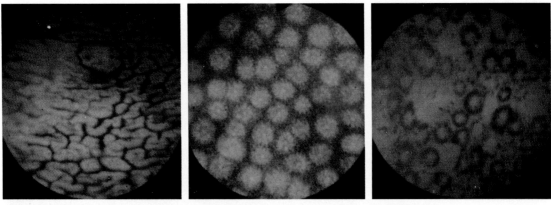

PLATE 10–22.   PLATE 10–23.   PLATE 10–24.

PLATE 10–22. Chromoscopy with 0.5% indigo carmine solution demonstrates fine colon areae and minute polyp too difficult to observe by conventional colonoscopy.
PLATE 10–23. Magnified view of normal colon mucosa using a CF–HM endoscope (x35). Mucosa stained by 1.0% methylene blue. Minute round pits arranged regularly.
PLATE 10–24. Magnified view of mucosa in quiescent stage of ulcerative colitis. No erosions are observed; various-sized pits are arranged irregularly.

TABLE 10–5. **Classification of Minute Mucosal Structures in Ulcerative Colitis**

Endoscopic Findings	Grade III	Grade II	Grade I	Grade 0
Color	Redness (+ +)	Redness (+ to −)	Normal	Normal
Depression	(+ +)	(+ to −)	(± to −)	None
Colonic Area				
Shape	Disappear or abnormal	Abnormal	Almost normal	Normal—spiral, oval
Arrangement	Irregular	Irregular	Almost regular	Regular
Margin	Unclear or irregular	Irregular	Regular	Regular
Colonic Pit				
Shape	Disappear or abnormal	Abnormal	Almost normal	Normal—round, oval
Arrangement	Irregular	Irregular	Almost regular	Regular

sprayed on the surface, the grooved pattern is observable without difficulty (Plate 10–22). Several normal variations in the shape of the colonic mucosal areas defined by the grooves can be seen: spindle, oval-form, and so on.

Diagnosis of Colonic Diseases

In the active stage of ulcerative colitis, the regular spindle-shaped appearance of the colonic area is lost, and irregular ulceration or erosions become evident.[11] When ulcerative colitis enters an inactive phase, and the mucosal inflammation begins to recede, the fine network-like pattern of mucosal areas is recovered little by little. In the recovering stage, minute depressions in the mucosal surface may still be found in a sporadic distribution. These prove to be either microerosions or their scars, or both, when observed with the high-magnification colonoscope. Even though standard endoscopic observation appears to indicate that the process is completely quiescent, high-magnification chromoscopy clearly demonstrates in some cases that the inflammation has not receded completely.

The minute structures of the colonic mucosa demonstrated by chromoscopy may be classified into four grades (0, I, II, and III) by reference to four endoscopic findings. These are: color; the presence of depressions in the mucosa; the shape, arrangement, and the condition of the margins of the colonic areas formed by the nonspecific furrowing of the mucosa; and the shape and arrangement of the minute colonic pits (Table 10–

5). In ulcerative colitis this grading system corresponds closely to histologic study of the mucosa (Table 10–6). All mucosa graded as III and 58% graded as II by chromoscopic observation prove histologically to be in an active stage of the disease. If graded I by chromoscopy, the mucosa is almost always in a healed stage, and microscopic study always indicates healing and quiescent disease if the chromoscopic findings are in Grade 0.

Early in the course of ulcerative colitis, the mucosa may revert to a nearly normal appearance as inflammation subsides and the disease enters a quiescent phase. At this stage, endoscopic diagnosis may be difficult. However, minute mucosal changes (Grade I) may be observed using chromoscopy. Although the normal shape and arrangement of the colonic areas may be recovered almost completely, scattered minute depressions may still be detected. Histologically these prove to be

TABLE 10–6. **Grading of Minute Mucosal Structures Versus Histologic Stage in Ulcerative Colitis**

	Histologic Stage			
Grade	*Active*	*Almost Healed*	*Healed*	Total
III	18 (100)*			18
II	29 (58)	21 (42)		50
I		13 (35)	24 (65)	37
0			14 (100)	14

*( ) Indicates percentage.

TABLE 10–7. Classification of Minute Features of Polypoid Lesions of the Colon

Category	Characteristics
Round (circular)	Regular, round or very nearly round pits; slightly larger than normal mucosal pits
Tubular	Various patterns, from circular to elliptical and oval
Sulcus	Sinus formation resembling cerebral gyrus; no pits
Irregular	Cauliflower-like, rough, irregular surface; no regular structural pattern

microerosions or small scars. Microscopic examination of the mucosa surrounding these depressions always reveals nearly normal findings except for a slight incremental increase in inflammatory cells and fibrosis. Thus, colonoscopic observations in ulcerative colitis are more reliable and accurate when the techniques of chromoscopy are applied. A minor level of disease activity may be recognized, or the disease may be categorized with greater certainty as quiescent.

The characteristics of minute polypoid colonic lesions may also be studied more thoroughly using chromoscopy than is possible with conventional colonoscopic observation.

Magnified Observation

Magnifying endoscopes (CF-MB-M and CF-HM, see Table 10–4) add another dimension to chromoscopy: they provide images that are magnified about 10 to 35 times. The CF-UHM has two optical systems, one of which is a conventional type. The second is a magnifying system that has a field of view 0.213 mm in diameter, a range of observation from 0.095 to 0.105 mm, and a magnification of 170×. The two systems can be interchanged while the endoscope is in use by means of a control on the instrument, which therefore provides "ultra high" magnification with ease.

When chromoscopy is combined with high-magnification endoscopy, it is not difficult to study the fine details of the colon. The numerous minute pits which can be seen superimposed on the furrowing pattern and colonic areas are the crypts of Lieberkühn (Plate 10–23). These minute pits are regularly arranged and are round or oval. The diameter of each pit is about 50 microns.

In the active stage of ulcerative colitis, the mucosa is not stained by methylene blue because it cannot absorb the dye. The mucosa is also eroded in this stage and the pits are obscured. Therefore, it is not possible to observe the crypts by high-magnification endoscopy in the active stage of the disease. However, during the healing process, the mucosal architecture recovers gradually. As healing progresses, the pits may again be seen (Plate 10–24). There may be slight mucosal staining in which the pits, nevertheless, are clearly outlined. However, the arrangement of the pits is usually irregular, and their diameter varies. Observations such as the

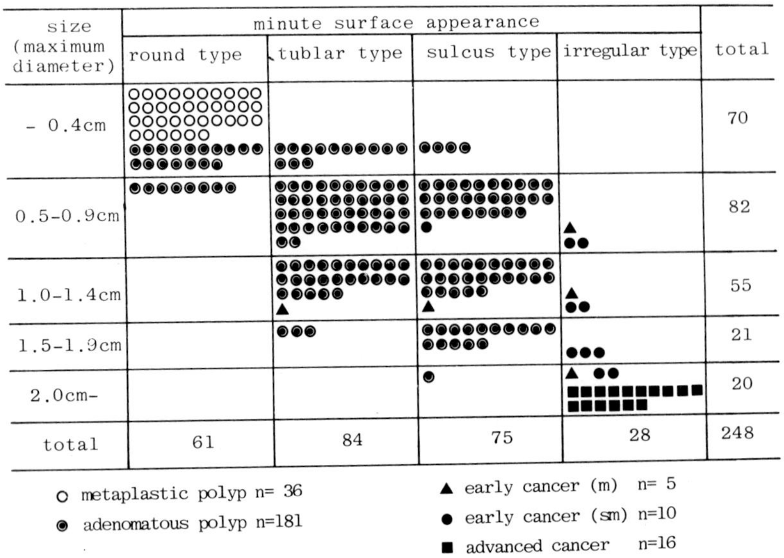

size (maximum diameter)	minute surface appearance				total
	round type	tublar type	sulcus type	irregular type	
– 0.4cm	○○○○○○○○○○ ○○○○○○○○○○ ○○○○○○ ◉◉◉◉◉◉◉◉◉◉ ◉◉◉◉◉◉◉	◉◉◉◉◉◉◉◉◉◉ ◉◉◉	◉◉◉◉		70
0.5–0.9cm	◉◉◉◉◉◉◉◉	◉◉◉◉◉◉◉◉◉◉ ◉◉◉◉◉◉◉◉◉◉ ◉◉◉◉◉◉◉◉◉◉ ◉◉	◉◉◉◉◉◉◉◉◉◉ ◉◉◉◉◉◉◉◉ ◉	▲ ●●	82
1.0–1.4cm		◉◉◉◉◉◉◉◉◉◉ ◉◉◉◉◉ ▲	◉◉◉◉◉◉◉◉◉◉ ◉◉◉◉◉ ▲	▲ ●●	55
1.5–1.9cm		◉◉◉	◉◉◉◉◉◉◉◉◉◉ ◉◉◉◉◉	●●●	21
2.0cm–			◉	▲ ●● ■■■■■■■■■ ■■■■■■	20
total	61	84	75	28	248

FIGURE 10–55. Correlation between minute surface appearance and histologic findings of small polypoid lesions of the colon.

○ metaplastic polyp n= 36
◉ adenomatous polyp n=181
▲ early cancer (m) n= 5
● early cancer (sm) n=10
■ advanced cancer   n=16

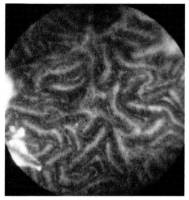
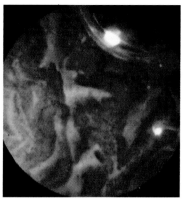
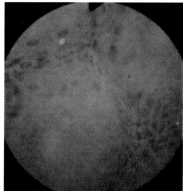

PLATE 10–25.   PLATE 10–26.   PLATE 10–27.

PLATE 10–25. Minute mucosal pattern of polypoid lesions of colon, sulcus type (adenomatous polyp).
PLATE 10–26. Irregular mucosal pattern of early cancer.
PLATE 10–27. Ultra-magnified view of normal colon mucosa, using a CF–UHM endoscope.

return of this feature in the normal mucosa allow a more precise estimate of the activity of the mucosal inflammatory process.

Minute polypoid lesions can be classified into four categories according to the shape or arrangement of the pits (Table 10–7). Their shapes are termed circular or round, tubular, sulcus (Plate 10–25), and irregular (Plate 10–26). The correlation in our series between the minute mucosal detail of these polypoid structures with their size and histologic characteristics is illustrated in Figure 10–55. The smaller metaplastic polyps are classified as having circular pits. The pits of adenomatous polyps are circular, tubular, or sulcus in type and are regular in shape and arrangement. All advanced cancers have irregular pits. About 80% of early cancers have irregularly shaped pits and can be recognized easily with this technique. However, 20% of early cancers have pits of the tubular or

sulcus type, and therefore their appearance overlaps with that of benign adenomas. Small early cancers such as these are often misdiagnosed, and their recognition remains problematic.

The newly designed ultra high-magnification colonoscope, the CF-UHM, was introduced in 1982 to improve the recognition of small colonic cancers.[12] With this instrument it is possible to observe cellular features such as the nucleus. The minute appearance of the colonic pits in normal, flat mucosa can be inspected at magnifications of 170× (Plate 10–27). The pits are round or somewhat oval. The small nuclei of cells are arranged peripheral to the opening into the pit. Each nucleus is round and regular in size. The pits of an adenomatous polyp are enlarged and have an elliptical shape in comparison (Plate 10–28). The nuclei are arranged in a peripheral position around the pit as occurs in flat,

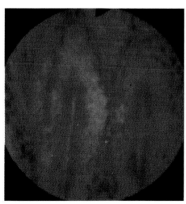
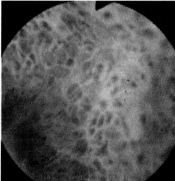

PLATE 10–28. Mucosal pattern of adenomatous polyp (x170). Pits are enlarged and have elongated oval shape.
PLATE 10–29. Mucosal pattern of early cancer (x170). Pits are not clearly defined and are displaced by regular sulcus formation. Nuclei are irregular in size and arrangement.

PLATE 10–28.   PLATE 10–29.

normal mucosa; each nucleus is regular in its arrangement and size. In early cancer, pits are indistinct and are displaced by the formation of regular furrows (Plate 10–29). The nuclei are also irregular in shape and can be differentiated without difficulty from those found in benign polyps. It appears that colon cancer can be diagnosed in an early or diminutive stage by observation with the CF-UHM. It may also be possible to recognize cellular atypism prior to the appearance of structural changes.

References

1. Yamakawa K, Naito S, Kanai J, et al. Superficial staining of gastric lesions by fiberscopy. Proceedings of the First Congress of the International Society of Endoscopy. Tokyo; 1966; 586–90.
2. Ida K, Misaki J, Kohli Y, Kawai K. Fundamental studies on the dye scattering method for endoscopy. Jpn J Gastroenterol Endosc 1972; 14:261–6.
3. Ida K, Hashimoto Y, Kawai K. In vivo staining of gastric mucosa. Its application to endoscopic diagnosis of intestinal metaplasia. Endoscopy 1975; 7:18–24.
4. Schiller W. Early diagnosis of carcinoma of the cervix. Surg Gynecol Obstet 1933; 56:210–22.
5. Nothmann BJ, Wright JR, Schuster MM. In vivo vital staining as an aid to identification of esophagogastric mucosal junction in man. Am J Dig Dis 1972; 17:919–24.
6. Okuda S, Saegusa T, Ito T, et al. An endoscopic method to investigate the gastric acid secretion. Proceedings of the First Congress of the International Society of Endoscopy. Tokyo, 1966; 221–6.
7. Ida K, Kohli Y, Shimamoto K, et al. Endoscopical findings of fundic and pyloric gland area using dye scattering method. Endoscopy 1973; 5:21–6.
8. Ida K, Hashimoto Y, Takeda S, et al. Endoscopic diagnosis of gastric cancer with dye scattering. Am J Gastroenterol 1975; 63:316–20.
9. Ida K, Kubota Y, Okuda J, et al. Differential diagnosis of gastric polypoid lesion by the application of methylene blue staining. J Kyoto Pref Univ Med 1979; 88:291–8.
10. Tada M, Misaki F, Kawai K. Endoscopic observation of villi with magnifying enterocolonoscopes. Gastrointest Endosc 1982; 28:17–9.
11. Tada M, Misaki F, Shimono M, et al. Endoscopic studies on the minute structures of colonic mucosa in the follow-up observation of ulcerative colitis. Gastroenterol Japonica 1978; 13:72–6.
12. Tada M, Kawai K. A new method for the ultramagnifying observation of the colon mucosa. J Kyot Pref Univ Med 1982; 91:349–54.

Part 3

HIGH–MAGNIFICATION ENDOSCOPY

TADAYOSHI TAKEMOTO, M.D.
NOBUHIRO SAKAKI, M.D.

High-magnification endoscopy is a diagnostic endoscopic system used to observe various changes occurring in the pits or villi of the gastrointestinal mucosa. Conceptually, it is intermediate between macroscopic and microscopic observation. The unit of reference in magnification endoscopy is the fine mucosal pattern which consists of pits (colon and stomach) or villi (small intestine).

Although all fiberscopes provide some magnification, the power of standard instruments in this respect is insufficient for observation of the finer details of the gastric and colonic mucosa. However, special fiberscopes have been produced in Japan since 1967 for the purpose of high-magnification endoscopy. In recent years, after many trials, fiberscopes with a magnification capacity as great as $35\times$ have been developed.

We have created a diagnostic system for magnification endoscopy of gastric mucosa using the most recent magnifying fiberscopes. The instrumentation and this diagnostic system will be introduced, focusing on gastroscopy.

HISTORY

The origin of high-magnification endoscopy—that is, the first attempt to observe

TABLE 10–8. **Development of Magnifying Endoscopes**

Area of Use	Instrument	(Mag)*	Developed by (Year)
Stomach	FGS-ML, Type 1	(3×)	Okuyama (1967)
	MGF-I	(15×)	Suzaki and Miyake (1969)
	FGS-ML, Type 2	(15×)	Maruyama and Takemoto (1971)
	GIF-M	(15×)	Ida and Kawai (1975)
	FGS-ML (II)	(30×)	Sakaki and Takemoto (1978)
	GIF-HM	(35×)	Ooida and Okabe (1980)
Colon	CF-MB-F	(10×)	Tada and Kawai (1975)
	FCS-ML (II)	(30×)	Nishizawa and Kobayashi (1976)
	CF-HM	(35×)	Tada (1979)

*Magnification capability.

gastric pits—dates to the period of gastroscopy with rigid instruments. In 1954, Gutzeit and Teitige[1] observed foveoli in the body of the stomach and published their findings. Subsequently, a diagnostic system based on the shapes of the gastric pits was developed in the field of pathology. This made use of the dissecting microscope. Salem and Truelove[2] in 1964 stressed the value of this system for examination of gastric biopsies, especially in the diagnosis of gastritis. Matsumoto[3] reported that normal papillary patterns are destroyed and replaced by regenerated pseudopapillary patterns in cases of gastric ulcer and gastric cancer. Yoshii[4] reported that normal gastric mucosal patterns, which were divided into foveolar, foveolar-sulciolar and sulciolar patterns, changed to various characteristic patterns under disordered conditions. This work was also carried out using dissecting microscopes, and in fact this type of investigation provides the basis and background for the diagnostic system of high-magnification endoscopy.

The development of magnifying fiberscopes is outlined in Table 10–8. Many prototype fiberscopes were produced, but detailed study of the patterns of gastric or colonic pits awaited the development of the most recent magnifying fiberscopes such as the ML (Machida Corp.) and HM (Olympus Corp.) series.[5–8]

INSTRUMENTATION

High-magnification gastroscopy is performed using the FGS-ML II and GIF-HM instruments. For high-magnification colonoscopy, the FCS-ML II (Machida) and CF-HM (Olympus) instruments are also used. The specifications for these endoscopes are given in Table 10–9. In general, they are forward-viewing fiberscopes, with magnification capabilities ranging from 30 to 35×.

TABLE 10–9. **Specifications of Magnifying Fiberscopes**

	FGS-ML II	FCS-ML II	GIF-HM	CF-HM
Bending Angle (in degrees)				
Up	180	120	180	180
Down	60	120	90	180
Right and left	90	120	100	160
Dimensions (in mm)				
Total length	1272		1330 / 1670	
Working length		1045	1135	1420
Diameter of:				
Distal tip		15.0	13.0	14.6
Insertion tube		12.4	12.5	14.4
Biopsy channel		2.6	2.8	2.8
Optical System				
Angle of view	65 Degrees		70 Degrees	
Observation	Forward		Forward	
Range	0.5 mm–∞		2.3–100 mm	
Magnification	30×		35×	

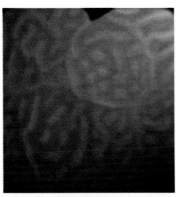

PLATE 10–30. View of fine structure of gastric mucosal surface using the ML II endoscope (30x).

The techniques for performance of endoscopy with these instruments are almost the same as those for endoscopy with a conventional fiberscope.

In our experience, photographs taken with the FGS-ML II and FCS-ML II (Machida) are superior to those obtained with other instruments. This is because these instruments have an obliquely oriented light supply for magnified observation. When magnification is required, the light guide connector is changed from straight illumination to oblique, and the focus is adjusted after contact with the mucosa. However, the GIF-HM and CF-HM instruments (Olympus) are easier to use because they have a wider field of view and the capability to zoom in close to the mucosa. This means that the endoscopist can change readily from ordinary observation to high magnification by means of the close-up and focus controls. This capability makes these instruments superior for clinical use because magnified observations may be made at any time and as necessary during the course of a standard endoscopic examination.

These magnifying endoscopes provide a capacity for excellent observation of fine mucosal patterns, although they have some limitations in handling. Certain conventional fiberscopes, the GIF-D series (Olympus) for example, have a close-up focus, and are therefore occasionally useful for magnified observation of the mucosa, although they only resolve relatively coarse mucosal features and patterns.

Dye-spraying (chromoscopy) techniques are occasionally used in conjunction with high-magnification endoscopy (discussed in Part 2 of this chapter).

HIGH-MAGNIFICATION GASTROSCOPY

Classification of Fine Gastric Mucosal Pattern

The gastric mucosal surface, when observed with a magnifying endoscope, displays a complicated pattern composed of variously shaped gastric pits (Plate 10–30). Slightly reddish areas are elevated parts of the mucosal surface, and whitish-yellow areas are depressions, the latter being the gastric pits. We named this appearance "the fine gastric mucosal pattern." When this is observed, the field of view takes in an area that is smaller than one area gastrica. The fine gastric mucosal pattern is therefore the substructure of the areae gastricae. (Areae gastricae are small subdivisions, 1 to 5 mm in diameter, superimposed on the gastric mucosa by a system of furrows. They are often visible at endoscopy and may sometimes be defined by double contrast radiography.) The fine gastric mucosal pattern is altered in various disease states.

The classification of the fine gastric mucosal pattern used in high-magnification endoscopy is based on characterization of the shapes of the gastric pits. There are 7 types: A, AB, B, BC, C, CD, and D (Fig. 10–56 and Plate 10–31). Type A is characterized by dotted gastric pits, Type B by short, linear pits; Type C by winding and striped grooves, and Type D by mesh-like grooves. Types AB, BC, and CD are intermediate or mixed patterns of A and B, B and C, and C and D, respectively.[9]

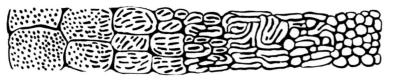

A   AB   B   BC   C   CD   D

FIGURE 10–56. Classification schema for high magnification endoscopy of the fine gastric mucosal pattern.

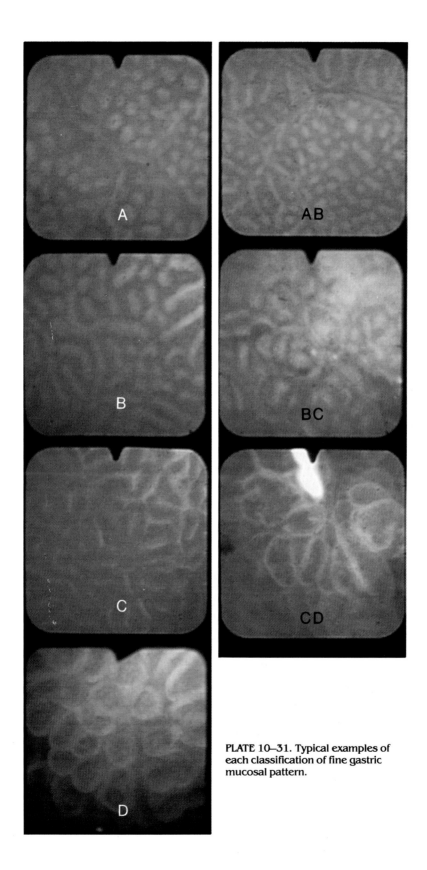

PLATE 10–31. Typical examples of each classification of fine gastric mucosal pattern.

Chronic Gastritis

Early in our investigations, the relationships between fine gastric mucosal patterns and histologic findings were studied by means of endoscopic and surgical biopsies. These were examined histologically after observation under the dissecting microscope. It was found, for example, that Type A was characteristic of normal fundic mucosa, but that with atrophic gastritis this changed to Type AB. With continuous high magnification from corpus to antrum, serial changes of classification from A through AB, B, BC, and C are frequently observed in normal or slightly atrophic gastric mucosa (Plate 10–32). Types AB and B are found mainly at the junction of the fundic and pyloric (antral) glandular areas. After spraying a 0.3% solution of congo red on the mucosa, this border is definable between a black metachromatic area (fundic mucosa) and a red area (pyloric mucosa) (Plate 10–33).

Methylene blue staining can be combined with high-magnification endoscopy to demonstrate gastric mucosal intestinal metaplasia. A 0.5% solution is sprayed onto the mucosa and then washed away with water. Intestinal metaplasia appears as blue dots when observed by high magnification (Plate 10–34).

Localized Gastric Lesions

Basis of High-Magnification Endoscopy

In the application of high-magnification endoscopy to clinical diagnosis, the basic classification of fine gastric mucosal pattern is used. However, to give detailed expression to the various characteristic patterns of localized lesions, types C, CD, and D are divided into two subtypes, regular and irregular, according to the shape and size of the elevated portions of the mucosa surrounding the grooves that are the openings into the gastric pits (Fig. 10–57).

During high-magnification endoscopy of depressed gastric lesions, flat, shapeless areas, which indicate a mucosal deficit, were occasionally observed in the central portion of the lesion. No fine mucosal pattern is observable in these areas. In such cases, attention is directed to the mucosa adjacent to flat areas.

Gastric Ulcer

The basic fine gastric mucosal patterns which indicate benign gastric ulcers are regular C, CD, and D types. However, it must be emphasized that transformations in the fine pattern occur throughout the process of ulcer healing, as reported by Miyake et al.[10] in their investigations using dissecting microscopy.

At the onset of gastric ulceration, the mucosa adjacent to the ulcer has the same fine mucosal pattern as the surrounding mucosa (Plate 10–35).

Characteristic fine mucosal patterns are seen in the regenerated mucosa that appears as the ulcer heals. In the early stage, a narrow band with a C-type pattern is found surrounding a white coating. A palisade-like, coarse Type-C pattern extending radially from the center of an ulcer is observed during almost all stages of the healing process (Plate 10–36).

During the initial stages of scar formation, the fine mucosal pattern is that of a radiating, palisade-like Type C, with associated reddening. Later, Type CD and D patterns (Plate 10–37) replace Type C, as described by Miyake et al.[10] A Type BC pattern may occasionally appear after the scar has been present for a long time. A gastric ulcer that underwent a typical healing process over the course of one month is illustrated in Plate 10–38.[11] A long-standing chronic ulcer may have a Type D pattern even during healing. The persistence of Type D is suspected to be evidence of a recrudescence or an interruption of the healing process.

Gastric Polypoid Lesions

Gastric polyps that are histologically hyperplastic have mainly a coarse Type BC or CD fine mucosal pattern, characteristically with a soft, swollen appearance (Plate 10–39). Elevated "borderline lesions," that is, those that are histologically hyperplastic but contain areas of atypia, have complicated fine mucosal patterns (Plate 10–40). The fine pattern of the mucosa covering submucosal tumors does not, as expected, differ from the pattern in the surroundng mucosa.

Gastric Carcinoma

Advanced gastric cancer is diagnosed without difficulty by conventional endoscopy alone. Early gastric cancer (as defined by the Japan Gastroenterological Endoscopy Society) should be studied by high magnification to increase the accuracy of endoscopic assessment and diagnosis. Under high magnification, a cancerous ulceration or erosion appears as a whitish or reddish flat, shapeless area with no particular pattern. Therefore,

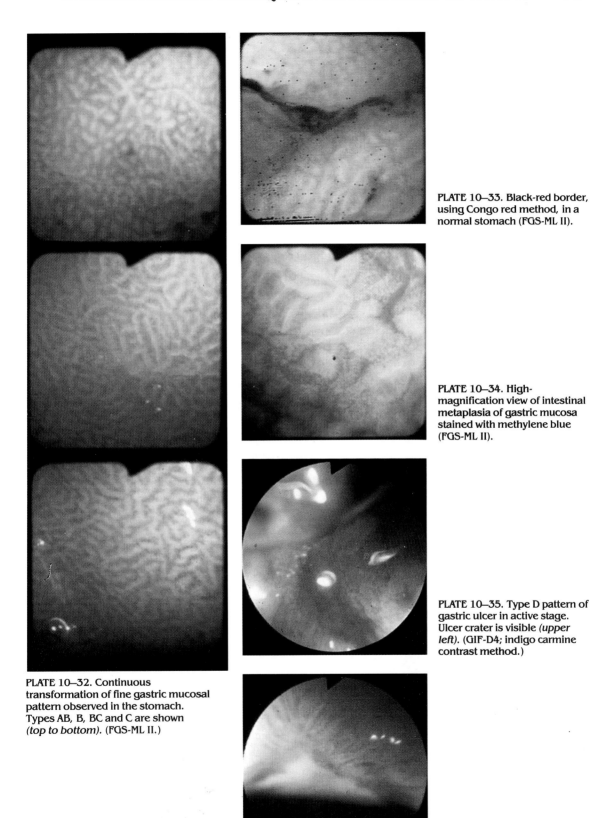

PLATE 10–33. Black-red border, using Congo red method, in a normal stomach (FGS-ML II).

PLATE 10–34. High-magnification view of intestinal metaplasia of gastric mucosa stained with methylene blue (FGS-ML II).

PLATE 10–35. Type D pattern of gastric ulcer in active stage. Ulcer crater is visible *(upper left)*. (GIF-D4; indigo carmine contrast method.)

PLATE 10–32. Continuous transformation of fine gastric mucosal pattern observed in the stomach. Types AB, B, BC and C are shown *(top to bottom)*. (FGS-ML II.)

PLATE 10–36. Coarse type C pattern of a healing gastric ulcer with palisade-like feature (GIF-D4).

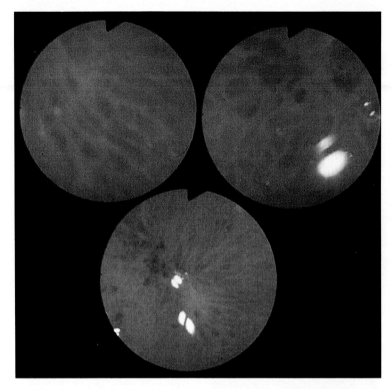

PLATE 10–37. Scar of gastric ulcer showing type CD pattern (GIF–HM).

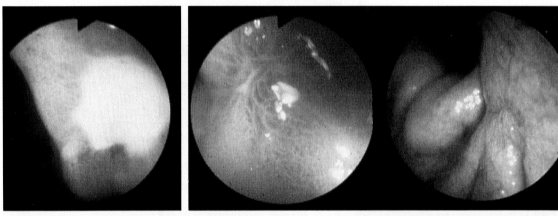

PLATE 10–38. Typical healing process of gastric ulcer. *Left,* Active stage; *center,* 2 weeks later; *right,* 4 weeks later (GIF–D4).

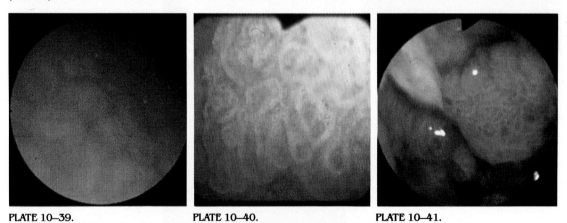

PLATE 10–39.   PLATE 10–40.   PLATE 10–41.

PLATE 10–39. Typical BC pattern of a hyperplastic polyp with a softly swollen appearance (GIF–HM).
PLATE 10–40. Finely complex BC pattern of elevated "border-line" lesion (FGS–ML II).
PLATE 10–41. Cancerous erosion bordered by regular C and irregular D fine mucosal patterns (GIF–HM).

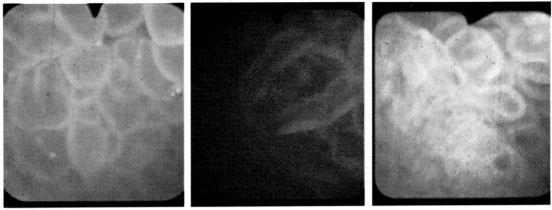

PLATE 10–42.   PLATE 10–43.   PLATE 10–44.

PLATE 10–42. Irregular D pattern characteristic of early gastric cancer. Note slight, various-shaped elevations of the surface (FGS–ML II).
PLATE 10–43. Irregular C pattern of type IIa elevated, early gastric cancer (FGS–ML II).
PLATE 10–44. Flat, shapeless area without pattern due to thick mucus *(lower left)* observed in elevated gastric cancer (FGS–ML II).

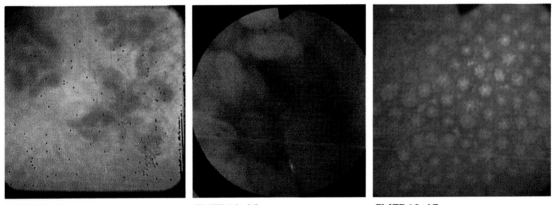

PLATE 10–45.   PLATE 10–46.   PLATE 10–47.

PLATE 10–45. High-magnification view of localized capillary dilations (GGS–ML II).
PLATE 10–46. Type D pattern observed with microerosion (GIF–HM, indigo carmine).
PLATE 10–47. Type A pattern of normal colonic mucosa stained with methylene blue (FCS–ML II).

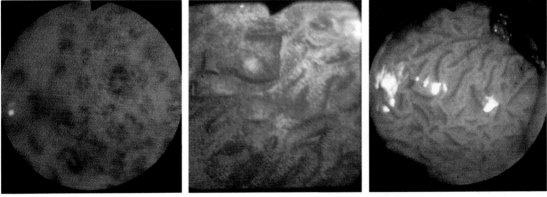

PLATE 10–48.   PLATE 10–49.   PLATE 10–50.

PLATE 10–48. Type AB pattern and flat, reddish area of ischemic colitis (CF–HM, methylene blue stain).
PLATE 10–49. Type BC pattern of healing mucosa in ulcerative colitis (FCS–ML II, methylene blue stain).
PLATE 10–50. Fine colonic mucosal pattern of tubular adenoma (CF–HM, methylene blue stain).

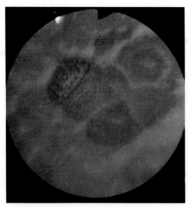

PLATE 10–51. Deeply staining, coarse colonic mucosal pits (CF–HM, methylene blue stain).

diagnosis depends on assessment of the fine mucosal pattern of the mucosa surrounding depressed-type early gastric cancers. Ooida et al.[11] reported that early gastric cancers of the erosive type occasionally exhibit transformations of the fine mucosal pattern during their evolution into a malignant ulcer (Plate 10–41).

Recognition of an irregular Type D pattern is very important in the investigation of a depressed lesion that might be an early gastric cancer. The irregular Type D pattern consists not only of irregular elevations of various sizes but is also a mixture of various other patterns (Plate 10–42).

In contrast to early carcinomatous lesions, which are depressed, elevated early gastric cancers are characterized by the irregular Type C pattern, with rigid linear grooves in a disorderly arrangement (Plate 10–43). In some cases of elevated early cancers, the fine

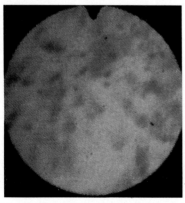

PLATE 10–52. Ultra-high magnification (100x) of gastric mucosal intestinal metaplasia after spraying methylene blue solution (FGS–ML).

gastric mucosal pattern is obscured by a thick coating of mucous (Plate 10–44).

Data from our high magnification observations using FGS-ML II and GIF-HM instruments with small localized gastric lesions are given in Table 10–10. Based on these data, we believe that the differential diagnosis of small gastric lesions by high-magnification endoscopy is reliable, and that the diagnosis of early gastric cancer is highly accurate.

Minute Gastric Lesions

High-magnification endoscopy may have its greatest usefulness in the differential diagnosis of minute gastric lesions.

The red mucosal spots or linear red mucosal streaks of superficial gastritis appear as reddish mucosa with a normal fine gastric mucosal pattern under high magnification endoscopy. The red spots, which are due to localized capillary dilation, are distinguished as dilated vessels without difficulty under high magnification (Plate 10–45).

Minute polypoid lesions are diagnosed without difficulty by high-magnification endoscopy. Minute polyps have a slightly coarse fine mucosal pattern that is similar to the pattern of the mucosa in the vicinity of the lesion. Areas of intestinal metaplasia may be elevated, and by high-magnification endoscopy these appear as multiple elevations with flat surfaces and a Type C fine mucosal pattern.

High-magnification endoscopy discloses minute gastric erosions in an acute stage as flat areas without pattern surrounded by mucosa with a fine mucosal pattern that is normal for the given area of the stomach. During healing, the transformations in the fine mucosal pattern are similar to those occurring with healing of an ulcer. The scar produced by a minute erosion has a regular Type D pattern (Plate 10–46). It is important to determine whether the Type D pattern is regular or irregular, since this differentiates the lesion as benign or malignant. For example, minute Type IIc early gastric cancer may have an irregular Type D pattern.

HIGH-MAGNIFICATION COLONOSCOPY

Normal Findings and Inflammatory Bowel Disease

The diagnostic unit for high-magnification colonoscopy is the colonic pit. These structures are actually the orifices of the crypts of

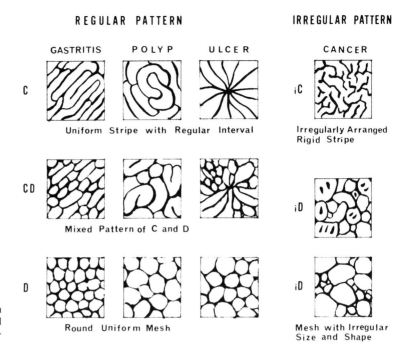

FIGURE 10–57. Classification schema for fine gastric mucosal pattern of localized gastric lesions.

Lieberkühn. To observe the colonic pits, it is necessary to use the techniques of chromoscopy as outlined in Part 2 of this chapter. The normal colonic mucosa, stained deeply with methylene blue, is illustrated in Plate 10–47.

The shape of the colonic pit changes under the influence of certain diseases. For example, the normal round shape changes to elliptical, tubular, and other configurations in colitis. In order to express pathologic changes with a standard nomenclature, we have applied the magnification classification used earlier to describe the fine gastric mucosal pattern.

Normal colonic pits are characterized by a Type A pattern. In ischemic colitis, a flat, shapeless area is surrounded by colonic mucosa with a Type AB pattern (Plate 10–48). Types B or C are occasionally observed with various inflammatory bowel diseases. The changes that occur in the high magnified features of colonic mucosa in inflammatory diseases are thought to be nonspecific. The various patterns relate to the differences in the severity of the inflammatory process.

Nishizawa et al.[6] and Watanabe[12] used high-magnification colonoscopy to investigate the process of healing in ulcerative colitis. Stages in the clinical course can be classified by changes observed in the fine colonic mucosal pattern. In the active stage of the disease, the mucosa is flat and shapeless and there is no discernible pattern. Abnormal pits appear during the healing process, and fine colonic mucosal patterns such as AB, B, BC, and C will be found. Gradually the normal Type A pattern returns as healing becomes nearly complete. A Type BC pattern characteristic of healing ulcerative colitis is illustrated in Plate 10–49.

Localized Colonic Lesions

The fine colonic mucosal pattern of a polyp, diagnosed as a tubular adenoma after polypectomy, is shown in Plate 10–50. Adenomas, as shown in the example, have a Type BC or C fine colonic mucosal pattern. Tada et al.[13] have shown that advanced cancers have an irregular, cauliflower-like, rough, non-structured appearance. They also have reported that early cancers have mixed features: fine mucosal patterns of the type associated with advanced cancer as well as patterns characteristic of benign adenomas. This is problematic. As a result of this mixed appearance, the differential diagnosis between an adenoma and early cancer, especially an adenoma with a focus of cancer, is difficult by high-magnification endoscopy of the fine colonic mucosal pattern.

Occasionally a few coarse, deeply stained pits will be observed by high-magnification

TABLE 10–10. **Fine Gastric Mucosal Pattern of Localized Lesions**

	Regular Pattern							Irregular Pattern			Total	% Irregular
	A	AB	B	BC	C	CD	D	C	D	F*		
Depressed Gastric Lesion												
Advanced cancer		1			2	2			18		23	78
Early cancer						1	2	1	14		18	83
Gastric ulcer			4	22	18	24			2		70	3
Gastric erosion			3	15	2	30			2		52	4
Elevated Gastric Lesion												
Advanced cancer										5	5	100
Early cancer								5	3	2	10	100
Borderline lesion				1	2	3	1	2			9	22
Gastric polyp	2	2	3	14	3	15	6		2		47	4

*Flat, shapeless pattern.

colonoscopy (Plate 10–51). Nishizawa et al.[14] regard this as indicative of an incipient hyperplastic or adenomatous polyp.

ULTRA HIGH-MAGNIFICATION ENDOSCOPY

Further advances in magnification endoscopy appear possible as technologic improvements are achieved. A new magnifying colonoscope (CF-UHM, Olympus), with a magnifying capacity of 170×, has been developed by Tada et al.[15] Thus, ultra high-magnification endoscopy is now possible in which the units of diagnostic reference are considered to be cellular features and the nucleus.

Another system we developed is the FGS-SML (Machida) ultra high-magnification endoscope, which also has a magnification capability of 170×. An ultra high-magnification view of gastric intestinal metaplasia is shown in Plate 10–52. Ultra high-magnification is also discussed with reference to chromoscopy in Part 2 of this chapter.

References

1. Gutzeit H, Teitige H. Die gastroskopie, Lehrbuch und Atlas. Munchen: Urban & Schwarzenberg, 1954.
2. Salem SN, Truelove SC. Dissection microscope appearance of the gastric mucosa. Br Med J 1964; 2:1503–4.
3. Matsumoto M. Dissecting microscopic study of gastric ulcer and gastric cancer. Gastroenterol Endosc (Tokyo) 1973; 15:639–65.
4. Yoshii T. Staining dissecting microscopic observation and its application for endoscopy. In: Takemoto T, Kawai K, eds. Gastrointestinal Endoscopy with Application of Dye. Tokyo: Igaku Shoin, 1974; 11–20.
5. Sakaki N, Iida Y, Okazaki Y, et al. Magnifying endoscopic observation of the gastric mucosa, particularly in patients with atrophic gastritis. Endoscopy 1978; 10:269–74.
6. Nishizawa M, Kariya A, Kobayashi S, Shirakabe H. Clinical application of an improved magnifying fiber-colonoscope (FCS-ML II), with special reference to the remission features of ulcerative colitis. Endoscopy 1980; 12:76–80.
7. Ooida M, Igarashi M, Kumano S, et al. Magnifying fiberscopic study about the course of various gastric mucosal lesions. Part 1: Specification and endoscopic feature of magnifying fiberscope, GIF-HM. Gastroenterol Endosc (Tokyo) 1980; 22:227–34.
8. Tada M, Suyama Y, Shimizu T, et al. Magnifying observation of the colonic mucosa by means of a newly developed colonoscope, type CF-HM (Olympus). Gastroenterol Endosc (Tokyo) 1979; 21:1178–89.
9. Sakaki N, Iida Y, Saito M, et al. New magnifying endoscopic classification of the fine gastric mucosal pattern. Gastroenterol Endosc (Tokyo) 1980; 22:377–83.
10. Miyake T, Suzaki T, Oishi M. Correlation of gastric ulcer healing features by endoscopy, stereoscopic microscopy, and histology, and a reclassification of the epithelial regeneration process. Dig Dis Sci 1980; 25:8–14.
11. Ooida M, Kubo K, Katsumata T, et al. Studies on depressed type of gastric cancer using magnifying endoscopy. Special reference to the life cycle of malignant ulcer. Gastroenterol Endosc (Tokyo) 1981; 23:1246–55.
12. Watanabe M. Classification of the stages due to magnifying colonofiberscopy in ulcerative colitis. Gastroenterol Endosc (Tokyo) 1979; 21:1178–89.
13. Tada M, Misaki F, Kawai K. A new approach to the observation of minute changes of the colonic mucosa by means of magnifying colonoscope, type CF-MB-M (Olympus). Gastrointest Endosc 1978; 24:146–7.
14. Nishizawa M, Okada T, Sato F, et al. A clinicopathological study of minute polypoid lesions of the colon based on magnifying fiber-colonoscopy and dissecting microscopy. Endoscopy 1980; 12:124–9.
15. Tada M, Nishimura S, Watanabe Y, et al. A new method for the ultra-magnifying observation of the colon mucosa. J Kyoto Pref Univ Med 1982; 91:349–54.

Part 4

PERORAL CHOLANGIOSCOPY AND PANCREATOSCOPY

MASATSUGU NAKAJIMA, M.D.
SOTARO FUJIMOTO, M.D.
KEIICHI KAWAI, M.D.

Advances in fiberoptic duodenoscopy with retrograde cannulation of the papilla of Vater have greatly improved the management of diseases of the bile and pancreatic duct systems. Endoscopic retrograde cholangiopancreatography (ERCP) and endoscopic sphincterotomy are major diagnostic and therapeutic advances. A logical extension of these techniques is the noninvasive direct endoscopic visualization of the biliary and pancreatic ductal systems. Peroral cholangiopancreatoscopy (PCPS) is now possible because of the recent development of very small caliber fiberoptic instruments.

DEVELOPMENT OF INSTRUMENTS AND TECHNIQUES

Takekoshi and Takagi[1] and Nakamura et al.[2] introduced the master duodenoscope and a thin subendoscope designed for passage through the master instrument. Visualization of the ducts was poor, however, and damage to the instruments occurred in the course of only a few procedures.

We developed new endoscopic instruments in conjunction with Olympus, Tokyo.[3] These provided reasonably good visualization of both the bile and pancreatic ducts, which led to interesting findings not previously reported.[4-6] However, frequently it was not possible to examine the ductal systems completely because the prototype subendoscopes had neither a tip deflection mechanism nor an effective accessory channel for instrumentation and irrigation.[4] These major difficulties were later resolved by the development of a subendoscope with two-way tip control. Endoscopic sphincterotomy has become an acceptable alternative to surgery for treatment of various biliary tract diseases, especially stones.[7-9] The enlarged orifice of the distal common bile duct after endoscopic sphincterotomy allows passage of a larger-caliber subendoscope which has a controlla-

ble tip as well as a satisfactory channel for instrumentation and irrigation. Urakami et al.[10] reported a case of biliary endoscopy in which a small-caliber end-viewing upper gastrointestinal endoscope (Olympus, GIF-P) was used, but only the distal portion of the common bile duct was entered. New instruments and techniques have been developed for peroral cholangioscopy (PCS) and transendoscopic instrumentation of the biliary tract. We have developed instruments for PCS that are used in a sliding tube guidance technique,[11] and have reported the effectiveness of this technique for diagnosis and management of biliary tract diseases.[12, 13] Kimura et al.[14] also reported the results of their technique for PCS, which employs a specially designed cholangioscope and balloon-tipped catheter guidance.

INSTRUMENTS

The instruments for PCPS and PCS described in this section of Chapter 10 were made by Olympus Optical Co. according to the specifications and recommendations of the authors.

Peroral Cholangiopancreatoscopy Under Duodenoscopic Guidance (Master and Subendoscope System)

This procedure is made possible by the combined use of a master duodenoscope and a small-caliber subcholangiopancreatoscope that can be passed through the accessory channel of the master instrument (Fig. 10–58). Two standard, cold-light sources are required. The master endoscope, a modified side-viewing duodenoscope, resembles the Olympus standard duodenoscopes used for ERCP except for the larger sizes of the insertion tube (12.0 mm) and accessory channel (3.7 mm). The most improved subendoscope designed for passage through the master endoscope is an end-viewing instrument with a working length of 1850 mm and an external diameter of 3.2 mm. It has a mechanism for two-way tip deflection (90 degrees up and down) and no instrument channel.

Peroral Cholangioscopy Under Sliding Tube Guidance (Single Endoscope System)

In this system, a small-caliber cholangioscope and a sliding tube are used (Fig. 10–59). The cholangioscope, designed for passage through the sliding tube, has end-viewing optics, a working length of 1745 mm, and an external diameter of 5.7 mm. Its controllable tip can be deflected in four directions (130 degrees up, 100 degrees down, right and left), and it has an instrument channel, 2.0 mm in diameter, which permits insufflation, washing, and suction. The sliding tube is 1100 mm long with an external diameter of 12.0 mm and an internal diameter of 6.0 mm. It also has a mechanism for four-way tip deflection (120 degrees up, 90 degrees down, right and left). Note that in Figure 10–59 the sliding tube resembles an endoscope and has some of the mechanical features of an endoscope, but it has no optical or light guide bundles.

TECHNIQUES

Both PCPS and PCS are performed in a room equipped for fluoroscopy after ERCP with or without prior endoscopic sphincterotomy. Two endoscopists are required; one operator manipulates the controls of the master duodenoscope or the sliding tube for entry into the duodenum, for identification of the papilla of Vater, and insertion of the small-caliber endoscope into the biliary and pancreatic ducts. The second operator controls the small-caliber subendoscope for visualization and in some cases transendoscopic instrumentation of the ducts. The endoscopic image of the ducts can be viewed by the operator of the master endoscope or sliding tube my means of a lecturescope ("teaching attachment") attached to the subendoscope.

Peroral Cholangiopancreatoscopy Under Duodenoscopic Guidance

Most aspects of this technique are similar to those of ERCP. Under topical pharyngeal anesthesia and intravenous premedication for sedation and duodenal atony, the master duodenoscope is introduced into the descending duodenum. After the papilla of Vater is identified, the tip of the subcholangiopancreatoscope is guided from the master instrument into the ampulla of Vater. Once inserted into the papilla, the tip of the subendoscope may be introduced into either the bile duct or the pancreatic duct. It is then carefully and gently advanced toward the liver or the tail of the pancreas under endoscopic and fluoroscopic guidance (Plate 10–53 and Fig. 10–60). The ducts are visualized while the subendoscope is advanced and withdrawn through bile or pancreatic juice (Plates 10–54 and 10–55).

Peroral Cholangioscopy Under Sliding Tube Guidance

The technique of PCS under sliding tube guidance is illustrated in Figure 10–61. The procedure is done after endoscopic sphincterotomy. The technique for reaching the second portion of the duodenum is almost identical to that of conventional upper gastrointestinal endoscopy with a forward-viewing instrument. After standard pharyngeal anesthesia and intravenous premedication, the sliding tube containing the cholangioscope is introduced into the descending duodenum by the combined manipulations of the two endoscopists. The deflection controls of both instruments are employed to gain an *en face* orientation to the papilla of Vater. The cholangioscope is then advanced into the biliary tract through the incised papilla, with the tip of the sliding tube acting as a prop. The cholangioscope is then selectively advanced from the common bile duct into the intrahepatic ducts under direct vision, using the maneuverable tip to advantage, and fluoroscopic control (Fig. 10–61B). The entire ductal system can be visualized with the aid of tip deflection and the automatic irrigation system of the cholangioscope (Plate 10–56). If necessary, transendoscopic instrumentation of the biliary tract can be performed under direct vision, using various accessory instruments such as biopsy forceps or basket catheters.

RESULTS

Peroral Cholangiopancreatoscopy Under Duodenoscopic Guidance

This procedure was successful in 70 of 78 patients (89.7%); there were no significant

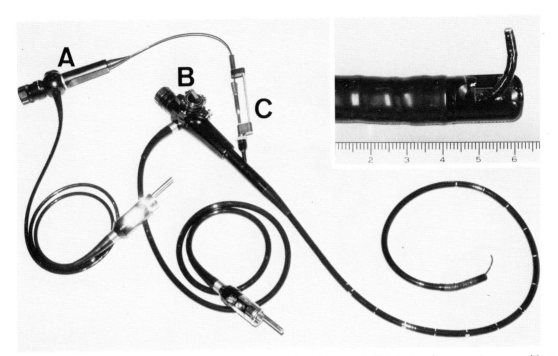

FIGURE 10–58. Instruments for PCPS under duodenoscopic guidance. *A*, Subcholangiopancreatoscope with a mechanism for two-way tip control. *B*, Master duodenoscope for retrograde cannulation. *C*, Subscope thrusting device, which protects the small caliber subcholangiopancreatoscope from damage. Inset, Distal aspect of the insertion tube of the master duodenoscope showing deflected exit of the subendoscope.

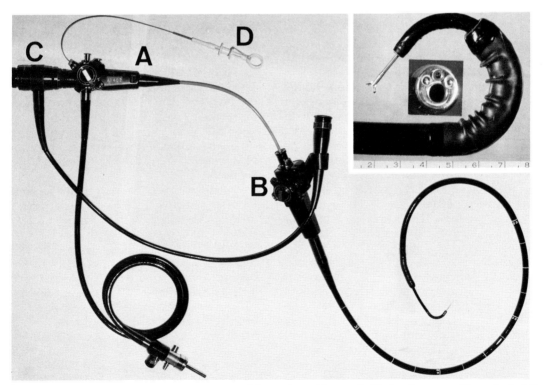

FIGURE 10–59. Instruments used for PCS under sliding tube guidance. *A*, Cholangioscope with controlled tip deflection and instrument channel. *B*, Sliding tube with mechanism for tip control. *C*, Supplemental lecturescope (teaching attachment). *D*, Biopsy forceps passed through cholangioscope. Inset, Distal aspect of the sliding tube showing exit of the cholangioscope. A standard biopsy forceps has been passed through the accessory channel of the cholangioscope.

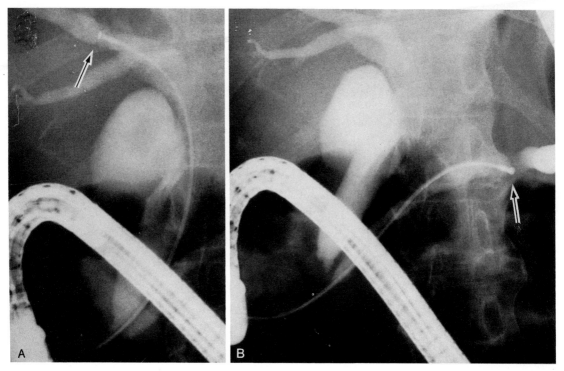

FIGURE 10–60. Radiographs depicting PCPS under duodenoscopic guidance. *A*, Subendoscope (*arrow*) in right hepatic duct. *B*, Subendoscope (*arrow*) in pancreatic duct in tail of gland.

complications (Table 10–11). In the remaining 8 patients the subendoscopic cholangioscope could not be introduced into the papilla because of technical or anatomical limitations. The technique was successful in many patients with an intact papilla, as well as in some patients with fistulas at the choledochoduodenal junction that were created either surgically or by endoscopic electrosurgery. The image provided by both instruments was bright enough for examination, and the lumen of both the bile and pancreatic ducts was inspected without the use of an irrigation system. The cholangioscope was durable enough for this examination despite its small diameter.

The bile duct was successfully entered in 54 of 78 patients (69.2%); in 35 patients, inspection of the intrahepatic tree in addition to the extrahepatic duct was possible. Adequate visualization of the bile duct was achieved in 46 of 55 patients (83.6%) with biliary tract diseases. The normal appearance of the bile ducts (see Plate 10–54) is as follows: The mucous membrane appears yellow when seen through bile. The bifurcation of the common hepatic duct is recognized as a carina similar to the tracheobronchial bifurcation; and the hepatic ducts divide into

two or three segments. Biliary endoscopy was accomplished in 33 of 36 patients (91.7%) with choledocholithiasis; stones were visualized directly in all cases (Plate 10–57 and Fig. 10–62). Inspection of tumors protruding into the lumen of the bile duct was possible in 5 of 9 patients with this disease; in the remaining 4, the duct could not be entered with the tip of the subendoscope because of technical problems related to the lack of a prior sphincterotomy.

Peroral pancreatoscopy was performed in 58 of 78 patients (74.4%); in 10 patients, this included visualization of the entire main pancreatic duct, with observation of the main duct in the head and body in the others. The duct was adequately inspected in 18 of 23 patients with pancreatic diseases (78.3%). The wall of the main duct was pale pink, with a delicate submucosal vascular reticulum; the orifices of the main pancreatic duct branches can sometimes be recognized as pinholes (see Plate 10–55). In patients with pancreatic calcification, pancreatic stones were white or whitish-yellow (Plate 10–58 and Fig. 10–63). Close inspection of calculi was often difficult because pancreatic fluid within the duct was turbid and contained mucous or fibrinous plaques.

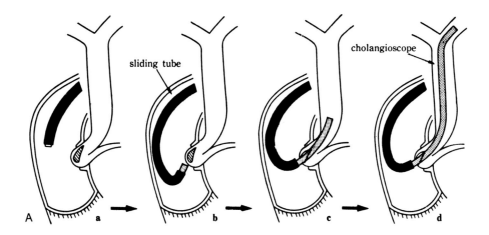

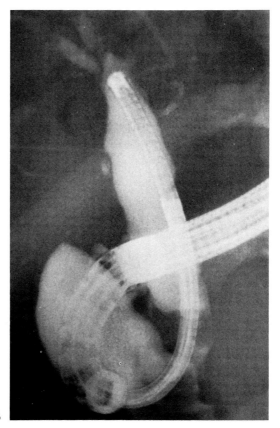

FIGURE 10–61. A, Schemata illustrating techniques of PCS under sliding tube guidance. B, Radiograph demonstrating PCS under sliding tube guidance.

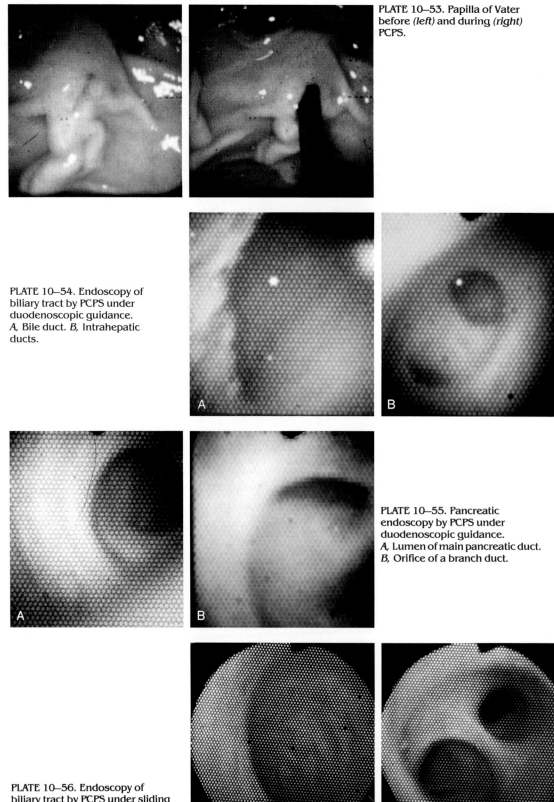

PLATE 10–53. Papilla of Vater before *(left)* and during *(right)* PCPS.

PLATE 10–54. Endoscopy of biliary tract by PCPS under duodenoscopic guidance. *A,* Bile duct. *B,* Intrahepatic ducts.

PLATE 10–55. Pancreatic endoscopy by PCPS under duodenoscopic guidance. *A,* Lumen of main pancreatic duct. *B,* Orifice of a branch duct.

PLATE 10–56. Endoscopy of biliary tract by PCPS under sliding tube guidance. *A,* Lumen of common bile duct. *B,* Intrahepatic ducts.

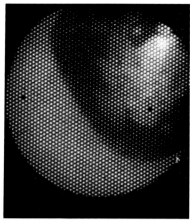

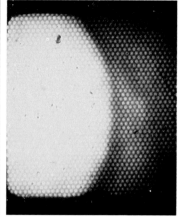

PLATE 10–57. Endoscopy of the common duct stone shown in Figure 10–62. The stone is viewed through bile.

PLATE 10–58. Pancreatic endoscopy of patient in Figure 10–63 demonstrating yellowish-white stone within main pancreatic duct.

PLATE 10–57.

PLATE 10–58.

PLATE 10–59. Endoscopy of pancreas of patient in Figure 10–64, demonstrating a polypoid tumor with papillary growth.

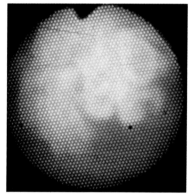

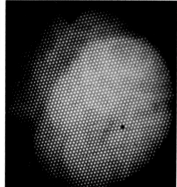

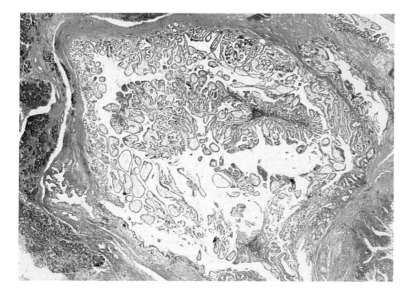

PLATE 10–60. Photomicrographs of pancreatic duct tumor of patient in Plate 10–59 and Figure 10–64, revealing papillary adenoma with focal atypical glands.

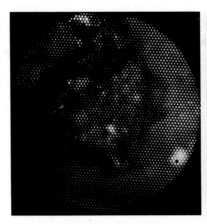
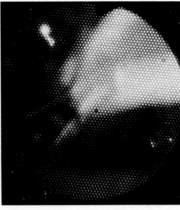

PLATE 10–61. Endoscopy with removal of intrahepatic stone in patient in Figure 10–65.

Pancreatoscopy in patients with tumors, which was possible in 6 of 8 cases, revealed an abrupt stricture or obstruction of the duct at the point of which the mucosa was reddish and the subendoscope could not be advanced toward the tail of the pancreas. The retrograde pancreatogram of 1 patient demonstrated a round, radiolucent shadow within a dilated main duct in the region of the head of the gland. This suggested the presence of a polypoid tumor or stone (Fig. 10–64). Pancreatoscopy in this patient revealed a polypoid, papillary tumor, not a stone, within the duct (Plate 10–59). Microscopic study of the resected specimen disclosed a papillary adenoma of the pancreas with focal atypism (Plate 10–60).

Peroral Cholangioscopy Under Sliding Tube Guidance

This procedure was attempted in 64 patients with various biliary tract diseases who had undergone endoscopic sphincterotomy (Table 10–12). Biliary endoscopy was successful in 47 of these patients (73.4%). Complete inspection of the intrahepatic tree and extrahepatic ducts was possible, except for patients with tumors that occluded the lumen. There were no complications. In the remaining 17 patients, the cholangioscope could not be inserted into the biliary tract because of technical limitations, even though the papilla of Vater was directly visualized. Illumination within the bile duct was excel-

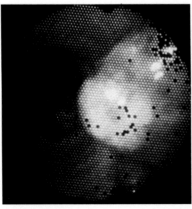
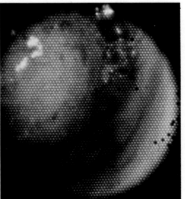

PLATE 10–62. Endoscopy of patient in Figure 10–66, demonstrating irregularly shaped tumor with erosions. PLATE 10–63. Biliary endoscopy of patient in Figure 10–68 reveals polypoid tumor; there is no stone within duct.

PLATE 10–62.   PLATE 10–63.

TABLE 10–11. **Results of PCPS Under Duodenoscopic Guidance**

| Diseases | No. | Successful Visualization | | | Fail |
		BD	PD	Both	
Biliary tract					
Choledocholithiasis	36	4	3	29	0
Tumor	9	3	0	2	4
Others	10	3	1	5	1
Subtotal	55	10	4	36	5
Pancreas					
Stones	8	1	5	1	2
Tumor	8	1	4	1	1
Others	7	0	3	4	0
Subtotal	23	2	12	6	3
Total	78	12	16	42	8

No. = number of patients; BD = bile duct; PD = pancreatic duct; Both = both ducts; Fail—failure.

lent. For this reason, and because of the excellent maneuverability and automatic irrigation system of the instrument (Fig. 10–61B), the bile ducts could be thoroughly examined. Moreover, removal of gallstones or biopsy under direct vision was easily performed with accessories passed through the instrument channel.

In patients with choledocholithiasis or papillary stenosis who had undergone endoscopic sphincterotomy, no additional abnormalities of the bile ducts were noted endoscopically, except for some erosions or redness of the mucosa suggestive of the chronic inflammation of the duct. Intrahepatic stones located near the hepatic hilus could be visualized clearly and removed under direct vision by employing a grasping forceps or basket catheter (Plate 10–61 and Fig. 10–65). Biliary endoscopy was also effective in patients with primary tumors or postoperative granulomas. Direct endoscopic inspection and optimal biopsy of the lesions confirmed the diagnosis. PCS in a patient with early carcinoma of the common bile duct and orifice of the cystic duct is shown in Figure 10–66. The endoscopic appearance is that of an irregularly shaped tumor with some erosions (Plate 10–62); biopsy specimens revealed atypical glands of the ductal mucosa. The resected specimen proved to be a mucosal adenocarcinoma with villous hyperplasia of the duct (Fig. 10–67). In another patient, ERCP demonstrated a round, radiolucent shadow within the dilated common bile duct, this suggesting a stone or small polypoid tumor; PCS under sliding tube guidance was performed for differential diagnosis (Fig. 10–68). This showed a reddish,

polypoid tumor rather than a stone within the lumen (Plate 10–63), and directed biopsy revealed a malignant tumor. The resected specimen also showed that histologically the 10 × 10 mm tumor was a well-differentiated adenocarcinoma that was limited to the muscular layer of the bile duct and without lymph node metastasis (Fig. 10–69).

COMMENTS

Direct observation of any phenomenon is always preferable to the use of indirect methods. The ability to visualize the lumen of the bile and pancreatic ducts results in a level of diagnostic precision that is not attainable by other means. In recent years, operative biliary endoscopy through a choledochotomy incision and postoperative choledochoscopy through a T-tube track have been valuable diagnostic tools in biliary tract disease, especially for management of biliary neoplasms as well as identification and retrieval of retained stones[15–18] (see Chapter 34). Intraoperative pancreatic endoscopy has also been found to be valuable in a few cases.[19, 20]

TABLE 10–12. **Results of PCS Under Sliding Tube Guidance**

Diseases	No. of Patients	No. Examined Successfully
Choledocholithiasis	40	31
Intrahepatic stones	9	6
Biliary tract tumor	7	5
Papillary stenosis	4	2
Others	4	3
Total	64	47

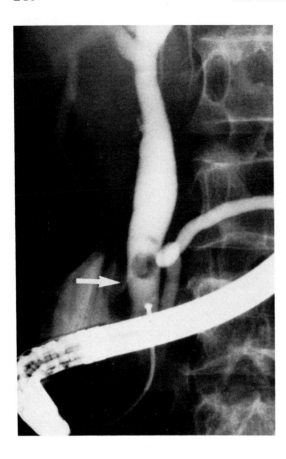

FIGURE 10–62. Radiograph of PCS under duodeno-scopic guidance in patient with choledocholithiasis. Tip of subendoscope approaches a common duct stone.

FIGURE 10–63. ERCP shows stones (*arrow*) within dilated main pancreatic duct in head of pancreas.

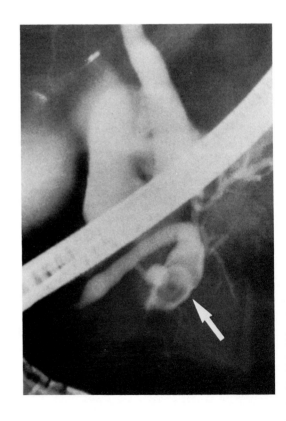

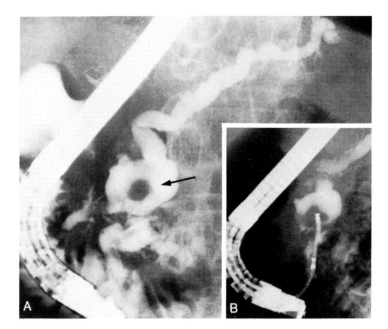

FIGURE 10–64. ERCP (*A*) and PCPS (*B*) in patient with pancreatic duct tumor, which is manifest as a radiolucent shadow (*arrow*) within the dilated main pancreatic duct.

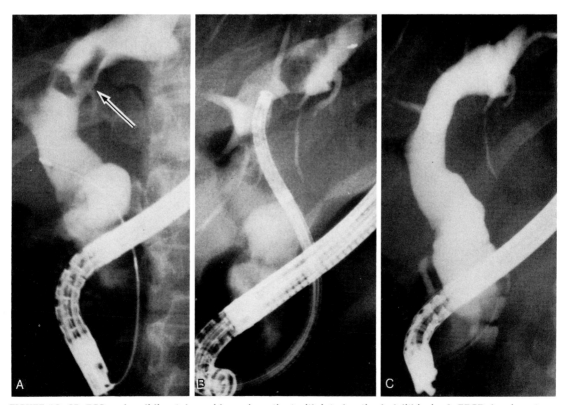

FIGURE 10–65. PCS under sliding tube guidance in patient with intraheptic cholelithiasis. *A*, ERCP showing stone impacted in left intrahepatic duct (*arrow*). *B*, PCS with direct extraction of the stone. *C*, ERCP demonstrating no stones within the ducts after PCS.

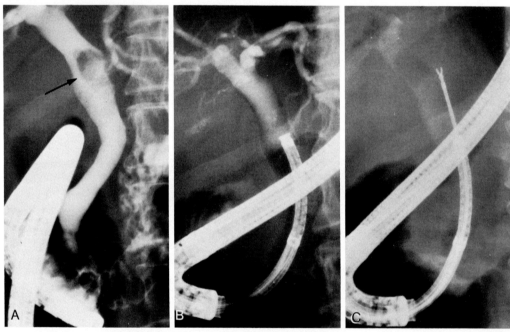

FIGURE 10–66. Early carcinoma of the common bile duct. *A*, ERCP showing a radiolucent shadow (*arrow*) in bile duct, which suggests a polypoid tumor of the duct. *B*, Direct endoscopy of the tumor by PCS after endoscopic sphincterotomy. *C*, Biospy of lesion under direct PCS visualization.

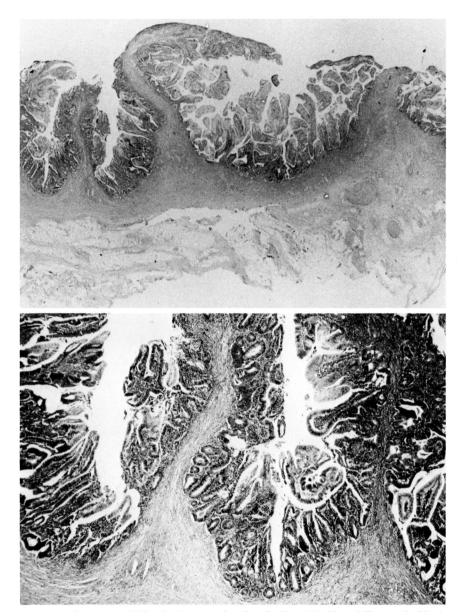

FIGURE 10–67. Photomicrograph of bile duct tumor of patient in Plate 10–62 and Figure 10–66, demonstrating mucosal carcinoma with villous hyperplasia.

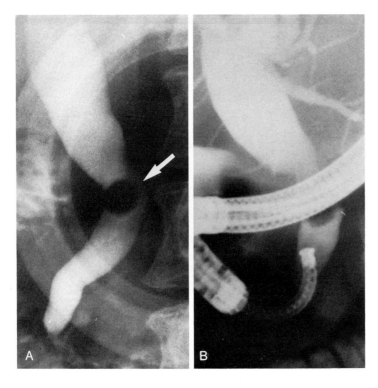

FIGURE 10–68. Small polypoid cancer of common bile duct. *A*, ERCP demonstrates a round shadow (*arrow*) within the dilated common bile duct, suggestive of tumor or stone. *B*, PCS shows a cholangioscope approaching the lesion.

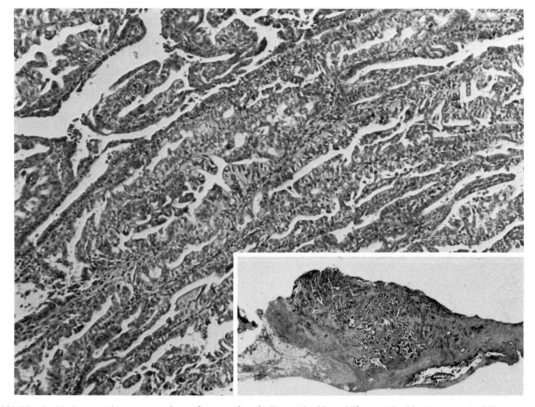

FIGURE 10–69. Resected tumor specimen from patient in Plate 10–63 and Figure 10–68, shows well-differentiated adenocarcinoma limited to the muscular layer of the common duct.

PCPS is a new concept in gastrointestinal endoscopy, which has resulted from major advances in the design of small-caliber fiberoptic instruments. It offers a new dimension for evaluation of the bile and pancreatic ducts, and can improve the management of a variety of diseases.[5, 12–14] The authors began to investigate the possibilities with this technique using master and subendoscope systems.[3, 4] Despite early enthusiasm and reasonably favorable results,[5] the method did not gain wide acceptance because of technical limitations, especially the lack of controlled tip deflection and an effective accessory channel with prototype instruments. However, this technique of PCPS under duodenoscopic guidance has the following advantages:

1. The procedure is not difficult for those experienced in ERCP.

2. The technique is almost the same as that of duodenoscopy with retrograde cannulation of the papilla of Vater.

3. This method can be applied safely, even in patients without prior endoscopic sphincterotomy.

4. The use of very small diameter subendoscopes allows visualization of the lumen of the pancreatic and bile ducts even in the absence of duct dilation.[4, 5]

5. The recently improved subendoscope has a two-way tip deflection capability which permits improved inspection of both duct systems.

Based on our experience, further refinements in instrumentation will increase the usefulness of this endoscopic procedure.

Efforts toward an improved instrument system have also led to development of another system that consists of an improved cholangioscope and a sliding tube for guidance. Prior endoscopic sphincterotomy is required in this technique. However, this system overcomes some of the shortcomings of the earlier systems. It provides excellent visualization of the lumen of the biliary tract. Although experience with this system to date is limited, the technique will most probably become the definitive diagnostic and therapeutic method for noninvasive cholangioscopy and transendoscopic instrumentation of the biliary tract. Although certain technical difficulties must be resolved, this method expands the diagnostic and therapeutic indications for endoscopic sphincterotomy in the management of biliary tract diseases.

Prior to development of PCPS, preoperative diagnosis of bile and pancreatic diseases depended on various radiographic procedures. The radiographic features of the duct systems are easily and clearly defined with a variety of direct approaches, including ERCP and percutaneous transhepatic cholangiography (PTC). These special procedures permit a high degree of confidence in the diagnosis and management of diseases of the bile and pancreatic ducts. However, there are still problems in interpretation of cholangiograms and pancreatograms that usually relate to the uncertain nature of filling defects, ductal deformity, obstruction to the flow of contrast medium, poor quality radiographs, or to technically inadequate studies.[21, 22]

The precise observation possible with peroral cholangioscopy and pancreatoscopy can be valuable in numerous ways. The nature of doubtful, suspicious, and uncertain ERCP and PTC x-ray findings can be resolved. A varying degree of cholangitis is often encountered in ducts harboring stones. This may vary from mild congestion and edema to marked ulceration with fibropurulent exudate. Stones within the intrahepatic ducts or main pancreatic duct can be visualized and removed under visual control. Biliary tract tumors can be identified and biopsies obtained. Diagnosis of biliary tract and pancreatic tumors at an early stage is possible, sometimes as a result of investigation of findings that appear to be minimal by conventional methods.

CONCLUSION

Peroral cholangioscopy and pancreatoscopy have been developed for noninvasive, direct endoscopic examination of the bile and pancreatic duct systems. The atraumatic nature of the procedures is demonstrated by the absence of injury to the ducts and the low incidence of complications. Although there are still certain technical or mechanical limitations to the successful use of the prototype instruments, they provide satisfactory visualization of the ducts. With the expected improvements in instrument design, PCPS promises to be the most reliable method for diagnosis and management of a variety of biliary and pancreatic diseases.

References

1. Takekoshi T, Takagi E. Retrograde pancreatocholangioscopy. Gastroenterol Endosc (Tokyo) 1975; 17:678–83.
2. Nakamura M, Toki F, Ohi I, et al. The research of transduodenoscopic pancreatocholedochoscopy. Gastroenterol Endosc (Tokyo) 1976; 18:152–8.

3. Kawai K, Nakajima M, Akasaka Y, et al. Eine neue endoskopishe Technik: Die perorale Choledocho-Pankreatikoskopie. Leber Magen Darm 1976; 6:121–4.
4. Nakajima M, Akasaka Y, Fukomoto K, et al. Peroral cholangiopancreatoscopy (PCPS) under duodenoscopic guidance. Am J Gastroenterol 1976; 66:241–7.
5. Nakajima M, Akasaka Y, Yamaguchi K, et al. Direct endoscopic visualization of the bile and pancreatic duct systems by peroral cholangiopancreatoscopy (PCPS). Gastrointest Endosc 1978; 24:141–5.
6. Rösch W, Koch H, Demling L. Peroral cholangioscopy. Endoscopy 1976; 8:172–5.
7. Safrany L. Endoscopic treatment of biliary tract diseases. An international study. Lancet 1978; 2:983–5.
8. Demling L, Classen M, eds. Endoscopic Sphincterotomy of the Papilla of Vater—International Workshop, Munich. Stuttgart: Georg Thieme, 1978.
9. Nakajima M, Kizu M, Akasaka Y, Kawai K. Five years' experience of endoscopic sphincterotomy in Japan: a collective study from 25 centres. Endoscopy 1979; 11:138–41.
10. Urakami Y, Seifert E, Butke H. Peroral direct cholangioscopy (PDCS) using routine straight-view endoscope: first report. Endoscopy 1977; 9:27–30.
11. Nakajima M, Kizu M, Akasaka Y, et al. Peroral cholangioscopy (PCS) under sliding tube guidance—A preliminary report of the instruments and techniques. In: Classen M, Greenen J, Kawai K, eds. International Workshop—the Papilla Vateri and Its Diseases. Baden-Baden: Gerhard Witzstrock, 1979; 99–102.
12. Nakajima M, Fujimoto S. Peroral cholangioscopy (PCS) under sliding tube guidance. In: Kawai K, ed. Frontiers of GI Endoscopy. Tokyo: Olympus Optical Co., 1982; 43–8.
13. Nakajima M, Fujimoto S, Kawai K. Peroral cholangioscopy (PCS) and transendoscopic instrumentation of the biliary tract. In: Demling L, Classen M, eds. International Symposium—Endoscopic Papillotomy (EPT) Now 10 Years Old. 1986. In press.
14. Kimura K, Sakai H, Yoshida Y, et al. Development of a new peroral cholangioscope (FDS-CP). Am J Gastroenterol 1982; 77:580–4.
15. Shore JM, Berci G, Morgenstern L. The value of biliary endoscopy. Surg Gynecol Obstet 1975; 140:601–5.
16. Tompkins RK, Johnson J, Storm FK, Langmire WP Jr. Operative endoscopy of biliary tract neoplasms. Am J Surg 1976; 132:174–82.
17. Yamakawa T, Mieno K, Nogucki T, Shikata J. An improved choledochofiberscope and non-surgical removal of retained biliary calculi under vision control. Gastrointest Endosc 1976; 22:160–7.
18. Murata T. Treatment of intrahepatic lithiasis using the choledochofiberscope. Endoscopy 1981; 13:240–4.
19. Nakamura M, Hamano K, Endo H, et al. Endoscopic study of pancreatic diseases. Gastroenterol Endosc (Tokyo) 1971; 13:426–8.
20. Classen M, Schwemmule K, Demling L. Endoscopy of the pancreatic duct. Endoscopy 1972; 4:221–3.
21. Block MA, Schuman BM, Weckstein ML. Interpretive problems in endoscopic retrograde cholangiopancreatography. Am J Surg 1975; 129:29–33.
22. Kittredge RD, Baer JW. Percutaneous transhepatic cholangiography; problems in interpretation. Am J Roentgenol 1975; 125:35–46.

Part 5

PERCUTANEOUS ENDOSCOPIC GASTROSTOMY

JEFFREY L. PONSKY, M.D.

A feeding gastrostomy is an effective means for providing long-term enteral alimentation in patients who are unable to swallow. Candidates for a feeding gastrostomy include patients with severe facial trauma, mentally retarded infants, those with severe neurological impairment, and individuals with tumors of the oral cavity. Heretofore, placement of a gastrostomy required laparotomy, often under general anesthesia. For those patients in whom general anesthesia represents a significant risk, gastrostomy can be performed using local anesthesia, although it may then be difficult because of poor exposure or lack of patient cooperation.

Percutaneous endoscopic gastrostomy is a simple, safe, and rapid endoscopic method for the placement of a gastrostomy tube that requires neither general anesthesia nor laparotomy.[1-4]

TECHNIQUE

Enteral feedings are withheld for 8 hours prior to the procedure, and a single preoperative intravenous dose of a cephalosporin antibiotic is administered. The gastrostomy tube should be prepared before beginning the procedure. Although the necessary items of equipment are commercially available in

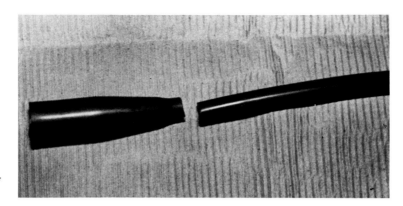

FIGURE 10–70. The flared end of the mushroom catheter is cut off.

kit form, the procedure may also be performed using readily available materials as follows.[1-3] A standard 16 French mushroom tip catheter is modified to serve as the gastrostomy tube. The flared end opposite the mushroom tip is cut off (Fig. 10–70) and discarded, a stitch of strong suture material is placed through the cut end of the catheter, and then the suture is threaded through a tapered intravenous cannula (Fig. 10–71). The rubber catheter is stretched, using the suture, so that the end opposite the intravenous cannula begins to decrease in diameter, at which point the catheter is pulled inside the intravenous cannula. When tension on the suture is released, the cut end of the rubber catheter will remain snugly within the cannula. The tapered end of the cannula will later function as a dilator. A crossbar is fashioned by cutting small side holes in a 2-inch piece of soft rubber tubing. The crossbar is threaded onto the catheter and positioned behind the mushroom tip (Fig. 10–72). A second crossbar is prepared in the same fashion for use later in the procedure.

The patient is placed in the supine position and the posterior pharynx anesthetized with a topical agent. Intravenous drugs may also be administered for sedation. The abdomen is cleansed with an antiseptic solution and the patient is draped in sterile fashion. The endoscope is introduced. After inspection of the stomach, it is maximally distended with air by insufflation with the endoscope. This displaces the liver in a cephalad direction, and the colon toward the pelvis. Also, as a result of maximum distention the anterior wall of the stomach now lies in contact with the peritoneal surface of the anterior abdominal wall. The light of the endoscope may cause transillumination of the abdominal wall, which is observable when the endoscopy room light is dim. A site for the gastrostomy is chosen at this point. It should lie on an imaginary line at approximately one third of the distance from the mid-point of the left costal margin to the umbilicus (Fig. 10–73).

As the endoscopist observes the wall of the stomach, an assistant applies gentle external pressure with one finger at the site chosen. This causes an indentation of the gastric wall, which can be seen by the endoscopist, and identifies the point within the stomach at which a puncture will be made. This point

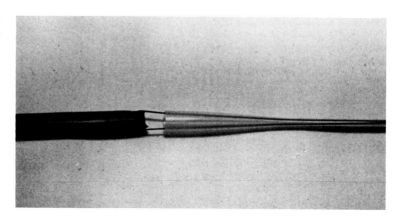

FIGURE 10–71. A simple stitch of a strong suture material is placed through the cut end of the catheter and threaded through a tapered intravenous cannula.

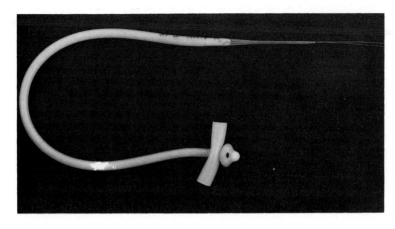

FIGURE 10–72. The completed catheter with a crossbar behind the mushroom tip.

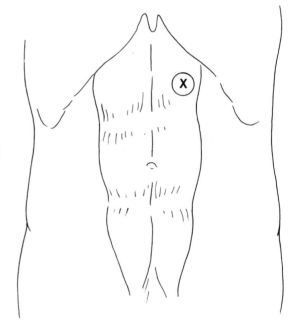

FIGURE 10–73. The site chosen is approximately one third the distance from the midpoint of the left costal margin to the umbilicus.

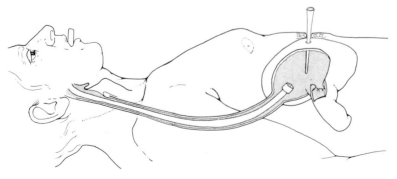

FIGURE 10–74. The endoscopist will observe the cannula entering the stomach and pass the snare around the cannula.

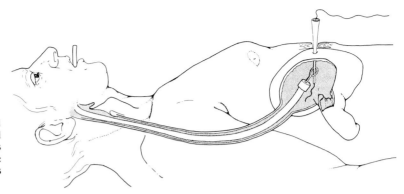

FIGURE 10–75. After several inches of suture have passed into the stomach, the snare is loosened and allowed to slide down around the silk itself. It is then tightened again.

should be well visualized endoscopically before attempting a puncture. The skin at the selected site is then anesthetized with several milliliters of a local anesthetic agent, and a 0.5 cm incision is made in the skin. The endoscopist maintains gastric inflation and closely observes the area of anticipated puncture. A polypectomy snare is passed through the accessory channel of the endoscope and held in readiness. A large-bore, tapered intravenous cannula with a metal stylet is now inserted into the incision and thrust through the abdominal and gastric walls. The endoscopist will see the cannula enter the stomach (Fig. 10–74). If the polypectomy snare is open and in proper position, the cannula may actually enter the snare loop. In any case, the endoscopist must be sure that the snare loop is closed snugly around the cannula at the point that it passes through the gastric mucosa before the assistant removes the stylet from the cannula.

Upon removing the stylet a piece of #2 silk suture, 60 inches in length, is threaded through the cannula into the stomach. The endoscopist will observe the silk suture as it exits the intragastric tip of the cannula. After several inches of the suture have passed into the stomach, the endoscopist loosens the polypectomy snare loop from around the cannula and allows the loop to slide off the cannula and onto the silk suture (Fig. 10–75). The snare loop is now reclosed tightly around the silk suture (Fig. 10–76). The assistant now releases the silk suture, and the endoscopist removes the gastroscope with polypectomy snare and thereby brings the entrapped suture out through the patient's mouth. The silk suture now passes across the abdominal and gastric walls, upward through the esophagus and out the patient's mouth (Fig. 10–77). The cannula, which traversed

the abdominal and gastric walls, is removed, leaving the silk suture in place.

The suture emerging from the patient's mouth is tied securely to the suture attached to the previously modified mushroom catheter (Fig. 10–78). Recall that the suture attached to the catheter runs through the tapered intravenous cannula which will shortly assume its dilating role. The gastrostomy tube is well lubricated and traction is applied to the silk suture at the abdominal wall site. A slow, steady pull is maintained as the mushroom catheter moves through the patient's mouth, esophagus, and stomach (Fig. 10–79). Eventually, the tapered end of the gastrostomy tube (the intravenous cannula) will exit through the puncture site (Fig. 10–80). The tapered cannula at the leading end of the gastrostomy tube should not be grasped, lest this disconnect from the gastrostomy tube

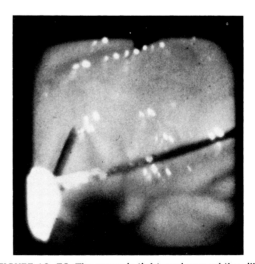

FIGURE 10–76. The snare is tightened around the silk suture.

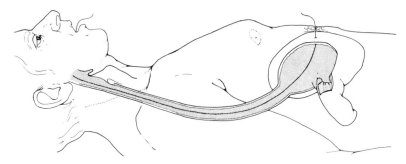

FIGURE 10–77. The silk suture is pulled up through the esophagus and out of the patient's mouth.

proper. Rather, traction on the silk suture is maintained until the rubber catheter itself exits through the incision. The catheter may now be grasped and pulled outward. After pulling several inches of the gastrostomy tube through the abdominal wall, the endoscope is passed again. The mushroom head of the catheter is visualized and the assistant is directed to pull the gastrostomy tube outward until there is gentle contact of the catheter's inner crossbar, which was positioned behind the mushroom head, and the gastric mucosa

(Fig. 10–81). Once this is accomplished, the endoscope is removed.

The second rubber (external) crossbar is now threaded along the exposed length of the gastrostomy tube until it touches the skin. Excessive tension should be avoided, because it will cause necrosis of underlying tissue and possibly extrusion of the tube. The crossbars (inner and outer) serve to hold the gastric and abdominal walls in contact (Fig. 10–82). A simple suture is placed through the skin at each end of the outer crossbar and tied to

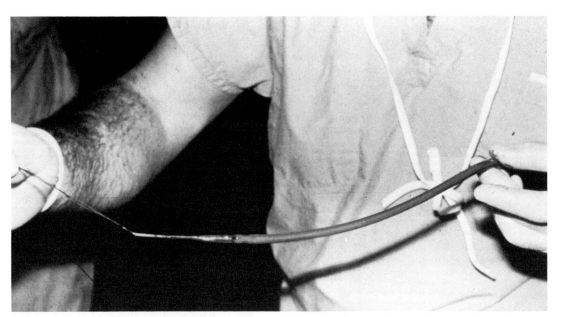

FIGURE 10–78. The silk emerging from the patient's mouth is tied to the suture attached to the gastrostomy tube.

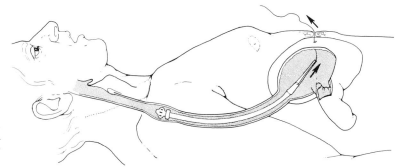

FIGURE 10–79. As traction is applied to the abdominal end of the silk suture, the gastrostomy tube moves in a retrograde fashion downward through the esophagus and into the stomach.

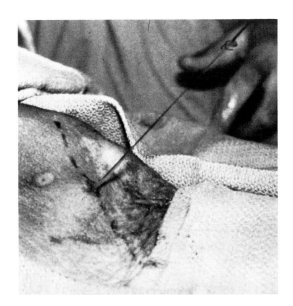

FIGURE 10–80. Continued traction is applied as the gastrostomy tube emerges from the abdominal wall.

FIGURE 10–81. The inner crossbar should lie in contact with the gastric mucosa.

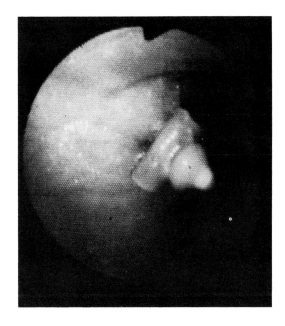

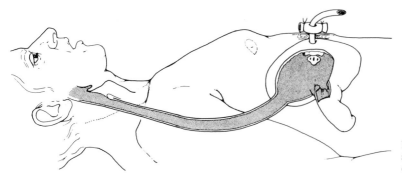

FIGURE 10–82. The crossbars serve to hold gastric and abdominal walls in close contact.

each end. The "dilator-like" end (intravenous cannula) is removed by cutting the rubber catheter near the junction point, and a plastic adapter is inserted into the end of the gastrostomy tube (Fig. 10–83).

Antibiotic ointment or a small dressing may be applied. Gastrostomy feedings are begun in 24 hours, starting with dextrose in water and progressing to a standard feeding preparation within a day.

COMMENT

Percutaneous endoscopic gastrostomy has been performed safely in patients ranging from small neonates to the aged. Complications have been infrequent and include superficial wound infections, early extrusion of the tube, pneumoperitoneum, and gastrocolic fistula.[5] Superficial wound infections are usually caused by bacteria from the mouth flora, presumably carried by the catheter as it is pulled through the puncture site. This occurrence can be greatly reduced by administering a penicillin or cephalosporin antibiotic immediately prior to the procedure.

Early extrusion of the tube may be the result of excessive tension applied to the catheter as it is secured in place. Care should be exercised that the gastrostomy tube is pulled outward until the inner crossbar just meets the gastric mucosa. No additional tension is required. Should extrusion occur shortly after gastrostomy tube placement, the procedure may be repeated immediately using the same site for replacement of the catheter.

Pneumoperitoneum is not unusual after this procedure, and may signify the escape of air around the puncture site. In the early period after the procedure this is of no concern, but if discovered several days after placement of the gastrostomy tube it may signify an incomplete seal between the stomach and the abdominal wall. In this case, the tube should be pulled outward with slight tension, and a water-soluble radiographic contrast agent should be instilled into the stomach via the gastrostomy tube. If contrast extravasates into the peritoneal cavity, additional tension may be added, followed by repetition of the contrast study. If there is persistent leakage, laparotomy is indicated to secure a permanent seal.

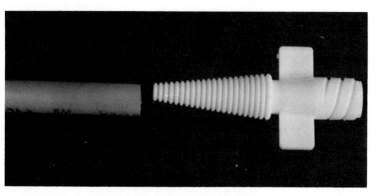

FIGURE 10–83. A plastic adapter is inserted into the end of the gastrostomy tube.

Gastrocolic fistula has been reported in two patients after percutaneous gastrostomy. In both patients this was due to entrapment of the colon between the gastric and abdominal walls. After removal of the gastrostomy tube the fistulas in both cases resolved spontaneously within days.

Gastrostomy tubes may be required for a number of years in some patients, whereas improvement in clinical status may permit early removal in others. When removal or replacement of a percutaneous gastrostomy tube is required, this can be accomplished easily by applying steady and gentle external traction. The mushroom tip will come out without difficulty, although the inner crossbar will remain in the stomach. This will pass without harm in the stool. The remaining opening through the anterior abdominal wall is small and will close rapidly if another gastrostomy tube is not inserted. If tube replacement is desired, an equivalent size Foley catheter may be inserted through the opening and its balloon then inflated, or another mushroom catheter may be inserted using a stylet to straighten the mushroom tip until it is within the stomach. No inner crossbar is necessary on the replacement catheter.

Percutaneous endoscopic gastrostomy has proven to be a safe, simple, and effective method for establishing a gastrostomy. It avoids laparotomy and general anesthesia in debilitated patients. It may become the procedure of choice when a feeding gastrostomy is required.

Editor's note: Information continues to accumulate as knowledge of this technique increases. References 6, 7, 8, 9, and 10 are of interest.

References

1. Gauderer MW, Ponsky JL. A simplified technique for constructing a tube feeding gastrostomy. Surg Gynecol Obstet 1981; 152:82–5.
2. Ponsky JL, Gauderer MW. Percutaneous endoscopic gastrostomy: A nonoperative technique for feeding gastrostomy. Gastrointest Endosc 1981; 27:9–11.
3. Gauderer MW, Ponsky JL, Izant RJ Jr. Gastrostomy without laparotomy: A percutaneous endoscopic technique. J Pediatr Surg 1980; 15:872–5.
4. Larson DE, Fleming CR, Ott BJ, Schroeder KW. Percutaneous endoscopic gastrostomy. Simplified access for enteral nutrition. Mayo Clin Proc 1983; 58:103–7.
5. Ponsky JL, Gauderer MW, Stellato TA. Percutaneous endoscopic gastrostomy: review of 150 cases. Arch Surg 1983; 118:913–4.
6. Greif JM, Ragland JJ, Ochsner MG, Riding R. Fatal necrotizing fasciitis complicating percutaneous endoscopic gastrostomy. Gastrointest Endosc 1986; 32:292–4.
7. Kozarek RA, Ball TJ, Ryan JA Jr. When push comes to shove: a comparison between two methods of percutaneous endoscopic gastrostomy. Am J Gastroenterol 1986; 81:642–6.
8. Ruge J, Vazquez RM. An analysis of the advantages of Stamm and percutaneous endoscopic gastrostomy. Surg Gynecol Obstet 1986; 162:13–6.
9. Jonas SK, Neimark S, Panwalker AP. Effect of antibiotic prophylaxis in percutaneous endoscopic gastrostomy. Am J Gastroenterol 1985; 80:438–41.
10. Stellato TA, Gauderer MW, Ponsky JL. Percutaneous endoscopic gastrostomy following previous abdominal surgery. Ann Surg 1984; 200:46–50.

Part 6

VIDEO ENDOSCOPY

JOHN L. PETRINI, JR., M.D.

Fiberoptic technology has progressed in two distinct areas. There has been a steady improvement in the optics provided to the observer. Image clarity, field of vision, and depth of field have gradually improved since the first flexible instruments of the early 1960's. Each step has been marked by a perceptible change in image, enough to warrant the purchase of new instruments. In addition, the mechanics of the instruments have also steadily improved, so that today's fiberoptic endoscopes are narrower in diameter, more flexible, and have larger accessory channels for biopsy and therapy work. The major limitation to fiberoptic technology has been the inability to provide "hard copy" documentation for the patient, referring physician, consultants, housestaff, nursing personnel, insurance companies, peer review boards, and other interested persons. Currently available photographic and video equipment fall short of providing high resolution, inexpensive, and manipulable data to meet these needs.

At the Digestive Disease Week in Washington, DC, 1983, Welch Allyn, Inc, made a dramatic announcement. They combined the capabilities of a remote video camera with the mechanical delivery system of the flexible endoscope. Using a charge-coupled device (CCD) video camera, they were able to present near–fiberoptic quality images via a television monitor, opening the door to several possibilities for information modification and storage. Data could be stored on video tape; transmitted through television wires; be computer enhanced, augmented, modified, or stored; and instant hard copy images could be made directly from the TV monitor. In addition, the theoretic resolution of the CCD image was sharper than that of the fiberoptic bundles. Finally, the durability of the video system should be much greater than that of the fiberoptic system, with its sensitivity to water, x-radiation, and torque damage.

Although the device was heralded as the next step in endoscopic technology, sales of the instruments and their use are still far behind that of conventional endoscopes. The computer-generated signal has not yet achieved its potential for improved image. Most endoscopists still consider the CCD image as inferior to that provided by fiberoptic bundles. Unfortunately, the video endoscope system is not compatible with fiberoptic light sources and vice versa, requiring that endoscopists wishing to use the CCD endoscopes purchase a second complete system. Furthermore, Welch Allyn was a relative late comer to the endoscope market, and the mechanical aspects of their instrument were considered by most endoscopists to be less desirable than those provided by the three major instrument manufacturers. The gap is narrowing, however, and endoscopists must decide whether to buy into the video endoscope market. An understanding of the device and its potential uses will help the consumer avoid hasty and costly mistakes.

CHARGE-COUPLED DEVICE TECHNOLOGY

The charge-coupled device was developed at Bell Laboratories in 1969 by Willard S. Boyle and George E. Smith as an extension of semiconductor technology. CCDs have been used in video cameras and remote cameras, such as on space probes and deep-sea cameras, for several years. The first black and white camera was developed in 1971 and the first color camera in 1972. There are two functions for such a device. First, light emanating from an object must somehow be captured unequivocally. Second, the captured light must be read-out from the device and displayed at a distant monitor.

The CCD consists of a photosensitive silicon wafer grid that generates current through light activation and an array of electrodes placed over the grid. Photons striking the silicon grid generate electrons or positively charged electron holes, an area in the grid where an electron is absent. Each photon generates one electron and one positively charged hole. To prevent ions from moving in the silicon, the wafer is divided into a grid (potential wells) by nonconducting buffers. By adjusting the depth of the potential wells, charges of varying sizes can be stored (from zero to some theoretic maximum). An image from an object gives off light in a characteristic spatial relationship—brighter light from some areas, less light from others. This light can be focused through the use of lenses onto the silicon grid. The grid, therefore, has the capability of generating electrical charges corresponding to the amount of light striking the grid, thus forming an electrical image of the object generating the light. The smaller the potential wells (i.e., pixels), the more accurately the light coming from the object can be interpreted and reproduced.

Generation of the image is of little use unless the charges in the wells can be read off the grid. This is accomplished by transferring the information (charges) from the potential wells sequentially across the grid. It is useful to visualize the grid as a series of small buckets arranged in rows on parallel conveyer belts. These buckets can each contain a unique amount of charge. The charge in the last bucket on each belt can be determined by "dumping" the charge through a circuit, giving a column of individual charges. The next series of buckets can then be moved into the reading area and dumped. In this fashion, the value of the charges in each well of the grid can be determined (Fig. 10–84).

In actuality, the charges in each row of potential wells are moved to the adjacent row by sequential changes in the voltage of electrodes placed across the grid. Each electrode

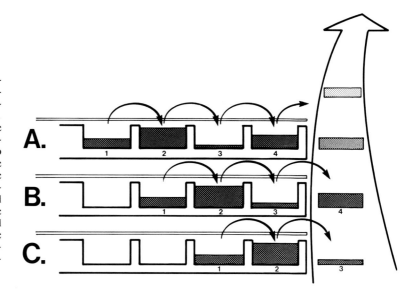

FIGURE 10–84. Schematic diagram of CCD imaging technology. *A,* The light generates pixels of varying intensity (1–4), which electrically represents the image of the object. *B,* The pixels are electrically "shifted" to the reading register by charge coupled technology; as one pixel leaves the reading register, the adjacent pixel is moved to the vacant spot. *C,* The entire row of pixels can thus be moved to the reading register, where the information can be amplified and depicted on the monitor.

controls the flow of one row of wells. The charges are thus coupled to one another (i.e., charge-coupled device) as they move across the grid. At the top of the grid, the charge in each well is moved to a transfer register. Using the same type of sequential or gated electrodes, the information is converted to a shift register, which moves the information in each row horizontally to the amplifier. At this point it becomes useful to consider the individual wells as pixels, with the charge giving some value to the pixels. The summation of the pixels forms the image that can be seen on the monitor.

CCDs cannot simultaneously collect and read the information. Therefore, several types of technology are employed to transfer the collected information. The first is the frame transfer method, which is the simplest to construct. This method uses two separate CCD chips, the first to collect the information and the second to accept the collected data for reading. The collection or integration phase takes only a fraction of a second. The data are then transferred to the storage chip approximately 60 times a second, where the information is read out in the manner described above.

In the second method, the interline transfer method, each row of collecting wells is adjacent to a shift register. After the integration phase, the data are moved to the shift register by the gated electrode technology, where the information can be read. This frees the photosensitive area to again begin collecting information. Since each row of collecting wells has a parallel row of shift registers, the chip's surface area is divided between collecting and storage wells.

A third system relies on transferring the data to the storage register during the time when the illuminating light is off. For color photography, this involves reading the pixels after the red, the blue, and the green lights have been projected. The image can then be compiled by the video processor as the sum of the data for the individual lights, generating the red/green/blue (RGB) monitor image. Most endoscope manufacturers use this type of system, whether the image is read using the frame transfer, shift register, or direct reading technique.

Each method has advantages and disadvantages. The frame transfer method is simpler to construct and is more sensitive to light. It requires a larger area, however, since the positioning of chips alongside one another requires more space. The minimum size for a frame transfer chip with enough pixels to be acceptable for endoscopic work is about 10 mm by 20 mm. This places certain constraints on the minimum diameter of endoscopes. There is some compensation by placing the chip obliquely in the tip of the endoscope, but the minimum width cannot be further reduced without advances in chip construction. The interline transfer method uses less of its surface area for the collection of light, so it is less sensitive to low levels of light. It is also more difficult and expensive to construct. The advantage is that it can be made smaller, with an acceptable image from a chip 8 mm by 10 mm.

Other design characteristics must be also

taken into account in the construction of the CCDs. The most important aspect is that of the standard cathode ray tube (CRT) that is used in television monitors. The image on a television screen is composed of pixels arranged in parallel horizontal rows. The image is composed of about 500 lines, each of which contains 300 to 400 pixels. The full screen image would be a mosaic of 150,000 to 200,000 pixels. The CCD imager must contain an equivalent number of potential wells to produce a sharp image. The production of a color image would require at least twice as many pixels, half for the green or luminance signal and half for the red-blue or chrominance signal.

A major limitation to the production of smaller CCDs is the minimum size required to construct a grid with adequate pixels and electrodes. The actual size of the grid is related to the resolution of the lenses in the system and the sensitivity to light required for the imager. For the lens system of an upper endoscope, a grid of approximately 196×165 pixels is used, or approximately 32,000 pixels. The Fujinon chip uses approximately 56,000 pixels.

There are other design characteristics that play a role in the selection of these solid-state imagers. They are so sensitive to light that imaging of distant stars by this system is superior to that of other photographic methods. For the endoscopist, however, bright light may play a role during the procedure, such as in defining location in the abdomen during colonoscopy and in selecting a site for percutaneous feeding gastrostomy tube placement. Problems arise in CCD technology when excess light is applied.

The potential wells can accept a finite number of electrical charges. As the amount of light striking a given area exceeds the capacity of the well to store charges, the electrons and electron holes can spill over into adjacent wells. This effect, called blooming, is clearly visible in the CCDs used for the production of video endoscopes. Blooming results in the production of a white area on the screen whenever the ambient light overwhelms the capacity of the potential wells. This is most apparent when viewing close objects and in the slide-by technique during colonoscopy, but also can occur in the duodenal bulb. Blooming may also become a problem if the instrument is used for laser work, as the light from the laser may obliterate the monitor image. Circuit designs contain anti-blooming

mechanisms, but they are inadequate to eliminate the problem completely. Another method for correcting this problem is to alter the aperture used on the focusing lens. If a smaller aperture is used, there are two distinct advantages. First, the light produced by the light source can be increased and the amount of light that strikes the collecting area will still be acceptable. Second, the smaller the aperture, the greater the focal length. This permits objects at various distances to be in focus at the same time, which is extremely important in endoscopy. Current flexible fiberoptic endoscopes have a focal length of 3 mm to 100 mm. That is, objects within these distances are in focus. In practicality, objects are rarely beyond 100 mm from the tip of the endoscope. Closer objects can be brought into focus by varying the focus at the head of the instrument. Most video endoscopes have lenses with a larger aperture, which has given them a slightly narrower focal length (5 mm to 100 mm). In addition, there is no mechanism for altering the focal length, so that objects very close are seen more clearly with the fiberoptic endoscopes.

Silicon photosensitive crystals are variably sensitive to individual wavelengths of light. They absorb more light from the red and infrared spectra than from the ultraviolet range. The lenses on the system may be treated with special coatings that increase or decrease the sensitivity to various wavelengths, such as to protect the chip from Nd-YAG laser light. This may prove useful for endoscopes that could utilize characteristic wavelengths of light emitted by photoactive compounds. Such compounds might be used to identify a given population of cells or tissue type, such as dysplastic or malignant cells in specific disease states.

The standard upper gastrointestinal fiberoptic endoscope contains approximately 22,000 to 30,000 bundles to recreate the image. The CCD, with its 32,000 to 56,000 pixels, has the potential to produce an image nearly twice as sharp. It is clear that improvements in the CCDs and circuitry will enhance the visual image provided by the video endoscopes and that the image may ultimately be a better endoscopic image.

THE VIDEO ENDOSCOPE SYSTEM

Video endoscope systems require at least three components: the endoscope, a video

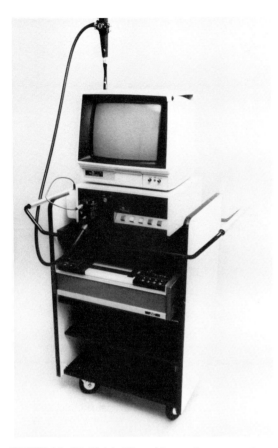

FIGURE 10–85. Welch Allyn video endoscopy system. The prototype system includes the monitor seated atop the video processor. The endoscope is suspended from a holder mounted at the left of the cart. A 3/4-inch video tape recorder is also on the cart.

processor, and a television monitor (Fig. 10–85). The instrument itself is nearly identical to standard flexible fiberoptic instruments, except that the objective lens is not present. The control valves for suction and air/water insufflation, as well as the accessory channel, are in standard locations. The position of the objective lens has been replaced by control buttons for freezing/unfreezing the image for photographing from the monitor on the Olympus model and by the biopsy port on the Welch Allyn model (Fig. 10–86). The insertion tube looks nearly identical to the standard instrument until the light source is activated. The light bundles are then seen to produce red/green/blue light for color television imaging in rapid sequence. This occurs too quickly for the eye to interpret and gives a strobe light–type effect. The lens has been modified to focus the light on the CCD and resembles the standard distal objective lens of a standard fiberoptic endoscope (Fig. 10–

87). The actual position of the components differs slightly between the manufacturers' models.

The first time an endoscopist handles the video endoscopes there is a distinct novelty that can be appreciated. Instead of holding the instrument at eye level, the hand is positioned just above the waist. The hand grasps the head of the endoscope at right angles, a different feel from the near parallel grasp on a standard fiberoptic endoscope. The controls and locking mechanism, as well as the valve controls, operate identically to the standard endoscopes. Within a short time, a skilled endoscopist adjusts hand-eye coordination to read the screen rather than the objective lens. More than once, however, the endoscope will be brought to the eye out of conditioned response. The optimum position for the head would probably be at or below the waist, but this would require significant modifications of the control mechanism. A "joy-stick" steering mechanism might be acceptable if endoscopists would be willing to make the adjustment in their mental set.

Other components of the handle include buttons to freeze/unfreeze the image and to activate the photographic equipment. Some require a significant adjustment in grip for activation, and production models of video endoscopes may have alternate locations for these buttons.

The actual mechanics of the insertion shaft and deflection section are largely dependent upon the manufacturer. These prototype instruments are retoolings of standard flexible instruments, so that the Olympus and Fujinon video endoscopes have the same characteristics as their fiberoptic counterparts. These manufacturers have a significant head start in the internal components and produce a mechanically more acceptable instrument. The actual image is a function of the CCD and the processor. The Welch Allyn chip has improved the light sensitivity so that the depth of field and transillumination properties have improved. In addition, the smaller CCD permits the development of a narrower instrument.

The image generated at the tip of the endoscope by the CCD is in analog form, i.e., contains varying amounts of information (charge) for each pixel. It is carried to the video processor by wire, theoretically improving the durability of video endoscopes over conventional fiberoptic scopes. The video processor has two functions. It provides the controlled split color light necessary for the

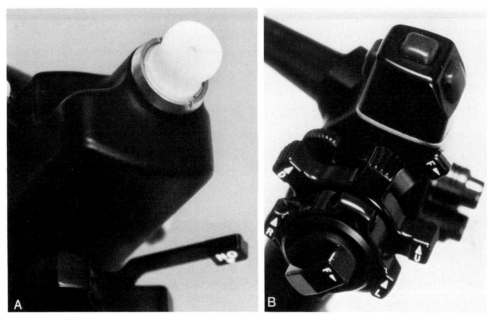

FIGURE 10–86. Top of Welch Allyn (*A*) and Olympus (*B*) video endoscopes showing replacement of objective lens by the biopsy port (Welch Allyn) or control buttons for freezing the monitor image and still photography (Olympus).

CCD and hence is the light source for the endoscope. In addition, it contains the circuitry that enables conversion of the endoscope signal to the standard binary code for projection to the video monitor. The data produced by the CCD in analog form must be converted to a binary system for use with the CRT. Once converted, however, the image can be stored on video tape, computer

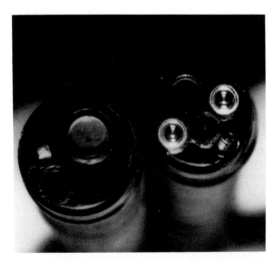

FIGURE 10–87. Distal tip of standard fiberoptic endoscope (*right*) and Welch Allyn video endoscope (*left*). When activated, the light for the video endoscope emanates from the viewing lens on this instrument.

disc, laser disc, or other media for binomial storage. The data could also be used to produce instant hard-copy images, employing the same technology used to print pictures in newspapers. Furthermore, binary information can be easily retrieved and compared with past or future images. It is these applications that hold the greatest promise for the video endoscopes (see Data Storage and Retrieval).

The video or television monitor is the most critical component for clarity of image. The data that can be projected are keyed to the number of pixels that the monitor can accept. Standard TV monitors can image 150,000 to 200,000 pixels. Some new monitors have the capacity to image over a million pixels, but these are beyond the imaging circuitry of standard endoscopic CCDs. Current video endoscopes are designed to produce television signals for use with standard RGB monitors. To rectify the difference between the number of pixels on the monitor and the number generated by the CCD, manufacturers have resorted to two techniques. One is to interlace the image into two identical lines; i.e., the first row of pixels is identical to the second row, the third to the fourth, etc. This reduces the number of pixels required to 75,000 to 100,000. The second technique is to reduce the area of the screen devoted to the image. By devoting 32,000 of the remain-

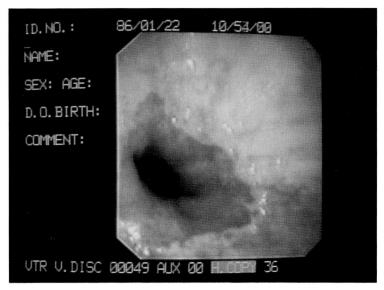

PLATE 10–64. Photograph of the monitor image from the Olympus video endoscopy system. The gastroesophageal junction can be seen on the monitor, and space for identification data is on the left.

ing pixels to the CCD-generated image, 32/75 of the screen (42%) is used for the picture and the remainder is either black or devoted to text.

The text can include the name of the patient, physician, date, time, and additional pertinent comments (Plate 10–64). The manufacturers have individualized the screen display to their specifications. The Welch Allyn display includes a second page for more text than can be displayed when the endoscopic image is not needed. Text data are entered from a keyboard that is attached to the video processor. Although a standardized keyboard would be ideal, each company uses a different layout. The keyboard may also control additional storage mechanisms, such as entering directly to an endoscopic database or to a laser disc writer.

Each manufacturer has attachments for the monitor that will permit use of a 35-mm or instant camera for photographing the image off the screen (Fig. 10–88). The image is first frozen on the screen, and the camera is then activated. Images produced by this method are considerably sharper than those with the standard flexible fiberoptic instruments (Plate 10–65). The reason appears to be the

PLATE 10–65. Vocal cords and arytenoid cartilages as seen on the Olympus video endoscopy monitor.

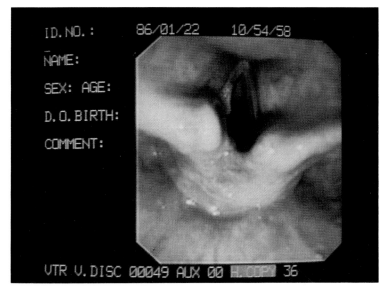

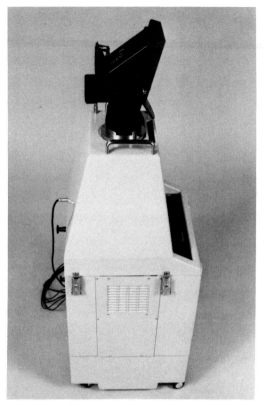

FIGURE 10–88. Accessory monitor for endoscopic photography for the Olympus video endoscopy system. A Polaroid instant camera is mounted face down atop the monitor.

fixed image, which can be exposed to the photographic medium for the long period of time required for the film.

The video endoscope system must be considered to operate as a unit. It is not possible presently to separate the various components from each other by distance. The entire set-up must be housed in the endoscopic unit or on a cart (Fig. 10–89). Each manufacturer has produced a cart to store and transport the system should it be needed outside the unit. None is ideal, but the portability of the system should be considered before purchase.

A final component of the video endoscope system is the adapter that permits use of a standard fiberoptic instrument with the video processor. This consists of a chip that fits on the head of a standard endoscope. Fujinon has been the most aggressive at adapting their system to all the standard instruments, but the image offered by the Welch Allyn adapter is the sharpest. These adapters allow use of standard endoscopic equipment with the data storage and retrieval systems afforded by the video endoscopes. If the tech-

nology of the video endoscopes can be improved, however, the use of the fiberoptic technology will be less desirable.

Cleaning of the video endoscope system is the same as with the standard fiberoptic endoscopes. The scopes will tolerate 2% glutaraldehyde and ethylene oxide gas, but may be damaged in glutaraldehyde/surfactant solutions. As yet, none of the instruments is fully immersible.

DATA STORAGE AND RETRIEVAL

Current information obtained at endoscopic procedures relies on the subjective information provided by the observer. The information is then given to the patient and referring physician orally or by a written report. The "data" from the procedure are not transmitted and become the exclusive domain of the endoscopist. The value of the written report is dependent upon the skill and experience of the endoscopist. The ability to observe and accurately convey the information (as well as the accuracy of the observation) varies, even for experienced endoscopists.

In addition to the implications for the patient and referring physician, the lack of objective data has consequences that extend to the medicolegal and scientific communities. It is clear that the likelihood of accurate interpretation of the data would be increased if the data could be re-examined by colleagues and compared with a reference source. Video cameras that mount to the endoscope are available, but their use is limited at this time. The positioning of the video camera between the fiberoptic bundle and the eye reduces the light and clarity of the image. The mechanics of mounting the camera can be cumbersome, with booms, pulleys, and other annoying contraptions. The amount of video tape necessary to provide for storage of the procedure data in busy endoscopy units is prohibitive. Cameras that mount directly to the endoscope are also available, but again, the pictures produced are inferior to the direct image. The best photographs are those obtained with standard 35-mm film. The availability of photographic data is limited by the time required for development and review. The quality of instant photographs is inferior owing to the large amount of light required to produce a clear image, a factor that prolongs the shutter speed. Motion in the gastrointestinal tract

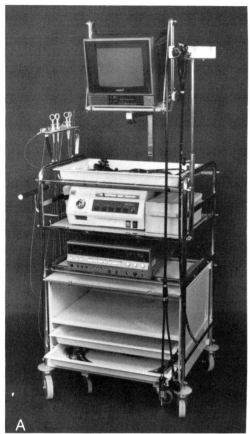 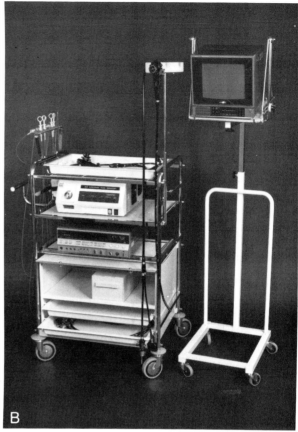

FIGURE 10–89. Fujinon video endoscopy cart. The monitor can be pushed with the cart as a unit (A) or separated for easier viewing during the procedure (B).

usually blurs the photograph, and often several photographs of the same area are needed to obtain a clear print. Even if high quality pictures could be produced, storage and retrieval of the pictures would be a time-consuming and expensive undertaking. The availability of the data to others outside the endoscopic unit or storage area would also be a problem.

By reducing the data from endoscopic procedures to binary code, the door has been opened to a wide variety of methods to store and retrieve data. The image from the system arrives at the monitor in a binary form and could be split off to a video tape without loss of quality. The same data can be frozen on the monitor and instant or 35-mm photographs taken directly from the monitor. This eliminates the motion artifact, and the clarity of the photograph becomes a function of the resolution of the monitor. The data could also be coded onto computer tape or disc, but the large number of bits of information required to reproduce the monitor image exceeds the capacity of available computer storage systems. A more useful system is that of laser disc storage. The laser disc writer uses a plastic disc that costs about $300 and has the capability to store approximately 24,000 images for the monitor (Fig. 10–90). By interfacing the writer to a computer, additional information regarding the nature of the image, the name of the patient, data, etc., can be coded, with the image permitting unlimited recall and comparison. Images can be examined simultaneously from previous and current endoscopic procedures by projecting split-screen images. Follow-up for healing, tumor growth or regression, and effectiveness of medication can thus be facilitated. The information can also be assimilated into a computer-generated database for the procedure. This information is available to generate reports, compare populations, study disease trends, and improve endoscopic skills.

The data are also transmissible via telephone lines or even satellite. Thus, the data could be brought to a distant colleague for review or to an instructional conference. The

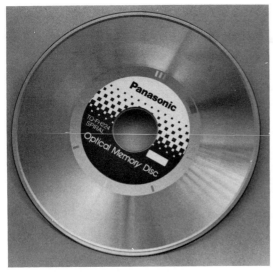

FIGURE 10–90. Laser disc for use with Olympus video endoscopy system laser writer.

AVAILABLE VIDEO ENDOSCOPE SYSTEMS

Endoscopists at the Cleveland Clinic have had the opportunity to examine and use each of the video endoscopy systems. Video endoscopes are manufactured by Welch Allyn, Inc., Fujinon, Inc., and Olympus Optical Co. Each of the instruments, except the Welch Allyn scopes, is a prototype and not a production model. The design of the endoscope is likely to undergo some changes before it is available commercially, but the system should be similar to the systems we tested. Tables 10–13 to 10–16 list some of the characteristics of the instruments. It would be unfair to judge the finished production endoscopes on the basis of our experience with these prototypes, and we offer comparisons only to guide critiques of the final product. Except for minor differences, the image obtained from all the instruments is similar.

In general, we found the image to be of lower quality than that of the standard Olympus OES fiberoptic endoscope. Many of the instruments have smaller biopsy channels

than are required for therapeutic work, especially in the biliary tree. In addition, several of the electrical devices used in the same room, such as in electrosurgical units, would cause interference with the image momentarily. The endoscopes functioned without flaw, although several of the video processors and accessory photographic devices would require servicing. This is assumed to be a function of their developmental stage rather than the video technology. It was apparent, however, that the nurses and patients were much more interested in the procedure when the findings could be shared over the monitor.

Welch Allyn System

Welch Allyn was the first company to market video endoscopes, and they are currently working on the second generation of scopes.

TABLE 10–13. **Upper Gastrointestinal Electronic Video Endoscopes**

	Welch Allyn	Fujinon	Olympus
Model	81205	EVG-F	GIF-VIO
Diameter (mm)	9.5	11.4	10.5
Accessory channel diameter (mm)	3.0	2.8	2.8
Depth of field (mm)	3–100	3–100	5–100
Angle of view (degrees)	120	105	120
Deflection (degrees)			
Up/down	210/90	210/90	210/90
Left/right	100/100	90/90	100/100

TABLE 10–14. **Video Colonoscopes**

	Welch Allyn	Fujinon	Olympus
Model	82156 (82176)	EVC-M (EVC-L)	CF-VIOI (CF-VIOL)
Length (cm)	150 (170)	150 (167)	132.5 (163.5)
Diameter (mm)	13.5	13.5	13.8
Accessory channel diameter (mm)	4.2	3.7	3.2
Depth of field (mm)	3–100	4–100	5–100
Angle of view (degrees)	130	125	140
Deflection (degrees)			
Up/down	180/180	180/180	180/180
Left/right	160/160	160/160	160/160

TABLE 10–15. **Video Duodenoscopes**

	Fujinon	Olympus
Model	EVD-XL	JF-VIO
Length (cm)		124.5
Diameter (mm)	12.2	12.5
Accessory channel diameter (mm)	2.8	2.8
Depth of field (mm)	3–100	5–60
Angle of view (degrees)	90	100
Deflection (degrees)		
Up/down	120/120	120/90
Left/right	100/100	90/110

The characteristics of their upper gastroscope, colonoscope, and sigmoidoscope are listed in Tables 10–13 and 10–14.

The company has adapted a new CCD into the second generation of endoscopes that has reduced the size of the chip without reduction in pixels. It is also more sensitive to light, which has allowed reduction in the aperture of the objective lens. The result has been the production of a smaller caliber gastroscope (9.5 mm) with a greater depth of field. The previous depth of field was 5 mm to 100 mm, which is virtually the same as the instruments from the other manufacturers. The newer scopes have a focal length of 3 mm to 100 mm, which is virtually the same as fiberoptic endoscopes. Anti-blooming circuits have been improved and there is a marked reduction in glare. The output from the light source has also been increased, so that it now produces a continuous lamp of 300 watts, a 16-fold increase in the available amount of light. This allows for transillumination through the abdominal wall during procedures.

The Welch Allyn system is mounted on a cart that is fully self-contained (Fig. 10–91). The monitor is not easily viewed during the procedure when on the cart and is best moved across from the cart. It is mobile, however, and can be transported for emergency endoscopy outside the unit. The keyboard is a pressure-pad type board with auditor que to input (Fig. 10–92). The data are clearly displayed on the screen and mastering the keyboard is quite simple. A second screen is available for additional information, but it cannot be displayed while viewing the procedure. The cart has space for a video tape recorder and set-up is relatively simple.

The model 81205 upper gastrointestinal endoscope is the thinnest available. It has a large biopsy port (3.0 mm) and a replaceable valve over the channel to circumvent leakage. The image produced is of good quality ex-

TABLE 10–16. **Current Prices for Video Endoscopy Equipment (in U.S. Dollars)**

	Welch Allyn	Fujinon	Olympus
Gastroscope	7,900	10,500	9,400
Colonoscope	9,525	11,500	9,850
Duodenoscope		11,500	10,400
Sigmoidoscope	5,875		6,500
Video processor/ light source	5,915	11,000	8,900*
Keyboard	400	750	
Cart	1,060	1,995	
Monitor	850	(1,595)†	
Fiberscope module		4,000	

*Includes video processor and keyboard, light source, and mobile cart.
†Panasonic.

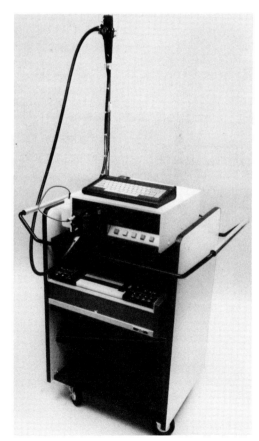

FIGURE 10–91. Welch Allyn cart with monitor removed. The keyboard can be placed atop the video processor for easier data entry.

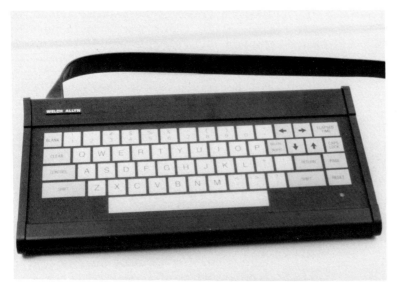

FIGURE 10–92. Pressure keyboard used with Welch Allyn video endoscopy system.

cept at the cricopharynx and in the duodenal bulb. Here the focal length and limited light-adjusting circuits prevent accurate evaluation of the mucosa, a problem that is still not adequately resolved. Welch Allyn measures the angle of view diagonally across the picture. The older endoscopes had a 90-degree angle, but the newer instruments have a viewing angle of 120 degrees.

The mechanics of the upper gastrointestinal endoscope are somewhat less acceptable than that of the other manufacturers, but have been greatly improved over the first generation instruments. We found that the scope would not respond well to torquing maneuvers, which made visualization of the descending duodenum difficult. Further improvements in aperture size and the insertion shaft should result in an excellent endoscope.

The colonoscope comes in two lengths: model 82156 (150 cm) and the longer model 82176 (170 cm). These instruments also utilize the smaller and more light sensitive CCD. This allows a large accessory port (4.2 mm) without increasing scope diameter. The deflection section has also been improved. By shortening the bending section by 1 cm, the turning radius has been reduced (Fig. 10–93). The angle of view for the colonoscopes is 130 degrees.

Mechanically, the colonoscopes function well. The previous model was studied extensively at the Cleveland Clinic and was given a satisfactory review.[1] One problem, the overhanging plastic cap that extends out over the tip of the colonoscope, is currently being revised. This overhang frequently collects fluid or stool and causes distortion in the light and image.

We also tested a prototype adapter that fits over the head of standard fiberoptic instruments. It produced a remarkably clear picture that was indistinguishable from the fiberoptic instrument alone. The manufacturer is also producing laser-compatible instruments that will use an infrared filter to reduce blooming and protect the CCD. Photographs can be made directly off the monitor by the use of special adapters. A sigmoid-

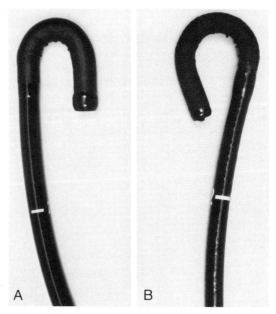

FIGURE 10–93. Turning radius of Welch Allyn video colonoscope (A) and upper endoscope (B).

oscope, model number 80065, is also available.

Fujinon System

The second manufacturer of video endoscopes was Fujinon. This company had the advantage of greater experience in the flexible endoscope market and has recently produced three instruments: a gastroscope, colonoscope, and duodenoscope. As with their previous products, compatibility with a wide variety of instruments has been a major objective.

The Fujinon system is mounted on a well-designed cart (Fig. 10–89). It is the most mobile and functional of any cart produced by the three companies and incorporates a separate stand for the monitor that securely attaches to the main cart. The design of the monitor stand allows it to be conveniently placed opposite the endoscopist, and it slides under a bed or examining table to minimize space requirements. When attached to the main cart, the unit is easily maneuverable by one person.

Fujinon video endoscopes are modified versions of their standard fiberoptic instruments and are identical mechanically. The head contains buttons for freezing/unfreezing the monitor image and for photography. With the left hand in the standard position on the control section, the buttons can be activated with the ring and little fingers, but this does take time to master. Hard-copy images (35 mm or instant) can be added by purchasing a separate camera-monitor system that is activated by these buttons. Alternatively, a hood-type camera mount for the monitor can be purchased, as for the Welch Allyn system.

The video processor for the Fujinon system (model EPX-301) contains a 300-watt xenon light source (Fig. 10–94). It will also accept standard Fujinon fiberoptic endoscopes. The monitor is a 13-inch red/green/blue (RGB)

FIGURE 10–94. Video processor for use with Fujinon system. The upper port is a standard fiberoptic endoscope umbilical cord port (A); the video endoscope image is entered by the lower port (B).

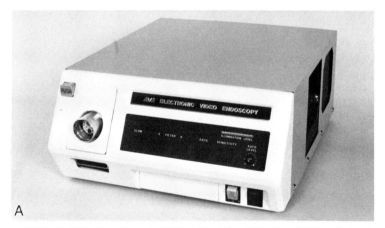

A

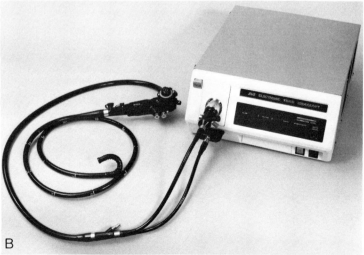

B

Sony. The image produced is of good quality, but the same difficulties with close-ups and blooming occur. The focal length of the Fujinon CCD is 3 mm to 100 mm, which is similar to standard fiberoptic endoscopes and the Welch Allyn video endoscopes.

The upper gastrointestinal video endoscope is the EVG-F, a 11.4-mm diameter endoscope (Fig. 10–95). It has a standard 2.8-mm accessory channel and an angle of view of 105 degrees. Its chip is composed of 56,000 pixels, nearly twice that of the Welch Allyn and Olympus chips. The colonoscopes are available in two lengths: 150 cm (EGC-M) and 167 cm (EGC-L). Each has an insertion tube diameter of 13.5 mm and a 3.7-mm diameter accessory channel. The angle of view is 125 degrees, with a 96,000 pixel chip. The duodenoscope is 12.2 mm in diameter with a 2.8-mm accessory channel. It has an angle of view of 90 degrees.

Fujinon has approached the problem of compatibility aggressively and manufactures a number of adapters that will fit standard Fujinon and Olympus fiberoptic endoscopes, as well as some rigid laparoscopy instruments (Fig. 10–96). The adapters attach to the video processor and produce an image that is projected on the monitor. The objective lens is not visible with the adapter in place. Each adapter costs about $500 and is specific for the instrument (i.e., one adapter will fit all Olympus OES endoscopes but not older Olympus models).

Olympus System

We are currently testing three prototype instruments from the Olympus Optical Co. They are adaptations of OES model instruments that share the maneuverability and smooth operating internal deflection system of those instruments. In addition, they are coupled to a laser disc writer that enables storage and retrieval of nearly 24,000 images per disc, a system that is extremely useful for data storage, although somewhat expensive to purchase (Fig. 10–97).

The Olympus system consists of the video endoscope with the objective lens replaced by buttons that operate the freeze/unfreeze mechanism, laser writer, photography system, and monitor. The video processor has adjustable brightness and hue controls and a control section to define output to the monitor, laser writer, video tape recorder, and photography system (Fig. 10–98). The hardcopy photography system has a separate monitor with cameras for instant and 35-mm pictures. Photographs can also be taken directly off the monitor with an attachable hood mount.

The keyboard can be used to input data to the screen, but the area for display is limited. It is possible to input directly to the laser writer for more complete information regarding stored data. Images can be stored from the instrument, from the keyboard, or from a hand-held remote unit. Each image

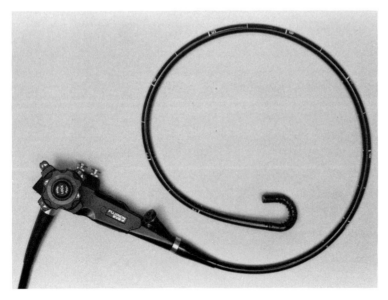

FIGURE 10–95. Fujinon video upper endoscope.

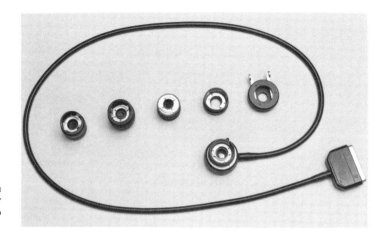

FIGURE 10–96. Adaptors for Fujinon system to convert standard rigid or fiberoptic endoscope images to video endoscopic images.

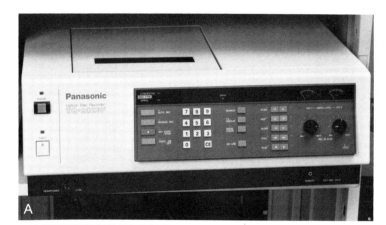

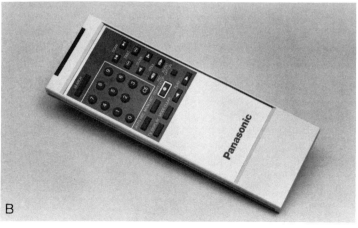

FIGURE 10–97. Laser writer (A) for Olympus video endoscopy system. Data can be entered directly or by use of a hand-held remote control (B).

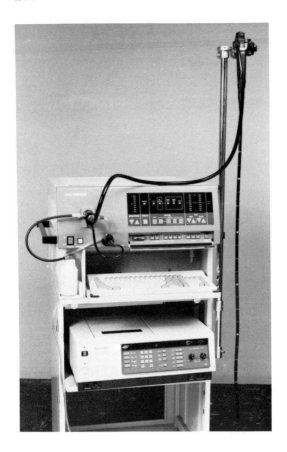

FIGURE 10–98. Prototype Olympus video endoscopy system. The video processor (*top*), keyboard, and laser writer are shown on the mobile cart.

FIGURE 10–99. Distal tip of Olympus video duodeno-scope.

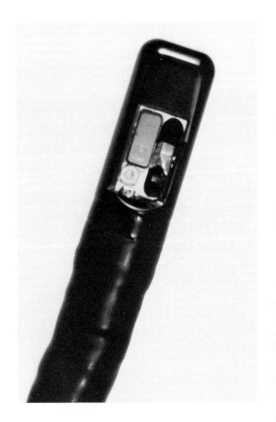

frozen from the monitor is given a sequential number as well as other definable characteristics. Thus, images can be recalled by the number, by patient name, or by name of the image (e.g., "polyps" or "polyps, cancer, with polypectomy"). Recall of data is also available in slow or fast frame advance or by single frame advance. The possibility of interfacing the laser writer to a defined database, such as the ASGE database, is an exciting prospect.

The system is mounted on a cart, but with the attachments is somewhat cumbersome to move. There is no separate monitor mount, but a somewhat less sophisticated system could be easily adapted for transport. There is an attachment for standard fiberoptic endoscopes similar to those made by the other manufacturers.

The CCD used in the Olympus video endoscopes has a shorter focal length than either of the other endoscopes, and the effective field of focus is 5 mm to 100 mm. Aside from minor differences, the image produced is similar.

The upper gastrointestinal endoscope, the GIF-VIO, is 10.5 mm in diameter with a 2.8-mm diameter accessory channel. The angle of view is 120 degrees. Two colonoscopes are available. The CF-VIOI is 132.5 cm long and the CF-VIOL is 163.5 cm in length. The diameter of the insertion tube is 13.8 mm with a 3.2-mm diameter accessory port. The angle of view is a wide 140 degrees. A duodenoscope is also available with the familiar 15-degree retroflexed view. It is 12.5 mm in diameter with a 2.8-mm diameter biopsy channel (Fig. 10–99). The angle of view is 100 degrees. The image from these instruments is of good quality, with the same exceptions for close objects. The attachment for adapting standard fiberoptic endoscopes is less satisfactory.

SUMMARY

The major advantage of video endoscope technology is clearly its capacity to provide image storage and dispersal of data to other observers. The image can be coded in binary or analog fashion and stored on photographic medium, floppy or hard disc, tape, laser disc, and as yet undiscovered means. The possibility of coupling endoscopic database recordings to the image could be an invaluable aid to retrospective and prospective study. Presently, at this point we are comparing fourth and fifth generation fiberoptic instruments with first and second generation video endoscopes. The gap is not appreciably large, and if refinements in video endoscope technology continue, the CCD endoscope may live up to its potential and replace fiberoptic instruments.

Reference

1. Sivak MV, Fleischer DE. Colonoscopy with a VideoEndoscope (tm): preliminary experience. Gastrointest Endosc 1984; 30:1–5.

Section II

UPPER GASTROINTESTINAL ENDOSCOPY

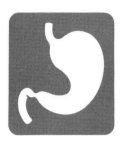

Chapter 11

TECHNIQUE OF UPPER GASTROINTESTINAL ENDOSCOPY

MICHAEL V. SIVAK, JR., M.D.

Upper gastrointestinal endoscopy, one of the most fundamental methods of investigating the gastrointestinal tract, is a well established, indispensable procedure. This chapter is concerned with the technical points of maneuvering an endoscope through the pharynx, esophagus, stomach and duodenum. In esophagogastroduodenoscopy (EGD) the ability to manipulate an endoscope within a patient is essential but second in importance to observation.

As the beginner learns to perform EGD, the ability to maneuver the endoscope is almost always attained before the capacity for endoscopic diagnosis. The thought processes of the novice are more concerned with moving the instrument from one point to another. Thus preoccupied, the beginner frequently does not observe all that may be seen. In contrast, the required maneuvers are second nature to the expert; they are performed in a natural, flowing manner that requires minimal conscious attention. The expert thus becomes more cognizant of what can be seen.

The word "see" can have many connotations. It is never enough that an endoscopist simply collects observations in a mechanistic manner. Rather, observations must be synthesized with relation to a clinical problem and compared with prior experience. Because many disorders affect the upper gastrointestinal tract, there is much to be seen. Experience, therefore, has an important place in upper gastrointestinal endoscopy.

Upper gastrointestinal endoscopy extends the sense of sight through the use of a device. It is, in a very real sense, physical diagnosis

for the gastroenterologist and the gastrointestinal surgeon.

The indications, contraindications, and complications of endoscopy are discussed elsewhere (see Chapter 12). Endoscopic diagnosis, or the things to be "seen," is discussed throughout this book.

PREPARATION FOR EGD

Every endoscopy procedure includes many steps, with the actual performance of the procedure being only one of these (see Chapters 3 and 5).

Assessment of the Patient

There is a tendency, greater now, to lessen contact with the patient during the preparation process. When the patient's physician is also the endoscopist, this is usually not a problem. However, patients are often referred to the endoscopist or the endoscopy unit for a procedure alone. Frequently this type of referral is for a special therapeutic procedure, but the use of primary diagnostic gastrointestinal endoscopy is also increasing (see Chapter 3). This method of referral does not diminish the responsibility of the endoscopist with respect to the indications, contraindications, and safety of the procedure.

Gastrointestinal endoscopy has value in many clinical situations. It is impractical to require that every patient with an indication for endoscopy be completely evaluated by the endoscopist who will perform the procedure. Nevertheless, the indications for the procedure must be well defined and carefully reviewed by the endoscopist. The endoscopist must also be satisfied that there are no contraindications. These aspects of preparation for EGD can be problematic when the patient has been referred specifically for endoscopy.

To some degree the endoscopist must rely on the thoroughness and ability of the referring physician in determining the fitness of the patient for the procedure. This is less difficult when there is an established professional relationship with the referring physician, such as exists in a closed group practice of medicine where complete case records are also available to the endoscopist. It is more problematic when there is no existing relationship with a referring physician. In addition to establishing the indication for the procedure, it must be verified that a patient has no associated illnesses that will compromise the safety of the procedure. This often requires a more formal evaluation of the patient prior to the procedure in which the emphasis should be focused on disorders that have a direct bearing on the procedure, such as a history or evidence of cardiovascular illness, hypertension, and respiratory disorders, especially respiratory insufficiency. A complete history of medications, including drug allergies, should be obtained to avoid drug interactions, but also because many drugs affect the gastrointestinal tract in either beneficial or adverse ways.

Preprocedure Instruction

Patients should be advised in advance of the time of the EGD that they will not be able to drive, operate machinery, or perform intricate mental tasks for a number of hours afterward, and that it is necessary that another person accompany them after the procedure. The patient must be given the reason for undergoing the procedure, a brief description of EGD, and be apprised of the remote possibility of a complication including the most common untoward events. An informed and motivated patient generally allows the procedure to be performed in an equable manner that assures safety and thoroughness. Although a written description of the procedure is often advantageous, it remains necessary to review the important points with the patient. Because of the lingering effects of sedative drugs, patients undergoing EGD should also be given postprocedure instructions before the procedure, including directions in the event of a delayed complication. Written instructions are again advantageous.

Preparation

General

Patients must fast for 6 hours prior to EGD. When there is delayed or defective gastric emptying, the required period of fasting may be longer, and in some cases it may be necessary to aspirate gastric contents in order to perform EGD. Dentures and eyeglasses should be removed. Other steps in the process of preparing the patient, the procedure room, and endoscopic equipment for EGD are discussed in Chapter 5.

Premedication

Three basic types of drugs are used in EGD: medications that produce sedation, drugs that affect gastrointestinal motility, and topical anesthetic agents. The two drugs most widely used for sedation are meperidine (pethidine) and diazepam. I prefer a combination of these two drugs for most endoscopic procedures.

Upper gastrointestinal endoscopy can be performed without pharmacologic preparation. This may be done in highly motivated patients, especially those who are fearful of the effects of sedative drugs. In clinical situations of an emergency nature, it may be advisable to avoid the use of drugs that depress respiration or to use these agents in very small doses.

There are certain practical advantages to endoscopy without the use of sedative drugs: the risk of a complication is reduced, virtually no time is required for postprocedure recovery, and postprocedure monitoring is minimized. The use of endoscopes with smaller insertion tube diameters is thought to facilitate EGD without sedation. Those with diameters of 1.0 cm or less are easier to pass and are thought to be better tolerated by patients. Although there are these advantages to eliminating premedication for EGD, the procedure is nevertheless better tolerated by patients if some form of sedation is administered.[1]

There may be cultural differences from country to country with respect to the need for sedation during EGD. In some countries I have observed that the procedure is performed with minimal or no sedation without undue difficulty, whereas in others the need for medication appears to be greater. Webberley and Cuschieri[2] studied personality traits of patients in relation to their tolerance of EGD. Traits characterized as neuroticism were associated with a poor tolerance to the procedure and unacceptance of future procedures. These authors suggested that a patient's need for sedation can be assessed by reference to their Eysenck personality inventory.

Many of the pharmacologic agents used in endoscopy are administered parenterally, intravenous administration being preferred because of the rapid action of most agents given by this route. Whether it is necessary to maintain access to the vascular system during endoscopy is a matter of preference. Since diagnostic EGD is a relatively short procedure, an indwelling needle or catheter is usually unnecessary. If further sedation or additional drugs might be needed during a procedure, or if some hazard such as bleeding is anticipated, then maintaining a route for rapid intravenous administration of drugs may be prudent.

Topical Pharyngeal Anesthesia

Opinions diverge concerning the use of a local anesthetic agent for EGD. Topical pharyngeal anesthesia may be obtained by administration of one of several different agents by spray, gargle, painting, or lozenge. Topical anesthetics are known to be absorbed into the systemic circulation.[3] These agents are often regarded as innocuous, although in the past they have been implicated in endoscopic complications including death.[4, 5] Most such accidents appear to have been related to overdosage.

There are relatively few controlled studies, from the viewpoint of the endoscopist and/or the patient, of the value of topical pharyngeal anesthesia. Buchanan[6] considered only the endoscopist's assessment of the ease of the procedure and concluded that topical anesthesia did not significantly influence the course of the procedure, although the gag reflex of the patients receiving topical anesthesia was abolished. In this study patients also received meperidine intramuscularly and intravenously as well as phenobarbital intramuscularly. The opinions of both patients and endoscopists were considered in the trial of Sparberg and Knudsen.[7] Meperidine and atropine given intramuscularly were also used. They concluded that topical anesthesia was of no importance in EGD. Gordon et al.[8] performed a double-blind study in 111 consecutive elective EGDs of the efficacy of topical lidocaine anesthesia in addition to meperidine and atropine intramuscularly plus diazepam intravenously. EGD was significantly easier for both patients and endoscopists in the group who received topical lidocaine compared with those who received a placebo. There were no significant differences between the lidocaine and placebo groups with respect to age, sex, prior endoscopy, method of explanation of the procedure, familiarity with the endoscopist, or the dosage of diazepam.

It is difficult to draw conclusions from available data regarding the value of topical pharyngeal anesthesia. There are many variables that cannot be accounted, including the endoscopist's skill, the type of endoscope used, and the method of passing the endoscope. In the report by Gordon et al.,[8] for example, the method of passing the endoscope and the experience of the endoscopists are not mentioned. Furthermore, the controlled studies are based on subjective grading of the degree of difficulty encountered by the endoscopist and/or the patient. There are discrepancies between the assessment of the endoscopist and patient in some cases. As noted above, personality traits are probably a significant factor in a patient's reaction to EGD. Therefore, double-blind studies of the efficacy of topical anesthesia should match patients according to personality, which might be exceedingly difficult. The question of value must also be related to the use of other drugs for sedation. Virtually every study includes sedative drugs, and these tend to mask differences in response to topical anesthesia depending on what degree of sedation the investigators consider appropriate. However, this also suggests that topical anesthesia may not add much to the patient's comfort or the ease of endoscopy for the endoscopist if the patient is properly sedated. The converse opinion, that topical pharyngeal anesthesia is effective and also permits a reduction in the dosage of sedative drugs, may also be valid. My personal opinion is that local pharyngeal anesthesia adds little when EGD is performed in an adequately sedated patient using direct vision passage of a small diameter (1.0 cm) endoscope.

Benzodiazepine Drugs

Diazepam is widely used as a sedative drug for EGD. It is generally given intravenously, slowly, and by titrating the dosage according to a patient's responses. Mildly dysarthric speech and ptosis are good end points. Nystagmus may also be observed especially when the drug is used in combination with meperidine. Although diazepam given intravenously is relatively safe, there is a wide range in the response of individual patients that is dependent on age and weight and on chronic use of benzodiazepine drugs.[9] Small dosages, even less than 5 mg, may produce serious respiratory depression in the elderly and in patients with concomitant pulmonary and/or hepatic insufficiency.[10] Patients who routinely take diazepam or similar drugs[11] and those whose consumption of alcohol is excessive may have a high tolerance for diazepam.[9] Longstreth et al.[12] studied the factors influencing the intravenous dose of diazepam required by 100 consecutive patients undergoing EGD on an outpatient basis. The dosage required in 11 patients who used two or more doses of a benzodiazepine drug per week was significantly higher than that required in other patients. There were inverse and positive correlations between the age and weight of the patient, although no relation to alcohol consumption was found in this study. In the study of Cook et al.,[9] however, there was a significant correlation between the dose of diazepam required for sedation and consumption of more than 40 g of alcohol per day.

Amnesia for the EGD procedure is thought to occur as a result of intravenous administration of diazepam. Whether the drug also produces retrograde amnesia for events prior to the procedure is a cause for concern, since the patient may not remember important instructions and conversations. However, Liu et al.[13] were unable to demonstrate the occurrence of significant retrograde amnesia after intravenous diazepam. With higher doses of diazepam, patients may also not recall events that occur immediately after EGD, even though they appear to be awake and alert.

Pain at the injection site and thrombophlebitis are relatively common sequelae of intravenous administration of aqueous diazepam preparations. Extravasation of the drug can cause tissue injury and even necrosis. The risk of thrombophlebitis can be decreased by using a large vein and flushing it with saline after injection of the diazepam.[14]

Midazolam, a relatively new imidazobenzodiazepine drug, has undergone investigation as a sedative for endoscopy. Midazolam is more potent than diazepam and has a shorter duration of action. In addition, it is reported to have a lower incidence of postprocedure thrombophlebitis.

Cole et al.[15] randomized 40 patients undergoing EGD to receive either midazolam or diazepam. Induction time was significantly decreased in patients who received midazolam. The time required for recovery after sedation was similar for both drugs, as was the level of patient and endoscopist satisfaction with the procedure. Amnesia for the EGD was significantly greater in patients receiving midazolam. Although there were fewer instances of thrombophlebitis in the midazolam group, the difference between the two groups was not statistically significant. In a similar study by Magni et al.,[16] 185 patients were randomized to receive either diazepam (in an emulsion) plus meperidine, or midazolam plus meperidine. The levels of sedation were the same for both groups although midazolam produced more amnesia. Midazolam also received a higher rating in terms of patient satisfaction with the procedure. The lipid emulsion of diazepam used in this study was compared with midazolam; the latter was associated with a slight but insignificant increase in thrombophlebitis. Sensory-motor performance was assessed and found to be defective at 2 hours after the procedure in the case of both drug regimens. Al-Khudhairi et al.[17] compared midazolam in a dose of 0.1 mg/kg body weight with diazepam 0.15 mg/kg in patients undergoing gastroscopy. The level of sedation at the conclusion of the procedure was greater in patients who received midazolam, as was the length of time needed for recovery. Midazolam was found to have a faster onset of action and to provide better amnesia for the procedure. Thrombophlebitis with midazolam was found to be uncommon. Whitwam et al.[18] compared midazolam (0.07 mg/kg) with diazepam (0.15 mg/kg) in 100 patients undergoing upper gastrointestinal endoscopy. The level of sedation, ease of the procedure, and recovery period were comparable for both drugs. These authors also found that midazolam had a faster onset, provided a greater degree of amnesia, and did not produce pain during injection.

Narcotic Agents

Meperidine (also known as pethidine in some countries) is frequently used for sedation for endoscopic procedures. It is generally administered intravenously and is often used in combination with diazepam. One of the attractive aspects of the use of meperidine is that the effects of the drug, particularly respiratory depression, are reversible by intravenous administration of naloxone (Narcan).[19] Because the duration of action of naloxone is shorter than that of meperidine, an additional intramuscular dose of naloxone should be given in cases of serious respiratory depression. Fentanyl, a short-acting narcotic, has also been effective in producing sedation for EGD.[20]

Drugs That Suppress Gastrointestinal Motility

Various agents may be used to suppress gastrointestinal motility, including atropine, glucagon, and hyoscine-N-butyl bromide (Buscopan).

The anticholinergic agent atropine, given either intramuscularly or intravenously, is an effective suppressant of gastrointestinal motility. It has the added advantage of reducing the production of secretions such as saliva. However, the side effects of atropine include abdominal and bladder distention, and furthermore, there is no evidence that atropine makes endoscopy easier for the endoscopist or patient. Cattau et al.[21] assessed the efficacy of atropine as premedication for endoscopy in a double-blind study of 196 procedures in 189 patients. One group of patients received meperidine alone, and another received meperidine plus atropine. Although there was a significant reduction in oral secretions and gastric motility in patients who received atropine, there were no differences with respect to the ease of endoscopy or acceptance of the procedure by patients.

There should be no need to suppress gastrointestinal motility for the majority of diagnostic endoscopic procedures, including EGD with or without biopsy. In some technical situations, however, it may be desirable or necessary to suspend gut motion. Hyoscine-N-butyl bromide (Buscopan, 20–40 mg) given intravenously, with a duration of action of about 5 minutes, is suitable for this purpose, although this agent is not available in the United States. Glucagon given intravenously is also effective and has a somewhat longer duration of action at about 15 to 20 minutes, but it is more expensive.

General Anesthesia

Except for infants and for some small children (see Chapter 13), general anesthesia is almost never necessary for EGD. On very rare occasions a patient may insist on being "put to sleep" for the procedure. The reasons for this aversion to the procedure are usually difficult to comprehend, a fact often readily admitted by the patient. When the information to be gained by EGD is vitally important, for example, the differential diagnosis of a benign from a malignant gastric ulcer, then general anesthesia may be justified. When a decision for surgery depends on the outcome of EGD, it is advisable that the operation, if indicated, be performed under the same general anesthetic.

ENDOSCOPIC INSTRUMENTS

The Upper Gastrointestinal Panendoscope

The standard upper gastrointestinal panendoscope for diagnostic EGD should be about 1 meter long, have four-way distal tip deflection with at least 180 degrees of upward deflection, independently locking deflection controls, air/water and suction capability, an accessory channel with a diameter of at least 2.0 mm and preferably larger, and forward-viewing optics. There are other desirable but not essential characteristics. Instruments that are fluid-tight and immersible are easier to clean. The design of the endoscope should also permit various types of endoscopic photography.

There is a general trend toward instruments with small diameter insertion tubes. Decreases in instrument caliber often require some compromise in the performance capabilities of the instrument. Marked reductions in diameter necessitate corresponding reductions with respect to other features such as accessory channel diameter and illumination (see Chapter 2). However, advances in instrument design and manufacturing technology have reduced the forfeiture of other instrument functions in exchange for smaller diameter insertion tubes.

There is a general impression, probably correct, that smaller diameter endoscopes are easier to pass and are better tolerated by patients. However, it is difficult to determine the ideal diameter. There is a theory that progressively reducing insertion tube diameter is accompanied by better and better patient tolerance, even to the point that no sedation will be needed. Thus, diagnostic EGD with ultra-thin (less than 8 mm diameter) endoscopes and without sedation has been proposed. However, it has not been demonstrated that patient acceptance of an 8 mm (or less) diameter endoscope is any better than tolerance of a 10 mm instrument. Furthermore, many features of the standard panendoscope such as the presence of an accessory channel must be sacrificed in exchange for thinness. In my view, the loss of standard features outweighs the potential benefit of ultra-small diameter. In terms of patient tolerance and ease of the examination, the differences between an endoscope of 10 mm diameter and one of 7 or 8 mm diameter are not great enough to justify the loss of standard features.

A wide variety of upper gastrointestinal endoscope models, all with the basic features described above, are offered by endoscope manufacturers. The general design of all of these instruments is the same. However, there will also be subtle differences in the handling characteristics of the insertion tube. Some will have greater torque and longitudinal stability than others. There are also minor differences in viewing angle, deflection capability, and accessory channel diameter, and the design of the control section differs slightly among the various manufacturers. Although these minor variations are not markedly important with respect to the adequacy and safety of EGD, one tends to become accustomed to the design of one or another company. Changing to an instrument made by another manufacturer usually entails a slight period of adjustment and can be distracting. Minor differences in the stiffness characteristics of the insertion tube, the shape of the deflection controls and the control section itself, the position of the accessory channel valve, weight, location of the air/water and suction valves, length of the bending section of the insertion tube, tightness of the deflection angle, and so forth, may be nettlesome at a minimum and may even necessitate a change in examination technique. It is advisable, therefore, to use endoscopes made by a single company.

The Side-viewing Endoscope

A thorough examination of the entire upper gastrointestinal tract may not be possible with a forward-viewing endoscope. Because of anatomic features, certain regions cannot be viewed well or may not be seen at all. These "blind areas" include the medial wall of the descending duodenum, the area of the duodenal bulb immediately beyond the pylorus, and the region of the small bowel just beyond a gastroenterostomy stoma.

Approximately 80% to 90% of the duodenal bulb can be seen with a forward-viewing endoscope. Even though the recesses of the bulb beyond the pylorus may be difficult to view, a lesion in this area usually produces other secondary findings that may give a clue to its presence. An ulcer in this hidden area, for example, may produce edema, spasm, and deformity of the pylorus as well as erythema of the bulbar mucosa that may be noted even though the crater itself cannot be seen.

The medial duodenal wall, including the duodenal papilla, is more problematic as a blind area. This region can only be viewed tangentially with a forward-viewing endoscope, so that a lesion in this area, particularly one involving the duodenal papilla, may be overlooked. An instrument with side-viewing optics provides a much more satisfactory view of the medial aspect of the descending duodenum, and for this reason it is sometimes necessary to use both types of instruments to accomplish a thorough and complete examination of the upper gastrointestinal tract.

Care and Handling

Gastrointestinal endoscopes are both useful and expensive. With proper care a panendoscope can be used to perform hundreds, even thousands of procedures. In addition to the correct methods of cleaning and storage, proper care also applies to methods of handling the instrument. The distal deflecting section of the insertion tube should not be bent with the hand. Serious damage will result if the distal tip strikes a hard surface such as may occur if it is dropped into a sink. The insertion tube should never swing about freely when the instrument is transported. A straight, outward pull should be used to disconnect the endoscope from the light source. A rocking or twisting motion during the disconnection will throw the connecting pins (including the light guide bundle) out of alignment and may result in even more serious damage.

An endoscope should always be checked to assure that it is in working order before use. A quick view through the objective lens will reveal any clouding of the field that may indicate improper cleaning or that water has entered the insertion tube as a result of damage or mishandling. The instrument tip should be deflected through its full range of motion using the deflection controls to determine that the controls are not only functional, but also that the degree of tip angulation in each direction is reasonably close to that specified by the manufacturer. Over the course of time the cables that control tip deflection will become stretched so that the degree of tip angulation will decrease. This loss of function may compromise the endoscopist's ability to maneuver the instrument in subtle but significant ways. The distal end of the insertion tube may be held in a small basin of clean water to check the function of the air/water and suction systems. The accessory channel may be lubricated by passing a biopsy forceps through the channel, placing a drop of silicon lubricant on the end of the forceps after it exits the distal end of the instrument, and then withdrawing the forceps back through the channel. This provides lubrication of the channel within the distal bending section of the insertion tube where an accessory passing through the channel encounters the greatest friction. There are several kinds of accessory channel valves, many of them being diaphragm-type devices. The competence of the valve should be checked since repeated passage of accessories wears out the diaphragm, allowing fluid to leak. Newer endoscopes allow for periodic replacement of the valve and/or diaphragm.

Other steps preliminary to the actual EGD, such as positioning the patient on the procedure table in the left decubitus position, are discussed in Chapter 5.

TECHNIQUE OF UPPER GASTROINTESTINAL ENDOSCOPY

Every beginning student of endoscopy is anxious to take hold of an endoscope, insert it into a patient, and begin work. However, two preliminary and vitally important points must be understood to acquire a long-range foundation for expertise in endoscopy: (1) the method of holding the instrument, and (2) the endoscope–body position relationship.

Holding the Instrument

The first and most important lesson in endoscopy occurs when the novice picks up the instrument with the left hand for the first time. Initial experience plays an important part in establishing a correct method of holding the instrument. This method, once adopted, determines the "style" of endoscopy in large measure. It should be clearly understood that the method of holding the instrument either facilitates or hinders the development of expertise, particularly in other procedures such as ERCP and colonoscopy.

The many methods for holding the endoscope can be classified into two general types: the two-finger and the three-finger grips.

From a human engineering standpoint, the control section of any endoscope appears to be uniquely designed to fit the left hand. In reality, the design of any instrument is a crude approximation because of the great differences in the size of the human hand and finger length. In practice, the hand in many cases must compensate for the characteristics of the instrument.

Two-finger Grip

All currently designed endoscopes are made to be held in the left hand. With most, but not all endoscopes, two coaxial deflection control knobs are placed near the eyepiece objective. The control section nearest the insertion tube is usually smaller than the upper part that houses the deflection controls and air/water and suction valves.

Since there are two valves, it would seem desirable to place one finger (index and middle) on each valve. As the instrument is grasped, the thumb, index and middle fingers come into relation to the valves and control knobs, leaving the fourth and fifth fingers to hold the lower part of the control section tightly (Fig. 11–1). An endoscopist with short fingers will find that this grip places the tips of the second and third fingers on the valves. For most people, however, the second and third fingers come to lie across the valves. If so, there is no point in attempting to place the fingertips squarely on the

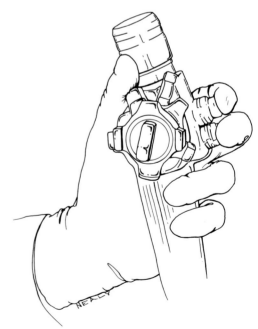

FIGURE 11–1. "Two-finger" method of holding the control section of an endoscope. Note position of the left index and middle fingers across the suction and air/water valves, respectively.

corresponding valves, since this loosens the grip of the fourth and to some degree the fifth fingers.

Exceptionally long fingers may reach the control knobs when the two-finger grip is used. This has an advantage in that the knobs may be operated with the index and middle fingers as well as the thumb. Lateral finger motion is limited, however, and extension of the fingers across the valves toward the control knobs provides only the small benefit of holding a knob in place after it has been turned with the thumb. In any case, the fingers of most individuals are not long enough to take advantage of this without some compromise.

When the index and middle fingers are placed across the air/water and suction valves, the instrument is being held for the most part by the fourth and fifth fingers, and thus the term "two-finger grip." The top of the control section of many endoscopes is contoured in such a way that it comes to rest against the lateral aspect of the fourth finger, which thus supports some of the weight of the instrument. This reduces the degree of grip strength needed to hold the instrument.

Millions of years of evolution have made the thumb a most important appendage. Deflection of the insertion tube is controlled for the most part by turning the deflection knob with the left thumb. Although it is possible for a few endoscopists to reach either of the two coaxial control knobs comfortably with the thumb, the left thumb of most endoscopists is only long enough to reach the inner of the two knobs ("up/down"). Since the distal tip of the endoscope must not only be deflected but also at times held in position as the endoscope is maneuvered, and since it is not possible to operate the locking mechanisms for each of the control knobs with one hand alone, no matter its size or the dexterity of the endoscopist, the ability to reach both control knobs with the left thumb is not a marked advantage. Since use of the thumb is so important, the guiding principle in developing a method of holding the endoscope is the ability to use this appendage.

The main disadvantage of placing the second and third fingers across the valves is a partial loss of function of the thumb. This method of grasping the instrument tends to move the thumb upward along the control section in the direction of the objective lens. The usual result is that the left thumb contacts the inner control knob near the distal interphalangeal joint rather than at the tip

of the thumb (Fig. 11–1). The knob is then moved mainly by opposition rather than flexion of the thumb, which provides a range of motion of the knob that is less than that possible when the tip of the thumb is on the control knob and a combination of flexion and opposition of the thumb is used to turn the control.

It takes some time to become accustomed to holding an endoscope in the left hand for prolonged periods. Until this becomes habitual, the student usually finds that the grip strength of his or her fourth and fifth fingers gradually decreases through the course of several procedures. The control section tends to drop downward in the hand so that eventually it may be supported almost entirely in the groove between the thumb and index finger (Fig 11–2). This greatly compromises the use of the left thumb so that the novice increasingly employs the right hand to turn both control knobs. This slovenly use of the left thumb as a "hanger" for the instrument is deplorable.

Three-finger Grip

Another method of holding the instrument involves shifting the control section upward in the hand so that the narrower lower part of the control section is grasped with the

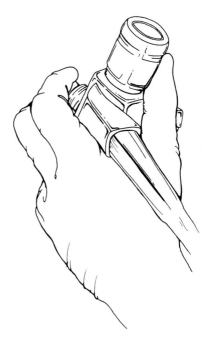

FIGURE 11–2. Downward displacement of the control section in the left hand. The instrument is now supported mainly in the groove between the left thumb and index finger. Use of the left thumb in this position is ineffective.

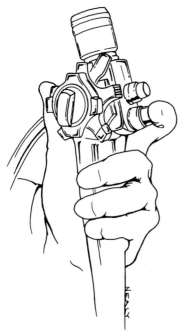

FIGURE 11–3. "Three-finger" method of holding the control section of an endoscope. Note the position of the left index finger on the air/water valve. The index finger can also be used to operate the suction valve.

third, fourth and fifth fingers, thus the term "three-finger grip" (Fig. 11–3). This has two effects: the middle finger is no longer available to operate the air/water insufflation valve, but the tip of the thumb can now be placed on the inner deflection knob (Fig. 11–4). With this method, the left index finger must be used to operate both the air/water and suction valves (Fig. 11–3). This is not especially difficult, although it poses a slight disadvantage in that simultaneous operation of both the air/water and suction valves can only be accomplished by shifting the instrument downward in the left hand, or by using the fingers of the right hand to operate one or both valves, the latter being the preferred method. In practice, simultaneous depression of both valves very often is not necessary, except to clean material from the tip of the instrument.

The advantage of the three-finger grip is that it permits greater use of the left thumb. However, it also means that the instrument must be held entirely with the third, fourth, and fifth fingers. The location of the accessory channel valve may compromise this method of holding the instrument. On older instruments this valve was placed above the suction valve near the eyepiece (Fig. 11–5A and B). However, any fluid leaking from the

valve tended to run down over the other parts of the control section as well as over the endoscopist's hand. This placement of the valve was uncomfortably close to the endoscopist's face. A sudden increase in intra-abdominal pressure, as occurs when a patient retches, could cause the valve to "spit back" gastrointestinal contents. These problems were circumvented by relocating the valve below the hand and nearer the insertion tube. When the three-finger grip method of holding newer-model instruments is employed, the accessory channel valve may lie under the fifth finger, depending on the size of the endoscopist's hand, a factor that tends to make this method of grasping the instrument more difficult.

Lateral Deflection

Both deflection control knobs cannot be operated with any degree of skill with the left hand alone regardless of the method used for holding the instrument. It is especially difficult to rotate the two control knobs in opposite directions. Manipulation of both knobs in addition to the suction and air/water valves with one hand becomes extremely clumsy and ineffective except for a few unusually dexterous individuals. For practical purposes, the lateral deflection control knob, the outermost of the two on coaxial systems, is turned with the right hand.

The other function of the right hand is

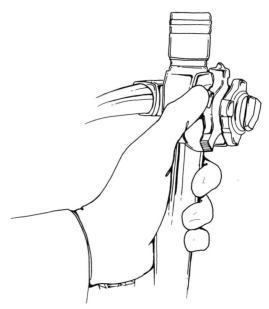

FIGURE 11–4. The position of the tip of the left thumb on the up/down deflection control when the "three-finger" method of holding the control section is used.

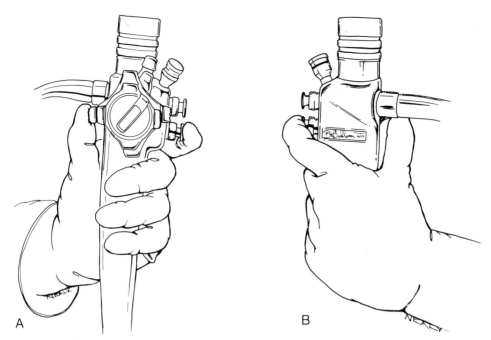

FIGURE 11–5. A and B, The "three-finger" method of holding an older model endoscope with the accessory channel valve near the eyepiece.

advancement and withdrawal of the insertion tube. Because the lateral deflection knob must also be operated with the right hand, it is not possible to laterally deflect and advance the instrument at the same time. This would seem to make a case for allowing an assistant to advance the instrument while the physician steers with both hands at the control section. However, this two-man method is never as quick or precise as when endoscopy is performed by one individual. As will be described below, the technique of rotating or torquing the insertion tube eliminates or greatly decreases any disadvantage inherent in the inability to laterally deflect and advance the instrument at the same time. In fact, it should not be necessary to remove the right hand from the insertion tube until after the tip of the instrument has reached the apex of the duodenal bulb. As will also be described, it is entirely possible to use both deflection controls simultaneously while withdrawing the insertion tube.

The Endoscope-Body Position Relationship

The endoscope-body position relationship refers to the configuration of the insertion tube outside the patient. This is determined entirely by the position of the endoscopist or, more precisely, the position of the control section of the endoscope, relative to the point of entry of the endoscope into the patient. The expert endoscopist determines the configuration and position of the insertion tube external to the patient and takes advantage of this relation in maneuvering the instrument. Concentrating on what seems to be occurring within the patient, the novice allows the insertion tube to assume any number of configurations and is unaware that this greatly influences the ability to maneuver in both positive and negative ways.

Although all modern endoscopes are considered flexible, they also have certain degrees of stiffness. Resistance to deforming force is most evident in an instrument's torque stability. This means that a twisting motion applied to the insertion tube at one end will be transmitted along its long axis to the other end with little or no loss of motion provided the insertion tube is straight. When the instrument is straight, rotatory motion also has fidelity, that is, any degree of rotation at one end will be reproduced promptly and equally at the opposite end. When the insertion tube is in a looped configuration, a twisting force applied at one end will be absorbed to some degree by the loop and the rotatory motion at the opposite end will be diminished. The degree of transmission of the rotatory motion will also be less predictable or may not occur at all, and the quick

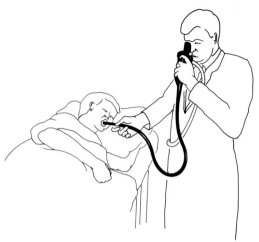

FIGURE 11–6. Endoscopist is standing too close to the procedure table. The loop in the instrument between the endoscopist and the table will damp attempts at rotation of the instrument except for rotation performed with the right hand.

response at the distal end of the instrument will also be lost.

The behavior of the insertion tube in response to rotary motion gives rise to a guiding principle for all endoscopic procedures: the straighter the instrument the more precise will be the control. The gastrointestinal tract is obviously not straight, but neither is it a rigid tube. Some degree of straightening is therefore possible during virtually any endoscopic procedure. Furthermore, only part of the insertion tube is within the patient at any given time, and it is obviously possible to control the configuration of that part which is outside the patient.

All of the tip motions that are possible by combined use of the up/down and lateral deflection controls can be reproduced by rotation of the insertion tube (torque) and movement of the up/down deflection control with the left thumb. This almost completely removes the disadvantages associated with the inability to advance and laterally deflect at the same time. As noted, however, this only works if the instrument is in a relatively straight configuration. Thus, coiling or looping of the section of the insertion tube external to the patient should be avoided (Fig. 11–6). In order to do this, it is usually necessary to stand back somewhat from the patient. For some unexplained reason, most beginning students of endoscopy tend to stand too close to the patient, leftward from the patient's mouth (i.e., in the direction of the patient's feet), and to lean forward, sometimes almost to the point of hovering over the patient. This "novice crouch," as body language, communicates intense concentration and forewarns of life-long lower back pain as well, but it allows little or no effective rotation of the insertion tube. There are also methods, as will be discussed, of keeping the insertion tube relatively straight within the patient.

There are three ways to rotate the insertion tube of the endoscope during EGD: (1) turning the control section clockwise or counterclockwise by flexion or extension of the left wrist, (2) turning the entire body left or right beginning from a position facing the patient (Fig. 11–7A and B), and (3) raising or lowering the left shoulder (Fig. 11–8). Torquing the insertion tube with the right hand is ineffective if the control section is held in a

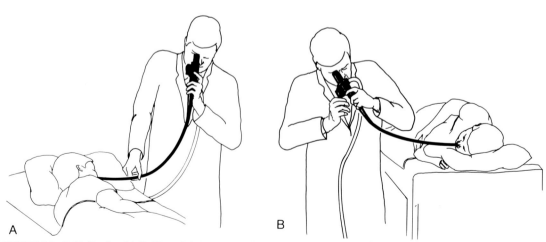

A   B

FIGURE 11–7. Methods of left (A) and right (B) rotation of the insertion tube. A, The endoscopist turns to the left and lowers the left shoulder slightly to obtain rotation to the left. B, The endoscopist turns to the right to obtain rightward rotation.

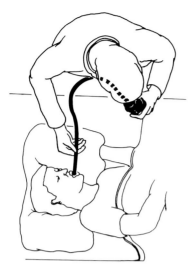

FIGURE 11–8. Left rotation of the insertion tube by leaning forward and lowering the left shoulder is shown. Note the position of the endoscopist slightly to the left of the patient's mouth.

fixed position and may damage the instrument. Up to 90 degrees of rotation to the right occurs with flexion of the left wrist, and a small degree of rotation to the left can be achieved by wrist extension. If the endoscopist simply turns from a position facing the patient to the left or right, the result will be a corresponding rotation of the insertion tube in the same direction. Finally, a significant degree of left rotation occurs if the endoscopist moves his or her left shoulder downward, forward, and slightly to the left. A small degree of right rotation also occurs by raising the left shoulder.

When the insertion tube is straight, the position of the endoscopist relative to the point of entry into the patient has added importance. When the endoscopist's position is moved to the left of the patient's mouth, the instrument as well rotates to the left (Fig 11–9). Since the insertion tube is held with the right hand, there is a natural tendency to stand slightly to the left of the patient's mouth. A similar but opposite change occurs if the endoscopist's position is changed to the right relative to the patient's mouth.

Rotation of the insertion tube is accomplished in practice by some combination of the various maneuvers described above. Flexion of the left wrist and a right turn by the endoscopist toward his or her right is most effective when right (clockwise) torque is desired. Lowering the left shoulder is usually satisfactory when left (counterclockwise) torque is called for.

EGD may be performed in either a standing or sitting position. It should be clear, however, from the above discussion that a sitting endoscopist is less mobile and therefore less able to rotate the insertion tube properly. Conversely, a standing endoscopist is in a much better position to take advantage of the various methods of instrument rotation.

The behavior of the instrument in response to the maneuvers described can be demonstrated by standing at an empty procedure table in the usual position for EGD with the instrument laid out on the table as if it were in a patient's stomach. It is helpful if the instrument is passed through a mouthguard, and the guard is held by an assistant at a point that approximates its usual location between a patient's teeth. The distal tip should be deflected upward to a slight degree so as to better appreciate the motion imparted to the distal end of the instrument in response to the various maneuvers. The rotation maneuvers are then performed while observing the behavior of the deflected tip of the instrument.

Conventions

Certain conventions have been adopted with respect to deflection of the tip of the endoscope.

Deflection of the tip is usually referred to as upward or downward, and left or right. These terms have no meaning with respect to common reference points (e.g., the sky is up). The easiest way to understand the terminology of tip deflection is to relate the motion of the tip to the control section of the

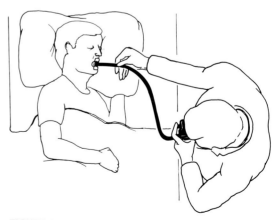

FIGURE 11–9. Endoscopist is to the left of the patient's mouth. In this position the insertion tube is necessarily rotated to the left.

instrument when the insertion tube is perfectly straight. In this configuration the air/water and suction valves face upward (toward the ceiling). Thus, upward deflection of the tip bends it backward along the insertion tube in the direction of the valves; downward deflection is away from the valves. Left deflection is to the left, and right toward the right, from a vantage looking along the length of the insertion tube from the control section. The actual motion of the tip within a patient upon upward deflection, for example, may be something entirely different from upward in relation to our physical surroundings.

Terms that describe the directions in which the control knobs are turned to deflect the tip are also relative. For the purpose of description, the control section will be viewed on the side that has the deflection knobs. Each knob may then be considered as moving in either a clockwise or counterclockwise direction. Thus, counterclockwise rotation of the innermost control knob deflects the tip upward. A counterclockwise turn of the outer knob deflects the tip to the left. Clockwise rotation of the inner and outer knobs results in downward and right tip deflection, respectively.

The endoscopic visual field may be divided in a clockface fashion, the 12 o'clock position being at the top of the field, 3 o'clock to the right, and so forth. Some endoscopes have a small marker in the visual field at the 12 o'clock position. As the endoscopist looks through the instrument, upward tip deflection causes the visual field to move toward the 12 o'clock position, right lateral deflection toward 3 o'clock, and so forth.

Passing the Endoscope

As the endoscope is passed, the patient should be in the left lateral position on the procedure table, left hand under a pillow, right hand at the side, knees drawn up at a right angle to the torso, and the neck slightly flexed. The mouthguard should be in place between the patient's teeth. The gastrointestinal assistant (GIA) has certain specific and important functions during passage of the instrument (see Chapter 5).

There are two methods of passing the endoscope: blind and direct vision. The most basic rule of safe and effective endoscopic practice is that the instrument should not be advanced when the endoscopist is unable to see ahead. There is no reason to discard this rule for passage of the instrument, and therefore direct vision is unarguably the best method of insertion.

Blind Passage

The blind method of passing the endoscope requires that the endoscopist place two fingers (generally the index and middle fingers of the left hand) in the patient's mouth and over the back of the tongue. Ideally the space between the fingers will lie in the midline and form a groove to guide the instrument downward into the pharynx. Some physicians guide the instrument tip with the index finger if the tip strays from between the fingers as the insertion tube is being advanced with the right hand.

Once within the space between the fingers, the instrument may be advanced into the posterior pharynx. Note that the deflection controls should be unlocked and are not used during this process. Resistance to further advancement of the instrument is encountered as the tip reaches the level of the cricopharyngeus. This muscle is usually located at about 15 to 18 cm from the incisor teeth (or mandibular ridge) so that it is easy to anticipate the point at which the resistance offered by the closed cricopharyngeus will be encountered. The right hand should be just behind the 20-cm mark (at about 22 or 23 cm) on the insertion tube. If placed distal to the 20-cm mark it will often be necessary to shift its position backward so that an adequate length of instrument will be available to reach the esophagus. This may result in a momentary loss of control. When the instrument tip reaches the cricopharyngeus, gentle forward pressure is maintained as the patient is asked to swallow. There is a distinct sensation as the cricopharyngeus opens and the instrument moves forward without resistance. As this last action is being performed the endoscopist withdraws his or her fingers from the patient's mouth.

There are numerous disadvantages to blind instrument passage. The endoscopist and/or the endoscope is more likely to be bitten. Sedated patients have greater difficulty in controlling their reactions and are slower in their response to commands. Placing two fingers and an endoscope in the posterior pharynx is much more likely to cause gagging than will the instrument alone. The patient is less able to initiate a swallow when barely able to move the tongue. The glottis, pyriform sinuses, larynx, cricopharyngeus, and even the proximal several centimeters of the esophagus are not examined, and these structures are also more likely to be traumatized in this method. Trauma to these tissues may create the appearance of an abnormality. Certain abnormalities such as an esophageal web may be overlooked. Blind passage of the instrument is contraindicated in patients with dysphagia that suggests a proximal esophageal lesion, especially if a Zenker's diverticulum is suspected or known to be present (see Chapter 15).

Direct Vision Passage

Observation begins and continues throughout the examination in the direct vision method of insertion as the instrument tip passes the back of the tongue. All of the structures of the posterior pharynx and larynx are noted, and observation guides the advancement of the endoscope.

The endoscopist must actively manipulate the tip of the endoscope when using the direct vision method. It is impossible to use the lateral deflection knob during this maneuver, since this would require that the right hand be shifted from the insertion tube to the control knob. This shift almost always results in loss of control of the instrument tip. Steering the tip to the left or right is accomplished by torquing the insertion tube with the right hand. Since the cricopharyngeus will be located about 15 to 18 cm from the incisor teeth, and since it is necessary to maintain control of the insertion tube with the right hand at all times during insertion, the thumb of the right hand should be placed at about the 23-cm level on the insertion tube to begin with and kept in this place until the instrument tip reaches the upper esophagus. Up and down deflection is by means of the left thumb. Fortunately, most of the necessary movements are relatively fine and no marked degrees of twisting or turning are required.

Before the instrument is passed, the lateral deflection control should be locked with the tip in a straight, neutral position. The endoscopist then stands slightly to the left of the patient's mouth with both hands at about the level of the mouth. The instrument is inserted to the back of the patient's tongue, whereupon the tip is deflected upward with the left thumb as the objective lens is brought up to the endoscopist's eye. If this maneuver has been performed properly, it will generally result in a view of the patient's epiglottis (Plate 11–1). If this is not seen then the instrument should be withdrawn slightly

while it is rotated left and right slightly with the right hand. Generally this reveals an identifiable structure. Sometimes the instrument tip will end up in the left or right vallecula of the epiglottis. This may give the mistaken impression that the tip is in one of the pyriform sinuses. However, this is easily recognized by the fact that the instrument has not been advanced far enough to reach the pyriform sinus and by the paler yellow color of the mucosa in this area.

Once the epiglottis is visualized, the tip of the instrument is advanced. Some downward deflection and slight rotation to the left or right may be necessary at this point to steer the tip around the epiglottis. As the instrument is advanced, the next structures visualized will be the larynx and vocal cords and the pyriform sinuses (Plate 11–2). If the patient swallows and the cricopharyngeus relaxes at this point, the esophageal lumen will be seen between the pyriform sinuses and posterior to the larynx (Plate 11–3). Ideally, the instrument should be advanced in this direction, keeping to the midline by means of small degrees of rotation of the insertion tube with the right hand, and directed posteriorly away from the larynx. The latter is accomplished by downward deflection with the left thumb. The patient is asked to swallow as the rosette of the closed cricopharyngeus is encountered, and then the tip of the instrument is advanced into the esophagus a few centimeters as the cricopharyngeus relaxes.

It is difficult in practice to perform the last part of the direct vision method perfectly since the instrument must be kept precisely in the midline as it is advanced toward the cricopharyngeus, and the advancement must be perfectly timed to the patient's swallow. Therefore, the tip often ends up in one of the pyriform sinuses, frequently the left because of its dependent position, and the endoscopist encounters resistance to forward motion. There are two options at this point.

The instrument tip can be withdrawn 1 or 2 cm and another attempt to pass the cricopharyngeus can be made as above. Alternately, the endoscopist may rotate the instrument slightly toward the midline. If the tip is in the left pyriform sinus, right rotation is needed. Small adjustments can also be made with the up/down control as the patient is asked to swallow while the endoscopist maintains gentle forward pressure. The required rotation and adjustment of the up/down deflection are very slight. Generally, the instru-

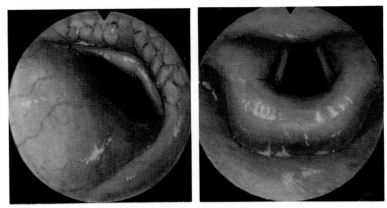

PLATE 11–1.   PLATE 11–2.

PLATE 11–1. The first view of the epiglottis during insertion of the endoscope under direct vision. The epiglottis is the wedge-shaped structure in the upper right aspect of the field.

PLATE 11–2. Endoscopic view of the vocal cords and pyriform sinuses (left and right edges of the field).

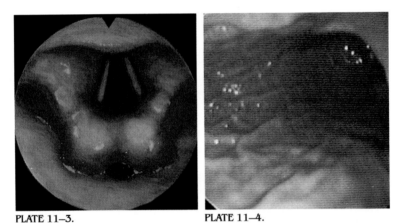

PLATE 11–3.   PLATE 11–4.

PLATE 11–3. The location of the esophagus as the cricopharyngeus relaxes (6 o'clock position in the field).

PLATE 11–4. View of the stomach as the endoscope is advanced and rotated toward the right. The gastric rugal folds at the lower left of the photographs are on the greater curvature. The lesser curvature near the angulus is seen in the upper right.

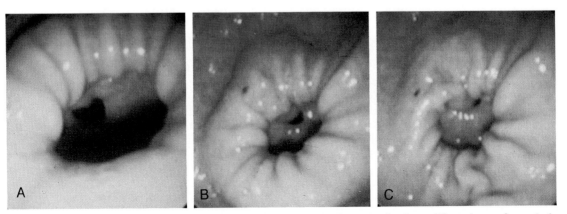

PLATE 11–5. *A-C*, Endoscopic photographs showing development and progression toward the pylorus of an antral peristaltic wave.

ment does not immediately enter the esophagus, but each swallow reveals some clue as to the location of the cricopharyngeus and thus allows for further and more directed adjustments of the position of the tip. There are small capillary vessels in the mucosa near the cricopharyngeus that run longitudinally, and if these are visible they also indicate the direction of the lumen.

Esophagus

Once within the esophagus, the instrument can be advanced easily. Direct vision should be used at all times. The surface mucosa is pale pink, smooth and flat, and glistens somewhat. Small vessels are usually visible in the mucosa, especially in the distal esophagus. These are oriented longitudinally with the long axis of the esophagus.

The esophagus is essentially a straight tube. Although it possesses no landmarks, certain structures external to the esophagus may sometimes be noted (see Chapter 18). As the instrument is advanced through the esophagus, intermittent air insufflation may be used to keep the lumen open. Peristaltic motion may or may not be evident. Some patients may retch and vomit as the endoscope enters the esophagus. This may cause small amounts of gastric contents to flow upward toward the pharynx. Quick use of the suction will prevent fluid from gaining access to the pharynx and further coughing and gagging.

Normally, the gastroesophageal mucosal junction should be clearly evident as a color change occurring at about 38 to 40 cm from the incisor teeth (or mandibular ridge). The pale pink mucosa of the esophagus contrasts sharply with the red or deep orange color of the stomach. The mucosal junction forms a line around the inner circumference of the lumen. This usually follows an undulating course so that the junction is often referred to as the "Z line." Normally, the diaphragmatic constriction of the gut lumen should be noted within 2 cm of the Z line. The position of the diaphragm is more evident during inspiration. Its constriction of the esophagus may be exaggerated by asking the patient to sniff.

Entering the Stomach

If only anterior and posterior directions are considered, the course of the endoscope through the upper gastrointestinal tract will

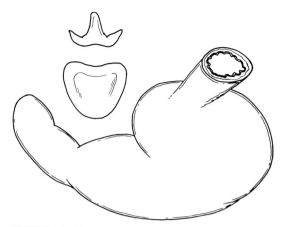

FIGURE 11–10. Transverse view from above showing the relative positions of the esophagus, stomach, and duodenum. Note that the stomach lies anteriorly in relation to the other two structures.

be from posterior to anterior to posterior. The esophagus is essentially a posterior organ, whereas the stomach lies in a more anterior plane. Viewed from above, the stomach is largely anterior in position to the esophagus so that it can swing over the spine (Fig. 11–10). This means that a turn in an anterior direction is often needed to advance the endoscope from the distal esophagus through the cardia and into the proximal stomach. This may be accomplished by rotation to the left (anterior) with upward deflection as the endoscope passes the Z-line (Fig. 11–11). The easiest method of left rotation

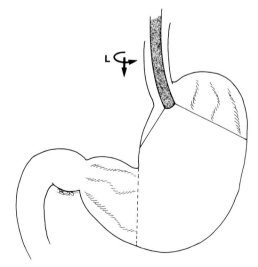

FIGURE 11–11. Diagrammatic representation of the method of passing the endoscope from the esophagus through the cardia and into the stomach proper. Left rotation and upward deflection of the tip are required as the instrument is advanced.

is to lower the left shoulder in a slightly forward direction (Fig. 11–7A) (see above).

An unsatisfactory alternative to direct vision passage of the tip through the cardia is to advance the endoscope without rotation or deflection. It will pass through this segment and usually stop against the posterior aspect of the lesser curvature.

As the instrument tip enters the stomach, the rugal folds, generally on the greater curvature of the body, will be seen. There is often a small pool of fluid in this dependent location. This observation is useful because it identifies the greater curvature of the stomach and so also the opposite lesser curvature, and the anterior and posterior walls. If only a small amount of fluid is present, aspiration of the gastric contents is probably not necessary. If, however, the pool obscures the rugal folds beneath, then it is advisable to aspirate the gastric contents. This should be done as much as possible with the instrument tip lying parallel to the mucosal surface and with alternating suction and air insufflation. Applying suction with the instrument tip perpendicular to the mucosa frequently draws a portion of the mucosa into the accessory channel. This delays aspiration, and in addition the mucosa, once freed, will be red, perhaps slightly raised, and/or bleeding.

If in passing the instrument through the esophagus only a small volume of air was insufflated, then the stomach may still be collapsed or partially collapsed. The initial view of the stomach may then be unsatisfactory and it is necessary to pause and insufflate air. The ideal degree of gastric distention is a matter of judgment. Generally, the distention should be to the point that the rugal folds should just begin to separate. Later in the procedure it may be necessary to distend the stomach to a greater degree to thoroughly examine all of the mucosa of the body of the stomach, especially if small mucosal abnormalities such as vascular malformations may be present. Patients differ with respect to the degrees of gastric distention they will tolerate. Some will belch uncontrollably in response to small volumes, and it may be necessary to accept less than ideal distention. Excessive air insufflation almost always causes the patient some discomfort and should be used only briefly if at all. Furthermore, excessive insufflation will markedly flatten the rugal folds and may lead to the mistaken impression that there is evidence of gastric atrophy.

Body of the Stomach

The endoscope will be in a position of left rotation with upward tip deflection as a result of advancing from the esophagus through the cardia and into the stomach. To bring the tip through the body and toward the pylorus it will be necessary to rotate to the right as the insertion tube is advanced (Plate 11–4). If the left shoulder was lowered to rotate to the left, then the insertion tube external to the patient will be oriented mostly along the length of the patient's body, i.e., it will be rotated about 90 degrees to the left. To accomplish the necessary right rotation as the instrument is advanced through the stomach, over the spine, and toward the pylorus, it is only necessary to bring the left shoulder back to the normal position so that the external part of the insertion tube follows a straighter line of entry at the patient's mouth. This usually requires that the endoscopist stand slightly back from the table. The advancement and right rotation of the insertion tube through the stomach should be a coordinated, smooth maneuver. Small adjustments of the up/down deflection will also be needed, especially additional upward deflection as the tip advances through the body of the stomach.

Paradoxic Motion

The esophagus and duodenum are relatively fixed, narrow, and inelastic structures. The stomach, however, will stretch considerably to accommodate intralumenal forces. As the tip of the instrument is advanced toward the antrum and pylorus, the insertion tube invariably comes to lie along the greater curvature. Because of the elasticity of the stomach, a considerable part of the forward force will be absorbed by the greater curvature so that the curvature is pushed toward the pelvis and a lower position within the abdomen as a loop forms along the curvature. Endoscopically it may appear that the instrument tip is not moving forward or even that the tip is moving away from the pylorus during this maneuver, and thus the term "paradoxic motion." It is necessary to continue to advance the instrument until the greater curvature loop is fully formed and the instrument tip begins to move forward again (Fig. 11–12). Generally this will also require additional upward deflection of the tip with the left thumb.

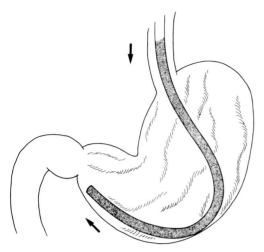

FIGURE 11–12. Diagram showing formation of the greater curvature loop. The point of paradoxic motion has been passed and the instrument is being advanced toward the pylorus as the greater curvature loop continues to develop.

Antrum

There are two obvious differences between the antrum and the body of the stomach: rugal folds are present in the body but not the antrum, and peristaltic contractions are not noted in the body but are readily observed in the antrum. At this point in the examination the tip of the instrument is probably at the midpoint of the greater curvature or slightly beyond. Full upward deflection of the tip will often reveal a view of the angulus of the stomach, although this depends on the overall configuration of the stomach itself. Some endoscopists perform the retroverted view of the fundus and proximal stomach at this point.

If the endoscope has been advanced to the antrum quickly, smoothly, and with minimal air insufflation, there may be no observable contractions. It can be advantageous at this point to proceed directly to the pylorus. The physiologic function of the pylorus is to close in response to gastric distention so that repetitive antral peristaltic contractions grind the food against the pylorus and progressively reduce the size of the intragastric food particles. When gastric distention has been kept to a minimum and there are no antral contractions, the pylorus is in a relatively lax state.

It is also desirable to observe the antral peristaltic contractions, since a disturbance in the normal pattern usually indicates past or present disease. The antral peristaltic waves are seen as round and symmetrical rings that form in the proximal antrum and move as a rolling wave toward the pylorus (Plate 11–5 A–C). The frequency of the waves is usually about 3 to 4 per minute. The amplitude and speed of the waves increase as they approach the pylorus.

Pylorus

The previous left rotation of the insertion tube will have been largely corrected as the tip of the instrument passes along the greater curvature, into the antrum, and toward the pyloric ring, and the external section of the insertion tube between the patient's mouth and the endoscopist's left hand will be relatively straight. As the tip advances through the antrum, the pylorus should be kept in the middle of the endoscopic field. This will require small adjustments of the up/down deflection and minor degrees of rotation to the left and/or right. Small left/right corrections can be made with the left hand and wrist alone provided the external portion of the insertion tube is relatively straight.

The endoscope tip can be passed through the pyloric ring without difficulty in most patients. In other cases, however, the pylorus may be closed and offer resistance to advancement into the bulb. This can also be an indication of disease in the region of the pylorus, which may itself be strictured. A certain amount of judgment must be exercised based on experience as to how hard to push the instrument tip against the pyloric ring. If considerable resistance is encountered and the view of the ring at a distance in the antrum suggests deformity, then it may not be possible to enter the bulb.

The cardinal rule in negotiating a "spastic" or persistently closed pylorus is to keep the ring in the center of the endoscopic field as the instrument is advanced. This may require momentary adjustments of the lateral deflection. However, it may be difficult to maintain forward pressure with the right hand while changing the lateral deflection. One way to maintain a gentle forward pressure is to rest the insertion tube on a pillow near the patient's mouth. It may be necessary that the endoscopist bend forward slightly to press the insertion tube gently against the pillow. This maneuver preserves forward pressure and prevents the instrument from falling back into the antrum as the right hand is moved to the lateral deflection control. A

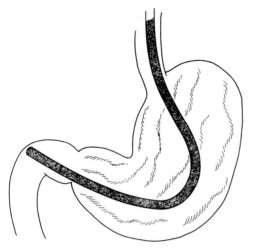

FIGURE 11–13. Diagram showing insertion of the tip of the insertion tube to the region of the apex of the duodenal bulb and the superior angle of the duodenum.

distinct sensation is often felt by the right hand on the insertion tube as the pylorus relaxes and allows the endoscope to enter the bulb. Passage of the endoscope through the pyloric ring produces a peculiar sensation, sometimes discomfort, in some patients.

Duodenal Bulb

The bulb is a relatively small structure. The forward force exerted on the pylorus to gain entry to the bulb usually carries the instrument tip to the apex (Fig. 11–13). As a result, most of the bulb may not have been observed. The instrument should therefore be withdrawn slightly to view the bulb. This examination proceeds in a circumferential manner using both deflection controls. The mucosa of the bulb has a slightly irregular, villous surface and the color is a pale tan in comparison with the color of the stomach.

The novice may be anxious that the instrument not return to the stomach, especially if difficulty was encountered in inserting it into the bulb. This tendency to fall back into the antrum can be countered to some degree by keeping the right hand on the insertion tube. If the instrument does return to the stomach, the pyloric ring should be observed closely for any evidence of ulcer or other disease process, especially if it was difficult to pass the ring. It is almost always easier to pass the endoscope through the pyloric ring after one successful passage.

Descending Duodenum

The endoscopic view of the apex of the duodenal bulb usually discloses no obvious lumen (Plate 11–6) because of the acute angulation at the superior angle between the bulbar apex and the proximal descending duodenum. Sometimes a valvular fold or two may be visible and a portion of the lumen may be noted, but this is unusual.

Because the lumen ahead is not clearly defined, insertion of the tip of the instrument into the descending duodenum is a partially blind maneuver. First it is necessary to place the tip at the apex of the bulb. In most cases the course of the lumen will be directed superiorly and posteriorly. In the endoscopic field this will be upward and to the right. Once in position, therefore, the tip is deflected almost fully upward and fully or almost fully to the right while the insertion tube is rotated 90 degrees or more to the right (Fig. 11–14). The latter rotation is best accomplished by a combination of flexion of the left wrist and turning toward the right (Fig. 11–7B). This maneuver will hook the superior angle, and if performed properly it will provide a view of the descending duodenum (Plate 11–7). Toward the end of this maneuver it is often necessary to make minor adjustments in tip deflection in order to provide a tubular view of the duodenum.

Another method of insertion into the proximal descending duodenum also begins by positioning the tip at the apex of the bulb. The tip is then deflected to the right and the insertion tube is advanced while the tip is deflected sharply downward. In this maneuver the degree of downward deflection required may be as much as 150 degrees. Some endoscopes, however, do not provide this much tip angulation in the downward direction.

After the instrument tip is in the proximal descending duodenum, the next step is to withdraw the instrument. Since it may be necessary to further correct tip deflection, the withdrawal maneuver should be performed with both hands at the control section (Fig. 11–7B). This is not difficult and can be done by simply lifting the left wrist upward and stepping back a slight distance from the procedure table.

Withdrawal of the insertion tube at this point takes up the greater curvature loop in the stomach and causes the tip to move forward in a paradoxic fashion (Fig. 11–15).

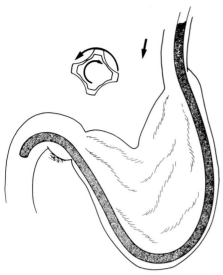

FIGURE 11–14. Diagram showing maneuvers to deflect the instrument tip from the apex of the bulb into the proximal descending duodenum. Right rotation of the insertion tube is required (Fig. 11–7B) in addition to full upward and right tip deflection.

This will straighten the configuration of the insertion tube within the stomach and bulb and generally results in advancement of the instrument to the inferior angle of the descending duodenum. The amount of instrument that must be withdrawn in this "straightening maneuver" varies, but is often 30 cm or more. When the instrument is straight, only 55 to 60 cm remain within the patient. This can be noted by referring to the distance marks on the insertion tube.

When the endoscope is deeply inserted and there is a large loop on the greater curvature of the stomach, the degree of responsiveness of the insertion tube to rotation is greatly diminished, as described above. Once the straightening maneuver is accomplished, however, the response to rotation returns.

At the conclusion of the straightening maneuver, the instrument tip will be near the inferior duodenal angle, the insertion tube will be relatively straight, and the endoscopist should have both hands at the control section. The instrument should then be slowly withdrawn from the duodenum by making use of both rotation and tip deflection to gain the best possible view. The difficulty this presents is that the tip may suddenly fall back a considerable distance, even into the stomach, before an adequate examination can be made. This occurs as the tip becomes hooked,

especially at one of the duodenal angles or at any point in a duodenal lumen that is more tortuous than usual.

The tendency for the insertion tube to slide suddenly back toward or into the stomach can be anticipated by noting any resistance to withdrawal. This indicates that the tip has come to a turn in the lumen and that by maintaining a view of the lumen with the deflection controls the endoscopist is also maintaining a hook at the end of the endoscope. The tip should be deflected, usually with loss of the view of the lumen, to release this hook. Further withdrawal is then possible without abruptly sliding backwards.

Once the instrument tip is in the descending duodenum, it is often possible to advance the instrument by allowing a larger greater curvature loop to form. This often gives a somewhat different view of the descending duodenum and may allow observation of areas that were not seen well during the straightening/withdrawal maneuver. However, the formation of a large greater curvature loop may also cause the instrument tip to move in a paradoxical, backward direction as the insertion tube is advanced.

In practice, it is often necessary to resort to both the withdrawn/straightened and greater curvature looped positions as well as intermediate combinations of these two extremes in order to piece together a more complete picture of the descending duodenum. But even with maximum use of these maneuvers, certain parts of the descending

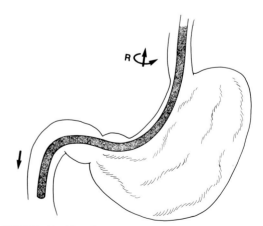

FIGURE 11–15. Diagram showing straightening maneuver. When performed in conjunction with the maneuvers illustrated in Figure 11–14, right rotation and withdrawal of the instrument cause the tip of the insertion tube to move farther into the duodenum.

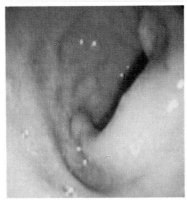

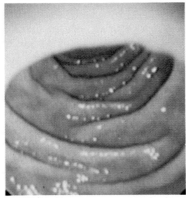

PLATE 11–6. Endoscopic photograph of the apex of the duodenal bulb. The direction of the lumen is not evident.
PLATE 11–7. Endoscopic view of the proximal descending duodenum upon completion of the maneuver illustrated by Figure 11–14.

PLATE 11–6.

PLATE 11–7.

duodenum, particularly the medial wall, may not be seen satisfactorily. The maneuvers used in EGD for examination of the duodenum are very similar to those of ERCP (see Chapter 25).

Distal Duodenum

Upper gastrointestinal endoscopy is usually considered complete if the examination is carried out to the level of the inferior duodenal angle. It can be difficult to insert the instrument tip into the third part of the duodenum and extremely difficult or even impossible to reach the ligament of Treitz. The reason for this is again the formation of the greater curvature loop in the stomach.

Usually, it is possible to obtain a view of the third portion from the inferior angle. When it is essential to advance the tip into the third portion it is usually necessary to form a loop of considerable proportions in the stomach. This has several limitations. It usually causes discomfort to the patient, and the standard panendoscope is not long enough to take great advantage of the forward motion achieved at the expense of loop formation. In thin patients with lax abdominal wall muscles, the formation of the greater curvature loop may be partially controlled by exerting external, upwardly directed pressure in the left upper quadrant of the abdomen. Repeated straightening and loop formation may gradually advance the instrument toward the ligament of Treitz in some cases.

Retroversion (Retroflexion)

The instrument can be withdrawn from the level of the pylorus while the endoscopist keeps both hands at the control section. This is done by simply lifting the left hand upward while gradually stepping back from the procedure table in slight increments. Keeping the right hand at the lateral deflection knob

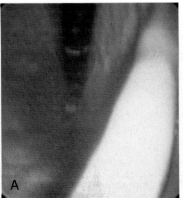
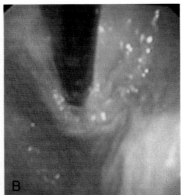
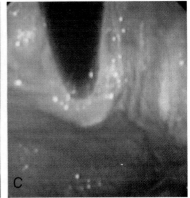

PLATE 11–8. Endoscopic views in the direction of the proximal stomach as the retroversion maneuver is performed. A, Initial view showing angulus at right of photograph. B, View at the midpoint of the withdrawal segment of the maneuver. C, View of the cardia and fundus after maximum withdrawal of the insertion tube.

allows the endoscopist to manipulate the distal tip in wide, circumferential arcs in order to view all areas of the wall of the stomach. It is really not necessary to place the right hand back on the insertion tube until the instrument has reached the cardia, unless the retroversion maneuver is to be performed during this part of the EGD.

The importance of the retroversion maneuver is that it provides an en face view of the angulus and the fundus of the stomach. The region of the angulus is seen only tangentially on forward view. The fundus is not seen at all.

To provide a view of the angulus, the retroversion maneuver must be initiated at a point opposite the angulus. This is facilitated by a partial loop on the greater curvature, which allows maximum upward tip deflection without encountering the lesser curvature of the stomach with the tip of the instrument.

Once in position opposite the angulus, the instrument tip is deflected upward as far as possible with the left thumb. Generally, at least 180 degrees of tip deflection will be required. Many instruments permit an even greater degree of upward deflection. The instrument is then withdrawn while the tip is kept in this attitude (Fig. 11–16). This provides a retroverted view of the instrument entering the stomach through the cardia (Plate 11–8A). In addition to withdrawing the instrument it is also necessary to add a significant degree of rotation, as much as 180 degrees. This can be done to the left or right, but it is easier to accomplish this degree of rotation if to the left. If left rotation is selected, the lateral deflection should be set and locked full left (Fig. 11–17).

Rotation and withdrawal should be accomplished simultaneously by degrees. The insertion tube must be withdrawn with the right hand. In order to rotate to the left simultaneously, the left shoulder can be brought forward and downward (Fig 11–8). If at the same time the left hand (holding the control section) is brought toward the right hand, and if the right hand simultaneously lifts the insertion tube upward toward the oncoming left hand, then a loop will form in the external configuration of the instrument (Fig. 11–18). When this occurs, the insertion tube has in effect been rotated 180 degrees to the left.

The left rotation retroversion maneuver provides an excellent view of the fundus and cardia (Plate 11–8B and C). This can be augmented by deflecting the tip to the left and right by using the right hand to operate

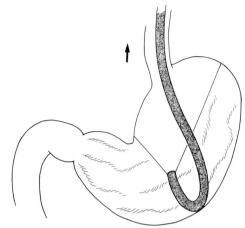

FIGURE 11–16. Initial steps in the retroversion maneuver. The instrument tip has been deflected fully in the upward direction. Note position of the instrument tip at the midpoint of the greater curvature as this maneuver is initiated.

the lateral deflection knob. However, this view may still be incomplete and it may be necessary also to rotate the insertion tube to the right to complete the assessment of the area. This can be done by simply undoing the 180-degree external left loop. To do so, it is necessary to raise the left shoulder to the normal position, to step back from the procedure table, and to turn to the right (Fig. 11–7B). This must be done without further withdrawal (or advancement) of the insertion tube. Since the right hand remains on the insertion tube throughout the retroversion maneuver, it is not difficult to keep the insertion tube in place with respect to forward

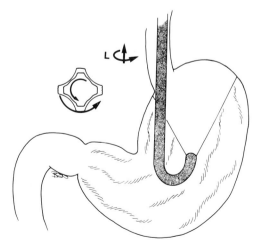

FIGURE 11–17. Additional steps in the retroversion maneuver. The lateral deflection has been set and locked full left and the insertion tube has been rotated 180 degrees to the left.

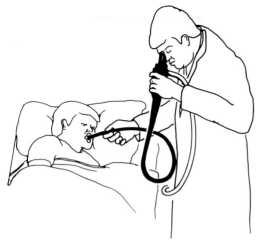

FIGURE 11–18. Diagram showing formation of a full external left loop. Seen from above, the loop is nearly closed. Formation of this loop results in rotation of the portion of the insertion tube within the patient 180 degrees to the left.

and backward motion even as it is being rotated through 270 degrees or more.

The retroversion maneuver can be completed by simply moving the deflection controls to a neutral position while the instrument tip is still in the proximal stomach. However, it is also advantageous to return the tip to the proximal antrum while maintaining the retroverted view. This provides an additional and somewhat different view of the proximal stomach and lesser curvature. To accomplish this it is only necessary to unrotate the instrument back to its usual position while advancing. When the view of the angulus is again obtained, the lateral deflection is returned to the neutral position with the right hand and the tip is deflected downward with the left thumb to obtain a view of the pylorus. Withdrawal to the level of the cardia then proceeds as described above.

Withdrawal of the Endoscope

When the tip of the instrument is returned to the cardia, it becomes more difficult to continue withdrawing the instrument without placing the right hand on the insertion tube. The distance between the endoscopist and the procedure table has become greater and the weight of the insertion tube across this distance tends to cause it to slip backward out of the esophagus. Therefore, withdrawal of the endoscope through the esophagus is performed by the right hand on the insertion tube. This still allows a satisfactory range of

tip motion by means of slight degrees of rotation with the right hand in combination with up/down deflection by the left thumb. This provides very precise control of the tip and allows reexamination of the structures of the posterior pharynx and larynx.

Air Insufflation and Suction

Deflation of the stomach as the instrument tip approaches the cardia during withdrawal diminishes the patient's postprocedure discomfort.

Air insufflation of the upper gastrointestinal tract should be controlled precisely during EGD. A common misconception of the beginning student is that further air insufflation is the answer to all maneuvering problems. This may become so automatic and unconscious that the instrument's air insufflation mechanism is activated throughout the procedure.

Overdistention of the bowel tends to make it difficult to view certain surfaces that are seen tangentially. Suction and air insufflation can actually be used to manipulate the wall of the gut. By collapsing the gut, areas that are seen poorly because of a tangential alignment with the instrument tip may be seen more en face.

POSTPROCEDURE RECOVERY

Some aspects of the patient's recovery after a procedure are discussed in other chapters (see Chapter 5). The length of time required depends on the type and dosage of sedation. Most patients rest or sleep for about 30 minutes after the intravenous administration of meperidine and/or diazepam. If a topical anesthetic was applied to the posterior pharynx, the patient should not attempt to drink fluid until the effect of the agent dissipates. Generally, the patient may be discharged after about 1 hour. He or she should be reminded not to drive or operate machinery for the rest of the day.

References

1. Thompson DG, Lennard-Jones JE, Evans SJ. Patients appreciate premedication for endoscopy. Lancet 1980; 2:469–70.
2. Webberley MJ, Cuschieri A. Response of patients to upper gastrointestinal endoscopy: effect of inherent personality traits and premedication with diazepam. Br Med J [Clin Res] 1982; 285:251–2.
3. Adriani J, Zepernick R, Arens J, et al. The comparative potency and effectiveness of topical anesthetics in man. Clin Pharmacol Ther 1964; 5:49–62.

4. Palmer ED, Wirts CW. Survey of gastroscopic and esophagoscopic accidents; report of committee on accidents of the American Gastroscopic Society. JAMA 1957; 164:2012–5.
5. Jones FA, Doll R, Fletcher CM, Rodgers HW. The risks of gastroscopy: a survey of 49,000 examinations. Lancet 1951; 1:647–51.
6. Buchanan DP. Topical anesthesia for esophagogastroscopy. Am J Dig Dis 1960; 5:121–5.
7. Sparberg M, Knudsen KB. Is local anesthesia necessary in fiberoptic esophagogastroscopy? A controlled study. Am J Dig Dis 1967; 12:1131–4.
8. Gordon MJ, Mayes GR, Meyer GW. Topical lidocaine in preendoscopic medication. Gastroenterology 1976; 71:564–9.
9. Cook PJ, Flanagan R, James IM. Diazepam tolerance: effect of age, regular sedation, and alcohol. Br Med J [Clin Res] 1984; 289:351–3.
10. Hall SC, Ovassapian A. Apnea after intravenous diazepam therapy. JAMA 1977; 238:1052.
11. Giles HG, MacLeod SM, Wright JR, Sellers EM. Influence of age and previous use on diazepam dosage required for endoscopy. Can Med Assoc J 1978; 118:513–4.
12. Longstreth GF, O'Brien PM, Youkeles LF. Determinants of the intravenous diazepam dose required for gastroscopy. Gastrointest Endosc 1980; 26:92–4.
13. Liu S, Miller N, Waye JD. Retrograde amnesia effects of intravenous diazepam in endoscopy patients. Gastrointest Endosc 1984; 30:340–2.
14. Dutt MK, Thompson RP. Saline flush: a simple method of reducing diazepam-induced thrombophlebitis. J R Soc Med 1982; 75:231–3.
15. Cole SG, Brozinsky S, Isenberg JI. Midazolam, a new more potent benzodiazepine, compared with diazepam: a randomized, double-blind study of preendoscopic sedatives. Gastrointest Endosc 1983; 29:219–22.
16. Magni VC, Frost RA, Leung JW, Cotton PB. A randomized comparison of midazolam and diazepam for sedation in upper gastrointestinal endoscopy. Br J Anaesth 1983; 55:1095–101.
17. Al-Khudhairi D, Whitwam JG, McCloy RF. Midazolam and diazepam for gastroscopy. Anaesthesia 1982; 37:1002–6.
18. Whitwam JG, Al-Khudhairi D, McCloy RF. Comparison of midazolam and diazepam in doses of comparable potency during gastroscopy. Br J Anaesth 1983; 55:773–7.
19. Handal KA, Schauben JL, Salamone FR. Naloxone. Ann Emerg Med 1983; 12:438–45.
20. Stephens MJ, Gibson PR, Jakobovits AW, et al. Fentanyl and diazepam in endoscopy of the upper gastrointestinal tract. Med J Aust 1982; 1:419–20.
21. Cattau EL Jr, Artnak EJ, Castell DO, Meyer GW. Efficacy of atropine as an endoscopic premedication. Gastrointest Endosc 1983; 29:285–8.

Chapter 12

INDICATIONS, CONTRAINDICATIONS, AND COMPLICATIONS OF UPPER GASTROINTESTINAL ENDOSCOPY

WILLIAM D. CAREY, M.D.

Endoscopy of the proximal gastrointestinal tract using fiberoptic instruments has taken an increasingly dominant role in diagnosis and therapy since the introduction of the first panendoscope by Hirschowitz in 1963.[1] During its early development, fiberoptic esophagogastroduodenoscopy (EGD) was principally an adjunct to other diagnostic methods, especially x-ray contrast studies with barium. However, in recent years many physicians and surgeons interested in the upper gastrointestinal tract have come to regard EGD as the primary method of diagnosis when symptoms suggest a pathologic process of the esophagus, stomach or duodenum. This has resulted in a substantial increase in the use of EGD in many hospitals (Fig. 12–1) that corresponds with a decrease in the performance of upper gastrointestinal x-ray series.[2]

The increasing use of EGD is not without controversy, particularly concerning questions of cost and the lack of specifically effective methods of treatment for many disorders discoverable by endoscopy.[3, 4] There is little question that endoscopy increases diagnostic yield in comparison to roentgenographic studies of the gastrointestinal tract.[5, 6] However, at the present time the diagnostic precision of EGD has outpaced its therapeutic capability. Nevertheless, as this superior diagnostic capability becomes more widely available, considerations of cost will undoubt-

edly be the only factor preventing the wider utilization of EGD.[7, 8]

The success of EGD is readily explained. Most of the commonly encountered disorders of the upper gastrointestinal tract either involve the mucosa of the organ in question or deform mucosal anatomy. With certain exceptions, EGD permits unparalleled observation of the esophageal, gastric and duodenal mucosa. Endoscopic biopsy and collection of cytology specimens add a further dimension by providing rapid and reliable assessment of many disorders. Furthermore, most patients do not find the examination too uncomfortable.[9] The patient

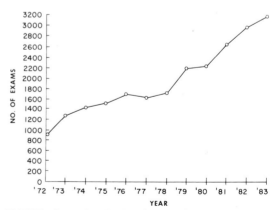

FIGURE 12–1. Graph showing the increase between 1972 and 1984 in the use of fiberoptic esophagogastroduodenoscopy (EGD) at the Cleveland Clinic.

296

TABLE 12–1. **Therapeutic Uses of EGD in Gastrointestinal Abnormalities**

Site of Abnormality	Use of EGD
Esophageal	Dilation
	Sclerotherapy
	Placement of stents
	Laser treatment of obstructing cancer
	Foreign body removal
Gastric	Coagulation of bleeding lesions
	Feeding gastrostomy tubes
	Polypectomy
	Foreign body removal
Duodenal	Coagulation of bleeding lesions
	Polypectomy
	Manipulation of or through ampulla of Vater (e.g., sphincterotomy, placement of nasobiliary tube or stent)

who, for whatever reason, requires a second examination will almost always consent to the EGD procedure. Finally, as the therapeutic dimension of EGD continues to evolve, many therapeutic endoscopy techniques have replaced older, more cumbersome and time-consuming approaches, with the advantages of lower cost and greater safety (Table 12–1). Therapeutic endoscopy is discussed in numerous chapters in this volume. Most of the remainder of this chapter will focus on the diagnostic features of EGD.

INDICATIONS FOR AND LIMITATIONS OF DIAGNOSTIC EGD

The clinical utility of EGD in diagnosis is very broad. Well-established indications for the use of EGD for diagnosis are compiled in Table 12–2. Other chapters in this volume consider most of these in great detail. However, at this point a few general statements will be of value.

Diagnosis of Esophageal Abnormalities

In the esophagus, as elsewhere in the gastrointestinal tract, endoscopy is most effective for detection of mucosal abnormalities. Thus, inflammatory, neoplastic and certain infectious processes involving the esophageal mucosa are well seen and their diagnosis is reasonably precise. With regard to the most common esophageal inflammatory condition, reflux esophagitis, the sensitivity of endoscopy in diagnosis is less than that for other diseases. In one study of patients with un-

TABLE 12–2. **Gastrointestinal Disorders Amenable to Diagnosis by EGD**

Site of Disorder	Type of Disorders			
	Inflammatory	*Infectious/Immunologic*	*Anatomic*	*Neoplastic**
Esophageal	Esophagitis, reflux Chemical injuries (acid, alkali)	Candida esophagitis Viral esophagitis Graft versus host disease	Strictures—benign and malignant Hiatus hernia Esophageal varices Barrett's esophagus	Squamous cell carcinoma Adenocarcinoma Polyps (rare) Metastases (rare) Cancer screening (e.g., Barrett's esophagus)
Gastric	Gastritis Ulcer—benign and malignant Chemical injuries		Atrophic gastritis Postoperative deformities Gastric varices Hypertrophic gastropathies	Adenocarcinoma Lymphoma Leiomyosarcoma Metastatic lesions Cancer screening—high risk populations (e.g. pernicious anemia, post-gastrectomy)
Duodenal	Duodenal ulcer Duodenitis		Postoperative deformities Duodenal webs	Adenocarcinoma Lymphoma Leiomyosarcoma Metastatic polyp

*Duodenal neoplasms cited are uncommon.

equivocal chronic reflux esophagitis by clinical assessment, the diagnosis was suggested by endoscopy in only 61% of cases. A better correlation with symptoms of reflux is obtained with pH probe monitoring combined with suction biopsy of the distal esophagus. However, certain findings at endoscopy are specific for reflux esophagitis.[10] (Peptic disease of the esophagus is considered in Chapter 18.)

Motor disturbances of the esophagus, achalasia for example, may occasionally be recognized in their later stages by endoscopy; however, other methods of investigation, such as esophageal manometry or cine esophagoscopy, are more sensitive and specific. The most common esophageal motor disturbance, decreased lower esophageal sphincter pressure, can be inferred at EGD from the presence of reflux esophagitis. Occasionally, difficulty may be encountered with endoscopic diagnosis of esophageal strictures. This is compounded by more frequent use of endoscopes with small diameter insertion tubes that may pass without resistance through a symptomatic stricture.

Diagnosis of Gastric Abnormalities

Gastroscopy mainly defines abnormalities of the gastric mucosa, but it may also reveal distortion of the stomach's normal anatomic relationships by displacement or extrinsic compression as a result of enlargement of a contiguous organ or the presence of a mass. The latter is sometimes difficult to appreciate, and a diagnosis of this type should be made with caution. Many factors may interfere with adequate visualization during gastroscopy.

The main requirement for a successful gastroscopic examination is that the stomach is empty. However, under certain circumstances fasting alone is insufficient to ensure an empty stomach. If gastric emptying is significantly impaired, because of either obstruction (e.g., pyloric outlet obstruction due to peptic disease) or abnormal gastric motility (e.g., diabetic gastroparesis or postgastrectomy stasis), then significant amounts of food and debris may compromise the adequacy of the examination. There may be a problem during EGD determining a source of bleeding; blood and clots in the stomach severely restrict the ability to identify the exact source of bleeding. Copious irrigation through a large-bore tube with multiple side ports is necessary in such circumstances before introduction of the endoscope.

The ability to diagnose alkaline reflux gastritis, except perhaps in its most florid form, by EGD is also limited. The difficulty is that varying degrees of erythema are present in most patients after gastric surgery, and diagnosis depends to some extent on the degree of mucosal abnormality present. The endoscopic assessment is often overly sensitive, and therefore nonspecific, and may correlate poorly with symptoms. (Postoperative reflux alkaline gastritis is discussed in greater detail in Chapter 24.)

Because biopsies obtained with standard endoscopic biopsy forceps are relatively small, sufficient tissue is sometimes unavailable for confident diagnosis. This may occur with certain processes that begin extramucosally, such as lymphoma, even when the mucosa is obviously involved by tumor. In lymphoma the accuracy of endoscopic observation is reportedly as low as 62%, with endoscopic biopsies being positive in not more than 87% of cases, in constrast to an accuracy of more than 95% for endoscopic biopsy in gastric adenocarcinoma.[11] This problem may be minimized by use of large biopsy forceps or electrosurgical snare excision to obtain a larger piece of tissue.[12] Results of recent studies indicate that higher diagnostic yields in gastric lymphoma are possible.[13, 14] Differentiation by EGD and endoscopic biopsy of lymphoma, which is relatively uncommon, from the rare gastric pseudolymphoma is particularly difficult. (Benign and malignant tumors of the stomach are discussed in Chapter 22.)

Diagnosis of Duodenal Abnormalities

The duodenum is usually well visualized during endoscopy unless some pathologic process, such as antral or pyloric strictures from prior peptic disease or tumor, prevents passage of the instrument into the duodenum. Because nearly all endoscopes used in diagnostic EGD have forward-viewing optics, visualization of the mucosa immediately beyond the pylorus may be difficult. Furthermore, certain portions of the duodenum, e.g., the medial wall of the descending segment, are only observed tangentially. The significance of this is best illustrated by the excellent views of the papilla and medial wall obtained with side-viewing duodenoscopes in contrast to forward observation with standard diagnostic instruments. When it is imperative that this area be examined thoroughly, it is frequently necessary to use both types of instrument. The duodenum cannot be seen in certain postoperative circumstances—for example, after Roux-Y anastomosis. Active motility distal to the duodenal bulb may occasionally impair observation. The administration of pharmacologic agents such as glucagon to reduce motility may sometimes be necessary. The use of EGD to obtain small bowel biopsies in suspected sprue or other diffuse mucosal disorders of the small intestine has recently been reported.[15, 16]

Diagnosis of Upper Gastrointestinal Bleeding

Endoscopy in upper gastrointestinal bleeding is considered in detail in Chapter 6. Notwithstanding the controversy surrounding the observation that precise diagnosis of bleeding lesions has, in general, not been shown to have a substantial impact on outcome (mortality, length of hospital stay, transfusion requirement, need for surgery), it is well established that if one wishes to know the source and cause of bleeding, early endoscopy (within 12 hours of the onset of bleeding) is the method of choice.[17, 18] However, the risk of a complication as the result of EGD in the bleeding patient is nearly 10 times that for the non-bleeding patient.[19] (Aspects of endoscopic therapy of upper gastrointestinal bleeding lesions are considered in Chapters 8 and 9.)

CONTRAINDICATIONS TO EGD

Many contraindications to the performance of EGD are relative rather than absolute (Table 12–3). Adults who refuse the examination should not be coerced, both on ethical grounds and because the risks of the examination are greater in uncooperative patients. However, it is very uncommon to encounter a patient who will not consent to EGD when the purpose and nature of the examination is carefully explained. The psychologic preparation of the patient is equal in importance to the pharmacologic preparation.

In general, the use of higher than usual doses of sedative drugs to obtain satisfactory cooperation in a reluctant patient is unacceptable since it increases the risk of oversedation and cardiorespiratory compromise. However, this must be balanced carefully when diagnostic endoscopy is required for patients who are unable to cooperate because their clinical condition has resulted in disorientation, confusion, or other mental disturbance.

Since ectopic cardiac rhythms can be precipitated by EGD, unstable, life-threatening arrhythmias should be corrected before undertaking endoscopy. Many less threatening cardiac rhythm disturbances constitute only a relative contraindication, particularly if the information required from EGD is critical to early therapeutic decisions. This is true also when dealing with patients with precarious pulmonary function. If the information to be obtained by EGD is vital, then intubation and mechanically controlled ventilation of such a patient may provide sufficiently controlled conditions for endoscopy.

Insufflation of air into a perforated viscus will speed contamination of the peritoneal cavity and may even convert a sealed-off perforation into free perforation. EGD is not likely to disclose the source of a perforation in any event, and perforation is an indication for surgical exploration rather than endoscopy.

Because the technique of EGD is relatively easy for experienced endoscopists, and because the vast majority of examinations are performed without incident, the endoscopist may become complacent with regard to the

TABLE 12–3. **Contraindications to Performance of EGD**

Absolute	Relative	Controversial
Adult patient refuses examination	Large Zenker's diverticulum	Repeat endoscopy for uncomplicated benign conditions that have responded to therapy (e.g., duodenal ulcer, esophagitis, gastritis)
Patient is moribund	Severe respiratory insufficiency	
Known or suspected perforation	Diagnosis already established by alternative testing modalities	
Unavailability of resuscitation equipment and personnel	Massive bleeding in suspected aortoduodenal fistula	Dysphagia when no esophagogram is available
Life-threatening instability of cardiac or pulmonary function		

rare occurrence of potentially fatal respiratory arrest. Many endoscopists, because of lack of practice, may no longer be proficient in cardiopulmonary resuscitation. Therefore, it is important that procedures are established for resuscitation and monitoring, whether the endoscopy suite is located in a hospital or in an office. Every effort must be made to avert complacency with respect to the possibility of respiratory depression.

Relative Contraindications to EGD

There is a danger of perforation if the tip of an endoscope passes into a large diverticulum. This is usually minimal unless the endoscopist fails to recognize that the endoscope has entered a diverticulum. With a Zenker's diverticulum there is abundant opportunity for perforation, since intubation of the proximal esophagus is often done blindly, or at least with less than ideal visualization. There is also a risk of perforation of the proximal esophagus with intubation in the presence of a high stricture, either benign or malignant. For these reasons it has been suggested that dysphagia constitutes a contraindication to endoscopy unless a roentgenogram is available to point out potential hazards.[20] The author intubates the esophagus under constant visual control (see Chapter 11) and, using this method, does not consider dysphagia in the absence of a prior esophagogram a contraindication.

Endoscopy in the Bleeding Patient

Aortoduodenal fistula may present with self-limited (sentinel) bleeding or with life-threatening hemorrhage. If bleeding is persistent and of major proportions in a patient with an aortic graft, surgical intervention should not be delayed by an attempt at EGD. Despite the possibility of visualizing the graft eroding into the duodenum in some cases, the price of this information is delay in definitive surgery. When bleeding is intermittent and has stopped in a patient with an aortic graft, prompt, accurate diagnosis is essential, and thus EGD is the procedure of choice. Even if erosion of the graft into the duodenum is not found, the absence of any other source of hemorrhage in the upper gastrointestinal tract usually warrants surgical exploration, since virtually all aortoduodenal fistulas end in death unless treated surgically,

a fact that renders the surgical risk relatively insignificant. Although aortoenteric fistulas usually involve the duodenum, especially the third portion, they are known to communicate to other segments of the intestine as well, which must be kept in mind during the endoscopic examination.

The most difficult situation arises when other potential sources of blood loss are discovered. If active bleeding is observed or there are signs of recent hemorrhage, or of a visible vessel in an ulcer, it can usually be concluded that an aortoduodenal fistula is not present. When such clues are absent, the management decisions become very difficult. Angiography may be of assistance; however, if the bleeding has stopped, a large hematoma will be present in the region of the leak and the fistula may not be visualized. Generally speaking, any suspicion of aortoduodenal fistula warrants surgical exploration.

Repeat Diagnostic EGD

Although not strictly contraindicated, repeat diagnostic EGD is generally not indicated in uncomplicated benign conditions that have responded to therapy. It is easy to become convinced that it is in the patient's interest to verify the resolved or resolving status of a pathologic process previously diagnosed at EGD, such as duodenal ulcer; however, the utility of this practice has not been established. It has been argued with a certain logic that verification of healing, even of mundane lesions such as a duodenal ulcer, is beneficial.[7] In the case of duodenal ulcer this is based on the poor correlation between symptomatic response and the presence or absence of a crater that has been documented in clinical trials of pharmacologic agents. Because of this, endoscopic verification of healing may be the best basis for the decision to stop ulcer therapy.

This view has not been widely accepted for three reasons: (1) it is an expensive undertaking; (2) in patients with healed duodenal ulcer, it logically leads to regular endoscopic surveillance for asymptomatic recurrence; and (3) there is no evidence that this policy modifies the complications of duodenal ulcer. In general, a good clinical response to treatment of conditions that are certainly benign, such as uncomplicated duodenal ulcer, erosive gastritis, and peptic esophagitis, makes repeat endoscopy superfluous.

COMPLICATIONS OF EGD

General

Although EGD is reasonably safe, it is not perfectly so. The incidence of untoward events varies somewhat, depending on methods of collecting data (survey, institutional or personal series, retrospective study or prospective analysis). Three relatively large series representing experience from the United States, Great Britain and Denmark are summarized in Table 12–4.[21–23] In more than 250,000 EGD procedures, the incidence of a fatal complication was 3 per 10,000. The commonest complications (13 per 10,000) were aspiration or cardiac problems, or both, that were often related to the effects of sedative drugs. Major morbid events occurred in 20 per 10,000 cases; in addition, minor complications were associated with nearly 1% of procedures. Such problems as phlebitis at the injection site, dental injuries, minor drug reactions, and prolonged obtundation, constituted these minor complications. Although it is possible that there may be underreporting of complications to some degree in the American and British surveys, the smaller Danish study,[22] from a single center, avoided many of the inaccuracies inherent in surveys and systematically recorded untoward events. In addition the Danish study used a mail survey to assess side-effects that occurred after the patient left the endoscopy unit. It is remarkable that the incidence and proportions for major morbid events are similar in all series.

Pulmonary Complications

The physiologic effects of EGD upon respiratory function have been extensively studied. Hypoxemia, usually mild in degree,

occurs regularly. Four factors contribute to its occurrence: (1) the endoscope itself, which may partially impede air flow into the trachea; (2) the oropharyngeal topical anesthetic (usually lidocaine); (3) the muscle relaxant (usually diazepam); and (4) the narcotic (usually meperidine). The relative contributions of the endoscope and lidocaine topical anesthetic to hypoxemia can be inferred from a study of 81 patients whose blood gases were determined 2 minutes after gargling 40 ml of 2% lidocaine. This group was compared with a group of 33 patients who did not gargle. The partial pressure of oxygen in the blood was significantly higher in the group who used the gargle. Thus, lidocaine does not cause hypoxemia by itself.[24] EGD in 15 patients who underwent the procedure with only oropharyngeal anesthesia (lidocaine) produced a decrease of approximately 15% in the partial pressure of oxygen with no corresponding rise in the partial pressure of carbon dioxide. This suggests that the presence of the endoscope itself in the hypopharynx contributes to hypoxemia. This group of patients was then compared with another group of 50 who underwent EGD after receiving intravenous diazepam in addition to oropharyngeal anesthesia. There was a comparable fall in the partial pressure of oxygen in this latter group.[25]

In another study, 114 patients undergoing endoscopy received atropine plus diazepam (10 mg), or atropine, diazepam (10 mg) and meperidine (50 mg) or fentanyl (0.05 mg). Although there was a slight fall in the partial pressure of oxygen in all groups, only with inclusion of a narcotic (meperidine or fentanyl) did the immediate decline reach statistical significance. Fourteen minutes after administering the drugs, the partial oxygen pressure was still depressed in subjects who

TABLE 12–4. **Retrospective Surveys of Complications of EGD**

Country	No. of Procedures	No. of Endoscopists	Complications*				Major Morbidity (%)	Death (%)	Reference
			Infection	Cardio-respiratory	Bleeding	Perforation			
U.S.	211,410	404	17 (0.008)	129 (0.06)	63 (0.03)	70 (0.03)	0.2	0.006	21
Britain	23,500	63	NR	16 (0.07)	6 (0.03)	26 (0.01)	0.2	0.012	22
Denmark	995	NR	0	2 (0.20)	NR	1 (0.10)	0.2	NR	23

NR = not reported.
*Numbers in parentheses indicate percentages. U.S. study included pneumonia in cardiorespiratory group instead of in infection group.

received meperidine or fentanyl. An increase in the partial pressure of carbon dioxide was observed in the groups receiving narcotics.[26] It has been shown by others also that diazepam alone does not produce hypoxemia.[24]

Hypoventilation, comparable to that occurring during EGD, also occurs after the same premedication is given to patients undergoing colonoscopy,[27] indicating that this is an effect of the narcotic agents that is independent of any effect of the presence of the endoscope in the hypopharynx. It has been suggested that the presence of the endoscope results in low-grade aspiration that may contribute to hypoxemia.[28] The degree of hypoxemia that occurs during EGD is of greater significance and risk for the individual with preexisting obstructive airway disease.

Thus it appears that mild hypoxemia is a regular occurrence during EGD and that this is produced by at least two factors: (1) the presence of the endoscope in the hypopharynx (possibly allowing for subclinical aspiration) and (2) hypoventilation caused by the use of narcotic agents as premedication. These observations describe events during the usual endoscopic procedure. However, not addressed in these studies is the recognized but fortunately small risk of apnea after intravenous administration of diazepam, particularly in the elderly patient given the "standard or usual dose" without consideration of drug effect on an individual basis. Despite studies that demonstrate relative freedom from respiratory depression in the great majority of patients given diazepam, many endoscopists fear this drug more than the narcotic component of the premedication. This may be explained by the fact that narcotics in the doses used for endoscopic procedures rarely if ever produce total apnea. More importantly, their effects can be rapidly reversed by intravenous narcotic antagonists. However, diazepam cannot be pharmacologically neutralized.

Respiratory embarrassment may occasionally be caused by frank aspiration.[29] Adequate suction capability, an attentive endoscopy assistant, and avoidance of over-sedation will minimize this problem. Other mechanisms of respiratory embarrassment have been encountered rarely, such as ventilatory compromise from massive abdominal distention as a result of insufflation distal to an esophageal obstruction.[29]

Cardiac Complications

Clinically serious cardiac complications during endoscopy are very uncommon. In 211, 410 EGD procedures, only 6 myocardial infarctions (0.002%) were recorded by the American Society for Gastrointestinal Endoscopy (ASGE).[21] Nevertheless, if monitoring is performed routinely, arrhythmias are found during 33% to 35% of EGD procedures.[30–32] Commonly encountered arrhythmias include premature ventricular contractions, multiple premature atrial beats, and atrial fibrillation. It is rarely necessary, according to published reports, to terminate an EGD procedure because of such rhythm abnormalities.

Factors increasing the likelihood of an arrhythmia during EGD are ischemic heart disease (55%), chronic lung disease (89%), and old age. The mechanism by which EGD produces arrhythmias is not fully understood, but a relationship between hypoxemia and the incidence of arrhythmias has been reported. Anxiety may also be a factor, since in one study the onset of ectopic beats was found to precede the introduction of the endoscope in 22% of cases.[31] A significant serum concentration of lidocaine has been demonstrated after administration of this drug as a topical pharyngeal anesthetic, and this may actually modulate the appearance of serious arrhythmias.[33] Mexiletine, an antiarrhythmic agent, has been shown to decrease the incidence of arrhythmias during endoscopy by 50%.[31]

Considering the frequency with which arrhythmias occur during EGD, it is interesting that clinically adverse cardiac events are encountered so rarely. In the majority of patients, no routine recommendations for cardiac monitoring or prophylaxis with antiarrhythmic drugs are warranted for EGD.

Perforation

Perforation during EGD was the second commonest major complication in the ASGE survey, occurring once in every 3300 endoscopies.[21] The proximal esophagus and pharynx are the most common sites of perforation, over 50% occurring in these areas. Perforations are usually attributed to a lack of patient cooperation or difficulty in intubating the esophagus. Anatomic abnormalities that increase the risk of perforation include Zenker's diverticulum, stricture, cancer, and hypertrophic spur formation of the cervical spine.[20] At the Mayo Clinic, 7 of 47 endoscopy-related esophageal perforations occurred during fiberoptic endoscopy; the remainder occurred during rigid endoscopy.[34] The predilection for these to occur in the cervical esophagus (43%) was apparent in this series as well. Severe pain was the most common symptom and usually occurred immediately after endoscopy. It was usually localized to the cervical region, upper back or epigastrium. The diagnosis was delayed more than 8 hours in 64% of cases, usually because the symptoms were misinterpreted. Crepitus was present in 60% and was frequently elicited if the cervical esophagus had been perforated; however, it was uncommon after perforation of the distal esophagus. Objective evidence of esophageal perforation was obtained radiographically. Fever and leukocytosis were present in two thirds of patients. Characteristic findings were cervical and mediastinal emphysema, pleural effusions, and extravasation of contrast material. Surgery is the usual treatment.

Nonesophageal perforations during EGD occur mainly in the stomach, although a few perforations of the duodenum or afferent limb after Billroth II gastrectomy have been recorded. Gastroduodenal perforations are often related to endoscopic biopsy.

Occasional reports document events that mimic free perforation following EGD. Excess insufflation of air into the bowel may produce marked abdominal distention with tenderness and even rebound tenderness. Plain x-ray films of the abdomen confirm the intraluminal location of the gas.[35] This problem is self-limiting. Pneumomediastinum, pneumoperitoneum, and submucosal air dissection have been reported without identification of free perforation at surgery.[36–38] In a prospective study of 124 patients who underwent either EGD or colonoscopy, 3 patients (2.4%) had intramural air on plain x-ray films of the abdomen performed immediately after the endoscopy.[38] This resolved spontaneously in all cases. It is hypothesized that air introduced under high pressure (up to 800 cc of water) during endoscopy may occasionally pass through a weak point in the mucosa in the absence of a frank perforation. If this air in the wall of the bowel then dissects to the serosa, blebs

may form and rupture, resulting in free intra-abdominal or mediastinal air.[39] Air dissection mimicking free perforations may explain why some patients with apparent perforation do well without surgical intervention.[21]

Infection

Diagnostic EGD–Related Infection

The most common infection resulting from diagnostic EGD is aspiration pneumonia. In a British survey, this was found in 0.07% of patients with upper endoscopies,[23] a figure somewhat higher than that recorded in the ASGE survey.[21] The main factor promoting aspiration is over-sedation.[28, 40, 41] (Of course, the patient with a stomach full of food or blood is highly likely to vomit during EGD.) It is worth re-emphasizing that the presence of a trained gastrointestinal endoscopy assistant, adequate suctioning equipment, and careful titration of sedative and narcotic medication will minimize this problem.

Bacteremia has been found during and immediately after diagnostic EGD in some[42–44] but not all[45] studies. The presence of bacteremia has serious implications for patients with prosthetic heart valves or joints and possibly for patients with rheumatic valvular heart disease. The prevalence of positive cultures after EGD varies from 0% to 10%. The level of bacteremia as estimated by pour plate techniques is very low. The likelihood of bacteremia, which is transient, does not correlate with the performance of biopsy or the type of mucosal abnormality seen.[42] Organisms encountered include *Neisseria* species, *Perflava*, streptococcal species including *Streptococcus pneumoniae*, *Staphylococcus epidermidis*, and *Acinetobacter calcoaceticus*.

Prophylactic antibiotics for diagnostic EGD are not routinely used even in patients with prosthetic heart valves.[46] For patients at risk for infective endocarditis, antibiotic prophylaxis has been recommended for the following procedures: esophageal dilation, sclerotherapy of esophageal varices, colonoscopy, upper gastrointestinal endoscopy with biopsy and proctosigmoidoscopy with biopsy.[47] Diagnostic upper gastrointestinal endoscopy and proctosigmoidoscopy without biopsy were not included. Many physicians consider antibiotic prophylaxis to be prudent for all types of gastrointestinal endoscopy in patients with prosthetic devices such as a heart valve since such patients appear to be at especially high risk for infective endocarditis.[47] The demonstration of *Pseudomonas aeruginosa* sepsis in 3 patients with acute nonlymphoblastic leukemia following EGD is of concern and may indicate another group of patients in whom antibiotic prophylaxis should be considered, especially if the granulocyte count is very low.[48] However, reports confirming this observation are not available. Currently the Cleveland Clinic Section of Endoscopy does not routinely employ antibiotic prophylaxis in these patients, although many of them are already on a regimen of antibiotics for established or suspected sepsis.

Therapeutic EGD–Related Infection

Patients undergoing therapeutic EGD may be at higher risk for infection; one recent study, for example, demonstrated transient bacteremia in 50% of patients undergoing endoscopic sclerotherapy for bleeding varices.[49] In patients at high risk for endocarditis, the use of prophylactic antibiotics during therapeutic endoscopy procedures remains controversial.[50, 51] Antibiotic prophylaxis as it relates to specific problems encountered in endoscopy, particularly therapeutic endoscopy, is discussed in various other chapters in this text.

Hepatitis B Infection

The spread of hepatitis B from patient to patient via contaminated endoscopes is a potential complication that is frequently a cause for concern, particularly in light of the fact that it is not known whether routinely employed decontamination and sterilization techniques eradicate hepatitis B virus from endoscope surfaces and channels. (It should be noted that biopsy forceps are one of the most difficult endoscopic accessories to clean and decontaminate.) However, some data are available. According to one report, 4 individuals were examined with an endoscope shortly after it had been used for ERCP in a jaundiced patient who subsequently was found to have acute hepatitis B. These 4 patients were followed for 6 months, during which time no laboratory or clinical evidence of hepatitis B developed.[52] In a somewhat larger series from Nigeria,[53] the investigator assumed that the instrument used for EGD was contaminated by hepatitis B, since it had been in widespread use in a country where the carrier rate for hepatitis B is between 5% and 10%. No cases of clinical hepatitis developed in 57 patients who had no serologic evidence of hepatitis B prior to endoscopy and who were followed for 1 year after endoscopy. In 21 patients, serial biochemical tests of liver function and HBsAg testing were obtained. None developed abnormal liver tests or converted to HBsAG positivity.

In an endoscopy unit in Italy the carrier rate for HBsAg positivity in 678 patients undergoing EGD was 8%.[54] A follow-up study of 298 patients who had no markers of hepatitis B infection prior to endoscopy was carried out. Of the 80% who were available for serologic testing, none developed HBsAG. One patient developed anti-HB and anti-HBs but not clinical hepatitis. In a concomitant control group (no endoscopy) serologic evidence of hepatitis developed in one patient.[54]

The available data indicate that the risk of contracting hepatitis B infection from a contaminated endoscope is remote; however, a recent case report[55] of hepatitis developing 2 months after endoscopy suggests that transmission may rarely be possible. In the subject of this report, an EGD instrument was used that had been used the previous day in a bleeding man who died of fulminant hepatitis. The serologic subtype of the B virus was identical in both patients.

Risk of Infection for Endoscopist

Infection may rarely be a risk for the endoscopist, excluding the obvious risk inherent in frequent contact with blood and secretions. Inadvertent inoculation of the conjunctiva by fluid contaminated by herpes simplex virus from a patient with herpes esophagitis resulted in recurrent herpetic conjunctivitis in an endoscopist.[56]

SUMMARY

Esophagogastroduodenoscopy is a commonly employed diagnostic procedure of high utility. There are few contraindications to the procedure. Although many types of complications have been reported, these are infrequent, and the safety of this examination can be defined with a high degree of precision. Because major morbidity rarely occurs, the endoscopist must maintain a high level of awareness of these potential complications to minimize their occurrence and to take corrective action when they occur.

References

1. Hirschowitz BI. A fibre optic flexible oesophagoscope. Lancet 1963; 2:388.
2. Jacobs WH. Cost benefit and cost containment. (Editorial) Gastrointest Endosc 1982; 28:110–1.
3. Showstack JA, Schroeder SA, Steinberg HR. Evaluating the costs and benefits of diagnostic technology: the case of upper gastrointestinal endoscopy. Med Care 1981; 19:498–509.
4. Almy TP. The role of the primary physician in the health care "industry." N Engl J Med 1981; 304:225–8.
5. Tedesco FJ, Griffin JW Jr, Crisp WL, Anthony HF. "Skinny" upper gastrointestinal endoscopy—the initial diagnostic tool: a prospective comparison of upper gastrointestinal endoscopy and radiology. J Clin Gastroenterol 1980; 2:27–30.
6. Martin TR, Vennes JA, Silvis SE, Ansel HJ. A comparison of upper gastrointestinal endoscopy and radiology. J Clin Gastroenterol 1980; 2:21–5.
7. Fleshler B, Achkar E. An aggressive approach to the medical management of peptic ulcer disease. Arch Intern Med 1981; 141:848–51.
8. Schuman BM. Upper gastrointestinal endoscopy—is it a first-line diagnostic service? Gastrointest Endosc 1981; 28:213–4.
9. Lichtenstein JL, Feinstein AR, Suzio KD, et al. The effectiveness of panendoscopy on diagnostic and therapeutic decisions about chronic abdominal pain. J Clin Gastroenterol 1980; 2:31–6.
10. Behar J, Biancani P, Sheahan DG. Evaluation of esophageal tests in diagnosis of reflux esophagitis. Gastroenterology 1976; 71:9–15.
11. Nelson RS, Lanza FL. The endoscopic diagnosis of gastric lymphoma. Gastrointest Endosc 1974; 21:66–8.
12. Martin TR, Onstad GR, Silvis SE, Vennes JA. Lift and cut biopsy technique for submucosal sampling. Gastrointest Endosc 1976; 23:29–30.
13. Spinelli P, Lo Gullo C, Pizzetti P. Endoscopic diagnosis of gastric lymphomas. Endoscopy 1980; 12:211–4.
14. Prolla JC, Reilly RW, Kirsner JB, Cockerham L. Direct-vision endoscopic cytology and biopsy in the diagnosis of esophageal and gastric tumors: current experience. Acta Cytol 1977; 21:399–402.
15. Scott BB, Jenkins D. Endoscopic small intestinal biopsy. Gastrointest Endosc 1981; 27:162–7.
16. Parker HH, Agayoff JD. Enteroscopy and small bowel biopsy using peroral colonoscope. Gastrointest Endosc 1983; 29:139–40.
17. Roth HP. Endoscopy—what is its role in upper GI bleeding? (Suppl) Dig Dis Sci 1981; 26:15–55.
18. Eastwood GL. Does the patient with upper gastrointestinal bleeding benefit from endoscopy? Reflections and discussion of recent literature. (Suppl) Dig Dis Sci 1981; 26:225–65.
19. Gilbert DA, Silverstein FE, Tedesco FJ. National ASGE survey on upper gastrointestinal bleeding. Complications of endoscopy. (Suppl) Dig Dis Sci 1981; 26:55S–95S.
20. Vennes JA, Silverstein FE. Upper gastrointestinal fiberoptic endoscopy. In: Sleisenger JS, Fordtran MH, eds. Gastrointestinal Disease. Philadelphia: W. B. Saunders Co., 1983; 1599–1617.
21. Mandelstam P, Sugawa C, Silvis SE, et al. Complications associated with esophagogastroduodenoscopy and with esophageal dilatation. Gastrointest Endosc 1976; 23:16–9.
22. Andersen KE, Clausen N. Outpatient gastroscopy risks. Endoscopy 1978; 10:180–3.
23. Schiller KF, Cotton PB, Salmon PR. The hazards of digestive fibre-endoscopy: A survey of British experience. (Abstr) Gut 1972; 13:1027.
24. Rostykus PS, McDonald GB, Albert RK. Upper intestinal endoscopy induces hypoxemia in patients with obstructive pulmonary disease. Gastroenterology 1980; 78:488–91.
25. Whorwell PJ, Smith CL, Foster KJ. Arterial blood gas tensions during upper gastrointestinal endoscopy. Gut 1976; 17:797–800.
26. Rozen P, Fireman Z, Gilat T. The causes of hypoxemia in elderly patients during endoscopy. Gastrointest Endosc 1982; 28:243–6.
27. Rozen P, Oppenheim D, Ratan J, et al. Arterial oxygen tension changes in elderly patients undergoing upper gastrointestinal endoscopy. I. Possible causes. Scand J Gastroenterol 1979; 14:577–81.
28. Prout BJ, Metreweli C. Pulmonary aspiration after fibre-endoscopy of the upper gastrointestinal tract. Br Med J 1972; 4:269–71.
29. Abou-Madi MN, Yacoub JM. An unusual complication of fiberoptic esophagoscopy. Anesthesiology 1974; 41:504–5.
30. Fugita R, Kumura F. Arrhythmias and ischemic changes of the heart induced by gastric endoscopic procedures. Am J Gastroenterol 1975; 64:44–8.
31. Pristautz H, Biffl H, Leitner W, et al. Influence of an antiarrhythmic premedication and the development of premature ventricular contractions during fiberoptic gastroduodenoscopy. Endoscopy 1981; 13:57–9.
32. Mathew PK, Ona FV, Damevski K, Wallace WA. Arrhythmias during upper gastrointestinal endoscopy. Angiology 1979; 30:834–40.
33. Van Durme JP, Elewant A, Rosseel MT, et al. Electrocardiographic changes during oesophagogastro-duodenoscopy. (Letter to editor) Endoscopy 1974; 6:134.
34. Rastogi H, Brown CH. Pseudoacute abdomen following gastroscopy. Gastrointest Endosc 1967; 14:16–8.
35. Mann NS, Sachdev AJ. Transient megacolon after gastroscopy. South Med J 1977; 70:755–6.
36. Katz D, Cano R, Antonelli M. Benign air dissection of the esophagus and stomach at fiberesophagoscopy. Gastrointest Endosc 1972; 19:72–4.
37. Lezak MB, Goldhammer M. Retroperitoneal emphysema after colonoscopy. Gastroenterology 1974; 66:118–20.
38. Glouberman S, Craner GE, Ogburn RM, Burdick GE. Radiographic survey from extraluminal air following gastrointestinal tract fiberendoscopy. Gastrointest Endosc 1976; 22:165–7.
39. Fierst SM, Robinson HM, Lasagna L. Interstitial gastric emphysema following gastroscopy; its relation to the syndrome of pneumoperitoneum and generalized emphysema with no evident perforation. Ann Intern Med 1951; 34:1202–12.
40. Taylor PA, Cotton PB, Towey RM, Gent AE. Pulmonary complications after oesophagogastroscopy using diazepam. Br Med J 1972; 1:666.
41. Cotton PB. Pulmonary aspiration after fibre-endoscopy. (Letter) Br Med J 1972; 4:491–2.
42. Shull HJ Jr, Greene BM, Allen SD, et al. Bacteremia with upper gastrointestinal endoscopy. Ann Intern Med 1975; 83:212–4.
43. Stephenson PM, Dorrington L, Harris OD, Rao A. Bacteraemia following oesophageal dilatation and

oesophago-gastroscopy. Aust NZ J Med 1977; 7:32–5.

44. Graham JR. Pneumococcal septicaemia after endoscopic gastric polypectomy. (Letter) Med J Aust 1980; 2:457–8.

45. Linnemann C, Weisman E, Wenger J. Blood cultures following endoscopy of the esophagus and stomach. South Med J 1971; 64:1055–62.

46. Meyer GW. Prophylaxis of infective endocarditis during gastrointestinal procedures: report of a survey. Gastrointest Endosc 1979; 25:1–2.

47. Shulman ST, Amren DP, Bisno AL, et al. Prevention of bacterial endocarditis. A statement for health professionals by the committee on rheumatic fever and infective endocarditis of the council on cardiovascular disease in the young. Circulation 1984; 70:1123A–27A.

48. Greene WH, Moody M, Hartley R, et al. Esophagoscopy as a source of Pseudomonas aeruginosa sepsis in patients with acute leukemia: the need for sterilization of endoscopes. Gastroenterology 1974; 67:912–9.

49. Cohen LB, Korsten MA, Scherl EJ, et al. Bacteremia after endoscopic injection sclerosis. Gastrointest Endosc 1983; 29:198–200.

50. Camara DS, Gruber M, Barde CJ, et al. Transient bacteremia following endoscopic injection sclerotherapy of esophageal varices. Arch Intern Med 1983; 143:1350–2.

51. Simon GL. Transient bacteremia and endocarditis prophylaxis. Arch Intern Med 1984; 144:34–5.

52. McDonald GB, Silverstein FE. Can gastrointestinal endoscopy transmit hepatitis B to patients? Gastrointest Endosc 1976; 22: 168–70.

53. Ayoola EA. The risk of type B hepatitis infection in flexible fiberoptic endoscopy. Gastrointest Endosc 1981; 27:60–2.

54. Villa E, Pasquinelli C, Rigo G, et al. Gastrointestinal endoscopy and HBV infection: no evidence for a causal relationship. A prospective controlled trial. Gastrointest Endosc 1984; 30:15–7.

55. Birnie GG, Quigley EM, Clements GB, et al. Endoscopic transmission of hepatitis B virus. Gut 1983; 24:171–4.

56. Kaye MD. Herpetic conjunctivitis as an unusual occupational hazard (endoscopists' eye). Gastrointest Endosc 1974; 21:69–70.

Chapter 13

ESOPHAGO-GASTRODUODENOSCOPY IN THE PEDIATRIC PATIENT

ROBERT WYLLIE, M.D.

During the past two decades, esophagogastroduodenoscopy in infants and children has become a safe, well-established diagnostic procedure for gastrointestinal disease. Smaller diameter, more flexible endoscopes with wider angles of view have been of major importance in the evolution of endoscopy as a routine outpatient procedure in pediatric patients. The approach to the patient, technique of the procedure, and spectrum of disease, however, are different from that for the adult patient.

FACILITIES

Preprocedure anxiety and fear are significant problems for young children and their parents. The physical surroundings of the endoscopy unit and waiting area are important and must be as relaxing as possible. Toys and books should be available. A recovery area that is separate from that for seriously ill adults is also important in reducing fear.

A "familiar face" also decreases the anxiety of young patients. An endoscopy assistant who works with pediatric patients is ideal for this purpose. This individual should orient children to the procedure. Dolls are useful for illustrating the procedure, and this is most effective if done well in advance of the actual endoscopy. The same assistant can greet the patients before the procedure and accompany them from the waiting area into the endoscopy suite.

There should be two endoscopy assistants if general anesthesia is not used. One holds and reassures the patient while the other performs the usual functions associated with endoscopy in adults. The presence of parents at the actual procedure depends on the endoscopist's preference and also on assessment of the personalities of the patient and parent(s). A thorough explanation of the procedure and a gentle manner usually allow endoscopy to proceed without difficulty in older children and teenagers. Adequate supervision after the procedure usually requires the presence of a nurse and the parent(s).

INSTRUMENTS

The esophagus in the term infant is 9 to 10 cm in length and 4 to 6 mm in diameter.[1] These dimensions require instruments specifically adapted to pediatric patients. The smallest upper gastrointestinal endoscopes currently available have an insertion tube diameter of approximately 7 mm. These have been used without trauma to the esophagus, stomach, or duodenum in neonates and infants. In premature neonates, a fiberoptic bronchoscope with an insertion tube diameter of 4 to 5 mm is the instrument of choice. However, this type of instrument lacks a simultaneous suction and air insufflation capability. Most have only bidirectional tip deflection, making examination of the entire stomach and duodenal bulb more difficult even with torquing of the insertion tube. In older children and teenagers, standard endoscopes may be used.

PREMEDICATION

The goals of premedication in pediatric patients are different from those for the adult. Sedation is titrated not only to minimize discomfort but also to provide amnesia for the procedure. This permits several procedures in sequence when necessary and ensures that the child will not become fearful of contact with the physician. The latter goal is particularly important in pediatric patients with chronic conditions that may require repeated procedures.

During the early and mid-1970's most endoscopists relied on general anesthesia for sedation so that the patient would experience no discomfort during the procedure. General anesthesia also had advantages for the endoscopist, for example, a quiet patient and ancillary personnel to monitor cardiorespiratory functions. Greater attention to the special problems of pediatric anesthesia have decreased morbidity and mortality, although in a collaborative study from seven institutions published in 1975 there was 1 death in every 3600 pediatric patients undergoing general anesthesia.[2] Cardiac and respiratory factors contributed equally to morbidity. Preoperative anemia was a major risk factor with respect to cardiac arrest. Fever, debility, and immaturity were other contributing factors.[3] At Children's Hospital Medical Center in Boston the death rate from anesthesia during the 1970's was 0.8% to 1.3%, although the mortality for relatively uncomplicated operations such as tonsillectomy and/or adenoidectomy was negligible.[4] Anesthesia-associated mortality remains highest in the first decade of life, particularly during the neonatal period.

Endoscopy in neonates may be performed with or without sedation depending on the indication for the procedure. Sedation is helpful when the presence of a foreign body is suspected or there is gastrointestinal hemorrhage and the procedure may be prolonged. A more routine examination by an experienced pediatric endoscopist may be performed without sedation during the first few months of life.

In most infants and children endoscopy is now performed with intravenous sedation. The many medications and methods of administration include intramuscular promethazine, chlorpromazine, and meperidine or a sedative such as chloral hydrate given orally. These medications, however, produce unpredictable levels of sedation and have a delayed onset of action.

Many pediatric endoscopists now use a combination of meperidine and diazepam. After venous access is established, 1 to 2 mg/kg to a maximum of 100 mg meperidine is administered by slow infusion, followed by 5 to 15 mg diazepam. Meperidine is given first to decrease the discomfort associated with intravenous diazepam. The dose of diazepam is titrated to allow a comfortable examination. Younger children may require more diazepam per kilogram of body weight than children older than 10 years.[5] Occasionally it may be necessary to administer additional amounts of these drugs during the procedure.

Reactions at the site of medication administration with the above method of sedation are common, and include cutaneous erythema distal to the site of injection. This type of reaction is transient and not associated with clinically significant thrombophlebitis. Other reactions include coughing and a strange taste if the meperidine is infused rapidly. In a prospective evaluation of this method of sedation in 100 pediatric procedures at the Cleveland Clinic, approximately 50% of the patients had generalized cutaneous flushing, and urticaria without audible wheezing developed in 12. Rechallenge with the same sedative in 2 patients did not result in a more severe reaction.

Neurologically impaired patients often have gastrointestinal problems that require endoscopy. Sedation in these patients is unpredictable and respiratory depression is common. The dosage of meperidine is therefore reduced to 0.5 to 1.0 mg/kg and the dosage of diazepam, if this drug is used, is titrated very slowly. Careful and attentive monitoring of the cardiorespiratory status is essential.

Resuscitation equipment in sizes appropriate for small patients should be readily available, including an Ambu bag and mask and endotracheal tubes along with drugs for resuscitation. Suction equipment, oxygen, and naloxone to reverse meperidine-induced respiratory depression should be immediately available. Intravenous access should be maintained during the procedure in infants or in any case in which the procedure will be lengthy, so that ancillary medication or drugs for resuscitation may be given expeditiously. Naloxone is indicated only for narcotic-induced respiratory depression because its use is usually associated with marked irritability in infants and young children.

PREPARATION

Infants less than 6 months of age are not fed for 2 to 4 hours prior to endoscopy. Children over 2 years of age fast for 6 to 8 hours and receive intravenous medication just prior to the procedure.

TECHNIQUE

The technique of upper gastrointestinal endoscopy in pediatric patients is generally similar to that in adults (see Chapter 11). The endoscope should only be advanced under direct vision. In young children, and when general anesthesia is used in any patient, overinsufflation should be avoided.

The introduction of an endoscope in neonates and young infants may cause tracheal compression and compromise the airway. Additional personnel must therefore monitor the cardiorespiratory status of the patient during the procedure and assist in resuscitation if necessary. In older children with teeth, additional assistance is also needed to keep the bite block in proper position during the procedure.

COMPLICATIONS

There have been few reports of complications associated with fiberoptic examination of the upper gastrointestinal tract in children. In young infants, transient bradycardia has been noted secondary to vagal stimulation or airway compression.[6] Stridor after introduction of the endoscope, probably related to tracheal compression, has been described. In reported cases, this was reversible with the removal of the endoscope.[7] Mucosal tears may occur in patients who are not well sedated or have a paradoxical excitability reaction to diazepam.[8] As in adult patients, the risk of perforation or aspiration should be small, although this has not been studied prospectively.

Bacteremia was reported in 1 of 50 children undergoing upper endoscopy and biopsy.[9] The organism was a group A streptococcus. The patient had no clinical signs of infection and was not given antibiotics. Until the exact risks are defined, however, the use of antibiotics as a prophylactic measure is currently recommended only for patients with congenital or vascular heart disease, central venous or hyperalimentation catheters, and ventricular shunts.

INDICATIONS

Hemorrhage

Prior to the widespread use of endoscopy in pediatric patients, the cause of upper gastrointestinal hemorrhage was not identified in at least one third of patients.[10–13] During the first 6 months of life, a source of bleeding was found in less than one half of the patients.[14] With endoscopic evaluation, the source of bleeding is identified in 75% to 95% of patients with gastrointestinal bleeding.[15] In more recent studies, the source has been identified in almost all patients including young infants.[6, 16]

The most common causes of upper gastrointestinal hemorrhage vary with age. In children less than 1 year old, esophagitis, gastric and duodenal ulcers, and gastric erosions comprise the majority of lesions (Table 13–1).[6, 7, 16–19] In older children, gastrointestinal bleeding is often associated with drug ingestion or life-threatening illness (Table 13–2); between 12% and 25% had taken aspirin; 40% to 75% had another associated severe illness.[6, 7, 16–18, 20] Gastric ulcer is the major cause of bleeding in children from 1 to 6 years of age followed by inflammation of the duodenum or esophagus. Varices also occur in this age group and are usually associated with cirrhosis or portal vein obstruction. Duodenal ulcer is the most common cause of bleeding between the ages of 7 and 18 years, followed by gastric erosions, varices, and esophagitis (Table 13–3).[7, 16–18]

Foreign Bodies

The peak incidence of foreign body ingestion is from 6 months to 3 years. In older children, ingestion is usually accidental, except for mentally incompetent individuals.

In pediatric patients, there is often a witness to the act. In other patients the presence of a gastrointestinal foreign body may only be inferred from the disappearance of an object and the acute onset of symptoms. Older children, when questioned, will often admit the ingestion or proudly volunteer the information to their parents.

TABLE 13–1. Source of Upper Gastrointestinal Bleeding in 1-Year-Old Infants*

Series	N	DU	Duod	GU	GE	Esoph
Gleason et al.[18]	2			2		
Cox and Ament[16]	17	3		1	4	4
Graham et al.[7]	3		1			
Liebman et al.[19]	1				1	
Gryboski[17]†	2				2	
Hargrove et al.[6]	5	4	1			
Total	30	7	2	3	7	4

N = Number of patients; DU = duodenal ulcer; Duod = duodenitis; GU = gastric ulcer; GE = gastric erosions; Esoph = esophagitis.
*Adapted from Gryboski.[17]
†Unpublished observation quoted by Gryboski.[17]

Most foreign bodies traverse the gastrointestinal tract without difficulty. Those that fail to do so usually lodge in the esophagus (Plate 13–1). Common presenting symptoms in infants and young children include choking, excessive drooling, and poor feeding. Older children often complain of substernal pain and dysphagia. Occasionally, patients may present only with respiratory symptoms such as stridor, wheezing, or chronic pneumonia.

Once in the stomach, 95% of all ingested objects pass uneventfully through the remainder of the gastrointestinal tract.[21, 22] If an object does become lodged, it is usually at an anatomic or physiologic sphincter such as the pylorus or ileocecal valve, at a fixed bend in the course of the bowel such as occurs with the duodenum, at a surgical anastomosis, or at the level of a congenital malformation such as a web, diaphragm, or diverticulum.

Most foreign bodies are radiopaque, and plain radiographs should be obtained routinely to demonstrate their location, nature, and number. Radiolucent objects are often more difficult to detect.

The most common site of impaction in the esophagus is just below the cricopharyngeal sphincter at the thoracic inlet.[23, 24] Radiopaque foreign bodies are easily identified by soft-tissue lateral neck and chest radiographs. Flat objects tend to lie in the coronal plane in the esophagus and in the sagittal plane in the trachea. It is often necessary to use contrast material or fluoroscopy of the hypopharynx, larynx, and trachea to demonstrate radiolucent objects.

Respiratory symptoms arise from compression of the soft posterior tracheal wall, recurrent aspiration, or by direct extension of an associated inflammatory process from the esophagus to the larynx or trachea, which results in stridor and occasionally tracheoesophageal fistula.[25, 26] It is not uncommon for children less than 3 years of age with radiolucent esophageal foreign bodies to have presenting symptoms of asthma, croup, bronchitis, or bronchopneumonia.[27] The normal diet at this age consists largely of liquids and puréed food that will pass around an impacted object so that dysphagia is less evident than in older children and adults.

Conservative management on an outpatient basis is indicated in almost all instances in which the foreign body has entered the stomach. Most objects will be passed in 4 to 6 days; however, some may take as long as 3 to 4 weeks.[28] Failure to progress over a 3- to

TABLE 13–2. Source of Upper Gastrointestinal Bleeding in Children 1 to 6 Years Old*

Series	N	DU	Duod	GU	GE/U	Esoph	Var
Gleason et al.[18]	1			1			
Cox and Ament[16]	15	1		6	1	3	3
Graham et al.[7]	8	1		2	1		
Gryboski[17]†	8	2	1	1	1	2	1
Hargrove et al[6]	1		1	1			
Total	33	4	2	11	3	5	4

N = Number of patients; DU = duodenal ulcer; Duod = duodenitis; GU = gastric ulcer; GE/U = gastric erosions and ulcer; Esoph = esophagitis; Var = varices.
*Adapted from Gryboski.[17]
†Unpublished observation quoted by Gryboski.[17]

TABLE 13–3. **Source of Upper Gastrointestinal Bleeding in Children 7 to 18 Years Old***

Series	N	DU	Duod	GU	GE	Esoph	Var
Gleason et al.[18]	7	2			2	1	2
Cox and Ament[16]	36	10		5	4	3	4
Graham et al.[7]	8	3		2	1		1
Gryboski[17]	7	3	1		1	2	
Total	58	18	1	7	8	6	7

N = Number of patients; DU = duodenal ulcer; Duod = duodenitis; GU = gastric ulcer; GE = gastric erosions; Esoph = esophagitis; Var = varices.
*Adapted from Gryboski.[17]

4-week period seldom implies an impending complication but may be associated with a congenital or acquired bowel abnormality.[29, 30] While waiting for the object to pass, parents are usually instructed to have the child continue a regular diet and observe the stools for the appearance of the ingested object. Cathartics should be avoided. The progress of unusually long or sharp objects should be observed radiographically. Metal detectors have been used to follow metallic bodies through the colon and to screen stools for their presence.[31] Parents and patients should be instructed to report immediately abdominal pain, vomiting, persistent temperature elevation, hematemesis, or melena.

Patients with foreign bodies lodged in the esophagus are usually hospitalized. Fiberoptic endoscopy is routinely employed to snare and remove such objects under direct visualization. Blind removal with Foley catheters has been recommended in the past, but this does not allow visualization of the esophageal mucosa and has the added risk of perforation while inflating the balloon. Metallic objects have occasionally been retrieved by magnets passed under fluoroscopic guidance.[32] Meat tenderizers have been used for esophageal meat impaction but have been associated with hypernatremia and erosion of the esophageal mucosa.[33]

Conservative management is contraindicated for objects that are potentially corrosive or whose shape or sharpness makes perforation more likely. An estimated 500 to 800 small batteries are ingested each year, with more than 200 cases reported.[30, 34–39] Two fatalities have been reported that occurred when the batteries became lodged in the esophagus with subsequent perforation.[40, 41] Tracheoesophageal fistula and rupture of a Meckel's diverticulum have also been reported.[42, 43] Other potential complications include gastric perforation and mercury poisoning. The mechanism of injury is thought to be either the leakage of alkaline electrolyte solution from the battery or direct current flow through adjacent tissue.[28, 44]

Management following battery ingestion remains controversial. There are advocates of immediate endoscopic or surgical removal, as well as those who recommend cautious observation.[34, 45] Considering the reported fatalities, all batteries lodged in the esophagus should be immediately removed. Definitive management of a battery in the stomach is less certain. Until the true risks are known for each type of battery, our present policy is to observe the patient for 24 hours. If the patient becomes symptomatic or the battery has not exited from the stomach at the end of the observation period, then it is removed endoscopically.

Sharp objects, such as razor blades and open safety pins, and those that are unlikely to pass through the pylorus are also removed. Most children will require general anesthesia unless the objects can be quickly grasped and withdrawn. The use of an overtube may also be beneficial since it protects the esophagus during extraction. Techniques for removal of foreign objects are discussed in Chapter 14.

The physical properties of a foreign body must also be considered. Lead is rapidly leached by gastric acid, and lead-containing objects should probably be removed if they fail to leave the stomach within 1 week of ingestion or the lower gastrointestinal tract within 2 weeks of ingestion.[46]

The complications of foreign body ingestion are infrequent but dramatic. Perforation of the intestinal lumen by a foreign body with generalized peritonitis is unusual. Most objects that puncture the bowel wall are slowly extruded into the peritoneal cavity. The area is usually isolated by adjacent loops of intestine and omentum and a localized inflammatory mass is formed. Mechanical obstruction may result from trapping or sharp angulation of the involved bowel. The most common site of perforation is the ileocecal area, particularly the appendix.[47] Duodenal perforation occasionally occurs when objects greater than 5 to 6 cm in length fail to negotiate the duodenal loop. Urinary tract complications have been reported with duodenal perforations directed toward the patient's right side.[47] Surgical or endoscopic intervention with urinary tract evaluation is indicated if such a foreign body remains within the duodenum beyond 5 or 6 days.

Caustic Ingestion

Gaudreault et al.[48] reported a retrospective series of 378 children who had ingested caustic substances. These authors attempted to relate the severity of the patient's symptoms and the presence of oropharyngeal damage to the presence of esophageal or gastric injury. Eight percent of the children were between 1 and 3 years of age. The most common symptoms associated with severe burns were vomiting, fever, excessive salivation, abdominal pain, and dysphagia. Eighty-six percent of the patients had swallowed alkali; acid was ingested by 14%. There was no difference in the incidence of esophageal injury between symptomatic and asymptomatic patients. The severity of esophageal injury was comparable for alkali and acid ingestion. Strictures developed in only 2% of the patients, and then only after alkali ingestion. All strictures responded satisfactorily to esophageal dilation. The low frequency of esophageal stricture in this study was thought to be related to a decrease in the strength of caustic products, introduction of safety caps, and greater awareness of parents to the danger of the substances.

In another study of 176 patients over a 10-year period, all but 12 had ingested an alkaline substance.[49] The mean age of patients in this series was 2 years, although 44 patients were over 10 years old. In 34 cases ingestion of a caustic substance was a suicide attempt. There were no complications of early esophagoscopy; the results of the procedure also eliminated the need for prolonged therapy in more than half the patients. An esophageal stricture developed in 24%; 8 patients responded to dilation and 7 required colonic interposition. When esophageal injury was identified, patients were treated with antibiotics and corticosteroids, and either an esophageal stent or a luminal string was left in the esophageal lumen.

The management of caustic ingestion remains controversial. Various combinations of antibiotics, corticosteroids, and esophageal stents have been used in an attempt to control secondary infection and stricture formation. The role of early endoscopy is to define the extent and severity of injury and separate those patients who can be managed by observation alone from those who will require aggressive therapy. Endoscopic complications have usually been related to the use of rigid endoscopes in uncooperative patients.[50, 51] This led to the routine use of general anesthesia during the examination. With currently available fiberoptic instruments, a complete examination of the esophagus, stomach, and duodenum can be safely performed with sedation even in young children. Barium studies, particularly during the acute stages, usually are not sensitive enough to delineate the severity and extent of injury.[52–56]

Many schemes have been devised to grade the severity of injury.[49, 57–60] Most of these attempt to differentiate mucosal injury from extensive necrosis of the esophagus and stomach. Uncomplicated mucosal inflammation is usually identified easily by the presence of erythema, edema, and focal hemorrhage. The prognosis for these patients is good, and they do not require specific therapy.

More severe injury is characterized by hemorrhage, ulceration, and focal necrosis. The depth of injury may be difficult to determine, particularly if an exudate covers the involved area.[58] Circumferential areas of inflammation should be noted, since stricture formation is more likely in such areas.[53, 61, 62] Patients with these findings require more aggressive therapy, including the use of total parenteral nutrition. Serial endoscopic examination is useful in defining the extent of healing. Oral nutrition can be started in many patients within 2 to 4 weeks, although severe esophageal burns may take as long as 3 months to heal.[60]

Stricture formation is a late complication that may involve the esophagus or gastric antrum (Plate 13–2). The role of corticosteroids and early dilation remains controversial, since no prospective controlled studies have been performed that demonstrate their benefit. In the case of severe burns, consensus of opinion favors the use of antibiotics and corticosteroids. The use of agents that

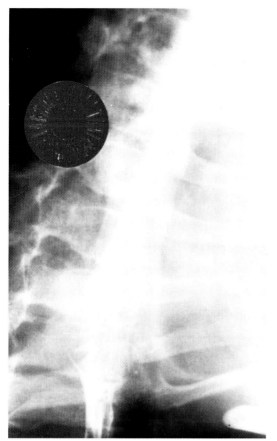

PLATE 13–1. Poker chip lodged in the upper esophagus of a 1-year-old infant. Red poker chip is shown in upper left for comparison.

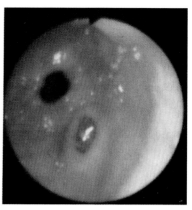

PLATE 13–3. Pancreatic rest in 3-year-old child with recurrent abdominal pain and vomitting.

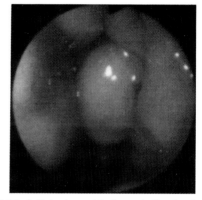

PLATE 13–4. Ectopic gastric tissue in the duodenum of a 14-year-old patient with chronic abdominal pain and anemia.

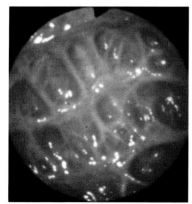

PLATE 13–2. Severe scarring of the gastric antrum in a 16-year-old patient following ingestion of concentrated acid.

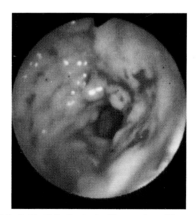

PLATE 13–5. Gastric Crohn's disease in a 12-year-old girl with abdominal pain.

reduce gastric acid secretion also seems reasonable. At the present time, esophageal dilation is usually deferred until a stricture has been demonstrated.

Carcinoma of the esophagus and of the stomach have been reported following caustic ingestion, although the association with gastric carcinoma has not been firmly established.[63-67] In patients who have sustained caustic injury to the esophagus, it is estimated that carcinoma will occur at a rate 1000 times greater than the expected incidence.[68] The interval between injury and the development of carcinoma varies between 1 and 7 decades. A formal screening procedure has not been adopted, but routine evaluation should probably be carried out to identify dysplasia prior to the development of carcinoma.

Peptic Ulcer Disease in Children

Peptic ulcer disease in pediatric patients was first recognized in 1826 when the German physician Von Siebold[69] reported the case of a 2-day-old infant with a perforated gastric ulcer. Peptic ulcers in children were considered unusual until 1941, when 119 cases of children requiring surgery were described by Bird et al.[70] Seven hundred ninety-one cases were reported to the Childhood Registry for Peptic Ulcers and reviewed by Tudor in 1974[71]; this author also described a personal experience of 168 cases. Reports of peptic ulcer disease in children in North America are listed in Table 13-4.[72-82]

Peptic ulcers in children can be divided into primary and secondary categories. Primary ulcers occur in otherwise healthy patients, the ulcer itself being the principal pathologic lesion. A peptic ulcer may be a secondary occurrence in association with other concomitant diseases. Examples are

Curling's ulcer, which occurs in association with severe cutaneous burns, and Cushing's ulcer, which is associated with intracranial lesions. Many other conditions including sepsis, hypoglycemia, shock, and respiratory failure predispose to peptic ulcer formation. Approximately 80% of ulcers in infancy can be considered secondary; more than 70% are primary in older children and adolescents.

Several series from pediatric centers in North America have been reported, but few of these are concerned with incidence. Sultz et al.,[83] reviewing experience in Erie County, New York, demonstrated an increasing incidence from 0.5 per 100,000 to 3.9 per 100,000 between 1947-1949 and 1956-1958, respectively. Sixty-eight peptic ulcers occurring from 1964 to 1968 in 21,565 students were reported by Miranti,[84] an incidence of 67 per 100,000. In a large pediatric practice in Texas (over 7000 patients), 123 ulcers were reported by Nickey et al.,[85] a prevalence of 1.7%. All were diagnosed radiographically.

Primary ulcers in children are more common in males and are predominantly duodenal. In a series of 377 ulcers reported by Prouty,[78] all but 6 were duodenal. In children below age 6, however, gastric ulcers appear to be at least as common as duodenal ulcers. Deckelbaum et al.[80] described 48 ulcers in children less than 6 years old, and all were gastric.

Genetic factors seem to play a role in childhood peptic ulcer disease. Studies in twins have shown a concordance rate of 50% in monozygous twins and only 14% in dizygotic twins. Tudor[71] noted a positive family history in approximately 20% of his patients. A similar observation was made by Deckelbaum et al.[80] for duodenal ulcer disease, but a positive family history was not a frequent occurrence in association with primary gastric ulcers.

TABLE 13-4. **Peptic Ulcers in Infants and Children in North America**

Author	Pub	N	Yr	Location
Ramos et al.[72]	1960	32	22	Chicago, IL
Michener et al.[73]	1960	108	28	Rochester, MN
Schuster and Gross[74]	1963	28	32	Boston, MA
Thompson and Jewett[75]	1964	50	—	Buffalo, NY
Gieske and Storey[76]	1966	62	8	Baltimore, MD
Rosenlund and Koop[77]	1970	27	20	Philadelphia, PA
Prouty[78]	1970	337	16	Madison, WS
Seagram et al.[79]	1973	144	20	Toronto, Canada
Deckelbaum et al.[80]	1974	73	11	Montreal, Canada
Grosfeld et al.[81]	1978	29	11	Indianapolis, IN
Nord and Lebenthal[82]	1981	22	4	Buffalo, NY

Pub = Year that report was published; N = number of patients; Yr = years.

Blood type O is also more common in children with duodenal ulcer.[86]

Studies of gastric acidity demonstrate that children with duodenal ulcer, like adults, tend to be hypersecretors of gastric acid. Christie and Ament[87] studied acid secretion in ulcer patients and controls. Children with active ulcers had a greater increase in maximal and basal acid output than control subjects. Excessive acid output has also been demonstrated in children with Zollinger-Ellison syndrome.[88] Clinically these cases were characterized by recurrent multiple ulcers with frequent perforation. In all reported cases, the patients have been older than 6 years.

Psychologic studies of children and adolescents with peptic ulcer disease have not demonstrated a consistent personality profile that might predispose them to the development of ulcers.

The symptoms that accompany primary ulcers are age-dependent. Newborns usually present with perforation, bleeding, or both. Older infants may have poor feeding, vomiting, and growth failure. In children under age 6, vomiting is common but pain is infrequent. When a young child complains of pain, the pain is usually poorly localized. Up to one third of these patients will present with bleeding. In older children, pain is the most common symptom, but this often has no relation to meals. Bleeding occurs in half the older children. In adolescence, pain is similar to that for peptic ulcer in adults; it is periumbilical and relieved by food or antacids.

Peptic ulcer can be diagnosed by upper gastrointestinal x-ray study or endoscopy. Deckelbaum et al.[80] reported that a second radiologic procedure was required in one fourth of their patients for confirmation of the diagnosis. In one of the early reports of pediatric endoscopy, Tedesco et al.[20] included 17 patients with peptic ulcer disease. When compared with endoscopy, radiologic diagnosis was accurate in less than half the cases. Most studies suggest that radiographic investigation detects from 50% to 75% of the ulcers that are visualized at endoscopy. Endoscopy may also allow identification of various other diseases that may mimic peptic ulcer disease (Plates 13–3, 13–4, and 13–5).

Treatment is with antacids, cimetidine, ranitidine, or sucralfate and is based on experience in adults. No controlled studies have been undertaken to determine the superiority of one regimen over another in children.

Anecdotal reports suggest H2 blockers are as safe and effective as in adults. Bland diets have not been helpful and are no longer prescribed. In those patients with recurrent ulcers, Zollinger-Ellison syndrome and hypercalcemia must be considered.

In the series reported by Tudor,[71] 7.5% of pediatric patients with peptic ulcer disease required surgery; none of the 337 patients in the series of Prouty[78] underwent operation. As in adult patients, surgery is reserved for patients with perforation, obstruction, uncontrolled hemorrhage, and intractable ulcers.

Portal Hypertension

Extrahepatic Portal Hypertension

The most common cause of portal hypertension in childhood is obstruction of the portal vein. This may be due to thrombosis, fibrosis, or congenital malformation of the portal or splenic vein.

Portal vein thrombosis is often a complication of umbilical vein catheterization (Fig. 13–1). This procedure is performed in the

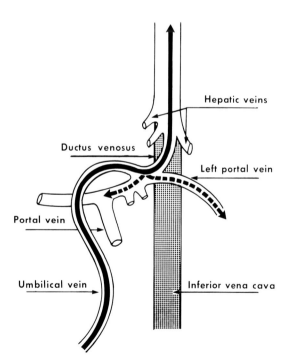

FIGURE 13–1. The catheter in the umbilical vein normally must go through the canal of Arantius to the inferior vena cava (*solid arrow*). Sometimes it follows the left branch or rarely the right branch of the portal vein (*broken arrows*). (From: Alagille D, Odievre M. Liver and Biliary Tract Disease in Children. New York: John Wiley and Sons, Inc., 1979; 272.)

neonatal period for fluid administration or exchange transfusions. Hyperbilirubinemia is the usual reason for the latter, although other indications include hyperviscosity syndromes and disseminated intravascular coagulation. Septic thrombosis of the portal vein is a consequence of an infectious process and is usually associated with omphalitis, peritonitis, or sepsis. "Bland thrombosis" is the term given to portal vein obstruction that follows dehydration. Forty percent of children with obstruction of the portal vein and no history of any of the above causes will have other congenital abnormalities. This suggests a congenital insult or maldevelopment.[89]

Patients with portal vein obstruction have presenting features of portal hypertension, i.e., hemorrhage or hypersplenism. There are no stigmata of cirrhosis, jaundice is absent, and bleeding does not precipitate hepatic coma. There is usually nothing in the clinical history of infants with portal venous obstruction during the neonatal period to suggest the diagnosis until the occurrence of hematemesis, this being the most frequent presenting symptom. The onset of hemorrhage in children with portal vein thrombosis is earlier than in those with cirrhosis, but this usually does not occur before 3 or 4 years of age (Fig. 13–2). Bleeding episodes are often associated with febrile illnesses and seem to be precipitated by aspirin administration. Less frequent presenting signs and symptoms include splenomegaly, collateral circulation over the anterior abdomen, ascites, hepatomegaly, and clubbing. Occasionally, an infant will have growth retardation.

Extrahepatic portal hypertension is one of the few causes of varices in the pediatric age group in which liver function tests are normal. When abnormal biochemical tests are discovered, diseases to be considered in the differential diagnosis include cystic fibrosis, Wilson's or Gaucher's diseases, congenital hepatic fibrosis, and cirrhosis due to primary hepatic diseases and biliary causes. These diseases account for approximately one third of the cases of varices occurring in childhood.

The diagnosis of extrahepatic portal hypertension is usually suggested by esophageal varices with normal liver function tests. About one third of the patients will have a clinical history compatible with omphalitis or manipulation of the umbilical vein. Currently, the most useful studies in establishing the diagnosis are endoscopy, ultrasonography, splenoportography, and measurement of the portal pressure.[90, 91]

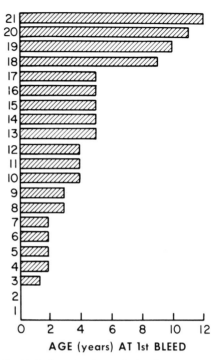

FIGURE 13–2. Portal vein occlusion in neonates. Age at first hemorrhage in 21 patients in whom portal vein blockage occurred in neonatal period. (From: Webb LJ, Sherlock S. The aetiology, presentation and natural history of extra-hepatic portal venous obstruction. Q J Med 1979; 48:633.)

Endoscopy in patients with extrahepatic portal venous obstruction may also identify causes of hemorrhage other than varices. Five of 81 children with extrahepatic portal hypertension and gastrointestinal hemorrhage reported by Alvarez et al.[90] were found to have bleeding sites other than varices. Gastric varices were demonstrated in 16 of 56 (28%) of the children examined.

Variceal bleeding will often stop by the time the child receives medical attention. Hemorrhage decompresses the portal system, and with normal clotting function bleeding usually stops spontaneously. Intravascular volume expansion should be judicious, as rapid elevation of portal pressure may precipitate further bleeding. Antacids are routinely used to buffer gastric acid. If significant bleeding persists or recurs, vasopressin at a dose of 2 to 4 mU/kg/min in 5% dextrose can be administered intravenously over 15 to 20 minutes. The dose may be repeated as needed. A constant superior mesenteric artery infusion of vasopressin at 0.2 to 0.4 unit/min has also been used, although investigations in adults suggest that this is no more effective than the peripheral intravenous route of administration.

If bleeding persists, balloon tamponade or palliative surgery may be necessary. The aim of immediate surgical therapy is control of bleeding until the child grows and has vessels of adequate size for a portosystemic shunt procedure. Transesophageal or transgastric ligation is followed by bleeding-free periods of 3 to 36 months. Esophagogastrectomy with resection of the lower esophagus and colonic interposition has been advocated, but this has a high surgical mortality and is associated with postoperative reflux esophagitis.

Shunting procedures are less difficult technically in children 5 to 6 years old (60 to 70 pounds). If the splenic vein measures at least 1 cm in diameter, a splenorenal shunt may be performed. If the anastomosed veins are small, thrombosis of the shunt occurs in the majority of cases. Furthermore, such an anastomosis may not effectively reduce portal pressure in those children in whom the shunt remains patent. The portacaval shunt is associated with encephalopathy in adults and children.[5, 92] In portal vein thrombosis, the splenic vein may be small or occluded, making shunting difficult.[93] A shunt in these children has been made by anastomosis of the superior mesenteric vein to the inferior vena cava or mesocaval anastomosis, or more recently by jugular vein interposition.[94]

The natural history of portal vein thrombosis was described in 1974 by Fonkalsrud et al.[95] They documented two important features: the failure rate for a wide variety of surgical procedures is high, and there is a distinct tendency for episodes of variceal bleeding to become less frequent with increasing age in children who have not undergone surgery. Other investigators have reached similar conclusions.[96] Alvarez et al.[90, 91] regard portosystemic shunting as the surgical procedure of choice, and in some patients they propose this as a prophylactic measure before the onset of bleeding. However, since cavernous transformation and collateral circulation may develop, a procedure to produce temporary variceal ablation should be the initial operative approach.

Endoscopic injection sclerosis of esophageal varices is now practiced widely for the control of variceal hemorrhage. Sclerotherapy has also been used for control of variceal hemorrhage in children.[97, 98] Although experience in children is limited, variceal sclerosis should be at least as successful in children as in adults. In the case of extrahepatic portal hypertension, it might be anticipated that the results might be even better since clotting function is normal and because of the tendency for development of collateral circulation. Esophageal variceal sclerotherapy is discussed in Chapter 16.

Cirrhosis

Cirrhosis with portal hypertension and esophageal varices is less common in the pediatric age group than extrahepatic portal hypertension. Liver disease in childhood may be due to infectious, metabolic, and structural problems. The most common causes include postnecrotic cirrhosis following chronic active hepatitis, biliary atresia, and progressive familial cirrhosis such as Byler's disease. Metabolic disorders include cystic fibrosis, alpha-1-antitrypsin deficiency, Wilson's disease, hereditary fructose intolerance, galactosemia, tyrosinemia, and glycogen storage diseases. Congenital hepatic fibrosis, like schistosomiasis, causes presinusoidal intrahepatic portal hypertension and secondary esophageal varices.

The prognosis for most pediatric patients with cirrhosis is poor. Even in biliary atresia where portoenterostomy has been advocated to stop the progression of liver damage, the long-term prognosis is poor for most patients.[99–102] In view of the recent advances in liver transplantation, sclerosis of esophageal varices may become a valuable procedure for control of hemorrhage prior to transplantation.

Esophagitis

Gastroesophageal reflux and esophagitis are common problems in the pediatric age group. Reflux is particularly common during the first 6 months of life, during which time the lower esophageal sphincter undergoes a functional maturation. Children with esophagitis will often complain of "atypical" pain rather than the characteristic "heartburn" that is usually described by adults.

Comparative analysis of the methods for identification of reflux in pediatric patients suggests that the best single test is prolonged pH monitoring.[103–105] Gastroesophageal scintiscanning, esophageal motility, and barium contrast x-rays identify from 50% to 75% of the patients as compared with pH monitoring. However, pH studies do not identify inflammatory mucosal changes that may occur with reflux or as sequelae of reflux, conditions that may require careful follow-up. Likewise, barium contrast radiography does not reliably detect mucosal lesions.[106] For example, barium x-rays demonstrated reflux in 65% of 470 children with and without esophageal disease.[107] Aside from the question of whether or not a barium meal is analogous to ingestion of milk or solid food, radiography frequently gave a false positive result in this study. Double contrast radiography is more sensitive, but less specific because of a higher rate of false-positive examinations.[108]

Endoscopy will provide evidence of gastroesophageal reflux disease in approximately three fourths of the children with positive pH tests.[103] The yield is increased by biopsy of the esophageal mucosa.[109] In a study of 103 children who were being evaluated for gastroesophageal reflux, 13 cases of Barrett's esophagus were discovered.[110] The long-term consequences of this finding are unknown. However, the possibility of carcinoma must be considered until long-term follow-up studies clarify the implications of Barrett's esophagus in pediatric patients.

Editor's note: References 111 and 112 are recent publications of interest.

References

1. Freeman NV. Clinical evaluation of the fiberoptic bronchoscope (Olympus BF 5B) for pediatric endoscopy. J Pediatr Surg 1973; 8:213–20.
2. Salem MR, Bennett EJ, Schweiss JF, et al. Cardiac arrest related to anesthesia. JAMA 1975; 233:238–41.
3. Greenberg HB. Cardiac arrest in 20 infants and children: causes and results of resuscitation. Dis Chest 1965; 47:42–6.
4. Smith R. Anesthesia for infants and children. Mortality in pediatric anesthesia. St. Louis: C.V. Mosby, 1980; 653–61.
5. Hassall E, Benson L, Hart M, Krieger D: Hepatic encephalopathy after portacaval shunt in a noncirrhotic child. J Pediatr 1984; 105:439–41.
6. Hargrove CB, Ulshen MR, Shub MD. Upper gastrointestinal endoscopy in infants: diagnostic usefulness and safety. Pediatrics 1984; 74:828–31.
7. Graham DY, Klish WJ, Ferry GD, Sabel JS. Value of fiberoptic endoscopy in infants and children. South Med J 1978; 71:558–60.
8. Ament ME, Christie DL. Upper gastrointestinal fiberoptic endoscopy in pediatric patients. Gastroenterology 1977; 72:1244–8.
9. Byrne WJ, Euler AR, Campbell M, Eisenach KD. Bacteremia in children following upper gastrointestinal endoscopy or colonoscopy. J Pediatr Gastroenterol Nutr 1982; 4:551–3.
10. Collins REC. Some problems of gastrointestinal bleeding in children. Arch Dis Child 1971; 46:110–2.
11. Spencer R. Gastrointestinal hemorrhage in infancy and childhood: 476 cases. Surgery 1964; 55:718–34.
12. Raffensperger JG, Luck SR. Gastrointestinal bleeding in children. Surg Clin North Am 1976; 56:413–24.
13. Berman WF, Holtzapple PG. Gastrointestinal hemorrhage. Pediatr Clin North Am 1975; 22:885–95.
14. Sherman NJ, Clatworthy HW Jr. Gastrointestinal bleeding in neonates: A study of 94 cases. Surgery 1967; 62:614–9.
15. Hyams JS, Leichtner AM, Schwartz AN. Recent advances in diagnosis and treatment of gastrointestinal hemorrhage in infants and children. J Pediatr 1985; 106:1–9.
16. Cox K, Ament ME. Upper gastrointestinal bleeding in children and adolescents. Pediatrics 1979; 63:408–13.
17. Gryboski JD. The value of upper gastrointestinal endoscopy in children. Dig Dis Sci 1981; 26:17s–21s.
18. Gleason WA, Tedesco FJ, Keating JP, et al. Fiberoptic gastrointestinal endoscopy in infants and children. J Pediatr 1974; 85:810–3.
19. Liebman WM, Thaler MM, Bujanover Y. Endoscopic evaluation of upper gastrointestinal bleeding in the newborn. Am J Gastroenterol 1978; 69:607–8.
20. Tedesco FJ, Goldstein PD, Gleason WA, et al. Upper gastrointestinal endoscopy in the pediatric patient. Gastroenterology 1976; 70:492–4.
21. Stevenson EO, Hastings N. Foreign bodies in the gastrointestinal tract of infants and children. Am Surg 1968; 34:151–8.
22. Daseler EH. Foreign bodies in the gastrointestinal tract. Calif Med 1969; 111:19–22.
23. Jackson C, Jackson CL. Bronchoesophagoscopy. Philadelphia: W. B. Saunders Co., 1950; 13.
24. Grekin TD, Musselman MM. The management of foreign bodies in the alimentary tract. Ann Surg 1952; 135:528–35.
25. Pasquariello PS, Kean H. Cyanosis from a foreign body in the esophagus. Clin Pediatr 1975; 14:223–5.
26. Friedberg SA, Bluestone CD. Foreign body accidents involving the air and food passages in children. Otolaryngol Clin North Am 1970; 3:395.
27. Newman DE. The radiolucent esophageal foreign body: an often-forgotten cause of respiratory symptoms. J Pediatr 1978; 92:60–3.
28. Lewis SR. New use of a metal detector. Pediatrics 1980; 65:680–1.
29. Kassner EG, Rose JS, Kottmeier PK, et al. Retention of small foreign objects in the stomach and duodenum. Radiology 1975; 114:683–6.
30. Mofenson HC, Greensher S, Caraccio TR, et al. Ingestion of small flat disc batteries. Ann Emerg Med 1983; 12:88–90.
31. Benson CD, Lloyd JR. Foreign bodies in the gastrointestinal tract. In: Ravitch RM, Welch KJ, Benson CD, et al., eds. Pediatric Surgery. Chicago: Year Book Medical Publishers, 1979; 897–902.
32. Equen M, Roach G, Brown R. Magnetic removal of foreign bodies from the esophagus, stomach and duodenum. Arch Otolaryngol 1957; 66:698–706.
33. Mandell GA, Rosenberg HK, Schnaufer L. Prolonged retention of foreign bodies in the stomach. Pediatrics 1977; 60:460–2.
34. Litovitz TL. Button battery ingestions: A review of 56 cases. JAMA 1983; 249:2495–500.

35. Janik JS, Burrington JD, Wayne ER, et al. Alkaline battery ingestion. Colo Med 1982; 79:404–5.

36. Kulig K, Rumack CM, Rumack BH, et al. Disc battery ingestions: Elevated urine mercury levels and enema removal of battery fragments. JAMA 1983; 249:2502–4.

37. Votteler TP, Nash JC, Rutledge JC. The hazard of ingested alkaline disc batteries in children. JAMA 1983; 249:2504–6.

38. Beyer P, Muhlendahl KE, Krienke EG. Ingestion von kleinen Queck silberbatterien (Knopfbatterien): Mögliche Komplikationer. Pediatr Prax 1981; 24:455.

39. Litovitz TL. Battery ingestions: Product accessibility and clinical course. Pediatrics 1985; 75:469–76.

40. Blatnik DS, Toohill RJ, Lehman RH. Fatal complication from an alkaline battery foreign body in the esophagus. Ann Otol 1977; 86:611–5.

41. Shabino CL, Feinberg AN. Esophageal perforation secondary to alkaline battery ingestion. JACEP 1979; 8:360–3.

42. Votteler TP. Warning: ingested disc batteries. Tex Med 1981; 77:7 (Feb).

43. Willis GA, Ho WC. Perforation of Meckel's diverticulum by an alkaline hearing aid battery. Can Med Assoc J 1982; 126:497–8.

44. Litovitz T, Butterfield AB, Holloway RR, et al. Button battery ingestion: assessment of therapeutic modalities and battery discharge state. J Pediatr 1984; 105:868–73.

45. Temple DM, McNeese MC. Hazards of battery ingestion. Pediatrics 1983; 71:100–3.

46. Biehusen FC, Pulaski EJ. Lead poisoning after ingestion of foreign body contained in the stomach. N Engl J Med 1956; 254:1179–81.

47. Pellerin D, Fortier-Beaulieu M, Quequan J. The fate of swallowed foreign bodies: experience of 1250 instances of subdiaphragmatic foreign bodies in children. Prog Pediatr Radiol 1969; 2:286.

48. Gaudreault P, Parent M, McGuigan MA, et al. Predictability of esophageal injury from signs and symptoms: a study of caustic ingestion in 378 children. Pediatrics 1983; 71:767–70.

49. Symbas PN, Vlasis SE, Hatcher CR Jr. Esophagitis secondary to ingestion of caustic material. Ann Thorac Surg 1983; 36:73–7.

50. Chung RS, DenBesten L. Fiberoptic endoscopy in treatment of corrosive injury of the stomach. Arch Surg 1975; 110:725–8.

51. Welsh JJ, Welsh LW. Endoscopic examination of corrosive injuries of the upper gastrointestinal tract. Laryngoscope 1978; 88:1300–9.

52. Buttross S, Brouhard BH. Acute management of alkali ingestion in children: a review. Tex Med 1981; 77:57–60 (Nov).

53. Webb WR, Koutras P, Ecker RR, Sugg W. An evaluation of steroids and antibiotics in caustic burns of the esophagus. Ann Thorac Surg 1970; 9:95–102.

54. Haller JA Jr, Andrews HG, White JJ, et al. Pathophysiology and management of acute corrosive burns of the esophagus: results of treatment in 285 children. J Pediatr Surg 1971; 6:578–84.

55. Marchand P. Caustic strictures of esophagus. Thorax 1955; 10:171–81.

56. Stannard MW. Corrosive esophagitis in children. Am J Dis Child 1978; 132:596–9.

57. Hawkins DB, Demeter MJ, Barnett TE. Caustic ingestion: controversies in management: a review of 214 cases. Laryngoscope 1980; 90:98–109.

58. Kirsh MM, Ritter F. Caustic ingestion and subsequent damage to the oropharyngeal and digestive passages. Ann Thorac Surg 1976; 21:74–82.

59. Holinger PH. Management of esophageal lesions caused by chemical burns. Ann Otol Rhinol Laryngol 1968; 77:819–29.

60. Di Costanzo J, Noirclerc M, Jouglard J, et al. New therapeutic approach to corrosive burns of the upper gastrointestinal tract. Gut 1980; 21:370–5.

61. Messersmith JK, Oglesby JE, Mahoney WD, Baugh JH. Gastric erosion from alkali ingestion. Am J Surg 1970; 119:740–1.

62. Middlekamp JN, Ferguson TB, Roper CL, et al. The management and problem of caustic burns in children. J Thorac Cardiovasc Surg 1969; 57:341–7.

63. Appelgvist P, Salmo M. Lye corrosion carcinoma of the esophagus: a review of 63 cases. Cancer 1980; 45:2655–8.

64. Hopkins RA, Postlethwait RW. Caustic burn and carcinoma of the esophagus. Ann Surg 1981; 194:146–8.

65. Maull KI, Scher LA, Greenfield LJ. Surgical implications of acid ingestion. Surg Gynecol Obstet 1979; 148:895–8.

66. Eaton H, Tennekoon GE. Squamous carcinoma of the stomach following corrosive acid burns. Br J Surg 1972; 59:382–7.

67. Benirschke K. Time bomb of lye ingestion? (Editorial) Am J Dis Child 1981; 135:17–8.

68. Kiviranta UK. Corrosion carcinoma of the esophagus: 381 cases of corrosion and nine cases of corrosion carcinoma. Acta Otolaryngol 1952; 42:89–95.

69. Von Siebold AE. Brand in der Kleinen curvatier des Mageseines atrophischen Kindes. J Geburtsh Frauenzimmer Kinderkr 1826; 5:3.

70. Bird CE, Limper MA, Mayer JM. Surgery in peptic ulceration of the stomach and duodenum in infants and children. Ann Surg 1941; 114:526–42.

71. Tudor RB. Letter to the editor. Peptic ulcer in childhood. Lancet 1974; 2:219.

72. Ramos AR, Kirsner JR, Palmer WL. Peptic ulcer disease in children. Am J Dis Child 1960; 99:135–9.

73. Michener WM, Kennedy RLJ, Dujhare JW. Duodenal ulcer in childhood. Am J Dis Child 1960; 100:814–7.

74. Schuster SR, Gross RE. Peptic ulcer disease in childhood. Am J Surg 1963; 105:324–33.

75. Thompson NB, Jewett TC. Peptic ulcers in infancy and childhood. JAMA 1964; 189:539–42.

76. Gieske JP, Storey B. Duodenal ulcer in infants. Bull John Hopkins Hosp 1966; 118:499–506.

77. Rosenlund ML, Koop CE. Duodenal ulcer in childhood. Pediatrics 1970; 45:283–6.

78. Prouty M. Juvenile ulcers. Am Fam Physician 1970; 2:66–71.

79. Seagram CGF, Stephens CA, Cumming WA. Peptic ulceration at the Hospital for Sick Children, Toronto, during the 20 year period, 1949–1969. J Pediatr Surg 1973; 8:407–13.

80. Deckelbaum RJ, Roy CC, Lussier-Lazaroff J, et al. Peptic ulcer disease: a clinical study in 73 children. Can Med Assoc J 1974; 111:225–8.

81. Grosfeld JL, Shipley F, Fitzgerald JF, et al. Acute peptic ulcer disease in infancy and childhood. Am Surg 1978; 44:13–9.

82. Nord KS, Lebanthal E. Peptic ulcer in children. Am J Gastroenterol 1980; 73:75–80.

83. Sultz HA, Schlesinger ER, Feldman JG, et al. The epidemiology of peptic ulcer in childhood. Am J Public Health 1970; 60:492–8.

84. Miranti JP. A review of experience with peptic ulcer in adolescents and young adults in a university health service. J Am Coll Health Assoc 1970; 18:381.

85. Nickey LN, Huchton P, Campbell JJ. Childhood peptic ulcer—a common entity in our turned on world. Tex Med 1972; 68:80–3.

86. Habbick BF, Melrose AC, Grant JC. Duodenal ulcer in childhood. Arch Dis Child 1968; 43:23–7.

87. Christie DL, Ament ME. Gastric acid hypersecretion in children with duodenal ulcer. Gastroenterology 1976; 71:242–4.

88. Buchta RM, Kaplan JM. Zollinger-Ellison syndrome in a nine-year-old child: a case report and review of the entity in childhood. Pediatrics 1971; 47:594–8.

89. Alagille D, Odievre M. Liver and biliary tract disease in children. New York: Wiley-Flammarion, 1979.

90. Alvarez F, Bernard O, Brunelle F, et al. Portal obstruction in children I. Clinical investigation and hemorrhage risk. J Pediatr 1983; 103:696–702.

91. Alvarez F, Bernard O, Brunelle F, et al. Portal obstruction in children II. Results of surgical portosystemic shunts. J Pediatr 1983; 103:703–7.

92. Voorhees AB, Chaitman E, Schneider S, et al. Portal-systemic encephalopathy in the noncirrhotic patient: effect of portal-systemic shunting. Arch Surg 1973; 107:659–63.

93. Maksoud JG, Miles S, Carvalho Pinto V. Distal splenorenal shunt in children. J Ped Surg 1978; 13:335–40.

94. Altman RP, Potter BM. Portal decompression in infants and children with the interposition mesocaval shunt. Am J Surg 1978; 135:65–9.

95. Fonkalsrud EW, Myers NA, Robinson MJ. Management of extrahepatic portal hypertension in children. Ann Surg 1974; 180:487–93.

96. Mikkelsen WP. Extrahepatic portal hypertension in children. Am J Surg 1966; 111:333–40.

97. Lilly JR. Endoscopic sclerosis of oesophageal varices in children. Surg Gynecol Obstet 1981; 152:513–4.

98. Dall' Oglio L, Bagolan P, Ferro F, et al. Endoscopic injection sclerosis of oesophageal varices in children—indications and techniques. Endoscopy 1984; 16:98–100.

99. Kasai M. Results of surgery for biliary atresia. In: Javitt NB, ed. Neonatal hepatitis and biliary atresia. Bethesda, MD: U.S. Department of Health, Education and Welfare, 1979; 417–33.

100. Berenson MM, Garde AR, Moody FG. Twenty-five year survival after surgery for complete extrahepatic biliary atresia. Gastroenterology 1974; 66:260–3.

101. Arima E, Kikuchi J, Sakoguchi Y, Atika K. Surgically correctable biliary atresia—A follow-up study. Acta Med Universitat Kogoschimaensis 1976; 18:39–45.

102. Psacharopoulos HT, Howard ER, Portmann B, et al. Extrahepatic biliary atresia: Preoperative assessment and surgical results in 47 consecutive cases. Arch Dis Child 1980; 55:851–6.

103. Arasu T, Wyllie R, Fitzgerald JF, et al. Gastroesophageal reflux in infants and children—comparative accuracy of diagnostic methods. J Pediatr 1980; 96:798–803.

104. Boix-Ochoa J, Lafuente JM, Gil-Vernet JM. Twenty-four hour esophageal pH monitoring in gastroesophageal reflux. J Pediatr Surg 1980; 15:74–8.

105. Fink S, McCallum RW. The role of prolonged esophageal pH monitoring in the diagnosis of gastroesophageal reflux. JAMA 1984; 252: 1160–4.

106. Gyepes MT, Smith LE, Ament ME. Fiberoptic endoscopy and upper gastrointestinal series: Comparative analysis in infants and children. Am J Roentgenol 1977; 128:53–6.

107. Cleveland RH, Kushner DC, Schwartz AN. Gastroesophageal reflux in children: results of a standardized fluoroscopic approach. AJR 1983; 141: 53–6.

108. Creteur V, Thoeni RF, Federle MP, Allred EN. Role of single- and double-contrast radiography in the diagnosis of reflux esophagitis. Radiology 1983; 147:71–5.

109. Biller JA, Winter HS, Grand RJ, et al. Are endoscopic changes predictive of histologic esophagitis in children? J Pediatr 1983; 103:215–8.

110. Barrett Dahms B, Rothstein FC. Barrett's esophagus in children: a consequence of chronic gastroesophageal reflux. Gastroenterology 1984; 86: 318–23.

111. Shub MD, Ulshen MH, Hargrove CB, et al. Esophagitis: a frequent consequence of gastroesophageal reflux in infancy. J Pediatr 1985; 107:881–4.

112. Hassall E, Weinstein WM, Ament ME. Barrett's esophagus in childhood. Gastroenterology 1985; 89:1331–7.

Chapter 14

FOREIGN BODY EXTRACTION IN THE GASTROINTESTINAL TRACT

ROBERT A. SANOWSKI, M.D.

Ingestion of a foreign body is a common occurrence. Fortunately, most foreign objects will pass without causing symptoms. Only 10% to 20% fail to traverse the entire gastrointestinal tract.[1] In a Swedish study, the incidence of hospitalization for foreign body ingestion was 122 per million population per year.[2] A high mortality rate is reported in psychotic patients who ingest foreign objects because of the bizarre objects swallowed and difficulty encountered in making the diagnosis.[3] In the United States, approximately 1500 deaths occur each year as a consequence of foreign body ingestion.[4]

Because of the remarkable variety of articles eaten, the endoscopist must be able to use various instruments to remove objects that impact the esophagus, stomach, and duodenum. The imagination of the physician is often tested by the variation in size, shape, and potential for damage to the alimentary tract of ingested material. The decision to remove an object will be influenced by a number of factors, including the age and clinical status of the patient; the size, shape, and nature of the material ingested; the anatomic area in which the object is lodged; and the technical ability of the endoscopist. Fiberoptic instruments with minor modifications, and using the available accessories, facilitate removal with minimal mortality and morbidity.

Those who swallow foreign objects are most commonly children, psychotic patients, accidental swallowers, or manipulative swallowers. Smooth, round objects will usually pass through the alimentary tract, but hospitalization for endoscopic removal of the object is required when a foreign body has lodged proximal to the diaphragmatic hiatus.[5] Psychotic and mentally retarded patients may ingest great quantities of bizarre materials, necessitating endoscopic or surgical removal.[6] Prisoners may swallow foreign bodies as a manipulative measure. In this group, diagnosis is not difficult since the patient is aware of the occurrence and communicates the fact for the purpose of obtaining secondary gain (e.g., a hospital stay with endoscopic therapy is preferable to prison). Alcoholism, both acute and chronic, is frequently associated with foreign body ingestion and food bolus impaction.

Elderly individuals with dentures may have poor gingival sensation and thus be unable to detect swallowed bones. Loose or broken dentures may become dislodged and impact in the upper gastrointestinal tract. Poor vision and rapid eating associated with poor mastication can compound the problem.

The materials that are ingested consist of a wide variety of substances limited only by human imagination and the size of the oropharyngeal cavity. Generally, three types of material can lodge in the gastrointestinal tract: bezoars consisting of hair or vegetable matter; food impactions; and true foreign bodies such as bones, coins, dentures, and pins. The types of true foreign body ingested vary according to the patient's age, occupation, and dietary habits. Fish and chicken bones are a common source of impaction in Oriental populations.[7] Dentures, toothpicks, wire, pins, and tacks may be swallowed accidentally by the older patient or by those whose occupation involves use of any of these objects. The majority of patients ingesting true foreign bodies are younger than age 40. Food impaction usually occurs in those older than 60 years.[8]

ANATOMY OF IMPACTION

The sites of impaction in the gastrointestinal tract are the normal anatomic as well as pathologic points of narrowing. Once beyond the oropharynx, pointed objects lodge in the pyriform sinuses and valleculae. Approximately 50% to 80% of esophageal foreign bodies are arrested in the cervical esophagus, and the remainder lodge in the upper thoracic and distal esophagus.[7] The normal anatomic points of narrowing at the level of the cricopharyngeus muscle, aortic arch, left main stem bronchus, and cardioesophageal junction entrap sharp foreign bodies. Objects impacted at the aortic arch may perforate into the aorta, leading to an aortoesophageal fistula and exsanguination.[7]

After passing through the esophagus, most foreign bodies will clear the remainder of the alimentary tract. However, if the objects are long (such as spoons, wires, springs) or hair or other material that will not pass the pylorus, impaction and obstruction may occur at this level. Other points of anatomic narrowing are the duodenum, ileocecal valve, Meckel's diverticulum and anus.

Impaction and obstruction may occur at pathologic points of narrowing in the stomach, duodenum, and ileum. Esophageal stricture, hiatal hernia, and tortuosity of the cardioesophageal junction are frequently associated with food impaction. Carcinoma of the esophagus uncommonly results in the arrest of a foreign body.[7] This may be explained by the gradual development of stenosis caused by the growing tumor, and the resultant caution exercised by patients to avoid obstruction. Obstruction of stents placed in the esophagus to palliate encroaching carcinoma occasionally occurs. Stenosis of the pylorus, alterations in the stomach after operation, and impaired gastric emptying are associated with retention of foreign bodies. Ileal strictures can trap swallowed materials.

The alimentary tract is capable of passing 90% of sharp objects, including needles. This is explained by a hypothesized reflex of mural relaxation of the intestinal musculature. Axial flow in the intestinal lumen, combined with reflex relaxation and slowing of peristalsis, tends to turn these objects around, thus making the sharper end trail rather than lead.[1] In the colon, foreign objects become covered with fecal material which protects the bowel wall.

CLINICAL FEATURES

Presenting symptoms resulting from a gastrointestinal foreign body vary. The presentation may be acute, and the patient may recall in detail the time and type of foreign body ingestion. However, in children, the mentally deranged or retarded, or those ingesting objects for secondary gain, complications related to the presence of a foreign body may bring the patient to the physician.

Symptoms vary depending on the area of lodgement. In adults, foreign bodies in the esophagus cause pain and discomfort on swallowing. There may be a persistent sensation or awareness, on swallowing, of a foreign body (such as a fish bone). The saliva may become blood-stained, and there may be a history of gagging or choking during meals. Children, on the other hand, may refuse to take feedings, have increased salivation, pain and discomfort on swallowing and vomiting. Fever, pain, and tenderness in the neck may indicate perforation, and a high index of suspicion of foreign body ingestion must be considered for patients with severe psychotic or emotional problems or mental retardation.

Sudden onset of dysphagia after eating or drinking indicates lodgement of a foreign body or impacted food. Impacted food is commonly roast beef, steak, chicken, or other meat with a stringy texture. A patient with symptoms of esophageal reflux and a history of foreign body ingestion or food bolus impaction is a prime candidate for a repetition of this problem. Gastric foreign bodies are frequently associated with partial or complete outlet obstruction with accompanying characteristic symptomatology.

Physical findings are not remarkable unless the foreign body can be palpated in the pharynx or a mass is present in the abdomen, such as occurs with a trichobezoar. Nonspecific, mild abdominal tenderness and a decrease in bowel sounds may be present.

DIAGNOSTIC EVALUATION

A plain roentgenogram should be the first study if the object is thought to be radiopaque, since it may be localized easily with anteroposterior and lateral views. Care must be taken to ascertain whether the object is in the airway or extraluminal air is present. Objects such as fish and chicken bones, glass, wood, and plastic are not radiopaque. Special radiographic techniques for viewing the soft tissues of the neck may be necessary to outline thin metallic objects.

If impaction has occurred in the esophagus, a contrast study is required. To avoid aspiration, a small amount of barium should be used which can be suctioned from the esophagus after definition of the object and anatomic circumstances. If there is evidence of perforation, a water-soluble agent such as Gastrografin is preferred. Since Gastrografin is irritating to the tracheobronchial tree, its use should be avoided whenever aspiration is a possibility. Chicken bones and other nonopaque foreign bodies may be found only by endoscopy.

COMPLICATIONS OF FOREIGN BODY INGESTION

In a review of more than 2000 cases of esophageal foreign bodies,[7] 24 serious complications, including three deaths, occurred. Perforation and abscess formation in the neck were the most common complications; mediastinitis, lung abscess, and esophageal-aortic fistula also occurred. Probably less than 1% of all ingested foreign bodies cause a perforation.[8] Esophageal and gastric foreign bodies may be vomited and aspirated. Gastric perforation can result from ingestion of metal wires and paper clips.[9] On leaving the stomach, a foreign body may impact and perforate the appendix, a Meckel's diverticulum, the ileum, cecum, and various locations in the colon.[10] Problems with swallowed dental materials, including fatal ingestion of a dental prosthesis, have been reported.[11, 12]

Systemic toxicity may be associated with ingestion of certain foreign bodies. Small disc batteries that are used as an energy source for watches, hearing aids, and cameras are easily swallowed by small children. These contain alkali, such as potassium hydroxide, and the heavy metals mercury and cadmium.[13–16] Endoscopic or surgical removal is mandatory if the battery remains in the stomach for more than 24 hours or lodges in other parts of the intestine. Toxicity depends on leakage from the casing, duration of contact with the mucosa, and the inherent toxicity of the chemicals themselves. Alkali in

significant quantities can produce a local caustic action and perforation. The heavy metals may be absorbed, producing systemic toxicity.

Cocaine and other narcotics may cause toxicity in "body packers" who attempt to smuggle illicit drugs by swallowing drug-filled condoms and balloons.[17–20] Intestinal obstruction, respiratory depression, and death may be associated with this practice if impaction and rupture of the latex container occur.

GASTRIC BEZOARS

Gastric bezoars are substances which impact in the stomach. These are classified as phytobezoars, composed of vegetable and fruit fiber, and trichobezoars, consisting of hair; others may be concretions of various materials such as shellac, sand, and medications. Trichobezoars were thought to be the most common. However, phytobezoars are frequently seen in the postgastrectomy stomach and in other conditions associated with gastric stasis or obstruction.[21–24]

Trichobezoars

Trichobezoars are most commonly seen in women with long hair who are younger than 30 years. These patients may ingest not only their own hair but also that of other persons and animals and also carpet fibers and other synthetic or natural fibers.[21] Evidence of hair loss may be present, and an abdominal mass is sometimes palpable. Upper gastrointestinal roentgenographic series will demonstrate a large, irregular, intraluminal filling defect. The trichobezoar will be visible endoscopically as a dark, hairy mass with intermeshed food materials and debris.[24]

Phytobezoars

Phytobezoars frequently develop following partial gastric resection, in association with disturbances of gastric emptying, or with gastric atony of any cause. The chief component of these bezoars is the fibrous, pithy material of vegetables and fruits, particularly oranges. Upper gastrointestinal roentgenograms will demonstrate an intragastric mass, and the endoscopist will visualize clumps of white or orange-colored food material and identifiable food stuffs such as celery, carrots, and vegetable leaves. Ingestion of unripened persimmons is associated with phytobezoar formation.

Symptoms may be absent or nonspecific; occasionally gastric obstruction develops. Complaints relating to the presence of a trichobezoar may be mild, but complications such as ulceration, bleeding, and perforation may occur.[21]

TREATMENT OF INGESTED FOREIGN BODIES

After the diagnosis of foreign body ingestion has been made and the object located radiographically, the necessity for removal is considered. Since 90% of such objects will pass spontaneously, observation is indicated in the case of small objects such as coins, nails, and pins and objects which are round or have smooth edges. Cathartics and other medications that increase peristalsis should be avoided. Objects lodged in the hypopharynx should be removed as soon as possible. When impaction has occurred, it is unlikely that the object will pass spontaneously. Edema and local trauma tend to lessen the possibility of spontaneous passage. In general, objects lodged in the stomach for more than 72 hours will not pass.

A wide variety of foreign body grasping devices are available commercially along with improvised types to effect removal (Fig. 14–1). Objects trapped above the cricopharyngeal muscle or in the pyriform sinuses should be removed under direct vision with a laryngoscope. Impactions below the cricopharyngeal muscle are removable with a fiberoptic endoscope. Rigid endoscopy is rarely needed, since fiberoptic endoscopy is safer and may be performed without general anesthesia.

Prior to endoscopy, adult patients and older children can be sedated with intravenous meperidine and diazepam.[25] Children less than 2 years of age require general endotracheal anesthesia. Intubation is necessary to avoid sudden aspiration of the foreign body as it is being removed and to prevent tracheal compression.

The endoscope should be passed under direct vision to view the entire circumference of the lumen and visualize a foreign body located in the most proximal segment of the esophagus. The majority of esophageal foreign bodies are arrested immediately distal to the cricopharyngeus.[7] If contraction of the cricopharyngeal muscle causes difficulty, the endoscope is removed and inserted into an

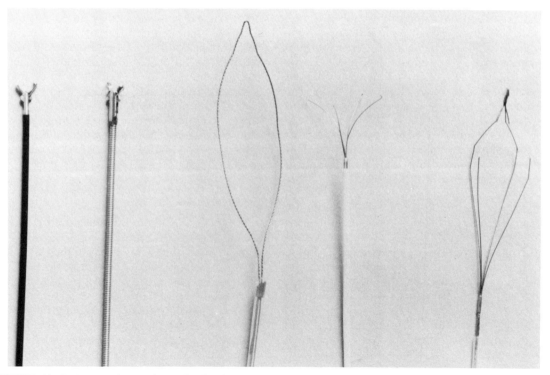

FIGURE 14–1. Accessories available for foreign body removal. Foreign body forceps, biopsy forceps, polyp snare, polyp retriever, retrieval basket (*left to right*).

overtube. The endoscope and overtube are then passed together. An overtube has proved to be useful for removing impacted objects from the esophagus, stomach, and duodenum. One can be made simply from polyvinyl tubing, which should be long enough to reach the foreign body and extend out of the patient's mouth.[26] The overtube affords better visualization of the area immediately distal to the cricopharyngeus, aids in keeping this area open, and protects the patient from aspiration. Suction and lavage are easily performed through the overtube without damage to mucosa. Sharp objects such as glass, needles, pins, or dental bridges lodged at any point in the esophagus may be withdrawn into the overtube with a forceps or other suitable instrument, thus avoiding laceration of the mucosa (Fig. 14–2). Should esophageal spasm inhibit removal, 1.0 mg of intravenous glucagon may induce relaxation.

A polypectomy snare can be used to remove large foreign bodies such as chicken bones.[27] Smooth, round objects can be retrieved with a stone basket. Coins can be removed easily with a foreign body forceps. (Various types of foreign bodies are shown in Plate 14–1.)

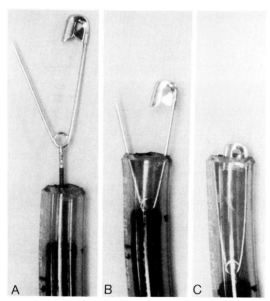

FIGURE 14–2. Overtube-endoscope technique for removal of safety pin from stomach. A, The safety pin is grasped at the blunt end with a foreign body forceps which has been passed through the accessory channel of the endoscope. Note the endoscope within the transparent overtube. B, The safety pin is pulled into the overtube with the grasping forceps. C, The endoscope is withdrawn into the overtube which pulls the safety pin further into the overtube. The overtube and endoscope may be withdrawn safely at the same time.

The endoscopist must be certain that perforation has not occurred. Follow-up plain roentgenograms of the mediastinum to assess for extraluminal air may be indicated, as well as barium contrast studies. Nasogastric suction and broad-spectrum antibiotics are required if there is evidence of a perforation, and surgical intervention must be considered.

METHODS FOR FOOD BOLUS REMOVAL

Several common abnormalities that alter normal anatomy can lead to meat impaction in the esophagus. Most common are hiatal hernia with an associated Schatkzi ring, peptic esophageal stricture, and carcinoma. Long-standing intermittent dysphagia is characteristic. Many of these patients wear dentures or have no teeth. Frequently there is a history of overindulgence in alcoholic beverages during the time that the impaction occurred.[28, 29]

A number of therapeutic modalities have been developed over the years to treat the problem of food bolus removal. The procedure has been simplified by the development of fiberoptic endoscopy and the use of the overtube.

At the initial examination an esophagram should be performed to locate the site of bolus obstruction. Since abnormalities such as hiatal hernia, lower esophageal Schatzki ring, and concomitant esophageal spasm may be the cause of the esophageal obstruction, 1.0 mg of glucagon should be given intravenously. A barium swallow can then be repeated after several minutes, at which time the bolus may have passed into the stomach.[30] If this is unsuccessful, endoscopic extraction is indicated.

In the past, enzymatic digestion of meat impactions using papain has been advocated.[31, 32] However, its effectiveness and safety are questionable, since perforation, aspiration, and death have occurred with its use.[28–33]

Removal of the obstructing mass should be performed on an emergency basis if there is associated discomfort or pain, straining, salivation, or aspiration.[34] The bolus may have been present for hours or days, in which case it is not likely to be dislodged easily. Prompt removal is necessary to avoid the complications of aspiration and a Mallory-Weiss laceration secondary to vomiting.

Fatal esophageal perforation by direct instrumental trauma during endoscopic extrac-

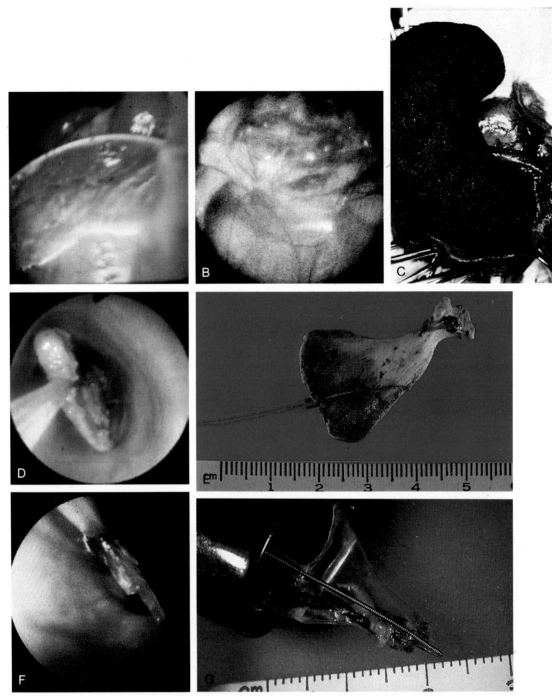

PLATE 14–1. *A,* Endoscopic view of a swallowed penny in a 53-year-old patient with partial gastric outlet obstruction. Coin removed with foreign body forceps. *B,* Endoscopic view of a hairy, foul-smelling mass in the stomach of a 15-year-old girl who had been ingesting her hair. *C,* Gross surgical specimen, a large trichobezoar, removed from the stomach of the same patient as in *B. D,* Endoscopic view of a bone impacted proximal to the cardioesophageal junction in a 60-year-old woman with dysphagia and chest pain. She had ingested fried chicken the previous night. *E,* Large chicken bone seen in Fig. 14-3D has been removed with a polypectomy snare. *F,* Endoscopic view of a piece of glass ingested by a 72-year-old woman. A polypectomy snare encircles the broken glass. *G,* The piece of glass shown in *F* is seen grasped in its long axis a snare at the edge of a black overtube.

Illustration continued on opposite page

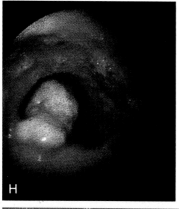

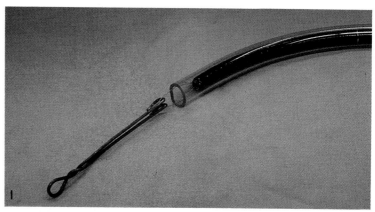

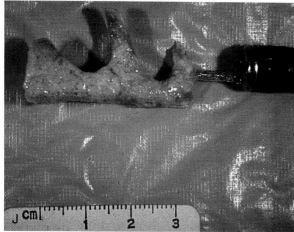

PLATE 14–1 Continued. H, Endoscopic view in an 84-year-old man with meat impacted proximal to the cardioesophageal junction. A four-pronged polyp grasper was used to remove the impaction. I, Pieces of bedspring removed from the stomach of a 40-year-old prisoner. The endoscope-overtube technique was used. J, Large bone removed from the esophagus of a 43-year-old man. (F, G, H and J courtesy of Dr. R. McCray.)

tion has been reported; however, use of an overtube will protect the esophageal mucosa and airway during removal.[8, 26, 35] After passage of the overtube and endoscope, the bolus can be identified and may be removed piecemeal with foreign body forceps or a polypectomy snare. Lavage and suction may also be performed through the overtube without fear of aspiration. After the bolus has been reduced in size, it will generally slide into the stomach, or it can be removed easily through the overtube. Intravenous administration of glucagon during the endoscopic extraction may shorten the procedure.

A quick method for removal of a meat bolus has been described that uses a modified gastric lavage tube and aspiration syringe. This simple aspiration technique has been used as an outpatient procedure to remove soft meat impactions and has proved to be safe and effective.[28] This suction maneuver also may be used through the overtube, avoiding possible aspiration as the meat is pulled past the airway (Fig. 14–3). In general,

use of an overtube is advised for removal of most foreign bodies from the esophagus.

REMOVAL OF GASTRODUODENAL FOREIGN BODIES

Impaired progression of a foreign body through the stomach will necessitate its removal, especially if the object is large, long, sharp, or potentially toxic. The techniques used in conjunction with fiberoptic endoscopy described above can also remove most gastroduodenal foreign bodies. In preparation for endoscopic removal, it may be helpful to practice grasping objects similar to those that have been ingested. Determination of the best endoscopic accessory for grasping the object prior to the actual attempt will shorten the procedure and increase safety.

The overtube is especially useful when several objects must be recovered (Fig. 14–4). Small objects can be grasped and pulled into the overtube. For larger ones, such as pens, pencils, spoons, and wires, which are more difficult to remove, a snare or a special grasp-

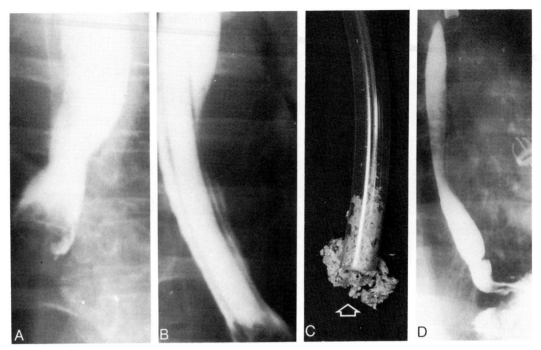

FIGURE 14–3. Rapid suction method for removing impacted meat. *A*, Barium swallow demonstrating bolus impacted in hiatal hernia. *B*, Radiograph showing large-bore tube passed into the esophagus with suction applied. *C*, Suction tube after removal from patient. Meat was suctioned into distal end (*arrow*). *D*, Follow-up barium swallow showing hiatal hernia and Schatzki ring.

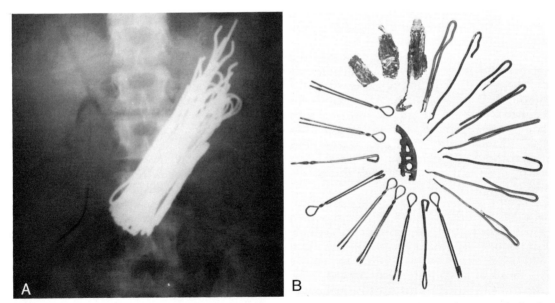

FIGURE 14–4. *A*, Plain roentgenogram of the abdomen of a 40-year-old prisoner with multiple metallic foreign bodies in stomach. *B*, Twenty-one pieces of bedsprings, wires, toothpaste tubes and shower grating removed endoscopically without complications from the patient described in *A*.

ing or foreign body forceps should be passed ahead of the endoscope; if grasped properly, the object can frequently be pulled into the overtube. It may be necessary to hyperextend the patient's neck to bring a large foreign body through the posterior hypopharynx.

The use of a polypectomy snare to grasp and remove large, irregular objects such as peach pits, metallic rings, springs, hat pins, and a coat hanger has been reported.[36–38] Open safety pins in the stomach pose a potential hazard of mucosal injury during removal. This may be reduced by using a polypectomy snare to close the pin prior to removal or by retracting it into an overtube.[39]

The use of magnets for removal of metallic foreign bodies has been successful. However, the endoscopic-overtube method is more precise and obviates loss of an object at points of anatomic narrowing or in the airway.[40]

Objects that lodge in the duodenum should be pulled back into the stomach using a polypectomy snare and then removed as a gastric foreign body. Glucagon can be used to achieve relaxation of the antrum and pylorus. A long overtube may be used to keep the pylorus open while extracting the object from the duodenum with a polypectomy snare.

REMOVAL OF GASTRODUODENAL BEZOARS

In the past, bezoars were considered omens of good luck and were thought to have medicinal qualities. However, it is now known that, as gastric foreign bodies, they can cause bleeding, obstruction, perforation, and death.[21]

Enzyme therapy is ineffective and contraindicated for trichobezoars, which must be removed surgically. Treatment of phytobezoars consists of disruption of the bezoar at endoscopy, followed by lavage of the stomach through an overtube with large amounts of water. Most phytobezoars can be cleared from the stomach in this manner. The use of enzymes to chemically break up phytobezoars has been unsuccessful. Those that obstruct the small intestine must be removed surgically. Patients with partial gastric resections should be advised of the nature of phytobezoar formation, especially in regard to the foodstuffs that are responsible. Metoclopramide is useful in some instances of disordered gastric motility.

Almost anything that can be swallowed can be removed endoscopically.[41] Recent studies

report few complications associated with endoscopic removal.[8] The success rate for endoscopic removal of foreign bodies is about 85%. Advances in instrument technology have helped to make this approach a safe, widely used therapeutic modality.

FOREIGN BODIES IN THE RECTUM

Foreign bodies in the colon and rectum are becoming a common problem because of changing customs, mores, and social milieux and an increase in the number and variety of objects used for transrectal sexual gratification. The types of foreign bodies encountered in a recent review included vibrators, rubber and metal balls, rubber phalluses, screwdrivers, paperweights, and a cucumber.[42]

When objects are introduced into the anal canal they slip into the rectum, and because of sphincter spasm, may not be retrieved by the patient. Usually, the foreign body remains in the rectum or sigmoid, but occasionally may advance into the descending colon. Rectal and anal injury may occur from inserting the object or from attempts to remove it by the patient or physician.

Patients generally complain of abdominal pain, rectal bleeding, or discharge. The history may be limited because of patient embarrassment.

Management

If a rectal foreign body is suspected, a rectal examination may reveal its presence. A plain radiographic examination of the abdomen is required to locate metallic objects and check for signs of a perforation. If perforation exists, the problem becomes a surgical one.

Most objects can be removed in the emergency room, and standard rigid proctosigmoidoscopy should be performed routinely if a foreign body is suspected. If lacerations are noted, or if bleeding or perforation is present or suspected, the patient should be hospitalized. Increased experience in removal of rectal foreign bodies with the flexible fiberoptic colonoscope has decreased the need for surgical intervention[43]; however, surgery may be necessary for removal of large objects.

Endoscopic removal is indicated if the foreign body is small and can be withdrawn through a rigid sigmoidoscope or removed with a colonoscope. Biopsy forceps, polypectomy snares, or other surgical instruments may be used for extraction. Objects such as balloons have been removed from the transverse colon with the colonoscope without complications.[44]

Topical anesthesia may be used to induce anal sphincter relaxation if larger objects are to be removed. Bottles may create suction in the bowel when they are turned upward. A Foley catheter passed around the object may relieve the suction and facilitate removal.[45] Obstetrical forceps may be of assistance in removal, but caudal or general anesthesia is necessary for this procedure. Light bulbs, bottles, and vibrators may be difficult to extract because of their size, but under spinal anesthesia the anus can be satisfactorily dilated and the object removed[46] (Fig. 14–5).

After removal, sigmoidoscopy should be performed to assess for laceration of the bowel wall. Patients should be observed for 24 hours to be certain that a perforation has not occurred. Perforation, a serious complication, occurred in 6 of 36 patients in a well-studied series.[42]

Editor's note: References 47 to 50 are recent publications of interest.

References

1. Davidoff E, Towne JB. Ingested foreign bodies. NY State J Med 1975; 75:103–7.
2. Haglund S, Haverling M, Kuylenstierna R, Lind MG. Radiographic diagnosis of foreign bodies in the esophagus. J Laryngol Otol 1978; 92:1117–25.
3. Teimourian B, Cigtay AS, Smyth NP. Management of ingested foreign bodies in the psychotic patient. Arch Surg 1964; 88:915–20.
4. Devanesan J, Pisani A, Sharma P, et al. Metallic foreign bodies in the stomach. Arch Surg 1977; 112:664–5.
5. Erbes J, Babbitt DP. Foreign bodies in the alimentary tract of infants and children. Appl Ther 1965; 7:1103–9.
6. Bitar DE, Holmes TW Jr. Polybezoar and gastrointestinal foreign bodies in the mentally retarded. Am Surg 1975; 41:497–504.
7. Nandi P, Ong GB. Foreign bodies in the oesophagus: review of 2,394 cases. Br J Surg 1978; 65:5–9.
8. Vizcarrondo FJ, Brady PG, Nord HJ. Foreign bodies of the upper gastrointestinal tract. Gastrointest Endosc 1983; 29:208–10.
9. Sartory A, Trabant G. Endoscopic extraction of a perforating paperclip from the stomach. Endoscopy 1978; 10:217–8.
10. MacManus JE. Perforations of the intestine by ingested foreign bodies; report of 2 cases and review of the literature. Am J Surg 1941; 53:393–402.
11. Raff L, Kalish SB, Vye M. Wolff MP. Fatal ingestion of a radiolucent dental prosthesis. South Med J 1981; 74:900–1.
12. Makrauer FL, Davis JS. Gastroscopic removal of a partial denture. J Am Dent Assoc 1977; 94:904–6.
13. Mofenson HC, Greensher J, Caraccio TR, et al. Ingestion of small flat disc batteries. Ann Emerg Med 1983; 12:88.
14. Janik JS, Burrington JD, Wayne ER, Foley LC. Alkaline battery ingestion. Colo Med 1982; 79:404–5.
15. Kulig K, Rumack CM, Rumack BH, Duffy JP. Disk battery ingestion. Elevated urine mercury levels and enema removal of battery fragments. JAMA 1983; 249:2502–4.
16. Votteler TP, Nash JC, Rutledge JC. The hazard of ingested alkaline batteries in children. JAMA 1983; 249:2504–6.
17. Suarez CA, Arango A, Lester JL III. Cocaine-condom ingestion. Surgical treatment. JAMA 1977; 238:1391–2.
18. Seaman WB. The case of the abdominal smuggler. Hosp Pract 1982; 17:74–9 (Dec.).
19. Weber F, Williams G, Swartz MA. Effect of ipecac in "body packers." Ann Emerg Med 1982; 11:699.
20. Fainsinger MH. Unusual foreign bodies in bowel. JAMA 1977; 237:2225–6.
21. Deslypere JP, Praet M, Verdonk G. An unusual case of the trichobezoar: the Rapunzel syndrome. Am J Gastroenterol 1982; 77:467–70.

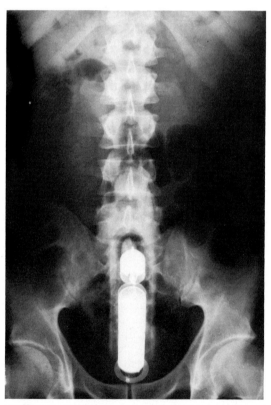

FIGURE 14–5. Plain roentgenogram of the pelvis and abdomen in a 34-year-old male with 23 cm battery-powered vibrator in rectum. The vibrator was removed with the aid of a speculum, with the patient under general anesthesia.

22. Edell S, Wagner DK. Duodenal stenosis contributing to bezoar formation. Clin Pediatr 1971; 10:543–5.

23. Buchholz RR. Phytobezoars following gastric surgery. Med Times 1976; 104:82–9 (Aug).

24. Sanowski RA, DiBianco J Jr. Pseudotumors of the stomach. Am J Dig Dis 1966; 11:607–14.

25. Christie DL, Ament ME. Removal of foreign bodies from esophagus and stomach with flexible fiberoptic panendoscopes. Pediatrics 1976; 57:931–4.

26. Rogers BHG, Kot C, Meiri S, Epstein M. An overtube for the flexible fiberoptic esophagogastroduodenoscope. Gastrointest Endosc 1982; 28:256–7.

27. Tedesco FJ. Endoscopic removal of foreign bodies using fiberoptic instruments. South Med J 1977; 70:991–2.

28. Kozarek RA, Sanowski RA. Esophageal food impaction: description of a new method for bolus removal. Dig Dis Sci 1980; 25:100–3.

29. Hargrove MD Jr, Boyce HW Jr. Meat impaction of the esophagus. Arch Intern Med 1970; 125:277–81.

30. Ferrucci JT Jr, Long JA Jr. Radiologic treatment of esophageal food impaction using intravenous glucagon. Radiology 1977; 125:25–8.

31. Cavo JW, Koops HJ, Gryboski RA. Use of enzymes for meat impactions in the esophagus. Laryngoscope 1977; 87:630–4.

32. Richardson JR. A new treatment for esophageal obstruction due to meat impaction. Ann Otol 1945; 54:328–48.

33. Goldner F, Danley D. Enzymatic digestion of esophageal meat impaction. (Abstr) William Beaumont Gastrointestinal Symposium, 1983.

34. Palmer ED. Backyard barbecue syndrome. Steak impaction in the esophagus. JAMA 1976; 235:2637–8.

35. Sawyer JL, Lane CE, Foster JH, Daniel RA. Esophageal perforation. An increasing challenge. Ann Thorac Surg 1975; 19:233–4.

36. Griffiths WJ, Bird PC, Zantout I, et al. Fiberoptic endoscopic retrieval of swallowed intragastric foreign objects. J Okla State Med Assoc 1979; 72:67–71.

37. Brady PG, Johnson WF. Removal of foreign bodies: the flexible fiberoptic endoscope. South Med J 1977; 70:702–4.

38. Puppala AR, Cheng JC. Fiberendoscopic extraction of a coiled spring from the stomach. Am J Gastroenterol 1977; 67:278–80.

39. Altman AR, Gottfried EB. Intragastric closure of an ingested open safety pin. Gastrointest Endosc 1978; 24:294–5.

40. Himadi GM, Fischer GJ. Magnetic removal of foreign bodies from the upper gastrointestinal tract. Radiology 1977; 123:226–7.

41. Dunkerley RCD, Shull HJ, Avant GR, Dunn GD. Fiberendoscopic removal of large foreign bodies from the stomach. Gastrointest Endosc 1975; 21:170–1.

42. Barone JE, Yee J, Nealon TF. Management of foreign bodies and trauma of the rectum. Surg Gynecol Obstet 1983; 156:453–7.

43. Oehler JR, Dent TL, Ibrahim MA, Gracie WA Jr. Endoscopic identification and removal of an unusual symptomatic colonic foreign body. Dig Dis Sci 1979; 24:236–9.

44. Wolf L, Geraci K. Colonoscopic removal of balloons from the bowel. Gastrointest Endosc 1977; 24:41.

45. Martin DW, Jr, Naughton JL, Smith LH Jr. Venereal aspects of gastroenterology. West J Med 1979; 130:236–46.

46. Graves RW, Allison JE, Bass RR, Hunt RC. Anal eroticism: two unusual rectal foreign bodies and their removal. South Med J 1983; 76:677–8.

47. Webb WA, McDaniel L, Jones L. Foreign bodies of the upper gastrointestinal tract: current management. South Med J 1984; 77:1083–6.

48. Caruana DS, Weinbach B, Goerg D, Gardner LB. Cocaine-packet ingestion. Diagnosis, management, and natural history. Ann Intern Med 1984; 100:73–4.

49. Nehme-Kingsley A, Abcarian H. Colorectal foreign bodies. Management update. Dis Colon Rectum 1985; 28:941–4.

50. Selivanov V, Sheldon GF, Cello JP, Crass RA. Management of foreign body ingestion. Ann Surg 1984; 199:187–91.

Chapter 15

ESOPHAGEAL MOTILITY AND MISCELLANEOUS DISORDERS*

DAVID A. PEURA, M.D.
LAWRENCE F. JOHNSON, M.D.

This chapter deals with the endoscopic evaluation of esophageal motility disorders and other miscellaneous conditions which involve the esophagus. Although these may be associated with symptoms such as chest pain, dysphagia, and regurgitation, the symptoms are nonspecific. Thus, most patients with these disorders undergo endoscopy to exclude benign and malignant obstructive and mucosal diseases that cause similar symptoms. Endoscopy is very effective as a diagnostic tool to exclude obstructive and mucosal abnormalities, but is of limited value in assessing disorders of esophageal peristalsis and emptying. Therefore, the evaluation of these conditions should include other investigative techniques such as a barium esophagram, esophageal scintigraphy, and esophageal manometry.

ESOPHAGEAL MOTILITY DISORDERS

Achalasia

Achalasia is an esophageal motility disorder characterized by loss of peristalsis and a hypertensive lower esophageal sphincter that relaxes incompletely with swallowing, both of which result in impaired esophageal emptying.[1,2] To some degree, the clinical presentation of patients with achalasia varies according to the point at which medical attention is sought in the course of the disease.[3] Dysphagia and chest pain occur early, whereas regurgitation and weight loss are more prom-

inent with long-standing disease. Our clinical observations of 34 patients with newly diagnosed achalasia who were studied at Walter Reed Army Medical Center between 1977 and 1981 reflect the clinical experience of others, and also provide further insight.[4] All patients had dysphagia for solid food, and the majority also had dysphagia for liquids. Noted by 66% was regurgitation of undigested food that had neither the acidic taste of gastric contents nor the bitter taste of bile. Substernal chest pain was noted by 42%. Interestingly, 42% complained of pyrosis despite the absence of objective evidence of gastroesophageal reflux. Unlike the pyrosis associated with reflux, there was a tendency for that associated with achalasia to occur at times other than the immediate postprandial period, to be unrelieved by antacid, and frequently to awaken patients at night.

Weight loss, a finding previously emphasized in secondary achalasia,[5,6] was seen in 84% of patients. We believe that weight loss was the best parameter for assessment of the chronicity and severity of the disease. It directly correlated with the degree of abnormal esophageal emptying as assessed by radionuclide esophageal transit. Effective treatment, which resulted in decreased symptoms and improved esophageal emptying, was always accompanied by subsequent weight gain.

Diagnosis

Barium swallow x-rays, radioisotope scintigraphy, esophageal motility and esophagoscopy are complementary in the investigation for suspected achalasia. Characteristic roent-

---

*The opinions and assertions contained herein are the private view of the authors and are not to be construed as official or as reflecting the views of the Department of the Army or the Department of Defense.

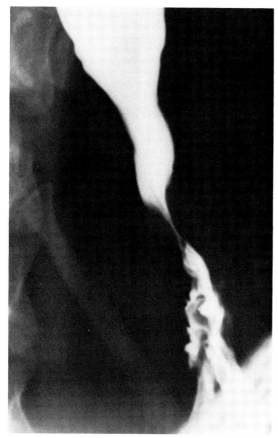

FIGURE 15–1. Barium swallow x-ray demonstrates tapering "bird beak" configuration of distal esophagus in achalasia.

genographic findings include symmetric dilation and tortuosity of the esophagus. The distal esophagus tends to be smooth and symmetric, tapering to a "bird beak" configuration (Fig. 15–1). At fluoroscopy, there is no peristalsis in the body of the esophagus, although repetitive nonperistaltic contractions may be observed. The esophageal mucosa should appear smooth; if surface irregularity or nodularity is present, malignancy should be considered.

Radioscintigraphy performed with various isotope meals demonstrates a dilated adynamic esophagus.[7] In addition, esophageal transit time of the isotope is markedly prolonged, indicative of the impaired esophageal emptying that is characteristic of this disease.[8]

Esophageal manometry should be performed to confirm the diagnosis. There are several characteristic findings:[1, 2] (1) hypertensive lower esophageal sphincter pressure, (2) incomplete relaxation of the sphincter with swallowing, (3) absence of esophageal peristalsis, and (4) resting pressure in the esophageal body that is greater than gastric pressure.

Endoscopic Findings

Prior to endoscopy in patients with achalasia, lavage using a large-bore tube may be necessary since retained solid and liquid material may be present in the esophagus despite prolonged fasting (Fig. 15–2). Lavage decreases the chance of pulmonary aspiration of this retained material during the procedure.

The dilated esophagus in the patient with long-standing achalasia may appear cavernous, simulating the appearance of the colon at colonoscopy (Plate 15–1A to C). In patients with a tortuous "sigmoid" esophagus, endoscopy may prove difficult because of the numerous bends and turns. Most patients with achalasia have normal esophageal mucosa. However, as the esophagus dilates, mild diffuse erythema may be noted distally. Whitish mucosal plaques, erosions, and discrete ulcers, presumably the result of stasis of ingested material, may also be seen. Air insuf-

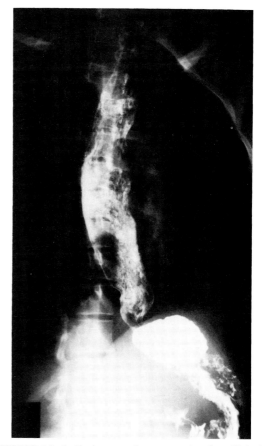

FIGURE 15–2. Barium swallow x-ray showing dilated tortuous esophagus containing food and debris.

flation may initiate distal esophageal contractions.

As the endoscope is advanced into the gastroesophageal segment, mild resistance is often encountered. However, with gentle forward pressure this can be overcome, and the instrument should readily "pop" into the stomach. Undue difficulty in traversing the gastroesophageal junction suggests the presence of underlying malignancy or benign stricturing. After esophageal dilation, the gastroesophageal junction may occasionally become eccentrically positioned, thereby preventing easy intubation of the stomach.

The endoscopist should conduct a precise appraisal for a hiatal hernia, even though this is unusual in achalasia, since esophageal perforation during pneumatic dilation is more common if a hiatal hernia is present.[9] The gastric cardia must be evaluated using forward and retroflexed views to exclude carcinoma of this area, a cause of secondary achalasia. Biopsies must be obtained of any mucosal abnormalities that are noted in the cardia, especially in patients over the age of 50 and those with progressive symptoms of short duration.

Endoscopy occasionally plays a role in the nonoperative treatment of achalasia. If the esophagus is tortuous and dilated, it may be difficult to position a pneumatic dilator properly at the gastroesophageal junction. This can be facilitated by passing the dilator over a guide wire previously placed in the stomach under endoscopic control.

Patients with long-standing achalasia possibly have an increased risk for squamous cell carcinoma of the esophagus.[10, 11] Characteristically, carcinoma occurs at the mid-esophageal level. The incidence and hence the importance of this problem is controversial. Periodic endoscopic surveillance has been suggested as a method to diagnose such tumors at potentially curable stages. However, our experience seems to indicate that the incidence of squamous cell carcinoma is quite low. Therefore, at this time we do not recommend routine surveillance for cancer in patients with achalasia.

Differential Diagnosis

Gastric adenocarcinoma with orad esophageal extension is the most common malignancy which mimics achalasia, termed secondary achalasia in such cases. Other tumors reported to cause secondary achalasia, either by direct esophageal involvement or as a paraneoplastic phenomenon, include oat cell carcinoma of the lung, reticulum cell sarcoma, prostatic carcinoma, and pancreatic cancer.[5, 6, 12]

Chagas' disease, caused by infection with *Trypanosoma cruzi,* is generally confined to South and Central America. Esophageal disease that is radiographically and manometrically indistinguishable from achalasia can develop in patients with chronic infection.[13] Unlike achalasia, however, megacolon, megaureter and myocardial disease may also develop in patients with Chagas' disease.[14]

Scleroderma and other connective tissue disease may be associated with a moderately dilated aperistaltic esophagus. Because these entities are not associated with a hypertensive lower esophageal sphincter or impaired esophageal emptying in the upright position, they may be differentiated from achalasia by esophageal manometry and barium swallow roentgenography performed with the patient in the upright position. Other conditions such as a peptic stricture, esophageal compression by a pancreatic pseudocyst, vagotomy, and anticholinergic therapy may occasionally produce esophageal dilation that can be confused with achalasia.

Treatment

Both medical and surgical methods of treatment are effective in achalasia.[15] Medical treatment with pneumatic dilation is easy to perform, usually well tolerated by the patient, and rarely associated with gastroesophageal reflux. However, this procedure may be complicated by esophageal perforation. Surgical esophageal myotomy generally results in longer and more complete relief of symptoms, but postoperative gastroesophageal reflux can be a major problem. With surgical myotomy the mortality is low, but the cost and perioperative morbidity are high. For these reasons, we initially recommend nonoperative therapy and refer patients for operation only if they remain symptomatic after three attempts at pneumatic dilation. The technique of esophageal pneumatic dilation described here is performed at our institution with the use of a Hurst-Tucker pneumatic dilator.

Prior to dilation, we inspect the dilator by inflating the bag to check its symmetry and measure its circumference and by submerging it under water to discover leaks. The entire procedure is performed under fluoroscopic control. Retained material is re-

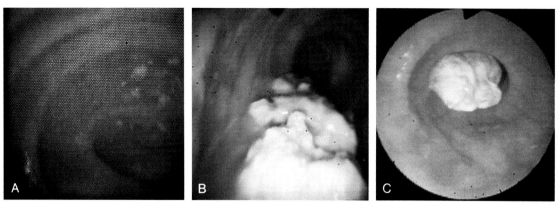

PLATE 15–1. *A,* Tortuous "sigmoid" endoscopic appearance. *B,* Dilated esophagus containing food material. *C,* Impacted food bolus in distal esophagus of patient with early achalasia. (*B, C,* Courtesy M.V. Sivak, Jr., M.D.)

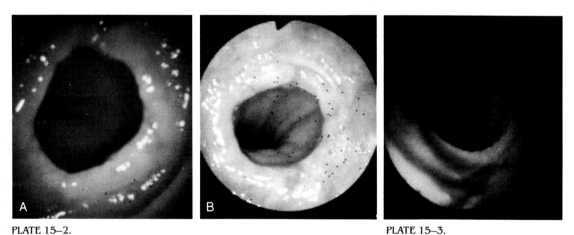

PLATE 15–2.   PLATE 15–3.

PLATE 15–2. *A & B,* Hiatal hernia with Schatzki ring. (Courtesy M.V. Sivak, Jr., M.D.)
PLATE 15–3. Multiple mid-esophageal webs.

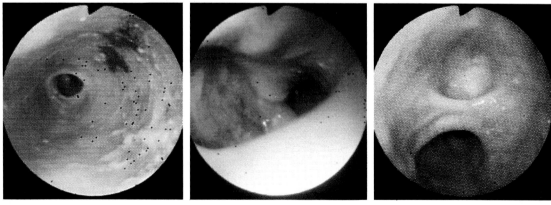

PLATE 15–4.   PLATE 15–5.   PLATE 15–6.

PLATE 15–4. Proximal esophageal web. Note traumatic area caused by instrument.
PLATE 15–5. Zenker's diverticulum (left side of field) containing food material. (Courtesy M.V. Sivak, Jr), M.D..
PLATE 15–6. Mid-esophageal diverticulum. (Courtesy M.V. Sivak, Jr., M.D.)

moved by esophageal lavage, and the patient, who has fasted for 12 hours, is then pre-medicated with topical oropharyngeal anesthetic spray and intravenous meperidine. A large-diameter bougie is passed under fluoroscopic guidance to insure that the patient does not have a stricture.

The pneumatic dilator is then passed into the esophagus and the radiopaque inflatable bag is centered lengthwise on the gastroesophageal junction. The bag is gradually inflated, taking care to maintain the indentation or waist deformity in the bag created by the lower esophageal sphincter at the midpoint of the bag. Insufflation is continued until the waist deformity is obliterated; pressure is then maintained for 30 to 60 seconds. The usual pressure required with this system to obliterate the waist is between 9 and 15 psi. The bag is then deflated and immediately re-inflated to determine the new pressure at which waist obliteration occurs. If the dilation has been effective, less pressure (3–6 psi) should be required for obliteration of the waist deformity. If no change in this pressure is noted, a second dilation can be performed, but no more than two should be performed at a single session.

After removal of the dilator, an esophagram with 1 to 2 ounces of barium is performed with the patient in the semi-upright position. If a small walled-off perforation is noted extending just beyond the lumen of the esophagus, the patient is not permitted any oral intake and is closely observed. If barium flows freely into the mediastinum or left chest, immediate surgery is indicated. The incidence of complications associated with pneumatic dilation ranges from 0 to 6%.[16–18] Small, walled-off esophageal perforations compose the majority of complications, and these can usually be managed with conservative methods without immediate surgical intervention.

Diffuse Esophageal Spasm (DES)

DES is a rare esophageal motility disorder characterized clinically by chest pain and dysphagia. Specific manometric abnormalities[19, 21] include repetitive simultaneous esophageal contractions of prolonged duration and occasionally of high amplitude. The lower esophageal sphincter may be hypertensive and may relax in an abnormal fashion in response to swallowing. Periods of normal peristaltic activity of varying length may be interspersed with these manometric abnormalities.

Endoscopy is indicated in DES only to exclude other lesions that mimic this disorder since there are no characteristic endoscopic abnormalities. Occasionally, air insufflation during endoscopy can induce nonperistaltic esophageal contractions and initiate chest pain. Endoscopic evidence of esophagitis suggests mucosal injury (pill-induced, infectious, superficial cancer, etc.) with esophageal spasm as a secondary phenomenon, since DES is infrequently associated with gastroesophageal reflux.

Various types of drugs including nitrates, anticholinergics, sedatives, calcium channel blockers, and antacids have been used to treat DES with varying degrees of success. Patients sometimes obtain relief of symptoms after peroral bougienage.[22] Individuals with well-documented manometric abnormalities characteristic of DES and with severe debilitating symptoms including weight loss can be treated by pneumatic dilation[23] or long surgical myotomy.[24]

Other Motility Disorders

Certain systemic disorders such as scleroderma and other collagen vascular diseases may have associated abnormalities of esophageal peristalsis and lower esophageal sphincter function.[21, 25] While symptoms of dysphagia and chest pain can be in part related to primary esophageal motor failure, most symptoms in these patients result from esophagitis and strictures related to the gastroesophageal reflux that complicates these conditions.

Endoscopic findings are generally related to underlying gastroesophageal reflux. For instance, severe erosive esophagitis with hemorrhage and stricturing is commonly encountered in patients with scleroderma. Occasionally, there may be endoscopic evidence of Candida esophagitis with its characteristic "cheesy" white, plaque-like membrane in a seriously ill patient with systemic symptoms.

Management involves the use of vigorous antireflux therapy, such as elevation of the head of the bed to promote esophageal acid clearance and H_2 receptor–blocking drugs to decrease acid secretion. Benign esophageal strictures respond to peroral bougienage while antifungal therapy should effectively eliminate associated esophageal candidiasis.

MISCELLANEOUS ESOPHAGEAL DISORDERS

Mucosal Esophageal Rings

Distal esophageal ring[26] (Schatzki's ring or B ring) is a common finding on barium swallow roentgenograms and at endoscopy. These rings consist entirely of mucosa and occur at the squamocolumnar mucosal junction of the esophagus and stomach. Although most B rings are asymptomatic, they may be associated with intermittent dysphagia or food impaction when they narrow the lumen to less than 12 mm in diameter.[27]

A thin, symmetric, circumferential membranous projection that partially occludes the distal esophageal lumen at the squamocolumnar junction is demonstrated at endoscopy (Plate 15–2). The ring has a fixed diameter as demonstrated by failure to obliterate the membrane with continuous air insufflation. If the diameter of the ring is less than the critical 12 mm, then slight resistance to passage of a standard diameter endoscope may be perceived as it enters the stomach. On occasion the ring will be ruptured during intubation of the gastroesophageal junction, resulting in a mucosal tear and slight bleeding. This may not be appreciated until the endoscope is withdrawn through the traumatized area. Small-caliber endoscopes can pass through a Schatzki's ring without difficulty; hence the lesion may be missed at endoscopy or its significance may be misjudged. If undue resistance is encountered during intubation of the gastroesophageal junction, or esophagitis is present, then a peptic stricture rather than a Schatzki's ring should be suspected.

Conventional endoscopes are not designed to dilate esophageal lesions. Forceful attempts at intubation of a fixed stenosis may result in instrument damage or, more importantly, in damage to the esophagus itself. Tight rings as well as benign and malignant strictures should be treated by manipulation with commercially available dilators according to established techniques. Peroral bougienage is effective therapy for most rings.[26] A single passage of a large-caliber mercury-filled bougie will rupture the ring and usually alleviate symptoms permanently. Occasion-

ally, recurrent symptoms may necessitate repeat bougienage.

Muscular Esophageal Rings

Muscular esophageal rings most commonly occur several centimeters proximal to the squamocolumnar junction.[28] When observed during radiologic examination or at endoscopy, this type of ring changes in appearance as the esophageal musculature contracts and relaxes. This dynamic feature, the characteristic location, and the lack of resistance to passage of the endoscope help to differentiate a muscular ring from a mucosal ring or a peptic stricture. Muscular rings rarely cause symptoms, but if dysphagia is present in a patient with such a ring, peroral bougienage may be helpful.

Esophageal Webs

Esophageal webs are membrane-like structures, completely covered by squamous epithelium, that may focally narrow the esophageal lumen. They may be solitary or multiple (Plate 15–3).[29] Webs usually occur in the cervical esophagus in the immediate postcricoid area, but can be found at any level of the esophagus. They are usually diagnosed first by barium swallow radiographs (Fig. 15–3). Symptoms are variable, although most often an esophageal web is asymptomatic and represents only an incidental radiographic finding. However, some patients complain of severe dysphagia localized most often in the cervical area.[30] An association between webs and iron deficiency anemia has been described (Plummer-Vinson or Patterson-Kelly syndrome), but probably they usually occur without other associated conditions.

Endoscopists frequently overlook the presence of cervical esophageal membranes, since they may inadvertently rupture them during blind intubation of the hypopharynx and cervical esophagus. Careful endoscopic intubation under direct vision occasionally permits the demonstration of a thin, often transparent, postcricoid membrane (Plate 15–4). More often, the torn membrane is visualized during withdrawal of the endoscope. Endoscopic evaluation should include thorough examination of the cervical esophagus and hypopharynx, since carcinoma in this region is more common in patients with webs asso-

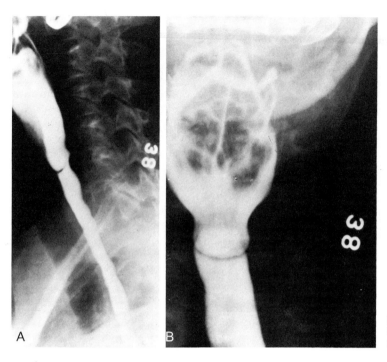

FIGURE 15–3. Lateral (*A*) and anterior-posterior (*B*) barium swallow x-rays of esophageal web.

ciated with iron deficiency anemia.[31] Since the web is usually ruptured with the endoscope, further treatment is rarely required. In patients with persistent symptoms after endoscopy, or in those with multiple webs, peroral bougienage is effective therapy.

Extrinsic Compression of the Esophagus

Abnormal structures, aberrant vessels, and neoplasms adjacent to the esophagus may produce symptoms due to compression or deviation of the esophageal lumen.[32, 33] Examples include large osteophytes of the cervical spine, cardiac chamber enlargement, tortuous or aneurysmal deformity of the thoracic aorta (dysphagia aortica), aberrant right subclavian artery (dysphagia lusoria), lung cancer, and enlarged mediastinal lymph nodes. The exact location of extrinsic esophageal narrowing is best identified by barium swallow roentgenograms. Endoscopy generally will demonstrate deviation or tortuosity of the esophageal lumen or the smooth rounded deformity of extrinsic compression without disruption of the mucosa. On occasion, mucosal abnormalities indicative of esophageal invasion by an extrinsic lesion may be noted. Endoscopy is contraindicated if a thoracic aortic aneurysm is suspected. Endoscopy with a rigid instrument is hazard-

ous in patients with posterior compression of the cervical esophagus by osteophytes because of possible esophageal damage during intubation. Extrinsic compression of the esophagus does not usually cause symptoms except in malignancy. Peroral bougienage to treat dysphagia due to an extrinsic process is generally not successful because the esophageal wall quickly collapses when the dilator is removed.

Pharyngeal Esophageal Diverticulum (Zenker's Diverticulum)

A pharyngeal esophageal diverticulum occurs when the hypopharyngeal mucosa forms a posteriorly directed pouch by protruding between the inferior pharyngeal constrictor muscle and the cricopharyngeal muscle in an area of junctional muscle weakness (Kilian's dehiscence).[34] Symptoms from a Zenker's diverticulum are usually related to the size of the pouch. A small diverticulum is often asymptomatic or associated only with a sensation of a foreign body in the back of the throat. As the diverticulum enlarges, it can cause unexplained regurgitation of undigested food or nocturnal aspiration. An extremely large diverticular sac can compress and deform the esophageal lumen, resulting in severe dysphagia and weight loss.

Pharyngeal esophageal diverticulum is usually diagnosed by barium swallow roentgenography (Fig. 15–4). Endoscopy is not required, and because the diverticulum is located in the cricopharyngeal area it is usually not visualized during endoscopy. If endoscopy is undertaken in a patient with a Zenker's diverticulum to exclude another cause of symptoms or to evaluate another lesion, it should be done cautiously. During blind intubation, the endoscope can inadvertently enter and perforate the diverticulum, whose thin wall consists entirely of mucosa. Endoscopic intubation under direct vision or over a previously placed guide wire can reduce this risk. Generally, one tends to enter the diverticular sac preferentially because this is proximal to the cricopharyngeus muscle and is easily inflated during the procedure. The esophageal lumen will always be found at or very close to the opening into the diverticulum, and therefore the tip of the endoscope need not be passed into the diverticulum itself (Plate 15–5).

Esophageal Diverticulum

Esophageal diverticula may be single or multiple and can occur in the mid-esophagus (traction) (Plate 15–6) or distal esophagus (epiphrenic) (Plate 15–7). It was formerly thought that a mid-esophageal diverticulum resulted from traction on the esophagus produced by inflammatory conditions (tuberculosis, fungal infection, etc.) in the mediastinum. Recent evidence, however, suggests that mid-esophageal as well as distal esophageal diverticula result from esophageal motility disorders.[35] A diverticulum of the esophageal body rarely produces symptoms, but occasionally it may bleed, perforate, or enlarge to such a degree that it compresses the esophageal lumen.

An esophageal diverticulum is usually diagnosed on barium swallow x-rays. Endoscopy is not required, but in patients undergoing endoscopy for other reasons, the opening of the diverticulum is often noted. If the diverticulum is extremely large and has a wide mouth, it may be difficult to determine which opening represents the esophageal lumen and which the diverticular lumen (Plate 15–8). An esophageal diverticulum does not preclude carefully performed endoscopy. However, during blind intubation of the esophagus, such as occurs with peroral bougienage or passage of a nasogastric tube, there is a chance of diverticular perforation. This risk can be reduced by performing dilation over an endoscopically placed guide wire.

Since esophageal diverticula are usually asymptomatic, no therapy is required. However, in the rare case of a diverticulum that bleeds, perforates, or causes esophageal obstruction, surgical treatment is indicated.

FIGURE 15–4. Lateral (A) and anterior-posterior (B) radiographs of Zenker's diverticulum.

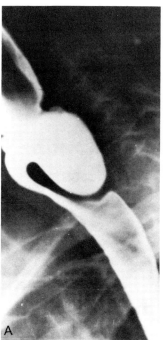
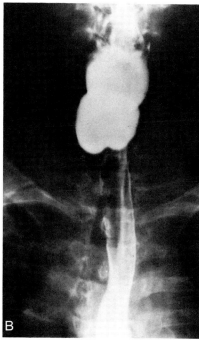

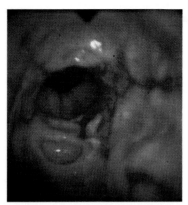

PLATE 15–7. Epiphrenic diverticulum, hiatal hernia, and severe esophagitis. (Courtesy M.V. Sivak, Jr., M.D.)

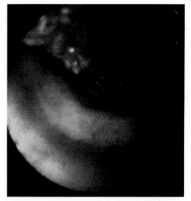

PLATE 15–9. Esophageal hematoma with mucosal irregularity simulating a a carcinoma.

Esophageal Hematomas

Esophageal hematomas result from submucosal bleeding that can occur spontaneously in patients with impaired hemostasis or after esophageal trauma such as that occurring, for example, with vigorous retching or an aborted sneeze.[36] Most hematomas due to trauma involve the distal esophagus but may extend in an orad direction within the esophageal wall to involve the entire organ. In patients with clotting abnormalities, hematomas may be multicentric. Symptoms include dysphagia, odynophagia, and hematemesis. The presence of an esophageal hematoma may be suspected on barium swallow x-rays. It appears as a submucosal mass indenting the barium column, often with occlusion of the esophageal lumen. In fact, it may simulate esophageal malignancy. However, radiographs several days later will show rapid resolution of the process.

At endoscopy a hematoma appears as a reddish-purple submucosal swelling that par-

tially occludes the esophageal lumen.[36, 37] A multicentric lesion can have the apearance of multiple, discrete submucosal ecchymoses. Mucosa overlying the hematoma is usually smooth, but occasionally it is disrupted and irregular and simulates malignancy (Plate 15–9). Patients with esophageal hematoma rarely require transfusion or surgical therapy, because most lesions resolve spontaneously over several days.

Glycogenic Acanthosis

Glycogenic acanthosis is a benign mucosal lesion of the esophagus commonly seen at endoscopy.[38, 39] This lesion is easily recognized as many small (<1 cm), pale or whitish papules usually found in the distal esophagus (Plate 15–10). Histologically, the lesion is characterized by hyperplastic squamous acanthotic epithelium with increased glycogen. Its clinical significance is unknown, although it has been suggested as an indicator of gastroesophageal reflux. Since this entity is com-

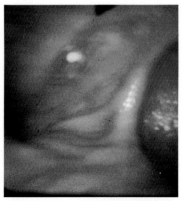

PLATE 15–8. Large, wide-mouthed esophageal diverticulum.

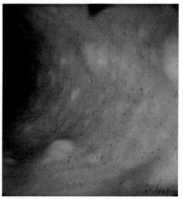

PLATE 15–10. Glycogenic acanthosis of the esophagus.

mon (15% of consecutive endoscopies),[40] it must be differentiated from other more significant lesions that can have a similar appearance, such as moniliasis, leukoplakia, and early esophageal carcinoma.

References

1. Cohen S, Lipshutz W. Lower esophageal sphincter dysfunction in achalasia. Gastroenterology 1971; 61:814–20.
2. Castell DO. Achalasia and diffuse esophageal spasm. Arch Intern Med 1976; 136:571–9.
3. Barrett NR. Achalasia of the cardia: reflections upon a clinical study of over 100 cases. Br Med J 1964; 1:1135–40.
4. Wong RKH, Johnson LF. Achalasia. In: Castell DO, Johnson LF, eds. Esophageal Function in Health and Disease. New York: Elsevier Biochemical, 1983:99.
5. Tucker HJ, Snape WJ Jr, Cohen S. Achalasia secondary to carcinoma: Manometric and clinical features. Ann Intern Med 1978; 89:315–8.
6. Sandler RS, Bozymski EM, Orlando RC. Failure of clinical criteria to distinguish between primary achalasia and achalasia secondary to tumor. Dig Dis Sci 1982; 27:209–13.
7. Russell CO, Hill LD, Holmes ER III, et al. Radionuclide transit: A sensitive screening test for esophageal dysfunction. Gastroenterology 1981; 80:887–92.
8. Gross R, Johnson LF, Kaminski RJ. Esophageal emptying in achalasia quantitated by a radioisotope technique. Dig Dis Sci 1979; 24:945–9.
9. Vantrappen G, Hellemans J. Diseases of the Esophagus. New York: Springer-Verlag, 1974; 341.
10. Lortat-Jacob JL, Richard CA, Fekete F, Testart J. Cardiospasm and esophageal carcinoma: Report of 24 cases. Surgery 1969; 66:969–75.
11. Wychulis AR, Woolam GL, Andersen HA, Ellis FH Jr. Achalasia and carcinoma of the esophagus. JAMA 1971; 215:1638–41.
12. Davis JA, Kantrowitz PA, Chandler HL, Schatzki SC. Reversible achalasia due to reticulum-cell sarcoma. N Engl J Med 1975; 293:130–2.
13. Bettarello A, Pinotti HW. Oesophageal involvement in Chagas' disease. Clin Gastroenterol 1976; 5:103.
14. Koberle F. Enteromegaly and cardiomegaly in Chagas disease. Gut 1963; 4:399–405.
15. Cassella RR, Brown AL Jr, Sayre GP, Ellis FH Jr. Achalasia of the esophagus: Pathologic and etiologic considerations. Ann Surg 1964; 160:474–87.
16. Kurlander DJ, Raskin HF, Kirsner JB, Palmer WL. Therapeutic value of the pneumatic dilator in achalasia of the esophagus: Long-term results in sixty-two living patients. Gastroenterology 1963; 45:604–13.
17. Sanderson DR, Ellis FH Jr, Olsen AM. Achalasia of the esophagus: Results of therapy by dilation, 1950–1967. Chest 1970; 58:116–21.
18. Vantrappen G, Hellemans J, Deloof W, et al. Treatment of achalasia with pneumatic dilations. Gut 1971; 12:268–75.
19. DiMarino AJ Jr, Cohen S. Characteristics of lower esophageal sphincter function in symptomatic diffuse esophageal spasm. Gastroenterology 1974; 66:1–6.
20. Mellow M. Symptomatic diffuse esophageal spasm: manometric follow-up and response to cholinergic stimulation and cholinesterase inhibition. Gastroenterology 1977; 73:237–40.
21. Cohen S. Motor disorders of the esophagus. N Engl J Med 1979; 301:184–92.
22. Goldin NR, Burns TW, Herrington JP. Treatment of nonspecific esophageal motor disorders. Beneficial effects of bougienage. (Abstr) Gastroenterology 1982; 82:1069.
23. Vantrappen G, Hellemans J. Treatment of achalasia and related motor disorders. Gastroenterology 1980; 79:144–54.
24. Leonardi HK, Shea JA, Crozier RE, Ellis FH. Diffuse spasm of the esophagus. Clinical, manometric, and surgical considerations. J Thorac Cardiovasc Surg 1977; 74:736–43.
25. Cohen S, Laufer I, Snape WJ Jr, et al. The gastrointestinal manifestations of scleroderma: Pathogenesis and management. Gastroenterology 1980; 79:155–66.
26. Goyal RK, Glancy JJ, Spiro HM. Lower esophageal ring. N Engl J Med 1970; 282:1298–305, 1355–62.
27. Schatzki R. The lower esophageal ring: Long term follow-up of symptomatic and asymptomatic rings. Am J Roentgenol 1963; 90:805–10.
28. Goyal RK, Bauer JL, Spiro HM. The nature and location of lower esophageal ring. N Engl J Med 1971; 284:1175–80.
29. Shiflett DW, Gilliam JH, Wu WC, et al. Multiple esophageal webs in adults. Gastroenterology 1979; 77:556–9.
30. Ekberg O. Cervical oesophageal webs in patients with dysphagia. Clin Radiol 1981; 32:633–41.
31. Chisholm M. The association between webs, iron and postcricoid carcinoma. Postgrad Med J 1974; 50:215–9.
32. Johnson LF, Moses FM. Endoscopic evaluation of esophageal disease. In: Castell DO, Johnson LF, eds. Esophageal Function in Health and Disease. New York: Elsevier Biomedical, 1983; 237.
33. Cattau EL Jr, Castell DO. Symptoms of esophageal dysfunction. Adv Int Med 1982; 27:151–81.
34. Knuff TE, Benjamin SB, Castell DO. Pharyngoesophageal (Zenker's) diverticulum: A reappraisal. Gastroenterology 1982; 82:734–6.
35. Kaye MD. Oesophageal motor dysfunction in patients with diverticula of the mid-thoracic oesophagus. Thorax 1974; 29:666–72.
36. Shay SS, Berendson RA, Johnson LF. Esophageal hematoma; Four new cases—a review, and proposed etiology. Dig Dis Sci 1981; 26:1019–24.
37. Tim LO, Segal I, Mirwis J. Intramural haematoma of the oesophagus. The role of endoscopy. S Afr Med J 1982; 61:798–800.
38. Bender MD, Allison J, Cuartas F, Montgomery C. Glycogenic acanthosis of the esophagus: A form of benign epithelial hyperplasia. Gastroenterology 1973; 65:373–80.
39. Clemencon G, Gloor F. Benign epithelial hyperplasia of the esophagus: Glycogenic acanthosis. Endoscopy 1974; 6:214.
40. Stern Z, Sharon P, Ligumsky M, et al. Glycogenic acanthosis of the esophagus. A benign but confusing endoscopic lesion. Am J Gastroenterol 1980; 74:261–3.

Chapter 16

ESOPHAGEAL VARICES

MICHAEL V. SIVAK, JR., M.D.

OVERVIEW

Esophageal varices are usually a consequence of portal hypertension. They produce no symptoms except hemorrhage. Although the causes of portal hypertension and attendant esophageal collateral venous channels are well known, the precise factors that initiate hemorrhage are not understood. Unfortunately, variceal hemorrhage is a difficult clinical problem for which there is no universally satisfactory solution. Management of varices is almost exclusively concerned with this complication; treatment is almost always after the fact.

Until recently, the role of endoscopy was differentiation of variceal hemorrhage from other gastrointestinal sources of bleeding. Renewed interest in injection sclerosis of esophageal varices has changed this role to diagnosis and therapy. Despite introduction of sclerotherapy over 40 years ago, less than 1000 cases are to be found in the literature prior to 1978. Since then there has been a remarkable increase in the literature on sclerotherapy. This curious disparity is usually attributed to the overriding attention devoted to portosystemic shunt surgery during the past 20 years.

Since shunt surgery has not proved as satisfactory as once anticipated, it is attractive to view the renaissance of sclerotherapy as a deliberately developed alternative rather than a procedure currently in vogue. Although sclerotherapy has assumed a dominant role in the management of esophageal variceal hemorrhage, experience with the procedure and an understanding of the favorable and unfavorable results are continuing to evolve.

VARICEAL ANATOMY

The esophageal venous system has three main components: intrinsic veins, associated veins, and extrinsic veins.[1]

The intrinsic component is made up of (1) a subepithelial plexus in the lamina propria and (2) a submucosal plexus deep to the muscularis mucosa. These two plexuses are interconnected. The intrinsic vessels are the ones observed at endoscopy. Proximally these anastomose with the pharyngeal-laryngeal venous plexus, distally to the subglandular plexus of the stomach. However, the connections between the subglandular gastric plexus and the intrinsic esophageal venous plexus are rudimentary or nonexistent in most individuals. The inconstant nature of this anastomosis may explain the fact that extensive gastric mucosal varices are usually not associated with esophageal varices and why gastric varices under certain circumstances may become large in the absence of correspondingly large esophageal varices.

Two longitudinal vessels on the external aspect of the esophagus compose the associated veins. These anastomose distally with the left gastric vein and proximally with the bronchial veins. The associated veins probably have no great importance with respect to endoscopy and sclerotherapy.

The left gastric vein anastomoses with the extrinsic system of esophageal veins. The extrinsic veins in turn empty into the azygous system and also anastomose proximally with the thyroidal and peritracheal venous plexuses, the anterior deep cervical veins, and a number of other venous structures.

The extrinsic and intrinsic esophageal venous systems are interconnected at frequent intervals along the length of the esophagus by perforating veins. The latter have valves that normally prevent blood flow from the extrinsic into the intrinsic plexuses.

ENDOSCOPIC APPEARANCE OF ESOPHAGEAL VARICES

The contour of the inner aspect of the esophagus is normally smooth except for occasional minor surface irregularities. Small longitudinal mucosal vessels are also discernible, but these are never more than a few millimeters in diameter. Esophageal varices have several characteristic endoscopic features, including shape, size, location, color, and surface features.

Endoscopically, an esophageal varix is an elongated structure arranged parallel to the long axis of the lumen. An isolated variceal vessel is unusual. Typically three or four columns are seen.

The most obvious characteristic of esophageal varices is their elevation above the mucosal surface (sometimes referred to in terms of size or diameter). Smaller varices tend to be relatively straight tubular structures that are separated from one another by intervening normal mucosa. Large diameter varices have an irregular, undulating configuration. The largest vessels distort a greater portion of the mucosal surface, so that little or no normal mucosa can be seen and the entire surface appears to be covered by varices (Plate 16–1).

Varices may have the color of surrounding mucosa, or they may have a slightly bluish tint, the latter being usual for those of large diameter. Red spots in various shapes are another surface feature. Generally not larger than a few millimeters, these "red color signs" may be slightly elevated above the variceal surface when seen in profile. They tend to occur on larger diameter variceal columns (see Plate 16–1).

When small, varices are typically located in the distal one third of the esophagus. Large diameter is usually associated with greater linear extent, so that larger vessels typically occupy at least the distal two thirds of the esophagus and the largest frequently encompass the entire length. Variceal diameter is usually greatest in the distal esophagus near the esophagogastric mucosal junction and tends to decrease in an orad direction.

Although varices are usually most prominent in the distal esophagus, there are exceptions. Rarely, esophageal varices will be located primarily in the proximal esophagus. Sometimes referred to as "downhill" esophageal varices, their pathogenesis differs from that of the more common distal vessels.[2]

Fully developed varices are not difficult to recognize endoscopically. However, size and linear extent of the columns are not static in a given patient. Distention of the esophagus by air insufflation reduces the prominence of the varices; they may be more apparent as the lumen is permitted to collapse. Length and diameter may also increase or decrease during the clinical course of the varices. Varices may be less prominent during and immediately after an episode of hemorrhage and decreased intravascular volume.

Variceal hemorrhage is often intermittent, so that it is unusual to actually see bleeding from a vessel during endoscopy (Plate 16–2). On occasion, a clot may be seen protruding from a varix. This is frequently unstable so that bleeding may resume at any time.

The initial management of a patient with upper gastrointestinal hemorrhage that might be due to esophageal varices is the same as other sources of bleeding and is discussed in Chapter 6. Endoscopic techniques for diagnosis of variceal hemorrhage do not differ from those for diagnosis of the source of upper gastrointestinal bleeding in general.

PATHOPHYSIOLOGY OF VARICEAL BLEEDING

Causes of Portal Hypertension

Some of the causes of portal hypertension are classified in Table 16–1 according to the anatomic site of increased resistance to blood flow. Some "causes" listed are merely categories that include a variety of diseases and conditions. Elucidation of the pathogenesis of portal hypertension in every patient is essential for proper management. Although the treatment of end-stage hepatic cirrhosis may have little relation to its primary cause, other causes of portal hypertension, such as a web in the inferior vena cava or thrombosis of the splenic vein, require differing treatments that are in some cases specific and effective. Sclerotherapy might be appropriate for variceal bleeding in relation to some "causes" but inappropriate for others.

One of the consequences of portal hypertension is that the collateral interconnections

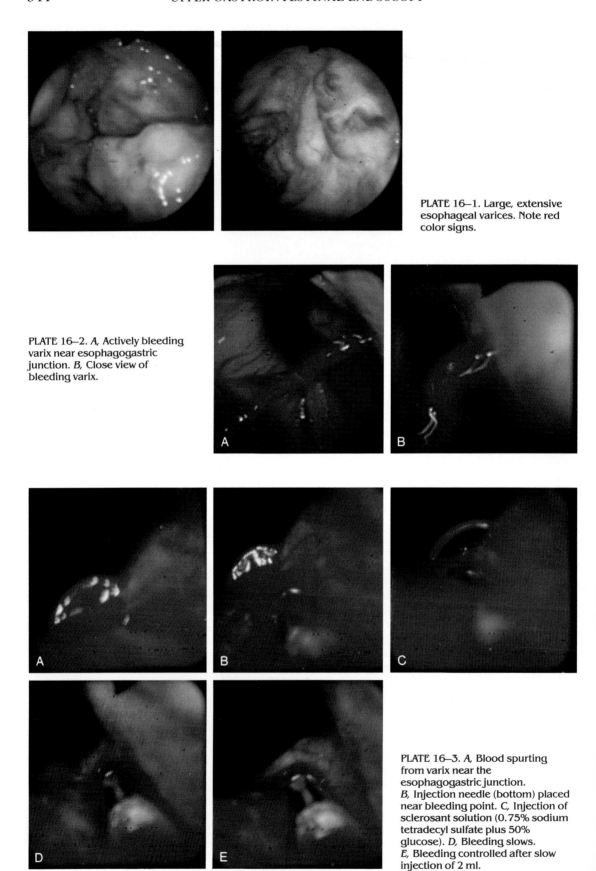

PLATE 16–1. Large, extensive esophageal varices. Note red color signs.

PLATE 16–2. *A,* Actively bleeding varix near esophagogastric junction. *B,* Close view of bleeding varix.

PLATE 16–3. *A,* Blood spurting from varix near the esophagogastric junction. *B,* Injection needle (bottom) placed near bleeding point. *C,* Injection of sclerosant solution (0.75% sodium tetradecyl sulfate plus 50% glucose). *D,* Bleeding slows. *E,* Bleeding controlled after slow injection of 2 ml.

TABLE 16–1. **Causes of Portal Hypertension**

1. Cardiac Diseases

2. Vascular Diseases
   Budd-Chiari syndrome
   Membranous obstruction of the inferior vena cava
   Thrombosis of the inferior vena cava

3. Acute and Chronic Liver Disease
   Cirrhosis
   Idiopathic portal hypertension
   Schistosomiasis
   Congenital hepatic fibrosis
   Exposure to environmental toxins
   Metastatic carcinoma

4. Venous Occlusion of Portal System
   Portal vein
   Splenic vein

between the portal and systemic venous systems become functional. There are numerous avenues for this blood flow, but the esophageal and gastric variceal vessels have the greatest clinical significance. Although hemorrhoidal bleeding and bleeding from varices elsewhere in the gastrointestinal tract and colon may occur, this is relatively rare. It appears that portal blood flow is not evenly distributed among the venous collateral channels. Rather, one or more of the possible channels become dominant. The reason(s) for this are entirely unknown, but the concept explains why for equal degrees of portal hypertension, some patients have large varices with bleeding and others do not.

The most common cause of proximal esophageal varices is obstruction of the superior vena cava in various diseases including metastatic carcinoma and mediastinal fibrosis.[3, 4] The obstruction must occur either at the junction of the azygous vein with the superior vena cava or proximal to this point. Theoretically, this should produce varices along the entire esophagus, but in most cases they are present only in the proximal aspect. This is thought to be related to the abruptness and duration of the venous obstruction; since the cause is malignancy in most cases, there may be insufficient time for the development of varices of maximal extension. When the underlying disease process is protracted, in mediastinal fibrosis for example, varices may extend over the length of the esophagus. A primary or idiopathic type of proximal esophageal varices without obstruction of the major venous system has also been described.[5]

Blood Flow in Esophageal Varices

Esophageal varices are usually thought of as simple conduits that transport portal blood from the gut to the systemic circulation. However, blood flow in these vessels is more complex. McCormack et al.[6] studied flow patterns by means of Doppler ultrasound and injection radiography in 18 and 34 patients, respectively. They found that the direction of blood flow was not always cephalad; that sometimes flow was toward the stomach, and that the direction might be reversed during the respiratory cycle; and that venous outflow from the stomach is not always via the esophageal varices. This latter point is in agreement with the anatomic observations of Butler[1] that the mucosal venous communications across the esophagogastric mucosal junction are either rudimentary or non-existent.

McCormack et al.[6] suggested that the perforating veins that connect the extrinsic and intrinsic venous systems are crucially important in the pathogenesis of variceal bleeding. They suggested that the valves of the perforating veins are incompetent and permit retrograde flow from the extrinsic veins to the intrinsic system. In this concept the extrinsic esophageal veins are the primary collateral vessels, and the intrinsic esophageal varices are actually a backwater or "cul de sac" for blood. Differences in the competence of the valves of the perforating veins account for the fact that determination of portal pressure alone does not predict size of variceal vessels nor the likelihood of bleeding.

Prediction of Variceal Hemorrhage

When cirrhosis is the cause of portal hypertension, there is no correlation between the severity of the hepatic parenchymal disease as related to clinical and biochemical parameters and the propensity for variceal hemorrhage.

Many investigators have attempted to correlate hepatic wedge pressure with variceal bleeding. A certain increase in portal pressure is required before esophageal varices are likely to be present; a portohepatic gradient of 10 to 12 mm Hg is required. At levels less than this, the presence of varices is unlikely.[7, 8] In patients with liver disease in an early stage, the presence of varices is related to the degree of portal hypertension.[9] However, in patients with established portal hypertension and esophageal varices there is no relation between variceal hemorrhage and the level of the portal venous pressure.[9]

Variceal Size in Relation to Hemorrhage

Although available data conflict, it appears there is no relation between the size and extent of variceal channels and the level of portal pressure. The existence of such a correlation is supported by the results of some investigations.[10–12] But other investigators have failed to find any relation.[8, 13–17] Lebrec et al.[8] suggested that these conflicting conclusions result from the inclusion of patients with normal or only slightly increased portal pressure in earlier studies that support a relation between variceal size and the level of portal pressure; if only patients with frankly elevated portal pressure are considered there is no relation.

Although the level of portal hypertension cannot be correlated with the likelihood of variceal bleeding or the size of the variceal channels, a relationship has been sought between variceal size and/or endoscopic appearance and the risk of bleeding. The results of the available investigations suggest that there is an imprecise relation between variceal size, especially diameter, and the variceal bleeding.

Baker et al.[18] studied 115 cirrhotic patients with varices but no prior bleeding. Variceal size was classified as Grade 0, no definite varices visible; 1+, one or more varices under 4 mm diameter and under 4 cm in length; 2+, multiple varices 4 to 10 cm in extent; and 3+, multiple varices over 10 cm long. During follow-up the frequency of bleeding was approximately the same in patients with 1+ and 2+ varices, but was twice as frequent in those with an initial classification of 3+. However, there was an inverse relation between the variceal grade and the severity of bleeding episodes. Twenty-eight patients underwent endoscopic follow-up; varices disappeared in 9, decreased in grade in 7, remained unchanged in 6, and became more extensive in 6 patients.

Palmer and Brick[19] measured variceal size and length in 201 patients with proved cirrhosis. Some patients had a history of variceal bleeding and others did not. Varices were classified as mild (less than 3 mm in diameter), moderate (3 to 6 mm in diameter), and severe (greater than 6 mm in diameter). The length of the columns was also measured as a fraction of the total length of the esophagus. Three fourths of the patients examined during active hemorrhage had varices that were classified as severe; one half of those examined during acute hemorrhage had varices that occupied the entire length of the esophagus. If endoscopy was performed shortly after an episode of bleeding, there was a tendency for vessel diameter and extent to be greater than in patients examined at a longer time interval after bleeding. The authors concluded that most patients have large-diameter varices that extend over a substantial length of the esophagus at the time of variceal hemorrhage, that small varices tended to enlarge just before the onset of bleeding, and that variceal size decreased during bleeding free intervals. Because transitions occurred in the graded severity, it was concluded that small variceal size alone offers no assurance that the chance for hemorrhage is small.

Dagradi[20] reported the results of a study of esophageal varices in patients with alcoholic liver disease. Varices were classified endoscopically into five grades based on diameter. For grade 1, small varices (2 mm in diameter) were noted upon compression of the esophageal wall with the semiflexible endoscope. Variceal diameters for grades 2, 3, and 4 were 2 mm, 3 to 4, and 5 mm or more, respectively. The diameters for grades 4 and 5 were identical, the difference between the two being the presence in grade 5 of "small varices on top of varices." The latter were bright red, small, telangiectatic vessels also described as "cherry-red" spots.

In 65% of patients who continued to drink alcohol during follow-up in this study by Dagradi,[20] there was a progressive transition toward variceal enlargement. An average of approximately 50 months was required to reach the most severe grade. Varices of a given caliber usually increased in length to varying degrees before their diameters increased to the next highest grade. Varices never disappeared in those who continued to consume alcohol, although a significant decrease in caliber and extent was noted in 80% of patients who stopped drinking. Dagradi concluded that variceal rupture was likely when varices reached a grade 4 or 5, especially when they were longer than 5 cm. Although bleeding occurred in one patient with grade 5 varices that were only 4 cm long, the average length found in association with bleeding varices of this grade was 11 cm.

Lebrec et al.[8] reported the results of a study of variceal size and the risk of bleeding in 100 patients; 47 had no prior bleeding and underwent evaluation for liver disease. The remaining 53 patients had a history of gastrointestinal bleeding; the source was variceal in 26 patients, and gastric erosions in 27 patients. Variceal size was classified using barium swallow x-rays in all patients. Varices were considered large or small according to whether or not a varix was less or greater than 5 mm in diameter. Additional endoscopic grading was carried out in the 53 patients who had prior bleeding. This was said to agree with the radiographic classification in all but one patient.

The prevalence of recent bleeding (i.e., prior to entry), whether due to varices or to acute gastritis, was significantly higher in those patients with large varices in this study by Lebrec et al.[8] During a one-year follow-up, bleeding occurred in 17 patients, 14 in the group with prior bleeding and 3 in the group that had only signs of liver disease at the outset. The incidence of gastrointestinal bleeding during follow-up was significantly greater in patients with large varices. Variceal size had been measured endoscopically in most patients with bleeding during follow-up, although in some cases the grading had been done radiographically. All patients who bled during follow-up had large varices. However, in some cases recurrent bleeding was due to acute gastritis and in others to varices.

The correlation between endoscopic and radiographic assessments of varices reported by Lebrec et al.[8] is considerably better than that reported by others.[21] The risk of variceal bleeding was significantly higher if varices were large, but the risk of bleeding from gastric erosions was also significantly increased. Lebrec et al.[8] theorized that this might be explained by the general increase in collateral circulation through gastric and esophageal veins in association with portal hypertension, and that this might favor bleeding from established gastric erosions.

Variceal Appearance in Relation to Bleeding

Some features of the endoscopic appearance of varices may correlate with the potential for hemorrhage. Dagradi[20] found that large varices were also distinguished by certain surface markings that he referred to as "varices on varices" or "cherry-red" spots (see Plate 16–1). The Japanese Research Society for Portal Hypertension has proposed a classification of esophageal varices based not only on size but also endoscopic appearance (Table 16–2).[22]

Although this classification appears complex its essential features are relatively uncomplicated. The basic observations relate to the color of the varices (that of normal mucosa versus a bluish tint), the presence of red color signs, the diameter of the vessels (form), their longitudinal extent (location), and the presence of any endoscopic evidence of associated esophagitis (adjunctive finding). Red color signs are subdivided into several types based on size and shape, although it is not certain that this is useful clinically. The distinction between a cherry-red spot and a hematocystic spot is mainly one of size, the latter being the larger. The term *red wale marking* refers to linear, slightly raised, red streaks on the surface of a variceal vessel, an appearance likened to ridges on the surface of cloth, corduroy for example. Red wale markings and cherry red spots are also graded 1+ to 3+, based on their size and number.

TABLE 16–2. **General Rules for Recording Endoscopic Findings on Esophageal Varices of the Japanese Research Society for Portal Hypertension**

1. Red Color Signs (RCS)* (small dilated vessels or microtelangiectasia on varix surface
   Red wale marking (RWM)
   Cherry-red spot (CRS)
   Hematocystic spot (HCS)
   Diffuse redness (DR)

2. Fundamental Color
   White (Cw)
   Blue (Cb)

3. Form
   Small, straight varices (F1)
   Enlarged, tortuous; occupy less than ⅓ of lumen (F2)
   Largest coil-shaped; occupy more than ⅓ of lumen (F3)

4. Location (longitudinal extent)
   Lower ⅓ (Li)
   Mid ⅓ below tracheal bifurcation (Lm)
   Upper ⅓ above tracheal bifurcation (Ls)

5. Adjunctive Finding
   Erosion (E+)

*The RWM and CRS are graded from 1+ to 3+ depending on number and extent.

Using this classification, Beppu et al.[23] carried out a retrospective analysis of 172 patients with varices to compare prior bleeding to the variceal classification.

In the group of patients with no red color signs (RCS), only 9.1% had prior bleeding. However, 58.7% of patients with RCS had a history of bleeding, a statistically significant difference. The majority of those with diffuse redness (DR) had prior bleeding, but most had other RCS, and there was no correlation between DR alone and bleeding.

With respect to color, 79.4% of patients with bluish varices (Cb) had prior bleeding, whereas 45.7% of those with whitish varices (Cw) had bleeding, a significant difference. It was concluded that patients with Cb had a greater risk of bleeding irrespective of the presence or absence or even the extent of RCS. If the varices were classified as Cw, bleeding appeared to depend on the presence of RCS. If there were none, the chance of bleeding was small.

The presence of large varices correlated with a history of prior variceal bleeding, but most large varices also had RCS, and the higher percentage of patients with large varices in the group with prior bleeding was attributed to this. There was no relation between prior bleeding and length of the variceal columns. Evidence of esophagitis was found in only 9 (3.2%) patients, but 7 of these had bled. The presence of esophagitis was believed to be a predictive factor, although the small number of patients with this finding precluded a definite conclusion.

Beppu et al.[23] concluded that RCS and bluish variceal color correlated with a history of bleeding. However, linear extent of the columns and variceal diameter did not correlate with bleeding. Other authors report similar findings.[22]

The Nature of RCS

Beppu et al.[23] regarded RCS as microtelangiectasias or small dilated vessels. Although the exact nature of these red spots is uncertain, there is evidence that they are not small vascular structures.

Spence et al.[24] studied esophageal tissue from 27 patients who underwent esophageal transection and reanastomosis for esophageal varices. These tissue rings were compared with ones from patients with other diseases. Dilated intraepithelial blood-filled channels were found in all of the rings from patients with varices. When studied by electronmicroscopy these channels were found to be lined by cells that were not typical endothelial cells. The authors suggested that these intraepithelial channels may correspond to the cherry-red spots seen endoscopically and that they may play a role in variceal hemorrhage.

Cause of Variceal Hemorrhage

Despite a greater understanding of the pathogenesis of esophageal varices, the immediate cause and events that lead to hemorrhage remain unknown. There is no correlation between the level of portal pressure and the risk of bleeding in patients with established portal hypertension. There have been attempts to implicate other factors such as the presence of ascites, changes in plasma volume, and reflux esophagitis. Although increases in portal flow and pressure were thought to occur in association with ascites, Iwatsuki and Reynolds[25] demonstrated that portal pressure and hepatic blood flow are unchanged after paracentesis. Esophageal erosions due to gastroesophageal reflux have been considered as a precipitating factor. However, esophageal function in patients with a history of variceal bleeding has been shown to be normal,[26, 27] and there is no histologic evidence of esophagitis.[28] Although plasma volume is known to be increased in cirrhosis, it is unlikely that sudden increases occur in the non-hospitalized patient, although loss of plasma volume may be a factor in the intermittent cessations of bleeding that occur in variceal hemorrhage.

Certain aspects of the endoscopic appearance of esophageal varices may have predictive value with respect to bleeding. Variceal diameter and/or linear extent have been suggested as predictive of hemorrhage, but it appears that variceal size may change over the course of time. There is some speculation that large variceal diameter plus red color signs may be reliable indicators of a high risk of bleeding.

CLINICAL ASPECTS OF VARICEAL HEMORRHAGE

Natural History of Variceal Bleeding

The frequency of esophageal varices in patients with cirrhosis varies from about 14% to 77%.[29] Many patients with portal hypertension and esophageal varices never develop variceal bleeding; this occurs in 12% to 70% of patients with cirrhosis.[29] An initial episode of bleeding appears in cirrhotic patients at a rate of about 10% per year, although the incidence of recurrent bleeding is 46%.[30] About two thirds of patients who are followed prospectively after recovering from an episode of bleeding will have recurrent hemorrhage.[31, 32] When variceal hemorrhage recurs in-hospital after discontinuance of tamponade, the mortality is very high.[33]

Variceal bleeding stops spontaneously in about 60% of patients, although bleeding will resume in about one third of these.[34] Variceal bleeding is, however, a frequent cause of upper gastrointestinal hemorrhage that is severe and persistent. Fleischer[35] found that about 20% of patients with upper gastrointestinal hemorrhage could be classified as having severe, persistent bleeding and that among these patients esophageal varices was the most common cause. Although this study suggests variceal bleeding is a likely cause of severe persistent bleeding, the nature of the patient population of the institution where this investigation was carried out was not defined and might have included a greater than usual percentage of patients with alcoholic cirrhosis.

The prognosis for patients with variceal bleeding depends significantly on the underlying cause of portal hypertension. The outcome for a group of patients having a high percentage with alcoholic cirrhosis will be markedly worse than that for a group in which presinusoidal portal hypertension predominates. Exsanguination is usually preventable, but patients may succumb to other complications of the underlying disease with hemorrhage being frequently an initial event that contributes in varying measure to other causes of death.

Despite the difficulties with establishing prognosis in variceal bleeding, the associated mortality is obviously high. In general, variceal hemorrhage has the worst prognosis of all causes of upper gastrointestinal bleeding with some exceptions such as an aortoduodenal fistula. The survey of the American Society for Gastrointestinal Endoscopy (ASGE) on gastrointestinal bleeding indicated that over 30% of patients with this diagnosis died.[36] Graham and Smith[34] determined that the mortality associated with variceal bleeding in patients with advanced cirrhosis is 42% at 6 weeks from onset.

Approximately three fourths of these deaths occurred during the first week after onset of hemorrhage, and almost two thirds of these are attributed to hemorrhage. In those patients that survive beyond 6 weeks, the causes of death were equally distributed among bleeding, hepatic failure, and other causes. Furthermore, survival is better in those patients alive at 6 weeks after an episode of variceal hemorrhage in comparison to the initial 6-week period after an episode of variceal hemorrhage. The survival curve for this select group actually approximates that for patients with similar liver disease who have not had any bleeding.

The long-term overall outcome for patients with cirrhosis and varices is poor and depends in greater measure on the severity of the underlying liver disease rather than the occurrence of variceal bleeding. For example, Garceau and Chalmers[37] studied survival in patients with cirrhosis and esophageal varices. The survival for a group of 288 patients with varices but without bleeding was compared with a group of 179 patients who had sustained variceal bleeding. Five-year survival was less than 10% for both groups.

Diagnosis of Esophageal Varices

There are three methods to diagnose esophagogastric varices: barium swallow radiography, percutaneous transhepatic portography, and gastrointestinal endoscopy. For practical purposes, gastrointestinal endoscopy is the primary method especially when a patient presents with acute variceal hemorrhage.

Although some reports indicate a close correlation between endoscopic and x-ray diagnosis,[8] the results of most comparative studies indicate that endoscopy is superior to radiography for recognition of varices unless the varices are large, in which case the two methods may be equal.[21, 38] Contrast radiography is seldom if ever used now as an initial procedure in the diagnosis of upper gastrointestinal bleeding.

Percutaneous transhepatic portography offers the best anatomic definition of the collateral circulation.[17] Gastric varices are often demonstrated to be more prominent than appreciated by endoscopy or contrast radiography. However, transhepatic portography is a highly invasive and technically complex procedure that has a significant complication rate. It is seldom performed.

Indications for Endoscopy

Early endoscopy is indicated for any patient with gastrointestinal hemorrhage and known or suspected esophageal varices. Certain measures that are relatively specific in the management of variceal bleeding are inappropriate or contraindicated in other causes of gastrointestinal hemorrhage. Therefore, accurate diagnosis is mandatory.

Upper gastrointestinal bleeding that occurs in patients with known varices may have many sources. Endoscopy has established that other causes of bleeding are frequent. Dagradi et al.,[39] for example, found that varices were the source of bleeding in only 41% of 121 patients with cirrhosis and large esophageal varices. Palmer[40] found a nonvariceal bleeding site in 37% of patients with known varices and upper gastrointestinal hemorrhage. Nonvariceal sites were found by McCray et al.[41] in 72% of patients, by Waldram et al.[42] in 40%, and by Novis et al.[33] in 34%.

Although most authors emphasize the possibility of nonvariceal sites in patients with hemorrhage and known varices others have found varices to be the most common source in such patients. For example, Dave et al.[43] reported 140 consecutive cases of patients with known varices and gastrointestinal bleeding. Esophageal varices were the source of bleeding in 90% regardless of whether liver disease was due to alcoholism or other causes. Schoppe et al.[44] found that esophageal varices were the source of bleeding in 86% of 28 episodes of bleeding in 20 patients with portal hypertension that was due to causes other than alcoholic cirrhosis. Mitchell et al.[45] prospectively studied 90 episodes of bleeding in 65 patients with known portal hypertension and esophageal varices. Twenty-four of 54 patients had cirrhosis that was due to alcohol. Endoscopy was performed within 24 hours of admission. Variceal bleeding was diagnosed in only 23.3% of patients and a coexistent lesion was found in 38.8%, although the latter was bleeding in only 5.6% of cases. Of the 64 patients that did not have acute bleeding at the time of endoscopy 60.9% had recurrent bleeding. Repeated endoscopy in these patients disclosed active variceal bleeding in 20 cases (74.1%).

Endoscopic Diagnosis of Variceal Hemorrhage

Four sets of circumstances are possible when endoscopy is performed in a patient with esophageal varices and gastrointestinal bleeding; active variceal bleeding, non-bleeding varices without any other lesions or sources of bleeding, non-bleeding varices with another lesion that is actively bleeding, and non-bleeding varices plus one or more other lesions that are not bleeding.

In more than one half of the patients who had variceal bleeding in the ASGE survey, there was no evidence of variceal bleeding at the time of endoscopy.[46] If recent bleeding is an established fact, or there is old or fresh blood in the upper gastrointestinal tract, the presence of varices in the absence of any other lesion can usually be accepted as evidence of variceal bleeding. However, the possibility of another occult lesion, such as a small vascular ectasia that might be overlooked in the presence of a quantity of blood in the upper gastrointestinal tract, cannot be eliminated entirely. Even when bleeding has stopped, there may nevertheless be endoscopic clues that indicate a variceal bleed. A clot may occasionally be found protruding from a varix. Generally this appears as a conical elevation with a red or brown tip on the surface of the varix.

In about 45% of patients with variceal bleeding there is evidence of variceal blood loss at the time of endoscopy.[46] This may be torrential hemorrhage that itself presents a diagnostic problem if the endoscopist is unable to clear the field of blood. Hemorrhage such as this occurred in less than 10% of cases in the ASGE survey. It is unusual to actually observe blood flowing or spurting from a varix at endoscopy. If a bleeding point is visualized, it generally has no distinguishing features and simply appears as blood flowing from a small rent or hole in the wall of a varix (see Plate 16–2). In patients who have not undergone prior sclerotherapy, such a bleeding point will characteristically be near the esophagogastric mucosal junction. Slow bleeding or oozing of blood or an adherent clot at the site of variceal bleeding are more common findings.

The presence of esophageal varices and a second potential source of blood loss presents one of the most difficult problems for the endoscopist, since it may be impossible to determine the source of bleeding. Careful evaluation may reveal some feature that incriminates one lesion, a visible vessel in an ulcer base for example. When this fails, the patient must be closely observed during the convalescent period. Lesions that have an acid-peptic etiology may be treated with appropriate measures, and endoscopy should be performed promptly if bleeding recurs. Generally, sclerotherapy should be postponed if it cannot be established that bleeding was variceal.

Variceal hemorrhage is typically intermittent. When bleeding has stopped, a question may arise concerning precipitation of further bleeding by an endoscopic examination. Although it is possible that passage of an endoscope may dislodge a clot, this is not a common complication. In the ASGE survey, 215 patients with variceal bleeding underwent endoscopy. Bleeding attributed to the procedure occurred in 1.4% of these patients. In one case this was said to have led to the patient's demise. Endoscopy in any patient with upper gastrointestinal bleeding, especially profuse bleeding, requires special skills and experience. The complication rate for this type of emergency procedure is significantly higher than that for routine diagnostic endoscopy. No matter what type of lesion is responsible for bleeding, it is possible that endoscopic manipulation may precipitate bleeding. Nevertheless, accurate diagnosis is the basis for many therapeutic decisions when variceal bleeding is a consideration.

MANAGEMENT OF VARICEAL HEMORRHAGE

Relation to the Natural History of Variceal Bleeding

Differences in the clinical course of patients before and after 6 weeks from the onset of variceal bleeding have important implications with respect to therapy. If therapy is delayed, survival beginning from the point of treatment appears to improve, irrespective of other variables, because a significant number of presumably poor risk patients will have died. Smith and Graham[47] demonstrated that varying the time of entry of patients into any study concerned with the outcome of variceal bleeding will in itself alter the survival curve. Many studies of various methods of treatment, including sclerotherapy, pertain to selected and more favorable patient populations, a fact that is sometimes not obvious. Since, in most instances, therapy is initiated in response to, and not in anticipation of, bleeding, and since mortality and

cause of death vary considerably before and after 6 weeks from onset, management must be divided into immediate and long-term measures.

The objectives of immediate therapy are to prevent exsanguination, stop bleeding, and prevent recurrent bleeding with a minimum of complications. The goals of long-term therapy are to prevent further hemorrhage, to favorably influence survival, and to do both with minimum complications and side effects.

Currently, it is not possible to attain all these objectives with a single approach. For example, for a given method a reduction in hemorrhage may entail an unacceptable decrease in survival or increased morbidity. The interrelationships of survival, reduction of hemorrhage, complications, and side effects are also influenced by the severity of the underlying liver disease. The latter, the single most important determinant in overall survival, further compounds the difficulty of evaluating the efficacy of any form of management. Severity of liver disease does not, however, predict the manner of death.

Non-endoscopic Management

Management of Acute Variceal Hemorrhage

In addition to sclerotherapy, the methods for immediate control of hemorrhage include balloon tamponade, intravenous vasopressin, and emergency portosystemic shunt surgery. The relatively simple measures of tamponade and intravenous vasopressin, while effective, can only be considered temporary.

Bleeding is controlled initially by intravenous vasopressin in 50% to 75% of cases. It decreases flow in the superior mesenteric artery and portal vein by approximately 40% and reduces portal pressure by about 25%. It also lowers cardiac output and raises blood pressure and must be used with care when cardiac ischemia may not be well tolerated.

Balloon tamponade is generally employed after or with vasopressin in patients with severe and/or persistent bleeding. Some earlier studies suggested that tamponade has a high complication rate.[48, 49] Other carefully performed trials demonstrate that it is not only effective in most patients but also reasonably safe.[50, 51] However, monitoring by experienced personnel is required.

It is difficult to evaluate the results of emergency portacaval shunting for acute bleeding. Operative mortality is high, but recurrent bleeding is reduced dramatically.[52] It does not appear that the outcome with this approach is much different from that for the natural history of varical bleeding. The event proportions have simply changed: i.e., death due to bleeding is replaced by death due to surgery.

Percutaneous transhepatic obliteration of varices has been used in some centers, and although there was initial enthusiasm, it appears to be unsatisfactory. Portal vein thrombosis developed in about one third of these patients, bleeding resumed in more than half, and the procedure cannot be repeated.[53, 54]

Long-Term Management After Variceal Hemorrhage

The only approach to long-term control of variceal bleeding, until the resurgence of sclerotherapy and perhaps the use of propranolol, has been surgery. There are substantial problems with interpretation of data from early studies.[55] Later trials generally demonstrate a decrease in bleeding, an increase in encephalopathy, and no marked survival advantage.[56, 57] Various modifications of the portosystemic shunt are designed to improve results.[58] Other operations have been devised, such as devascularization and/or transection-reanastomosis using the stapling gun.[59-61] In general, these procedures have not been evaluated in controlled trials.

Lebrec et al.[62, 63] reported a trial of propranolol in good-risk patients that demonstrated a significant decrease in repeated episodes of hemorrhage compared with a control group. However, this therapy did not prove to be of value in another trial in patients with more severe liver disease.[64]

Prophylactic Treatment of Esophageal Varices

Prophylactic therapy for variceal hemorrhage is inherently indiscriminate. Because it has not been possible to predict which patients will develop variceal bleeding, some patients will undergo unnecessary therapy. The results of prophylactic portosystemic shunt surgery have been unsatisfactory.[65-67]

Endoscopic Management of Variceal Bleeding

Non-Injection Methods

Although there are various endoscopic methods available for control of gastrointes-

tinal hemorrhage, few of these have been employed in large series of patients for bleeding esophageal varices.

Jensen et al.[68] compared the efficacy of sclerotherapy, ferromagnetic tamponade, argon laser, Nd:YAG laser, monopolar electrocoagulation, and the heater probe for control of variceal bleeding in an animal model. Sclerotherapy and Nd:YAG laser were more effective than other methods. Fleischer[69] was able to stop active variceal bleeding in 7 of 10 patients using the Nd:YAG laser, although bleeding recurred frequently.

Sclerotherapy of Esophageal Varices

Indications

Sclerotherapy can be employed as an initial measure for control of acute variceal hemorrhage, in which case a range of circumstances may be encountered. These include torrential hemorrhage, slower blood loss around a clot adherent to a varix, or no evidence of the actual bleeding point. Variceal sclerosis may also be initiated after attempting to stop or slow bleeding using vasopressin and/or tamponade, although this does not guarantee that active bleeding will not be encountered during the procedure. Sclerotherapy may also be used as long-term management in an effort to prevent recurrent bleeding by obliterating all variceal channels.

Variceal sclerosis is not indicated for all causes of portal hypertension and variceal bleeding. Although highly effective in thrombosis of the portal vein, it is inappropriate in membranous obstruction of the inferior vena cava. In patients with cirrhosis, there is a wide range of hepatic reserve. When liver function has deteriorated to a marked degree, therapeutic options are limited but usually include sclerotherapy. In patients with relatively good liver function, however, there will usually be more therapeutic choices. The efficacy and complications of sclerotherapy must then be weighed against the risk and benefit of other methods of management.

Therapeutic modalities may also be combined simultaneously or in sequence in the management of variceal bleeding. For example, sclerotherapy might be used for acute and early management and surgery for long-term treatment. Vasopressin and/or balloon tamponade are often used as adjunctive or initial therapy in reported series of patients undergoing sclerotherapy for acute hemorrhage. Therapeutic combinations such as these have not been specifically evaluated. When methods are combined it is possible that one method will complicate the use of another. For example, sclerotherapy might make certain surgical procedures more difficult technically. The use of more than one therapeutic modality in the treatment of any group of patients also makes the assessment of results more difficult.

Many questions concerning the indications for sclerotherapy cannot be answered by presently available information. There should be reasonably good evidence based on endoscopic assessment that bleeding is or has been variceal in origin. Beyond this, it is difficult to make precise recommendations for the use of sclerotherapy at this time, although some general recommendations can be based on reported experience and practice.

Sclerotherapy is difficult if there is active hemorrhage, since blood frequently obscures the field making precise injection difficult (Plate 16–3). Although this situation cannot always be avoided and active variceal bleeding can be controlled by sclerotherapy, the procedure should not be used as the first therapeutic measure if possible. Other measures such as intravenous vasopressin and/or tamponade are effective for the immediate control of bleeding, are more readily available, and permit a period of time in most cases, during which the patient can be stabilized and appropriate preparations made for the sclerotherapy. In many reported series in which sclerotherapy was used for acute control of bleeding, initial management included tamponade and/or vasopressin.[70–74] The complication rate associated with sclerotherapy for active hemorrhage may also be higher than that for procedures performed under more controlled conditions, although this point has not been addressed in the literature (Plate 16–4 and Fig. 16–1). Since recurrent bleeding carries a high mortality, variceal sclerosis should be instituted in the first few hours after initial control of bleeding.

Most endoscopists experienced in sclerotherapy use the procedure in the long-term management of patients after variceal bleeding in an effort to reduce recurrent bleeding. There are a number of trials that compare sclerotherapy to conservative "medical" management, and these generally indicate favorable results for sclerotherapy at least with respect to recurrent hemorrhage and blood loss. For selected, good-risk patients, surgery

may also be an option in long-term management, especially the selective shunt procedures. There are no reported trials of sclerotherapy versus this type of operation in good risk patients.

The relation of liver function status to the selection of patients for sclerotherapy is problematic. This is less an issue in the immediate management of persistent variceal hemorrhage, especially when tamponade and vasopressin fail to control bleeding. However, many episodes of variceal hemorrhage cease spontaneously. The risk-benefit ratio of sclerotherapy has not been studied in a select group of patients with good liver function and spontaneous cessation of bleeding. It cannot be stated on the basis of any published data that long-term sclerotherapy is superior to shunt surgery in a group such as this. When surgery cannot be considered, either because of poor liver function, prior operation, or technical reasons, there is a stronger

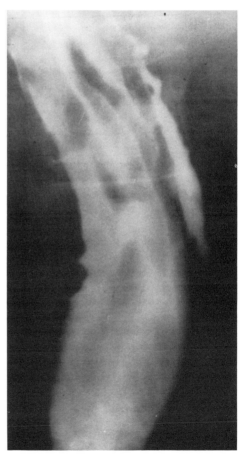

FIGURE 16–1. Barium swallow radiograph of same patient shown in Plate 16–4 demonstrates ulceration with extensive necrosis and walled-off perforation.

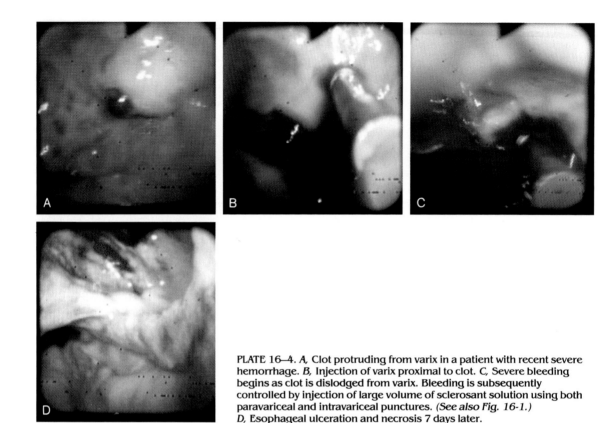

PLATE 16–4. *A,* Clot protruding from varix in a patient with recent severe hemorrhage. *B,* Injection of varix proximal to clot. *C,* Severe bleeding begins as clot is dislodged from varix. Bleeding is subsequently controlled by injection of large volume of sclerosant solution using both paravariceal and intravariceal punctures. *(See also Fig. 16-1.) D,* Esophageal ulceration and necrosis 7 days later.

argument for long-term sclerotherapy. The benefit of a protracted series of procedures, however, has not been confirmed by all investigators.[75]

A trial of prophylactic sclerotherapy that demonstrated that variceal sclerosis was superior to conservative management was reported by Paquet[76] in 1982. A similar study was reported by Witzel et al.[77] in 1985 in which 109 patients were randomized to

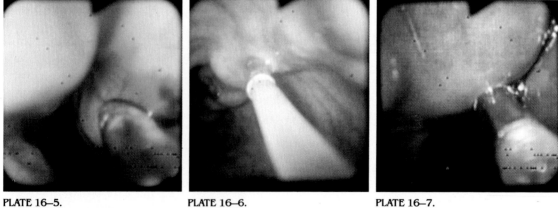

PLATE 16–5.   PLATE 16–6.   PLATE 16–7.

PLATE 16–5. Intravariceal injection of varix at esophagogastric junction.
PLATE 16–6. Intravariceal injection of esophageal varix. Injection needle is placed about 2 cm beyond the end of endoscope. In this position any sudden motion is absorbed by the injector's flexibility, and tearing of the varix is more easily avoided.
PLATE 16–7. Intravariceal injection of large varix near esophagogastric junction. Note characteristic grayish color change.

sclerotherapy or conservative management. In this study the endoscopically treated patients experienced not only a decreased frequency of variceal bleeding, but also a significantly better survival than the conservatively treated group. Although the outcomes of these two trials are favorable, there are not enough data at present to recommend sclerotherapy in patients without prior or ongoing bleeding.

Technique of Sclerotherapy

Virtually all techniques for endoscopic injection sclerosis are empiric, and there is great variability in methodology. This makes evaluation of results more difficult, since it is not known if a lower complication rate or better results are possible with one method compared with another. The variables include selection of sclerosing agent or agents, injection volume, pattern of injections, intravariceal versus paravariceal injections, schedule of procedures, choice of endoscope, and the use of various methods of compression.

Animal Experiments

Unfortunately, there are only a few experimental studies of sclerotherapy in animal models.

Sugawa et al.[78] demonstrated in an animal model that intravariceal injection of 5% sodium morrhuate produced intravenous thrombosis, perivenous fibrosis, and thickening of the intima of the veins. Injections were repeated an average of 3 times per animal, and endoscopy was performed at weekly intervals. Ulcers at injection sites were frequent, but these healed in about 3 weeks. It appeared that development of an ulcer depended to some degree on the injected volume of sclerosant.

Jensen et al.[68] compared the efficacy of sclerotherapy, ferromagnetic tamponade, argon and Nd:YAG laser photocoagulation, monopolar electrocoagulation, and a heater probe for control of variceal hemorrhage in an animal model. Intravariceal injections were made after bleeding was induced by puncture with a 19-gauge needle. An attempt was also made to reinduce bleeding by inflating a balloon proximal to the bleeding point after achieving control of bleeding. Nd:YAG laser photocoagulation and sclerotherapy were more effective in controlling bleeding, whereas all other methods were significantly less effective. Hemorrhage resumed after every method of treatment except Nd:YAG laser photocoagulation and sclerotherapy. The laser treatment was technically easier than injection sclerosis, but was associated with more frequent ulceration and nonobliteration of varices.

Instrumentation

A sclerosing agent or solution is injected with an injection device or injector. This accessory usually consists of a long, thin tube with a needle at the distal end and a connection for a syringe at the proximal end. A variety are available commercially. Some degree of flexibility is of assistance in avoiding laceration of a varix during a puncture as a result of motion caused by the endoscopist, esophageal contractions, or movement by the patient (especially by belching). The most flexible devices are simple tubular systems made of a synthetic material. These may potentially damage the fiberscope as they are passed through the accessory channel near the distal instrument tip. This can be avoided by being careful not to insert the injector through the channel when the bending section of the fiberscope is acutely angulated. Many injectors have a second outer sheath added, into which the needle is withdrawn when not in use. This increases the rigidity of the injector. Some retractable injectors have a spiral metal wire outer sheath. These tend to be even more rigid.

The advantages of a rigid endoscope have been stressed in some large series.[70, 79–81] Although large-caliber instruments can be used to compress varices and have excellent suction capability, use of a rigid endoscope frequently necessitates general anesthesia. This reduces some of the technical problems of sclerotherapy, lessens the danger of aspiration, and allows the endoscopist to focus attention on the injection procedure; it is an added risk for patients with poor liver function.

A higher incidence of instrument related perforation might be expected when a rigid endoscope is used, but this is not the case in reported series.[70, 79–81] However, it is difficult to extrapolate the work individuals skilled in rigid endoscopy to a prediction of general experience with this type of instrument. At present, few endoscopists are proficient with rigid endoscopes. Reilly et al.[82] initially used a rigid instrument, but they encountered problems, including difficulty with insertion, broken teeth, inability to inject gastric varices, pressure necrosis of the proximal esophagus, and problems related to general anesthesia. Fewer such problems were encountered when they changed to a fiberscope.

There are no data to indicate that use of one type of endoscope produces better results or is safer than others. Because of familiarity and ease of use, fiberscopes are preferred for sclerotherapy by most experienced endoscopists. Less than 1% of respondents in a survey of the ASGE indicated a preference for a rigid endoscope.[83] The main limitation of the fiberoptic instrument is its lesser degree of suction capability relative to that of various rigid instruments. Usually this is not a serious drawback unless hemorrhage is torrential. The fiberoptic instrument selected is a matter of personal preference. Double-channel fiberscopes or those with a single, large-diameter channel are probably more suitable.

Technique of Injection

Some sclerotherapy techniques incorporate various methods of variceal compression. Sclerotherapy is thought to be facilitated if compression of variceal columns is applied at a point proximal to an intended injection site. Theoretically, this retards disappearance of the sclerosant from the injection area and enhances its effect by virtue of more prolonged contact with the intima of the vein. Compression devices may also be used to control torrential bleeding when this is difficult or impossible to control by sclerotherapy alone.

Ease of variceal compression is a theoretical advantage of rigid instruments. These are sometimes modified by placing a slot at the distal end of the instrument. The varix to be injected protrudes into the slot to facilitate injection. Rotation of the instrument to the next puncture site produces compression of the previous site. Accessories and maneuvers have been devised for use with fiberscopes in an effort to retain this effect. These include balloon compression after completing injections, a balloon cuff attached to the endoscope, an overtube sheath, and a balloon fixed at the cardia of the stomach during injections.

A semi-flexible overtube sheath used in conjunction with a fiberscope was introduced by Williams and Dawson (Fig. 16–2).[84] This fits over the insertion tube of the flexible endoscope and has a window at its distal end through which successive varices can be injected as the device is rotated. The use of the overtube sheath was compared with free-hand injections in a study by Westaby et al.[85] Twenty-one patients underwent sclerotherapy using the overtube method, and 19 pa-

tients using free-hand injection. There was significantly less bleeding in the former group during the first 24 hours after sclerotherapy, but this was associated with a significant increase in esophageal stricture and postinjection pain. Bleeding recurred with the same frequency in both groups, although it was less severe in those treated by the sheath method. None of 11 bleeding episodes were fatal in the overtube treated group, compared with 5 of 15 fatal hemorrhages in the free-hand injection group. There was a trend toward earlier obliteration of varices when the overtube sheath was used.

Variceal compression can also be accomplished during sclerotherapy using various balloon devices. Usually this is done by placing a balloon cuff on the insertion tube of the endoscope at some location proximal to the distal tip.[86–88] There are also more complex methods. Takase et al.[89] used a balloon cuff on the insertion tube plus a balloon fixed in the cardia; in addition they performed injections under fluoroscopic control using a contrast agent in order to be certain of intravariceal injection. This method was successful even when there was active variceal bleeding. Wang et al.[90] combined the overtube method with a gastric balloon by using a modified orotracheal tube. This small-diameter device requires that a fiberoptic bronchoscope be used for injections.

The use of variceal compression should be considered in relation to variceal anatomy (vide supra) and, based on available data from human and animal studies, there is some doubt that the effect of the procedure is enhanced by promoting stasis and prolonged contact of the sclerosant with the veins.[91] Radiographic contrast agents have been combined with sclerosant in a few investigations to assess the movement of the sclerosing agent during and after injections. Silvis et al.[92] demonstrated that compression results in retention of active agent at the puncture site in an animal model. However, collateral vessels in the abdominal wall were used, and this is probably not analogous to the esophageal circulation. Grobe et al.[91] found that despite intended intravariceal injections, there was a local accumulation of the material at the puncture site in 44% of injections. In another 42% there was rapid clearance in a cephalad direction, and in 14% the injected material was rapidly cleared toward the gastric veins. Proximal compression with a balloon attached to the endoscope did not prevent cephalad movement of the injected material. A similar study by Barsoum et al.[93] also demonstrated rapid clearance toward the extrinsic veins. From both studies it can be concluded that the local accumulation of contrast medium is due to extravasation around the vein. This suggests that it is not always possible to position precisely the injection needle within the lumen of a varix, and/or that sclerosant will leak into the surrounding tissue via the needle track.

Since several reports demonstrate rapid clearance of injected substances in a cephalad direction in many patients, it is perhaps more likely that compression promotes clearance of sclerosant via the perforating veins to the extrinsic system rather than enhanced stasis-contact of the agent with the varix. Inflation of the balloon cuff before beginning injections may theoretically promote ongoing hemorrhage or dislodge a clot from a varix.

Free-hand injection is less complicated but requires quickness and skill when there is active bleeding (Plates 16–5, 16–6, 16–7, and 16–8). Some authors maintain that this is highly effective without resorting to compression.[94]

Injection sites may be placed paravariceally.[95–99] Injections may also be made by intravariceal puncture (Plates 16–5 through 16–8).[70, 71, 74, 80, 82, 86, 88, 94, 100–111] It is also possible to combine both methods of injection.[72, 112–114] Intravariceal injection appears to be the preferred method, based on descriptions in the current literature.

Rose et al.[115] reported that intravariceal injections were more thrombogenic than paravariceal injections in a study of 40 patients; a contrast agent was added to the sclerosant solution. The follow-up period was short, however, and the long-term effects of the two methods were not determined. Intravariceal punctures were accurately placed in only 75% of attempts on average. The accuracy was less if the varices were of small diameter, but somewhat greater if the diameters were large.

Multiple injections can be made over long segments of the esophagus, or the pattern can be limited to the distal few centimeters.[72, 116] There are no data to indicate that any approach is more satisfactory than another. It would be logical to inject vessels near the esophagogastric junction and within the cardia of the stomach, since variceal bleeding usually originates in the distal esophagus. After sclerotherapy, however, the original pattern of variceal blood flow is undoubtedly altered and bleeding prior to obliteration of the variceal columns can recur even in the mid-esophagus.

The volume injected per puncture and the volume used per procedure are other variables. A hypothetical ideal volume would be based on the concentration of the sclerosant, perhaps the type of agent, and the placement of injections, whether intravariceal or paravariceal.

Sclerosing Agents

There are little scientific data to guide the selection of a sclerosing agent or agents. The ideal agent should cause rapid thrombosis that is followed quickly by intimal damage to the vein. Fibrosis and obliteration of the vein with minimal damage to underlying esophageal muscle should then occur. It should be innocuous in the extra-esophageal vascular circulation, by means of which the substance may potentially reach other organs. A variety of agents have been used empirically or on the basis of information extrapolated from data and experience with sclerotherapy of

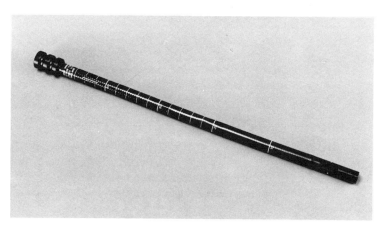

FIGURE 16–2. Williams overtube sleeve for injection of esophageal varices. Note window through which varices are injected (at right end of the device).

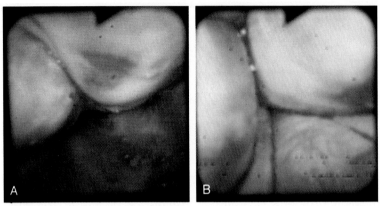

PLATE 16–8. *A,* Appearance of mid-esophageal varices a few moments after injection. Note distention and change to a "dirty" white color. *B,* Swollen distal esophageal varices after injection.

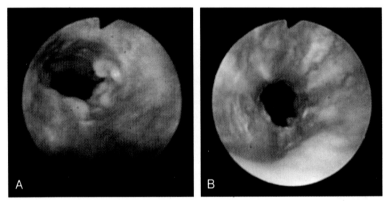

PLATE 16–9. *A,* Appearance of distal esophagus in another patient after 6 sclerotherapy sessions. *B,* Note residual vasa vasorum of the varices.

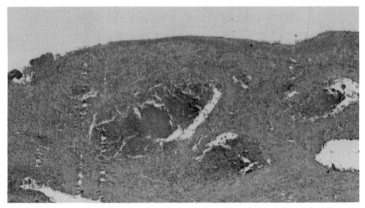

PLATE 16–10. Microscopic section of esophageal wall showing inflammatory reaction and fibrous obliteration of variceal channels as a result of sclerotherapy.

varicose veins in the lower extremities.[117] Agents with presumably different modes of action can be used together.[82, 94, 106, 107] The sequential use of different agents has also been proposed.

The many chemical agents that cause tissue damage and inflammation may be loosely classified according to their mode of action.[118] Those that react directly with tissue components include organic compounds such as salicylate quinine hydrochloride, heavy metal salts such as mercuric iodine, highly reactive halogens such as Lugol's solution, and virtually any strong alkaline solution. This group is unsuitable for esophageal sclerotherapy. The second broad category is composed of those agents whose action is physical rather than directly chemical. Included are the more familiar fatty acids such as sodium morrhuate and ethanolamine oleate. This category also contains aqueous solutions, such as the highly branched alkyl salt sodium tetradecyl sulfate and ethanol. Other empirically used agents include drugs such as cefazolin and topical bovine thrombin. Some agents, such as hypertonic glucose, act mainly through an osmotic and dehydrating effect.

According to one report, tetradecyl sulfate was superior to fatty acids (ethanolamine oleate, sodium morrhuate) because its action was more localized, an effect thought to be due to its neutral pH as opposed to the alkalinity of fatty acid solutions.[118] Blenkinsopp[119] in 1967 compared tetradecyl sulfate solutions with 5% ethanolamine in rats and found the 3% tetradecyl sulfate solution to be the most effective with respect to occlusion of veins and 5% ethanolamine the least effective. If injected paravariceally, all agents tested in this study were ineffective. No pathologic changes were found in the heart or lungs of the animals. In animal experiments Reiner[120] found tetradecyl more thrombogenic than morrhuate. Jensen et al.,[68] using an animal model, compared the efficacy of different agents including 5% sodium morrhuate, 5% ethanolamine oleate, 1.5% sodium tetradecyl sulfate, cefazolin, 95% and 45% ethanol, and a solution containing 0.5% tetradecyl and thrombin (50 U/ml) in 50% dextrose. With regard to hemostasis, all agents were equally effective. In another study by this group using a canine model, 1% tetradecyl plus 32% ethanol, 1.5% tetradecyl, and 5% morrhuate were more effective than cefazolin, 47% ethanol, 5% ethanolamine, and a combination of tetra-

decyl (0.5%) plus thrombin and 50% glucose.[121] There was a direct relationship between the degree of esophageal damage and effectiveness. The results of one study in humans suggested that 3% tetradecyl sulfate was less ulcerogenic than 5% morrhuate.[122]

It is difficult at present to recommend an agent or agents. Since all produce tissue damage, it is probable that within limits the end result achieved with different substances can be approximated by changing their concentrations. For example, the degree of tissue damage produced by a relatively destructive agent can be made to equal that of a less potent substance by decreasing the concentration of the former. For this reason, it is difficult to classify one substance as more "ulcerogenic" or more "effective" than another. The tissue reaction is also related to other factors such as the volume of sclerosant injected, perhaps the rate of injection, and the placement of the injections. It is possible that some substances may be more suitable for paravariceal injections compared with intravariceal injections and vice versa. Although the favorable and untoward results at an injection site may be nonspecific for the various agents, systemic side effects and complications occurring at sites removed from the esophagus could be related to the chemical composition of the agent in a more specific way. For example, the pattern and incidence of systemic complications for one sclerosant might be different from others. Many substances used for sclerotherapy are not available for worldwide use, or their use is restricted.

Schedule of Procedures

A single procedure is usually inadequate for the long-term prevention of recurrent bleeding. In the majority of reported series a sequence of injections was utilized to achieve variceal obliteration. Generally obliteration is judged by endoscopic assessment, although this may be imprecise.

If long-term control of recurrent hemorrhage is accepted as an indication, it is logical to perform a number of procedures at short intervals during the early period after onset of hemorrhage to prevent recurrent hemorrhage during this high mortality period. However, the most effective and safest schedule has not been established. This will undoubtedly vary according to the type of sclerosant, its concentration, the total volume injected per procedure, and the number and placement of injections. Each of these variables must be considered; excessiveness with respect to any one may lead to severe ulceration and necrosis. For example, an excessive number of injections of even a relatively unconcentrated and non-destructive agent may cause a degree of esophageal damage equal to that produced by a smaller number of injections of an excessively concentrated agent.

Westaby et al.[123] performed a randomized trial of sclerotherapy at 1-week and 3-week intervals in 55 patients. There was no difference between the two schedules with regard to efficacy, complications, or frequency of recurrent bleeding. However, in the group undergoing sclerotherapy at weekly intervals, it was often necessary to delay scheduled procedures because of ulceration. The time lapse to obliteration of varices was twice as long in the patients injected at 3-week intervals. Prior to obliteration, five deaths occurred in each group, one of five being due to bleeding in the group treated at weekly intervals and four of five due to bleeding in the 3-week interval group.

Obliteration of varices does not occur after a fixed number of procedures (Plate 16–9). Many injections in a long series of procedures may be required for large vessels, whereas smaller ones require only a few procedures.[115] It is possible to obliterate all variceal channels, but perhaps not in all patients. Thrombosed vessels may remain visible, although puncture of these does not produce any bleeding. After a series of injections, small, interrupted, nodular-appearing vessels may still be present. Intravariceal injection with assurance may become difficult. Further injection procedures may not increase effectiveness and may result in greater esophageal damage. It is sometimes difficult, therefore, to know when to conclude the series of procedures.

It would be advantageous to determine when and where blood flow persists after variceal sclerosis. Modification of the injection pattern according to these findings would permit fewer injections without loss of effect, but perhaps with less esophageal ulceration. Presclerotherapy intravariceal pressure was determined by Gertsch et al.[124] in 10 patients by a pressure sensor attached to the tip of an endoscope. Large-diameter varices were found to have the highest values, and a relation was found between this and recurrence of bleeding during or after sclerotherapy. The use of Doppler ultrasound devices with an endoscope may also prove beneficial in assessing variceal blood flow.[125] In animal models and in humans variceal pressure has been determined by direct puncture.[126, 127]

Results of Sclerotherapy

Sclerotherapy Reports Prior to 1978

Crafoord and Frenckner[128] performed the first endoscopic injection sclerotherapy procedure in 1939. Moersch[129] reported his results in 11 patients in 1941, and Patterson and Rouse[130] reported a series of 24 cases in 1947. Repeated injection procedures with sodium morrhuate were utilized in both series. Bleeding was controlled in a high percentage of cases, and the complication rate was less than 2% in each report. In 1942, Samson and Foree[131] reported a relatively long follow-up in one patient. However, variceal sclerotherapy was not adopted widely, and during the 1950s only a few reports were published.[132, 133] Fearon and Sass-Kortsak[134] described sclerotherapy in children in 1959.

Johnston and Rodgers[70] reported the first large series of 117 patients who underwent 217 procedures over a period of 15 years. Injections of ethanolamine were made by means of a rigid endoscope. Bleeding was controlled in 93% of patients, and the complication rate was 0.9%. The next reported large series of 640 was that of Paquet and Oberhammer in 1978.[79] Beginning with two publications by Terblanche et al.[71, 135] in the late 1970's, the number of reports concerned with sclerotherapy has increased dramatically. Terblanche et al. used a rigid endoscope and general anesthesia. However, the heightened interest in sclerotherapy is due in large measure to successful adaptation of the procedure to fiberoptic endoscopy.[84, 87, 94]

Review of Recent Literature

Sclerotherapy is reported to control acute variceal bleeding in about 75% of episodes.[71, 94, 102, 130, 134, 135] Palani et al.[74] reported definitive control in 79% of 24 hospitalizations of 22 patients (rigid endoscope, general anesthesia, and sodium morrhuate). In another report, acute hemorrhage was controlled for a period of 1 month in 16 of 19 patients (intravariceal injections, double channel fiberscope, 5% sodium morrhuate, balloon fixed in cardia).[73] Eight patients died during follow-up, primarily from causes other than variceal bleeding. Alwmark et al.[97] reported cessation of bleeding for at least 24 hours in 95% of 72 acutely bleeding patients (rigid endoscope, paravariceal injections, polidocanol). Sclerotherapy was begun within 8 hours of admission. Stray et al.[96] achieved hemostasis in 10 of 11 patients admitted for acute bleeding (paravariceal injection, polidocanol, single oblique channel or double-channel fiberscope). Kjaergaard et al.[98] reported 94% hemostasis in 29 patients (paravariceal injection, polidocanol). The median follow-up in this series was 17 months (range 1 to 48 months), and only 10% of the patients eventually bled to death during follow-up. Sclerotherapy was begun in the first 24 hours. Seventy-one cases of acute variceal hemorrhage were reported by Terblanche et al.[81] Sclerotherapy, combined with balloon tamponade, was effective in controlling 95% of episodes.

In nearly all of these series, tamponade and/or intravenous vasopressin were used to stabilize patients prior to sclerotherapy.[71, 74, 94, 96–98] There were, however, some exceptions.[73] The series reported by Fleig et al.[95] in which hemorrhage was controlled in 92% of cases was composed of patients with active hemorrhage unresponsive to balloon tamponade. Nevertheless, the use of temporary methods such as intravenous vasopressin and/or balloon tamponade for control of bleeding prior to sclerotherapy raises a question as to whether some patients in these series might have had no further bleeding without sclerotherapy. It is difficult to answer this question, based on available data.

A report by Barsoum et al.[112] is of interest with respect to the effect of additional hemostatic methods in conjunction with sclerotherapy. In this trial, 50 patients were randomized to balloon tamponade, and 50 to sclerotherapy. Absence of hemorrhage for 1 month after treatment was considered a satisfactory result. Sclerotherapy was successful in 74% of patients and tamponade alone in 42% of patients. Their technique utilized rigid endoscopy and general anesthesia. Although the sclerotherapy group contained a high proportion of Child's C patients, mortality was the same for both groups.

It is difficult to assess the incidence of recurrent hemorrhage during follow-up after sclerotherapy. Terblanche et al.[135] compared acute injection plus a long-term series of injections with acute sclerotherapy alone. There was a decrease in the number and severity of bleeding episodes in the former group. However, the numbers of patients in each group were small, and the groups were unevenly matched with respect to several parameters. Other investigators have also noted significant reductions in recurrent bleeding and transfusion requirements in response to chronic sclerotherapy,[86, 106, 136] although this has not been emphasized in all reports. Hennessy et al.,[80] for example, questioned the value of chronic sclerotherapy because of a rate of recurrent bleeding of 44% in an uncontrolled series. These authors did, however, conclude that sclerotherapy was effective for acute and emergent hemorrhage.

The results of an important trial of sclerotherapy in 36 patients compared with medical management in 28 patients were published in 1980 by Clark et al.[102] In this study bleeding recurred in about one-third of sclerotherapy patients versus about two-thirds of control patients. This difference was statistically significant at various intervals of follow-up. Survival at one year was 46% in the sclerotherapy patients, compared with 6% in the control population, a difference that was not statistically significant.

This work by Clark et al. was extended in a study by Macdougall et al.,[137] in which the recurrent bleeding rate for 51 sclerotherapy patients was 43% versus 75% for 56 control patients, a statistically significant difference. The risk of bleeding was reduced threefold by sclerotherapy for each month of follow-up.

The most remarkable aspect of the report by Macdougall et al.[137] was that survival at one year was better for sclerotherapy patients (75% versus 58%), and that this difference was statistically significant. The improvement in survival was thought to be directly related to obliteration of varices.

The work of other authors appears to support these conclusions,[88, 97, 107, 138] although some of these reports are of a preliminary nature. Goodale et al.,[88] for example, demonstrated a favorable effect on survival in 48 Child's B and C patients who underwent sclerotherapy in comparison with the outcome for a similar group of untreated patients reported elsewhere by Graham and Smith.[34] Larson et al.[138] reported results at 2 weeks' follow-up in a trial of sclerotherapy versus medical management. There was a decrease in the number of transfusions and episodes of bleeding as well as reduced mortality in treated patients, although the differences were not statistically significant and the number of patients in each group was small.

In another study by Alwmark et al.[97] hemostasis after sclerotherapy was maintained in 89% of 76 patients at 1 week. Injections were repeated at intervals from 3 to 6 months after the initial series. At 6 months and 1 year follow-up, 40% and 24%, respectively, of sclerotherapy patients had no further bleeding. However, 30% of the patients had died by 1 year, making assessment of these results difficult. Hepatic failure was the most common cause of death in Child's C patients, and hemorrhage the most common cause in Child's B patients.

Preliminary results from other trials are not in agreement with some of these conclusions. Trudeau et al.[139] found that sclerotherapy did not favorably influence transfusion requirements nor survival in 16 Child's C patients when sclerotherapy was compared with the untreated course of variceal hemorrhage as described by Graham and Smith.[34] In a later report by these investigators, however, it was concluded that sclerotherapy reduced bleeding in Child's C patients, although it did not increase survival.[140] Sclerotherapy was compared with esophageal transection in a small number of poor-risk patients by Cello et al.[109] They concluded that sclerotherapy was the superior procedure. There was no recurrent bleeding in the patients who had undergone surgery, although mortality was 83%. About one-third of patients treated by sclerotherapy had further bleeding; the mortality in this group was 67%.

Terblanche et al.[75] reported a trial of medical management in 38 patients and long-term sclerotherapy in 37 patients. Any patient in either group in whom recurrent bleeding developed underwent sclerotherapy on an acute basis. Varices were eradicated in nearly all patients in the sclerotherapy group, but there was a high rate of recurrence. The cumulative percentage chance of remaining free of recurrent bleeding was slightly higher in the sclerotherapy patients from 6 months onward, but the difference was not statistically significant. However, bleeding in the sclerotherapy-treated patients was usually mild, while that in control patients was frequently life-threatening. There was no difference in survival between the two groups. This work should be contrasted with that of Macdougall et al.[137] who found an increase in survival with long-term sclerotherapy and obliteration of varices. The contradictory results may relate to the fact that medically managed control patients in the trial by Terblanche et al. underwent sclerotherapy in response to all acute episodes of bleeding. Furthermore, there was a relatively frequent and unexplained reappearance of varices after eradication in the investigation reported by Terblanche et al.[75]

Cello et al.[141] reported a trial of sclerotherapy and emergency portacaval shunt in 52 patients with severe cirrhosis, each of whom had been transfused with at least 6 units of blood because of acute variceal hemorrhage. Twenty-eight patients were randomized to receive sclerotherapy (intravariceal 5% sodium morrhuate), and 24 to undergo operation. Recurrent bleeding was significantly more common in the sclerotherapy group, although the total amount of blood transfused was greater in surgically treated patients. With respect to long-term outcome, a significantly greater number of patients were rehospitalized for resumption of bleeding in the sclerotherapy group, and the total number of days spent in-hospital for bleeding was also significantly greater. However, total number of blood transfusions, number of patients rehospitalized for encephalopathy, total days in-hospital for encephalopathy, and the resumption of alcohol abuse did not differ between the two treatment groups.

Cello et al.[141] reported that survival at 30 days was about 40% for both groups. With regard to long-term outcome, univariate survival analysis (Kaplan–Meier) disclosed no significant difference between the two groups. Since a number of variables, such as the presence of ascites, shock, prolonged prothrombin time, and high serum bilirubin, may influence survival, the investigators also carried out a multivariate analysis (Cox proportional-hazards model) and found a significant improvement in survival for sclerotherapy patients by this statistical method. However, the number of patients included in this latter analysis was small and the number of variables large. Furthermore, there were more patients who had ceased alcohol ingestion in the sclerotherapy group, an occurrence that the authors attributed to chance. However, this may have biased the results with respect to multivariate analysis. The total financial cost of management was significantly greater for those patients who underwent portacaval shunt.

A large group of investigators reported their results with respect to survival and recurrent bleeding in a trial in which 187 unselected patients were randomized to either medical treatment, including tamponade, or medical treatment plus sclerotherapy (paravariceal polidocanol injections at intervals of 3 days).[142] Sclerotherapy appeared to have little effect on recurrent hemorrhage in the early follow-up period, although after 40 days there were significantly fewer patients with recurrent bleeding and fewer episodes of recurrent bleeding in patients treated by sclerotherapy.

Overall, survival in sclerotherapy treated patients in this trial was not better than medical treatment alone.[142] However, when other factors such as the presence of ascites and/or encephalopathy were considered, the overall survival in the sclerotherapy group was significantly better than that in the group treated medically. The difference in survival between the two treatment groups varied over the course of the trial. Generally, the improvement associated with sclerotherapy was attributed to better long-term survival. Although mortality was somewhat lower for sclerotherapy patients during the first 10 days, this was not statistically significant. At 10 to 40 days after randomization, mortality was higher in the sclerotherapy group.

Sclerotherapy for Variceal Hemorrhage Due to Portal Vein Obstruction

Portal vein obstruction due to thrombosis, fibrosis, or congenital malformation is the most common cause of variceal bleeding in children (see Chapter 13). Fearon and Sass-Kortsak[134] first described a favorable outcome for sclerotherapy in children with this disorder. Lilly et al.[143] treated 6 children by sclerotherapy (rigid endoscope, general anesthesia, 5% sodium morrhuate). There was no recurrent bleeding during a follow-up of up to 3½ years. Treatment was begun in 4 of these patients at the time of active variceal hemorrhage. Twenty-one children were treated by sclerotherapy in another study, although only 8 of these had portal vein obstruction.[111] The sclerosant was ethanolamine, and injections were made using a pediatric fiberscope. Difficulty was encountered using this small-diameter instrument when bleeding was brisk. Variceal obliteration was achieved in 18 patients after a mean of 3.5 procedures. There were no deaths due to hemorrhage. At 1 month, 24% of the patients had experienced recurrent bleeding. In a later report by these authors, 32 children were followed 6 months or more after obliteration of varices.[144] There was a substantial reduction in

the predicted rate of hemorrhage for patients with either extrahepatic portal vein obstruction or intrahepatic portal hypertension.

Postmortem Studies

There are several postmortem studies of sclerotherapy patients.[99, 104, 105, 145] The initial changes during the first few days after injection of a sclerosing agent include thrombus formation and intense inflammation. After a few weeks the inflammation subsides and the thrombus is well organized (Plate 16–10). It is uncertain when fibrosis begins, but this may be as early as 2 weeks,[99] or as late as several months.[145] A postmortem series of 8 patients who had undergone intravariceal sclerotherapy with tetradecyl sulfate and had died after varying periods of follow-up was reported by Evans et al.[104] Variceal thrombosis was present by 24 hours, and the onset of fibrosis occurred at 1 month, a time interval intermediate to that found in the two earlier investigations. An increase in the number and diameter of the veins in the deeper layers of the esophageal wall was demonstrated in one study.[146] This was regarded as evidence that blood was being shunted from the intrinsic plexus.

Summary of the Results of Sclerotherapy

Assessment of the overall effect of sclerotherapy is difficult because of the many variables involved. DiMagno et al.[146] have pointed out that treatment groups in many sclerotherapy trials contain mixtures of patients with differing causes of liver disease and portal hypertension and differing degrees of severity with respect to liver disease. These authors suggest that the results of some trials may have been influenced by these factors. There is evidence that sclerotherapy has a favorable effect on transfusion requirements in the early period after onset of hemorrhage and during extended follow-up. However, a significant number of treated patients, perhaps about 40%, experience further episodes of hemorrhage. There are data that indicate a survival advantage for patients undergoing sclerotherapy in comparison with patients managed by standard medical methods, but conclusions on this point must await further data.

Complications

The reported complication rate for endoscopic sclerotherapy ranges from 2% to 15% per patient.[70, 86, 94, 102, 129, 132, 141] Twenty-two major complications were encountered by Terblanche et al.[81] in 18 of 66 patients

(27%) treated over a period of 5 years. A complication occurred in 21 of 107 patients undergoing 240 procedures in the series reported by Macdougall et al.[137] The complication rate in the trial of prophylactic sclerotherapy reported by Paquet and Oberhammer[79] was 12.5%. A membership survey of the ASGE that pertains to experience before 1981 revealed a complication rate of 19% per patient or 9% per procedure.[83] This undoubtedly represents the early experience of a number of endoscopists. A similar survey of experience up to 1982 showed a decrease to 16.7% per patient and 6.4% per procedure (Sivak MV Jr. Unpublished survey in conjunction with ASGE Postgraduate Course, Chicago, May 1982).

Approximately 25% to 50% of patients have chest pain or discomfort after sclerotherapy. These symptoms are reported after paravariceal and intravariceal injections, as well as after combinations of both methods. The level of discomfort varies from mild to severe pain and is difficult to quantitate. These symptoms usually persist for 12 to 24 hours but may remain for longer periods of time.[88] Odynophagia may also occur.[88] Pain that occurs shortly after sclerotherapy does not usually indicate necrosis or perforation. These complications are usually more insidious and require several days to one week to become fully developed. An exception is chest pain occurring during and/or immediately after a procedure, which is due to an instrument-induced perforation. Two instances of this were included in the series of cases reported by Macdougall et al.[137] In one instance, an unsuspected esophageal diverticulum was perforated, and in the other perforation occurred during rigid endoscopy.

The cause(s) of postprocedure chest pain or discomfort are uncertain. Harris et al.[113] thought that these symptoms occurred more often when ethanolamine was used as the sclerosant and were less likely to occur with tetradecyl sulfate. However, it is not established that a specific sclerosant or its concentration or a pattern of injections are responsible. On the basis of analysis of barium swallow radiography in 11 patients, esophageal spasm has been suggested by Gebhard et al.[147] as an etiologic factor. Severe chest pain has been attributed to chemical mediastinitis, although it does not usually correlate with other expected signs of mediastinal irritation such as pleural effusion or fever.

Low-grade fever occurs after sclerotherapy in about 10% to 15% of patients, although Hughes et al.[86] reported temperature elevations in almost half of treated patients. This resolves spontaneously and without apparent sequelae in almost all cases after about 24 to 48 hours. It appears that postprocedure fever is not due to bacteremia in the majority of cases.[148] Antibiotic therapy should not be employed in response to this unless there is other evidence of sepsis. Abrupt, marked elevations and erratic fluctuations in temperature are not characteristic of post-sclerotherapy fever, and a fever curve of this type may indicate a more serious complication including sepsis.

The several studies of esophageal manometry in patients undergoing sclerotherapy offer differing results. Some investigators report no significant alterations in motility.[149, 150] However, a decline in lower esophageal sphincter (LES) pressure has been described.[151] In another study, a high percentage of simultaneous non-propulsive contractions, a decrease in amplitude of contractions, and delayed clearance were found in 19 patients who had undergone between 7 and 13 procedures.[114] A prospective study of esophageal manometry and esophageal pH monitoring in 22 patients was reported by Reilly et al.[152] Thirteen patients were studied both before and after sclerotherapy. Esophageal manometry was obtained after a mean of 2.9 injection procedures. Although LES pressure remained unchanged, there was a significant increase in abnormal motility patterns after sclerotherapy. An increase in gastroesophageal reflux was also documented, but this was not significant. Nevertheless, the authors concluded that reflux combined with defective esophageal motility and clearing was related to the pathogenesis of esophageal strictures. It is possible that some techniques, paravariceal injection for example, or some sclerosing agents, may have a greater effect on the esophageal musculature. Some degree of damage to the neuromuscular plexus and esophageal musculature seems likely after repeated sclerotherapy. This would account for alterations in esophageal function, but the clinical significance of this is unknown.

Chest x-ray may reveal pleural effusions in otherwise asymptomatic patients after sclerotherapy. This occurred in over half of the patients reported by Hughes et al.[86] Saks et al.[153] studied chest x-rays before and after sclerotherapy (intravariceal injections, 5% sodium morrhuate) in 38 patients and found various abnormalities in 79%. These resolved in all cases. Bacon et al.[154] found pleural effusions after 48% of sclerotherapy sessions in 30 patients. In this study postsclerotherapy chest pain correlated with the presence of an effusion, and the total volume of sclerosant (5% sodium morrhuate) injected was greater in patients with effusions. Infiltrates may also be found, and are a greater cause for concern in view of a report of serious pulmonary complications.[155] Although effusions resolve without apparent untoward effects, it is possible that permanent subclinical damage to the lungs and/or pleura may be occurring.

Acute respiratory failure has been reported in two patients in whom clinical signs and symptoms developed after sclerotherapy that in most respects resembled the adult respiratory distress syndrome.[155] Dyspnea, poorly responsive to oxygen, as well as bilateral alveolar infiltrates on chest x-ray developed after injections of sodium morrhuate. Monroe et al.[155] pointed out that sodium morrhuate is not homogeneous and contains elements toxic to the lungs. These authors demonstrated transient increases in pulmonary artery pressure and lymph flow in response to sodium morrhuate injections in an animal model but found no change in alveolar capillary permeability. Since substances injected into the esophageal venous system can be readily transported to the right heart and lungs via the azygous system, it is logical to expect that pulmonary complications may result from sclerotherapy, although the frequency of this is unknown. It is possible that some agents may be more hazardous with respect to the lungs than others, but this is also not established.

Esophageal stricture is estimated to occur in about 3% of patients after sclerotherapy.[83] Although acid reflux has not been eliminated as an etiologic factor, stricture is presumably a direct effect of the sclerosant. This complication could also be related to type and concentration of sclerosant and/or method of injection. A higher incidence might result with paravariceal injections; an incidence of 31% was reported in patients undergoing paravariceal injections of polidocanol.[98] In another series, stricture and/or dysphagia developed in 59%.[156] Most patients had stricturing and dysphagia, although a few had asymptomatic strictures and a few had dysphagia without evidence of a stricture. The method of sclerotherapy used by these inves-

tigators could be considered aggressive in that paravariceal injections of 3% polidocanol were carried out at intervals of 3 days until obliteration was achieved. Treatment was interrupted if ulceration or necrosis occurred. Patients with strictures had undergone a significantly greater number of procedures and received a greater volume of sclerosant. Recurrent bleeding was not less in those with a stricture compared with patients without this complication. Eleven patients underwent dilation using metal olives over a guide wire, and a fistula developed as a result of this in one patient. Although paravariceal injections should logically result in a higher incidence of stricture, there are no data to support this line of reasoning. Esophageal stricture has occurred with almost every agent and technique. Most can be managed by bougienage. Intermittent dysphagia without evidence of stricture usually resolves without treatment and is most likely due to transient spasm.

Esophageal perforation occurs in about 1% to 2% of patients[83] (Sivak MV Jr. Unpublished survey in conjunction with ASGE Postgraduate Course, Chicago, May 1982). Instrument perforations are rare with the use of fiberoptic endoscopes, but are reported with rigid instruments. Perforation related to the chemical action of the sclerosing agent usually requires 5 to 7 days to develop. The symptoms and clinical signs of this may be minimal. Carr-Locke and Sidky[157] described a patient with an esophageal-bronchial fistula who remained asymptomatic until 1 month after sclerotherapy. This patient was receiving corticosteroids, however, which may have been a contributing factor. Other reports emphasize the subtle nature and the delay that frequently occurs prior to the appearance of sclerotherapy-related esophageal perforation.[156, 158] Many perforations will wall off and remain localized, and in time they may heal. Conservative management is usually indicated and should include broad-spectrum antibiotics and chest tube drainage in some cases.

Esophageal ulceration may occur after sclerotherapy (Fig. 16–1; Plates 16–4 and 16–11). This has been regarded by some as a complication, although ulceration is extremely common after sclerotherapy, occurring in about 40% to 50% of cases.[83] Sanowski et al.,[159] for example, found ulcers in 57% of patients, as well as exudate adherent to the varices in one third, and variceal erosions in 14%. In our experience, yellowish, plaque-like lesions occur over variceal vessels in 45% of patients, and actual ulceration in about 30% (Plates 16–12 and 16–13). Most sclerotherapy-related esophageal ulcers heal spontaneously, although a permanent but clinically insignificant defect in the esophageal wall may remain[160] (Plate 16–14A). Healing of an ulcer undoubtedly interrupts variceal blood flow.

During the clinical course of a patient it may be difficult to distinguish between inconsequential or even beneficial ulcers and ones that must be considered complications. This generally must be related to the clinical course of the patient. Serious ulceration and esophageal necrosis may occur, sometimes as the forerunner of a perforation or hemorrhage (Fig. 16–1; Plates 16–4, 16–15, and 16–16). Although small ulcers have been incriminated as a source of hemorrhage,[161] they are probably not a common cause of resumed bleeding. However, large ulcers may result in severe persistent bleeding if nearby varices have been inadequately treated. Bleeding from such an ulcer may be impossible to control, since further sclerotherapy can be expected to cause additional tissue damage, and balloon tamponade and direct surgical attack would entail additional risks in an area of esophageal necrosis. In an uncontrolled study, Roark[162] treated a small number of patients with sclerotherapy-induced bleeding ulcers with a suspension of sucralfate, and reported this appeared to arrest bleeding perhaps by adherence of the drug to the ulcerated areas.

Ulceration, as with perforation, appears about 5 to 7 days after an injection procedure.[105] Whether certain agents or techniques are ulcerogenic to a greater extent than others is problematic. In a series of 122 injections in 53 patients using ethanolamine, thrombin, and cefazolin, no ulceration whatsoever was observed.[107] However, ulcers have occurred with the use of ethanolamine.[111] In one animal study there was little difference in the local toxicity of various agents tested.[163] Trudeau et al.[164] reported that a solution of 1% tetradecyl plus 33% ethanol was somewhat less ulcerogenic, but there was not much difference in local toxicity among the agents tested in this study. Brooks and Galambos[165] found that each of a variety of sclerosants produced ulceration in humans. They also concluded that significant ulceration occurred more often in patients with severe liver disease, a point not considered in other investigations.

The pathogenesis of large ulcers is uncertain. Since they occur with all agents, perhaps technique or the concentration of the sclerosant(s) is in some way related to their occurrence. Aside from the consideration of intravariceal versus paravariceal injection, ulceration could be related to the amount of active agent deposited at one location, either by an excess number of injections in a small area or by a smaller number of injections of a concentrated agent. This could occur, for example, when a large number of punctures are needed to control active bleeding.

Hemorrhage was the second most common complication in the survey of the ASGE membership in 1981.[83] However, in a similar survey one year later, precipitation of hemorrhage as a complication decreased by 28%, but there was an interesting reciprocal increase in ulceration (Sivak MV Jr. Unpublished survey in conjunction with ASGE Postgraduate Course, Chicago, May 1982). Perhaps better control of hemorrhage was achieved at the expense of increased damage to the esophagus.

Data on the occurrence of bacteremia during and after sclerotherapy are conflicting. Cohen et al.[148] found 14 episodes in 11 patients. Positive cultures were obtained mostly during the first 5 minutes after sclerotherapy, and oropharyngeal flora were predominant. Postprocedure chest x-ray abnormalities and fever did not correlate with bacteremia. Camara et al.[103] in a study of 40 procedures in 18 patients documented bacteremia in only 5% of cases. Brayko et al.[166] obtained positive blood cultures during 5 of 9 sclerotherapy sessions; a high percentage were *Pseudomonas aeruginosa*. These authors related bacteremia to contamination of the endoscopy equipment, especially the water bottle. No positive cultures occurred after improving disinfecting technique. Lange et al.[167] found a cumulative increase in the rate for septicemia but no relation to a lack of sterility. It appears that bacteremia occurs in association with sclerotherapy, but that its exact incidence is not established. Antibiotic prophylaxis does not appear to be indicated based on available data, although it would be prudent to consider this in patients with prosthetic heart valves.

Seidman et al.[168] reported the occurrence of spinal cord necrosis in a child who had undergone three sessions of sclerotherapy consisting of intravenous injections of ethanolamine. Irreversible paraplegia developed within 8 hours of the last injection procedure.

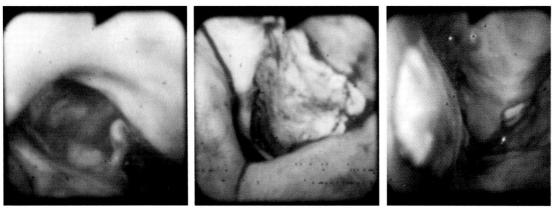

PLATE 16–11.   PLATE 16–12.   PLATE 16–13.

PLATE 16–11. Large, deep esophageal ulcer resulting from sclerotherapy.
PLATE 16–12. Yellow plaque over variceal injection site 5 days after procedure.
PLATE 16–13. Yellow plaques at variceal injection sites 5 days after procedure.

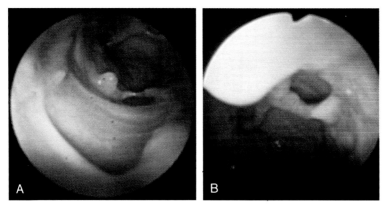

PLATE 16–14. A, Healed esophageal ulcer defect after 6 sclerotherapy sessions. B, Residual bridge of tissue after sclerotherapy.

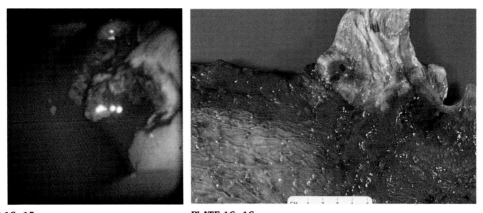

PLATE 16–15.   PLATE 16–16.

PLATE 16–15. Bleeding from yellow plaque over varix.
PLATE 16–16. Gross specimen of esophagus and stomach showing sclerotherapy-induced esophageal ulcer in area of partially thrombosed varices. Patient died because of exsanguination.

Intramural hematomas have occurred as a result of sclerotherapy, in one case leading to bacteremia and death, and in another to perforation.[74, 113] Gardner and Brooks[169] demonstrated that coagulopathy, disseminated intravascular coagulation, for example, did not occur with injections of a combination of 5% sodium morrhuate, 100 units of thrombin, and 2 ml of cefazolin in 50% dextrose. Two cases of portal vein thrombosis were reported by Goodale et al.,[88] and one case by Barsoum et al.[170] A bleeding duodenal varix post-sclerotherapy has been described.[171] Foutch and Sivak[172] have described the occurrence of hemorrhage from colonic varices in three patients undergoing sclerotherapy. Accidental contact of sclerosing agents with the eyes is injurious.[173, 174] Bradyarrhythmias have been reported in two elderly patients known to have cardiac conduction abnormalities prior to sclerotherapy with sodium morrhuate.[175] In one of the patients, the arrhythmia was noted after two separate procedures.

Editor's note: Information concerning sclerotherapy continues to accumulate at a rapid pace. References 176 to 180 are recent reports of interest.

References

1. Butler H. The veins of the oesophagus. Thorax 1951; 6:276–96.
2. Felson B, Lessure AP. "Downhill" varices of the esophagus. Dis Chest 1964; 46:740–6.
3. Fleig WE, Stange EF, Ditshuneit H. Upper gastrointestinal hemorrhage from downhill esophageal varices. Dig Dis Sci 1982; 27:23–7.
4. Glanz S, Koser MW, Dallemand S, Gordon DH. Upper esophageal varices: report of three cases and review of the literature. Am J Gastroenterol 1982; 77:194–8.
5. Palmer ED. Primary varices of the cervical esophagus as a source of massive upper gastrointestinal hemorrhage. Am J Dig Dis 1952; 19:375–7.
6. McCormack TT, Rose JD, Smith PM, Johnson AG. Perforating veins and blood flow in esophageal varices. Lancet 1983; 2:1442–4.
7. Viallet A, Marleau D, Huet M, et al. Hemodynamic evaluation of patients with intrahepatic portal hypertension. Relationship between bleeding varices and the portohepatic gradient. Gastroenterology 1975; 68:1297–1300.
8. Lebrec D, DeFleury P, Rueff B, et al. Portal hypertension, size of esophageal varices, and risk of gastrointestinal bleeding in alcoholic cirrhosis. Gastroenterology 1980; 79:1139–44.
9. Reynolds TB. Editorial. Interrelationships of portal pressure, variceal size, and upper gastrointestinal bleeding. Gastroenterology 1980; 79:1332–3.
10. Dagradi AE. Esophageal varices, splenic pulp pressure and "directional" flow patterns in alcoholic liver cirrhosis. A correlation study. Am J Gastroenterol 1973; 59:15–22.
11. Joly JG, Marleau D, Legare A, et al. Bleeding from esophageal varices in cirrhosis of the liver: hemodynamic and radiological criteria for the selection of potential bleeders through hepatic and umbilicoportal catheterization studies. Can Med Assoc J 1971; 104:576–80.
12. Willoughby EO, David D, Smith CW, et al. The significance of small esophageal varices in portal cirrhosis. Gastroenterology 1964; 47:375–81.
13. Greene L, Weisberg H, Rosenthal WS, et al. Evaluation of esophageal varices in liver disease by splenic-pulp manometry, splenoportography, and esophagogastroscopy. Diagnostic discrepancies. Am J Dig Dis 1965; 10:284–92.
14. Westaby S, Wilkinson SP, Warren R, Williams R. Spleen size and portal hypertension in cirrhosis. Digestion 1978; 17:63–8.
15. Palmer ED. On correlations between portal venous pressure and the size and extent of esophageal varices in portal cirrhosis. Ann Surg 1953; 138:741–4.
16. Simert G, Lunderquist A, Tylen U, Vang J. Correlation between percutaneous transhepatic portography and clinical findings in 56 patients with portal hypertension. Acta Chir Scand 1978; 144:27–34.
17. Smith-Laing G, Camilo ME, Dick R, Sherlock S. Percutaneous transhepatic portography in the assessment of portal hypertension. Clinical correlations and comparison of radiographic techniques. Gastroenterology 1980; 78:197–205.
18. Baker LA, Smith C, Lieberman G. The natural history of esophageal varices. A study of 115 cirrhotic patients in whom varices were diagnosed prior to bleeding. Am J Med 1959; 26:228–37.
19. Palmer ED, Brick IB. Correlation between the severity of esophageal varices in portal cirrhosis and their propensity toward hemorrhage. Gastroenterology 1956; 30:85–90.
20. Dagradi AE. The natural history of esophageal varices in patients with alcoholic liver cirrhosis. Am J Gastroenterol 1972; 57:520–40.
21. Conn HO, Mitchell JR, Brodoff MG. A comparison of the radiologic and esophagoscopic diagnosis of esophageal varices. N Engl J Med 1961; 265:160–4.
22. Fujita R. Endoscopic diagnosis and classification of esophageal varices in Japan. In: Sivak MV Jr, ed. Sclerotherapy of esophageal varices. New York: Praeger, 1984: 35–42.
23. Beppu K, Inokuchi K, Koyanagi N, et al. Prediction of variceal hemorrhage by esophageal endoscopy. Gastrointest Endosc 1981; 27:213–8.
24. Spence RAJ, Sloan JM, Johnston GW, Greenfield A. Oesophageal mucosal changes in patients with varices. Gut 1983; 24:1024–9.
25. Iwatsuki S, Reynolds T. Effects of increased intra-abdominal pressure on hepatic hemodynamics in patients with chronic liver disease and portal hypertension. Gastroenterology 1973; 65:294–9.
26. Eckardt V, Grace ND, Kantrowitz PA. Does lower esophageal sphincter incompetency contribute to esophageal variceal hemorrhage? Gastroenterology 1976; 71:185–9.
27. Eckardt VF, Grace ND. Gastroesophageal reflux and bleeding esophageal varices. Gastroenterology 1979; 76:39–42.

28. Ponce J, Froufe A, De La Morena E, et al. Morphometric study of the esophageal mucosa in cirrhotic patients with variceal bleeding. Hepatology 1981; 1:641–6.

29. Galambos JT. Esophageal variceal hemorrhage: diagnosis and an overview of treatment. Sem Liver Dis 1982; 2:211–26.

30. Resnick RH, Iber FL, Ishihara AM, et al. A controlled study of the therapeutic portacaval shunt. Gastroenterology 1974; 67;843–57.

31. Christensen E, Fauerholdt L, Schlichting P, et al. Aspects of the natural history of gastrointestinal bleeding in cirrhosis and the effect of prednisone. Gastroenterology 1981; 81:944–52.

32. Jackson FC, Perrin EB, Felix WR, et al. A clinical investigation of the portacaval shunt: V. Survival analysis of the therapeutic operation. Ann Surg 1971; 174:672–701.

33. Novis BH, Duys P, Barbezat GO, et al. Fibreoptic endoscopy and the use of the Sengstaken tube in acute gastrointestinal haemorrhage in patients with portal hypertension and varices. Gut 1976; 17:258–63.

34. Graham DY, Smith JL. The course of patients after variceal hemorrhage. Gastroenterology 1981; 80:800–9.

35. Fleischer D. Etiology and prevalence of severe persistent upper gastrointestinal bleeding. Gastroenterology 1983; 84:538–43.

36. Silverstein FE, Gilbert DA, Tedesco FJ, et al. The national ASGE survey on upper gastrointestinal bleeding. II. Clinical prognostic factors. Gastrointest Endosc 1981; 27:80–93.

37. Garceau AJ, Chalmers TC. The natural history of cirrhosis. Survival with esophageal varices. N Engl J Med 1963; 268:469–73.

38. Waldram R, Nunnerley H, Davis M, et al. Detection and grading of oesophageal varices by fibre-optic endoscopy and barium swallow with and without Buscopan. Clin Radiol 1977; 28:137–41.

39. Dagradi AE, Mehler R, Tan DTD, Stempien SJ. Sources of upper gastrointestinal bleeding in patients with liver cirrhosis and large varices. Am J Gastroenterol 1970; 54:458–63.

40. Palmer ED. The vigorous diagnostic approach to upper gastrointestinal tract hemorrhage. A 23-year prospective study of 14,000 patients. JAMA 1969; 207:1477–80.

41. McCray RS, Martin F, Amir-Ahmadi H, et al. Erroneous diagnosis of hemorrhage from esophageal varices. Am J Dig Dis 1969; 14:755–60.

42. Waldram R, Davis M, Nunnerly H, et al. Emergency endoscopy after gastrointestinal hemorrhage in 50 patients with portal hypertension. Br Med J 1974; 4:94–6.

43. Dave P, Romeu J, Messer J. Upper gastrointestinal bleeding in patients with portal hypertension: A reappraisal. J Clin Gastroenterol 1983; 5:113–5.

44. Schoppe LE, Roark GD, Patterson M. Acute upper gastrointestinal bleeding in patients with portal hypertension: a correlation of endoscopic findings with etiology. South Med J 1983; 76:475–6.

45. Mitchell KJ, Macdougall BRD, Silk DBA, Williams R. A prospective reappraisal of emergency endoscopy in patients with portal hypertension. Scand J Gastroenterol 1982; 17:965–8.

46. Gilbert DA, Silverstein FE, Tedesco FJ, et al. The national ASGE survey on upper gastrointestinal bleeding. III. Endoscopy in upper gastrointestinal bleeding. Gastrointest Endosc 1981; 27:94–102.

47. Smith JL, Graham DY. Variceal hemorrhage: A critical evaluation of survival analysis. Gastroenterology 1982; 82:968–73.

48. Conn HO. Hazards attending the use of esophageal tamponade. N Engl J Med 1958; 259:701–7.

49. Conn HO, Simpson JA. Excessive mortality associated with balloon tamponade of bleeding varices: a critical reappraisal. JAMA 1967; 202:587–91.

50. Pitcher JL. Safety and effectiveness of the modified Sengstaken-Blakemore tube: a prospective study. Gastroenterology 1971; 61:291–8.

51. Hunt PS, Korman MG, Hansky J, Parkin WG. An 8-year prospective experience with balloon tamponade in emergency control of bleeding esophageal varices. Dig Dis Sci 1982; 27:413–6.

52. Orloff MJ, Bell RH Jr, Hyde PV, Skivolocki WP. Long-term results of emergency portacaval shunt for bleeding esophageal varices in unselected patients with alcoholic cirrhosis. Ann Surg 1980; 192:325–40.

53. Smith-Laing G, Scott J, Long RG, et al. Role of percutaneous transhepatic obliteration of varices in the management of hemorrhage from gastroesophageal varices. Gastroenterology 1981; 80:1031–6.

54. Bengmark S, Borjesson B, Hoevels J, et al. Obliteration of esophageal varices by PTP. A follow-up of 43 patients. Ann Surg 1979; 190:549–54.

55. Conn HO. Therapeutic portacaval anastomosis: To shunt or not to shunt. Gastroenterology 1974; 67:1065–71.

56. Reuff B, Prandi D, Degos F, et al. A controlled study of therapeutic portacaval shunt in alcoholic cirrhosis. Lancet 1976; I:655–9.

57. Reynolds TB, Donovan AJ, Mikkelsen WP, et al. Results of a 12-year randomized trial of portacaval shunt in patients with alcoholic liver disease and bleeding varices. Gastroenterology 1981; 80:1005–11.

58. Warren WD, Millikan WJ Jr, Henderson JM, et al. Ten years portal hypertensive surgery at Emory. Results and new perspectives. Ann Surg 1982; 195:530–42.

59. Hassab MA. Nonshunt operations in portal hypertension without cirrhosis. Surg Gynecol Obstet 1970; 131:648–54.

60. Sugiura M, Futagawa S. Further evaluation of the Sugiura procedure in the treatment of esophageal varices. Arch Surg 1977; 112:1317–21.

61. Johnston GW. Six years' experience of oesophageal transection for oesophageal varices, using a circular stapling gun. Gut 1982; 23:770–3.

62. Lebrec D, Poynard T, Hillon P, Benhamou J. Propranolol for prevention of recurrent gastrointestinal bleeding in patients with cirrhosis, a controlled study. N Engl J Med 1981; 305:1371–4.

63. Lebrec D, Poynard T, Benhamou J, et al. A randomized controlled study of propranolol for prevention of recurrent gastrointestinal bleeding in patients with cirrhosis: a final report. Hepatology 1984; 4:355–8.

64. Burroughs AK, Jenkins WJ, Sherlock S, et al. Controlled trial of propranolol for the prevention of recurrent variceal hemorrhage in patients with cirrhosis. N Engl J Med 1983; 309:1539–42.

65. Resnick RH, Chalmers TC, Ishihara AM, et al. A controlled study of the prophylactic portacaval shunt; a final report. Ann Intern Med 1969; 70:675–88.

66. Jackson FC, Perrin EB, Smith AG, et al. A clinical

investigation of the portacaval shunt. II. Survival analysis of the prophylactic operation. Am J Surg 1968; 115:22–42.

67. Conn HO, Lindenmuth WW, May CJ, Ramsby GR. Prophylactic portacaval anastomosis. Medicine 1972; 52:27–40.

68. Jensen DM, Silpa ML, Tapia JI, et al. Comparison of different methods for endoscopic hemostasis of bleeding canine esophageal varices. Gastroenterology 1983; 84:1455–61.

69. Fleischer DE. Nd:YAG laser therapy for active variceal bleeding. (Abstr) Gastroenterology 1982; 82:1058.

70. Johnston GW, Rodgers HW. A review of 15 years' experience in the use of sclerotherapy in the control of acute haemorrhage for oesophageal varices. Br J Surg 1973; 60:797–800.

71. Terblanche J, Northover JMA, Bornman P, et al. A prospective evaluation of injection sclerotherapy in treatment of acute bleeding from esophageal varices. Surgery 1979; 85:239–45.

72. Soehendra N, de Heer K, Kempeneers I, Runge M. Sclerotherapy of esophageal varices: acute arrest of gastrointestinal hemorrhage or long-term therapy? Endoscopy 1983; 15:136–40.

73. Lewis JW, Chung RS, Allison JG. Injection sclerotherapy for control of acute variceal hemorrhage. Am J Surg 1981; 142:592–5.

74. Palani CK, Abuabara S, Kraft AR, Jonasson O. Endoscopic sclerotherapy in acute variceal hemorrhage. Am J Surg 1981; 141:164–8.

75. Terblanche J, Bornman PC, Kahn D, et al. Failure of repeated injection sclerotherapy to improve long-term survival after oesophageal variceal bleeding. A five-year prospective controlled clinical trial. Lancet 1983; 2:1328–32.

76. Paquet KJ. Prophylactic endoscopic sclerosing treatment of the esophageal wall in varices—a prospective controlled randomized trial. Endoscopy 1982; 14:4–5.

77. Witzel L, Wolbergs E, Merki H. Prophylactic endoscopic sclerotherapy of oesophageal varices. A prospective controlled study. Lancet 1985; 1:773–5.

78. Sugawa C, Okumura Y, Lucas CE, Walt AJ. Endoscopic sclerosis of experimental esophageal varices in dogs. Gastrointest Endosc 1978; 24:114–16.

79. Paquet KJ, Oberhammer E. Sclerotherapy of bleeding oesophageal varices by means of endoscopy. Endoscopy 1978; 10:7–12.

80. Hennessy TPJ, Stephens RB, Keane FB. Acute and chronic management of esophageal varices by injection sclerotherapy. Surg Gynecol Obstet 1982; 154:375–7.

81. Terblanche J, Yakoob HI, Bornman PC, et al. Acute bleeding varices. A five-year prospective evaluation of tamponade and sclerotherapy. Ann Surg 1981; 194:521–30.

82. Reilly JJ Jr, Schade RR, Roh MS, VanThiel DH. Esophageal variceal sclerosis. Surg Gynecol Obstet 1982; 155:497–502.

83. Sivak MV Jr. Endoscopic injection sclerosis of esophageal varices: ASGE survey. Letter. Gastrointest Endosc 1982; 28:41.

84. Williams KDG, Dawson JL. Fibreoptic injection of oesophageal varices. Br Med J 1979; 2:766–7.

85. Westaby D, Macdougall BRD, Melia W, et al. A prospective randomized study of two sclerotherapy techniques for esophageal varices. Hepatology 1983; 3:681–4.

86. Hughes RW Jr, Larson DE, Viggiano TR, et al. Endoscopic variceal sclerosis: A one-year experience. Gastrointest Endosc 1982; 28:62–6.

87. Brooks WS Jr. Adapting flexible endoscopes for sclerosis of oesophageal varices. (Letter) Lancet 1980; I:266.

88. Goodale RL, Silvis SE, O'Leary JF, et al. Early survival after sclerotherapy for bleeding esophageal varices. Surg Gynecol Obstet 1982; 155:523–8.

89. Takase Y, Ozaki A, Orii K, et al. Injection sclerotherapy of esophageal varices for patients undergoing emergency and elective surgery. Surgery 1982; 92:474–9.

90. Wang KP, Yang P, Hutcheon DF, et al. A new method of injection sclerotherapy of esophageal varices. Gastrointest Endosc 1983; 29:38–40.

91. Grobe JL, Kozarek RA, Sanowski RA, et al. Venography during endoscopic injection sclerotherapy of esophageal varices. Gastrointest Endosc 1984; 30:6–8.

92. Silvis SE, Sievert CE Jr, Wong N, et al. The disappearance of sodium morrhuate from a variceal injection site with and without compression. (Abstr) Gastrointest Endosc 1983; 29:167.

93. Barsoum MS, Khattar NY, Risk-Allah MA. Technical aspects of injection sclerotherapy of acute oesophageal variceal haemorrhage as seen by radiography. Br J Surg 1978; 65:588–9.

94. Sivak MV Jr, Stout DJ, Skipper G. Endoscopic injection sclerosis (EIS) of esophageal varices. Gastrointest Endosc 1981; 27:52–7.

95. Fleig WE, Stange EF, Ruettenauer K, Ditschuneit H. Emergency endoscopic sclerotherapy for bleeding esophageal varices: a prospective study in patients not responding to balloon tamponade. Gastrointest Endosc 1983; 29:8–14.

96. Stray N, Jacobsen CD, Rosseland A. Injection sclerotherapy of bleeding oesophageal and gastric varices using a flexible endoscope. Acta Med Scand 1982; 211:125–9.

97. Alwmark A, Bengmark, Borjesson B, et al. Emergency and long-term transesophageal sclerotherapy of bleeding esophageal varices. A prospective study of 50 consecutive cases. Scand J Gastroenterol 1982; 17:409–12.

98. Kjaergaard J, Fischer A, Miskowiak J, et al. Sclerotherapy of bleeding esophageal varices. Long-term results. Scand J Gastroenterol 1982; 17:363–7.

99. Helpap B, Bollweg L. Morphological changes in the terminal oesophagus with varices, following sclerosis of the wall. Endoscopy 1981; 13:229–33.

100. Lewis J, Chung RS, Allison J. Sclerotherapy of esophageal varices. Arch Surg 1980; 115:476–80.

101. Kirkham JS, Quayle JB. Oesophageal varices: evaluation of injection sclerotherapy without general anesthesia using the flexible fiberoptic gastroscope. Ann R Coll Surg Engl 1982; 64:401–5.

102. Clark AW, Westaby D, Silk DBA, et al. Prospective controlled trial of injection sclerotherapy in patients with cirrhosis and recent variceal hemorrhage. Lancet 1980; 2:552–4.

103. Camara DS, Gruber M, Barde CJ, et al. Transient bacteremia following endoscopic injection sclerotherapy of esophageal varices. Arch Intern Med 1983; 143:1350–2.

104. Evans DMD, Jones DB, Cleary BK, Smith PM. Oesophageal varices treated by sclerotherapy: a histopathological study. Gut 1982; 23:615–20.

105. Novis B, Bat L, Pomerantz I, Skemesh E. Endo-

scopic sclerotherapy of esophageal varices. Isr J Med Sci 1983; 19:40–4.

106. Ayres SJ, Goff JS, Warren GH. Endoscopic sclerotherapy for bleeding esophageal varices: effects and complications. Ann Intern Med 1983; 98:900–3.

107. Hedberg SE, Fowler DL, Ryan RLR. Injection sclerotherapy of esophageal varices using ethanolamine oleate. A pilot study. Am J Surg 1982; 143:426–31.

108. Yassin YM, Sherif SM. Sclerotherapy of oesophageal varices using the fiberoptic endoscope. J R Coll Surg Edinb 1981; 26:328–34.

109. Cello JP, Crass R, Trunkey DD. Endoscopic sclerotherapy versus esophageal transection in Child's class C patients with variceal hemorrhage. Comparison with results of portacaval shunt. Preliminary report. Surgery 1982; 91:333–8.

110. Lilly JR. Endoscopic sclerosis of esophageal varices in children. Surg Gynecol Obstet 1981; 152:513–4.

111. Stamatakis JD, Howard ER, Psacharopoulos HT, Mowat AP. Injection sclerotherapy for oesophageal varices in children. Br J Surg 1982; 69:74–5.

112. Barsoum MS, Bolous FI, El-Rooby AA, et al. Tamponade and injection sclerotherapy in the management of bleeding oesophageal varices. Br J Surg 1982; 69:76–8.

113. Harris OD, Dickey JD, Stephenson PM. Simple endoscopic injection sclerotherapy of oesophageal varices. Aust NZ J Med 1982; 12:131–5.

114. Sauerbruch T, Wirsching R, Leisner B, et al. Esophageal function after sclerotherapy of bleeding varices. Scand J Gastroenterol 1982; 17:745–51.

115. Rose JDR, Crane MD, Smith PM. Factors affecting successful endoscopic sclerotherapy for oesophageal varices. Gut 1983; 24:946–9.

116. Smith PM, Jones DB, Rose JDR. Simplified fibre endoscopic sclerotherapy for oesophageal varices. J R Coll Physicians Lond 1982; 16:236–8.

117. Brooks WS Jr. Variceal sclerosing agents. Am J Gastroenterol 1984; 79:424–8.

118. Cooper WM. Clinical evaluation of sotradecol, a sodium alkyl sulfate solution, in the injection therapy of varicose veins. Surg Gynecol Obstet 1946; 83:647–52.

119. Blenkinsopp WK. Comparison of tetradecyl sulphate in sodium with other sclerosants in rats. Br J Exp Pathol 1967; 49:197–201.

120. Reiner L. The activity of anionic surface active compounds in producing vascular obliteration. Proc Soc Exp Biol Med 1946; 62:49–54.

121. Silpa ML, Jensen DM, Machicado GA, et al. Efficacy and safety of agents for variceal sclerotherapy. (Abstr) Gastrointest Endosc 1982; 28:152–3.

122. Gibbert V, Feinstat T, Burns M, Trudeau W. A comparison of the sclerosing agents sodium tetradecyl sulfate and sodium morrhuate in endoscopic injection sclerosis of esophageal varices. (Abstr) Gastrointest Endosc 1982; 28:147.

123. Westaby D, Melia WM, Macdougall BRD, et al. Injection sclerotherapy for oesophageal varices: a prospective randomised trial of different treatment schedules. Gut 1984; 25:129–32.

124. Gertsch P, Loup P, Diserens H, et al. Endoscopic noninvasive manometry of esophageal varices: prognostic significance. Am J Surg 1982; 144:528–30.

125. McCormack T, Martin T, Smallwood RH, et al.

126. Matthew JS, Jensen DM, Tapia JI, et al. Portal pressure measurement via endoscopy. (Abstr) Gastrointest Endosc 1983; 29:190.

127. Staritz M, Poralla T, Meyer Zum Buschenfelde K-H. Intravascular oesophageal variceal pressure (IOVP) assessed by endoscopic fine needle puncture under basal conditions, Valsalva's manoeuvre and after glyceryltrinitrate application. Gut 1985; 26:525–30.

128. Crafoord C, Frenckner P. New surgical treatment of varicose veins of the oesophagus. Acta Otolaryngol 1939; 27:422–9.

129. Moersch HJ. Further studies on the treatment of esophageal varices by injection of a sclerosing solution. Ann Otol Rhinol Laryngol 1941; 50:1233–44.

130. Patterson CO, Rouse MO. The sclerosing therapy of esophageal varices. Gastroenterology 1947; 9:391–5.

131. Samson PC, Foree L. Direct injection of esophageal varices through the esophagoscope. West J Surg 1942; 50:73–7.

132. Macbeth R. Treatment of oesophageal varices in portal hypertension by means of sclerosing injections. Br Med J 1955; 2:877–80.

133. Kempe SG, Koch H. Injection of sclerosing solutions in the treatment of esophageal varices. Acta Otolaryngol (Suppl) 1955; 118:120–9.

134. Fearon B, Sass-Kortsak A. The management of esophageal varices in children by injection of sclerosing agents. Ann Otol Rhinol Laryngol 1959; 68:906–15.

135. Terblanche J, Northover JMA, Bornman P, et al. A prospective controlled trial of sclerotherapy in the long term management of patients after esophageal variceal bleeding. Surg Gynecol Obstet 1979; 148:323–33.

136. Sivak MV Jr, Williams GW. Endoscopic injection sclerosis (EIS) of esophageal varices: analysis of survival and transfusion requirement. (Abstr) Gastrointest Endosc 1981; 27:129.

137. Macdougall BRD, Westaby D, Theodossi A, et al. Increased long-term survival in variceal haemorrhage using injection sclerotherapy. Results of a controlled trial. Lancet 1982; 1:124–7.

138. Larson AW, Chapman DJ, Radvan G, Balart LI. Esophageal variceal sclerotherapy (EVS): acute phase results of a prospective controlled trial. (Abstr) Gastrointest Endosc 1982; 28:136.

139. Trudeau W, Gibbert V, Young W, et al. Child's C patients receiving endoscopic injection sclerosis of bleeding esophageal varices fare no better than patients receiving conventional therapy. (Abstr) Gastrointest Endosc 1982; 28:148.

140. Trudeau W, Prindiville T, Gibbert V, Siepler J. Endoscopic injection sclerosis in Child's C patients with bleeding gastroesophageal varices. (Abstr) Gastrointest Endosc 1983; 29:168.

141. Cello JP, Grendell JH, Crass RA, et al. Endoscopic sclerotherapy versus portacaval shunt in patients with severe cirrhosis and variceal hemorrhage. N Engl J Med 1984; 311:1589–94.

142. Copenhagen esophageal varices sclerotherapy project. Sclerotherapy after first variceal hemorrhage in cirrhosis. A randomized multicenter trial. N Engl J Med 1984; 311:1594–1600.

Doppler ultrasound probe for assessment of blood-flow in oesophageal varices. Lancet 1983; 1:677–8.

143. Lilly JR, Van Stiegmann G, Stellin G. Esophageal endosclerosis in children with portal vein thrombosis. J Pediatr Surg 1982; 17:571–5.

144. Howard E, Stamatakis JD, Mowat AP. Management of esophageal varices in children by injection sclerotherapy. J Pediatr Surg 1984; 19:2–5.

145. Hunt BL, Mitros FA, Lewis JW. Histologic changes in esophagus after injection sclerotherapy. (Abstr) Gastrointest Endosc 1982; 28:137.

146. DiMagno, EP, Zinsmeister AR, Larson DE, et al. Influence of hepatic reserve and cause of esophageal varices on survival and rebleeding before and after the introduction of sclerotherapy: a retrospective analysis. Mayo Clin Proc 1985; 60:149–57.

147. Gebhard RL, Ansel HJ, Silvis SE. Origin of pain during variceal sclerotherapy. (Abstr) Gastrointest Endosc 1982; 28:131.

148. Cohen LB, Korsten MA, Scherl EJ, et al. Bacteremia after endoscopic injection sclerosis. Gastrointest Endosc 1983; 29:198–200.

149. Larson GM. Esophageal motility after injection sclerotherapy. (Abstr) Gastrointest Endosc 1983; 29:164.

150. Simon C, Cohen L, Scherl E, et al. Esophageal motility and symptoms after endoscopic injection sclerotherapy. (Abstr) Gastrointest Endosc 1983; 29:192.

151. Ogle SJ, Kirk CJC, Bailey RJ, et al. Oesophageal function in cirrhotic patients undergoing injection sclerotherapy for oesophageal varices. Digestion 1978; 18:178–85.

152. Reilly JJ Jr, Schade RR, Van Thiel DS. Esophageal function after injection sclerotherapy: pathogenesis of esophageal stricture. Am J Surg 1984; 147:85–8.

153. Saks BJ, Kilby AE, Dietrich PA, et al. Pleural and mediastinal changes following endoscopic injection sclerotherapy of esophageal varices. Radiology 1983; 149:639–42.

154. Bacon BR, Bailey-Newton RS, Connors AF Jr. Pleural effusions after endoscopic variceal sclerotherapy. Gastroenterology 1985; 88:1910–4.

155. Monroe P, Morrow CF Jr, Millen JE, et al. Acute respiratory failure after sodium morrhuate esophageal sclerotherapy. Gastroenterology 1983; 85:693–9.

156. Sorensen T, Burcharth F, Pedersen ML, Findahl F. Oesophageal stricture and dysphagia after endoscopic sclerotherapy for bleeding varices. Gut 1984; 25:473–7.

157. Carr-Locke DL, Sidky K. Broncho-oesophageal fistula: a late complication of endoscopic variceal sclerotherapy. Gut 1982; 23:1005–7.

158. Soderlund C, Wiechel K-L. Oesophageal perforation after sclerotherapy for variceal haemorrhage. Acta Chir Scand 1983; 149:491–5.

159. Sanowski RA, Kozarek RA, Brayko C, Sarles H. Esophageal variceal sclerotherapy (EVS): course and complications. (Abstr) Gastrointest Endosc 1983; 29:193.

160. Scherl EJ, Fabry TL. Pseudodiverticula secondary to injection sclerotherapy. J Clin Gastroenterol 1983; 5:401–3.

161. Ayres SJ, Goff JS, Warren GH, Schaefer JW. Esophageal ulceration and bleeding after flexible fiberoptic esophageal vein sclerosis. Gastroenterology 1982; 83:131–6.

162. Roark G. Treatment of postsclerotherapy esophageal ulcers with sucralfate. Gastrointest Endosc 1984; 30:9–10.

163. Shepherd MM, Lee RG, Bowers JH. Local toxicity of sclerosing agents used in canine esophagus. (Abstr) Gastrointest Endosc 1983; 29:168.

164. Trudeau W, Prindiville T, Gibbert T, et al. An update on the safety of sclerosing agents used in endoscopic injection sclerosis. (Abstr) Gastrointest Endosc 1983; 29:168.

165. Brooks WS, Galambos JT. Sclerotherapy of esophageal varices: post injection ulceration. (Abstr) Gastrointest Endosc 1983; 29:191.

166. Brayko CM, Kozarek RA, Sanowski RA. Bacteremia during esophageal variceal sclerotherapy: its cause and prevention. (Abstr) Gastrointest Endosc 1983; 29:159–60.

167. Lange S, Laughlin B, Hughes RW, et al. Septic complications of variceal hemorrhage and ethanolamine sclerotherapy of varices. (Abstr) Gastrointest Endosc 1983; 29:191.

168. Seidman E, Weber A, Morin CL, et al. Spinal cord paralysis following sclerotherapy for esophageal varices. Hepatology 1984; 4:950–4.

169. Gardner EC, Brooks WS Jr. Absence of disseminated intravascular coagulation with endoscopic sclerosis of esophageal varices. Gastrointest Endosc 1982; 28:67–9.

170. Barsoum MS, Mooro HAW, Bolous FI, et al. The complications of injection sclerotherapy of bleeding oesophageal varices. Br J Surg 1982; 69:79–81.

171. Sauerbruch T, Weinzierl M, Dietrich HP, et al. Sclerotherapy of a bleeding duodenal varix. Endoscopy 1982; 14:187–9.

172. Foutch PG, Sivak MV Jr. Colonic variceal hemorrhage after endoscopic injection sclerosis of esophageal varices: a report of three cases. Am J Gastroenterol 1984; 79:756–60.

173. Bullimore DW. Sclerotherapist's eye. (Letter) Gastrointest Endosc 1982; 28:271.

174. Bat L, Shemesh E, Niv Y, Neumann G. More about sclerotherapist's eye. (Letter) Gastrointest Endosc 1982; 28:271.

175. Perakos PG, Cirbus JJ, Camara DS. Persistent bradyarrhythmia after sclerotherapy for esophageal varices. South Med J 1984; 77:531–2.

176. Warren WD, Henderson JM, Millikan WJ, et al. Distal splenorenal shunt versus endoscopic sclerotherapy for long-term management of variceal bleeding. Preliminary report of a prospective, randomized trial. Ann Surg 1986; 203:454–62.

177. Westaby D, Macdougall BR, Williams R. Improved survival following injection sclerotherapy for esophageal varices: final analysis of a controlled trial. Hepatology 1985; 5:827–30.

178. Kitano S, Terblanche J, Kahn D, Bornman PC. Venous anatomy of the lower oesophagus in portal hypertension: practical implications. Br J Surg 1986; 73:525–31.

179. Bailey-Newton RS, Connors AF Jr, Bacon BR. Effect of endoscopic variceal sclerotherapy on gas exchange and hemodynamics in humans. Gastroenterology 1985; 89:368–73.

180. Sauerbruch T, Moser E. Influence of long-term injection sclerotherapy on portal venous component of total liver perfusion measured by hepatosplenic radionuclide angiography. Hepatogastroenterology 1986; 33:17–9.

Chapter 17

BENIGN AND MALIGNANT TUMORS OF THE ESOPHAGUS

G. N. J. TYTGAT, M.D.

CLINICAL FEATURES

The presenting symptoms of benign esophageal tumors are dysphagia and bleeding; the latter is the result of central ulceration. The symptoms of esophageal malignancy include progressive dysphagia, first for solids then liquids; weight loss; regurgitation; alteration of voice; pain localized to the retrosternal, back or cervical regions; bronchopulmonary-related complaints such as coughing spells at night and symptoms of aspiration pneumonia and those resulting from a bronchopulmonary fistula; and supraclavicular lymph node enlargement. These classic symptoms usually indicate an advanced stage of the disease.

The most important symptom is dysphagia. The dysphagia that results from malignancy is usually of gradual onset and steadily increasing severity. At first the patient has difficulty with foodstuffs such as meat and apples. Dysphagia worsens until finally it may be impossible to swallow saliva. In other cases there may be sudden impaction of a bolus of food. Difficulty in swallowing usually develops long before the entire circumference of the esophageal lumen is compromised and often before there is radiologic evidence of impediment in the movement of barium. Rather, it begins when about half the intraluminal circumference has been invaded. Three different systems for classifying the severity of dysphagia are summarized in Table 17–1.[1-4]

Pain is not a prominent feature, except in the late stages when the tumor has spread locally. When present, pain is usually located in the area of the sternum and often radiates to the back.

Patients with early esophageal malignancy are either asymptomatic or may have characteristically vague complaints, such as an awareness of the passage of food through the esophagus; mild odynophagia with localized or radiating pain; mild, paradoxical dysphagia due to esophageal spasm proximal to the tumor; unilateral otalgia or pain in the jugular-carotid area; minimal dysphagia due to dysfunction of the upper esophageal sphincter; and, rarely, a discrete weight loss.

CLASSIFICATION, ETIOLOGY, AND PATHOGENESIS

Epithelial Tumors

Benign Epithelial Tumors

Squamous cell papilloma is a benign tumor composed of squamous cells covering finger-like projections of lamina propria. These lesions have a fibrovascular core without inflammatory cells, which is covered by an acanthoid epithelium of mature squamous cells. Squamous cell papillomas usually occur in elderly men. They perhaps have an inflammation pathogenesis that may be related to chronic esophageal reflux or prolonged nasogastric intubation, although infection with human papilloma virus has also been suggested.[5] Despite the fact that multiple squamous cell papillomas have been found in patients with tylosis and with acanthosis nigricans, available data do not on the whole suggest progression to malignancy.

Malignant Epithelial Tumors

Squamous Cell Carcinoma. Squamous cell carcinoma is by far the most common malig-

TABLE 17–1. **Scoring systems for dysphagia***

Stoller et al. 1977[2]
0: All foods
1: All soft foods
2: Blenderized foods
3: Clear liquids only
4: Nothing (not even saliva)

Atkinson et al. 1979[3]
0: Taking normal diet
1: Unable to swallow certain solids
2: Limited to semi-solid soft diet
3: Liquids only
4: Unable to swallow even liquids in
   adequate amounts; intravenous fluid
   needed

O'Sullivan et al. 1981[4]

None	0: No dysphagia
Minimal	1: Occasional episodes
Moderate	2: Requires liquids to clear
Severe	3: Episode of meat impaction, requiring medical treatment

*From: Tytgat GNJ, Bartelsman JFWM. Dysphagia—an overview. In: Salmon P, ed. Advances in Gastrointestinal Endoscopy. London: Chapman and Hall, Ltd., 1983.

nant tumor of the esophagus. Its frequency reaches epidemic proportions in Iran, China, and certain parts of Africa. The incidence in North American black men is increasing rapidly.[6]

Squamous cell carcinoma is usually graded microscopically as poorly, moderately, or well differentiated. Well-differentiated tumors are those with abundant keratin, easily demonstrated intercellular bridges, and minimal nuclear and cellular pleomorphism. A well-differentiated papillary growth is also termed a verrucous carcinoma. Poorly differentiated tumors are those which have marked cellular atypia, nuclear pleomorphism, and little or no keratin or intercellular bridges. Sometimes the malignant cells may appear spindle-shaped. Moderately differentiated tumors have a microscopic appearance that is intermediate to that of well- and poorly differentiated cancers.

Squamous cell carcinoma of the middle and distal esophagus shows a marked predilection for middle-aged and elderly men, especially those who use alcohol to excess and are heavy smokers. Carcinomas of the upper third of the esophagus account for approximately 10% of all squamous cell cancers. They develop almost exclusively in the region of the cricopharyngeus muscle, chiefly in young women.

Premalignant Conditions

A premalignant condition is an abnormal state or situation which creates an environment favoring the development of cancer. Several entities of differing etiology have been shown to be linked to malignant transformation of the esophageal epithelium. However, the proportion of esophageal cancer cases related to these conditions is very small.[7, 8]

Squamous cell carcinoma of the proximal esophagus, especially the postcricoid area, has been related to long-standing iron deficiency and is reported in as high as 15% of female patients with the Plummer-Vinson syndrome.[9] There are a number of other associated abnormal findings reported with this syndrome. The incidence of Plummer-Vinson syndrome has decreased considerably in recent decades, probably as a result of improved nutrition, although the deficiency state theory of pathogenesis does not explain all aspects of the syndrome. Esophageal webs may be found in the absence of any of the other findings usually associated with the Plummer-Vinson syndrome. However, it has not been established that isolated esophageal webs are associated with carcinoma. (Esophageal webs are discussed in Chapter 15.)

Tylosis (hyperkeratosis palmaris et plantaris) is a rare autosomal dominant genetic disorder associated with a striking susceptibility to esophageal cancer. The disease is characterized by thickening of the skin of the palms and soles. In the largest series published on this disorder, esophageal cancer developed in 37% of family members.[10]

The incidence of malignancy in patients with caustic burns of the esophagus, especially as a result of lye ingestion, varies from 0.8% to 5%. Usually there is a delay of over 20 years before the appearance of carcinoma, although exceptions occur. The older the patient at the time of lye ingestion, the earlier the carcinoma appears. Malignant transformation usually develops in areas of extensive scarring.[11]

Whether achalasia predisposes to esophageal cancer is less clear. Some investigators believe that patients probably have only a minimal, if any, increased risk of cancer. Others describe squamous cell carcinoma in approximately 3% of patients, with variations of 1% to 10%.[12–14] There is speculation that chronic irritation resulting from stasis is the etiologic mechanism. Because patients are accustomed to interference with the normal passage of food as a result of the underlying motility disorder, and because the enlarged esophagus will accommodate a rather bulky tumor, the carcinoma is usually advanced when detected. Cancer may occur in both surgically and non-surgically treated patients. (Achalasia is discussed in greater detail in Chapter 15.)

Contrary to the report of Joske and Benedict,[13] there are few data to support the concept that peptic stricture predisposes to esophageal malignancy.

Dysplasia. Certain pathologic changes in the esophageal mucosa are associated with a greater risk of cancer. Progressively worsening mucosal dysplasia is generally considered to be premalignant. Dysplasia is characterized by disruption of the normal epithelial architecture, with proliferation of atypical cells and partial loss of polarity. With severe dysplasia, the mucosa is totally replaced by dysplastic cells which, however, remain bounded by an intact, uninterrupted basal lamina. Early in the course of malignant lesions, when there is limited infiltration, it is often possible to discern evidence of a transition from normal mucosa through various degrees of dysplasia into focally invasive malignancy (Fig. 17–1).

Adenocarcinoma

Esophageal adenocarcinoma is a malignant tumor arising in glandular-type epithelium. Primary adenocarcinoma may develop either in heterotopic gastric mucosa or from submucosal mucous glands. At the gastroesophageal junction, adenocarcinoma is more common than squamous cell carcinoma. For adenocarcinoma to be accepted as esophageal in origin, it must lie entirely within the esophagus and be bounded by squamous cell epithelium on all sides, except in the case of adenocarcinoma arising in Barrett's epithelium. It may be very difficult if not impossible to distinguish adenocarcinoma found in the distal esophagus as being the result of proximal spread from the stomach or as arising as a true primary growth of the esophagus.

Premalignant Conditions

Most adenocarcinomas that develop within the esophagus are probably related to a transition to columnar-type esophageal mucosa known as Barrett's esophagus or endobrachyesophagus. The exact prevalence of this entity is unknown, but frequencies as high as 11.5% have been described in patients with symptoms and signs of esophageal reflux disease.[15, 16] The reported incidence of adenocarcinoma in patients with Barrett's esophagus varies from 2% to 9% but may be as high as 13%.[17, 18] Cancer usually occurs in the distal third of the esophagus, but may develop at more proximal levels, and it can be multifocal.

Dysplasia. Accumulating clinical experience indicates that severe dysplasia may be considered a reliable marker of impending adenocarcinoma (Fig. 17–2 and Plate 17–1).

Rare Epithelial Malignancies

Depending upon histologic characteristics, some rare forms of epithelial malignancy may be distinguished, such as adenoid cystic carcinoma, mucoepidermoid carcinoma,

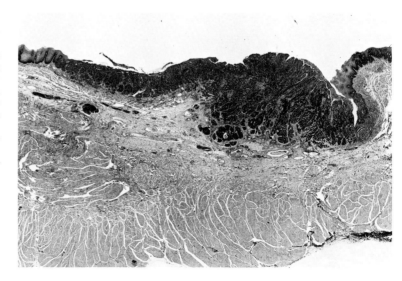

FIGURE 17–1. Microscopic appearance of early squamous esophageal cancer; normal mucosa merges via areas of severe dysplasia into early infiltrating malignancy. The finding of normal and dysplastic epithelium merging gradually with early invasive cancer is suggestive of a histologic sequence, that is, dysplasia developing into in-situ carcinoma, which, in turn, becomes superficial esophageal cancer.

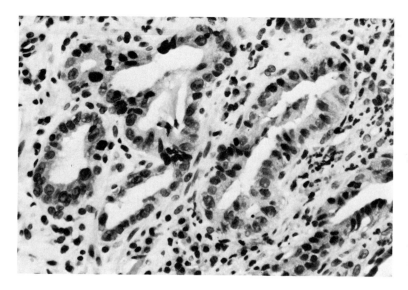

FIGURE 17–2. Example of severe dysplasia in Barrett's columnar-lined esophagus, characterized by architectural distortion, marked nuclear atypia, and cellular pleomorphism. Mitoses are abundant, and there is focal loss of polarity. The dysplastic cells are still bound by an intact basal lamina.

adenosquamous carcinoma (intermingled glandular and squamous components), undifferentiated carcinoma without recognizable glandular or squamous elements, and carcinosarcoma. A distinct but rare form of undifferentiated carcinoma referred to as oatcell carcinoma, sometimes associated with production of hormones, also has been described.[19]

A carcinosarcoma consists of an intimate mixture of carcinomatous elements (often as epithelial pearls and foci of highly anaplastic squamous cells) and sarcomatous cells growing together as a single tumor. Carcinosarcoma of the esophagus is usually a polypoid non-ulcerating lesion, only superficially invasive, that metastasizes comparatively late in its course (Plate 17–2).

Non-Epithelial Tumors

Benign Non-Epithelial Tumors

Leiomyoma is the most common type of benign non-epithelial tumor encountered in the esophagus. Usually found in the lower third of the esophagus, these lesions are mostly solitary, although multiple tumors have been encountered. In some rare cases of diffuse leiomyomatosis, the esophagus is studded throughout with these tumors.[20]

Other, rare, solid intramural tumors are the fibroma, lipoma, neurofibroma, osteochondroma, and glomus tumor. Lipomas usually develop in the cervical segment of the esophagus, although they may occur at any level. Granular cell myoblastoma, also called granular cell tumor (Abrikosov's tu-

mor), is characterized histologically by large polygonal cells with eosinophilic cytoplasm and eccentric nuclei. The great majority occur in women; most are located in the upper and lower thirds of the esophagus.[21] Multiplicity is possible. Although their origin is uncertain, they may arise from neural cells.

Hemangiomas are comprised of endothelium-lined spaces, varying in size from fine capillaries to larger cavernous structures. Hemangioma of the esophagus is a rare entity making up only 2% to 3% of benign esophageal neoplasms.[22] They are evenly distributed along the length of the esophagus. Size varies widely, the average diameter being 2 to 3 cm. Due to the propulsive effect of peristalsis, these lesions may develop long pedicles and become very mobile. Hemangiomas are usually considered to be vascular malformations (hamartomas) rather then true neoplasms. Most are probably congenital.

Malignant Non-Epithelial Tumors

Leiomyosarcoma is the most frequently encountered malignant non-epithelial tumor. Lymphomatous and leukemic involvement of the esophagus appears to be rare. Malignant melanoma of the esophagus is most commonly metastatic rather than primary. The very rare primary lesion usually presents as a large, polypoid pedunculated lesion. Metastasis of extraintestinal melanomas to the gastrointestinal tract usually produces numerous black, umbilicated nodules. Carcinoid tumors and choriocarcinoma have on rare occasions arisen in the esophagus. Occasionally biopsy specimens of an esophageal lesion will show large numbers of entero-

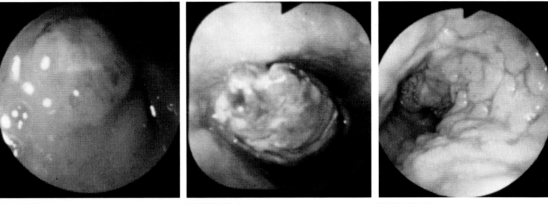

PLATE 17–1.   PLATE 17–2.   PLATE 17–3.

PLATE 17–1. Early malignant lesion, detected upon routine endoscopic screening, developed in an area where multiple previous biopsies (see Fig. 17–2.) had shown severe dysplasia. Biopsies in another area revealed foci of early multifocal invasive malignancy.

PLATE 17–2. Polypoid exophytic non-ulcerating carcinosarcoma obstructing the esophageal lumen.

PLATE 17–3. Nodular thickening of the esophageal squamous mucosa in longstanding stasis. The appearance of a single excresence is indistinguishable from that of a true papilloma.

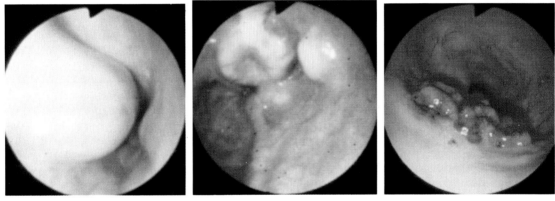

PLATE 17–4.   PLATE 17–5.   PLATE 17–6.

PLATE 17–4. Leiomyoma involving distal esophagus. The lesion is covered by normal mucosa, and it distorts the lumen in an extrinsic fashion.

PLATE 17–5. Two small nodular elevations (one is umbilicated), covered by normal appearing squamous mucosa, that proved to be granular myoblastomas.

PLATE 17–6. Early esophageal carcinoma of the papillary type (corresponding to Figure 17–1.).

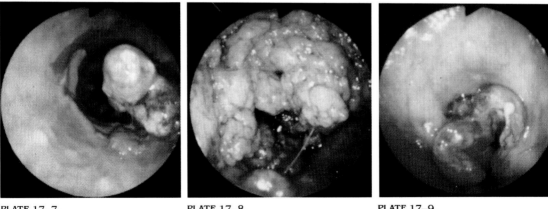

PLATE 17–7.   PLATE 17–8.   PLATE 17–9.

PLATE 17–7. Exophytic adenocarcinoma growing intraluminally in a columnar-lined esophagus. Note the sharply demarcated transition from columnar to squamous mucosa opposite the carcinoma.

PLATE 17–8. Bulky exophytic mass with coarsely nodular, hemorrhagic, focally eroded with ulcerated surface.

PLATE 17–9. Central malignant ulceration in a tumor that has the shape of a meniscus.

chromaffin carcinoid cells which, after detailed study of the resection specimen, are shown to accompany a deeply infiltrating, poorly differentiated adenocarcinoma.

Tumor-like Lesions

Heterotopias

Islands of gastric heterotopia may be found in the proximal esophagus as small elevated lesions. In the lower esophagus, heterotopic tissue is often more extensive and usually continuous with the normal glandular mucosa of the stomach. Gastric heterotopia in the lower esophagus, a subject of some debate, is either congenital or is associated with chronic reflux esophagitis.

Congenital Cysts

Congenital cysts are malformations lined entirely by epithelium that is ciliated, squamous, or gastric or is more than one of these types. They are usually the result of a developmental abnormality occurring during formation and differentiation of the lower respiratory tract, esophagus, and stomach.

Fibrovascular (Fibrous) Polyps

A fibrovascular polyp is a polypoid lesion composed of a core of fibrous or adipose connective tissue and blood vessels, covered by thickened but otherwise normal squamous epithelium.[23] This lesion may be differentiated from a myoma by its elasticity and tendency to develop a pedicle. When situated proximal to a sphincter, such polyps may acquire the shape of a bell clapper. Most fibrovascular polyps are located in the proximal one third of the esophagus and, because most are pedunculated, regurgitation with subsequent asphyxia may occur.

Glycogenic Acanthosis

The term glycogenic acanthosis has been applied to focal areas of excessive glycogen accumulation in the superficial squamous cells of the mucosa. Mucosal biopsy specimens reveal hyperplasia of the glycogen-rich intermediate squamous cells without cytologic atypia. This lesion, which has no known role as a cancer precursor, is discussed in Chapter 15.

Secondary Tumors

Tumors of adjacent organs, most commonly the bronchus or stomach, often invade the esophagus. Occasionally, mediastinal lymph nodes as a site of metastatic cancer from another organ will provide an avenue for esophageal involvement and obstruction. Metastatic esophageal involvement may also occur in patients with breast cancer, sometimes many years after treatment of the primary lesion.

DIAGNOSTIC TECHNIQUES

Endoscopy

Benign Lesions

Papillomas. A papilloma is an exophytic excrescence of the esophageal epithelium. Papillomas appear as small wart-like projections on the mucosal surface. They are preferentially located in the distal esophagus and are often multiple. Occasionally, large areas covered with plaques or verrucous projections consisting of epithelial hyperplasia and sometimes hyperkeratosis may be observed in association with chronic irritation such as occurs with long-standing achalasia. These areas have the endoscopic appearance of whitish, slightly elevated mucosal nodules (Plate 17–3). Papillomas must be distinguished from verrucous squamous cell carcinoma and proliferating granulation tissue. Verrucous squamous cell carcinoma is also papillary and well differentiated, but careful microscopic examination will reveal epithelial dysplasia and superficial carcinomatous invasion. Multiplicity, the usual case with papilloma, strongly favors a benign lesion. When there is doubt or uncertainty regarding the true nature of a papillomatous lesion based on endoscopic appearance and biopsy, endoscopic excision, if feasible, can be undertaken.

Leiomyomas. Esophageal leiomyomas exhibit great variation in size and shape. Most are spherical or ovoid, although many (25% in one study[24]) may be crescentic or even annular in configuration.[24] The most common shape is roughly oval, with dimensions of approximately 6 to 8 cm in length and 4 to 6 cm in width. The endoscopic appearance is that of a bulging mass with intact or focally ulcerated but freely movable mucosa stretched over the lesion (Plate 17–4). The surface may be regular and smooth or multilobulated. As leiomyomas are not infiltrative, the endoscope can usually pass these lesions without difficulty, unless the tumor is completely or almost completely annular. The endoscopist should be aware that the mobility of such intramural lesions may permit them to be displaced easily, and hence they can be overlooked at esophagoscopy. As a rule, biopsy is not advisable if the overlying mucosa is normal in appearance. Mucosal biopsies usually will not reveal the nature of the lesion except in some cases when they are taken from an ulcerated area. Biopsy is justified only if roughening, irregularity, or peculiar ulceration of the mucosa overlying the tumor suggests malignancy. The decision to perform extramucosal enucleation or partial resection is usually made at surgery, and there is a concern that multiple endoscopic biopsies can interfere with enucleation.

Myoblastomas. Granular cell tumors, or myoblastomas, appear endoscopically as tiny, sometimes slightly umbilicated, submucosal lesions in the distal esophagus (Plate 17–5). One might decide to remove such lesions endoscopically if this is feasible, when they are located within the lower esophageal sphincter zone, perhaps causing motility disturbances.

Hemangiomas. It may be possible to differentiate a hemangioma from other benign tumors at endoscopy if the lesion has a pale, bluish coloration and if it empties when pressure is applied with the endoscope. However, often the mucosa covering a hemangioma is indistinguishable from that of the surrounding esophagus. Usually hemangiomas are not sufficiently small or pedunculated to a degree that would make them suitable for removal by electrosurgical snare polypectomy. In principle, no biopsy should be taken of any vascular lesion because of the possibility of severe hemorrhage. This is problematic when the nature of the lesion is not obvious endoscopically and biopsy is contemplated to exclude malignancy. Data are limited on the consequences of endoscopic biopsy of such a lesion. The endoscopist must be prepared to deal with profuse bleeding. There are no reports of extensive experience in the endoscopic treatment of esophageal hemangiomas. If the lesion is large, attempted endoscopic control of bleeding could result in more profuse bleeding. Theoretically, such lesions might be treated by laser photocoagulation, but data are inadequate to support this point.

Polyps. Fibrovascular polyps appear endoscopically as oval-shaped or elongated sausage-like masses with a smooth or lobulated surface. The area of mucosal attachment of the stalk is usually identified without difficulty. Pedunculated intraluminal tumors should be removed, preferably at endoscopy if the lesion is not excessively voluminous.

Cysts. Congenital cystic lesions of the esophagus (teratoma, epidermoid cyst, duplication cyst, branchiogenic cyst, enterogenous cyst, coelom cyst, or others) usually have no characteristic endoscopic appearance. Such lesions manifest as a nonspecific, extrinsic compression, or as an intramural tumor. Retention cysts are round or fusiform structures which have a yellowish transparency and a smooth surface. They can be opened with a needle or biopsy forceps. This may result in the discharge of a mucous orange-yellow fluid. Retention cysts are usually solitary and have no preferential location. An isolated retention cyst is easily distinguished from polycystic chronic esophagitis (esophagitis cystica) in which the mucosal surface is covered by innumerable retention cysts. Microdiverticulosis and sometimes an inflammatory stricture may coexist with the latter entity.

Glycogenic Acanthosis. Glycogenic acanthosis (described in Chapter 15) is commonly noted at endoscopy and is usually easy to differentiate from other lesions and tumors. The plaques, usually less than 1 cm in diameter, sometimes tend to align along the longitudinal folds of the esophagus and will dye blue with application of 2% Lugol's solution because of their increased glycogen content.

Premalignant Lesions and Conditions

Endoscopic screening for severe dysplasia can be undertaken when conditions exist that predispose to esophageal malignancy. Preferably this should be done annually by endoscopy with multiple biopsies with or without brush cytology. However, the most efficacious schedule of procedures and methodology has not been established. Unfortunately, data concerning the outcome of this approach are limited. It is not known with certainty, for example, that such screening will result in curative treatment of significant numbers of patients. Furthermore, the exact risk of cancer is not established for all conditions that are considered to be premalignant. It is easy to justify this approach when the risk of malignancy is known to be high—when there has been a lapse of many years after lye ingestion, for example. Thus, screening should be decided on an individual case basis, since data accumulated from large series of patients undergoing endoscopic screening are not available as guidelines. Systematic endoscopy of the upper digestive tract is indicated in patients with squamous malignancy of the structures of the head and neck, and probably when mucosal dysplasia is discovered in this area, since such tumors are known to be associated with carcinoma of the esophagus.[25]

The endoscopic identification of dysplasia is problematic. Occasionally dysplastic areas may be visible endoscopically as whitish plaques, although most often such plaques consist of innocent-looking areas of mucosal thickening. In some patients, dysplasia may be discovered in areas that appear inflamed or manifest increased vascularity. In other patients, dysplasia may be present in areas that appear as shallow depressions of the mucosal surface. Despite these observations, no peculiar endoscopic features allow distinction between dysplastic and non-dysplastic mucosa.

Rarely, adenomatous polyps develop in the esophagus, especially in patients with columnar cell metaplasia. The significance of this finding is uncertain, but the occurrence of a benign neoplasm in Barrett's epithelium with its known premalignant potential should be regarded with circumspection. Rare instances of multiple adenomatous lesions in Barrett's esophagus have been reported.[26]

Early Esophageal Cancer

Early esophageal cancer can be defined as malignancy that is confined to the mucosa and submucosa and is without lymph node metastasis. Descriptions of the endoscopic appearance of early esophageal malignancy come mainly from China[27, 28] and Japan.[29]

Early esophageal malignancy may appear as a superficial erosion. Usually the cancerous mucosa is quite fragile and bleeds easily upon contact with the endoscope. The cancerous area appears slightly depressed, with gray erosive spots against a reddish background. These reddened areas usually have geographic shapes. Between the erosive defects, islands of whitish, normal-looking mucosa may be seen.

The endoscopic appearance may also be that of a plaque-like lesion in which the cancerous area appears slightly elevated, with a granular or coarse, knobby surface. Occasionally small plaques are scattered in the surrounding mucosa. In other areas these whitish plaques may be confluent, giving the surface an orange-peel appearance. The cancerous epithelium of plaque-like lesions is usually markedly thickened.

Sometimes early esophageal malignancy presents as a flat patch of localized edema and congestion (congestive type). Reddish spots may be found within and about the congested mucosal area. This localized mucosal roughening and hyperemia has been compared to tree bark. The abnormal mucosa tears easily and friability (bleeding that develops with slight trauma) is a prominent feature.

Early esophageal cancer may also look like a circumscribed polypoid or protruded lesion (papillary type) (Plate 17–6). The irregular, thickened mucosa will have a granular, nodular, papillary, or polypoid appearance. The diameter of this type of lesion is often less than 3 cm. The polypoid protrusion may have a relatively wide mucosal base, and occasionally friability or superficial erosive defects may be present.

In some patients, the only visible abnormality is either a circumscribed area of altered pliability or a circumscribed patch of mucosal discoloration (occult type). These early cancers are obviously difficult to detect. Only meticulous attention to detail, along with adequate biopsy sampling of any suspicious area, will detect these early cancers.

In the Japanese system of classification, early esophageal cancers are categorized as protruding, superficial, and ulcerating. This descriptive classification is in keeping with the accepted endoscopic nomenclature for early gastric cancer.[29] However, the term "erosive" would seem more appropriate than the term "ulcerated."

The plaque-like and erosive types of early cancer in the esophagus may be difficult to differentiate endoscopically from the mucosal changes resulting from reflux esophagitis. However, a zone of normal mucosa is usually found between the distal edge of the neoplastic lesion and the gastroesophageal junction. A normal mucosal segment is not a feature of reflux esophagitis, and this may be a useful differential criterion.

Early malignancy may also be difficult to detect in patients with a Barrett-type ulcer. The columnar epithelium surrounding the ulcer may be heaped up and polypoid, thus suggesting adenocarcinoma. However, the mucosal pattern of this polypoid mucosa can sometimes be distinguished from the more disorganized pattern with focal areas of discoloration seen in malignancy. Furthermore, fibroepithelial, inflammatory, pseudopolypoid projections may sometimes be present at the margins of a Barrett-type ulcer.[30] However, the true nature of lesions that are easily misinterpreted at endoscopy can only be determined by adequate biopsies.

Advanced Cancer

The macroscopic appearance of advanced cancer is traditionally of three main types, although many combinations and transitional forms exist. These types are (1) exophytic-polypoid, (2) ulcerative, and (3) diffusely infiltrating. The exophytic-polypoid growth is usually characterized as a bulky, cauliflower-like, wide-based lesion (Plate 17–7). The coarsely nodular surface is often hemorrhagic and may show additional erosive or ulcerative defects (Plate 17–8). The ulcerative type is characterized by central meniscoid-type necrosis (Plates 17–9 and 17–10) surrounded by heaped up edges (Plate 17–11). Usually a major part of the circumference of the esophageal lumen is involved by the tumor. A diffusely infiltrating scirrhous cancer is manifest as obvious thickening and rigidity of the esophageal wall of variable length, with fixation of the irregularly thickened, coarsely nodular, rarely ulcerated mucosa to the deeper layers. Luminal narrowing is often present (Plate 17–12). The most common and classic endoscopic appearance of advanced esophageal cancer is that of an eccentrically located ulcerated mass, with a projecting and overhanging margin located in a rigid, aperistaltic segment.

A peculiar form of presentation, referred to as "superficial spreading cancer," is defined as a lesion with an intramucosal extension of malignancy of at least 2 cm from the main portion of the cancer. The boundaries between involved and uninvolved mucosa may be indistinguishable.[31]

The endoscopist's impression may be inadequate for assessing the extent of disease in the esophagus. From an endoscopic standpoint it is important to realize that cancer has a tendency to spread submucosally and to establish satellite lesions at some distance from the obvious primary lesion (Plate 17–13). Tiny mucosal elevations proximal to a main lesion should be given special attention. These often have a somewhat yellowish hue. Biopsy usually proves these to be malignant (Plate 17–14). They probably are intramural

metastases, although some authorities contend that such apparent (sub)mucosal spread may actually be primary intramucosal carcinoma, with the intraepithelial changes representing a form of "field cancerization."

Careful endoscopic examination of the fundus and cardia of the stomach is mandatory. Detailed inspection after retroflexion of the endoscope assists in the detection of cancer that has extended proximally from the stomach into the esophagus.

According to Savary and Miller,[32] the following items compose the specified protocol for endoscopic assessment of esophageal cancer:

1. Location of the proximal margin, usually measured from the incisor teeth or mandibular ridge in the edentulous; extent and location longitudinally and circumferentially (tumor origin as from upper, middle, or lower thirds influences therapeutic decisions).

2. Position of the distal edge in relation to the cardia.

3. Type of tumor (exophytic, ulcerating, infiltrating, etc.).

4. Degree of mobility or fixation.

5. Diameter of the existing lumen.

6. Appearance of the mucosa proximal to the cancer.

7. Histologic type.

8. Status of the larynx, including recurrent laryngeal nerve function.

9. Tracheobronchoscopic examination, performed not only to detect tracheobronchial cancerous involvement or a tracheobronchial fistula (Plate 17–15) but also to detect (early) concomitant lesions in the respiratory tract.

Vital Staining (Chromoscopy)

Chromoscopy (in vivo dye staining, or dye scattering) is being used increasingly in some centers to facilitate detection of early esophageal malignancy. Although its application is not worldwide, those who have extensive experience with this method advocate its use for detection of small malignant lesions.[33] (Specific techniques for this method are discussed in Chapter 10, Part 2.)

The stains used most often are 1% to 2% Lugol's solution, 1% to 2% toluidine blue, and 1% to 2% methylene blue. Lugol's solution stains non-keratinized squamous epithelium in proportion to its intracellular glycogen content. Injured squamous epithelium

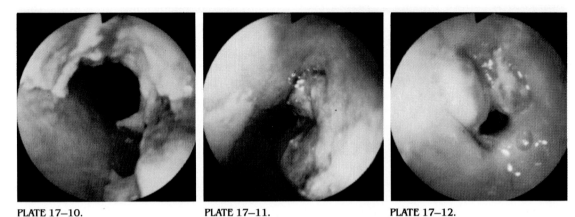

PLATE 17—10.   PLATE 17—11.   PLATE 17—12.

PLATE 17—10. Large central ulceration creates the radiologic appearance of a malignant meniscus sign.
PLATE 17—11. The proximal, heaped-up edges of the lesion with a central ulceration that is depicted in Plate 17-12.
PLATE 17—12. Diffusely infiltrating malignancy causing severe luminal constriction, surrounded by nodular elevations covered with discolored, partially necrotic mucosa.

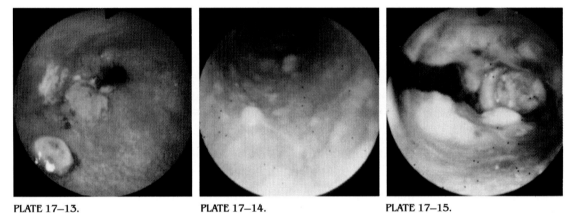

PLATE 17—13.   PLATE 17—14.   PLATE 17—15.

PLATE 17—13. Satellite lesion several centimeters proximal to a malignant stenosis caused by an infiltrating carcinoma.
PLATE 17—14. Small nodular elevations probably due to intramucosal metastases proximal to a distal malignant obstruction seen at the top of the figure.
PLATE 17—15. Large broncho-esophageal fistula at left. The original esophargeal lumen to the right is obstructed by an exophytic cancerous mass.

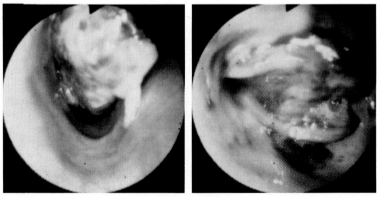

PLATE 17—16.   PLATE 17—17.

PLATE 17—16. Tumor simulating strongly adherent clot in a patient with an esophageal laceration due to vomitting.
PLATE 17—17. Vegetable material or fruit skin tightly impacted in.

or metaplastic columnar epithelium remains unstained or weakly stained, depending upon the severity of the mucosal injury. Early esophageal cancer consistently shows negative staining. Lugol's solution is not useful for isolating dysplastic areas because about 50% of such areas stain positively. Nuclear DNA has a much stronger affinity than cytoplasmic RNA for toluidine blue.[34] Dysplastic or neoplastic epithelium usually stains blue; the variable appearance includes tiny spots, interlacing stripes, irregularly shaped map-like areas, and extensive diffuse staining with sharp edges. Methylene blue can be used to stain columnar epithelium. It may be taken up by intestinalized cells and goblet cells but not by squamous epithelium. Methylene blue also accentuates mucosal relief, which differs for columnar and squamous epithelium.[35, 36]

Chromoscopy may facilitate detection and determination of the extent of cancerous lesions, including those not visible endoscopically. Multiple biopsies and cytologic specimens must be obtained from any suspicious area.

Biopsy and Cytology

A biopsy forceps with a central spike within the forceps' cups is probably the best instrument for biopsy of the esophagus. The spike is helpful in fixing the forceps on the mucosa when the surface of the area of interest is tangential to the trajectory of the biopsy forceps as it is advanced toward the lesion. Small forceps (7 Fr) do not permit full-thickness mucosal sampling. This may be a problem when carcinoma is infiltrating submucosally. In this circumstance, a larger forceps (9 Fr) may be useful. Repetitive biopsies in the same location can also be used to sample deeper submucosal layers.

The histologic diagnosis of polypoid and meniscoid tumors is not difficult when the proximal tumor margin is visible. Preferentially, biopsies should be taken from viable tumor tissue or from border areas between obvious proliferative growth and the area of invasion. Central necrotic, ulcerated areas and edematous adjoining walls should be avoided, because the yield will be lower in these regions. Cancer often extends proximally, and it may be useful to sample areas with mucosal pallor or tiny satellite nodules. Multiple biopsies in longitudinal sequence along the esophageal wall will aid in defining the proximal border of the cancer and in disclosing associated dysplasia. Contact be-

tween the endoscope and the tumor is often sufficient to cause bleeding. This may lead to imprecise biopsy localization and should be avoided if possible.

Esophageal cancer commonly presents as a stenotic lesion with apparently intact mucosa characterized by a moderately irregular surface. Infiltration of the esophageal wall usually provokes a fibrous reaction, this being perhaps the main cause of the stenosis. Moderately severe narrowing should be investigated with a small-caliber endoscope. Usually the endoscope may be passed through such a lesion, so that biopsies can be obtained not only from the proximal edge but also from within the tumor. Preferred biopsy sites include small nodular elevations, areas of whitish-yellowish discoloration, and the edges of eroded areas.

A malignant stenosis may be so tight that it is not possible to pass any endoscope beyond the lesion. Frequently, biopsy from within the stenosed segment is impossible, and tissue can be obtained only at a point proximal to the stenosis. In this circumstance it is not uncommon that biopsies, even in large numbers, fail to establish a diagnosis. Inflammatory changes or a nonspecific fibrous reaction are common microscopic findings. Diagnostic yield can be increased by introducing the forceps into the stricture to obtain tissue blindly. Unfortunately, it is difficult to obtain adequate tissue by this means, and the blind nature of the maneuver in itself lowers the incidence of positive results. In this circumstance it is especially important to obtain cytologic specimens from within the narrowed section. An alternative approach is to gently dilate the stricture to allow guided biopsies from within and from the distal border of the lesion, using a small-caliber endoscope. This maneuver—that is, dilation and immediate biopsy and/or cytology—has been shown to be practical and safe.[37] With any distal esophageal lesion it is essential that a retroflexed view of the gastroesophageal junction is performed from the gastric side to allow biopsy of this area.

Most endoscopists prefer a brush for obtaining cytology specimens. Generally, the type used has a plastic sheath into which the brush is withdrawn when not in use. This prevents contamination and loss of specimen material as the brush is withdrawn through the accessory channel of the endoscope. If both cytology and biopsy specimens are to be obtained, the cytology sample should be col-

TABLE 17–2. **Diagnostic Accuracy of Biopsy and Cytology in Malignancy of Esophagus and Cardia**

Authors	No. Patients	No. Bx	% Pos. Bx	% Pos. Cytol.	% Pos. Bx and Cytol.
Nakamura et al.[39]			85		
Kobayashi et al.[40]	8	>3	88	100	
Prolla[41]	25	3–4	72	92	
Bruni and Nelson[42]	103	6–8	94	87	
Seifert and Atay[43]	64		81		
Winawer et al.[44]	30	4	66	97	
Hishon et al.[45]	20		50	90	
Winawer et al.[46]					100
Witzel et al.[47]	47	6–10	77	89	
Prolla et al.[48]	73	6–8	78	89	
Eastman et al.[49]	69		71	76	
Gutz and Wildner[50]	75		93		
Mortensen and MacKenzie[51]	36		81	86	92
Graham et al.[52]	27	>7	96	88*	100
Yang et al.[28]†	115		80	88	
Wesdorp et al.‡	154	8–12	98		

*Salvage cytology.
†Early esophageal carcinoma.
‡Not published.
Bx = biopsies; Pos = positive; Cytol. = brush cytologic samples.

lected first. Otherwise blood in the area to be brushed will dilute the cytology sample. The brush should be swept over the slough from ulcerated and necrotic areas, the rim and margins of the lesion, and the surrounding tissue. Brush cytology is especially effective in the diagnosis of infiltrative lesions that produce severe lumenal narrowing, since the brush can be directed into the stricture. Positive samples can be obtained in cases in which biopsies of the proximal rim are negative.

Salvage cytology can be performed by aspirating the contents of the accessory channel of the endoscope into a mucus trap attached to the suction connector on the light guide section of the universal cord. Fluid aspiration between biopsies yields a pool of cytology material by recovery of material that clings to the biopsy forceps and is dislodged within the endoscope.[38]

In several studies reported, a correct biopsy diagnosis of esophageal carcinoma was obtained in over 90% of patients, provided that 6 or more biopsies were taken[28, 39–52] (Table 17–2). The higher the number of biopsies, the greater the chance of hitting non-necrotic tumor tissue. There is evidence that the yield of the first biopsy specimen is higher than that of following ones.[52] It is not uncommon, especially with distal infiltrating lesions, that more than 12 biopsies are needed to obtain a correct diagnosis; even with this number, a positive tissue diagnosis

occasionally may not be obtained. If, based on endoscopic assessment, esophageal cancer is suspected, but the diagnosis is not confirmed by cytologic and tissue sampling, then the procedure must be repeated. The false negative biopsy problem is most significant when the presence of carcinoma is not obvious. This pertains mostly to strictures that cannot be distinguished from those due to peptic reflux. The distinction between malignancy and florid proliferation of regenerating immature squamous cells in esophagitis may also be difficult for the histopathologist.

The diagnostic accuracy of cytology is high. In many series, brush cytology yielded a positive rate of diagnosis greater than 95% (see Table 17–2). When forceps biopsy and brush cytology are used in combination, a positive tissue diagnosis can be achieved in almost 100% of esophageal cancers; therefore, brush cytology and biopsy are considered complementary rather than mutually exclusive. The particular advantages of brush cytology when the luminal diameter through a tumor is only a few millimeters have been emphasized. A disadvantage, albeit small, of cytology is the small percentage of false positive results that have occurred in virtually all published series.[53]

ERRORS IN ENDOSCOPIC DIAGNOSIS

The endoscopic appearance of the esophagus may occasionally confuse the inexperienced examiner with respect to recognition of cancer. A classic error is misinterpretation of a strongly adherent clot which mimics an exophytic malignancy (Plate 17–16). Also deceptive is the appearance of food residue such as leguminous material impacted at a distal peptic stricture (Plate 17–17).

Submucosal malignancy that mimics achalasia can be problematic. The clinical and radiologic presentation of carcinoma of the gastric fundus and cardia encroaching on the gastroesophageal junction can be indistinguishable from that of primary achalasia. In rare cases, the esophageal manometric findings, including a positive Mecholyl test, truly mimic primary achalasia.[54, 55] Cancer should be suspected in patients with so-called secondary achalasia when the duration of symptoms is less than one year, the patient is older than 50, and there has been excessive and rapid weight loss. The ease with which a small-caliber endoscope may be passed through such a lesion, because of the lack of resistance to advancement of the instrument, may result in a serious oversight. Some au-

thorities recommend that a large-caliber dilator or large-diameter endoscope be passed through this segment prior to pneumatic dilation to be certain that the sphincter area is not mechanically constricted.[56] If a large-sized bougie will not pass or if it meets more than minimal resistance, it is likely that either a fibrotic stricture or an occult neoplasm is present, and pneumatic dilation should not be performed.

A carcinoma of the stomach with submucosal extension into the esophagus should be strongly suspected when the narrowed segment appears to be in a position proximal to the diaphragm, because the narrow segment in true achalasia almost always straddles the diaphragm. Frequently there are no visible abnormalities at endoscopy, and the usual small, superficial endoscopic biopsy specimens may reveal only normal squamous or gastric mucosa. The use of a large biopsy forceps is one approach to this problem; sampling is performed at the same site until tissue is obtained from the deeper layers of the submucosa[1, 57] (Fig. 17–3).

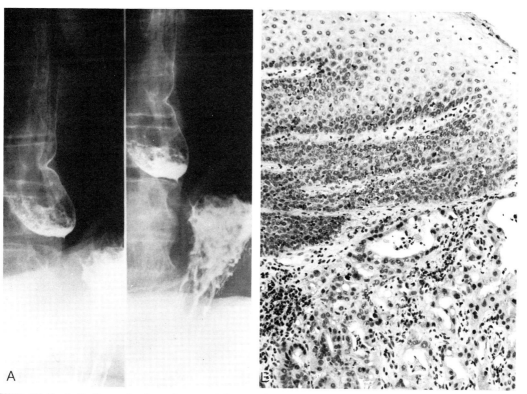

FIGURE 17–3. A, Radiograph of carcinoma at the cardia, infiltrating under normal squamous epithelium. B, Biopsy specimen obtained with large forceps in a patient with pseudoachalasia. Photomicrograph demonstrates squamous cell mucosa at the top of the figure and adenocarcinoma at the bottom.

PALLIATION OF MALIGNANT ESOPHAGEAL OBSTRUCTION

Despite several treatment modalities, survival of patients with esophageal carcinoma is usually short. Radiotherapy may be of temporary benefit in alleviating dysphagia, but unobstructed esophageal function may become difficult to maintain over the course of time. Of several methods of management of this problem, esophageal dilation and insertion of an endoprosthesis are discussed here. The relatively newer method of palliative laser photodestruction of obstructing gastrointestinal tumors is presented in Chapter 9. There are no comparative trials of laser treatment and endoprosthesis insertion. Each procedure has certain advantages, limitations, and specific complications, and both are effective. Experience with the endoprosthesis is greater than that with laser treatment. At the present time, therefore, the initial approach is discretionary when experience with both methods is equal. The two procedures are complementary in certain specific clinical situations.

Esophageal Dilation

Many patients with dysphagia due to carcinoma can be managed entirely by esophageal dilation. Initially it is advisable to introduce the dilating device over a guide wire, especially when the remaining lumen is narrow, tortuous or eccentric, or when there is a bronchoesophageal fistula. Several devices are available for guided dilation, such as the metal olives of the Eder-Puestow system, the stepwise enlarging Célestin type dilators,[58] and the gradually widening plastic bougies of the Savary type. The main advantages of the Savary-type dilators are easy passage through the pharynx and the gradual dilation produced.

The initial dilation is preferably done under fluoroscopic control, especially when difficulty is anticipated. Bougienage with mercury-weighted dilators is satisfactory, provided the dilation path is not too eccentric or tortuous. Repeated dilations are usually required; the interval between dilations varies considerably, depending on the procedure being used. A luminal diameter of 12 to 13 mm will usually eliminate dysphagia if the narrowed segment is short. For tumors of great longitudinal extension in the esophagus, dilation to a much larger diameter is usually necessary. In a high percentage of patients, a considerable symptomatic improvement is obtainable by dilation.[59]

Dilation can be continued as needed during radiation therapy. There is no evidence that properly performed dilation carries additional risk when performed in patients who have received or are receiving radiotherapy.[59] Dilation can also be accomplished safely in patients with a bronchoesophageal fistula. In some patients with bulky exophytic tumors, dilation may be ineffective because of recollapse of the tumor mass after the procedure. In others, dilation may be excessively painful or may be required too often to justify its continued use. In such circumstances, placement of an endoprosthesis may be more effective and acceptable. However, the success of peroral prosthesis insertion depends to a great extent upon adequate dilation of the malignant stenosis.

The rate at which dilators of increasing size should be passed is debatable. Some authors consider it safest to perform gradual dilations, using only a few successive dilators of increasing diameter in several sessions extending over 5 to 10 days.[56] Others prefer more rapid dilation, the rate for use of successive dilators being determined by the responsiveness of the malignant stenosis and the degree of resistance to passage of each dilator.

Peroral Endoprosthesis

Indications and Contraindications

Insertion of an endoprosthesis is the ultimate palliative measure for a malignant stricture when the possibilities for radiotherapy and surgery have been exhausted. Endoprosthesis insertion is indicated when dilation becomes ineffective, too many procedures are required, dilation becomes too difficult for the patient or physician, or the required frequency of dilations becomes unacceptable. Another well-accepted indication is a malignant bronchoesophageal fistula that results in incessant coughing and in aspiration pneumonia. Life expectancy should be at least 6 weeks except for patients with fistulas. Contraindications include location of the cancer within 2 cm of the pharyngeal-esophageal sphincter, short life expectancy excepting cases with a fistula, an uncooperative or unmotivated patient, and circumstances where there is no prospect of improving the quality of life, for example a patient with cerebral metastases.

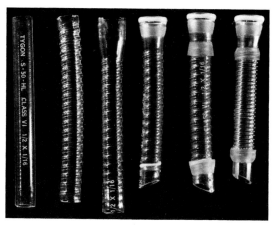

FIGURE 17–4. Various steps during manufacture of a custom-made endoprosthesis (*left to right*); original Tygon tubing; lateral spiral indentation, creation of a proximal funnel; addition of proximal and distal radiopaque lines; addition of proximal and distal shoulders to prevent migration; and addition of a plastic-embedded metal coil.

Types of Endoprostheses

Custom-Made Endoprostheses

It may be preferable to construct a prosthesis in order to meet special requirements for the length, stiffness, caliber, and other characteristics as the endoprosthesis is fashioned.[60, 61] Inexpensive polyvinyl tubing (Tygon) is useful for this purpose. Preferably this should have an outside diameter of 15.7 mm, an inside diameter of 12.5 mm, and a wall thickness of 1.6 mm. The length of the malignant segment is calculated in centimeters from endoscopic measurements. The prosthesis should be 5 to 6 cm longer than the stenotic segment, 2.5 to 3.0 cm longer than the stenosis at each end (Fig. 17–4). To make the tube less slippery, a spiral indentation may be created by softening the prosthesis in hot mineral oil and threading a wire spiral along its length. Next, the proximal end is widened into a funnel shape by heating the last 2.5 cm of the tube in mineral oil at 100 degrees for 30 to 60 seconds. This heated end is then forced into a funneling device (for example, a large glass centrifuge tube or an obturator) to stretch this end of the tube to a diameter of about 25 mm. A radiopaque line may be inserted in the everted ends of the flange and also added along the length of the tube, or a metal band may be incorporated in the phalanged portion as a radiopaque marker.[62] A proximal funnel-shaped phalange is essential to minimize leakage of liquids around the upper edge of the prosthesis and into fistulas. The opposite end of the tube is cut on a bevel and the rough edges are filed and smoothed. Retainer rings 5 to 8 mm in length are glued onto the prosthesis and filed in the desired direction to prevent migration of the device. To prevent displacement, a ring may be placed at positions corresponding to the proximal and distal margins of the stenotic segment. An additional retainer ring may be positioned at a point corresponding to a fistulous tract into the lung. To prevent kinking or collapse of the prosthesis in the case of sharp angulation or excessive scirrhous compression by the tumor, the wall of the prosthesis may be strengthened by adding a plastic-embedded metal coil to the outside of the prosthesis.

A section of polyvinyl tubing about 50 cm in length is prepared as a pusher tube by funneling one end as described previously. This will be used to drive the prosthesis into place. To prevent invagination of the pusher tube funnel into the prosthesis during insertion, the margin of the pusher funnel may be thickened by partially filling it in with rubber.

Commercially Available Endoprostheses

The Procter-Livingstone, Key-Med-Atkinson, and Medoc-Célestin models are commercially available endoprostheses that have been used most frequently[63] (Fig. 17–5). The Procter-Livingstone tube (Latex Products, Johannesburg) is an armored, soft latex rubber tube with an internal diameter of 12 mm and an outer diameter of 18 mm. The proximal end is expanded to an external diameter of 3.0 cm, which allows it to fit snugly above the tumor. To facilitate insertion and to prevent pressure necrosis of the esophageal wall, both

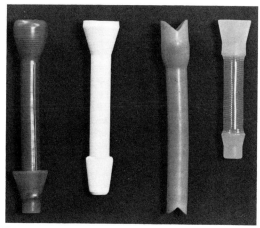

FIGURE 17–5. Commercially available prostheses (*left to right*): Célestin, Key-Med, Procter Livingstone, and Wilson-Cook.

the proximal and distal ends are shaped into two flanges and are not reinforced. This endoprosthesis is available in 10, 15, and 19 cm lengths.

The Key-Med-Atkinson prosthesis (Key-Med, Great Britain) is a radiopaque silicone rubber tube with an 11.7 mm bore with a nylon spiral incorporated in its wall to prevent kinking. A shoulder is attached to the distal end of the tube to prevent migration. This is available in lengths of 14 and 19 cm. The outer diameters of the tube and of the funnel are 16 and 29 mm, respectively.

The Medoc-Célestin type (Medoc, Great Britain) pulsion tube incorporates a distal collapsible flange to maintain position. Made of latex, the outer diameter of this prosthesis is 15 mm and the inner diameter is 12 mm. A nylon spiral is incorporated in the latex. The Medoc-Célestin tube fits snugly against the esophageal wall because of its tulip-shaped proximal end. The available lengths are 12.5, 15, and 21 cm.

Some authors prefer the Medoc-Célestin endoprosthesis to the Key-Med because of its greater internal diameter. Others prefer the Key-Med-Atkinson prosthesis because silicone rubber devices show less structural deterioration than latex tubes when exposed to hydrochloric acid, bile, and radiation.[64]

A 16 mm diameter prosthesis made by Wilson-Cook has also been introduced recently. It is made of silicone reinforced with a metal spiral and is available in prosthesis lengths of 4.4, 6.4, 8.4, 10.4, 12.4, 14.4, and 16.4 cm.

Introducing Devices

The endoprosthesis may be inserted over a flexible mercury-weighted bougie,[60] a small-caliber endoscope,[61, 65, 66] the Eder-Puestow dilator shaft,[67] a mandril set,[58] or the Nottingham Key-Med introducing device.[3, 68] The last-named device, which is probably used most frequently, consists of two stainless steel tubes; the outer tube terminates in a metal olive, and the inner tube has a detachable flexible tip that allows a plastic expansion cup to be inserted. When the outer tube is pushed forward on the inner, the metal olive is pushed into the plastic cup, causing it to expand and grip the prosthesis at the inside of its distal end. The outer and inner tubes are then locked in this position. This assembly is completed by a plastic pusher (rammer) tube which fits over the two steel tubes so that its distal end fits into the proximal funnel

of the prosthesis. The whole assembly is passed over a previously placed guide wire. When the funnel of the prosthesis rests on the proximal edge of the malignant stricture, the steel tubes are unlocked and removed with the guide wire while the rammer temporarily holds the endoprosthesis in place. Some authorities feel that the Nottingham introducer is superior to other pulsion systems, since its design causes the forward force to be applied to both the distal and proximal ends of the prosthesis. Recently, there has been an increasing interest in guiding a prosthesis over a 10.5 mm wide Savary-bougie and inserting the prosthesis with the help of a Dumon-Gilliard prosthesis pushing tube. Alternatively, one may use the Wilson-Cook prosthesis introducer, which consists essentially of a compression balloon catheter, which fixes the inner side of a prosthesis during insertion.

Placement of the Endoprosthesis

It is essential that a thorough explanation of the procedure be given to the patient and family before an endoprosthesis is placed.

The location of the tumor, including length and luminal diameter, must be accurately determined. Roentgenograms are of assistance in demonstrating the length and configuration of the tumor as well as fistula formation, but endoscopic measurement most reliably determines the distance from the incisor teeth to the upper edge of the tumor and the length of the cancerous segment.

The most essential step is dilation of the stricture to the appropriate diameter. Since the stenosis initially may be rigid and very narrow, this usually requires passage of a guide wire through the lumen of the tumor under endoscopic and, if necessary, fluoroscopic control. The number of dilators of increasing diameter passed over the guide wire depends entirely on the degree of narrowing, extent, and tortuosity of the lesion. A luminal diameter of about 15 mm (46–52 Fr) is usually required to accommodate a prosthesis. In general, soft, necrotic lesions require less dilation in comparison to scirrhous, tortuous malignancies, the latter sometimes requiring dilation to 18 to 20 mm. For easily dilated lesions, one dilation procedure may suffice. For scirrhous and tortuous lesions, usually not more than 3 or 4 sequential dilators are passed with each procedure. As dilation proceeds, a small-diameter endoscope should be passed to examine the regions within and distal to the tumor to determine carefully distal margin proximity to the cardia as well as exact distances from the teeth to proximal and distal margins. The endoscope itself serves as a convenient measuring device.

A measurement equal to that from the incisor teeth to the location point for the proximal funnel of the prosthesis is marked on the pusher tube, measuring from its forward end backward. The pusher tube and the prosthesis are lubricated well and positioned on an introducing device. As noted previously, this could be a small-caliber endoscope, a bougie, a special introducing device, or an Eder-Puestow dilator shaft.

Intravenous drugs should be administered for sedation. Meperidine (pethidine) plus diazepam, or Thalamonal (Innovar) (a combination of 2.5 mg droperidol and 0.05 mg fentanyl) plus diazepam are satisfactory. General anesthesia may be used as an alternative in some patients.

The introducing device carrying the endoprosthesis is passed over a guide wire under fluoroscopic control. After the tip of the endoscope (or other introducing device) has been advanced well past the distal margin of the tumor, the endoscope or the introducing device is held in a steady position while the pusher tube is advanced (using the inserting device as a guide) to the predetermined point marked on the pusher; the prosthesis should now be seated properly with its proximal funnel located above the proximal margin of the tumor. With the prosthesis in the proper position, the operator holds the pusher tube steady as the introducing device is quickly removed. Rotation of the pusher tube then disengages it from the prosthesis, whereupon the pusher is withdrawn. If the lesion has been dilated adequately, placement should require only a few minutes. The endoscope is then reinserted to check the position of the prosthesis. If it is seated too deeply, the prosthesis can be grasped with a foreign body retrieval forceps, grasping forceps, or polypectomy snare to gently pull it upward. When using the Key-Med-Atkinson system it is particularly important to be certain that the endoprosthesis is not displaced during withdrawal of the introducer. A small-caliber endoscope that will pass through the prosthesis should be used. Thereby, the position of the prosthesis, particularly the distal end relative to the cardia, can be determined, and the

presence of a patent channel to the stomach confirmed. Care must be exercised to avoid dislodgement of the prosthesis upon withdrawal of the endoscope. To avoid this, the pusher tube may be left in place to stabilize the prosthesis during this maneuver.

An endoprosthesis can be placed anywhere in the esophagus except near the proximal esophageal sphincter. When the funnel edge is located 2 cm or less from the cricopharyngeus, it is usually not tolerated by the patient. An endoprosthesis can be inserted in elderly and frail patients with marked kyphoscoliosis, and in those with limited respiratory function, provided the proximal funnel will not compress the upper respiratory tract. It can be introduced in patients with tumor recurrence after surgical resection or radiotherapy or both, and in patients with obstruction due to mediastinal spread of bronchial or other metastatic malignancy (Figs. 17–6 and 17–7). An endoprosthesis can

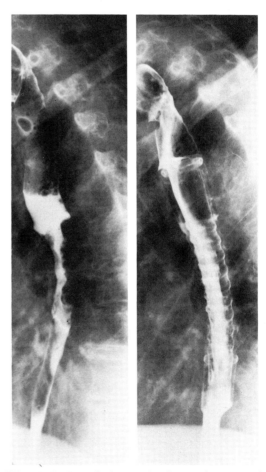

FIGURE 17–6. Typical example of extensive exophytic malignancy in the mid-esophagus (*left*), bypassed by an endoprosthesis (*right*).

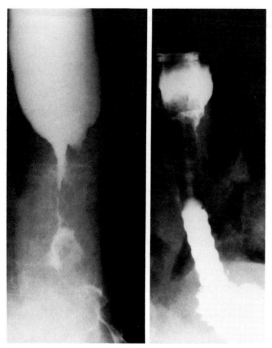

FIGURE 17–7. Typical example of a malignant narrowing of the distal esophagus, with marked proximal esophageal dilation (*left*). Luminal patency is established after bridging the stenosis with an endoprosthesis (*right*).

also be used to prevent pulmonary complications in many patients with esophagopulmonary fistulas.

The insertion of an endoprosthesis in a short, straight malignant stenosis is usually not difficult. The proximal tumor shelf must be adequate to anchor the device. Therefore, the preferential tumor configuration is concentric rather than a longitudinal growth that occupies only a portion of the circumference of the wall. If the cancer involves less than half the circumference, the stenosis is usually not adequate to hold the prosthesis in place.

Great care must be exercised in the presence of a malignant intramural sinus, because such tumors are usually very necrotic and easily allow the formation of a false passage into the lesion during manipulation. In these circumstances, the guide wire, once correctly positioned, should not be removed until the prosthesis is finally inserted into the correct luminal axis (Fig. 17–8).

The combination of cancer and a large hiatus hernia is not rare, and it is possible to insert a prosthesis correctly in most cases (Fig. 17–9). Depending upon the extent of the tumor and the size of the hernia, either a

short endoprosthesis can be introduced so that its distal end just enters the hernia, or a long tube can be used so that the hernia is bypassed and the distal end of the tube lies within the stomach and below the diaphragm. The latter is preferred in the majority of patients because a short prosthesis may become occluded by prolapsing mucosal folds at its distal end.

A chest x-ray should be obtained immediately after the procedure to exclude perforation, and before liquid intake is permitted. Preferably, luminal patency and function of the prosthesis should be studied radiologically at 24 hours, after the effects of sedating drugs have cleared. The first radiographic contrast study should be performed with water-soluble contrast; however, if no leakage occurs, a more satisfactory documentation of position and function, or in some cases ongoing leakage of contrast into a fistula, can be obtained by radiologic examination with a thin barium mixture.

When it has been established that displacement has not occurred and that the passage is adequate, the patient is ready to eat and can be discharged. Detailed instructions should be given concerning management of the prosthesis and diet. In general a regular diet is tolerated, provided dentition is adequate. The patient must be instructed to eat only in a bolt upright sitting position, to chew

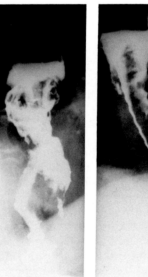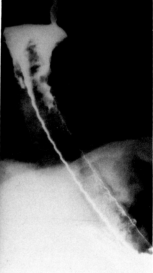

FIGURE 17–8. Extensive adenocarcinoma of the cardia, fixed to the descending aorta, with sinus tract formation (*left*). Bypass of the lesion by a prosthesis (*right*).

food carefully, and to take copious drafts of fluid during and after meals. Obstruction of the prosthesis of a minor degree may be relieved by taking carbonated beverages, which seem by their gaseous action to disrupt and eliminate accumulated debris.

When a prosthetic tube straddles the cardia, measures to control gastroesophageal reflux are required: sleeping with the head of the bed elevated, antacids after meals, and H_2 receptor blocker therapy at night if necessary. When the prosthesis is very long and broaches the cardia, it is appropriate to advise the patient that all meat should be finely chopped, crusts should be removed from breads, and all vegetables should be strained, in order to avoid episodes of blockage. These steps should be taken in addition to the antireflux measures. Taking large pills or capsules intact should also be avoided.

Results

The first successful palliation of an esophageal carcinoma by a combination of dilation and placement of a prosthetic device is usually attributed to Symonds in 1887.[69] In 1924, Souttar[70] used a prosthesis made of coiled silver that was inserted through a rigid endoscope in more than 300 patients. Nonsurgical insertion over a flexible mercury weighted bougie was revived by Boyce and Palmer.[60] Tytgat and colleagues[61] stressed the importance of guided insertion over an endoscope. Atkinson et al.[68] and Célestin and Campbell[58] developed similar methods for guided insertion.

The overall success rate for introduction of a prosthesis is greater than 90% in most series[66, 67, 71, 73–86] (see Table 17–3). Satisfactory

occlusion of fistulas can be achieved in the majority of patients with this type of lesion. The procedure is usually well tolerated and has an acceptable immediate mortality (that is, it is low in comparison to surgical alternatives). In a review published in 1974 by Girardet et al.,[87] the overall hospital mortality was 13.9% in 2459 patients who underwent palliative intubation either with a Mousseau-Barbin or Célestin tube introduced at laparotomy by pulling the device into the esophagus from proximal to distal, or by a pulsion technique through a rigid esophagoscope. There was a considerable difference in mortality for patients undergoing the traction technique (21.2%) and the pulsion method (5.6%), which probably reflects the mortality associated with laparotomy in debilitated patients.

Limitations of Non-Surgical Insertion of an Endoprosthesis

Difficulties with the introduction of an endoprosthesis can be expected when any of the following conditions exist:

1. There is complete luminal obstruction.

2. Tumor growth causes sharp angulation of the esophageal lumen (which may occur in cancer of the distal esophagus and cardia or after surgical resection).

3. A concomitant sliding or paraesophageal hernia is present.

4. The tumor is either unusually necrotic or excessively hard.

5. A fistula is present in the absence of appreciable luminal narrowing.

6. The origin of a fistula is located at the upper or lower end of a malignant stricture.

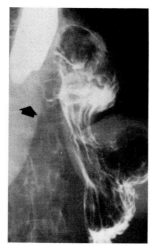 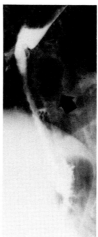 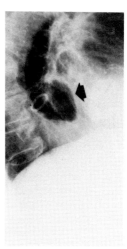

FIGURE 17–9. Malignancy of the cardia (left) involving the distal esophagus (arrow) in a patient with hiatal hernia, making insertion of the guide wire into the stomach difficult but not impossible. The prosthesis bypasses the hernia (middle and right) and enters the stomach. The upper rim of the endoprosthesis is clearly visible over the air pocket in the hernia pouch (arrows, middle and right).

7. The malignancy approaches the proximal esophageal sphincter.

Several of these problems may be solved, provided appropriate adaptations of both prosthesis and introducing device are effected. However, a considerable level of expertise and experience in insertion of these devices is required before attempting to deal with problems such as these. In addition, the capability for construction of specially formed endoprostheses must be acquired, since custom-made, specifically designed devices are frequently required to solve unique clinical problems. (See the section on custom-made endoprostheses on pg. 387.)

When obstruction is total, the operator can attempt to pass one of several types of tiny, flexible atraumatic lumen finders through the lesion. Alternately, an attempt may be made to inject a water-soluble contrast agent through a lumen after wedging a catheter at any point that looks like an opening; any remaining pathway through the tumor may sometimes be delineated fluoroscopically. When both approaches fail, pieces of tumor may be removed by endoscopic electrosurgical snare polypectomy, or laser photodestruction of the proximal tumor layers can be initiated. Ideally, radiologic demonstration of the location, longitudinal extent, tortuosity, angulation, and eccentricity of the mass should be available by reference to x-rays obtained prior to total obstruction. Upon reopening the lumen or creating an artificial path, an atraumatic lumen finder is passed, and then a sequence of catheters of increasing diameter are inserted over this wire until a point is reached at which a standard Eder-Puestow guide wire can be placed through the lumen. Metal olives or other dilation devices can be introduced along this guide to achieve proper progressive dilation.

If the cancer is located 2 cm or less from the cricopharyngeus, a foreign body sensation or stridor due to laryngeal compression, or both, can be expected if a regular prosthesis is employed. This problem can be circumvented only by inserting a prosthesis with a small, short funnel, or one without a funneling section, provided that this does not cause airway compression. The operator must be prepared to remove the prosthetic device immediately if acute stridor occurs after insertion. Astute inspection of lateral x-ray films may alert the endoscopist to the possibility of compression if the tumor and

airway are in close proximity, and this complication may thereby be avoided.

The presence of a large-diameter bronchoesophageal fistula in the absence of sufficient narrowing to anchor the prosthesis is notoriously difficult to treat. Widening the funnel to a maximum diameter of 30 mm may permit anchoring of the prosthesis, and may prevent leakage in some patients. Sometimes the endoprosthesis may be modified with an additional large shoulder or band placed on the device at a point which will correspond to the fistulous opening when the prosthesis is in proper position (Fig. 17–10).

It is not unusual to note persistent leakage of contrast medium when a fistulous tract begins at the proximal or distal end of a malignant stricture despite apparent satisfactory positioning of the prosthesis. In the case of a proximal fistula, the insertion of a device with an extra-wide funnel up to 30 mm in diameter, and a proximal wide shoulder may

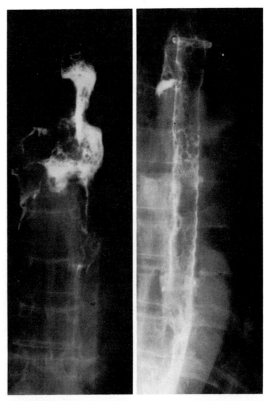

FIGURE 17–10. Large bronchoesophageal fistula (*left*) is visible in the left aspect of this x-ray film. Occlusion of the fistula (*right*) was achieved only after adding a wide shoulder (*arrow*) to the prosthesis. The segment with the shoulder is situated just proximal to the origin of the fistulous tract.

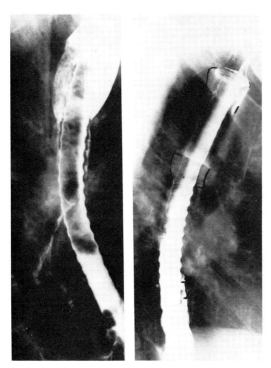

FIGURE 17–11. On-going leakage of contrast (*left*) into a bronchoesophageal fistula is not prohibited by the regular endoprosthesis. This problem was corrected (*right*) after widening the funnel and adding a large shoulder to the prosthesis (both outlined in black on the x-ray).

arrest leakage in some patients. An extra-large prosthesis with distal widening may be used to arrest distal leakage (Fig. 17–11). Fistulas with origins very close to the proximal sphincter cannot be treated with an endoprosthesis at present.

If cancer involves less than half the circumference of the esophageal wall, there is usually not enough of a stenosis to hold the prosthesis in place. Increasingly, laser photocoagulation is used to necrotize such malignancies.

Sharp angulation of the lumen may occur as a result of tortuous tumor growth, previous surgery, prior radiotherapy, severe kyphoscoliosis, or any combination of these. This may cause difficulty during dilation and insertion of the prosthesis. To transmit the dilating force to the tip of the dilating device, and to facilitate insertion of the prosthesis, devices with the capability to gradually stiffen and straighten the path for dilation and insertion are preferable. This thereby reduces the acuteness of the angulation.[88] With severely angulated lesions, compression and

kinking of the prosthesis may easily occur. This hinders the passage of food and predisposes to food impaction soon after insertion. Incorporation of a metal coil in the endoprosthesis prohibits kinking and may eliminate this problem. This type of strengthened prosthesis is also preferable in the case of very scirrhous tumors (Fig. 17–12).

Tumors with multiple stenotic segments that are sharply angulated to each other usually cannot be dilated properly with existing equipment. An attempt may be made to guide metal olives over an introducer that can be straightened and strengthened.[88]

Migration of the endoprosthesis may be expected, especially with a concomitant hiatal hernia, with tumors approaching or bridging the gastroesophageal junction, and in the case of extrinsic but eccentric compression. To obviate this, anchoring devices are usually required at variable points along the prosthesis, depending upon the anatomic circumstances. Upward dislodgement because of diaphragmatic movement may be prevented by adding a distal rim to the prosthesis. Downward migration, which can occur with a soft tumor or with eccentric compression due to invading pulmonary cancer, may be prevented by adding an extra flange at the proximal end just below the funnel.

Complications of Endoprosthesis Insertion

The most common complications of endoprosthesis insertion are perforation, dislocation, tumor overgrowth, stricturing due to reflux esophagitis, pressure necrosis, and blockage by food.

Perforation. Perforation is a major complication. In the majority of patients, it is evident immediately because of signs such as subcutaneous crepitation and pneumomediastinum. When recognized after the dilation procedure, insertion of the endoprosthesis is not necessarily precluded, since this may seal the perforation. Alternative conservative management consists of a 7 to 10 day regimen of no oral intake, adequate aspiration of the perforation site, and systemically administered antibiotics. Usually the perforation will seal and the prosthesis can be inserted successfully at a later time.

Blind insertion of a sump tube into the esophagus for aspiration is not advisable because it may enter the perforation. Rather, a guide wire should be positioned in the correct lumen under endoscopic control. In doing

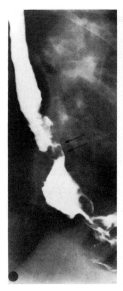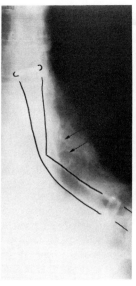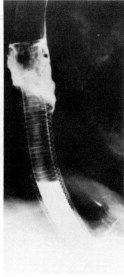

FIGURE 17–12. Linitis plastica (*left*) extending into the esophagus (*arrows, left*). Compression and kinking (*middle*) of a regular prosthesis due to angulation and the scirrhous character of the lesion. This problem was corrected using a prosthesis strengthened with a metal coil.

this, air insufflation with the endoscope must be avoided. Using the wire as a guide, a sump tube can be placed in correct position distal to the site of perforation. After removal of the guide wire, the proximal end of the sump tube may be rerouted from the throat to the nasopharynx and out the nostril. For the purpose of feeding, it is sometimes desirable to glue a second tube to the aspirating tube. The distal tip of the second tube should be positioned at the ligament of Treitz[89] (Fig. 17–13).

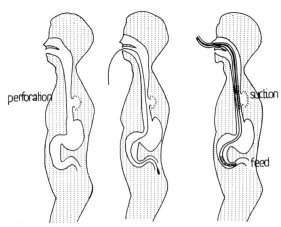

FIGURE 17–13. In a patient with iatrogenic perforation (*left*), one may elect first to insert a guidewire under endoscopic control up to the ligament of Treitz (*middle*). After removing the endoscope and rerouting the wire through the nose, a double catheter is inserted—the distal end of the first one being placed at the ligament of Treitz for feeding purposes, with the proximal tube being positioned at the perforation so that its aspiration holes are below, at, and above the previously determined level of perforation (*right*).

Whenever possible, surgical intervention should be avoided in frail preterminally ill patients.[90] It should not be assumed that perforation is synonymous with disaster. With conservative treatment, most patients will survive. Whether some perforations that occur with very narrow and necrotic strictures can be avoided through a more gradual approach to dilation is uncertain at present. It is, however, interesting that as yet a decrease in the perforation rate has not been observed with increasing experience.[86] The perforation rate varies among the series reported, although in most series it is approximately 10%. There appears to be a correlation between the degree of narrowing and the risk of perforation.

Dislocation. Dislocation may occur with any type of prosthesis. Usually a device with distal and proximal flanges will prevent further migration.

Tumor Overgrowth. Obstruction due to tumor overgrowth necessitates dilation of the recurrent stenosis with the original prosthesis in place before it can be removed and replaced by a longer one (Fig. 17–14). If an endoprosthesis has been in place for a long period of time, it will be difficult to remove. In the case of proximal overgrowth, a short funnel can be introduced into the original prosthesis to bypass the overgrowing tumor mass.

Stricture Due to Reflux Esophagitis. Fibrous stricturing related to severe reflux esophagitis may occur despite anti-reflux measures, although this is rare. This may be managed either by dilation with the original

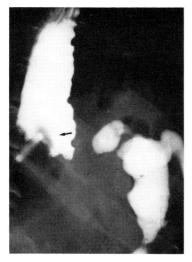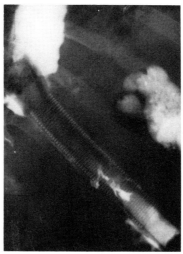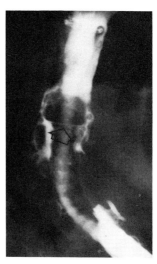

FIGURE 17–14. Tumor overgrowth (*left*) occurring just over 1 year after insertion of an endoprosthesis in a patient with extensive malignancy of the cardia (*arrow*). The prosthesis was removed and exchanged for a longer one, which did not function properly because of angulation between the funnel opening and the esophageal axis (*middle*). This problem was corrected (*right*) by using a longer prosthesis that was strengthened and stabilized with a wide shoulder (*arrow*).

prosthesis in place or by removal of the original prosthesis and introduction of a longer one.

Pressure Necrosis. Pressure necrosis caused by the funnel edge of the prosthesis usually occurs in an area of the wall that has been invaded by tumor or previously irradiated, or both. This causes pain and leads to formation of a mediastinal fistula. Deep pressure necrosis may extend to the aorta, with resultant exsanguination. The chance that pressure necrosis will occur is higher when there is marked angulation between the esophagus and the prosthesis, resulting in greater pressure along one portion of the circumference of the prosthesis. This may occur in patients with kyphoscoliosis or hiatal hernia, or when the axis of the prosthesis is in a transverse position relative to the long axis of the body, as in the case of tumors of the distal esophagus and cardia (Figs. 17–15 and 17–16).

Food Blockage. A common complication that occurs in the follow-up period after prosthesis insertion is blockage of the tube by food; this is usually the result of inadequate mastication or of dietary indiscretion. In the majority of patients the blockage can be cleared easily either by carefully passing a cytology brush through the endoprosthesis to push the food into the stomach or by gently moving a small-diameter endoscope up and down through the prosthesis to displace the impacted food bolus. Some physi-

cians have the patient drink a papain solution first (half an ounce of a 1 to 1 solution every half hour for 2 hours). The use of this enzyme is intended to loosen meat fibers. If all other measures fail, the prosthesis should

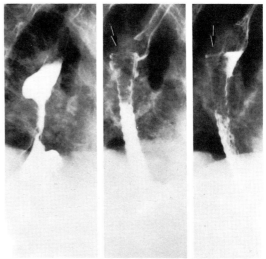

FIGURE 17–15. Esophageal cancer in a patient with kyphoscoliosis and a hiatal hernia (*left*). A barium swallow (*middle*) shortly after insertion of an endoprosthesis demonstrates an obvious eccentric indentation and compression of the esophageal wall (*arrow*). A barium swallow a few months later (*right*) demonstrates striking pressure necrosis of the esophageal wall and intramural migration of the funnel (*arrow*). This was corrected by insertion of a longer prosthesis.

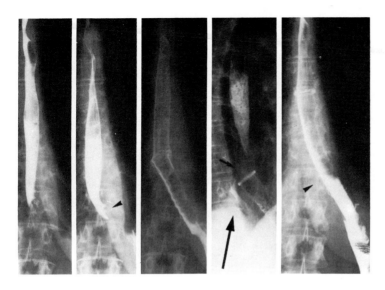

FIGURE 17–16. *From left to right:* The primary presenting esophageal cancer is 3 cm long, but distant metastasis is present; recurrence of the cancer (*arrow*) after radiotherapy; the first endoprosthesis has been inserted; pressure necrosis and leakage (*arrows*) due to asymmetric compression; correction of this problem (*arrow*) with longer prosthesis.

be removed and exchanged with a new one (Fig. 17–17).

Removal of the endoprosthesis may be necessary in the management of several of these complications. This can be carried out using a strong grasping forceps, polypectomy snare, the Key-Med Nottingham introducer, or a small-caliber endoscope. The latter functions as a hook after the tip of the instrument is deflected at a point below the distal edge of the prosthesis.

The overall complication rate for insertion of an esophageal prosthesis may be estimated from Table 17–3. Comparisons of procedure-related mortalities in populations with esophageal cancer with a high spontaneous mortality are of uncertain relevance because

procedure-related mortality depends to a large extent upon the underlying condition, timing of the introduction of the prosthesis, the degree of cachexia, and various other factors. Moreover, it is sometimes difficult to decide the extent to which the mortality is procedure-related or attributable to the underlying condition. The effort expended in searching for and treating complications is related to the general condition of the patient, in addition to the size and spread of the tumor, and probably biases such data. Unless all of these factors are standardized, comparisons between studies and with corresponding surgical series are probably irrelevant, the existing data merely giving an impression of the magnitude of the problem.

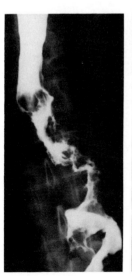
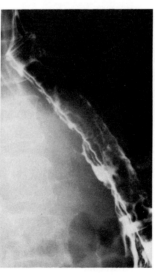
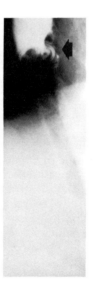

FIGURE 17–17. Adenocarcinoma of the cardia extending into the esophagus (*left*). The cancer is bypassed by an endoprosthesis (*middle*). Characteristic appearance of clogging (*see arrow, right*) due to poorly masticated meat.

TABLE 17–3. Non-surgical positioning of an endoprosthesis

Authors	No. of patients with esophageal cardiac malignancy	No. of patients with esophageal bronchial fistula	Successful intubation (%)	Perforation (%)	Hemorrhage (%)	Pressure necrosis + aorta fistula (%)	Prosthesis obstruction (%)	Migration (%)	Procedure-related mortality (%)	Type of prosthesis	Bougie	Small diameter endoscope	Key Med or EP guide	Medoc mandril set	Prost. individualized	General anesthesia
											Inserting device					
Weisel et al.[73]	103			16		1	2	1	0	Polyethylene	×				×	o
O'Conner et al.[74]	388	18	97	1.2	0		2	2	0.5	Polyethylene	×				×	o
Palmer[75]	75	49	100	1.3	0			0	0	Polyvinyl	×					o
Hegarty et al.[76]	181		94					8	16.6	Procter-Livingstone	×					×
Kairaluoma et al.[77]	108				8.5	1	8.6	14	16	Célestin						
Bergerault et al.[78]	35			5.5	1		6.6	7	14	Célestin				×		o
Célestin et al.[66]	91		87	8.3			6	8	12.5	Medoc-Célestin						o
Jones et al.[79]	55	3	100	10				10	3.3	Medoc-Célestin						o/×
Soehendra[80]	60	7	91		5.1		7.7	5.1	6	Célestin						o
Balmes et al.[81]	78		92	10.4	7.3	6.4	1.8	5.4	12.8	Häring			×			
van Blankenstein et al.[82]	119	19	100	0	0		—	—	0	Key-Med			×			o
Boyce[67]	41	5	85	11.8		2.4	20	13.5	3.4	Polyvinyl	×					o/×
Ogilvie et al.[83]	118		91	9.3			6	6	15.6	Key-Med			×		×	o
Watson[84]	32		94	9.1			8.3	18.6					×			o
den Hartog Jager and Tytga (1983)	600	55	82		1.3	2.0			4.2	Polyvinyl		×			×	
Lux et al.[85]	60	15		11	2.2		6.8	27	4.5	Key-Med/polyvinyl		×	×			o/×
Surveys																
Tytgat[71]	1847		97.8	8.4	1.2	0.9	5.0	9.7	4.5							o/×
Bennett[86]	820			9			8	10								

Conclusions

The insertion of an esophageal endopros-thesis through an inoperable carcinoma of the esophagus or cardia provides acceptable relief of dysphagia and usually allows a pa-tient to remain at home during the terminal stages of disease. Starvation is at least a com-mon contributing cause of death in untreated cancer of the esophagus and cardia. The insertion of an endoprosthesis combats this deterioration and often results in an imme-diate weight gain during the first few weeks after insertion. Outpatient supervision en-ables early detection of tube dysfunction that can usually be dealt with by endoscopic means. The essential value of an esophageal prosthesis lies in improvement in the quality of life that occurs with the elimination of dysphagia, thus allowing terminally ill pa-tients to remain at home.[91]

Editor's note: References 92 to 95 are of recent interest.

References

1. Tytgat GNJ, Bartelsman JFWM, Dysphagia—an overview. In: Salmon P, ed. Advances in Gastroin-testinal Endoscopy. London: Chapman & Hall Ltd., 1983.
2. Stoller JL, Samer KJ, Toppin DI, Flores AD. Car-cinoma of the esophagus: a new proposal for the evaluation of treatment. Can J Surg 1977; 20:454–9.
3. Atkinson M, Ferguson R, Ogilvie AL. Management of malignant dysphagia by intubation at endoscopy. J R Soc Med 1979; 72:894–7.
4. O'Sullivan GC, DeMeester TR, Smith RB, et al. Twenty-four hour pH monitoring of esophageal function. Arch Surg 1981; 116:581–90.
5. Syrjanen K, Pyrhonen S, Aukee S, Koskela E. Squa-mous cell papilloma of the oesophagus: A tumour probably caused by human papilloma virus (HPV). Diagn Histopathol 1982; 5:291–6.
6. Correa P. Precursors of gastric and esophageal can-cer. Cancer 1982; 50:2554–65.
7. Tytgat GNJ, Mathus-Vliegen EMH. Cancer Screen-ing. In: Hodgson HJF, Bloom SR, eds. Gastrointes-tinal and Hepatobiliary Cancer. London: Chapman & Hall, Ltd. 1983:157–87.
8. Tytgat GNJ, Mathus-Vliegen EMH, Offerhaus J. Value of endoscopy in the surveillance of high-risk groups for gastrointestinal cancer. In: Sherlock P, Morson BC, Barbara L, Veronesi V, eds. Precancer-ous Lesions of the Gastrointestinal Tract. New York: Raven Press, 1983:305–18.
9. Wynder EL, Hultberg S, Jacobsson F, Bross IJ. Environmental factors in cancer of upper alimentary tract. Swedish study with special reference to Plum-mer-Vinson (Patterson-Kelly) syndrome. Cancer 1957; 10:470–87.
10. Howel-Evans W, McConnell RB, Clarke CA, Shep-pard PM. Carcinoma of the esophagus with keratosis palmaris et plantaris (tylosis). Q J Med 1958; 27:413–29.
11. Lansing PB, Ferrante WA, Ochsner JL. Carcinoma of the esophagus at the site of lye stricture. Am J Surg 1969; 118:108–11.
12. Williams JL. Carcinoma of the oesophagus as a complication of achalasia of the cardia. Thorax 1956; 11:268–74.
13. Joske RA, Benedict EB. The role of benign esopha-geal obstruction in the development of carcinoma of the esophagus. Gastroenterology 1959; 36:749–55.
14. Just-Viera JO, Haight C. Achalasia and carcinoma of the esophagus. Surg Gynecol Obstet 1969; 128:1081–95.
15. Naef AP, Savary M, Ozzello L. Columnar-lined esophagus: An acquired lesion with malignant pre-disposition. Report on 140 cases of Barrett's esoph-agus with 12 adenocarcinomas. J Thorac Cardiovasc Surg 1975; 70:826–35.
16. Bozymski EM, Herlihy KJ, Orlando RC. Barrett's esophagus. Ann Intern Med 1982; 97:103–7.
17. Wesdorp ICE, Bartelsman J, Schipper MEI, et al. Malignancy and premalignancy in Barrett's esoph-agus: a clinical endoscopical and histological study. Acta Endosc 1981; 11:317–26.
18. Savary M, Monnier PH, Miller G: Diagnosis and pathophysiology of Barrett's oesophagus. In: Van Heukelem HA, Gooszen HG, Terpstra JL, Belsey RHR, eds. Pathological Gastro-oesophageal Reflux. Amsterdam: Zuid-Nederlandse Uitg Mij, 1983; 115–9.
19. Briggs JC, Ibrahim NBN. Oat cell carcinoma of the oesophagus: a clinicopathological study of 23 cases. Histopathology 1983; 7:261–77.
20. Seremetis MG, Lyons WS, deGuzman VC, Peabody JN Jr. Leiomyomata of the esophagus: an analysis of 838 cases. Cancer 1976; 38:2166–77.
21. Patel RM, DeSota-La Paix F, Sika JV, et al. Granular cell tumor of the esophagus: report of two cases and review of the literature. Am J Gastroenterol 1981; 76:519–23.
22. Hanel K, Talley NA, Hunt DR. Hemangioma of the esophagus: An unusual cause of upper gastrointes-tinal bleeding. Dig Dis Sci 1981; 26:257–63.
23. Stout AP. Tumors of the Soft Tissues. Sect II fasc 5. Washington DC: AFIP, 1953.
24. Totten RS, Stout AP, Humphreys GH, Moore RL. Benign tumors and cysts of the esophagus. J Thorac Surg 1953; 25:606–22.
25. Goldstein HM, Zornoza J. Association of squamous cell carcinoma of the head and neck with cancer of the esophagus. Am J Roentgenol 1978; 131:791–4.
26. McDonald GB, Brand DL, Thorning DR. Multiple adenomatous neoplasms arising in columnar-lined (Barrett's) esophagus. Gastroenterology 1977; 72:1317–21.
27. Wang GQ. Endoscopic diagnosis of early oesopha-geal carcinoma. J R Soc Med 1981; 74:502–3.
28. Yang G, Huang H, Qui S, Chang Y. Endoscopic diagnosis of 115 cases of early esophageal carci-noma. Endoscopy 1982; 14:157–61.
29. Ide H, Endo M, Kinoshika Y, et al. Clinicopatho-logical aspects of superficial esophageal cancer. Chir Gastroenterol 1976; 10:9–16.
30. Eller JL, Ziter FM Jr, Zuck TF, Brott LW. Inflam-matory polyp: a complication in esophagus lined by columnar epithelium. Radiology 1970; 98:145–6.
31. Soga J, Tanaka O, Sasaki K, et al. Superficial spread-ing carcinoma of the esophagus. Cancer 1981; 50:1641–5.
32. Savary M, Miller G. The Esophagus. Handbook and

Atlas of Endoscopy. Solothurn, Schweiz: Gassman, 1978.

33. Kawai K, Takemoto T, Suzuki S, Ida K. Proposed nomenclature and classification of the dye-spraying techniques in endoscopy. Endoscopy 1979; 11:23–5.

34. Yamakawa T, von Hofe FC, Kagan R, Morgenstern L. The use of tolonium in the diagnosis of malignant gastric lesions. Arch Surg 1972; 104:773–7.

35. Vicari F. Progress in the methods of endoscopic diagnosis in gastroenterology. (Suppl) Endoscopy 1980; 19–34.

36. Treille C, Aubert H, Rachail M. L'usage des colorants de muqueuze en endoscopie digestive hauts: intérêt, application pratique, perspectives. Acta Endosc 1981; 11:369–81.

37. Barkin JS, Taub S, Rogers AL. The safety of combined endoscopy, biopsy and dilatation in esophageal strictures. Am J Gastroenterol 1981; 76:23–6.

38. Graham DY, Spjut HJ: Salvage cytology. A new alternative fiberoptic technique. Gastrointest Endosc 1979; 25:137–9.

39. Nakamura Y, Arimori M, Kumagai Y. Examination with esophagoscopes: utilization of the fiberscope. Stomach Intestine 1968; 3:1361–7.

40. Kobayashi S, Prolla JC, Winans CS, Kirsner JB. Improved endoscopic diagnosis of gastroesophageal malignancy. Combined use of direct vision brushing cytology and biopsy. JAMA 1970; 212:2086–9.

41. Prolla JC. Cancer of the gastrointestinal tract. I. Esophagus—histopathology and cytology in detection. JAMA 1973; 226:1554–6.

42. Bruni HC, Nelson RS. Carcinoma of the esophagus and cardia. Diagnostic evaluation in 113 cases. J Thorac Cardiovasc Surg 1975; 70:367–70.

43. Seifert E, Atay Z. Maligne Tumoren des Gastrointestinaltraktes. Fortschr Endoskop. Stuttgart: Thieme, 1975.

44. Winawer SJ, Sherlock P, Belladonna JA, et al. Endoscopic brush cytology in esophageal cancer. JAMA 1975; 232:1358.

45. Hishon S, Lovell D, Gummer JWP, et al. Cytology in the diagnosis of oesophageal cancer. Lancet 1976; 1:296–7.

46. Winawer SJ, Melamed M, Sherlock P. Potential of endoscopy, biopsy and cytology in the diagnosis and management of patients with cancer. Clin Gastroenterol 1976; 5:575–95.

47. Witzel L, Halter F, Gretillat PA, et al. Evaluation of specific value of endoscopic biopsies and brush cytology for malignancies of the oesophagus and stomach. Gut 1976; 17:375–7.

48. Prolla JC, Reilley RW, Kirsner JB, Cockerham L. Direct vision endoscopic cytology and biopsy in the diagnosis of esophageal and gastric tumours: current experience. Acta Cytol 1977; 21:399–402.

49. Eastman MC, Gear MWL, Nicol A. An assessment of the accuracy of modern endoscopic diagnosis of oesophageal stricture. Br J Surg 1978; 65:182–5.

50. Gutz HJ, Wildner GP. Die diagnostische Sicherheit von Endoskopie und Biopsie bei stenosíerenden Prozessen in Osophagus und Kardia. Dtsch Z Verdau Stoffwechselkr 1978; 38:47–9.

51. Mortensen McCNJ, MacKenzie EF. Accuracy of oesophageal brush cytology: results of a prospective study and multicentre slide exchange. Br J Surg 1981; 68:513–5.

52. Graham DY, Schwartz JT, Cain GD, Gyorkey F. Prospective evaluation of biopsy number in the diagnosis of esophageal and gastric carcinoma. Gastroenterology 1982; 82:228–31.

53. Hughes HE, Lee FD, Mackenzie JF. Endoscopic cytology and biopsy in the upper gastrointestinal tract. Clin Gastroenterol 1978; 7:375–96.

54. McCallum RW. Esophageal achalasia secondary to gastric carcinoma. Am J Gastroenterol 1979; 71:24–9.

55. Tytgat GNJ, Bartelsman JFWM. Motility disorders of the oesophagus. In: Misiewicz JJ, Pounder RE, Venables CW, eds. Diseases of the Gut and Pancreas. London: Grant McIntyre Ltd., 1985.

56. Tulman AB, Boyce HW Jr. Complications of esophageal dilatation and guidelines for their prevention. Gastrointest Endosc 1981; 27:229–34.

57. Tucker HJ, Snape WJ Jr, Cohen S: Achalasia secondary to carcinoma: Manometric and clinical features. Ann Intern Med 1978; 89:315–8.

58. Célestin LR, Campbell WB. A new and safe system for oesophageal dilatation. Lancet 1981; 1:74–5.

59. Heit HA, Johnson LF, Siegel SR. Palliative dilation for dysphagia in esophageal carcinoma. Ann Intern Med 1978; 89;629–31.

60. Boyce HW Jr, Palmer ED. Techniques of Clinical Gastroenterology. Springfield: C Thomas, 1975.

61. Tytgat GN, Den Hartog Jager FCA, Haverkamp HJ. Positioning of a plastic prosthesis under fiberendoscopic control in the palliative treatment of cardioesophageal cancer. Endoscopy 1976; 8:180–5.

62. Sivak MV Jr: Therapeutic endoscopy of the esophagus. Surg Clin North Am 1982; 62:807–20.

63. Earlam R, Cunha-Melo JR. Malignant oesophageal strictures: a review of techniques for palliative intubation. Br J Surg 1982; 69:61–8.

64. Branicki FJ, Ogilvie AL, Willis MR, Atkinson M. Structural deterioration of prosthetic oesophageal tubes—an in vitro comparison of latex rubber and silicone rubber tubes. Br J Surg 1981; 68:861–4.

65. Etienne J, Celestin LR. Oesophageal intubation: past and present. Acta Endoscopica 1979; 9:235–9.

66. Célestin LR, Etienne J, Raimbert P, et al. Traitement endoscopique des sténoses oesophagiennes par prosthèse de Célestin. Nouv Presse Med 1980; 9:2155–7.

67. Boyce HW Jr. Medical management of esophageal obstruction and esophageal-pulmonary fistula. Cancer 1982; 50:2597–600.

68. Atkinson M, Ferguson R, Parker GC. Tube introducer and modified Celestin tube for use in palliative intubation of oesophagogastric neoplasms at fiberoptic endoscopy. Gut 1978; 19:669–71.

69. Symonds CJ. The treatment of malignant stricture of the oesophagus by tubage or permanent catheterism. Br Med J 1887; 1:870.

70. Souttar HS. A method of intubating the esophagus for malignant stricture. Br Med J 1924; 1:782–3.

71. Tytgat GN. Endoscopic methods of treatment of gastrointestinal and biliary stenoses. (Suppl) Endoscopy 1980; 12:57–68.

72. Tytgat GN: Diagnostik und differentialtherapie der malignen oesophagus-stenose. Der Internist 1982; 23:251–6.

73. Weisel W, Raine F, Watson RR, Frederick JJ. Palliative treatment of esophageal carcinoma: a method and its evaluation. Ann Surg 1959; 149:207–16.

74. O'Conner T, Watson R, Lepley D, Weisel W. Esophageal prosthesis for palliative intubation. Fur-

ther evaluation of 378 patients. Arch Surg 1963; 87:275–9.

75. Palmer ED. Peroral prosthesis for the management of incurable esophageal carcinoma. Am J Gastroenterol 1973; 59:487–98.

76. Hegarty MM, Angorn EB, Bryer JV, et al. Pulsion intubation for palliation of carcinoma of the oesophagus. Br J Surg 1977; 64:160–5.

77. Kairaluoma MI, Jokinen K, Kärkölä P, Larmi TKI. Celestin tube palliation of unresectable oesophageal carcinoma. J Thorac Cardiovasc Surg 1977; 73:3–6.

78. Bergerault P, Denez B, Mahe J, et al. Prostheses endo-oesophagiennes de Célestin posées par voie endoscopique. Experience de 35 cas de cancer de l'oesophage. Ann Gastroenterol Hepatol 1980; 16:37–40.

79. Jones DB, Davies PS, Smith PM. Endoscopic insertion of palliative oesophageal tubes in oesophagogastric neoplasms. Br J Surg 1981; 68:197–8.

80. Soehendra N. Endoskopisches Tubuseinfuhren bei malignen Osophagus und Kardiastenosen. Dtsch Med Wochenschr 1981; 106:504–6.

81. Balmes JL, Baghdadi H, Michel H. Palliative endoscopic treatment of malignant esophageal stenosis using a Häring prosthesis. Digestion 1982; 23:31–8.

82. Van Blankenstein M, Tan TG, Dees J. Fibreoptic intubation of malignant oesophago-gastric strictures by the Atkinson method. Neth J Surg 1982; 34:11–2.

83. Ogilvie AL, Dronfield MW, Ferguson, R, Atkinson M. Outcome of endoscopic intubation in 100 patients with oesophagogastric carcinoma. (Abstr) Gut 1981; 22:A414.

84. Watson A. A study of the quality and duration of survival following resection, endoscopic intubation and surgical intubation in oesophageal carcinoma. Br J Surg 1982; 69:585–8.

85. Lux G, Groitl H, Riemann JF, Demling L. Tumor stenosis of the upper gastrointestinal tract—nonsurgical therapy by bridging tubes. Endoscopy 1983; 15:207–12.

86. Bennett JR. Intubation of gastro-oesophageal malignancies: a survey of current practice in Britain, 1980. Gut 1981; 22:336–8.

87. Giardet RE, Randell HT, Wheat MW. Palliative intubation in the management of esophageal carcinoma. Ann Thorac Surg 1974; 18:417–30.

88. Den Hartog Jager FCA, Berkel J, Tytgat GNJ. Technique for endoscopic intubation of gastric cancer. In: Van Maercke YMF, Van Moer EMJ, Pelckmans PAR, eds. Stomach Diseases—Current Status. Amsterdam-Oxford-Princeton: Excerpta Medica, 1981; 86–95.

89. Mathus-Vliegen EMH, Tytgat GNJ. The role of endoscopy in the correct and rapid positioning of feeding tubes. Endoscopy 1983; 15:78–84.

90. Wesdorp ICE, Bartelsman JFWM, Huibregtse K, et al. Treatment of instrumental esophageal perforation. Gut 1984; 25:398–404.

91. Boyce HW Jr. Peroral prosthesis for palliating malignant esophageal and gastric obstructions. Gastroenterology 1979; 77:1141–3.

92. Froelicher P, Miller G. The European experience with esophageal cancer limited to the mucosa and submucosa. Gastrointest Endosc 1986; 32:88–90.

93. Leipzig B, Zellmer JE, Klug D. The role of endoscopy in evaluating patients with head and neck cancer. A multi-institutional prospective study. Arch Otolaryngol 1985; 111:589–94.

94. Jabbari M, Goresky CA, Lough J, et al. The inlet patch: heterotopic gastric mucosa in the upper esophagus. Gastroenterology 1985; 89:352–6.

95. Boulafendis D, Damiani M, Sie E, et al. Primary malignant melanoma of the esophagus in a young adult. Am J Gastroenterol 1985; 80:417–20.

Chapter 18

HIATAL HERNIA AND PEPTIC DISEASES OF THE ESOPHAGUS

H. WORTH BOYCE, JR., M.D.

ANATOMY OF THE DISTAL ESOPHAGUS AND GASTRIC CARDIA

Knowledge of the internal anatomy of the esophagus and the influences upon it by extrinsic contiguous structures is essential for accurate interpretation of endoscopic findings.

The importance of precise measurements of distance from a fixed point of reference, cannot be overemphasized. (In this chapter, the incisor teeth or alveolar ridge are used as the point of reference.) The evaluation of therapeutic response on repeat endoscopy depends upon precision in recording the findings at the prior endoscopic procedure. Measurement of lesion size and the accurate location within quadrants of the luminal circumference also are essential. Nowhere is this practice more important than in the case of the patient who has several esophageal biopsies, one of which reveals malignant change. Careful observation and recording of biopsy or lesion site reduces the risk of being unable to return to the same location for repeated biopsy or for assessment of the response to therapy.

The esophagus begins at the cricopharyngeus muscle in the neck at the level of the C5-C6 vertebral interspace about 16 cm distal to the incisor teeth (Fig. 18–1). In the adult it extends for approximately 25 cm, ending at its junction with the stomach 2 to 3 cm below the diaphragmatic hiatus. The potential diameter of the lumen is approximately 25 mm throughout its length. The first 3 to 4 cm in the cervical region are relatively collapsed because of pressure from surrounding structures. The esophagus enters the superior mediastinum at the 20 cm level and opens readily with air insufflation, this response being enhanced by the negative intrathoracic pressure. At 23 cm from the incisor teeth there is a visible arterial pulsation through the left anterior wall of the esophagus in the area of contact with the aortic arch. There may be slight compression of the esophageal wall at this level. At 26 to 27 cm it lies against the posterior wall of the left mainstem bronchus. Rarely is there any intraluminal evidence of this relationship. At about 30 cm, "a" and "v" waves transmitted by the left atrium through the left-anterior esophageal wall are easily detected. Contact with the left atrium extends from about 30 to 35 cm. At this level the distal esophagus curves gently leftward and anteriorly to the proximal end of the lower esophageal sphincter, which usually begins 37 to 40 cm from the incisor teeth. The esophagus in the average patient passes through the diaphragmatic hiatus at approximately 38 to 40 cm and ends distal to the squamocolumnar mucosal junction at about the 41 to 42 cm level. Distances measured with a rigid endoscope are 1 to 2 cm less than measurements made with flexible endoscopes.

The normal level of the squamocolumnar mucosal junction may vary 1 to 2 cm, depending on the type of endoscope being used and the care with which measurements are made. As the closed normal esophageal sphincter is approached with the endoscope it will relax with the gentle pressure, and with passage through the sphincter there is little or no detectable resistance. As the endoscope

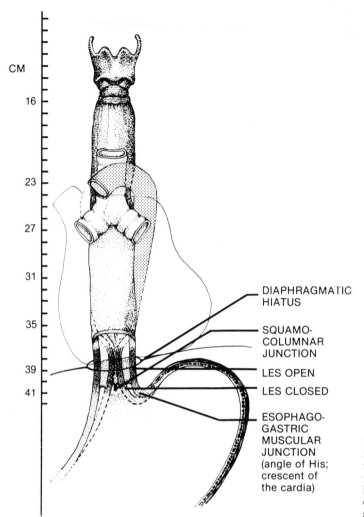

FIGURE 18–1. Esophageal anatomy and relationships with adjacent organs. Distances in centimeters are the average for an adult, as measured from the incisor teeth with a flexible fiberoptic endoscope. (LES = lower esophageal sphincter.)

is advanced 1 to 2 cm the lumen becomes widely patent, allowing visualization of the squamocolumnar mucosal junction and the most proximal segment of stomach (gastric cardia). If minimal air insufflation of the proximal and mid-esophagus is utilized during endoscopy, the closed lower esophageal sphincter region may be readily demonstrated. At the point of closure of the proximal end of the sphincter, several longitudinal, symmetric mucosal folds can be seen to disappear in the center of the lumen (Plate 18–1). This closure produces a rosette appearance, with the lumen being precisely centered at the point where these longitudinal folds converge. The tone of the lower esophageal sphincter relaxes with primary or secondary peristalsis and also opens in response to gentle insufflation. As the high-pressure sphincter zone relaxes, one can

identify the squamocolumnar mucosal junction and see into the tubular cavity of the proximal stomach, the cardia. The proximal end of the lower esophageal sphincter is most easily demonstrated in patients with achalasia because of the dilation of the body of the esophagus and typical hypertonicity of the closed sphincter.

The esophagus passes through the diaphragmatic hiatus in the adult 38 to 40 cm from the incisor teeth. The level of the hiatal margin is not as readily demonstrated in normal patients as in those who have a hiatal hernia; however, it is possible in most instances to determine the level with relative precision. As the lumen is gently insufflated with air, the patient is asked either to sniff or inhale rapidly, at which time the diaphragmatic hiatal margin moves inferiorly, either quickly or gradually depending upon the

Labels in figure:
CM
16
23
27
31
35
39
41

DIAPHRAGMATIC HIATUS
SQUAMO-COLUMNAR JUNCTION
LES OPEN
LES CLOSED
ESOPHAGO-GASTRIC MUSCULAR JUNCTION (angle of His; crescent of the cardia)

breathing maneuver used to demonstrate its location.

The squamous mucosal lining of the esophagus is pearly pink or pinkish-gray in color and contrasts sharply with the orange-red color of the gastric columnar epithelium (Plate 18–2). The esophageal mucosa is only slightly transparent and reflects light moderately. The gastric mucosa has a glistening surface because of the presence of mucus, but it is more transparent than the esophageal mucosa and consequently absorbs a great deal of light. For this reason gastric mucosa requires more light for adequate photography. The junction of the squamous and columnar epithelium appears after minimum inflation as a slightly irregular or undulating line, the so-called "Z" line. This line of demarcation between the two types of mucosa is readily identifiable in the absence of pathologic changes. In addition to surface characteristics and color, the distal extent of the esophageal squamous epithelium is also clearly demarcated by the presence of multiple, linear, frequently branching small blood vessels that abruptly disappear at the junction between squamous and columnar epithelium. If there is uncertainty about the location of this junction it can be dramatically demonstrated by application of several milliliters of Lugol's solution through an endoscopic catheter.[1] This will stain the esophageal mucosa in about 30 seconds. Chromoscopy is discussed in Part 2 of Chapter 10.

A crescent-shaped protrusion may be detected just distal to the squamocolumnar mucosal junction in the left lateral or greater curvature aspect of the cardia. This elevation has been called the semilunar-shaped fold or the crescent of the cardia and is believed to correspond to the horseshoe-shaped grouping of muscle fibers, the so-called sling muscle fibers, that are draped around the anatomic muscular union of esophagus and stomach forming the angle of His (see Fig. 18–1). This structure is usually located 39 to 41 cm from the incisor teeth, depending on the phase of respiration and the degree of bowing in a flexible endoscope.

After the endoscope is passed into the proximal stomach a retroversion maneuver should be performed to view the cardia and fundus from below (Plate 18–3). In the normal setting the insertion tube of the endoscope can be seen coming through a snugly fitting intra-abdominal segment of esophagus. The snug fit in this region is sustained throughout respiration and during moderate insufflation of the stomach, except that transient relaxation in response to primary or secondary peristalsis can be detected. The classic snug appearance of the region is always demonstrated in patients with achalasia because of the increased tone in the lower esophageal sphincter segment. During retroversion with insufflation, the squamocolumnar mucosal junction can be seen from several millimeters to 1 cm above the distal margin of this intra-abdominal segment (Plate 18–4). In patients with a hiatal hernia the area is patulous, the degree of this being dependent on the diameter of the esophageal diaphragmatic hiatus.

NORMAL ENDOSCOPIC AND RADIOLOGIC CORRELATIONS

The distal esophageal lumen fills evenly and symmetrically during contrast radiography.[2, 3] The column of barium begins to taper just proximal to the lower esophageal sphincter. With complete barium filling in the region of the esophagogastric junction, the proximal margin of the lower esophageal sphincter is demonstrated as a smooth narrowing of the barium column, beginning 1 to 2 cm above the diaphragmatic hiatus. After passage of barium through this region and complete closure of the lumen, a barium-free segment 3 to 4 cm long straddles the diaphragmatic hiatus; this segment corresponds to the closed lower esophageal sphincter. The angle of His on the greater curvature aspect demarcates the distal end of the sphincter region, also called the submerged or abdominal segment of the esophagus (Fig. 18–2A; see also Fig. 18–1). The normally located squamocolumnar mucosal junction cannot be identified radiographically. However, in patients with herniation of the proximal stomach through the hiatus, a lower esophageal ring can be demonstrated which represents the intrathoracically displaced squamocolumnar mucosal junction (Fig. 18–2B).

Earlier radiographic and anatomic studies have caused much confusion about this area relative to the structures that are seen in normal patients and in patients with hiatal hernias. In a normal individual there are no rings, no asymmetric bulges, and no bulbous contour of the distal esophagus. These alterations are seen only in patients with a hiatal hernia. Wolf[3] redefined the radiographic

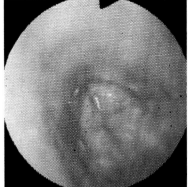

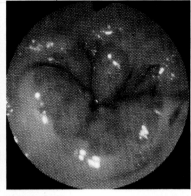

PLATE 18–1. Endoscopic view of upper limits of the closed lower esophageal sphincter, the so-called rosette.

PLATE 18–2. Endoscopic view of the squamocolumnar mucosal junction just proximal to the level of the diaphragmatic hiatus. The color difference between squamous and columnar epithelium is dramatic.

PLATE 18–1.

PLATE 18–2.

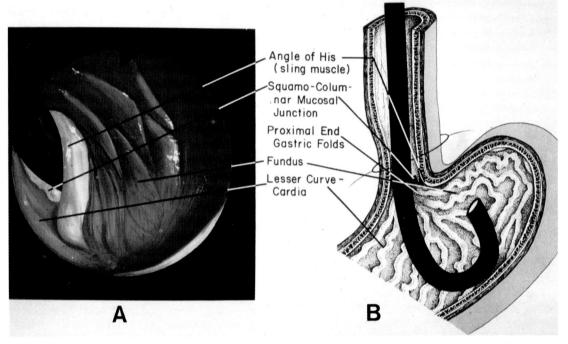

Angle of His (sling muscle)
Squamo-Columnar Mucosal Junction
Proximal End Gastric Folds
Fundus
Lesser Curve – Cardia

A   B

PLATE 18–3. Correlative drawings explaining anatomy in a retroverted view of the esophagogastric junction. A, Drawing from endoscopic photograph (Plate 18-4) of normal cardia region. B, Cross section showing endoscope position and sagittal view of esophagogastric junction region.

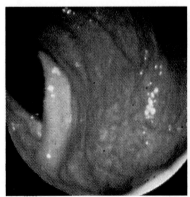

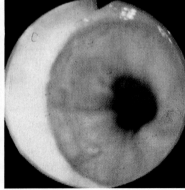

PLATE 18–4. Endoscopic retroverted view of esophagogastric junction and fundus of stomach. The distal margin of squamous epithelium is seen just below the endoscope.

PLATE 18–5. Endoscopic view of squamocolumnar mucosal junction displaced above the hiatus, representing a small hiatal hernia. The junction has straightened and a lower esophageal "B" ring has been formed under the influence of luminal distention with air.

PLATE 18–4.

PLATE 18–5.

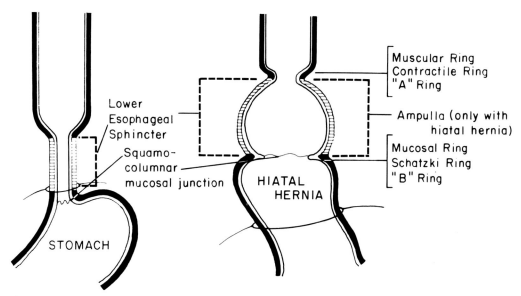

FIGURE 18–2. A, Profile of esophagogastric junction region, showing normal relationships and position of lower esophageal sphincter relative to the diaphragmatic hiatus. B, Profile of esophagogastric junction region herniated into the thorax via the esophageal hiatus of the diaphragm. The contour of the lower esophageal sphincter is readily altered by air or barium to produce this contour when it is displaced into the thorax above a hiatal hernia. (Modified from Goyal RK. Viewpoints on Digestive Dis: 1976; 8:1.)

anatomy of the esophagogastric region and clearly demonstrated the significance of the various radiographic contours that may be observed in this area. One of the reasons why there has been so much confusion concerning the normal anatomy is that the sliding hiatal hernia is so common in the population. Many radiologists have insisted on the classic definition of a hiatal hernia, the criteria for which are not present in patients with small hernias. It is imperative for the physician who performs endoscopy to understand the proper radiographic criteria for hiatal hernia as defined by Wolf, so that accurate endoscopic-radiographic correlations may be made.

ENDOSCOPIC DIAGNOSIS OF HIATAL HERNIA

The first step in endoscopic diagnosis of hiatal hernia is recognition of the important intraluminal landmarks utilized in defining this entity. There has been much argument over the criteria for endoscopic diagnosis, but there is a consensus at present with respect to the major diagnostic points.[4-9]

Under normal circumstances the squamocolumnar mucosal junction has been observed to migrate during swallowing and with respiration as much as 2 cm above the diaphragmatic hiatus. Dagradi et al.,[4, 9] Trujillo et al.,[5, 6] and others agree that displacement

of the squamocolumnar junction greater than 2 cm proximal to the diaphragmatic hiatus is abnormal. This opinion correlates well with the modern radiographic criteria for hiatal hernia as reported by Wolf.[3] In patients with hiatal hernia the diaphragmatic hiatus and cardia often are rather patulous so that the lumen opens with minimal insufflation. In many instances, this area is so widely patent that it can be seen from the proximal esophagus. The anatomic and radiologic correlation of findings at the esophagogastric junction are demonstrated diagramatically in Figure 18–2A and B, respectively.

Once the squamocolumnar junction is identified, the maneuvers as described above for localizing the diaphragmatic hiatus should be used. With minimal degrees of herniation, the displacement of the squamocolumnar junction proximal to the diaphragmatic hiatus by more than 2 cm is the primary endoscopic criterion for diagnosis of a hiatal hernia (Plate 18–5). A hernia pouch per se is not identifiable when this minimum criterion is applied. If, however, there is a moderately sized or large hiatal hernia, the gastric mucosal folds can be seen running proximally over the hiatal margin and lying in the bulbous cavity of the distended hernia pouch. When the patient inspires, the diaphragmatic margin moves downward to give the appearance of gastric mucosa gliding upward over this margin into the chest. If the patient sniffs, there is an abrupt, short, downward motion of the diaphragm, again producing a similar appearance of gastric mucosa gliding over the hiatal margin into the chest.

After observing the diaphragmatic hiatus from above, the endoscope should be passed into the proximal stomach and retroverted. In most instances of hiatal hernia the initial view from this vantage reveals a widened diaphragmatic hiatus with gastric mucosa lying loosely around the hiatal margin and gastric folds running upward well into the hiatal hernia pouch (Plate 18–6). If the patient is asked to sniff or take a deep breath, the diaphragmatic margin descends as the stomach glides in a proximal direction over its edge. In the herniated pouch several gastric folds usually can be seen running along its greater curvature or posterior wall aspects to terminate just distal to the squamocolumnar mucosal junction. These folds normally terminate within 5 to 10 mm of the normal location of the squamocolumnar mucosal junction. Therefore, this termination can be utilized endoscopically and radiographically as a marker for the approximate location of the normal squamocolumnar mucosal junction.

In some patients with a hiatal hernia and normal lower esophageal sphincter tone, the esophageal wall in the region of the esophageal sphincter will be closed snugly around the endoscope. Some relaxation may be apparent in relation to primary and secondary peristalsis or after greater degrees of air insufflation. In patients with reflux esophagitis—especially those with a columnar-lined esophagus, who tend to have the lowest sphincter pressures—there is considerable free space around the endoscope as it lies in the region of the lower esophageal sphincter just proximal to the hernia pouch.

When viewing the region of the squamocolumnar junction from below in patients with normal or slightly decreased lower esophageal sphincter pressure, the closure of the proximal end of the lower esophageal sphincter can be observed. The point of maximum closure in these cases appears 1 to 2 cm above the squamocolumnar junction (see Fig. 18–2B). This level of closure corresponds to the so-called esophageal "A" ring, or sphincter contraction ring, both in location and contour during radiography and endoscopy.

With a hiatal hernia of moderate or larger size, the retroverted endoscope can be pulled back to the level of the diaphragmatic hiatus or even a short distance into the hernia pouch, thus affording an examination of the squamocolumnar mucosal junction from below (Plate 18–7).

The lower esophageal "B" (Schatzki) ring may be clearly demonstrated during retroversion, using the same breathing maneuvers as previously mentioned, again illustrating the precise anatomic relationship between the squamocolumnar mucosal junction and the lower esophageal ring (see Plate 18–6).

It is important to observe carefully and record the characteristics of the distal esophagus and proximal stomach in patients with hiatal hernia who have no gastroesophageal reflux sequelae. The location of the diaphragmatic hiatus in relation to the proximal stomach, the level of the squamocolumnar mucosal junction, and the proximal extent of the gastric mucosal folds in the hernia pouch are characteristics utilized in the precise endoscopic diagnosis of hiatal hernia and reflux sequelae, including the earliest stages of a columnar-lined (Barrett's) esophagus.

In evaluating patients with a known or suspected hiatal hernia, it is appropriate to use more than minimal air insufflation. The radiologist makes use of changes in patient position and increased amounts of barium to demonstrate the same anatomy. Since patients with hiatal hernia tend to belch frequently, a considerable amount of insufflated air may be required to demonstrate adequately the landmarks as discussed. Sliding esophageal hiatal hernias are common, particularly in older patients. Nevertheless, it is important to demonstrate the presence of this entity by either radiography or endoscopy or both in all patients, and especially those with upper gastrointestinal or pulmonary symptoms. If the endoscopic criteria are utilized with the radiographic criteria of Wolf, it is not difficult to recognize the presence of a sliding hiatal hernia. It is the clinician's responsibility to determine whether this finding in the individual patient is significant. If neither radiologist nor endoscopic examining physician diligently reports the presence of this entity, the patient's physician may not suspect a reflux-related etiology for atypical or obscure complaints.

LOWER ESOPHAGEAL "B" (SCHATZKI) RING

With inflation of the distal esophagus the squamocolumnar mucosal junction gradually

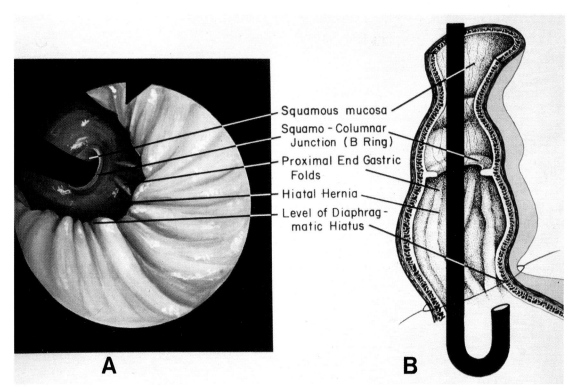

Squamous mucosa

Squamo - Columnar
Junction (B Ring)

Proximal End Gastric
Folds

Hiatal Hernia

Level of Diaphrag-
matic Hiatus

A   B

PLATE 18–6. *A,* Drawing of endoscopic retroverted view of a hiatal hernia. Note location of a lower esophageal "B" ring at level of squamocolumnar mucosal junction. *B,* Drawing of sagittal view of a hiatal hernia, showing endoscope position and correlative anatomy for the retroverted view shown in *A.*

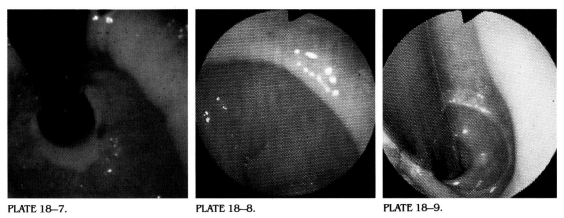

PLATE 18–7.   PLATE 18–8.   PLATE 18–9.

PLATE 18–7. Endoscopic retroverted view into a hiatal hernia, showing the squamocolumnar mucosal junction and patulous lower esophageal sphincter segment around the endoscope. The fold or ridge appearance in the right foreground is due to gastric mucosa lying over the margin of the diaphragmatic hiatus.

PLATE 18–8. Endoscopic view of small hiatal hernia and a lower esophageal "B" ring. There is a dramatic color difference between squamous and columnar epithelium.

PLATE 18–9. Endoscopic retroverted view into a distended hiatal hernia pouch that clearly demonstrates a lower esophageal "B" ring from below. The lighter color of the gastric mucosa compared to that shown on Plate 18-8 is due to the close proximity of the illuminating endoscope to the mucosa.

changes from its usual serrated appearance to a straight line (Fig. 18–3A–D). Adding a bit more air, or a Müller maneuver by the patient (inspiration against a closed glottis) to enhance negative intrathoracic pressure and thereby increase the effect of positive intraluminal pressure, maximally distends the distal hiatal hernia pouch and esophageal lumen proximal to the squamocolumnar junction (Fig. 18–3E). For some reason the line of junction between the two types of mucosa at the normal location has limited distensibility, and with optimal distention it often protrudes into the lumen as a perfectly straight, web-like elevation around the entire circumference of the lumen. This structure corresponds precisely to the lower esophageal or "B" ring. The radiologist can readily demonstrate this in patients with a hiatal hernia by distending this same region with an adequate quantity of barium. This "B" ring is diagnostic of hiatal hernia whether demonstrated by radiography or endoscopy.[3]

Close inspection reveals that the "B" ring forms precisely at the squamocolumnar junc-tion or within 3 mm proximal to the junction (Plate 18–8). When the hiatal hernia is examined from below using optimum inflation, the lower esophageal "B" ring is readily demonstrable (Plate 18–9; see also Plate 18–6). The fact that this ring occurs at the junction of the two types of mucosa suggests that its formation is dependent upon some anatomic feature of this contact point. This theory is supported by the finding that "B" rings do not occur in patients with a columnar-lined (Barrett's) esophagus. Apparently its absence is related to the proximal displacement of the squamocolumnar mucosal junction; it is not demonstrable in such cases, either because the more proximal esophagus cannot be adequately distended or because the unique anatomic characteristic that permits its development at the normally located mucosal junction is absent at the level of the displaced junction.

Our experience is in agreement with the observation of others that there appears to be a decreased frequency of reflux esophagitis in patients with a "B" ring. Whether a

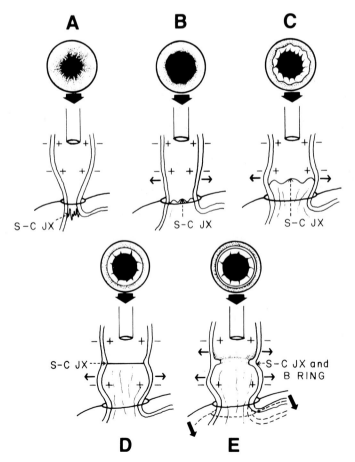

FIGURE 18–3. Schematic representation of the sequence of anatomic changes leading to demonstration of a hiatal hernia and a lower esophageal "B" ring by gradual inflation and luminal distention during endoscopy. A, View as sphincter region is first opened. B, Further inflation opens sphincter region and brings squamocolumnar junction to level of diaphragmatic hiatus. C, Further inflation brings squamocolumnar mucosal junction above hiatal margin. Negative intrathoracic pressure enhances luminal distention. D, With further inflation, the squamocolumnar mucosal junction changes from an irregular, serrated, or undulated contour to a straight line. A hiatal hernia pouch is now clearly visible. E, With further inflation or by having the patient sniff or perform a Müller maneuver (inspiration against a closed glottis), the combination of intraluminal positive pressure and intrathoracic negative pressure causes the mucosal junction to protrude into the lumen as a smooth, symmetric lower esophageal "B" ring.

"B" ring protects against esophagitis or whether esophagitis prevents development of a "B" ring is not known.

REFLUX ESOPHAGITIS

Endoscopic documentation of the presence of hiatal hernia correlates much better with the clinical syndromes of gastroesophageal reflux than does any other study, including manometric measurements of the lower esophageal sphincter.[10] Any study that purports to correlate reflux sequelae with hiatal hernia should primarily be based on endoscopic criteria and Wolf's radiographic criteria.[3]

The pathophysiology of gastroesophageal reflux, although investigated extensively by radiography, endoscopy, and manometry over the past two decades, is still poorly understood. It is becoming more and more apparent that reflux and reflux-related esophageal disorders result from a combination of anatomic and functional defects, of which sliding hiatal hernia and reduced lower esophageal sphincter pressure are only two.[11] The composition and quantity of refluxed material, its pH, and its duration of contact with the mucosa are likely important factors in the genesis of the endoscopic and histologic changes termed esophagitis.

Injury to the squamous epithelium of the distal esophagus seems to occur when there is a sufficient frequency and duration of exposure of this tissue to highly acid or alkaline material. The reason for this susceptibility to injury in certain patients and resistance in others is not understood. In general, it is accepted that the duration of acid or alkaline contact with the distal esophagus is a major factor in the genesis of the inflammatory changes recognized as reflux esophagitis. It has been suggested that the most injurious refluxant is a combination of acid-pepsin and bile acids.

The consequences of the inflammatory changes due to reflux may be so mild as to produce neither symptoms nor sequelae in some patients.[12-14] In others, esophagitis may proceed inexorably to produce mucosal friability, erosion, ulceration, and subsequently esophageal stricture. In an occasional patient, the changes are of sufficient chronicity and severity as to eventuate the development of a columnar-lined esophagus.[15-17] Since the radiographic findings in esophagitis are usually minimal or nonexistent, accurate diagnosis depends on esophagoscopy and biopsy.

Esophagitis secondary to reflux of gastric contents (i.e., hydrochloric acid, bile acids, or a combination of the two or possibly other substances) always involves the squamocolumnar mucosal junction at some point. The squamocolumnar junction becomes less distinct with the progression of hyperemia, erythema, and erosion. In some cases it is impossible to locate the junction with certainty because of the inflammation. The presence of tenacious exudate surrounded by a margin of hyperemia is typical for erosive esophagitis. Evidence of erosive esophagitis extending proximal to the squamocolumnar junction may appear either as proximally directed finger-like extensions or as isolated patches of eroded squamous mucosa. In all cases, however, the squamocolumnar junction will be diseased at some point (Plate 18–10). Esophagitis that is proximal to the squamocolumnar mucosal junction with no abnormality at the level of the junction should lead to a suspicion of another cause such as infection with monilia or herpes, drug-induced injury, or malignancy. These conditions are discussed in Chapter 19.

Reflux esophagitis is diagnosed endoscopically by the presence of friability (i.e., bleeding in response to gentle or minimal contact with the tip of the endoscope or closed biopsy forcep), erosion with exudate, or frank ulceration.[9, 14] Erosions may be linear (i.e., parallel to the long axis of the esophagus, starting from the squamocolumnar mucosal junction) or oval to round and surrounded by squamous epithelium (see Plate 18–10). The margins of erosions often are bright red. Mucosal friability often is present. Hyperemia and erythema are not reliable criteria for diagnosis, since such changes occur in the region of the squamocolumnar junction in patients without significant disease. Sonnenberg et al.[14] have devised a simple classification of erosive esophagitis as follows: grade 1 (mild)—isolated round or linear erosions; grade 2 (severe)—confluence of erosions involving the total luminal circumference; and grade 3 (complicated)—erosions as described for grades 1 and 2 plus deep ulcers, stenosis, or columnar-lined esophagus.

The biopsy studies of Ismail-Beigi et al.[12] showed that histologic changes occurring within 2 cm proximal to the lower esophageal sphincter may reflect acid injury in the absence of clinically significant disease. These histologic changes (i.e., lengthening of the rete pegs and thickening of the basal cell layer described by Ismail-Beigi et al.[12] and the increase in number of rete pegs described by Kobayashi and Kasugai[13]), if found more than 2 cm proximal to the lower esophageal sphincter, indicate clinically significant inflammation in symptomatic patients. The presence of polymorphonuclear leukocytes and edema of the esophageal mucosa are unequivocal signs of esophagitis and correlate with the classic endoscopic findings.[14] The finding of intraepithelial eosinophils has been proposed as a new diagnostic criterion for esophagitis.[18]

The histologic criteria of Ismail-Beigi and associates were established using manometric localization without direct endoscopic correlation; therefore, they must be modified to utilize standard endoscopic landmarks for accurate diagnosis. By most estimations the squamocolumnar junction normally lies within the region of the lower esophageal sphincter about 1 to 2 cm distal to the sphincter's proximal margin, as determined by manometry (see Fig. 18–2). Thus a mucosal biopsy taken 1 to 2 cm above the proximal margin of the lower esophageal sphincter would be about 3 to 4 cm proximal to the squamocolumnar mucosal junction. This location for biopsy in cases without visible diagnostic surface changes should meet most criteria for proper site selection.

When esophagitis is suspected in the absence of visible diagnostic changes in the mucosal surface, it is important that an adequate mucosal biopsy be obtained 3 cm or more above the squamocolumnar junction. Adequate implies full mucosal thickness—that is, to the level of the muscularis mucosa ideally or the full epithelial layer at a minimum. With proper technique adequate mucosal biopsies can be obtained with the standard flexible forceps.[19] Direct vision suction biopsies using a small bowel biopsy tube (Rubin-Quinton) are of excellent quality but are not often necessary for accurate diagnosis. Histologic changes diagnostic of acid-induced esophagitis appear before symptoms and endoscopically observable changes, and persist after the endoscopic indicators have disappeared in response to therapy.

An endoscopically demonstrable hiatal hernia is nearly always associated with reflux esophagitis (see Plate 18–10). In some instances circumferential exudate may be detected about the distal esophagus. This suggests the presence of chronic reflux esophagitis associated with stenosis (Plate 18–11). Stenosis of moderate degree may not be obvious to the casual observer and may go unrecognized at endoscopy using the newer small-diameter endoscopes, since no resistance to their passage will be encountered.

Over 90% of patients with symptoms of reflux esophagitis respond well to antireflux measures, antacids, and/or the H-2 receptor blockers cimetidine or ranitidine. Antireflux surgery is reserved for those who remain symptomatic despite optimal medical therapy.

ALKALINE REFLUX ESOPHAGITIS

Alkaline reflux esophagitis is most likely to result from two situations that may permit pure duodenal contents to enter the esophagus, that is, after total gastrectomy with esophagoduodenostomy or esophagojejunostomy,[20, 21] and in patients with hypochlorhydria or achlorhydria.[22] Undoubtedly some patients with a portion of the stomach remaining will have a combined acid-alkaline reflux. Nearly all patients with alkaline reflux esophagitis after partial gastrectomy have a hiatal hernia that likely plays a role in pathogenesis.

The term alkaline reflux esophagitis implies that the alkalinity of the refluxed material is the causative factor. This is misleading, since it is more likely that bile salts, proteolytic pancreatic enzymes, or a combination of the two or the presence of hydrochloric acid or some yet unidentified substances are responsible for injury of the esophageal squamous mucosa.

The usual clinical manifestations of pyrosis, retrosternal pain, or both, as well as bitter or sour-tasting regurgitant are identical to the symptoms of acid reflux esophagitis. Dysphagia, odynophagia, iron-deficiency anemia, or less often acute but severe hemorrhage may be presenting problems.

Barium contrast radiography is primarily helpful in confirming the altered postoperative anatomy. Strictures may be detected with proper technique or a solid bolus challenge, but as with acid-pepsin reflux esophagitis, the erosive diagnostic changes of reflux esophagitis rarely can be detected radiographically.

Esophagoscopy usually reveals mucosal erosions, hyperemic and friable mucosa, exudate, and in some cases, stenosis and stricture. These erosions may be single or multiple, but they always start at the squamocolumnar mucosal junction in the intact esophagus or at the site of esophagoduodenal or esophagojejunal anastomosis after total

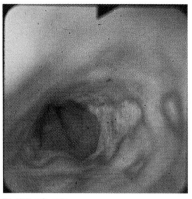

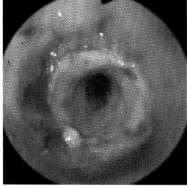

PLATE 18–10. Endoscopic view showing erosions of reflux esophagitis. A large erosion extending proximally from the squamocolumnar junction is shown at right, center. Isolated "islands" of erosion with central white exudate are present proximally. A hiatal hernia pouch is shown in the distance.

PLATE 18–11. Endoscopic view of severe distal reflux esophagitis with luminal stenosis and circumferential exudate within the stenosis.

PLATE 18–10.

PLATE 18–11.

PLATE 18–12. Endoscopic view of a severe reflux-related stricture. Circumferential exudate and a rim of hyperemia are seen at the margin of the stricture, with extension of these inflammatory changes proximally along one portion of the wall.

PLATE 18–13. Endoscopic view of a severe reflux-related stricture with residual esophagitis and gross mural deformity by fibrosis and formation of diverticula.

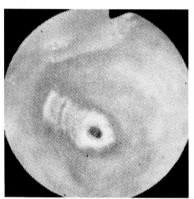

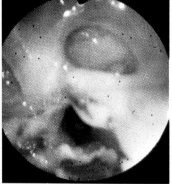

PLATE 18–12.

PLATE 18–13.

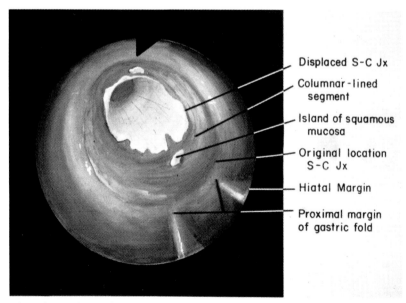

Displaced S–C Jx

Columnar-lined segment

Island of squamous mucosa

Original location S–C Jx

Hiatal Margin

Proximal margin of gastric fold

PLATE 18–14. Drawing of an endoscopic retroverted view of a hiatal hernia and displaced squamocolumnar mucosal junction, with an interposed segment of metaplastic columnar mucosa lining the distal esophagus. The endoscope was omitted from this drawing to permit a full view of the surface anatomy.

gastrectomy. The extent of mucosal injury is variable, but the endoscopic findings often are impressive. A columnar-lined esophagus may develop in some patients; therefore, the mucosal alterations of this condition should be searched for whether the reflux is predominantly alkaline or acid. The histologic changes found in the squamous mucosa on biopsy are indistinguishable from those attributed to acid reflux.[20, 21]

Management usually includes antireflux positional measures and bile acid binding with aluminum hydroxide or cholestyramine, but often the response is unsatisfactory. The use of a mucosal barrier–enhancing agent such as sucrose sulfate has been suggested, but no therapeutic benefit has been proved. Surgical management can be undertaken when patients fail to respond to medical therapy, the most effective procedure being diversion of the duodenal contents far enough distally into the small intestine to prevent esophageal reflux. This is usually accomplished with an isoperistaltic Roux-Y limb of jejunum at least 40 cm long.[21]

THE SENTINEL FOLD

The sentinel fold or polyp was first reported in 1973.[23] Some patients with a hiatal hernia shown by radiography, endoscopy, or both have a polypoid fold in the hiatal hernia pouch just distal to the mucosal junction, most often on the left or greater curvature aspect. This is a reliable indicator of significant inflammatory disease in the region of the squamocolumnar junction but must be differentiated from neoplasm by biopsy and from varices by inspection. The usual finding is an area of focal, severe erosion or ulceration or signs of prior ulceration between the proximal margin of the sentinel fold and the squamocolumnar mucosal junction only a few millimeters away. This fold has been variously described by others as a pseudotumor or inflammatory polyp, and according to several reports the lesion has been removed unnecessarily by electrosurgical snare polypectomy during endoscopy. Forceps biopsy reveals columnar epithelium with underlying acute and chronic inflammation.

DISTAL ESOPHAGEAL STENOSIS AND STRICTURE

When there is evidence of narrowing in the esophagus the term stenosis is appropri-

ate. Complete evaluation may reveal that this is caused by inflammation, spasm without evidence of fibrosis, or both. Peroral dilation is of little value in treating an inflammatory stenosis. The dysphagia produced by this lesion should respond to antireflux medical therapy. Actual fibrosis or cicatrix formation with narrowing should be designated a stricture. This requires peroral dilation in addition to antireflux medical therapy. Dysphagia for solid foods is always present when the lumen diameter is narrowed to 13 mm (39 French) or less. However, large swallowed boluses of solid food may elicit dysphagia with lesser degrees of narrowing. Dysphagia is always a significant symptom and requires evaluation by radiography with use of a bolus challenge as necessary to demonstrate the obstruction and, in all cases, evaluation by endoscopy.

For practical purposes a benign stricture at the squamocolumnar junction is related to reflux of gastric contents and is associated with a hiatal hernia. Reflux-related strictures always occur at the squamocolumnar junction regardless of its location. If the mucosal junction has been displaced proximally in a patient with a columnar-lined (Barrett's) esophagus the reflux-related stricture will occur at the squamocolumnar junction wherever it is located. Strictures related to reflux are less than 1 cm in length unless there has been some additional aggravating factor such as an indwelling nasogastric tube or secondary esophagitis related to superimposed injury by an impacted pill or tablet. The contour of the esophageal wall proximal to the stricture is usually smooth and tapered (Plate 18–12). As the degree of lumenal stenosis progresses, there will be less erosive esophagitis proximal to the stricture, because the stricture reduces the degree of reflux. If chronic submucosal injury has developed, fibrous bands or pseudodiverticula may be present proximal to the stricture (Plate 18–13). These structural alterations create a hazard during peroral dilation unless fluoroscopic control and a guide wire dilation system are used for initial therapy.

Treatment of Esophageal Stricture

A patient's quality of life is significantly affected by an esophageal stricture. Social activities may be restricted, nutrition and hydration are impaired, meals represent agony not pleasure, oral secretions cannot be handled adequately, and bronchopulmonary aspiration is common. These problems are intensified by the fact that most patients with esophageal obstruction produce large amounts of saliva (sialorrhea). Restoration of an adequate lumen relieves these symptoms of obstruction. The main goal of therapy is to establish and maintain a patent esophagus with the lowest risk and cost to the patient.[24]

Even after the diagnosis of an esophageal stricture is firmly established and a plan for dilation outlined, close follow-up and periodic re-evaluation of the stricture are in order. The frequency of dilation is determined by the etiology and characteristics of the stricture and the degree of remaining inflammation. The interval between dilations and evaluations must be determined individually for each patient.

Instruments for Peroral Esophageal Dilation

Two basic types of esophageal dilators are adequate for treating over 90% of esophageal strictures. The rubber, mercury-filled Hurst and Maloney dilators (Fig. 18–4A and B) are satisfactory for the most reflux-related strictures. The Savary tapered thermoplastic dilators (Fig. 18–4C) and the Eder-Puestow metal olive dilators (Fig. 18–4D) passed over a spring-tipped guide wire are ideal for initial dilation of very narrow, fibrotic strictures or strictures with associated diverticula, an eccentric or angulated lumen position, or an esophagopulmonary fistula. The interchangeable metal olives of the Eder-Puestow system were originally available in odd numbered French (Fr) sizes from 21 through 45, but currently are being manufactured in sizes up to 60 Fr. Extraordinary care should be taken when using Eder-Puestow olives above 50 Fr in size. Because of their metal construction and the mechanical advantage provided by their introduction on a flexible metal shaft, there is an increased hazard of overstretching with perforation at the stricture. Mural injuries during dilation are more often located above or below rather than within the strictured segment, suggesting that improperly controlled technique is the responsible factor and not the effect of stretching. Perforation of the esophageal or gastric wall is usually related to retroflexion and penetration by the spring tip rather than the stretching produced by the olives; thus, the importance of fluoroscopic control.[25]

The recently introduced Savary dilators (see Fig. 18–4C) combine features of the Maloney dilator (tapered tip) and the Eder-Puestow system (guide wire) and are marked with a 1 cm radiopaque band just proximal to the tapered tip. The Savary dilators are

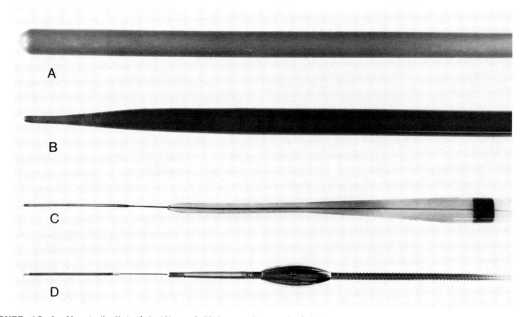

FIGURE 18–4. Hurst (bullet tip) (A) and Maloney (tapered tip) (B) rubber, mercury-filled dilators. Savary thermoplastic taper dilator (C) and Eder-Puestow metal olive dilator (D); both are used with spring-tipped guide wires that can be seen (left) exiting from the dilator.

constructed of a flexible thermoplastic material and contain a central channel. Successive dilators are passed over a properly positioned guide wire. The spring tip on the leading end of the guide wire has been modified to provide differential flexibility, this being maximal at the tip and minimal at the junction point with the wire. This modification reduces the tendency for the spring to become flexed and redirected 180 degrees in response to only minimal tip pressure, as may happen with the standard Eder-Puestow guide wire spring tip. Despite this modification, the safest method of dilation over a guide wire requires proper positioning with the aid of fluoroscopy as well as intermittent fluoroscopic observation of the guide wire throughout the procedure.

The spindle-shaped Tucker dilators, which have loops of silk thread at each end, are designed for retrograde passage via a gastrostomy using a pull-through technique with an indwelling heavy silk or nylon thread. These dilators are available in sizes 12 Fr through 40 Fr. Several dilators of successively larger sizes are connected at the thread loops and are pulled in tandem through the gastrostomy and then retrograde through the stricture.[24] The gastrostomy requirement is a major disadvantage, and this system is seldom used for peptic stricture. Tucker dilators are sometimes used with diffuse, severe stricturing of the esophagus, as may occur with ingestion of caustic substances such as lye, where repeated dilation may be required.

Pneumatic balloon dilators patterned after the Grundzig arterial balloon catheter are available. It has been claimed that pneumatic dilation of esophageal strictures is safer than other methods, but there is no proof for this claim as yet, nor is there any satisfactory evidence that this dilation method is more effective than any of the others. The balloon dilator is 8 cm long and has radiopaque limit markers at either end of the balloon portion, which is at the distal end of a catheter with a central channel. A very thin, flexible guide wire is first passed under fluoroscopic control well beyond the stricture. The dilator catheter is then passed over the guide wire and positioned across the stricture, using the radiopaque markers as reference points. Balloon sizes of 8 to 60 Fr are available. However, complete sets with sequentially increasing sizes are not available commercially, in contrast to other esophageal dilators. Consequently, there may be a tendency to

use available sizes and thereby attempt to dilate at a more rapid pace than ordinarily would be considered safe. The smaller-sized balloons are advantageous for dilation of the most severe strictures, provided that the guide wire can be passed and properly positioned first. If this is accomplished, the lumen diameter of the tightest strictures can be increased to 16 to 20 Fr with small balloon dilators, whereupon the Eder-Puestow or Savary dilators can be used over a guide wire to complete the therapy in a series of procedures.

Preparing the Patient and the Esophagus

Patients with esophageal obstruction severe enough to cause dysphagia for all solid foods should undergo dilation only after a 24-hour period on clear liquid intake to ensure that the esophagus is clean and empty.[24] This is important when endoscopy is planned for diagnosis or in conjunction with dilation.

Informed consent should be obtained from the patient after the procedure, its inherent risks, and alternative therapies are fully described. Premedication is used only in selected instances, depending on several factors including the patient's psychological state, the etiology and physical characteristics of the stricture, the customary dilation routine for referred patients, the presence of associated diseases, and anticipation of unusual degrees of discomfort during dilation.

Unfortunately, at times premedication is used for the benefit of the physician or surgeon who performs the dilation rather than the benefit of the patient. Most patients tolerate remarkably well the 10 seconds or so of mild to moderate discomfort associated with passage of each dilator. Omitting premedication makes it possible for the patient to depart after only brief observation and to function normally at home and work, including being able to drive shortly after the procedure; this is appreciated by most patients. Most prefer some form of oropharyngeal anesthesia, induced by either a gargle or spray, to reduce their gag reflex and discomfort of swallowing the dilator. A 1% Xylocaine gargle is effective and safe for this purpose.

The entire dilation procedure is infinitely more acceptable and tolerable if the physician who will perform the procedure explains the expected sensations to the patient, assures that breathing will be unimpaired, and continues comforting reassurance throughout the dilation. The equanimity, compassion, and honesty of the operator are reflections of his training and competence. Heavy-handedness and lack of skill and concern for the patient's comfort are readily sensed by the patient, and the end result may be a less than satisfactory and in some cases dangerous procedure.

Technique of Peroral Dilation

Little has been written regarding specific recommendations for techniques of dilating benign esophageal strictures. Consequently, there is no consensus on the principles of stricture management. Every esophageal stricture seems to have a "personality" of its own and variations in technique often are therefore necessary for successful therapy. However, several principles of peroral dilation technique merit consideration.[25]

The first principle of stricture management is to avoid a hurried approach to restoration of lumen patency. In many patients esophageal strictures require months to years to develop to the point of dysphagia. There is little need to attempt to return the stenotic lumen to normal diameter in a single sitting or within a few days. Second and subsequent dilations may be scheduled at intervals of one day to several weeks, depending on the response of the patient and of the stricture to the initial dilation. The ultimate success of therapy should not be a cause for concern, since essentially all benign esophageal strictures are successfully dilated over a period of time, on either an outpatient or inpatient basis.

A second principle is to pass no more than three dilators that meet with moderate or greater resistance at any one session. Often the proper size dilator is determined by passing smaller ones first to assess the degree of stricturing as well as the pathway to the stomach. The point at which resistance is encountered, and in some cases the characteristics of the stricture, can be sensed by a practiced operator; this is impossible when dilators are habitually passed with excessive force and abruptness. Dilators that meet minimal or no resistance and obviously produce no stretching of the strictured segment are not counted in the "rule of three." The principle is to limit the dilation session to passage of three dilators that encounter moderate or greater resistance. Only one or two dilators may be the appropriate number when the

stricture is extremely narrow, pain is severe, and bleeding occurs, or in severe strictures that have been symptomatic for years, such as those due to corrosive injury.

A third important principle is the use of fluoroscopy to monitor dilator position and path, especially during initial treatment sessions. The lumen axis for most typical benign esophageal strictures is directly in line with the axis of the proximal esophagus and distal stomach. Therefore, the rubber mercury-filled bougies (Maloney or Hurst) ordinarily used for simple strictures can be expected to pass safely into the strictured lumen and through it without appreciable lateral pressure on the wall except within the stricture. However, there are enough variations in these usual anatomic relationships that one is well advised to keep the dilator tip under control at all times. Fluoroscopy may be omitted with simple strictures that have been dilated under fluoroscopy initially and are known to have no associated anatomic factors that increase risk.

The guide wire of either the Eder-Puestow or Savary dilator sets is most safely passed under fluoroscopic control. The need for guide wire passage via the endoscope is uncommon. Precise fluoroscopic localization of the guide wire tip during dilation is believed to increase the safety of this technique. When the guide wire cannot be passed using fluoroscopic control alone, it can be inserted through the biopsy channel of a forward-viewing panendoscope. Some physicians who perform endoscopy prefer a combination of fluoroscopy and endoscopy for positioning the guide wire. This permits direct observation of the stricture just prior to each dilation procedure, and shortens the initial procedure, during which endoscopic evaluation is required prior to dilation in all cases. Even though the guide wire is being passed through the endoscope into the proximal end of the stricture under direct vision, its spring tip may become markedly angulated within the stricture or distal to it. This event may occur completely beyond the endoscopic view. Therefore, fluoroscopy should be used when attempting to pass the guide wire through the stricture either with or without direct endoscopic observation.

It is easier to prevent the development of a far-advanced stricture than to treat this condition. Therefore, the value of early treatment when the lumen is not markedly narrowed nor fibrosis very advanced cannot be overemphasized. Neglected esophageal narrowing is unfortunately still a dilemma and will remain so until the need for continuous effort at prophylaxis is better appreciated. All patients who have had dysphagia as a result of an esophageal stricture, even though this is adequately dilated initially, should undergo an evaluation at least once a year.

COLUMNAR-LINED (BARRETT'S) ESOPHAGUS

In the past few years columnar-lined, or Barrett's, esophagus has been recognized as more common than previously believed.[16, 17, 26] Since columnar-lined esophagus is a premalignant condition, early recognition of this high-risk state in patients is imperative. It is possible to recognize minimal degrees of columnar-lined esophagus, based on an understanding of the normal luminal topographic relationships.

Columnar-lined esophagus rarely, if ever, occurs without the presence of a hiatal hernia, and recognition of this relationship is of importance. When the squamocolumnar junction is displaced proximally 2 cm or more above the esophageal hiatus, one can readily recognize the gastric folds that extend through the hiatus into the hernia pouch. These folds stop at a point several millimeters to 1 cm distal to the squamocolumnar mucosal junction. Since a measurement of 1 cm above the proximal end of the gastric folds indicates the expected site of a normally positioned squamocolumnar mucosal junction in patients with a hiatal hernia, it is easy to determine whether the junction is displaced proximally (Plate 18–14). The endoscopic features that aid in diagnosis of columnar-lined esophagus include the transverse fold or ridge that marks the esophagogastric muscular junction, the patulous lower esophageal sphincter region, the dislocated squamocolumnar junction, and absence of a lower esophageal mucosal "B" (Schatzki) ring.

With the use of these endoscopic landmarks, minimal degrees of metaplastic epithelial change in the distal esophagus can be suspected and confirmed by biopsy.[15] It is, therefore, not necessary to await development of the classic squamocolumnar junctional midesophageal migration in order to diagnose this condition. Columnar-lined esophagus often exists in patients with minimal symptoms and will not be diagnosed in such cases if considered only in relation to severe reflux symptoms or a midesophageal stricture.

The squamocolumnar junction is normally located within 1 cm of the proximal end of the gastric mucosal folds in a hiatal hernia (see Plates 18–6 and 18–14). Another landmark that can be used to assess its proximal dislocation is the transverse mucosal fold, the luminal marker for the level of the angle of His (which also corresponds to the gastric sling muscle and the esophagogastric muscular junction). This region is always quite patulous and easy to examine in patients with columnar-lined esophagus. Endoscope withdrawal reveals the columnar-lined segment to be relatively dilated but responsive to peristalsis or tertiary contractions. The displaced squamocolumnar junction may be found at any level in the esophagus. Directing the retroverted tip of the endoscope into the columnar-lined segment will demonstrate the displaced squamocolumnar mucosal junction from a different perspective (see Plate 18–14).

Identification of the squamocolumnar mucosal junction in normal patients and in those with the typical columnar-lined esophagus usually is not difficult because of differences in mucosal color and texture. The mucosal color in the columnar-lined segment is orange-red to red; the color usually is more reddish than that of normal gastric mucosa and is distinctly different from the pinkish-gray color of normal esophageal squamous mucosa (Plate 18–15). It may be impossible to locate precisely the squamocolumnar junction in the presence of severe esophagitis or a stricture. Close-up observation of the texture of columnar mucosa will reveal a pitted or villoid pattern without the small blood vessels that are typical of esophageal mucosa. Several biopsies of suspected columnar metaplasia will provide histologic proof of the diagnosis.[15-17] The exact location of the biopsies and the relation of these sites to surrounding landmarks should be recorded when the samples are obtained. Normal squamous esophageal mucosa is characterized by a smooth surface and many small vessels oriented parallel to the long axis of the lumen. The latter disappear at the junction between squamous and columnar epithelium and are not observed in areas of severe esophagitis. Several milliliters of Lugol's solution can be instilled to stain squamous epithelium a brownish black when the location

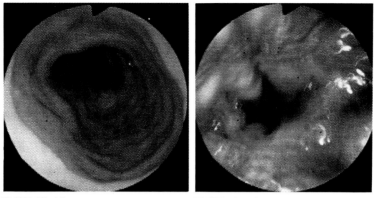

PLATE 18–15.   PLATE 18–16.

PLATE 18–15. Endoscopic view down columnar-lined esophagus from just proximal to the squamocolumnar mucosal junction, which was located at 23 cm. A portion of the displaced squamocolumnar mucosal junction is shown between the 6 and 9 o'clock positions.
PLATE 18–16. Lugol's iodine solution was used to stain the squamous side of the squamocolumnar junction in the patient shown in Plate 18-15. The mucosal junction is clearly demarcated at the junction of the reddish, unstained columnar epithelium with the darkly stained squamous epithelium. The lumen is narrowed somewhat by a tertiary contraction.

of the junction remains uncertain (Plate 18–16).[1]

The squamocolumnar mucosal junction can vary widely in location and appearance. It often has an undulating appearance with orange-red, finger-like cephalad extensions of metaplastic epithelium between downward directed peninsulas of squamous mucosa, the whole junction appearing asymmetric and interrupted (see Plate 18–14). There is a common tendency to attribute this appearance to esophagitis with erosion alone; however, in some cases the orange-red proximally directed streaks are due to metaplastic columnar epithelium at the site of previous linear erosions. On occasion isolated small islands of squamous epithelium will be scattered within the columnar-lined segment distal to the squamocolumnar mucosal junction (see Plate 18–14).

The endoscopic landmarks and topography described above should be used to avoid inaccurate diagnosis of columnar-lined esophagus. Over-diagnosis occurs when the mucosa in a hiatal hernia pouch is interpreted as being in the tubular esophagus. An adequate number of biopsy specimens and precise histologic interpretation usually avoid this misinterpretation. Under-diagnosis occurs with failure to recognize short segments of columnar mucosa lining the distal esophagus or failure to recognize the lining of most of the esophagus by columnar epithelium, the dislocated squamocolumnar junction being in the upper third of the esophagus.

This error is more likely when proximal esophagitis and stricture are absent, since when present these findings provide diagnostic clues to the location of the squamocolumnar junction.

ESOPHAGEAL ULCER

Deep, chronic ulcers of the esophagus in most instances indicate the presence of a columnar-lined esophagus. Such ulcers always occur at the squamocolumnar junction or distal to it and primarily involve the columnar epithelium. Instances of reflux-related ulceration in an esophageal segment totally lined by squamous epithelium have not been confirmed. Ulcers of this type in columnar-lined esophagus may have small islands of squamous mucosa located about their margins, but they are never surrounded entirely by squamous epithelium. Esophageal ulcers have the typical endoscopic features of a gastric ulcer and are prone to bleed or penetrate; these events often occur with minimal prior symptoms. Since adenocarcinoma occurs with increased frequency in columnar-lined esophagus, all ulcers and strictures should be evaluated with multiple biopsies and cytologic studies.[26, 27]

Stenosis due to reflux esophagitis is found in about 40% of patients with columnar-lined esophagus and always occurs at the squamocolumnar junction.[16, 17] However, stenosis is usually due to mucosal inflammation without submucosal injury and responds readily to peroral dilation. Because of this mucosal origin, a reflux stricture with columnar-lined esophagus can be observed to migrate over the years in the same way that the squamo-columnar mucosal junction migrates in a patient with inadequately treated reflux.

A stricture within the columnar-lined esophagus is uncommon but may be caused either by the fibrosis that results from ulcer healing or an invading carcinoma. It can occur at any level in the columnar-lined segment. The lumen of this segment typically is of normal or slightly larger diameter. Careful endoscopic observation permits detection of even minimal degrees of stenosis, mural rigidity, or asymmetry in lumen contour. Since reflux-related stricture occurs only at the squamocolumnar junction, any stenosis distal to the squamocolumnar junction in the columnar-lined segment can only be explained as secondary to submucosal fibrotic changes from a healed or active benign esophageal ulcer or as due to adenocarcinoma.

Since between 5% and 12% of patients with columnar-lined esophagus develop adenocarcinoma, most clinicians are recommending endoscopy screening examinations with biopsy and cytology at 1- to 2-year intervals.[16, 17, 26] Various aspects of this disorder are also discussed in Chapter 17.

Editor's note: References 28 and 29 are of interest in relation to peptic disease of the esophagus.

References

1. Nothmann BJ, Wright JR, Schuster MM. In vivo vital staining as an aid to identification of esophagogastric mucosal junction in man. Am J Dig Dis 1972; 17:919–24.
2. Gelfand DW, Ott DJ. Anatomy and technique in evaluating the esophagus. Semin Roentgenol 1981; 16:168–82.
3. Wolf BS. Sliding hiatal hernia: the need for redefinition. Am J Roentgenol Radium Ther Nucl Med 1973; 117:231–47.
4. Dagradi AE, Killeen RN, Schindler R. Esophageal hiatus sliding hernia: an endoscopic study. Gastroenterology 1958; 35:54–61.
5. Trujillo NP, Boyce HW Jr. Gastroscopy: aid to the detection of small sliding-type hiatal hernias. South Med J 1968; 61:1–4.
6. Trujillo NP, Slaughter RL, Boyce HW Jr. Endoscopic diagnosis of sliding-type diaphragmatic hiatal hernias. Am J Dig Dis 1968; 13:855–67.
7. Ortega JA. New criterion in the esophagoscopic diagnosis of sliding type hiatal hernia. Am J Gastroenterol 1972; 57:410–5.
8. Roesch W. Gastro-oesophageal reflux and hiatus hernia endoscopy. Postgrad Med J 1974; 50:199–201.
9. Dagradi AE. Endoscopic examination of the gastroesophageal area. Gastroint Endosc 1969; 15:175–7.
10. Jonsell G. The incidence of sliding hiatal hernias in patients with gastroesophageal reflux requiring operation. Acta Chir Scand 1983; 149:63–7.
11. Edwards DAW, Thompson H, Shaw DG, et al. Symposium on gastroesophageal reflux and its complications. Gut 1973; 14:233–53.
12. Ismail-Beigi F, Horton PF, Pope CE 2d. Histological consequences of gastroesophageal reflux in men. Gastroenterology 1970; 58:163–74.
13. Kobayashi S, Kasugai T. Endoscopic and biopsy criteria for the diagnosis of esophagitis with a fiberoptic esophagoscope. Am J Dig Dis 1974; 19:345–52.
14. Sonnenberg A, Lepsien G, Muller-Lissner SA, et al. When is esophagitis healed? Dig Dis Sci 1982; 27:297–302.
15. Paull A, Trier JS, Dalton MD, et al. The histologic spectrum of Barrett's esophagus. N Engl J Med 1976; 295:476–80.
16. Sjogren RW Jr, Johnson LF. Barrett's esophagus: a review. Am J Med 1983; 74:313–21.
17. Herlihy KJ, Orlando RC, Bryson JC, et al. Barrett's esophagus: clinical, endoscopic, histologic, manometric and electrical potential difference characteristics. Gastroenterology 1984; 86:436–43.
18. Winter HS, Madara JL, Stafford RF, et al. Intraepithelial eosinophils: a new diagnostic criterion for reflux esophagitis. Gastroenterology 1982; 83:818–23.
19. Johnson LF, DeMeester TR, Haggitt RC. Endoscopic signs for gastroesophageal reflux. J Clin Gastroenterol 1980; 2:387–99.
20. Wickbom G, Bushkin FL, Woodward ER. Alkaline reflux esophagitis. Surg Gynecol Obstet 1974; 139:267–71.
21. Pellegrini CA, DeMeester TR, Wernly JA, et al. Alkaline gastroesophageal reflux. Am J Surg 1978; 135:177–84.
22. Palmer ED. Subacute erosive ("peptic") esophagitis associated with achlorhydria. N Engl J Med 1960; 262:927–9.
23. Boyce HW Jr. Endoscopic diagnosis of hiatal hernia and related disorders. ASGE Postgraduate Course. Dallas, Texas, 1973.
24. Boyce HW Jr, Palmer ED. Techniques of clinical gastroenterology. Springfield: Charles C Thomas, 1975; 221–82.
25. Tulman AB, Boyce HW Jr. Complications of esophageal dilation and guidelines for their prevention. Gastrointest Endosc 1981; 27:229–34.
26. Naef AP, Savary M, Ozzello L. Columnar-lined lower esophagus: an acquired lesion with malignant predisposition. Report on 140 cases of Barrett's esophagus with 12 adenocarcinomas. J Thorac Cardiovasc Surg 1975; 70:826–35.
27. Haggitt RC, Tryzelaar J, Ellis FH, Colcher H. Adenocarcinoma complicating columnar epithelium-lined (Barrett's) esophagus. Am J Clin Pathol 1978; 70:1–5.
28. Kaul B, Halvorsen T, Petersen H, et al. Gastroesophageal reflux disease. Scintigraphic, endoscopic, and histologic considerations. Scand J Gastroenterol 1986; 21:134–8.
29. Berstad A, Weberg R, Fryshov-Larsen I, et al. Relationship of hiatus hernia to reflux esophagitis. A prospective study of coincidence, using endoscopy. Scand J Gastroenterol 1986; 21:55–8.

Chapter 19

SPECIAL VARIETIES OF ESOPHAGITIS

H. WORTH BOYCE, JR., M.D.

Esophagitis of varying degrees and clinical significance is caused by infections, chemical agents including drugs, and radiation injury and by epidermolysis bullosa, a rare hereditary disease. Idiopathic disorders such as eosinophilic gastroenteritis rarely have been associated with esophagitis. The more common of these relatively uncommon disorders will be discussed with emphasis on the role of endoscopy in their management.

Atypical cases of reflux esophagitis may cause confusion in diagnosis, especially when infection, chemical-induced esophagitis, or malignancy is superimposed upon changes caused by reflux. Reflux-related esophagitis is by far the most common inflammation of the esophagus. Its clinical, radiographic, and especially endoscopic-histologic features confirm the diagnosis without difficulty. A complete understanding and awareness of the spectrum of characteristic endoscopic changes of reflux as well as familiarity with important clinical clues are prerequisites for confirming the diagnosis of nonpeptic esophagitis. The endoscopic criteria for reflux-related acid-peptic and alkaline esophagitis are reviewed in Chapter 18.

ESOPHAGEAL INFECTIONS

Candida (Monilial) Esophagitis

The esophagus is the visceral organ most frequently infected by *Candida albicans*, and candidiasis caused by this agent is by far the most common infection of the esophagus. Kodsi et al.[1] reported a prospective study of the incidence of monilial esophagitis among 370 consecutive patients who underwent endoscopy for upper gastrointestinal symptoms. There were 27 cases (7%) of proved Candida esophagitis in this large series; 14 of these had symptoms of esophagitis. Others also have shown that this disease may appear without esophageal symptoms and various associated conditions considered in the past as necessary for the establishment of Candida infection.

The classic predisposing conditions for Candida infection include diabetes mellitus, malignancy and other chronic debilitating diseases, long-term therapy corticosteroids or antibiotics or both, and especially compromise of the immune system.[1, 2] In the absence of predisposing illness, Candida esophagitis is mainly a disease of the elderly. Kodsi's review suggests that any of three physiologic processes may play a role in the pathogenesis. The first is impaired immunity, the second is impaired esophageal motility, and the third is impaired carbohydrate metabolism associated with aging. Less than half the patients with esophagitis will have thrush, the oropharyngeal form of this infection.[3]

Dysphagia and odynophagia are the most common symptoms. Some patients complain only of an awareness of food passing down the esophagus; others have retrosternal pain with radiation to the scapular region or along the left of the lower thoracic spine. Malnutrition may result when these symptoms are severe or prolonged. The clinical syndrome plus findings on barium esophagram in the typical patient provide strong evidence for diagnosis. Although the barium esophagram is abnormal in many cases, the radiographic findings are variable and, by themselves, nondiagnostic.

It is surprising that the first report of the radiographic findings in Candida esophagitis was not published until 1956.[4] Radiographic abnormalities include motility disturbances manifested by diminished peristalsis, irritability, or spasm. The early mucosal changes of irregularity or granularity may progress to a shaggy appearance with edema and ulcerations. Focal accumulations of fungal debris may simulate varices or neoplasm. With progression of mural infection into the submucosa, edema becomes more apparent, ulceration may progress, and multiple sinuslike recesses or intramural pseudodiverticula may be demonstrated. This appearance has been likened to that of the colon wall in some severe cases of ulcerative colitis. Intramural infection may progress to stenosis due to edema and spasm or to frank fibrotic stricture.

The endoscopic appearance of Candida esophagitis ranges from an erythematous friable mucosa to complete covering of the mucosal surface by a heavy, shaggy, cream-colored to white pseudomembrane throughout the esophagus (Plates 19–1 and 19–2). The most common finding is the presence of cream-colored plaques scattered throughout the esophagus, usually with greater density in the lower two thirds. The mucosa just proximal to the squamocolumnar junction often is less involved. This plus the characteristic exudative plaques usually allow easy differentiation from reflux and other forms of esophagitis. However, when combined with other esophageal diseases, the endoscopic picture may not be typical.

The following grading scale for Candida esophagitis used by Kodsi and associates[1] nicely describes the stages of this infection: Grade I, a few raised white plaques up to 2 mm in size, with hyperemia but no edema or ulceration; Grade II, multiple raised white plaques greater than 2 mm in size, with hyperemia but no edema or ulceration (see Plate 19–1); Grade III, confluent linear and nodular elevated plaques, with hyperemia and frank ulceration; Grade IV, findings of Grade III plus increased friability of the mucous membranes and occasional narrowing of the lumen (see Plate 19–2).[1]

Because atypical surface changes often occur, direct smears of exudate from plaques or the mucosal surface as well as mucosal biopsies should be obtained for proper diagnosis. When ulcerations are present, mycelia usually can be demonstrated in biopsies of the ulcer base. Since routine hematoxylin and eosin stains demonstrate mycelia poorly, silver methenamine staining should be requested.

Esophagoscopy with collection of material using a brush-type endoscopic accessory for direct potassium hydroxide (KOH) smear is the procedure of choice for diagnosis.[1, 3] This rapid method for confirmation involves microscopic demonstration of mycelial forms in the exudate, which is mixed with a drop of 10% KOH solution under a cover slip. The pseudomycelia of Candida species also are readily identified on routinely stained cytology smears. Cultures do not differentiate between a commensal or infectious status for Candida and hence are of value only in species determination or for drug sensitivity testing. A serum agglutinin titer greater than 1:160 is considered confirmatory in patients with other evidence of Candida esophagitis.[1] This test is rarely positive at this titer in patients without other evidence of candidiasis.

Symptoms usually disappear with therapy, but clinical improvement does not necessarily indicate disappearance of the mucosal lesions. Endoscopy is necessary to confirm complete healing, although this is not essential in patients at average risk who have no residual symptoms after treatment.

Nystatin, 200,000 units, given as a combined gargle and swallow every 1 to 2 hours while the patient is awake has been the standard therapy and has had a good cure rate and low risk of side effects.[5] In patients not responding to nystatin, flucytosine has been used as a secondary drug at a dose of 100 mg per kg of body weight per day in divided doses after meals, for 4 to 6 weeks.

More recently, newer antifungal agents have been used successfully, especially in patients with severe nystatin-resistant infections or immunologic deficiency states. The latest preparation favored for this therapy is an imidazole compound, ketoconazole, which is said to be less toxic than amphotericin B, miconazole, and flucytosine.[6] However, there are several recent reports of anaphylaxis, some of which involved only a single dose of ketoconazole. Significant drug interactions also have been reported. Ketoconazole enhances the anticoagulant effect of coumadin-like drugs and increases blood levels of cyclosporin. For this reason, when ketoconazole is used with cyclosporin, blood levels of the latter should be monitored. The United States Food and Drug Administration (FDA)

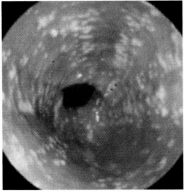 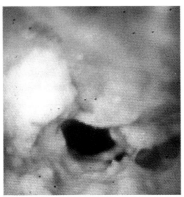 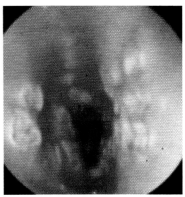

PLATE 19–1.   PLATE 19–2.   PLATE 19–3.

PLATE 19–1. Endoscopic view of monilial esophagitis showing typical focal, yellow-white plaques scattered over the mucosa. The degree of hyperemia around these plaques is highly variable.

PLATE 19–2. Endoscopic view of severe monilial esophagitis with thick exudate producing partial occlusion of the lumen.

PLATE 19–3. Multiple small ulcers typical of herpetic esophagitis are shown in this endoscopic view from the mid-esophagus. Two classic herpetic ulcers are shown to the left of the center, and multiple smaller ulcers in a linear orientation are shown on the opposite side. Distal to this level, small lesions have coalesced to form larger ulcers.

recently has stated that ketoconazole is valuable therapy for serious systemic fungal infections, provided that patients are carefully monitored. It is well absorbed when taken orally and is given as a single daily dose of 200 mg for 2 weeks. Ketoconazole should not be used for initial therapy of monilial esophagitis and is best reserved for cases associated with severe systemic disease that have not responded to nystatin.

Herpetic Esophagitis

Until recent years most reports of proven herpes virus (simplex or zoster) and cytomegalovirus infections of the esophagus ap-

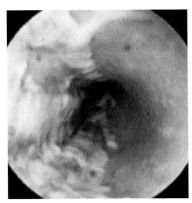 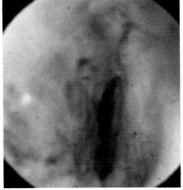 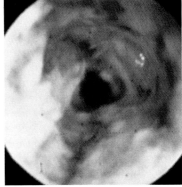

PLATE 19–4.   PLATE 19–5.   PLATE 19–6.

PLATE 19–4. Endoscopic view of corrosive injury of the esophageal mucosa due to lye ingestion. Hyperemia without exudate, erosion, or ulceration, visible on the right side, is compatible with first-degree injury. Exudate, patches of hyperemia, and some petechiae, seen on the left side, indicative of second-degree injury.

PLATE 19–5. Endoscopic view of severe inflammatory stenosis at the level atrium (30 to 35 cm) caused by potassium chloride formulated in a wax matrix (Slo K). The patient had cardiomegaly and left atrial enlargement that compressed the esophagus.

PLATE 19–6. Endoscopic view of severe inflammation, ulceration and fibrosis that resulted in a very tight stricture at the level of the aortic arch (23 cm). The squamous mucosa below the stricture was entirely normal to the squamocolumnar mucosal junction at 38 cm. Quinidine gluconate was the drug responsible.

peared in postmortem studies.[7-11] In the report of Nash and Ross[9] on 3000 consecutive autopsies, herpes esophagitis was found in 0.4%. When only patients with malignancy are considered, the overall incidence increases to almost 4%.[9]

Fiberoptic endoscopy is recognized as the most reliable diagnostic method for this condition, and there is an increasing number of reports of antemortem diagnosis of herpetic esophagitis.[12-16] When it occurs in an otherwise healthy person, the clinical course is so short that response to symptomatic therapy may occur before referral for endoscopic evaluation. Until the advent of fiberoptic endoscopy, relatively few cases were documented in persons without predisposing conditions.[12, 14] The most common occurrence is in hospitalized, immunosuppressed, and preterminal patients with or without malignancy.[7, 11, 17]

The classic presentation is that of a patient, gravely ill as a result of a malignancy, with severe dysphagia, odynophagia, and retrosternal pain. Usually monilial esophagitis is first suspected, but this diagnosis should be questioned when there is no response to nystatin or other antifungal therapy. Such patients should have further endoscopic and biopsy evaluation to confirm the etiology of the symptoms before proceeding to administration of the more toxic drugs used for resistant monilial esophagitis such as amphotericin B.

Physical examination may reveal either oral mucosal or vesicular skin lesions, or both, of herpes simplex or herpes zoster. Herpes simplex is much more commonly the infectious agent. When oral or cutaneous lesions are present, confirmation of their viral etiology should be attempted. Some patients may present with a mild, febrile, viral illness syndrome. Rosen and Hajdu[8] have reported that the esophagus was the only organ affected in 72% of cases.

Radiographic examination by barium esophagram is not adequate for specific diagnosis, although distinct abnormalities may be seen. Findings include multiple, diffuse, small, nodular filling defects; mucosal edema; numerous small ulcers; and irregular, vertically oriented plaque-like projections.[18, 19] These changes stop abruptly at the esophagogastric junction. Some radiologists regard air contrast esophagography as the preferred examination.[18] The radiographic findings may be identical to those of monilial

esophagitis. Further examination by esophagoscopy with cytologic study and biopsy is usually necessary for diagnosis.

Esophagoscopy may reveal diffuse, segmental, or focal involvement.[12, 14-16] The classic early lesion is a small (less than 5 mm) papule or vesicle that ultimately ulcerates (Plate 19–3). The mucosa surrounding this lesion is erythematous, but that between lesions may be normal in the early stages. The ulcers are round, with margins that are distinct and elevated above the plane of the mucosa. The base of the ulcer is covered with white to yellow exudate. As ulcers enlarge they may coalesce with the resulting larger ulceration, tending to be linear and oriented in the long axis of the esophagus. With severe involvement, part or all of the esophagus may be covered with a thick exudate, and therefore there may be no discrete ulcerations to provide a clue to the etiology. There is a tendency for ulcerations in the distal esophagus to be larger or to coalesce more readily than in other esophageal areas, suggesting a possible potentiation of the virus-induced ulceration by material refluxed from the stomach.

There is one report of severe bleeding from the distal esophagus in a patient with herpetic esophagitis proved by viral culture and cytology.[15] Esophageal manometry 4 weeks later revealed a hypotensive lower esophageal sphincter and absent peristalsis in the distal 7 cm of the esophagus. It was not determined whether the low sphincter pressure and abnormal motility permitted enhanced mucosal injury via reflux or whether viral esophagitis led to the reduced sphincter pressure and a motility disorder.

Active herpetic infection is best demonstrated in the relatively intact epithelium adjacent to the ulcer margin, and thus this area is the preferred site for biopsy.[9, 10, 14] The ulcers typically are shallow and do not penetrate the muscularis mucosa. The ulcer bed contains acute and chronic inflammatory cells, fibrin, and necrotic debris devoid of the microscopic findings characteristic of herpes infections. In some cases concomitant herpes and monilial invasion of the tissue may be demonstrated.[16]

Confirmation of viral esophagitis requires the use of accessory techniques. Positive viral culture of biopsy material, biopsy revealing the diagnostic eosinophilic intranuclear inclusions (Cowdry type A bodies), or cytologic smears showing multinucleated epithelial cells with ground glass changes in the nuclei will confirm the diagnosis of herpes simplex infection. The discrete intranuclear inclusions are often surrounded by a clear halo, intranuclear vacuoles may be present, and the nucleus may have a ground glass appearance, with disposition of chromatin beneath the nuclear membrane.[9, 10] Ultrastructural study by electron microscopy may demonstrate the virus within epithelial cells. Cytomegalovirus esophagitis is reported to have distinctive histologic features that permit differentiation from herpetic esophagitis.[20]

Serologic confirmation of acute herpetic infection also may be obtained by observing a fourfold rise in complement-fixing antibody to HSV-1 in the patient's serum. The opportunity for serologic, cytologic, or biopsy confirmation decreases rapidly 48 hours after the onset of the lesion.[14] Endoscopic observations may provide the only clue to the diagnosis in at least one half of the cases.

After confirmation of the diagnosis, appropriate therapy consists of supportive measures such as liquid-to-soft diet, topical anesthesia with viscous Xylocaine or an antacid-anesthetic combination, and analgesics as needed. The symptoms abate and the lesions heal within 7 to 21 days, usually in less than 14 days.[14] In severe cases of herpes simplex and herpes zoster infections diagnosed antemortem, especially in high-risk immunocompromised patients, the use of agents such as acyclovir and adenine arabinoside may prove effective.[17, 21]

Bacterial Esophagitis

Infectious esophagitis may be caused by a number of organisms and is an uncommonly suspected diagnosis.[22] The following organisms have been reported as responsible for acute esophagitis, usually in patients with other severe diseases: group A beta-hemolytic streptococcal infection as diffuse phlegmonous esophagitis when submucosa and muscularis propria are involved (also called esophagitis dissecans superficialis and esophagitis exfoliativa in older reports)[22]; mixed bacterial infections[23]; lactobacillus acidophilus infection.[24] Cultures should be taken in any case of esophagitis that is lacking the clinical and endoscopic criteria to satisfy the diagnosis of reflux or chemical injury. This practice is especially important in immunocompromised patients.

In the case of acute streptococcal esophagitis reported by Howlett,[25] barium radiography showed only some mucosal irregularity in the distal esophagus. Endoscopy revealed marked exudative inflammation throughout, which was more severe in the proximal esophagus. The response to penicillin therapy was dramatic and complete. According to the observations reported with these rare forms of bacterial esophagitis, there are no distinctive morphologic features to aid in endoscopic diagnosis.

CHEMICAL-INDUCED ESOPHAGITIS

Corrosive Esophagitis

Esophageal injuries due to corrosive ingestion, either accidental or suicidal, have been recognized for at least 200 years. Although once fashionable among those with suicidal intent, corrosive ingestion has become recognized as a poor method to end one's life. Often the consequence is either no esophageal damage at all or significant nonfatal esophageal injury that leads to chronic, painful, costly, and regrettable suffering for the patient.

In 1927 the United States Federal Caustic Act became law and has helped reduce accidental esophageal injury in the United States. However, potent corrosive chemical agents, although modified, and with improved labeling and packaging, still are readily available.[26] The stage is set for this horrible injury to occur if suicide is the goal, the patient is in an alcoholic stupor, or careless adults allow children access to toxic substances.

There has been much debate over the pathogenesis of and early therapy for corrosive injuries.[27-33] The site and extent of injury and the tissue effect produced by caustic agents vary primarily with the type of ingestant (liquid, paste, powder, or solid), the amount ingested, and the duration of tissue contact. Alkaline agents such as lye or concentrated sodium hydroxide dissolve tissues by liquefaction necrosis and may diffuse rapidly through several layers. In contrast, acids produce coagulation necrosis, a tissue response that tends to limit depth of penetration and possibly the risk of perforation. As a rule, alkaline agents tend to injure the esophagus more than the stomach, and vice versa for acid substances. Because of the ever-changing compositions of commonly used corrosive agents such as drain cleaners, it is recommended that physicians contact a poison control center for information before making major decisions on diagnosis and therapy for ingestion of a suspected corrosive substance.

Patients who claim or are suspected to have ingested a corrosive agent should be evaluated carefully. The clinical presentation varies from asymptomatic to profound shock, either severe chest or abdominal pain or both, and signs of infection. Chemical injury to the lips or oropharyngeal mucosa is not reliable, either by its presence or absence, as an indicator of the existence or extent of esophageal injury. Early endoscopy (within 24 hours) provides the most precise diagnosis. Older reports warn of perforation when rigid endoscopes are used, but recent experience with small-diameter, forward-viewing fiberoptic endoscopes does not indicate an increased risk when precautions are taken.

After initial assessment and supportive care, an esophagram should be obtained in patients suspected by history and physical examination of having esophageal or gastric injuries. A water-soluble contrast medium is generally recommended. Radiography alone is inadequate to assess such injury. When there is no clinical or radiographic evidence of perforation, mediastinitis, or peritonitis, it is reasonable to proceed with endoscopy unless contraindicated. In addition to signs of perforation, contraindications include severe respiratory distress with pharyngeal edema and necrosis, shock, and the nonavailability of a physician experienced in endoscopy.

Concern about proper therapy and potential complications can be resolved in many cases of questionable ingestion or minor injury by a complete endoscopic examination of the esophagus, stomach, and proximal duodenum. The procedure can be performed in nearly all adult patients and most older children, following the standard sedative-analgesic premedication for routine endoscopy. The endoscope should be passed under direct vision with careful examination of all visible mucosa from mouth to proximal duodenum, using as little insufflated air as possible to achieve an adequate examination. The location and extent of all injuries should be recorded with precision. Upon completion of the gastroscopy, as much air as possible should be aspirated via the endoscope.

The grading of degree of injury is difficult, especially when endoscopy is delayed beyond the first 24 hours. There are, however, some criteria that have proved helpful over the years.

Mucosal hyperemia and edema without exudate or ulcerations, exhibiting minimal or no friability upon contact with the endoscope, is classified as first-degree injury (Plate 19–4). Although a few small erosions may be present, there is no significant bleeding. This degree of injury is confined to mucosa and consequently not associated with stricture formation or other major complications.

The main difficulty in relating diagnosis to prognosis occurs with second-degree injuries (see Plate 19–4), in which inflammation with erosions, exudate, friability, bleeding, and esophageal spasm are seen more often. More advanced stages of second-degree injury show ulcers, more extensive bleeding and exudate, and areas suggestive of necrotic mucosa with impending mucosal slough. Differentiation between advanced second-degree and third-degree injuries is difficult. Prognosis is indefinite for this stage, but therapy probably should be the same as for third-degree injuries, since endoscopic interpretation of the precise depth of injury is imprecise.

The patient who has signs of mediastinitis, peritonitis, pneumomediastinum, pleural effusion, or tracheoesophageal fistula obviously has a third-degree injury. Other procedures, namely surgical-therapeutic maneuvers, may be more appropriate than endoscopy for acute management. Endoscopic findings include large areas of mucosal slough with hemorrhage and areas of gray to black membrane formation with the appearance of an eschar. The lumen may be almost completely closed by edema, or it can be dilated without evidence of tone or peristalsis, a sign of deep mural injury. There may be normal areas or the entire esophagus may be involved. When these ominous findings are first detected, the examiner may proceed cautiously, with minimal insufflation of air as long as visualization is adequate. It is helpful to know the precise extent of injury to stomach and duodenum as well, if complete endoscopic examination is possible. The object is to obtain a rapid but thorough assessment with minimal risk of endoscopic-related aggravation of the underlying pathologic process.

Radiographic contrast studies may be desirable after the patient's condition has stabilized during the first several days post-injury. Radiographic findings are not reliable with milder injury, but usually reveal to some extent abnormalities caused by second- and third-degree injuries. Detailed radiographic findings have been reviewed by Franken[34] and Muhletaler et al.[35]

Accurate diagnosis of the degree and extent of corrosive injury permit confident conclusions with regard to prognosis, natural history, and methods of therapy. Only supportive care and follow-up recommendations are needed for cases of accidental ingestion without any detectable mucosal injury. Patients with no mucosal injury who attempted suicide should be hospitalized for observation and psychiatric evaluation.

Patients with identifiable mucosal injury of the pharynx, respiratory tract, esophagus, stomach, or duodenum should be hospitalized. Supportive care should be consonant with the degree of injury, and early surgical consultation should be included as appropriate. A nasogastric tube, used early in the course for aspiration and later for enteric feeding, should be placed promptly after endoscopy. The duration of time the tube should remain in place and the appropriate time to begin feeding vary and should be determined according to the type of injury and the patient's general status. An indwelling nasogastric tube preserves access to the stomach for future dilation.

The role of corticosteroid and antibiotic therapy in corrosive injury has not been established by controlled studies in humans.[29, 30] Animal studies suggest that steroids might be helpful if given before the damaging agent is ingested;[36, 37] however, since corticosteroids cannot be given before injury in humans, are of unproven value, and may enhance the progression of septic complications, we avoid their use.

The use of antibiotics appears rational in patients with second- and third-degree injuries to minimize the risks of local and systemic sequelae of the bacterial infections that develop soon after these injuries. Various antibiotics have been recommended but no regimen has proved superior in humans. The goal is to provide antibiotic coverage initially for those organisms usually found in the oropharynx that will most likely contaminate the area of injury.

Once the extent and course of the injury is determined, early peroral dilation should be considered.[22, 27, 38] At the latest, this should be begun within 7 to 10 days post-injury in those patients without extraesophageal complications. Dilation should be performed under fluoroscopic control without force. The starting time for dilation in patients with complicated third-degree injuries must be determined on an individual basis. However, these patients are very likely to develop severe stricture, usually by the third week, so

that earlier rather than delayed dilation is desirable. The details of peroral dilation technique and frequency are reported elsewhere.[38, 39] In cases of severe or neglected esophageal injury, retrograde dilation with Tucker dilators is the safest and most effective therapy.[32, 38] Technical aspects of esophageal dilation are also discussed in Chapter 18. The use of esophageal stents has been evaluated for prevention of strictures in infants and children and appears to be effective in the small number of cases reported thus far.[31–33]

Long-term follow-up must take into consideration the tendency for severe strictures to recur and the increased risk of squamous cell carcinoma after many years.[40, 41]

Drug-Induced Esophagitis ("Pill Esophagitis")

Although more than 25 drugs are recognized as causes of over 220 reported cases of drug-induced esophagitis, this potentially lethal disorder is little known among primary care physicians and many specialists. Pill esophagitis was first reported in 1970 by Pemberton.[42] Kikendall et al.[43] have presented an excellent review of the subject.

Ordinarily, little thought is given to instructing patients in the proper way to swallow medications that are in solid form, either tablet or capsule. The delay in passage of tablets through the esophagus under the influence of recumbency and a small volume of fluid was amply demonstrated by Evans and Roberts.[44] They found a delay in passage of an aspirin-size barium tablet through the esophagus beyond 5 minutes in over 50% of subjects when in the recumbent position. The message is clear—avoid low fluid volume and recumbency when taking any solid form of medication.[45]

The more commonly used drugs that have caused esophageal injury include potassium chloride tablets (especially the wax matrix form such as Slo K), tetracycline, doxycycline, clindamycin, emepronium bromide, quinidine gluconate (Quinaglute), ferrous sulfate, and ascorbic acid.[42, 43, 46–50] The drug formulation appears to be an important factor in the potential for delayed passage and mucosal injury. For instance, doxycycline capsules have been shown to remain in the esophagus three times as frequently as tablets of the same compound.[49] The size of the tablet or capsule is important as well. Three of our last five cases of pill esophagitis have been severe esophageal strictures at the level of the aortic arch in patients taking quinidine gluconate. This tablet is 13 mm in diameter.

Common factors in the genesis of this form of esophagitis are esophageal "physiologic" narrowing at the level of the aortic arch, obstruction, disordered esophageal motility, or any combination of these. In the absence of obstruction, the patient usually gives a history of taking the medicine while in a recumbent position or without sufficient liquid just before retiring at night. The obstructive problem that seems to enhance the development of drug-induced injury most often is esophageal stenosis due to inflammation. Drug-induced esophagitis may also be associated with esophageal motor abnormalities such as esophageal spasm or with left atrial enlargement, which may cause compression and partial occlusion of the esophageal lumen. The most common contributory factors are ingestion of the drug without adequate fluid, recumbency immediately after ingestion, tablets or capsules of large size, and the chemical composition of the drug.

The pill-taking habits of the patient are a vital aspect of the history in suspected cases. Certain diseases and their related therapy suggest the diagnosis and site of injury. The patient with cardiomegaly and left atrial enlargement typically sustains esophageal injury from potassium chloride or quinidine at a level 30 to 35 cm from the incisor teeth, that is, at the level of esophageal compression by the enlarged left atrium (Plate 19–5). The person without intrinsic esophageal disease or cardiomegaly will more often develop pill esophagitis from transient impaction of drugs at the level of the aortic arch (22 to 24 cm) or proximally (Plate 19–6). The teenager with acne or the traveler (probably a physician) trying to prevent diarrhea typically presents with a lesion in the proximal esophagus caused by doxycycline. The patient with arthritis may develop esophagitis from aspirin, naproxen, indomethacin, or other anti-inflammatory drugs. In Great Britain a major cause of pill esophagitis is the drug emepronium bromide, an agent used to treat urinary frequency. In patients with reflux esophagitis, it is important to remember that drug-induced injury may aggravate, or render atypical, the lesions of this disorder.

Over 22 drugs have been reported to cause esophageal injury. It is likely that injury is asymptomatic in most cases. The classic symptoms are odynophagia (74%), continuous retrosternal pain (72%), dysphagia (20%), or combinations of these symptoms. Elderly patients may have dysphagia alone, and often drug-induced esophagitis and stenosis are never considered in the differential diagnosis. Our most recent five patients have complained of severe dysphagia without odynophagia or chest pain and were considered to be suffering from occult malignancy because of their ages and the location and radiographic appearance of the stenotic lesions. The history suggested the correct diagnosis in all five. Three were taking quinidine gluconate (Quinaglute) and had strictures at the aortic level; the fourth was taking potassium chloride and quinine sulfate in tablet form, and the fifth potassium chloride (Slo-K). The latter had a stricture at 30 cm, the level of his enlarged atrium. With continued ingestion of the offending drug, the esophageal injury may extend proximally from the original stenosis, thereby making diagnosis and therapy more difficult and increasing the risk of severe injury. Potassium chloride injury has been the most lethal, with at least nine deaths resulting from either ulceration with bleeding, perforation or mediastinal abscess, and from the long-term effects of severe esophageal stricture.[46]

Barium contrast radiography may provide clues by demonstrating esophageal stenosis or ulceration, but these findings are misleading unless drug-induced injury is suspected from the history. The atypical location of such injury in the region of the aortic arch or opposite an enlarged left atrium in patients without known prior esophageal disease should suggest drug-induced injury or malignancy. Reflux-related lesions do not occur at either of these levels unless a columnar-lined esophagus is present. Double contrast radiography may provide more detail, but without a proper history accurate diagnosis is unlikely.

Documentation of drug-induced esophagitis requires esophagoscopy. The findings vary but may include one or more of the following: a focal area of marked edema and erythema, usually with some degree of mucosal erosion covered by a pseudomembrane or exudative plaque; "punched out" ulceration, possibly with "kissing" type ulcers on opposite walls; and either inflammatory stenosis or stricture (see Plate 19–5). Instances of prolonged and repeated injury manifest longer segments of inflammation, ulceration, and fibrosis, findings most often diagnosed as probably malignant in nature but with negative findings by biopsy (see Plate 19–6). There are no endoscopic characteristics helpful for diagnosis other than the focal nature of the lesion, its atypical location, or its occurrence just proximal to an area of esophageal stenosis. Residual particles of the medication at a stricture may provide a clue to diagnosis.[47]

The chemical properties of the medication, as well as the duration of mucosal contact, are important factors in the degree of esophageal injury. In most cases therapy is simple. Ingestion of the possibly offending drug (tablet or capsule) should be stopped at least until the evaluation is completed. The medication may be resumed if neither stenosis nor motility disorder is present, provided the patient uses ample fluid and remains upright after swallowing and uses a liquid form, crushes the tablet, or empties the contents of capsules into a suitable liquid for ingestion. Inflammatory erosion and stenosis may resolve with such changes in dosing procedure, but strictures usually require peroral dilation over variable periods of time. A complete evaluation of strictures by endoscopy and biopsy to eliminate an occult neoplasm or other lesion as the reason for the pill impaction is absolutely essential.

All patients, especially those bedridden and those with esophageal motor disorders or esophageal stenosis of any type, must be warned regarding the danger of ingesting any medication in the recumbent position or with insufficient amounts of liquid immediately before going to bed. All patients should be advised to take all tablets or capsules with at least two ounces of fluid and then to remain in the upright position for at least 10 minutes. For patients who are bedridden, larger volumes of fluid should be given or liquid forms of drugs should be prescribed.

Radiation Esophagitis

Radiation-induced esophagitis is usually the result of mediastinal irradiation for bronchogenic carcinoma. Less common causes include irradiation for metastatic breast and testicular carcinoma, lymphoma, and primary squamous cell carcinoma. The dosage and rate of exposure that cause symptomatic esophagitis vary, but most patients have received between 2500 and 6000 rads. The natural history of this condition is not well understood.

The clinical syndrome associated with radiation injury is manifested primarily as dysphagia, odynophagia, and spontaneous chest pain. The barium contrast esophagram demonstrates no morphologic abnormality in most cases, and altered esophageal motility is the most frequently noted abnormality.[51, 52] Early in the course the dysphagia seems to be due primarily to edema and motor disturbances, but from 3 to 18 months after therapy a stricture usually will be found. The proximal end of the stricture typically is smooth and tapers gradually. Angulation of the lumen at the level of the stricture may be due to radiation effects, adherence of the esophagus to adjacent mediastinal structures, or recurrent neoplasm.

In some patients esophagoscopy may help to explain symptoms or uncertain findings on radiographic study. The nature of the mucosal changes found by endoscopy depends on the dosage, rate, and duration of therapy, and perhaps other factors such as prior or concomitant administration of chemotherapeutic agents that may enhance irradiation effects.[53] Infection by *Candida albicans* or herpes viruses may be superimposed. The endoscopic appearance of the mucosa may include hyperemia, friability, erosions, or ulceration and exudate. If the patient survives several years, telangiectatic vessels may be seen in the mucosa in the field of irradiation. Biopsy reveals nonspecific acute and chronic inflammation. Special stains for monilial pseudohyphae and a search for cellular changes of viral esophagitis should be included in the evaluation. The possibility of recurrent malignancy must always be considered when interpreting endoscopic findings.

When the condition is acute, therapy consists first of modifying the irradiation dosage and rate of subsequent treatments. Supportive care including dietary modifications with topical anesthetics and/or analgesics before meals and at bedtime usually is adequate for the limited course of this disorder.

The best therapy for post-irradiation stricture is peroral dilation.[38] A more gradual dilation program may be required for this type of stricture, because the esophageal stenosis is very firm and more elongated than strictures due to reflux. The Eder-Puestow or Savary dilators passed over a guide wire are the best instruments for the initial dilation program in such cases. Later, Maloney dilators usually are adequate for maintenance of patency. Nelson et al.[54] found intramural hydrocortisone injected via a transendoscopic needle to be helpful as a supplement to peroral dilation in more resistant cases.

Stasis Esophagitis

In some patients with chronic esophageal obstruction, a significant amount of residual food material and medications may remain in contact with esophageal mucosa for days. The classic example is achalasia. The mucosa becomes irritated to such an extent that visible changes are evoked. These appear as patchy areas of hyperemia, rarely with any erosion or ulceration. These findings may be widely scattered but tend to be prominent in the most distal esophagus, probably because retained material remains longest in contact with the mucosa in this region. Histologically, the alterations are non-specific, and biopsy is not helpful unless a more significant abnormality such as early malignancy is suspected.

NON-SPECIFIC ESOPHAGITIS

Eosinophilic Esophagitis

Eosinophilic esophagitis has been reported as a component of the eosinophilic gastroenteritis syndrome.[55–57] Eosinophilic gastroenteritis is an uncommon disorder characterized by peripheral eosinophilia, infiltration of the stomach or small intestine, and symptoms related to the site and severity of involvement. Up to one half the patients have either a history of allergy or specific food intolerance.[58] The clinical presentation correlates with the layer of the gut wall that is predominantly involved. Bleeding and malabsorption are prominent with mucosal disease; obstruction occurs with involvement of muscularis propria; and eosinophilic ascites, the rarest form, occurs with serosal disease. Dysphagia is the primary symptom associated with esophageal involvement and may be caused by disturbed motility or stenosis.[55, 57]

The diagnosis is suspected on the basis of symptoms plus peripheral eosinophilia. Barium contrast radiography reveals evidence of gut wall infiltration. Thickening and rigidity, mucosal nodules, and stenosis may be seen.[57]

In a case reported by Picus and Frank[57] there was a severe stricture at 24 cm from the incisors. A small-diameter pediatric endoscope would not pass the stricture. The mucosa at the proximal margin of the stricture was ulcerated, and a 3 mm polyp was removed at that level. Microscopic study of

this and the biopsy specimen revealed edema and eosinophilic infiltration of mucosa and submucosa.

Corticosteroid therapy usually provides objective and symptomatic improvement but may be required on a chronic basis. Residual stricture of the esophagus is managed by peroral dilation.

Epidermolysis Bullosa

Epidermolysis bullosa is an uncommon, inherited disorder that appears clinically in three forms. The simple type is transmitted as an autosomal dominant, is characterized by subepithelial bullae after minor trauma, rarely involves mucous membranes, subsides at puberty and makes up about 45% of cases. The hyperplastic dystrophic form is transmitted by a single autosomal gene of high penetrance and accounts for about 30% of cases. It is characterized by deep and superficial cutaneous bullae and involves mucous membranes in 20% of cases.[59] The most serious and least common form of this disease, polydysplastic epidermolysis bullosa, appears at birth and worsens with age as a mutilating and potentially fatal process. Any part of the body, including the esophagus, may be involved.

Esophageal involvement may occur at any time. It is more common in males than females and may result in aspiration, hemorrhage, malnutrition, perforation rarely, and possibly an increased risk of carcinoma with prolonged disease. Dysphagia and odynophagia, alone or together, are the prominent symptoms of esophageal involvement. Dysphagia does not necessarily indicate stricture and may be due to spasm and pain in the presence of vesicles, ulceration, or both.[60–62]

Barium contrast radiography can reveal disordered motility, mucosal nodules, ulcers, or stenosis. Stenosis, initially due to inflammation and later to true strictures, is found in the upper third of the esophagus in about half the cases, in the distal third in about 25%, and at multiple sites in 25%. Diffuse stricturing is distinctly uncommon. When multiple, the strictured segments usually are from 2 to 5 cm in length.

The indication for esophagoscopy should be carefully evaluated in each patient. Since there appears to be, based on older reports, an increased risk of perforation, it has been suggested that esophagoscopy is best performed when the disease is relatively quiescent or under control with corticosteroid therapy.[59] Such decisions depend to a great extent on the patient's need for relief of dysphagia.

Esophagoscopy should be performed with a flexible, small-caliber, forward-viewing fiberoptic endoscope, using direct observation throughout introduction and removal to minimize mucosal trauma. Multiple mucosal bullae of variable size are present in active disease and are easily ruptured. The mucosa is friable and granulation tissue may be seen at sites of earlier disease activity. With continued activity, the mucosa may become atrophic and scarred, such changes leading eventually to strictures that require dilation.

In addition to peroral dilation for strictures and topical anesthetics for relief of pain, dietary modifications minimize the inevitable malnutrition that will develop if these measures are not instituted. Corticosteroid therapy is helpful in some cases. Severe strictures may be unresponsive to peroral dilation. Esophagectomy with colon interposition has been reported as dramatically effective in two brothers with severe strictures.[63] Such treatment should only be advised when proper peroral dilation has failed and expert surgical help is available.

Editor's note: References 64 to 67 are recent publications that pertain to unusual types of esophagitis.

References

1. Kodsi B, Wickremesinghe PC, Kozinn PJ, et al. Candida esophagitis. A prospective study of 27 cases. Gastroenterology 1976; 71:715–9.
2. Eras P, Goldstein MJ, Sherlock P. Candida infection of the gastrointestinal tract. Medicine 1972; 51:367–79.
3. Sheft DJ, Shrago G. Esophageal moniliasis. The spectrum of the disease. JAMA 1970; 213:1859–62.
4. Andren L, Theander G. Roentgenographic appearances of esophageal moniliasis. Acta Radiol 1956; 46:571–4.
5. Kantrowitz PA, Fleischli DJ, Butler WT. Successful treatment of chronic esophageal moniliasis with a viscous suspension of nystatin. Gastroenterology 1969; 57:424–30.
6. Gregory DW, Blackburn WD, Madhavan SV, et al. Esophageal candidiasis: treatment with ketoconazole. South Med J 1983; 76:1307–8.
7. Pearce JA, Dagradi A. Acute ulceration of the esophagus with associated intranuclear inclusion bodies. Arch Pathol 1943; 35:889–97.
8. Rosen P, Hajdu SI. Visceral herpes virus infections in a patient with cancer. Am J Clin Pathol 1971; 56:459–65.
9. Nash G, Ross JS. Herpetic esophagitis. A common cause of esophageal ulceration. Hum Pathol 1974; 5:339–45.
10. Lasser A. Herpes simplex virus esophagitis. Acta Cytol 1977; 21:301–2.
11. Berg JW. Esophageal herpes: complication of cancer therapy. Cancer 1955; 8:731–40.
12. Depew WT, Prentice RSA, Beck IT, et al. Herpes simplex ulceration esophagitis in a healthy subject. Am J Gastroenterol 1977; 68:381–5.
13. Owensby LC, Stammer JL. Esophagitis associated with herpes simplex infection in an immunocompromised host. Gastroenterology 1978; 74:1305–6.
14. Springer DJ, DaCosta LR, Beck IT. A syndrome of acute self-limiting ulcerative esophagitis in young adults probably due to herpes simplex virus. Dig Dis Sci 1979; 24:535–9.
15. Fishbein PG, Tuthill R, Kressel H, et al. Herpes simplex esophagitis: A cause of upper-gastrointestinal bleeding. Dig Dis Sci 1979; 24:540–4.
16. Brayko CM, Kozarek RA, Sanowski RA, Lanard BJ. Type I herpes simplex esophagitis with concomitant esophageal moniliasis. J Clin Gastroenterol 1982; 4:351–5.
17. Whitley R, Barton N, Collins E, et al. Mucocutaneous herpes simplex virus infections in immunocompromised patients. A model for evaluation of topical antiviral agents. (Suppl) Am J Med 1982; 73:236–40.
18. Skucas J, Schrank WW, Meyers PC, Lee CS. Herpes esophagitis: a case studied by air-contrast esophagography. Am J Roentgenol 1977; 128:497–9.
19. Meyers C, Durkin MG, Love L. Radiographic findings in herpetic esophagitis. Radiology 1976; 119:21–2.
20. Toghill RJ, McGaughey M. Cytomegalovirus esophagitis. Br Med J 1972; 2:294.
21. Whitley RJ, Soong SJ, Dolin R, et al. Adenine arabinoside therapy of biopsy-proved herpes simplex encephalitis. National Institute of Allergy and Infectious Diseases collaborative antiviral study. N Engl J Med 1977; 297:289–94.
22. Palmer ED. The Esophagus and Its Diseases. New York: Hoeber, 1952; 242.
23. Givler RL. Esophageal lesions in leukemia and lymphoma. Am J Dig Dis 1970; 15:31–6.
24. McManus JPA, Webb JN. A yeast-like infection of the esophagus caused by Lactobacillus acidophilus. Gastroenterology 1975; 68:583–6.
25. Howlett SA. Acute streptococcal esophagitis. Gastrointest Endosc 1979; 25:150–1.
26. Leape LL. Liquid lye—still a hazard. (Correspondence) N Engl J Med 1971; 284:1443–4.
27. Salzer H. Frühbehandlung der Speiserohrenveratzung. Wien klin Wochenschr 1920; 33:307.
28. Palmer ED. Esophagitis due to corrosive agents. In: Palmer ED. The Esophagus and Its Diseases. New York: Hoeber, 1952; 288.
29. Webb WR, Koutras P, Ecker RR, et al. An evaluation of steroids and antibiotics in caustic burns of the esophagus. Ann Thorac Surg 1970; 9:95–102.
30. Haller JA Jr, Andrews HG, White JJ, et al. Pathophysiology and management of acute corrosive burns of the esophagus: results of treatment in 285 children. J Pediatr Surg 1971; 6:578–84.
31. Reyes HM, Lin CY, Schlunk FF, et al. Experimental treatment of corrosive esophageal burns. J Pediatr Surg 1974; 9:317–27.
32. Tucker JA, Yarington CT Jr. The treatment of caustic ingestion. Otolaryngol Clin North Am 1979; 12:343–50.
33. Hill JL, Norberg HP, Smith MD, et al. Clinical technique and success of the esophageal stent to

prevent corrosive strictures. J Pediatr Surg 1976; 11:443–50.

34. Franken EA Jr. Caustic damage of the gastrointestinal tract: roentgen features. Am J Roentgenol Radium Ther Nucl Med 1973; 118:77–85.

35. Muhletaler CA, Gerlock AJ Jr, deSoto L, Halter SA. Acid corrosive esophagitis: radiographic findings. AJR 1980; 134:1137–40.

36. Weisskopf A. Effects of cortisone on experimental lye burn of the esophagus. Ann Otol Rhinol Laryngol 1952; 61:681–91.

37. Rosenberg N, Kunderman PJ, Vroman L, Moolten SE. Prevention of experimental esophageal stricture by cortisone II. Control of suppurative complications of penicillin. Arch Surg 1953; 66:593–8.

38. Boyce HW Jr, Palmer ED. Techniques of Clinical Gastroenterology. Springfield: Charles C Thomas, 1975.

39. Tulman AB, Boyce HW Jr. Complications of esophageal dilation and guidelines for their prevention. Gastrointest Endosc 1981; 27:229–34.

40. Kiviranta UK. Corrosive carcinoma of the esophagus; 381 cases of corrosion and 9 cases of corrosion carcinoma. Acta Otolaryngol 1952; 42:89–95.

41. Appelqvist P, Salmo M. Lye corrosion carcinoma of the esophagus: a review of 63 cases. Cancer 1980; 45:2655–8.

42. Pemberton J. Oesophageal obstruction and ulceration caused by oral potassium therapy. Br Heart J 1970; 32:267–8.

43. Kikendall JW, Friedman AC, Oyewole MA, et al. Pill-induced esophageal injury. Case reports and review of the medical literature. Dig Dis Sci 1983; 28:174–82.

44. Evans KT, Roberts GM. Where do all the tablets go? Lancet 1976; 2:1237–9.

45. Applegate GR, Malmud LS, Rock E, et al. "It's a hard pill to swallow" or "Don't take it lying down." (Abstr) Gastroenterology 1980; 78:1132.

46. Collins FJ, Matthews HR, Baker SE, Stakova JM. Pill-induced oesophageal injury. Br Med J 1979; 1:1673–6.

47. O'Meara TF. A new endoscopic finding of tetracycline-induced esophageal ulcers. Gastrointest Endosc 1980; 26:106–7.

48. Mason SJ, O'Meara TF. Drug-induced esophagitis. J Clin Gastroenterol 1981; 3:115–20.

49. Carlborg B, Densert O. Esophageal lesions caused by orally administered drugs. An experimental study in the cat. Eur Surg Res 1980; 12:270–82.

50. Walta DC, Giddens JD, Johnson LF, et al. Localized proximal esophagitis secondary to ascorbic acid ingestion and esophageal motor disorder. Gastroenterology 1976; 70:766–9.

51. Seaman WB, Ackerman LV. The effect of radiation on the esophagus; a clinical and histologic study of the effects produced by the betatron. Radiology 1957; 68:534–41.

52. Goldstein HM, Rogers LF, Fletcher GH, Dodd GD. Radiological manifestations of radiation-induced injury to the normal upper gastrointestinal tract. Radiology 1975; 117:135–40.

53. Phillips TL, Fu KK. Quantification of combined radiation therapy and chemotherapy effects on critical normal tissues. Cancer 1976; 37:1186–1200.

54. Nelson RS, Hernandez AJ, Goldstein HM, Saca A. Treatment of irradiation esophagitis. Am J Gastroenterol 1979; 71:17–23.

55. Dobbins JW, Sheahan DG, Behar J. Eosinophilic gastroenteritis with esophageal involvement. Gastroenterology 1977; 72:1312–6.

56. Landres RT, Kuster GGR, Strum WB. Eosinophilic esophagitis in a patient with vigorous achalasia. Gastroenterology 1978; 74:1298–1301.

57. Picus D, Frank PH. Eosinophilic esophagitis. AJR 1981; 136:1001–3.

58. Goldberg HI, O'Kieffe D, Jenis EH, Boyce HW Jr. Diffuse eosinophilic gastroenteritis. Am J Roentgenol 1973; 119:342–51.

59. Manier JW, Kaplan AP. Polydysplastic epidermolysis bullosa with esophageal stricture. Gastrointest Endosc 1972; 19:19–20.

60. Nix TE Jr, Christianson HB. Epidermolysis bullosa of the esophagus: Report of two cases and review of the literature. South Med J 1965; 58:612–20.

61. Katz J, Gryboski JD, Rosenbaum HM, Spiro HM. Dysphagia in children with epidermolysis bullosa. Gastroenterology 1967; 52:259–62.

62. Warren RB, Warner TF, Gilbert EF, Pellet JR. Acquired double-barrel oesophagus in epidermolysis bullosa dystrophica. Thorax 1980; 35:472–6.

63. Absolon KB, Finney LA, Waddill GM Jr, Hatchett C. Esophageal reconstruction—colon transplant—in two brothers with epidermolysis bullosa. Surgery 1969; 65:832–6.

64. Feurle GE, Weidauer H, Baldauf G, et al. Management of esophageal stenosis in recessive dystrophic epidermolysis bullosa. Gastroenterology 1984; 87:1376–80.

65. Agha FP, Lee HH, Nostrant TT. Herpetic esophagitis: a diagnostic challenge in immunocompromised patients. Am J Gastroenterol 1986; 81:246–53.

66. McKenzie R, Khakoo R. Blastomycosis of the esophagus presenting with gastrointestinal bleeding. Gastroenterology 1985; 88:1271–3.

67. de Mas R, Lombeck G, Riemann JF. Tuberculosis of the oesophagus masquerading as ulcerated tumour. Endoscopy 1986; 18:153–5.

Chapter 20

PEPTIC DISEASES OF THE STOMACH AND DUODENUM

DAVID Y. GRAHAM, M.D.

Fiberoptic endoscopy has revolutionized our concepts of peptic diseases of the upper gastrointestinal tract mucosa. This includes major advances in diagnosis and knowledge of the prevalence and natural history of these diseases. However, the appropriate, cost-effective use of endoscopy in diagnosis and management of the dyspeptic patient remains unclear. Its primary use is as a diagnostic test, and considering that diagnostic testing constitutes a substantial portion of health care expenditures,[1, 2] it is important to assess the diagnostic value of endoscopy. Because most tests are performed on patients without the disease being sought, the calculation of their accuracy is often misleading. For example, if 100 patients with gastric ulcer, including five malignant ulcers, were evaluated, and four of the cancers were detected, the accuracy would be 99% (i.e., 99 of 100 correct diagnoses). The fact that 20% of the cancers were overlooked is obscured. A better measure of a test is its sensitivity for a given disease (i.e., the number of cases detected divided by total cases present in the population tested). Sensitivity and specificity are measurements with respect to single disease states and have less utility when the manifestations of a disease are variable.

Clinical utility is a subjective concept that measures the translation of a test result into a change in the patient's well-being. A finding may be clinically important (specifies or explains symptoms, is diagnostic, justifies therapy, or indicates further evaluation) or trivial. A negative result may also have clinical utility by redirecting the evaluation and reassuring the patient. With functional disorders, the principal value of diagnostic evaluation is the exclusion of disease or the reassurance of the patient, or both. One consideration with respect to the clinical utility, therefore, is the ability to exclude disease when there is a reasonable possibility that one is present.

EVALUATION OF THE DYSPEPTIC PATIENT

Barium contrast radiography has been the standard method for the evaluation of dyspeptic patients. There is a recent trend toward replacement of x-ray studies with fiberoptic endoscopy. Objective comparison of these two tests is difficult because there are few criteria or methods for assessment of data from either study that are independent of both.

Several reports indicate that double contrast radiography of the upper gastrointestinal tract is superior to single contrast studies.[3] Furthermore, it is suggested that double contrast radiography may rival endoscopy as the method of choice for evaluation of the stomach and duodenum.[4] A contrary report was offered by Gelfand and Ott[5] in a critical evaluation of reported statistics. Their analysis was confined to studies published in the radiology literature and excluded gastroenterology publications because the latter "tended to compare superb endoscopy to mediocre radiology." These authors found no increase in the sensitivity of double contrast compared to single contrast radiography for gastric or duodenal ulcers. The sensitivity of both was approximately 80% for gastric ulcers, indicating that 20% would be undetected. Based on these data, both tests were inferior to endoscopy.

Most reports reviewed by Gelfand and Ott[5] contained small numbers of patients. Their

431

conclusion that the radiologic techniques were equally sensitive is contrary to the general experience, this being a substantial decrease in the number of false negative x-rays after introduction of double contrast x-ray procedures. This might reflect the relatively poor quality procedures before radiologists became interested in double contrast studies; or those reporting no difference might have performed superb quality single contrast investigations; or both. Note also that most reports of single contrast studies predate endoscopy, so that false negatives were rarely found.

Is the question of differences in accuracy or diagnostic sensitivity between these two radiologic techniques important? No! The upper gastrointestinal x-ray series is inherently inaccurate; it is expensive, time-consuming, and over-utilized,[6, 7] being the second most frequently ordered diagnostic x-ray study in the United States.[6] It is unclear why the majority of these are ordered, especially since the examination may not result in a change in therapy regardless of the findings.[8] Marton et al.[8] documented that many upper gastrointestinal series are destined to be normal because most of the patients undergoing the procedure do not have symptoms, signs, or other indications of upper gastrointestinal disease. Presumably, a main indication for requesting the procedure is the reassurance provided to the patient or physician or both.

Many authors regard endoscopy and the upper gastrointestinal x-ray as complementary tests. I no longer support this view. The x-ray series may provide information not obtainable by endoscopy—observations pertaining to motility, for example—but it is best described as safe albeit inaccurate. Approximately 20% of patients with a variety of gastrointestinal complaints will be misdiagnosed by upper gastrointestinal radiography. The reported false negative rate is up to 32%, and the false positive rate ranges from 8% to 21%.[9–13] Double contrast studies tend to have fewer false negative results, but this is balanced by an increase in false positive tests. These figures apply not only to superficial inflammatory disease, but to advanced disease as well, including advanced gastric cancer and gastric ulcer. Endoscopy, more sensitive than standard or double contrast radiography, is now the diagnostic test of choice in patients with symptoms that may indicate upper gastrointestinal disease.

If the provisional diagnosis is functional disease, the primary goal of a diagnostic test is reassurance. Any reassurance derived by physicians from upper gastrointestinal radiography should be negligible given the magnitude of false negative and positive results. Although patients derive assurance that they do not have a serious disease, the upper gastrointestinal series has little or no effect on the management of disease;[8, 14] this suggests either that when functional disease is suspected physicians will embark on a course of therapy irrespective of test results or that patients believed to be suffering from a serious disease are referred for endoscopy instead of upper gastrointestinal x-rays.

If one accepts endoscopy as superior to upper gastrointestinal radiography, can endoscopy be recommended as the sole diagnostic technique for evaluation of patients with complaints pertaining to the upper gastroinestinal tract? Stevenson[12] has suggested that an internal audit compare the performances of the radiology and endoscopic services in each hospital, and that if a significant false negative rate is demonstrated for x-ray studies, this procedure should be abandoned. Potential problems with endoscopy as the sole diagnostic test are its complication rate (which, however, is low); the cost in terms of time, manpower, and expense; and the potential for over-utilization. Currently, the last does not appear to be a problem. For example, Beavis et al.[15] reported results from a one-visit endoscopy clinic for evaluation of patients with dyspepsia. Patients were referred by their practicing physicians and were examined by a gastroenterologist who determined if endoscopy was necessary (98%). Endoscopy was successfully performed in 186 patients (93%), and abnormal findings were observed in 70%. The frequency of significant peptic disease was over 50% (26.7% pyloric channel ulcer, duodenal ulcer, or scar; 17.7% esophagitis, 5.9% gastric ulcer, and 1% gastric cancer).

However, as more patients with functional complaints are referred for endoscopy, the percentage of false diagnoses may well increase. If the endoscopist were forced to examine a high volume of patients without organic disease, as is the case for the radiologist, the yield of true findings by endoscopy might also diminish. Note that half of radiologic "missed" diagnoses of gastric ulcer or cancer are clearly visible during retrospective evaluation of the x-ray films[16]; the abnormalities were overlooked in the context of the "routine exam."

The question remains whether endoscopy, as the only available diagnostic test, will be over-used. Although x-ray procedures are expensive, the cost pales in comparison to that of endoscopy. It is estimated that dyspeptic symptoms will develop in approximately 1% of a given population in the course of a year.[17, 18] The principal issue remains: how best to evaluate these patients. The appropriate approach is to choose the most sensitive and accurate test, currently fiberoptic endoscopy, and to apply this in those cases where signs and symptoms point to actual disease in the upper gastrointestinal tract.

FACTORS IN PEPTIC ULCER FORMATION

The pathogenesis of ulcer disease is not yet completely understood, and a detailed presentation of current knowledge is beyond the scope of this chapter. In a broad sense, ulcers are thought to be caused by an imbalance between aggressive and defensive factors. The aggressive factor may be endogenous (acid and proteolytic digestion by pepsin), exogenous (corrosive drugs or foods may be important in initiating or perpetuating the mucosal injury), or both. The recognized defensive factors include gastric mucus, bicarbonate secreted by cells of the gastric mucosal surface, epithelial cell regeneration, and gastric mucosal blood flow. The sequence of events leading to ulcer formation is thought to be submucosal hemorrhage followed by erosion, an increase in the depth of damage, and formation of an acute ulcer. The transition from acute ulcer to chronic ulcer is not understood and must be extremely rare. The natural tendency of erosions and acute ulcers is to heal. This has been documented by experimental studies in which acute ulcers were produced by cutting or injecting corrosive chemicals into the submucosa; these healed rapidly.[19]

The fact that gastric mucosa is not digested by acid and pepsin has fascinated and intrigued scientists since the 17th century, but the mechanism underlying this phenomenon is still not understood. Both acid and pepsin are required for rapid digestion to occur and pepsin is always found whenever gastric acid is present. Early workers were impressed with the concept of a "living principle," as living

tissue was discovered to be less rapidly digested than damaged or dead tissue. This theory was weakened when it was found that living tissue could be digested.[19] Gastric mucosa is digested whenever it is damaged. For example, topical application of concentrated ethanol or intramucosal injection of silver nitrate is followed by digestion of the damaged mucosa.

DEFINITION OF PEPTIC ULCER

Peptic ulcer is a generic term that signifies a break in any part of the gastrointestinal mucosa exposed to gastric acid and pepsin. It implies that the defect is caused by digestion of the gastric or duodenal mucosa by secreted acid and pepsin. An ulcer can also occur in an achlorhydric stomach, suggesting that another mechanism, or mechanisms, must be operative in such cases, e.g., the result of drug-induced corrosive injury. Gastric and duodenal mucosal disruptions are defined histologically as erosions, acute ulcers, or chronic ulcers.

PETECHIAE

Gastric petechiae are common and most often disappear without incident.[20, 21] They are thought to be precursors of erosions and ulcers, but they are also frequently observed in normal individuals who experience no known sequelae. Petechiae range in size from pinpoint to several millimeters in diameter and appear to be located in the submucosa (Plate 20–1). The intactness of the mucosa overlying petechiae can be ascertained from the appearance of mucosal highlights.

EROSIONS

An erosion is an epithelial defect that does not penetrate the muscularis mucosae and that heals spontaneously without scar formation usually within 2 to 8 days. The conversion of an erosion to a chronic gastric ulcer or gastric cancer must be extraordinarily uncommon. Erosions may be situated in either the acid- or non–acid-secreting mucosa and commonly occur at multiple sites. Schindler[22] first described endoscopically observed fundic erosions and noted that they resembled aphthous ulcers, having a grayish base and a red halo. Erosions are seen in 2% to 7% of routine autopsies, most commonly in the fundus, and are reported to occur in

10% to 80% of gastric specimens resected because of chronic gastric or duodenal ulcer.[23] Gastric erosions are observed in approximately 10% of patients undergoing endoscopy, about half of whom will have other demonstrable lesions, usually of peptic origin.[24, 25] The prevalence of erosion (determined as the percentage of those with erosion among those undergoing endoscopy) has been reported as 3% to 4%,[26, 27] 11%,[24, 28] and as high as 15%.[23] There seems to be a seasonal incidence, erosions being found most commonly from October through November and May through June.[24]

The actual incidence of erosions among Western populations is not known because there have been few studies of the gastric mucosa in normal, healthy individuals. Routine gastroscopy is performed on the general population of Japan to detect early gastric cancer; mucosal erosions are found in 3% to 4% of the population undergoing this screening procedure.[26] In the United States, gastroscopy is most often performed on normal individuals during clinical investigations of the effects of drugs on the gastric mucosa. We have observed mucosal abnormalities, most commonly submucosal hemorrhages (gastric petechiae), in approximately 10% of such procedures. Submucosal hemorrhages are usually located in the fundus and vary from few to many. They may also occur in a shower-like fashion immediately after retching or after the endoscope has been advanced over the mucosal surface. Gastric erosions are encountered occasionally but less frequently.

Volunteers for such drug studies refrain from alcohol use, spicy foods, and all drugs for at least two weeks prior to the gastroscopy. Without these restrictions, particularly that against aspirin usage, the percentage of individuals with mucosal abnormalities would presumably be greater.

The double contrast radiologic appearance of an erosion is a small filling defect surrounded by a halo.[29] Endoscopically the fully developed erosion is characterized by a central depression with or without a necrotic floor, a red rim, and prominent reaction in the surrounding mucosa (Plates 20–2 and 20–3). When the location of gastric and duodenal erosions was studied in 574 patients with acute or chronic lesions, the following results were obtained: in approximately 54% of patients, erosions were confined to the antrum, in 11% to the fundus, in 10% to the entire stomach, in 14% to the duodenal bulb, and in 8.4% to the antrum and duodenal bulb.[23]

Erosions are usually less than 0.5 cm in diameter; many investigators designate all lesions of greater diameter as acute ulcers. Endoscopically, it is impossible to tell if a small lesion extends through the muscularis mucosae. The estimation of depth is not reliable because swelling and edema at the edges of acute erosions may exaggerate the impression of depth. It is possible to determine if a lesion involves the deeper muscle layer (muscularis propria) by noting its effect on the normal muscular contraction waves that move through the antrum. If the deeper muscles are affected, the smooth peristaltic progression of these waves is altered. Roesch[23] suggested use of the biopsy forceps to determine whether the lesion (and the submucosa) can be pulled toward the lumen, apart from the gastric wall. This technique will reveal involvement of the muscularis propria but will not indicate a breach of the muscularis mucosae. Consequently, it cannot differentiate between a shallow acute ulcer and an erosion, but the distinction probably has little clinical significance.

It is difficult to discern whether erosions actually cause symptoms. They are usually associated with another disease which is responsible for the patient's discomfort. In addition, most patients undergo examination because of symptoms, and it is easy to incriminate gastric petechiae or erosions as the cause. The superficial mucosal lesions induced with aspirin during clinical investigations are usually asymptomatic; conversely, when symptoms are present, visible mucosal lesions are frequently absent.

Breach of the muscularis mucosae distinguishes an ulcer from an erosion. Erosions are shallow, circular or oval lesions, usually less than 0.5 cm in diameter, with sharply defined edges (see Plate 20–3). The defect does not penetrate the muscularis mucosae, so that glandular elements remain in the base and healing is rapid. Acute ulcers are commonly multiple, have the same general appearance and distribution as erosions, but are larger and penetrate through the muscularis mucosae. There is little or no fibrosis in the base of an acute ulcer, whereas chronic ulcers have underlying fibrous tissue. Chronic gastric ulcers are usually solitary, although they may be multiple in 6% to 10% of cases, recurrent clinically and histologi-

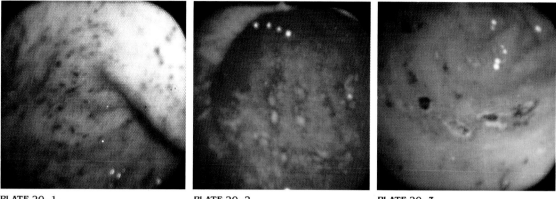

PLATE 20–1. PLATE 20–2. PLATE 20–3.

PLATE 20–1. Multiple gastric petechiae seen shortly after administration of aspirin to a normal, healthy volunteer.
PLATE 20–2. Gastric petechiae and erosions seen after approximately 24 hours of aspirin administration (2 tablets 4 times/day) to a normal, healthy volunteer showing the picture of "acute injury."
PLATE 20–3. Gastric petechiae and erosions seen after approximately 24 hours of aspirin administration (2 tablets 4 times/day) to a normal, healthy volunteer. This picture of "acute injury" shows more typical, well developed erosions.

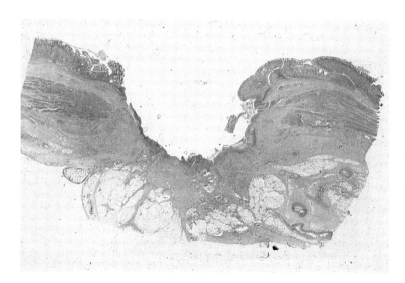

PLATE 20–4. Photomicrograph of a benign gastric ulcer. Note disruption of muscularis propria and intense fibrotic reaction in the ulcer base.

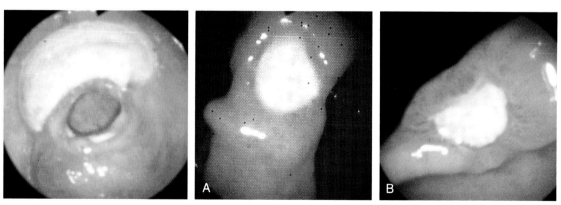

PLATE 20–5. PLATE 20–6.

PLATE 20–5. Giant prepyloric ulcer on lesser curvature in a patient taking aspirin on a chronic basis. Note normal appearance of surrounding mucosa. (Courtesy M.V. Sivak, Jr., M.D.)
PLATE 20–6. A, Acute ulcer at angulus of stomach. B, Acute ulcer at angulus, demonstrating early signs of healing. (Courtesy M.V. Sivak, Jr., M.D.)

435

cally, and are usually less than 2 cm in diameter. Large (giant) ulcers are usually benign chronic gastric lesions on the lesser curvature of the stomach.

HEALING OF ULCERS

If a piece of gastric mucosa is removed surgically, the mucosa rapidly regenerates to close the defect so that the site is not identifiable macroscopically. Regeneration can occur with remarkable rapidity, as demonstrated by healing of the mucosal surface within hours after acute superficial injury. Much of the available information concerning ulcer healing comes from carefully performed experimental studies in animals.[19, 30, 31]

Following acute gastric mucosal injury, or resection of a section of mucosa, the muscularis mucosae adjacent to the defect contracts and thereby invaginates the intact mucosal edge toward the base of the defect. In small defects such as erosions, adjoining mucosal cells rapidly migrate into the defect and cover the area. This is followed by invagination of the mucosa and restoration of normal glandular anatomy. In defects extending through the muscularis mucosae (acute ulcers), the ulcer base lacks a residuum of normal glandular elements, and healing is entirely dependent on the migration of adjacent cells to cover the defect. Although the normal glandular anatomy may be restored, the muscularis mucosae is not regenerated, and new glands lie on fibrous tissue instead of the muscularis mucosae. This is not evident by gross observation, and usually it can be detected only by histologic examination.

In chronic ulceration, the reparative processes are similar but the end result is different. The slow healing of a chronic ulcer implies either a defective or inhibited healing process or an imbalance in which the factors leading to ulcer formation and perpetuation are not overcome by reparative processes. A chronic ulcer is the summation of the simultaneous processes of mucosal destruction and regeneration. Fibroblastic proliferation, leading to a dense scar, occurs when the reparative processes are unable to restore epithelial continuity rapidly (Plate 20–4). The scar is initially covered by a single, fragile layer of gastric mucosal cells that can be easily removed. Later, the mucosal architecture may be largely restored, but the scar remains and is detectable both microscopically and ma-croscopically. An ulcer scar can be identified (and hence the fact that an ulcer is or was present can be verified) by simple palpation of the surface of the stomach. Endoscopy is restricted, however, to visual information; thus, it may be difficult for the endoscopist to distinguish accurately an ulcer as acute or chronic when visualized initially. The ulcer scar that remains after healing can often be defined by double contrast x-rays. It has been shown to change over time as the fibrous tissue contracts and becomes less apparent.[32]

The events of ulcer formation and healing are similar in the duodenum. As in the stomach, the muscularis mucosae does not regenerate and Brunner's glands, normally beneath the muscularis mucosae, become situated directly beneath the villous architecture after ulcer healing. However, this is not definite evidence of a previous ulcer, since the mucosa lies directly over Brunner's glands in some normal individuals.[33]

LOCATION OF ULCERS

Endoscopy is superior to x-ray studies in the identification of gastric and duodenal ulcers, but it is not perfect.[34] Some ulcers may not be seen, most often because of poor endoscopic technique. An ulcer should be suspected when there is gastric irritability, particularly as evidenced by general or localized muscle spasm. The majority of benign ulcers are located on the lesser curvature of the stomach near the angularis, an area that requires rigorous evaluation (Fig. 20–1).[19, 35, 36] An archlike deformity of the angulus (Henning's sign), the result of contraction of a healing ulcer, should arouse suspicion and occasion careful inspection. It is important to take advantage of gastric peristalsis to enhance examination of the lesser curvature of the antrum distal to the angularis. As peristaltic contractions move toward the pylorus, successive segments of mucosal surface can be observed on the contraction wave. This offers an *en face* albeit brief and constantly changing view of this part of the stomach, which is normally seen at a tangent with forward-viewing instruments.

On occasion, an ulcer is diagnosed when none is present. These phantom ulcers are caused by local muscular contractions that produce partially hidden or closed-over pockets. To avoid this error, it is important to wash such suspected lesions to remove trapped mucus.

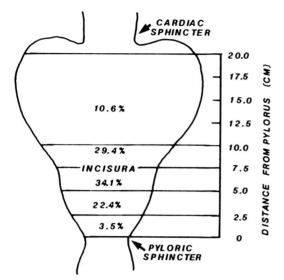

FIGURE 20–1. Location of benign gastric ulcers in relationship to the distance from the pylorus. The majority of benign ulcers will be found on the lesser curvature within 3 cm of the angularis. (Adapted from: Ivy AC, Grossman MI, Bachrach WH. Peptic Ulcer. Philadelphia: Blakiston Co. 1950; 509. With permission.)

Oi et al.[36] reported that benign gastric ulcers occur in mucosa with the histologic features of the pyloric gland-type of mucosa proximal to the normal junction between the pyloric and fundic (acid-secreting) types of mucosa. The anatomic extent of the pyloric mucosa was found to be variable. When ulcers were found in the proximal stomach, there was an associated cephalad extension of the pyloric gland mucosa, sometimes almost to the cardia. This hypothesis was consistent with previous data regarding ulcer location and explained the presence of ulcers high on the lesser curvature of the stomach. This concept has been challenged; whether the mucosa surrounding an ulcer is fundic mucosa altered by gastritis or is actually displaced pyloric gland mucosa is still a major issue.[37–40]

Endoscopic studies using the Congo red dye test[41] or indigo carmine[42] have investigated the nature of the gastric mucosa in which ulcers occur. With the Congo red test, mucosal areas that secrete acid (fundic mucosa) turn blue-black with application of the dye, whereas non–acid-producing mucosa (pyloric gland) does not change color. This type of chromoscopy is discussed in detail in Part 2 of Chapter 10. Tatsuta and Okuda[41] found a close correlation between the extent of gastritis and the location of gastric ulcers;

that is, fundal gastritis was extensive when the ulcer was located in the proximal stomach and less when the ulcer was located in the distal stomach. To determine the true ancestry of the non–acid-secreting mucosa, these authors also measured mucosal gastrin content and found that the gastrin content of the pyloric mucosa remained high even in severe antral gastritis (2096 ng/g versus 7557 ng/g in normal mucosa). Both normal fundic mucosa and mucosa adjacent to gastric ulcers occurring in the proximal stomach contained almost no gastrin (5.1 ± 4 ng/g), suggesting that gastric ulcers were located in altered fundal mucosa instead of antral (pyloric gland type) mucosa. Ulcers are focal defects, and the pathophysiologic reason for this is unknown. However, this does not mean that only the particular area of gastric mucosa containing the ulcer is abnormal. Recurrent ulcers (relapses) frequently develop apart from, and often proximal to the site of the original ulcer. These observations suggest that the mucosal defect is general rather than focal. It is also not clear whether the associated gastritis develops before or after the ulcer.

In countries where corrosive drugs such as aspirin are ingested in the form of tablets, large benign gastric ulcers in histologically normal mucosa on the greater curvature in the antrum have been reported, although this is based on limited data.[43] This area is the most dependent portion of the stomach of the normal, upright adult and it has been suggested that this type of ulcer (sump ulcer) is directly related to ingestion of corrosive drugs.[44] Although the surrounding normal gastric mucosa allows these ulcers to be differentiated histologically, they cannot be distinguished endoscopically from ulcers with other etiologies, since typical benign gastric ulcers also occur in this location (Plate 20–5). Location alone is insufficient for determining etiology.

Much of the data about the role of specific drugs in ulcer formation is anecdotal. The factors leading to chronicity in those who develop an ulcer are unknown. It is suggested that the frequency of ulcer formation is increased when drugs are administered at high doses for prolonged periods. Acute ulcers have been observed in endoscopic studies involving a variety of drugs; usually these ulcers are located on the greater curve of the antrum. It is often implied that there is a direct association between this type of mucosal damage, which heals rapidly, and the propensity to develop a chronic ulcer. No such association has been proved, and an attempt to predict the likelihood of development of a chronic ulcer, based on data obtained from acute drug administration studies, would be premature. Rather, available data suggest that there is no major difference between the principal nonsteroidal, anti-inflammatory drugs when evaluated according to the percentage of patients in whom a chronic ulcer develops.

ENDOSCOPIC APPEARANCE OF BENIGN ULCERS

Thorough evaluation of an ulcer includes analysis of the site, the shape, and the stage of a lesion. To identify and characterize ulcers, the stomach must be adequately distended so that the entire mucosal surface can be inspected. Ulcers on the lesser curvature of the proximal antrum and linear ulcers between folds on the greater curvature of the body of the stomach are particularly difficult to identify. Sometimes marked contraction of the gastric musculature causes an ulcer to be hidden within a deep crevice. Careful examination is essential when muscular contraction causes the stomach to have an abnormal or unusual shape. If it is impossible to sufficiently distend the stomach to efface large folds and visualize the mucosa, the intravenous administration of glucagon (1 mg) will usually relax the muscular contractions so that inspection of the entire mucosal surface is possible.

The basic shape of a gastric ulcer is round and discrete, although oval, oblong, or linear ulcers may occur. Most linear ulcers are positioned with their long axis parallel to the long axis of the stomach, although in the antrum the long axis may be transverse and have a saddle appearance (Plates 20–6 through 20–12). Linear ulcers are probably transformations of round or oval types that occur as part of the healing process. Insufflation of the stomach during gastroscopy separates the folds and spreads out the ulcer crater to permit detailed inspection of its edges and base and of surrounding mucosa. The edge of a typical ulcer is sharp and appears as if it were punched out; undermining of the border may also be discerned. The bottom or base of the ulcer is usually white, gray-white, or yellow-white, although it may become greenish because of bile-staining or

brown because of hemorrhage (see Plate 8–7). Particles of food or barium may adhere to the ulcer, and pinkish streaks occasionally are seen within the whitish floor. The ulcer base or floor has a smooth surface, except in large ulcers in which an uneven surface with nodes and ridges may be present.

Skilled endoscopists can usually estimate the diameter of an ulcer with reasonable accuracy. In addition, it is possible to use a reference scale, such as the ACMI measuring device (Plate 20–13) or open biopsy forceps, to estimate ulcer size. It is difficult to assess depth accurately using the endoscope, because the viewer is limited to monocular vision. However, the depth can be estimated by viewing the ulcer from different angles, with close observation of variations in illumination and shadow.

It is sometimes difficult to distinguish a chronic ulcer from an acute ulcer. When the ulcer is large, the distinction is easier. If restriction of gastric motility is evident, the presence of fibrosis may be inferred and this is, therefore, evidence of chronicity (see Plate 20–10). When mucosal biopsies are taken, the hard, gritty character of a fibrotic ulcer base can be appreciated, and the ulcer, as noted above, cannot be separated from the underlying musculature. In contrast, acute ulcers are soft and pliable, and shallow ones can be pulled away from the gastric musculature (muscularis propria) with the biopsy forceps.

In the acute stage, the mucosa surrounding an ulcer may be edematous with a mild slope upward toward the margin (see Plate 20–10). However, as the ulcer heals, this swelling disappears and the margin becomes flat (Fig. 20–2 and Plates 20–14 through 20–16; see also Plate 20–7). Most ulcers disappear without visible scar formation, although the mucosal surface at the site of healing may appear finely granular. Healing may be either symmetric or asymmetric, the latter leading to development of a linear scar. When asymmetric healing occurs, the ulcer may pass through a dumbbell shape (see Plate 20–8), with eventual division into two ulcers. The initial size of an ulcer is important as a determinant of whether a scar or gross deformity of the stomach will be produced by the healing process. Fortunately, scars are typically produced only by large chronic gastric ulcers. The scar of a healed gastric ulcer is identifiable as an arched deformity of the gastric lumen, as a collection of gently sloping

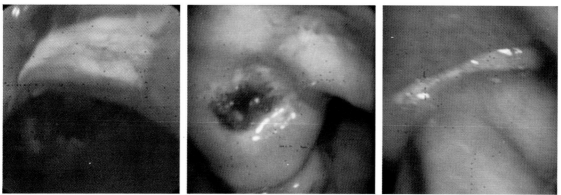

PLATE 20–7.   PLATE 20–8.   PLATE 20–9.

PLATE 20–7. Large benign gastric ulcer on lesser curvature near the angularis.

PLATE 20–8. Benign "dumbell" shaped gastric ulcer on anterior wall and lesser curvature at the angularis. The ulcer base is discolored by blood.

PLATE 20–9. Linear gastric ulcer located in the floor of the antrum.

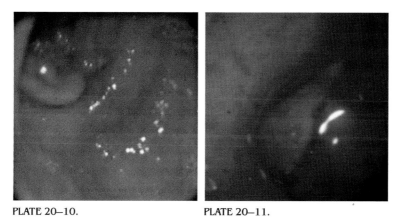

PLATE 20–10.   PLATE 20–11.

PLATE 20–10. Benign gastric ulcer in the "acute active stage", demonstrating edema of surrounding mucosa. Note that the peristaltic wave is deformed by the ulcer, indicating that the ulcer involves the muscularis propria.

PLATE 20–11. Deep benign gastric ulcer demonstrating erythematous ulcer margins.

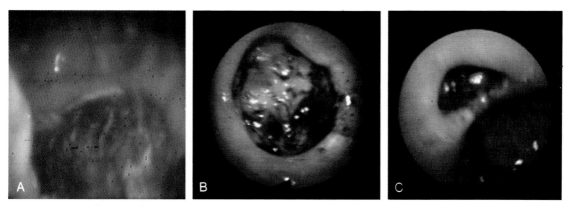

PLATE 20–12. A, Giant gastric ulcer on greater curvature, with penetration through gastric wall into mesentery and colon. B, En face view of large ulcer that has penetrated throught the gastric wall. C, Tangential view of ulcer shown in B.

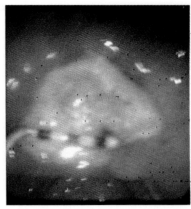

PLATE 20–13. Benign gastric ulcer, showing measurement of ulcer diameter using the ACMI measuring device. Each black or white bead measures 2 mm.

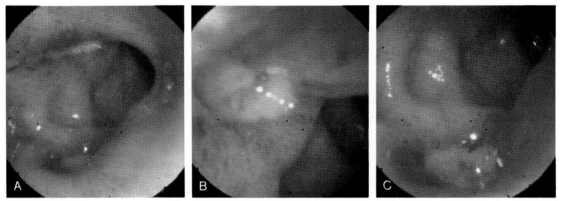

PLATE 20–14. *A*, Acute active antral ulcers on lesser and greater curvatures of antrum. *B*, Lesser curvature ulcer. *C*, Greater curvature ulcer. Note surrounding diffuse erythema.

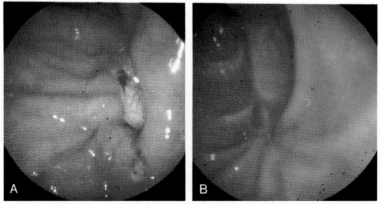

PLATE 20–15. Ulcer in early regressive or healing stage *(A)*, and later scarring stage *(B)* in same patient.

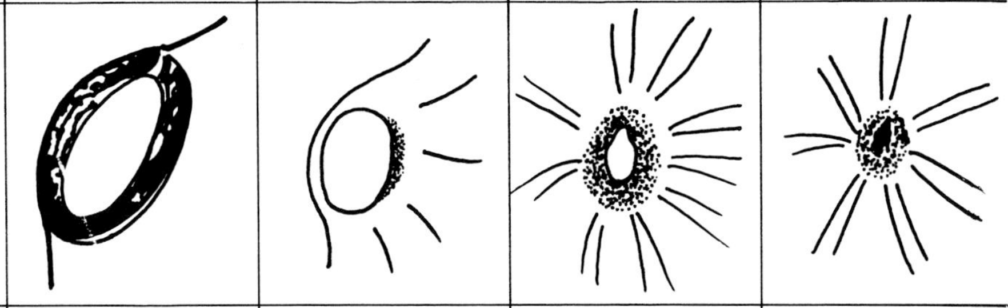

	Acute Active Stage	Regressive Stage	Healing Stage	Scarring Stage
Shape	Round or Oval	Round or Oval	Round, irregular linear, or dumbell shaped	Point, linear or irregular
Edema	++	+	−	−
Diffuse Erythema	+	−	−	−
Red Halo	−	+	++	++ − + − −
Overrriding of coating	+ (−)	−	−	−
Ulcer bottom	Thick white coating, occasionally mingled with brown or black tint	White or yellow coating	Thin grey or yellowish white coating	No coating
Convergence of folds	−	+	++	++ − +

FIGURE 20–2. Changes in endoscopic appearance of gastric ulcer. (From Tsuneoka K, Takemoto T, Fukuchi S, eds. Fiberscopy of Gastric Diseases. Tokyo: Igaku Shoin Ltd., 1973; 139. With permission.)

and converging folds accompanied at times by a central pit or depression, or as a localized regular mucosal depression without discoloration or hyperemia. Folds converging toward the edge of the ulcer are seen less frequently at endoscopy than in x-ray studies, although lessening gastric distention by removal of insufflated air may allow endoscopic visualization.

The time required for complete ulcer healing is related to the initial size of the ulcer. Large ulcers take longer to heal than small ulcers, a relationship that holds for both stomach and duodenal ulcers. With treatment, most gastric ulcers heal within 12 weeks; large ulcers, i.e., those with a diameter over 2.5 cm, are allowed 16 weeks of therapy before they are designated as "unhealed."[45, 46] Duodenal ulcers are generally smaller than gastric ulcers and most heal within 4 weeks of treatment.[47]

DIFFERENTIATION BETWEEN BENIGN AND MALIGNANT ULCERS

A final diagnosis with regard to a benign or malignant ulcer may be composed of a number of elements including clinical impression, radiologic assessment, endoscopic assessment and, finally, the interpretation of biopsy and the cytology specimens.

It is inappropriate to consider any factor exclusively.

The first goal of endoscopy is to find the cause of symptoms, e.g., the presence of a gastric ulcer. Once an ulcer has been identified, the next goal is to determine whether the ulcer is benign or malignant.[48–52]

Radiographically, the most reliable criteria for a benign ulcer are radiating folds, regular shape, a smooth base, and location of the base on or outside the stomach wall. The most significant radiographic criteria of malignancy are an adjacent mass, gastric wall rigidity, and failure of the ulcer base to project beyond the contour of the stomach.

The endoscopist has considerable advantage over the radiologist because of the ability to examine carefully a magnified image of the ulcer, including the margin, base, and surrounding mucosa. Furthermore, observations can be made repeatedly from different vantage points. Gastric carcinomas usually present as mass lesions and as such are easily diagnosed. An early gastric cancer may mimic a benign ulcer, although stigmata of cancer can usually be found by careful inspection. In the absence of a mass, endoscopic features that suggest carcinoma include a stepwise depression of the ulcer edge; small extensions of the crater that blur the ulcer's edge (the edge or margin of a benign ulcer is

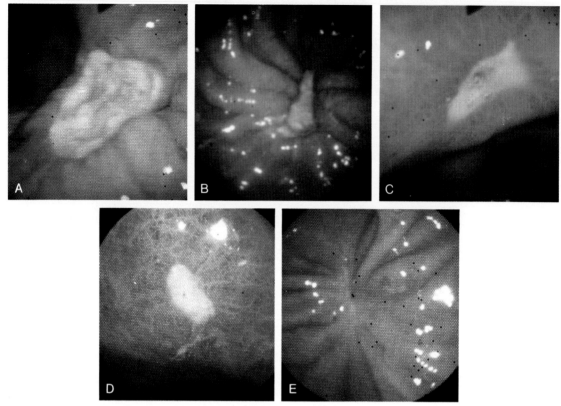

PLATE 20–16. Gastric ulcers in various stages of evolution. *A,* Regressive stage. Note converging folds. *B,* Late regressive or early healing stage. Note converging folds. *C,* Early healing stage. *D,* Healing stage. *E,* Scarring stage (Courtesy M.V. Sivak, Jr., M.D.)

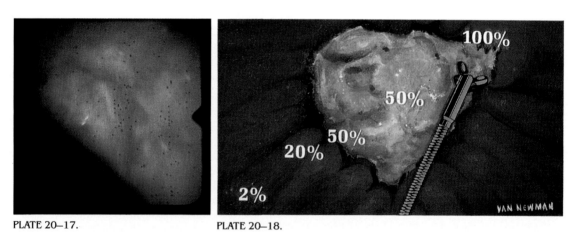

PLATE 20–17.   PLATE 20–18.

PLATE 20–17. Ulcerating gastric carcinoma demonstrating blurring of ulcer margins and moth-eaten appearance of surrounding mucosa.

PLATE 20–18. Percentage of positive biopsy specimens obtained in relation to site of biopsy of gastric carcinoma that simulates a benign gastric ulcer. The 100% yield is related to the fact that a skilled endoscopist can accurately identify the site that has the greatest likelihood of a positive biopsy.

usually sharply demarcated) (Plate 20–17); bleeding from the edge of the crater; a necrotic, "dirty" appearance of the crater itself; the presence of abnormal folds (clubbing or fusion of the tips) at the margin; disruption of the mucosal folds before they reach the crater; and an irregular or moth-eaten appearance of the surrounding mucosa.

Gabrielsson[49] compared gastroscopic and radiographic evaluations of 20 benign and 20 malignant gastric ulcers that were carefully selected as diagnostic problems. Each ulcer had been diagnosed by both x-ray examination and gastroscopy, and obvious carcinomas were excluded. The benign ulcers were large and scarred. In no case was carcinoma restricted to the mucosa or submucosa. The most distinctive x-ray signs were an incisura opposite a benign ulcer crater and abnormal and disrupted folds with malignant ulcers. The strongest endoscopic criterion for malignancy was a disruption (flattening) of the folds before they reached the ulcer margin or marginal wall, whereas blurring of the ulcer edge was the next most reliable endoscopic marker (found in 50% of those with malignancy). Obviously, absence of the latter sign is meaningless unless the entire circumference of the ulcer margin can be inspected. A marginal wall that rose steeply from the surrounding mucosa was a strong indication for malignancy but also occurred in a benign ulcer. No conclusions could be drawn from a regular ulcer shape, whereas an asymmetric shape strongly indicated malignancy. In spite of these guidelines, this study conclusively demonstrated that neither x-ray examination nor endoscopic inspection alone was adequate to differentiate between benign and malignant gastric ulcers.

BIOPSY OF GASTRIC ULCERS

The purpose of endoscopic biopsy is to confirm the clinical impression of the nature of a lesion and to exclude other diseases that have a similar endoscopic appearance. The diagnosis is rarely in doubt with a large polypoid or ulcerating tumor. A sufficient number of biopsies will ensure that the cell type of the tumor is identified correctly and the diagnosis confirmed. In the event that all biopsies are negative, the procedure will be repeated or the patient will be referred for laparotomy. The real problem is the cancer which appears to be a benign gastric ulcer

endoscopically. Although endoscopic appearance alone is not reliable in the differentiation of benign from malignant ulcers, some endoscopists nevertheless use clinical judgment exclusively and do not obtain biopsies. An accuracy of 95% is assured with this approach simply because only 5% of benign-appearing gastric ulcers are actually malignant (diagnostic accuracy, 95%; sensitivity, 0%). Whether all patients with radiographically "benign" ulcers should undergo endoscopy for the purpose of biopsy remains controversial. If the ulcer is diagnosed first by endoscopy, hopefully the usual case in the future, the question is moot. The ulcer first diagnosed by roentgenography is the problem. In this circumstance, if the ulcer is judged radiographically to be benign, endoscopy can be delayed until the first follow-up evaluation at 4 or, preferably, 8 weeks. This allows time for healing, a factor that helps distinguish benign from malignant lesions. If there is any degree of uncertainty as to whether or not a lesion is radiographically benign, it is prudent to proceed immediately with endoscopy and biopsy. The primary indication for endoscopy in a patient with a radiologically identified ulcer is to exclude cancer. As a general rule, patients with gastric ulcers should be followed until healing has been confirmed endoscopically.

The endoscopist must develop a routine to ensure that a sufficient number of biopsies are obtained to exclude a small cancer. The prognosis of these "early" cancers is much better than that for advanced gastric carcinoma; thus their detection is imperative. Unfortunately, there have been few studies that address the question of where to direct the biopsy forceps.

I believe that endoscopists can specifically recognize abnormal anatomic features and direct the biopsy to the area most likely to contain a carcinoma. In fact, the experienced endoscopist proves to be quite skillful at correct identification of the area most likely to contain a cancer. For example, we obtained a positive diagnosis with the first biopsy specimen in 70% of those cases ultimately proven to have cancer.[53]

Hatfield and coworkers[54] have provided the best guidelines for placement of biopsies. They performed an in vitro study in which they obtained biopsies from freshly resected, ulcerating carcinomas and then compared the biopsy site with the frequency of positive biopsy specimens. Fifty percent of the biopsies obtained from either the margin or the base of the ulcer yielded a diagnosis of cancer. There was a marked reduction in the percentage of positive specimens when the biopsies were obtained beyond the inner edge of the ulcer (Plate 20–18). This study also emphasizes the value to the endoscopist in personally reviewing the biopsy slides. This permits an ongoing critique of biopsy technique. If a large number of slides contained normal gastric epithelium, the ulcerating lesion was missed too often and the evaluation was inadequate. Depending upon the clinical situation, repetition of the procedure may be required.

How many biopsy specimens are sufficient to ensure that a seemingly benign lesion is truly benign? When an obvious cancer is present, the endoscopist is likely to take many biopsies. In this situation, "more is better," and at least 7 or 8 biopsy specimens should be obtained. The endoscopist may be less inclined to obtain an adequate number of specimens from benign-appearing ulcers. At a minimum, 4 biopsies (3 from the margin and 1 from the base) should be obtained along with directed cytology specimens. If cytology specimens are not collected, it is prudent to increase the number of biopsies from an apparently benign ulcer to 7 or 8.

It is a good rule not to place more than 4 or 5 biopsy specimens in a single bottle of fixative. When a large number are pooled, they are often embedded at different levels within the paraffin block and, consequently, some may be lost during the initial sectioning process or remain unsectioned deeply within the block. Another important point is that the physician should personally review the biopsies to ensure that all the obtained specimens were examined by the pathologist.

Biopsy forceps in various sizes, with biopsy cups of different shapes and configurations (solid vs. fenestrated), are available (Fig. 20–3). The forceps may also contain a spear or bayonet, which permits several biopsies without withdrawing the forceps. Although there are few controlled studies comparing biopsy forceps, we have found that there is little difference in terms of positive yield with respect to the type of forceps used. We have obtained a high yield of positive biopsies with the small forceps designed for pediatric instruments, as well as with large instruments designed for new wide-channel gastroscopes. Large biopsy forceps are particularly useful when detailed histology of the duodenal, gas-

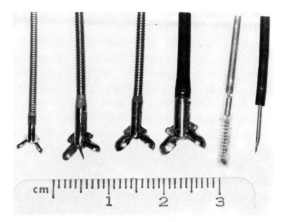

FIGURE 20–3. Various types of instruments used to obtain biopsy material from mucosal lesions via the fiberscope.

tric, or esophageal mucosa is desired. Forceps with fenestrated (open) cups probably reduce the problem of "crush artifact," but there is no evidence for a significant increase in the yield for cancer. I personally find little use for forceps with a bayonet because I withdraw the forceps after each biopsy. A bayonet-type forceps can aid in acquisition of biopsies from lesions that are difficult to reach; the bayonet impales the lesion, thus ensuring that a biopsy is obtained from the correct site.

A "lift and cut" technique, which utilizes a twin-channel endoscope and electrosurgical snare excision of a piece of mucosa held in the grasp of a biopsy forceps (Fig. 20–4), has been suggested for submucosal lesions,[55] but this has not achieved wide usage. Recently, endoscopists have begun using needles (similar to sclerotherapy injection needles but with a larger internal diameter) for needle biopsies of infiltrating or submucosal lesions (see Fig. 20–3).[56] This is a limited but useful technique.

The collection of cytology specimens in addition to biopsy generates more controversy than the issue deserves. Cytology specimens slightly improve the diagnostic accuracy of endoscopy at the risk of an occasional false positive result. Cytology specimens are frequently not collected, probably because this lengthens the procedure; breaks the endoscopic routine; and is inconvenient. There are two efficient ways to obtain specimens: brushing and salvage cytology technique. A type of cytology brush that is protected by a plastic over-tube, the sheathed brush, was introduced as a replacement for the simple, unsheathed brush without any preliminary

LIFT AND CUT BIOPSY TECHNIQUE

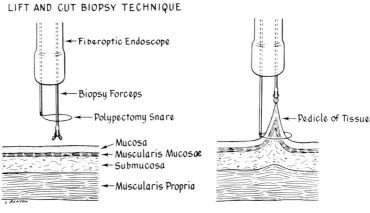

FIGURE 20–4. Technique of lift and cut biopsy of submucosal lesions (Adapted from Martin TR, Onstad GR, Silvis SE, Vennes JA. Lift and cut biopsy technique for submucosal sampling. Gastrointest Endosc 1976; 23:29. With permission.)

STEP 1   STEP 2

studies to show that the sheathed brush increased the diagnostic yield. Recent studies in our unit suggest that both types of brush yield similar results. We rarely perform brush cytology, except when anatomic features of a lesion preclude collection of adequate biopsy specimens, e.g., a very narrow stricture of the esophagus, stomach, or colon. It has been suggested that the yield of positive results from brush cytology is better if the samples are obtained before biopsy.[57] Although it has not been demonstrated directly that brushing influences the diagnostic yield of subsequent biopsies, brushing often causes bleeding that obscures the lesion and interferes with the aiming of the forceps. It is our intuitive opinion that positive biopsy yield is less after brushing because of a reduced ability to carefully pinpoint the cancer.

We prefer the salvage cytology technique because it is rapid, does not require an additional instrument, and can be performed as part of the routine biopsy technique.[58] A mucous trap is attached between the fiberscope and the suction line. The contents of the biopsy channel are aspirated between the collection of each biopsy specimen. The result is about 5 to 20 ml of fluid. This is diluted with alcohol or another suitable fixative and submitted for cytologic examination. This technique salvages malignant cells remaining within the accessory channel and those that fall from the biopsy forceps. Salvage cytology has a relatively high positive diagnostic yield; its advantage is that it does not interrupt the endoscopic routine.

DUODENAL ULCER

Duodenal and gastric ulcers are similar endoscopically. The average duodenal ulcer is round and located in the duodenal bulb (Plates 20–19 through 20–23). Ulcers appear with equal frequency on the anterior and posterior aspects of the bulb. Since they are found uncommonly in the second or third portion of the duodenum, postbulbar occurrence suggests a high level of acid secretion and the Zollinger-Ellison syndrome.

When the duodenum is irritable or markedly scarred, it may be difficult to exclude the presence of an ulcer. The entire duodenal bulb must be inspected to ensure that an ulcer is not overlooked. As in the stomach, administration of glucagon will abolish duodenal muscular activity and facilitate examination of the mucosal surface when there is excessive irritability. Marked scarring is a more difficult problem, particularly because food particles and other material may be trapped within mucosal folds (Plates 20–24 and 20–25). A small diameter (pediatric) endoscope is ideally suited for examination of the scarred duodenal bulb because its small diameter and flexibility permit examination of each recess. Post-bulbar ulcers, particularly those on the medial wall just beyond the junction of the first and second portions, may be particularly difficult to identify; adequate examination of this area may require a pediatric or side-viewing instrument.

Ulcers within the pyloric channel or within 1 cm of the pyloric channel (prepyloric ulcers) (Plate 20–26) behave clinically as duodenal ulcers with the exception that symptoms of gastric outlet obstruction due to edema, deformity, and narrowing of the pylorus are more common. Ulcers within, or just beyond, the pyloric channel may be difficult to observe. One useful technique to avoid missing an ulcer in these locations is to examine the area carefully while withdrawing

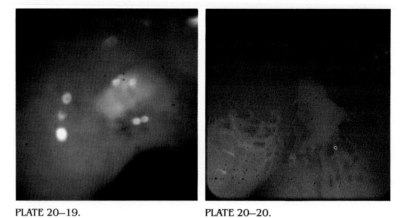

PLATE 20–19.   PLATE 20–20.

PLATE 20–19. Duodenal ulcer in apex of bulb.
PLATE 20–20. Benign duodenal ulcer with erythematous rim, marked muscular contraction, and duodenal deformity.

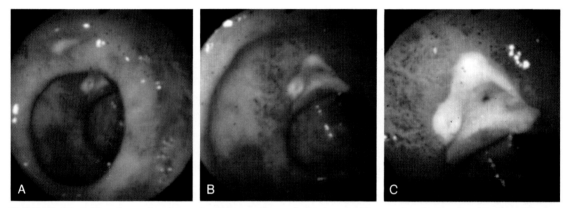

PLATE 20–21. A, View through pylorus showing small prepyloric ulcer and larger ulcer in duodenal bulb. B, Closer view of duodenal ulcer as instrument tip passes through pylorus. C, Close-up view of acute duodenal ulcer. Note inflamed and edematous surrounding mucosa and small amount of fresh blood in the ulcer crater. (Courtesy M.V. Sivak, Jr., M.D.)

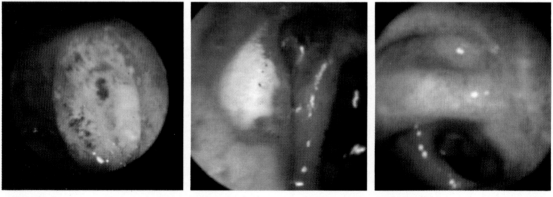

PLATE 20–22.   PLATE 20–23.   PLATE 20–24.

PLATE 20–22. Acute duodenal ulcer. The red spot in the center of the crater proved to be a visable vessel. (Courtesy M.V. Sivak, Jr., M.D.)
PLATE 20–23. Acute duodenal ulcer in a deformed bulb.
PLATE 20–24. Marked duodenal deformity. It is difficult to be certain that an ulcer is not present unless care is taken to distend, and often wash out each of the crevices.

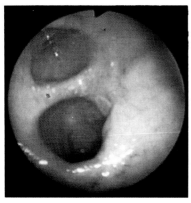
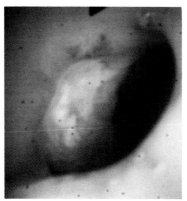
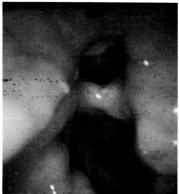

PLATE 20–25.   PLATE 20–26.   PLATE 20–27.

PLATE 20–25. Pseudodiverticulum of duodenal bulb, due to chronic peptic ulcer disease.
PLATE 20–26. Ulcer in pyloric channel.
PLATE 20–27. Double pylorus with an ulcer in channel between stomach and duodenum.

the endoscope from duodenum to stomach. The fiberscope is passed into the duodenum, the tip is deflected into one quadrant with reference to the pyloric ring, and then the endoscope is slowly withdrawn while maintaining the tip deflection in order to examine the bulbar mucosa immediately distal to the pylorus. This will also flatten out spastic folds in the pyloric valve itself. The endoscope is then reintroduced and the technique repeated for each of the other quadrants.

When duodenal ulcers are very large, they are designated "giant" ulcers. Ulceration of the entire duodenal bulb may not be appreciated by upper gastrointestinal radiography. The radiographic clue is that the bulb remains large and its outline does not change through multiple films, that is, no muscular contractions are evident. Most giant ulcers will heal with H_2-receptor antagonist therapy, but because of their large size, healing is

delayed in comparison with that of typical small ulcers. Considerable duodenal deformity usually accompanies healing.

An interesting complication of pyloric or prepyloric ulceration is the development of a double pylorus (Plate 20–27).[59] In this instance, the ulcer deepens, penetrates the wall, and eventually perforates into the duodenum. The remaining column of tissue between the two channels may be a thick muscular band or a thin band that is easily torn and removed as the endoscope enters the duodenum.

The patient with a duodenal ulcer may present with a variety of symptoms. Many times the young patient with typical symptoms can be managed without precise endoscopic diagnosis. When a diagnosis is needed, duodenoscopy is clearly more accurate than roentgenography in recognizing the presence of an ulcer and in distinguishing various

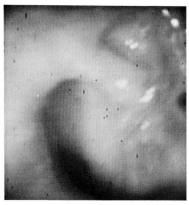
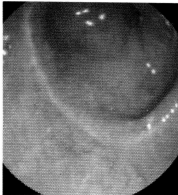

PLATE 20–28. Duodenal mucosal diverticulum that trapped barium and simulated a duodenal ulcer radiographically.
PLATE 20–29. Scar that resulted from healing of a duodenal ulcer. (Courtesy M.V. Sivak, Jr., M.D.)

PLATE 20–28.   PLATE 20–29.

anatomic abnormalities that simulate an ulcer (Plate 20–28). Endoscopy should be performed in the older patient who is more likely to have another cause for symptoms such as gastric ulcer or cancer, and in any patient with complicated disease or disease significant enough to require the consultation of a subspecialist. Endoscopy serves not only to confirm the clinical diagnosis but also to exclude other disorders in the stomach or esophagus. Other indications for duodenoscopy in suspected duodenal ulcer disease include complications such as symptoms of gastric outlet obstruction (regular nausea and vomiting), intractability, and/or bleeding. The diagnosis of duodenal ulcer should always be confirmed endoscopically when surgery is considered.

The natural tendency of the duodenal ulcer is to heal (Plate 20–29), so that follow-up endoscopy to assess healing is not particularly important after a course of adequate therapy and control of symptoms. Likewise, repetition of endoscopy is not necessary in every patient to confirm that recurrence of typical symptomatology is indeed due to an active ulcer. Rather, the use of endoscopy in follow-up of the duodenal ulcer patient should be individualized.

DRUG-INDUCED GASTRIC MUCOSAL DAMAGE

The sequence of events leading to ulcer formation is thought to be submucosal hemorrhage, erosion, increasing depth of damage, and finally formation of an acute ulcer. This sequence is illustrated best by drug-induced gastric mucosal damage, and aspirin-induced injury is probably the most thoroughly understood.[60, 61] The initial event in humans is unknown. In the mouse and rat, it is damage to single cells or to small groups of superficial gastric epithelial cells.[62, 63] The initial event is probably analogous in humans. Acetylsalicylic acid, or aspirin, was introduced by Bayer in 1899. Currently, more than 300 proprietary preparations contain aspirin, and the yearly consumption is in excess of 20 billion tablets. The current hypothesis for aspirin-induced gastric mucosal damage is related to the fact that un-ionized aspirin (pKa 3.5), the favored form in an acid environment, is lipid-soluble.[60] Aspirin is absorbed into gastric mucosal cells, where it becomes ionized because of the higher

intracellular pH and damages the cell. Based on this concept, the concentration of un-ionized aspirin in gastric juice is the prime determinant of whether injury occurs. Methods designed to prevent injury attempt to reduce the amount of un-ionized aspirin in the stomach.

The first endoscopic evidence of the adverse effects of aspirin on the gastric mucosa was reported in 1939 by Douthwaite and Lintott.[64] Recent studies confirm that oral ingestion is important. Intravenous or rectal administration is not associated with increased gastric blood loss or gastric mucosal changes, as evidenced by endoscopy, biopsy, and measurement of potential difference.[65] Ultrastructural changes occur within 3 minutes of oral aspirin administration, and the potential difference across the gastric mucosa changes immediately. Endoscopically, the first evidence of damage is red, brown, or black pinpoint dots on and within the mucosa, often associated with streaking of blood on the surface (see Plate 20–1). This change may be visible within 30 minutes after aspirin ingestion. Within 1 to 2 hours, submucosal hemorrhages ranging from 2 to several millimeters in diameter appear, and by 8 hours small erosions may be evident (see Plates 20–1 through 20–3). By 24 hours, erosions ranging in size from 3 to 5 mm may be seen, as well as larger acute lesions that are either erosions or small acute ulcers.[66, 67] Erosions may be induced by a single dose of aspirin. Any area of the stomach may be involved, and crossover studies reveal that location is neither consistent nor predictable.[66]

With continual aspirin administration, the gastric mucosa adapts, previous lesions heal, and the evidence of damage resolves.[66, 68, 69] We compared the extent of gastric mucosal damage associated with 7 days versus 1 day of aspirin therapy.[66] The degree of mucosal injury reached a maximum early during therapy and then decreased despite continued aspirin administration. Gastric mucosal healing took longer after a single day of aspirin therapy (median 10 days) than it did after 7 days of aspirin therapy (median 4 days). Thus, the gastric response to continuous aspirin injury is to heal and to do so at an accelerated rate. The mechanism of this compensation is as yet unclear. It is also probable that this compensatory adaptation is variable, because delayed healing occurred in some patients, and there is a definite association between chronic aspirin ingestion (more than

15 tablets or capsules per week) and the occurrence of chronic gastric ulcer.[70]

Endoscopic studies of the effect of nonsteroidal anti-inflammatory drugs (NSAID) on the gastric mucosa represent situations that are partially artificial and contrived, since most were designed to evaluate the stomach at the point of maximum aspirin-induced injury without consideration of the process of gastric adaptation. Studies that have compared aspirin with other NSAID assumed a time course of injury and adaptation similar for all the various drugs. This hypothesis requires verification. The results of many endoscopic studies comparing the effects of aspirin and other drugs have been described. Comparison is difficult because rating scales used to quantify gastric mucosal injury differ markedly.

Rating scales can be grouped into two types: those that count lesions and those that assess both the severity and distribution of lesions. Gastric damage is not linear, i.e., a grade 4 lesion is not simply twice as severe as a grade 2 lesion. Therefore, each scale results in a generalized classification of damage from mild to severe. It is assumed that acute ulcers are a more severe injury than erosions, and erosions are more severe than submucosal hemorrhages.

We have employed a variety of scales ranging from complex to simple (Fig. 20–5) and find that the simple scoring system modified from that of Lanza et al.[71] provides the same overall score as more complicated systems. The conclusions of comparative studies may be tenuous since, as stated, most investigators have tended to disregard the fact that gastric mucosal injury is a dynamic process and have equated aspirin damage with that caused by other drugs. Recent studies of gastric mucosal damage have been single time-point studies, usually designed to compare the effect of aspirin with those of other NSAID.

Published data[71-76] and unpublished studies (Graham DY; Smith JL; and Lanza JL) that compare the frequency of apparent gastric mucosal injury after acute drug administration (1 to 14 days) with that noted after chronic use (months) are shown in Table 20–1. These data are presented without regard to the severity of mucosal injury. In each study the proportion of patients demonstrating injury after chronic drug administration is less than after acute administration.

All known NSAID have the potential for acute damage to the gastric mucosa. Table 20–2 ranks a number of such drugs in order of propensity to cause acute gastric mucosal injury. Reported damage ranges from mild

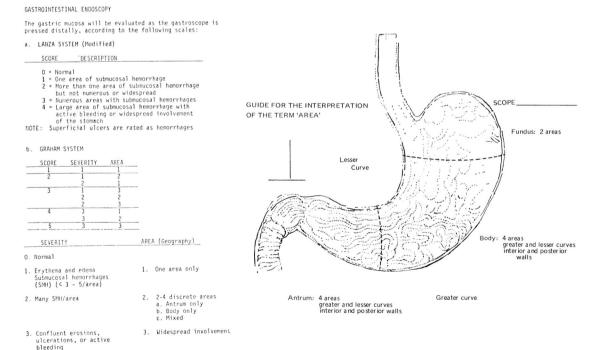

GASTROINTESTINAL ENDOSCOPY

The gastric mucosa will be evaluated as the gastroscope is pressed distally, according to the following scales:

a. LANZA SYSTEM (Modified)

SCORE   DESCRIPTION

0 = Normal
1 = One area of submucosal hemorrhage
2 = More than one area of submucosal hemorrhage but not numerous or widespread
3 = Numerous areas with submucosal hemorrhages
4 = Large area of submucosal hemorrhage with active bleeding or widespread involvement of the stomach
NOTE: Superficial ulcers are rated as hemorrhages

b. GRAHAM SYSTEM

SCORE	SEVERITY	AREA
1	1	1
2	1	2
	2	1
3	1	3
	2	2
	2	3
4	3	1
	3	2
5	3	3

SEVERITY

0. Normal

1. Erythema and edema Submucosal hemorrhages (SMH) (< 3 - 5/area)

2. Many SMH/area

3. Confluent erosions, ulcerations, or active bleeding

AREA (Geography)

1. One area only

2. 2-4 discrete areas
   a. Antrum only
   b. Body only
   c. Mixed

3. Widespread involvement

GUIDE FOR THE INTERPRETATION OF THE TERM 'AREA'

SCOPE_____

Fundus: 2 areas

Lesser Curve

Body: 4 areas greater and lesser curves interior and posterior walls

Antrum: 4 areas greater and lesser curves interior and posterior walls

Greater curve

FIGURE 20–5. Two rating scales used for evaluation of drug-induced gastric mucosal damage. a, Modified Lanza system; b, Graham system. Each gives similar results.

TABLE 20–1. **NSAID: Potential for Gastric Mucosal Injury from Acute and Chronic Drug Administration**

Drug	Frequency (%) of Gastric Mucosal Injury	
	Acute Admin.*	Chronic Use†
Placebo	10	10
Aspirin	100	50
Indomethacin	100	30
Ketoprofen	100	27
Naproxen	100 (40)‡	27
Diclofenac	—	20
Ibuprofen	100 (40)§	18
Oxyphenbutazone	—	15
Corticosteroids	—	14
Sulindac	35	10
Fenbufen	35	—
Diflunisal	—	10

*Drug administration for 1 to 14 days.
†Drug use for month(s).
‡2,400 mg vs 1,600 mg.
§750 mg vs 500 mg.

(barely distinguishable from that associated with placebo administration) to severe mucosal changes similar to those mediated by aspirin. In comparison with available NSAID, aspirin is consistently associated with the most severe lesions. It is postulated that NSAID-associated damage is related to the anti-inflammatory properties of the drugs, as neither acetophenonin nor codeine (drugs with only analgesic properties) cause visible mucosal injury. Comparative studies in both animals and humans have been undertaken to identify the parameters associated with the production and prevention of mucosal damage. Two NSAID (fenbufen and sulindac) that are administered as pro-drugs (i.e., anti-

TABLE 20–2. **NSAID: Potential for Acute Gastric Mucosal Damage**

Potential Damage	Drug
None	Enteric-coated aspirin
Mild	Fenbufen Sulindac
Moderate	Naproxen Tolmetin Zomepirac Ibuprofen
Severe	Aspirin High Dose: Naproxen Tolmetin Ibuprofen Indomethacin

inflammatory activity requires absorption and metabolism) are associated with a low frequency of minimal gastric changes when administered acutely. The reduced tendency for acute gastric injury may not be a direct reflection of the inactive nature of the administered compound, since the gastric mucosal response is identical when the active metabolite of sulindac (sulindac sulfide) is administered orally to normal volunteers.[77] However, both drugs are nearly insoluble in gastric contents; solubility may be a more important factor than their inactive metabolic state. Another explanation for these results is that any drug absorbed in the stomach may be converted to an active metabolite within the gastric mucosa.

The acute administration of aspirin is associated with endoscopically identifiable lesions in approximately 100% of recipients.[66, 67, 71, 72, 78, 79] In contrast, only 20% to 25% of rheumatology patients who have taken aspirin daily for many months have mucosal injury.[80, 81] The gastric erosions associated with a given drug should not cause excessive concern, since there is no evidence that the acute endoscopic findings precede or predict the development of an ulcer or hemorrhage. Although the increased incidence of gastric ulcer in association with chronic aspirin ingestion is accepted, there is no way to identify susceptible subgroups of patients.

SPICES AND GASTRIC MUCOSAL DAMAGE

The ability of spicy foods to cause gastric mucosal damage has not been carefully investigated. It is our impression that the use of chili peppers (jalapenos) and Indian curry is associated with mucosal lesions similar to those induced by aspirin.

Spices that appear to be associated with symptoms of gastric distress when taken with food are black pepper, chili pepper, mustard seed, and cloves.[82] In humans, mustard and paprika have been shown to affect gastric acid secretion; mustard (1 gm) has a depressive action, whereas paprika (0.5–1 gm) may cause an increase in gastric acidity.[83] Celery salt, nutmeg, sage, cinnamon, cloves, and pepper have no apparent effect on gastric secretion.[83] Chili pepper has been shown to increase gastric mucosal epithelial cell turnover, as evidenced by an increase in DNA content of gastric aspirates.[84]

In one study,[82] several spices were studied; endoscopy was performed after each spice ($2\frac{1}{2}$ times the amount ordinarily used in highly spiced foods) was allowed to remain in the stomach for 10 minutes. No significant change in the gastric mucosa was observed in patients who received cinnamon, nutmeg, allspice, thyme, black pepper, chili pepper, cloves, or paprika. Thyme and mustard seed produced mild erythema, but no symptoms. Chili pepper produced moderate mucosal hyperemia and black pepper produced severe hyperemia, although neither elicited symptoms. The interval between spice administration and endoscopy may have been too short to allow mucosal damage to become visible. It should be noted that administration of large doses (3 to 6 gm daily) of paprika, mustard, pepper, and cloves to dogs (along with histamine-in-beeswax) produced marked changes in the gastric mucosa, including ulceration, after 4 to 5 days.[83]

Editor's note: References 85 to 90 are recent publications pertaining to endoscopy and gastric ulcer.

References

1. Conn RB. Clinical Laboratories. Profit center, production industry, or patient care resource? N Engl J Med 1978; 298:422–7.
2. Griner PF, Liptzin BJ. Use of the laboratory in a teaching hospital: Implications for patient care, education, and hospital costs. Ann Intern Med 1971; 75:157–63.
3. Goldberg HI. Radiographic evaluation of peptic ulcer disease. J Clin Gastroenterol 1981; 3:57–65.
4. Salter RH. X-ray negative dyspepsia. Br Med J 1977; 2:235–6.
5. Gelfand DW, Ott DJ. Single- vs. double-contrast gastrointestinal studies: Critical analysis of reported statistics. Am J Roentgenol 1981; 137:523–8.
6. Population Exposure to X-rays. U.S. 1940. Publication (FDA) 73–8047. U.S. Department of Health, Education and Welfare, 1973.
7. Revesz G, Shea FJ, Ziskim MC. Patient flow and utilization of resources in a diagnostic radiology department. Radiology 1972; 104:21–6.
8. Marton KI, Sox HC Jr, Wasson J, Duisenberg CE. The clinical value of the upper gastrointestinal tract roentgenogram series. Arch Intern Med 1980; 140:191–5.
9. Tedesco FJ. Endoscopy in the evaluation of patients with upper gastrointestinal symptoms: indications, expectations, and interpretation. J Clin Gastroenterol 1981; 3(Suppl 2):67–71.
10. Cotton PB. Upper gastrointestinal endoscopy. Br J Hosp Med 1976; 16:7–15.
11. Cotton PB. Fibreoptic endoscopy and the barium meal: results and implications. Br Med J 1973; 2:161–9.
12. Stevenson GW. Who needs radiology? Gastrointest Endosc 1980; 26:119–25.
13. Wormsley KG. Diagnostic Procedures. In: Horrobin DE, ed. Annual Research Reviews. Vol 2, Duodenal Ulcer. Edinburgh: Churchill Livingstone, 1979; 88.
14. Bulpitt CJ, Rowntree RK, Semmence A. A randomised controlled trial of the effects of screening for ulcer-type dyspepsia. J Epidemiol Comm Health 1982; 36:172–5.
15. Beavis AK, La Brooy S, Misiewicz JJ. Evaluation of one-visit endoscopic clinic for patients with dyspepsia. Br Med J 1979; 1:1387–9.
16. Gelfand DW, Ott DJ, Tritico R. Causes of error in gastrointestinal radiology. I. Upper gastrointestinal examination. Gastrointest Radiol 1980; 5:91–7.
17. Gear MW, Ormiston MC, Barnes FJ, et al. Endoscopic studies of dyspepsia in the community: an "open-access" service. Br Med J 1980; 280:1135.
18. Gear MW, Barnes RJ. Endoscopic studies of dyspepsia in a general practice. Br Med J 1980; 280:1136–7.
19. Ivy AC, Grossman MI, Bachrach WH. Peptic Ulcer. Philadelphia: Blakiston Co., 1950.
20. Palmer ED. Whatever happened to gastric petechiae? Gastrointest Endosc 1974; 21:80–1.
21. Dagradi AE, Stempien SJ, Lee ER, Juler G. Hemorrhagic-erosive gastritis. Gastrointest Endosc 1968; 14:147–50.
22. Schindler R: Lehrbuch und Atlas der Gastroskopie. Munchen: Lehmann, 1923; 220.
23. Roesch W. Erosions of the upper gastrointestinal tract. Clin Gastroenterol 1978; 7:623–34.
24. Karvonen AL. Occurrence of gastric mucosal erosions and their association with other upper gastrointestinal disease: A study of patients examined by elective gastroscopy. Ann Clin Res 1981; 13:159–63.
25. Karvonen AL. Occurrence of gastric mucosal erosions in association with other upper gastrointestinal diseases, especially peptic ulcer disease, as revealed by elective gastroscopy. Scand J Gastroenterol 1982; 17:977–84.
26. Kawai K, Shimamoto K, Misaki F, et al. Erosion of gastric mucosa—pathogenesis, incidence and classification of the erosive gastritis. Endoscopy 1970; 3:168–74.
27. Roesch W, Ottenjann R. Gastric Erosions. Endoscopy 1970; 2:93.
28. Soehendra N, Rehner M, Sternberg N, Lietzke C. Die chronischen (kompletten) Erosionen des Magens. Munch Med Wochenschr 1972; 114:1857–60.
29. Catalano D, Pagliari U. Gastroduodenal erosions: radiological findings. Gastrointest Radiol 1982; 7:235–40.
30. Magnus HA. The pathology of peptic ulceration. Postgrad Med J 1954; 30:31–136.
31. Morson BC, Dawson IMP. Peptic ulceration. In: Gastrointestinal Pathology. Oxford: Blackwell Scientific Publications, 1972:110–27.
32. Gelfand DW, Ott DJ. Gastric ulcer scars. Radiology 1981; 140:37–43.
33. Kreuning J, Bosman FT, Kuiper G, et al. Gastric and duodenal mucosa in "healthy" individuals. An endoscopic and histopathological study of 50 volunteers. J Clin Pathol 1978; 31:69–77.
34. Martin TR, Vennes JA, Silvis SE, Ansel HJ. A comparison of upper gastrointestinal endoscopy and radiology. J Clin Gastroenterol 1980; 2:21–5.
35. Thomas J, Greig M, McIntosh J, et al. The location of chronic gastric ulcer. A study of the relevance of ulcer size, age, sex, alcohol, analgesic intake and smoking. Digestion 1980; 20:79–84.

36. Oi M, Oshida K, Sugimura S. The location of gastric ulcer. Gastroenterology 1959; 36:45–56.

37. Ruding R. Gastric ulcer and antral border. Surgery 1967; 61:495–7.

38. Thomas E, Hall P, Hislop IG. Observations on the histology of the gastric mucosa in chronic gastric ulcer. Am J Dig Dis 1972; 17:683–8.

39. Gear MWL, Truelove SC, Whitehead R. Gastric ulcer and gastritis. Gut 1971; 12:639–45.

40. Mackay IR, Hislop IG. Chronic gastritis and gastric ulcer. Gut 1966; 7:228–33.

41. Tatsuta M, Okuda S. Location, healing, and recurrence of gastric ulcers in relation to fundal gastritis. Gastroenterology 1975; 69:897–902.

42. Ida K, Kohli Y, Shimamoto K, et al. Endoscopical findings of fundic and pyloric gland area using dye scattering method. Endoscopy 1973; 5:21.

43. MacDonald WC. Correlation of mucosal histology and aspirin intake in chronic gastric ulcer. Gastroenterology 1973; 65:381–9.

44. Kottler RC, Tuft RJ. Benign greater curve gastric ulcer: The "sump-ulcer." Br J Radiol 1981; 54:651–4.

45. Lewis JH. Treatment of gastric ulcer. What is old and what is new. Arch Intern Med 1983; 143:264–74.

46. Scheurer U, Witzel L, Halter F, et al. Gastric and duodenal ulcer healing under placebo treatment. Gastroenterology 1977; 72:838–41.

47. Graham DY, Schwartz JT, Sabesin SM, et al. Double-blind multicenter comparison of 1,200 mg. and 1,000 mg. cimetidine in hospitalized and ambulatory duodenal ulcer patients. Am J Gastroenterol 1981; 76:500–5.

48. Chang FM, Saito T, Ashizawa S. Follow-up endoscopic study of gastric mucosal changes secondary to gastric ulcer. Endoscopy 1978; 10:33–40.

49. Gabrielsson N. Benign and malignant gastric ulcers. Evaluation of the differential diagnostics in roentgen examination and endoscopy. Endoscopy 1972; 4:73.

50. Kawai K, Akasaka Y, Kohli Y. Endoscopical approach to the "malignant change of benign gastric ulcer" from our follow-up studies. Endoscopy 1973; 5:53.

51. Keller RJ, Wolf BS, Khilnani MT. Roentgen features of healing and healed benign gastric ulcers. Radiology 1970; 97:353–9.

52. Salter RH, Gill DK, Girdwood TG, et al. Gastric ulcer: Is endoscopy always necessary? Br Med J 1981; 282:2097.

53. Graham DY, Schwartz JT, Cain GD, Gyorkey F. Prospective evaluation of biopsy number in the diagnosis of esophageal and gastric carcinoma. Gastroenterology 1982; 82:228–31.

54. Hatfield ARW, Slavin G, Segal AW, Levi AJ. Importance of the site of endoscopic gastric biopsy in ulcerating lesions of the stomach. Gut 1975; 16:884–6.

55. Martin TR, Onstad GR, Silvis SE, Vennes JA. Lift and cut biopsy technique for submucosal sampling. Gastrointest Endosc 1976; 23:29–30.

56. Raskin JB, Welch P, Nadji M, Gould E. Transendoscopic needle aspiration cytology in the diagnosis of gastrointestinal malignancies. (Abstr) Gastrointest Endosc 1980; 26:75.

57. Keighley MR, Thompson H, Moore J, et al. Comparison of brush cytology before or after biopsy for diagnosis of gastric carcinoma. Br J Surg 1979; 66:246–7.

58. Graham DY, Spjut HJ. Salvage cytology. A new alternative fiberoptic technique. Gastrointest Endosc 1979; 25:137–9.

59. Hansen OH, Kronborg O, Pedersen T. The double pylorus. Scand J Gastroenterol 1972; 7:695–6.

60. Cooke AR. The role of the mucosal barrier in drug-induced gastric ulceration and erosions. Am J Dig Dis 1976; 21:155–64.

61. Pfeffer CJ, ed. Drugs and Peptic Ulcer. Vol 2, Pathogenesis of Ulcer Induction Revealed by Drug Studies in Humans and Animals. Boca Raton: CRC Press, Inc., 1982.

62. Harding RK, Morris GP. Cell loss from normal and stressed gastric mucosae of the rat. An ultrastructural analysis. Gastroenterology 1977; 72:857–63.

63. Hingson DJ, Ito S. Effect of aspirin and related compounds on the fine structure of mouse gastric mucosa. Gastroenterology 1971; 61:156–77.

64. Douthwaite AH, Lintott GAM. Gastroscopic observation of the effect of aspirin and certain other substances on the stomach. Lancet 1938; 2:1222–5.

65. Ivey KJ, Paone DB, Krause WJ. Acute effect of systemic aspirin on gastric mucosa in man. Dig Dis Sci 1980; 25:97–9.

66. Graham DY, Smith JL, Dobbs SM. Gastric adaptation occurs with aspirin administration in man. Dig Dis Sci 1983; 28:1–6.

67. O'Laughlin JC, Hoftiezer JW, Ivey KJ. Effect of aspirin on the human stomach in normals: endoscopic comparison of damage produced one hour, 24 hours, and 2 weeks after administration. Scand J Gastroenterol (Suppl) 1981; 67:211–4.

68. Hurley JW, Crandall LA Jr. The effect of various salicylates upon the dog's stomach: A gastroscopic photographic evaluation. In: Dixon A–St J, Martin BK, Smith MJH, Wood RHN, eds. Salicylates, An International Symposium. Boston: Little, Brown and Co., 1963; 213–6.

69. Eastwood CL, Quimby GF. Effect of chronic aspirin ingestion on epithelial proliferation in rat fundus, antrum, and duodenum. Gastroenterology 1982; 82:852–6.

70. Cameron AJ. Aspirin and gastric ulcer. Mayo Clin Proc 1975; 50:565–70.

71. Lanza F, Royer GL Jr, Nelson RS. Endoscopic evaluation of the effects of aspirin, buffered aspirin, and enteric-coated aspirin on gastric and duodenal mucosa. N Engl J Med 1980; 303:136–8.

72. Lanza FL, Royer GL, Nelson RS, et al. The effects of ibuprofen, indomethacin, aspirin, naproxen, and placebo on the gastric mucosa of normal volunteers. A gastroscopic and photographic study. Dig Dis Sci 1979; 24:823–8.

73. Lanza FL, Royer GL Jr, Nelson RS, et al. A comparative endoscopic evaluation of the damaging effects of nonsteroidal anti-inflammatory agents on the gastric and duodenal mucosa. Am J Gastroenterol 1981; 75:17–21.

74. Caruso I, Fumagalli M, Montrone F, et al. Controlled double-blind study comparing acetylsalicylic acid and diflunisal in the treatment of osteoarthritis of the hip and/or knee; Long-term gastroscopic study. In: Diflunisal in Clinical Practice, Proceedings of a Special Symposium, San Francisco: XIV Congress of Rheumatology, 1977; 63–73.

75. Caruso I, Bianchi Porro G. Gastroscopic evaluation of anti-inflammatory agents. Br Med J 1980; 280:75–8.

76. Irani MS. The effects of anti-inflammatory agents on the gastric mucosa in patients with osteoarthritis:

preliminary report of a randomised study. J Int Biomed Inform Data 1980; 1:21.

77. Graham DY, Smith JL, Holmes GI, Davies RO. Relationship between nonsteroidal anti-inflammatory effect and gastric mucosal injury. (Abstr) Gastroenterology 1983; 84:1173.

78. Thorsen WB Jr, Western D, Tanaka Y, Morrissey JF. Aspirin injury to the gastric mucosa. Gastrocamera observations of the effect of pH. Arch Intern Med 1968; 121:499–506.

79. Edmar D. The effects of acetylsalicylic acid on the human gastric mucosa as revealed by gastrocamera. Scand J Gastroenterol 1975; 10:495–9.

80. Sun DCH, Roth SH, Mitchell CS, Englund DW. Upper gastrointestinal disease in rheumatoid arthritis. Am J Dig Dis 1974; 19:405–10.

81. Silvoso GR, Ivey KJ, Butt JH, et al. Incidence of gastric lesions in patients with rheumatic disease on chronic aspirin therapy. Ann Intern Med 1979; 91:517–20.

82. Schneider MA, DeLuca V Jr, Gray SJ. The effect of spice ingestion upon the stomach. Am J Gastroenterol 1956; 26:722–32.

83. Sanchez-Palomera E. The action of spices on the acid gastric secretion on the appetite and on the caloric intake. Gastroenterology 1951; 18:254–68.

84. Desai HG, Venugopalan K, Antia FP. Effect of red chili powder on DNA content of gastric aspirates. Gut 1973; 14:974–6.

85. Davenport PM, Morgan AG, Darnborough A, DeDombal FT. Can preliminary screening of dyspeptic patients allow more effective use of investigational techniques? Br Med J [Clin Res] 1985; 290:217–20.

86. DiFebo G, Miglioli M, Calo G, et al. *Candida albicans* infection of gastric ulcer: frequency and correlation with medical treatment. Results of a multicenter study. Dig Dis Sci 1985; 30:178–81.

87. Tragardh B, Haglund U. Endoscopic diagnosis of gastric ulcer. Evaluation of the benefits of endoscopic follow-up: observation for malignancy. Acta Chir Scand 1985; 151:37–41.

88. Tatsuta M, Iishi H, Okuda S. Location of peptic ulcers in relation to antral and fundal gastritis by chromoendoscopic follow-up examinations. Dig Dis Sci 1986; 31:7–11.

89. Jorde R, Bostad L, Burhol PG. Asymptomatic gastric ulcer: a follow-up study in patients with previous gastric ulcer disease. Lancet 1986; 1:119–21.

90. Shike M, Gillin JS, Kemeny N, et al. Severe gastroduodenal ulcerations complicating hepatic artery infusion chemotherapy for metastatic colon cancer. Am J Gastroenterol 1986; 81:176–9.

Chapter 21

GASTRITIS AND INFLAMMATORY DISORDERS OF THE STOMACH

WILFRED M. WEINSTEIN, M.D.

The past decade has witnessed a considerable expansion in our knowledge of gastritis. Yet, many regard this topic as obscure, a prime reason for there being confusion concerning terminology. Gastritis is one of the most loosely used terms in gastroenterology. Clinicians without endoscopic expertise may use "gastritis" as a synonym for nonulcer dyspepsia. Many endoscopists use the term in a global sense to describe any variety of mucosal appearances ranging from erythema or swelling to discrete erosions. Unfortunately, some investigators in this field continue to define gastritis poorly or do not define it at all.

Another source of misunderstanding results when clinicans and pathologists use the same terms to mean different things. For example, to the endoscopist "acute gastritis" may denote the erosions and hemorrhages commonly observed in critically ill patients or in patients who are receiving nonsteroidal anti-inflammatory drugs. The connotation is temporal, i.e., these lesions are more evanescent than chronic ulcers. To the pathologist the term "acute gastritis" may signify a histologic pattern of inflammation with prominent neutrophilic infiltrates.

CLASSIFICATION

An overview classification of gastritis is given in Table 21–1. The two major categories are erosive/hemorrhagic and nonerosive. Erosive/hemorrhagic patterns refer to endoscopically visible lesions, as defined below. Nonerosive gastritis refers to histologic inflammatory changes. In nonerosive gastritis the endoscopic appearance of the mucosa does not reliably predict the presence, absence, or severity of the gastritis. Within each of the two major categories of gastritis, the histology may be either nonspecific or specific (Table 21–1). Nonspecific histology refers to a pattern of inflammation that is common to a variety of disorders. The histologic appearance is not diagnostic of any single disorder or even a narrow group of disorders. Specific histology refers to distinctive histologic features that are either diagnostic for a disorder or markedly narrow the differential diagnosis. Most of the specific types of gastritis are uncommon. They include Crohn's disease, Ménétrier's disease, and certain infections.

This chapter will consider gastritis in three major groupings. The first two will be the nonspecific types, with separate consideration of the erosive/hemorrhagic and nonerosive varieties. The third group will be the specific types of gastritis, combining the erosive and nonerosive types.

TABLE 21–1. **Overview Classification of Gastritis**

Erosive/Hemorrhagic
Nonspecific histology*
Specific histology†
Nonerosive
Nonspecific histology
Specific histology

*Pattern of inflammation that is not diagnostic for a disorder or group of disorders.

†Distinctive histologic features that are diagnostic for a disorder or a limited group of disorders.

EROSIVE/HEMORRHAGIC GASTRITIS: NONSPECIFIC TYPES

Nomenclature

Erosions and hemorrhages were defined in Chapter 20 and will also be defined briefly here. These lesions commonly coexist.

Erosion

The classic definition of an erosion is a shallow defect in the mucosa that does not extend through the muscularis mucosae into the submucosa (Fig. 21–1). A typical lesion is a flat or minimally depressed tiny white spot surrounded by a red halo. These aphthous-type lesions are usually multiple (Plate 21–1). If there has been recent bleeding from an erosion, its base may be black (Plate 21–2). For larger (e.g., 5 to 10 mm) flat or minimally depressed lesions containing exudate, the distinction between an erosion and an ulcer is arbitrary because depth of penetration into the mucosa cannot be assessed accurately at endoscopy.

Hemorrhage

The term hemorrhage refers to the endoscopic appearance of discrete petechiae or fire-engine red confluent streaks and patches unassociated with any visible breaks in the mucosa (Plate 21–3). Some use the term submucosal hemorrhage to describe these lesions, but this is purely speculative because the actual location of these lesions is not known. Subepithelial hemorrhage is a better descriptive term because it leaves open the possibility that the lesion is located in either mucosa or submucosa, deep to the lining epithelium.

Appearances that do not qualify as either erosions or hemorrhages include the following: erythema, mucosal swelling, friability (petechiae or oozing blood) induced by passage of the endoscope over a segment of mucosa, adherent white patches of exudate or plaques, and cherry-red spots resembling vascular lesions. These qualifications may sound pedantic. However, some continue to equate subjective findings[1] of dubious significance (such as erythema) with erosions.[2] This can only perpetuate misguided concepts and may even misdirect therapy.

Sometimes it is difficult to distinguish between subepithelial hemorrhages and other types of lesions. In this circumstance, the endoscopist should state the uncertainty in his report so that it leaves less room for clinical misinterpretation. For example, it is sometimes difficult to distinguish between a subepithelial hemorrhage and erythema, with or without accompanying friability. Similarly, it is not always easy to determine whether an isolated bright red spot represents an area of subepithelial hemorrhage or a tiny angioma. Furthermore, even extensive areas of apparent subepithelial hemorrhage may on occasion represent submucosal vascular ectasia with only minimal involvement

EROSION   ULCER

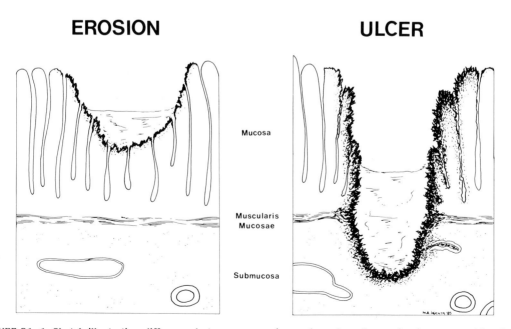

FIGURE 21–1. Sketch illustrating difference between an erosion and an ulcer. An erosion is a mucosal break that does not penetrate the muscularis mucosae, whereas an ulcer does.

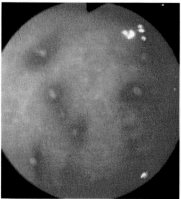 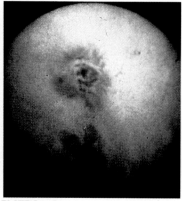 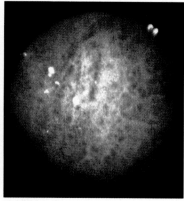

PLATE 21-1.   PLATE 21-2.   PLATE 21-3.

PLATE 21-1. Multiple white-based aphthous gastric erosions surrounded by red halos.
PLATE 21-2. Black-based gastric erosion in a patient with hematemesis.
PLATE 21-3. Diffuse subepithelial hemorrhages.

of the overlying mucosa (Plate 21-4). This can occur as an unexplained isolated event[3, 4] or in association with portal hypertension.[5]

Histology

Although gastric mucosal erosions and hemorrhages are classified as types of gastri- tis, it is important to stress that inflammatory cell infiltrates are often minimal or even absent histologically. Erosions and hemor- rhages may resemble ischemic lesions.[6, 7] Even in animal experiments in which condi- tions are highly controlled, the microscopic distinction between red, hemorrhagic, or ne- crotic lesions is subjective.[8] The histologic

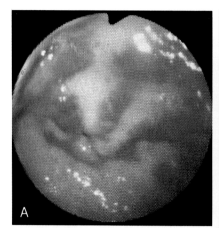

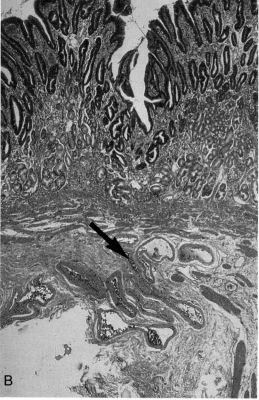

PLATE 21-4. Submucosal vascular ectasia. A, Broad red streaks in antrum radiating to pylorus. B, Antrectomy from A. There is extensive mucosal vascular ectasia (arrow) with only minimal hemorrhage in the overlying mucosa.

appearance of many of these experimentally induced lesions does not make it possible to predict whether the naked-eye appearance is due to simple vascular congestion, surface cell loss, or a deeper necrotic lesion.[8]

In clinical practice there is rarely any reason to obtain biopsies of erosions and hemorrhages, especially those seen in the most common settings, i.e., in critically ill patients or patients on nonsteroidal anti-inflammatory drugs. In a few studies, biopsies of erosions and subepithelial hemorrhages have been reported. However, there is no study that details the histology in such a way that the findings can be assessed in relation to all the lesions seen and in which the histology of the target lesions can be compared with the histology of the adjacent intact mucosa.

Our own anecdotal experience with random biopsies of erosions and hemorrhages, as well as information gleaned from published reports, indicates that biopsies of these lesions generally reveal a wide spectrum of change. In part, this may reflect various stages in the evolution and healing of these lesions. Fully developed erosions or hemorrhages may reveal partial or full-thickness mucosal necrosis with minimal inflammation (Plates 21–5 and 21–6). Some biopsies reveal an intact epithelium with foveolar hyperplasia[9] or abnormal cytologic changes of the surface epithelium and foveolae.[7] Biopsies from grossly hemorrhagic areas or from erosions commonly reveal no histologic abnormalities!

If an apparent subepithelial hemorrhage is theoretically due to an angioma or vascular ectasia, mucosal biopsy may be inadequate

with respect to verification of this possibility.[10] One reason is that small ectatic mucosal vessels may shrink in fixatives and thus not be apparent in the histologic sections. Another explanation is that vascular ectasia may predominate in the submucosa and involve the overlying mucosa in only a spotty fashion.[3, 4, 11] There are instances when red swollen areas of mucosa raise the question of mucosal congestion, as in portal hypertension.[5] Unfortunately, mucosal congestion is difficult to prove as the underlying basis for hemorrhagic lesions because histologic "congestion" is a common finding in many endoscopic biopsies. This is because of the pinch-avulsion forces exerted with endoscopic biopsy forceps.

Clinical Settings

The clinical settings in which nonspecific erosions and hemorrhages may be found are outlined in Table 21–2.

Stress Lesions

The incidence of erosions and diffuse hemorrhages approaches 100% in critically ill patients.[6] Frank gastrointestinal bleeding develops in only a small percentage of these patients, usually without abdominal pain. The lesions heal if the patient's underlying disease(s) improves. The pathogenesis of these lesions has been reviewed in detail.[12] Gastric acid is a prerequisite for their development, but mucosal ischemia and mucosal acidosis are considered the critical factors in pathogenesis.[12]

The subepithelial hemorrhages and erosions occur primarily in the body of the stomach. It is sometimes stated that the lesions are located in the fundus, but this is a terminologic misconception. The lesions occur in the fundic gland zone of the stomach where acid and pepsin are secreted. This zone occupies both the fundus and the body of the stomach.

The lesions that occur in burn patients, especially those with more massive burns, have a similar pattern.[13] However, in burn patients the antrum seems to be involved more commonly, i.e., in almost half the patients.[13] In burn patients erosive duodenitis and duodenal ulcers may be more common accompaniments than in comparably ill patients from other causes.[14] However, if antral or duodenal lesions are present, they are always accompanied by lesions in the gastric body.

TABLE 21–2. **Clinical Settings for Nonspecific Erosive/Hemorrhagic Gastritis**

Stress Lesions
Seriously Ill Patients

Localized Gastric Trauma
    Mechanical: Nasogastric tubes, retching
    Endoscopic treatment: Laser, electrocoagulation, thermal devices
    Corrosives
    Radiation

Drugs
    Nonsteroidal anti-inflammatory drugs
    Alcohol
    Other

Discrete Ischemic Insult

Postgastrectomy

Idiopathic "Chronic" Erosions

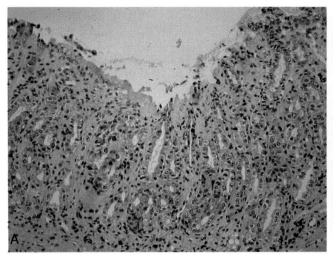
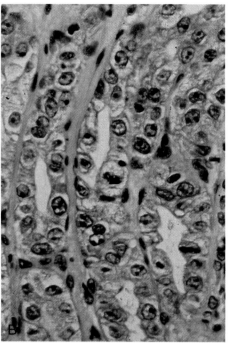

PLATE 21–5. Histology of an erosion. A, Low-power magnification shows shallow erosion with pink hyaline material at the luminal surface. B, High-power magnification shows marked epithelial abnormalities in the base of this erosion. Cells vary in size, and chromatin patterns in nuclei vary in density. Note the absence of inflammatory cells.

Lesions associated with cerebral trauma are often excluded from discussions of stress lesions because they are often deep ulcers that may perforate.[12] However, erosions have also been described in these patients.[15]

Localized Gastric Trauma

In patients with gastrointestinal bleeding who have had nasogastric tubes in place, it is sometimes impossible to determine whether mucosal hemorrhages were induced by the suction trauma of the nasogastric tube. If the hemorrhages are arranged in a linear or geometric pattern, nasogastric tube trauma becomes more likely as a cause.

Retching is another form of trauma that may induce petechiae. Major subepithelial hemorrhage in the proximal stomach induced by forceful retching has been termed "prolapse gastropathy."[16]

The endoscopic techniques used to obliterate vascular lesions also create erosions or ulcers.[17]

Corrosive injury to the stomach can occur with ingestion of either strong alkalis or acids.

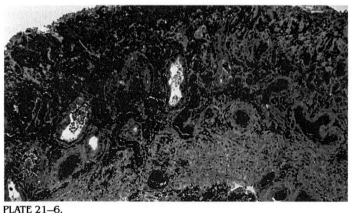
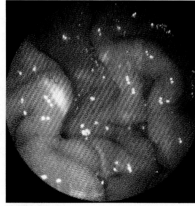

PLATE 21–6.   PLATE 21–7.

PLATE 21–6. Histology of an erosion. Contrast with Plate 21–5. Here there is extensive mucosal hemorrhage and virtually no residual glands.

PLATE 21–7. Idiopathic "chronic" erosions. There are multiple white-based erosions at crests of prominent folds in the body of the stomach.

The latter more commonly cause gastric damage, especially in the antrum. Early endoscopy is important to help stage the degree of injury. The finding of a black gangrenous slough generally indicates the need for early surgery.[18-20]

Radiation may induce gastric erosions and ulcers and result in the delayed formation of antral strictures. This form of gastritis is included here largely for historical interest. Primary irradiation of the stomach for peptic ulcer is obsolete, and secondary damage from massive abdominal irradiation is uncommon.[21]

Drugs

The relation of nonsteroidal anti-inflammatory drugs to gastric mucosal injury is discussed in Chapter 20. Heavy alcohol ingestion is well known to result in gastric erosions and hemorrhages and to carry the risk of bleeding.[22] Portal hypertension may contribute to the development of these lesions in the alcoholic patient.[5] For obvious reasons, the sequence of development of lesions after the acute administration of alcohol to volunteers has not been studied nearly as extensively as that for nonsteroidal anti-inflammatory drugs.[23, 24]

A recent preliminary report documented the development of gastric ulcers and erosions in patients receiving hepatic arterial chemotherapy with floxuridine.[25]

Discrete Ischemic Insult

There have been isolated reports of apparent ischemic erosions due to diverse causes, ranging from atheromatous embolization[26] to vasculitis.[27]

Postgastrectomy

Abnormalities of the gastric mucosa after gastric resection are also considered in Chapter 24. Erosions, especially near the stoma, may be seen in symptomatic as well as asymptomatic patients after surgery for peptic ulcer.[28]

Idiopathic "Chronic" Erosive Gastritis

Isolated erosions are occasionally encountered, even in asymptomatic individuals (see Chapter 20).

Idiopathic "chronic" erosive gastritis is an uncommon syndrome. It has also been termed "diffuse varioliform gastritis."[9] Patients with this syndrome have multiple persistent or recurrent gastric erosions. To qualify as idiopathic there should be no history of known risk factors such as nonsteroidal anti-inflammatory drug ingestion or alcohol abuse. In the largest published series it is not always clear whether all patients fulfilled this criterion.[7, 9, 29, 30]

The patients often have endoscopy because of dyspepsia, sometimes with accompanying weight loss. Massive hematemesis is rare, although occult bleeding with anemia is not uncommon. The lesions and the symptoms may wax and wane, often independent of each other. A variety of therapies has been employed with variable success.[31]

The erosions have a rather distinctive appearance. They are several millimeters in size and are found in the center of raised "nodules" of mucosa that are sometimes evident even on double contrast radiographs.[30] The lesions are often present in both the body and the antrum, especially along the greater curvature. In the body they may be aligned along the crests of prominent rugae (Plate 21–7). If the rugal folds are especially prominent, an underlying lymphoma or infiltrative carcinoma must be considered.[9] The biopsies of these lesions may show prominent foveolar (pit) hyperplasia[7, 9] and variable amounts of inflammation.

Clinical Implications

Endoscopists should describe what they see rather than use blanket terms such as "gastritis." A precise description permits others to interpret the findings. Lesions should be described as either erosions or hemorrhages. Some estimate of numbers and distribution should be given. Other more subjective mucosal appearances such as erythema, friability, and mucosal swelling may be noted separately.

Uniform descriptions of location are useful, especially if patients require repeated endoscopy. The location designations I use are fundus, body (proximal, mid, or distal), and antrum (proximal, mid, or distal). For lesions in the body and antrum I also designate location according to the curvature or wall. It is preferable to provide orientation in relation to the curvatures if possible, since there is no uniformity among endoscopists with regard to the anterior or posterior walls as landmarks.

Gastrointestinal bleeding can be attributed to erosions and subepithelial hemorrhages if there is active oozing of blood from these lesions. In the absence of active oozing, the finding of numerous black-based erosions (see Plate 21–2) is strongly suggestive of recent hemorrhage. Clinical judgment must often be used in deciding the significance of erosions or subepithelial hemorrhages. A patient receiving nonsteroidal anti-inflammatory drugs for a rheumatic disorder who also has melena or occult gastrointestinal tract blood loss would be an example. Should the evaluation reveal gastric erosions or hemorrhages that are quiescent and without evidence of bleeding, a clinical decision must be made whether to provisionally attribute the bleeding to the "inactive" gastric lesions or to pursue other possible causes.

An even greater challenge is to discern whether the finding of erosions or subepithelial hemorrhages accounts for a patient's dyspepsia. With the earlier use of endoscopy in the evaluation of dyspeptic symptoms, gastric erosions, especially antral, have been described in considerable numbers of patients. In one study from Norway, discrete erosions in the prepyloric region were found in approximately 14% of patients.[2] It is not known how many of those individuals were habitual users of nonsteroidal anti-inflammatory drugs or alcohol. When isolated erosions, subepithelial hemorrhages, or just a significant degree of erythema alone is encountered, it is frequently tempting to regard such findings as the basis of a patient's dyspepsia. However, this intuitive enthusiasm must be restrained based on the knowledge that many seriously ill patients and numerous patients receiving nonsteroidal anti-inflammatory drugs commonly have such findings and yet are asymptomatic. It is common practice to treat dyspeptic patients with such visible gastric lesions with the same drugs used for conventional peptic ulcer; however, these lesions will not disappear in some patients. In others, dyspepsia persists even though the lesions have vanished.

When erosions or hemorrhages are found on a recurring basis in symptomatic patients, every attempt should be made to determine whether there is clandestine ingestion of nonsteroidal anti-inflammatory drugs or alcohol.

Biopsies and smears of erosions are mainly indicated when opportunistic infection is suspected in the immunocompromised host. In idiopathic "chronic" erosive gastritis, biopsies are often obtained because such cases are baffling. However, the biopsy findings rarely help to refine the diagnosis or therapy.

NONEROSIVE NONSPECIFIC GASTRITIS

Nonerosive nonspecific gastritis is a histologic diagnosis that is often referred to as "chronic gastritis." It is common in the general population but is more prevalent or severe in patients with the disorders outlined below.

Histology

The histologic zones of the stomach are defined by their gland types. Apart from the narrow cardiac gland region located at the gastroesophageal junction, the stomach consists of two major histologic zones. The fundic gland mucosa occupies both the fundus and the body of the stomach. The glands consist mainly of acid-secreting parietal cells and pepsinogen-secreting chief cells. The antral (pyloric) gland mucosa occupies all of the gastric antrum. Its glands are of the mucus type. Between these two major gland zones are transition zones that combine features of the adjacent gland types. The antral-fundic transition zone is often more extensive along the lesser curvature of the stomach.

Nonerosive nonspecific gastritis may be confined primarily to the antral gland mucosa or the fundic gland mucosa, or it may occur in both areas. Combined involvement is common, but one zone is usually more severely affected than the other. The predominant pattern of inflammation is mononuclear, i.e., with plasma cells and lymphocytes. Sometimes neutrophilic infiltrates are prominent, and pathologists may use the descriptive terms "acute" or "active chronic" to emphasize this feature.

Nonerosive nonspecific gastritis is traditionally divided into superficial and atrophic patterns, depending on its severity. In a given patient both patterns may be present. In superficial gastritis inflammatory cells are confined to the regions of the pits or foveolae (Plate 21–8). Atrophic gastritis is characterized by variable degrees of gland loss and associated encroachment of inflammatory cells into the gland zones. The severity of the superficial or atrophic gastritis is often graded further as mild, moderate, or severe. Severe atrophic gastritis would represent full-thickness mucosal involvement with disappearance of much of the gland mass.

A common accompaniment of nonerosive nonspecific gastritis is intestinal metaplasia. Intestinal-type goblet cells and even absorptive cells may be found in a "patchy" distribution. In severe cases of atrophic gastritis, intestinal metaplasia may replace the full thickness of the mucosa, with minimal residual inflammation, making the mucosa vir-

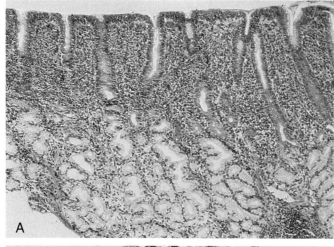

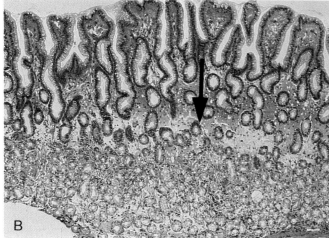

PLATE 21–8. *A,* Biopsy showing severe superficial antral gastritis. There are numerous inflammatory cells in pit (foveolar) regions. The clear-staining antral glands are preserved. Contrast with *B. B,* Normal antral gland biopsy. The black arrow spans some "edema" and hemorrhage, common findings in pinch biopsies.

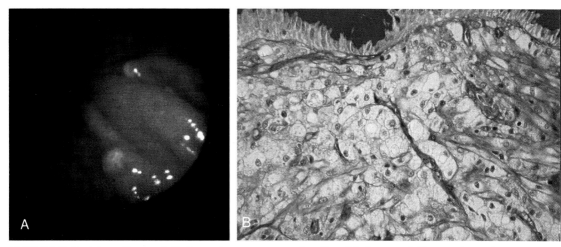

PLATE 21–9. Gastric xanthoma. *A,* Endoscopic appearance — two tiny white bumps. *B,* Biopsy of one of the bumps. The lamina propria is filled with ballooned clear-staining fat-laden histiocytes (PAS stain).

tually indistinguishable from that of the small bowel.

Gastric xanthomas, xanthelasma, or lipid islands are lesions that may represent idiosyncratic reactions that are part of the spectrum of nonerosive nonspecific gastritis. These are flat or slightly raised white or yellow-white lesions that range from pinpoint size to several millimeters in diameter (Plate 21–9). They have been observed with a frequency ranging from less than 1% to 58%[32, 33] and occur more commonly in the postoperative stomach.[34] Histologically, these lesions consist of accumulations of foamy, fat-laden histiocytes (Plate 21–9).

Endoscopy-Biopsy Correlations

The only instance in which endoscopic appearance predicts the severity of histologic change is when the mucosa, especially in the gastric body, exhibits a thin, parchment-like appearance with prominent visible vessels (Plate 21–10). In this circumstance, severe atrophic gastritis is likely to be present.[1, 35] Otherwise, there is a very poor correlation between endoscopic and microscopic appearances. Severe nonerosive gastritis may be found in endoscopically normal-appearing stomachs,[1] and, conversely, changes such as mucosal erythema and friability often correlate poorly with the degree of histologic abnormality.[1, 36]

What then do the endoscopic appearances of mucosal swelling, erythema, etc. represent if there is such a poor correlation with histologic evidence of gastritis? The answer is not known. Certain mucosal appearances may reflect functional changes such as alterations in blood flow, which cannot be detected using conventional morphologic techniques.

Endoscopic chromoscopy with Congo red–methylene blue dyes has been used in Japan for large surveys of nonerosive nonspecific gastritis in various disorders.[37] These techniques are discussed in Part 2 of Chapter 10.

Clinical Associations

Clinical conditions associated with nonerosive nonspecific gastritis are outlined in Table 21–3.

Health

Nonerosive nonspecific gastritis is a common finding in healthy asymptomatic persons. Surveys are available from a number of

TABLE 21–3. Clinical Associations with Nonerosive Nonspecific Gastritis

Association	Comment
Healthy Asymptomatic	Antral gland inflammation usually more severe than fundic gland inflammation
Peptic Ulcer	In contrast to gastric ulcer, the fundic gland mucosa is usually spared in duodenal ulcer
Adenocarcinoma	Exclusive of adenocarcinoma of the cardia region
Pernicious Anemia	Some patients have concomitant antral gland gastritis
Postgastrectomy	Severe gastritis not inevitable in all patients
Infectious "Epidemic" Gastritis	Spontaneous hypochlorhydria; organisms not identified
Campylobacter-like Organisms	Cause and effect not established

countries[38–41] but not from North America. The prevalence of gastritis may be greater in populations in whom the prevalence of gastric ulcer and gastric cancer is also increased.

Population surveys indicate that the gastritis begins in the third or fourth decade and progresses with time. Nonerosive nonspecific gastritis of the antrum usually predominates over fundic gland gastritis and is generally more severe on the lesser curvature.

Although there appears to be an age-dependent progression from superficial to more atrophic forms of gastritis, this process is not inevitable. Reversibility has been documented.[42] Furthermore, a recent endoscopic biopsy re-evaluation of a Finnish population[43] and an autopsy study from Japan[44] suggest that there may be a decrease in the prevalence of atrophic gastritis, especially in the antrum. This may be due to changing environmental factors such as diet and other habits. It has been suggested that these may be the same factors accounting for the decreasing incidence of gastric ulcer and gastric cancer.[44]

Peptic Ulcer

Nonerosive nonspecific gastritis, especially of the antrum, appears to be more severe and prevalent in both gastric and duodenal ulcer disease. It is not known whether the modern-day drugs used to treat peptic ulcers reduce the severity of this associated gastric inflammation.

Gastric Ulcer. Chronic gastric ulcers are

associated with a diffuse antral gland gastritis[45-47] that is more severe and more prevalent than in the general population. This observation has led to the notion that the basic defect in gastric ulcer disease is the extensive antral gland inflammation. The mucosa of the gastric body is commonly inflamed also, but usually to a lesser extent. However, in a recent follow-up study of patients who had previous gastric ulcers, it appeared that the antral gland gastritis actually improved but that there was a more striking progression of inflammation in the fundic gland mucosa.[47] This may not be unique to gastric ulcer patients but may actually reflect the changing environmental influences referred to earlier.

One important exception to the antral gland gastritis–gastric ulcer association occurs in some patients who habitually use aspirin. In some of these individuals there is no associated diffuse antral gland gastritis.[48]

Duodenal Ulcer. The association between antral gland gastritis and duodenal ulcer has not been studied as extensively as that with gastric ulcer. Nevertheless, it appears that nonerosive antral gland gastritis is more severe and more prevalent in patients with duodenal ulcers than in control populations.[49, 50] However, in contrast to gastric ulcer, the fundic gland mucosa of the stomach in duodenal ulcer patients remains more "juvenile" and appears to be less susceptible to the nonerosive nonspecific gastritis that occurs in healthy older persons.[50]

Adenocarcinoma

Adenocarcinomas of the gastric antrum and body are frequently associated with a severe antral gland and fundic gland gastritis with prominent accompanying intestinal metaplasia.[51-54] Most data in this regard come from countries or population groups in which the endogenous prevalence rates for gastric carcinoma are much higher than in North America. Adenocarcinomas of the gastric cardia region differ, however, in that the fundic gland mucosa is usually normal or only mildly inflamed.[55, 56]

Pernicious Anemia

In pernicious anemia there may be accompanying moderately severe antral gland gastritis.[57] For this reason, and because a combination of antral and fundic gland gastritis occurs so frequently in other settings. the popular terms type A (fundic gland) and type B (antral gland) gastritis[58] should be regarded as overly simplistic.

The gastric mucosa in pernicious anemia may also contain a variety of other findings. There is the well-recognized increased risk of gastric adenocarcinoma, which may be as great as three times that of the general population.[59, 60] In assessing cancer risk, the intrinsic prevalence of gastric carcinoma in a given country must be taken into account. Polyps of the inflammatory or hyperplastic type may occur.[61, 62] Inflammatory polyps may appear and disappear.[61] Hyperplasia of mucosal endocrine cells has been recognized in patients with pernicious anemia for some time,[57] but there has been more recent recognition of carcinoid polyps and tumors in small numbers of patients.[62, 63]

Endoscopic biopsy is not generally required to establish a diagnosis of pernicious anemia in clear-cut cases. If for some special reason histologic verification of severe atrophic fundic gland gastritis is required, the specimens should be obtained from the mid-body greater curvature. This is the zone where the fundic glands are normally thickest. Even in the presence of absolute achlorhydria there are often tiny residual nests of parietal and chief cells.[57]

The yield from repeated endoscopic surveillance for carcinoma is likely to be minimal. However, a recent recommendation from a group in England seems reasonable concerning the initial evaluation of these patients.[62] Specifically, they should have endoscopy with multiple biopsies at least once after pernicious anemia has been diagnosed. This serves to detect the very small group who might have adenomatous polyps, carcinoma, or gastric carcinoids. Follow-up thereafter is restricted to those patients with unusual findings.

Postgastrectomy

Postgastrectomy disorders are considered in detail in Chapter 24. Nonerosive nonspecific gastritis may develop after gastric surgery for peptic ulcer, especially antrectomy. The rate of development is accelerated in the first 2 years after the operation and then appears to proceed at the same rate as in the general population.[64] It should be stressed, however, that severe nonerosive gastritis is not inevitable in all patients. In some there is minimal or no inflammatory change with just a thinner fundic gland mucosa in the gastric remnant.[36] The stomal region often exhibits the most impressive changes on endoscopic examination. Histologically it has the most marked epithelial changes but contains fewer inflammatory cells than the rest of the gastric remnant.[36, 65]

Infections

Epidemic Gastritis. There have been two accounts of mini-epidemics of nonerosive nonspecific gastritis detected in volunteers for secretory studies.[66, 67] These individuals had short-lived upper abdominal complaints and developed hypochlorhydria. Endoscopy findings in one of the studies were reported to be normal.[67] The hypochlorhydria appeared to be due to severe functional impairment of the parietal cells, since the severity of the fundic gland gastritis histologically was not sufficient to account for the observed reduction in acid secretory potential.

Campylobacter-like Organisms. There has been a surge of interest in finding *Campylobacter*-like organisms in association with nonerosive nonspecific gastritis, especially in the antrum.[68, 69] The organisms have been detected in individuals who have histologic evidence of inflammation, independent of whether they are symptomatic. The bacteria appear to cluster more often on the surface epithelium and pits of biopsies in which neutrophils are more prominent. These mucosa-related bacteria have not been fully characterized, nor is it known whether they cause inflammation or simply nestle in areas that are already inflamed.

Clinical Implications

Dyspepsia

Does nonerosive nonspecific gastritis cause dyspepsia? If it does, it is likely that a cause and effect relation occurs only in a subset of individuals who have yet to be identified and that proving the connection represents a formidable challenge. The challenge begins with the reality that there is no easy way to define nonulcer dyspepsia. Also, one would have to demonstrate that some form of therapy improves both symptoms and mucosal inflammation in parallel.

From studies utilizing conventional grading of nonerosive nonspecific gastritis it has been concluded that there is no correlation between dyspepsia and nonerosive nonspecific gastritis.[70, 71] Other investigators have sought to determine whether density of neutrophils might correlate with dyspepsia. The results of one study suggested that this might be the case.[72] However, in a study of patients after gastric surgery, although therapy was associated with a reduction in density of neu-

trophils, there was no significant improvement in symptoms compared with controls.[73]

Thus, at present there is no clinical indication to take biopsies from patients with dyspepsia in order to determine whether they have nonerosive nonspecific gastritis.

Surveillance for Carcinoma in Severe Atrophic Gastritis

Are endoscopic surveillance biopsies for carcinoma beneficial in severe atrophic gastritis? At present the general answer is no. Patients with severe atrophic gastritis, especially with extensive accompanying intestinal metaplasia, have a statistically greater risk of adenocarcinoma developing in the stomach.[74] There is no way to select a smaller subset of these patients who are truly at risk, compared with the huge numbers in whom adenocarcinoma will never develop in their lifetime. In addition, such potential risk factors for gastric adenocarcinoma may be of less importance in countries with low incidence rates of gastric cancer.[74-76]

Endoscopy surveillance with multiple biopsies is reasonable in individuals with severe atrophic gastritis only if they have other risk factors such as a strong family history of gastric adenocarcinoma or a history of adenomatous polyps. In addition to biopsies of any discrete lesions, multiple random biopsies should be obtained in these settings. There is no uniform practice or guidelines. My approach is to take 12 biopsies, 6 each from the antrum and body respectively, half from each curvature or wall. In these super-selected high-risk groups there are no guidelines as to frequency of endoscopic biopsy surveillance, but a reasonable interval would be 3 to 5 years. This arbitrary interval is derived by analogy from the experience of European investigators who engaged in endoscopic biopsy surveillance studies of the postoperative stomach.[77, 78]

Endoscopic biopsy surveillance for adenocarcinoma must be tempered with a note of caution concerning the interpretation of the finding of dysplasia. Severe or high-grade dysplasia is an ominous lesion and is considered a precursor for invasive carcinoma. However, its natural history in terms of progression to invasive carcinoma is unknown. Its interpretation requires an experienced pathologist. If high-grade dysplasia is found in an area unassociated with an obvious mass lesion, a second biopsy should be undertaken immediately to determine how extensive the process is and whether microinvasive carcinoma is already present. Thereafter, a decision concerning surgery, which may entail partial or total gastrectomy, must be highly individualized. If faced with this problem, it is worthwhile soliciting an opinion from one of the handful of experts who have experience with the interpretation of high-grade dysplasia.

SPECIFIC TYPES OF GASTRITIS: EROSIVE AND NONEROSIVE

Specific types of gastritis are uncommon. Sometimes the gross endoscopic appearance is distinctive, as in Ménétrier's disease. More often it is the histologic changes that are either diagnostic or highly compatible with a limited group of disorders. Table 21–4 outlines the specific types of gastritis that will be discussed in this section.

Ménétrier's Disease

A synonym for this entity is idiopathic hypertrophic gastropathy. Since there are even rarer and more enigmatic syndromes that qualify as idiopathic hypertrophic gastropathy (to be discussed), the term Ménétrier's disease is preferred.

This syndrome generally occurs in older adults whose presenting symptoms are weight loss and abdominal pain. Hypoproteinemia is a prominent feature.[79, 80] A similar condition has been described in children but is potentially reversible and probably has a different pathogenesis.[81]

Many of these patients are referred for endoscopy because massively enlarged gastric folds are detected with barium upper gastrointestinal x-rays during initial investigation. The fundus and body (especially the greater curvature) are commonly affected, but there may be concomitant involvement of the antrum. Occasionally the antrum is selectively involved.[80]

The endoscopic findings are striking, with massively heaped-up folds, sometimes associated with erosions or ulcers. The folds may be pliable, but they are not fully effaced with air insufflation (Plate 21–11A). The crests of folds sometimes have a confluent polypoid appearance.

The histology is characterized by markedly elongated gastric pits and cysts with an edematous stroma (Plate 21–11B). Normal fundic gland elements are replaced in the gastric body; this accounts for the associated hypochlorhydria.

Surgical resection was formerly employed in most cases. This had two purposes: to confirm the diagnosis and to control the symptoms. If patients' symptoms can be controlled, surgery is not indicated to establish a primary diagnosis if the findings are otherwise compatible with Ménétrier's disease.[80] Biopsies obtained with pinch forceps at endoscopy provide a clue to the diagnosis, since marked foveolar cell hyperplasia will be present, but the relatively superficial endoscopic biopsy cannot establish the diagnosis with certainty. A more definitive diagnosis can be made with a full-thickness mucosal biopsy, but this requires special techniques at endoscopy such as an excisional electrosurgical snare biopsy.[82]

There are a few random reports of adenocarcinoma occurring in Ménétrier's disease.[79, 83] It has been recommended that periodic endoscopy surveillance be performed in patients who have not had resections and that biopsies be taken from the hypertrophied folds as well as the uninvolved areas.[83] This may be difficult to accomplish with such a massive degree of fold enlargement. Nevertheless, periodic endoscopy with multiple biopsies at 2- to 3-year intervals does seem reasonable. The rarity of Ménétrier's disease may never permit establishment of definitive risk data for adenocarcinoma.

If the differential diagnosis of Ménétrier's disease is viewed broadly from the perspective of all causes of thickened gastric folds, it ranges from "pseudo-thickened" folds seen on barium x-ray to infections and neoplasms. In reality, however, the main disorders to exclude by evaluation of these patients are

TABLE 21–4. **Specific Types of Gastritis: Erosive and Nonerosive**

Confined to Stomach
    Ménétrier's disease*
    Pseudolymphoma
    Isolated unexplained granulomas†

In Gastrointestinal Tract
    Crohn's disease
    Eosinophilic gastritis

In Systemic Disease
    Sarcoidosis

Infections and Infestations

*The text includes a discussion of other types of idiopathic hypertrophic gastropathies as part of the differential diagnosis of Ménétrier's disease.

†Table 21–5 contains a list of other disorders in which granulomas may be found.

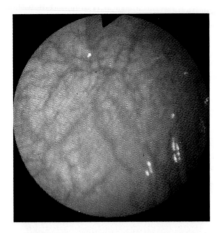

PLATE 21–10. Thin-appearing mucosa. Note the prominent vascular pattern. This endoscopic appearance in the gastric body on greater curvature suggests that there is severe atrophic gastritis.

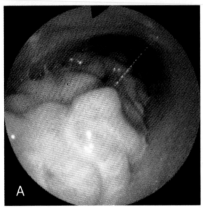

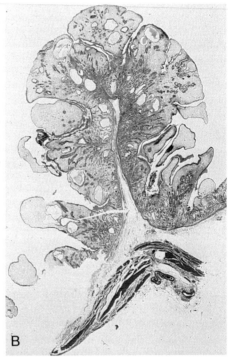

PLATE 21–11. Ménétrier's disease. A, Endoscopic view of raised polypoid folds on greater curvature of stomach. (Courtesy of Prof. G.N. Tytgat.) B, Snare biopsy of Ménétrier's disease. The polypoid lesion contains numerous cysts with a loose stroma (Courtesy of K. Lewin, M.D.)

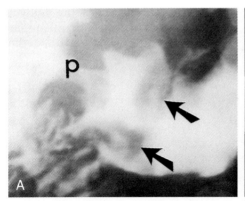

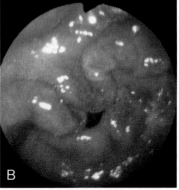

PLATE 21–12. Localized idiopathic antral hypertrophy. A, Barium x-ray, close-up view. There are nodular-type filling defects (arrows) for several centimeters proximal to pylorus (P). B, Red, raised serpentine folds radiating into the pylorus. Snare biopsy revealed only nonerosive nonspecific gastritis.

neoplasms, especially lymphomas and diffusely infiltrative carcinomas. Other conditions in the differential diagnosis are rarer than Ménétrier's disease itself and include hypertrophic hypersecretory states that may be accompanied by protein-losing gastropathy but in which parietal and chief cell numbers are not reduced.[84, 85] The Zollinger-Ellison syndrome may also be associated with giant gastric folds, but clinically this is not a problem in differential diagnosis. The endoscopy and biospy appearances in the Cronkhite-Canada syndrome[86] are very similar to the findings in Ménétrier's disease. Localized hypertrophic gastropathy of the antrum has been reported. Its histology is characterized by very prominent hyperplasia of surface and pit epithelium.[87] Underlying neoplasms must be excluded when this localized form of hypertrophic gastropathy is encountered (Plate 21–12).

Gastric Pseudolymphoma

Gastric pseudolymphoma refers to localized areas of lymphoid hyperplasia.[88–90] Sometimes these lesions are detected in biopsy specimens from the margins of gastric ulcers. In other instances the lesions may display a mass or plaque-like effect in the stomach. Histologically, there is massive lymphoid hyperplasia that may extend through the full thickness of the gastric wall (Plate 21–13). Endoscopic biopsies obtained with conventional forceps are inadequate to gauge depth or to exclude lymphoma satisfactorily. In a small area such as one surrounding an apparently benign gastric ulcer, a snare biopsy might be attempted for diagnosis. When gastric pseudolymphoma produces a mass-like lesion, however, surgical resection is necessary to exclude lymphoma completely. Some cases of gastric pseudolymphoma may represent precursor lesions for lymphoma,[89] whereas others are probably an atypical response to benign gastric ulceration. Prior to obtaining operative biopsies in these patients, the pathologist should be consulted to ensure that a part of the specimen is prepared for immunocytochemistry to aid in the differential diagnosis of lymphoma and the very rare syndrome of lymphomatoid granulomatosis.[91] Gastric pseudolymphoma is also discussed in Chapter 22.

Isolated (Unexplained) Granulomatous Gastritis

Isolated (unexplained) granulomatous gastritis is a term of exclusion that refers to the finding of isolated granulomas in the absence of any specific disease. It is not at all uncommon to find isolated granulomas in gastric biopsies taken for a variety of reasons (Plate 21–14). Some of these granulomas are of the foreign body type, containing debris, and are presumed to represent a reaction to some form of prior mucosal injury.

The term isolated granulomatous gastritis is used to describe granulomatous inflammation associated with striking structural changes in the stomach, especially the antrum. These findings may mimic gastric carcinoma with marked antral narrowing,[92] mass lesions,[93] and ulcerative lesions that may even perforate.[94, 95]

Before isolated granulomatous gastritis is diagnosed, other conditions in which granulomas may be found, especially infections, must be excluded. Some of these are outlined in Table 21–5.

Crohn's Disease

Gastroduodenal Crohn's disease is uncommon but not rare. The antrum is the main site affected in the stomach, and disease here usually coexists with involvement of the proximal duodenum. One should be extremely wary of the diagnosis of isolated Crohn's disease of the stomach in the absence of involvement in the more customary sites.

TABLE 21–5. **Conditions That May Be Associated with the Finding of Gastric Granulomas***

Isolated (Unexplained) Granulomas
    Foreign-body type
    As mass, ulcer, or in normal-appearing mucosa

Noninfectious
    Crohn's disease
    Sarcoidosis
    Chronic granulomatous disease (childhood)
    Allergic granulomatosis

Infectious
    Tuberculosis
    Histoplasmosis
    Late syphilis
    Parasitic

*Modified from Weinstein WM.[31]

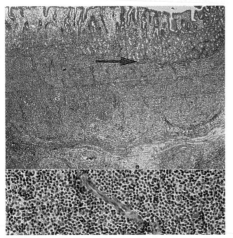

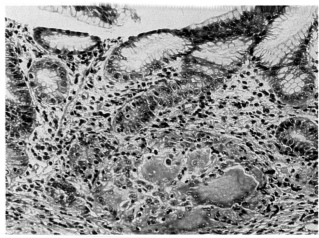

PLATE 21—13.   PLATE 21—14.

PLATE 21—13. Gastric pseudolymphoma resection specimen. The low-power view in the top panel shows a dense infiltrate beneath the gland zone, as demarcated by the arrow. The higher-power view in the lower panel shows a benign-appearing homogeneous cellular infiltrate.

PLATE 21—14. Isolated unexplained antral granuloma with pink-staining giant cells.

Patients may have presenting symptoms of delayed gastric emptying because of a narrowed gastroduodenal region or dyspepsia associated with mucosal lesions. Other complications include fistulas to the small bowel or colon. Transmural narrowing or fistulas are best evaluated radiographically.[96] The mucosal involvement of gastroduodenal Crohn's disease is best assessed by endoscopy.[96, 97] Gastroscopic findings attributable to Crohn's disease are similar to those seen elsewhere in the gastrointestinal tract, including fine nodularity, serpiginous ulcers, and aphthoid lesions (Plate 21—15). Biopsies of target lesions may reveal granulomas in up to two-thirds of patients.[96] Areas of normal-appearing mucosa may also contain granulomas.[98]

When patients seriously ill with Crohn's disease undergo endoscopy for gastrointestinal tract bleeding or severe ulcer-type symptoms and erosions or ulcers are seen, it may be impossible to differentiate between lesions that are intrinsically those of Crohn's disease and stress erosions or ordinary peptic ulcers. In this setting opportunistic infections should also be considered in patients who have been receiving immunosuppressive therapy.

Eosinophilic Gastritis

In this rare condition the stomach and usually some other part of the gastrointestinal tract, especially the small bowel, are infiltrated by eosinophils and there is accompanying peripheral blood eosinophilia.[99, 100]

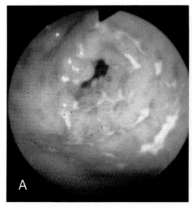

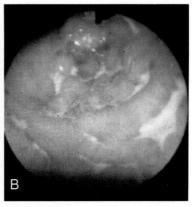

PLATE 21—15. Endoscopic views of Crohn's disease of the stomach. A, Erythema and serpiginous ulcers in prepyloric antrum. B, Closer view of serpiginous ulcers and nodularity. (Courtesy of M.V. Sivak, Jr., M.D.)

When the eosinophilic infiltrates predominate in the mucosa, malabsorption is the primary clinical problem. If the muscle layers are involved, obstructive symptoms predominate.

Symptoms from gastric involvement are those of delayed gastric emptying or gastrointestinal bleeding. Endoscopy during the active stage, when there is mucosal involvement, may reveal nodularity and sometimes persistent pyloric outlet obstruction.[101, 102] The diagnosis is not always easy, and in children it has been shown that random biopsies from the gastric antrum may reveal eosinophilic infiltrates.[103] The main differential diagnosis of eosinophilic gastritis is infestation with parasites. The relationship, if any, to the rarer disorder of allergic granulomatosis is unclear.[104]

The entity eosinophilic granuloma is sometimes confused semantically with eosinophilic gastroenteritis. A more appropriate term for this lesion is inflammatory fibroid polyp.[105] These are solitary lesions, either sessile or on a stalk, that are more commonly found in the ileum but may occur in the stomach. These lesions are not accompanied by peripheral blood eosinophilia, and their main histologic features are prominent vascularity and broad zones of connective tissue in the stroma.[105] These fibroid polyps have no relationship to eosinophilic gastritis. In the stomach the diagnosis may be established with endoscopic polypectomy, thus avoiding the need for surgery.[106]

Sarcoidosis

In this condition granulomas may be found in endoscopically normal mucosa[107] as well as adjacent to areas of antral narrowing, thickened folds in the gastric body, and gastric ulcers.[108–110] If granulomas are detected in the course of evaluating a patient with known sarcoidosis, other causes, specifically infections, should be ruled out. When there is marked wall narrowing or thickened folds, infiltrative neoplasms must be excluded.

Infections and Infestations

The most important infections of the stomach to consider are the opportunistic types. The two most treatable are *Candida* and perhaps herpes. Parasitic infestation of the stomach is rare in North Americans, but it should be considered in evaluating patients from some other countries. If parasitic infestation of the stomach is ever a consideration, duodenal aspirates for examination should be obtained at the same endoscopy session.

Phlegmonous and Emphysematous Gastritis

Phlegmonous and emphysematous gastritis are life-threatening entities in which extensive bacterial inflammation of the submucosa of the stomach is associated with perforation.[111] Emphysematous gastritis is a variant of phlegmonous gastritis in which gas-forming organisms form blebs in the submucosa.[112] Patients present with an acute abdomen. Plain and barium x-ray films suggest massive thickening of the gastric wall, sometimes with intramural air. Various organisms have been recovered,[111] including some exotic ones.[112, 113] Not surprisingly, this condition has now been reported in acquired immune deficiency syndrome (AIDS).[114] Endoscopy has no role because these patients require prompt laparotomy, although one patient did survive without surgery after a snare biopsy established the diagnosis.[115] Endoscopic procedures with polypectomy[116] and India ink marking of the stomach[117] have been reported to cause phlegmonous gastritis.

Tuberculosis

The stomach is only rarely involved in abdominal tuberculosis.[118, 119] The localization is similar to that of Crohn's disease, and the delayed development of pyloroduodenal obstruction may occur.

The main role of the endoscopist in a suspected case is to obtain biopsies to search for caseating granulomas and to submit biopsy tissue for culture.

Syphilis

Syphilis may rarely involve the stomach and present as thickened or deformed gastric folds or as erosions and ulcers.[120–122] The histologic findings may be nonspecific, and proof that syphilis causes gastric lesions rests with demonstration of the organism in gastric tissue and with serologic testing.

Fungal Infections

Candida albicans

If searched for, *Candida albicans* is found commonly in association with erosions, ulcers, and tumors in the immunocompromised as well as the immunocompetent host.[123–126] Because it is a common commensal organism, it can be cultured more often than it can actually be seen in tissue specimens.[126] Recognition of the presence of this fungus is of value mainly when plaques, erosions, or ulcers are encountered in the immunocompromised patient. Even in this setting, *Candida* may not be a major contributor to the mucosal injury. However, the diagnosis of *Candida*-associated mucosal disease may raise the possibility of more widespread dissemination. The simplest method of diagnosis is to prepare a dry smear on glass slides for examination. Often biopsies are obtained to determine if there is evidence of invasion. Clinical judgment, not histologic demonstration of tissue invasion in tiny biopsy specimens, should be the basis for treatment with local or systemic antifungal therapy. If cultures are taken, other species of *Candida* may be found, as well as other fungi such as *Torulopsis glabrata*.[126]

Histoplasmosis

When disseminated *Histoplasmosis* infection involves the stomach, it is usually characterized by large gastric ulcers or erosions associated with gastric rugal hypertrophy.[127] Histology may reveal the granulomas containing the fungus, but the definitive diagnosis requires culture of biopsy specimens.

Other Fungi

Phycomycetes produces the disease mucormycosis, an infection that is rare in North America. When this infection occurs in the stomach, there is a high mortality rate. Typical lesions are characterized by deep ulcers with black edges. In suspected cases biopsies and smears should be obtained to search for the typical-appearing hyphae.[128] Comparably rare involvement of the stomach occurs in actinomycosis.[129]

Viral Infections

Herpes Simplex Virus

Gastric erosions associated with herpes simplex virus infection in the stomach have been described.[130–132] With greater awareness of this association, it is likely that this virus will be identified more frequently in the stomach, especially in immunocompromised patients. This is an important consideration because of available antiviral therapy. The best approach to diagnosis in erosions or ulcers is a smear for cytologic examination to look for

the typical cells, another smear for culture, and several biopsies for culture and histology.[133] The exudate in lesions caused by herpes is the most productive source for diagnosis.[133]

Cytomegalovirus

Cytomegalovirus is commonly found in the stomach, as well as the rest of the gastrointestinal tract, in immunosuppressed patients.[134–136] Morphologic evidence on biopsy, i.e., large cells with typical intranuclear inclusions, may be seen in areas that are not inflamed or eroded. Therefore, it is difficult to know whether the finding of cytomegalovirus adjacent to an area of ulceration really means that the lesion was caused by the virus. The answer to this question of potential for mucosal damage awaits effective therapy for this virus. Sometimes documentation of gastric cytomegalovirus infection may be the first sign of generalized disease.[134] Recently, large nodular folds associated with erosions and ulcerations were described in the fundus or antrum of AIDS patients.[136] Biopsy specimens suggested cytomegalovirus infection. We have also observed this finding. The main considerations when these endoscopic findings are noted in a patient with AIDS, independent of whether or not cytomegalovirus is present, are underlying lymphoma or Kaposi's sarcoma.

Parasites

Anisakiasis

The thread-like nematode *Anisakis* is present in some raw fish and produces a dramatic syndrome of severe abdominal pain. The impressive radiologic and endoscopic findings are those of the worm protruding from a swollen or eroded gastric mucosa.[137] This is a self-limited illness, in which symptoms disappear within several days, and the worms disappear within several weeks. In Japan some of these patients are treated with endoscopic removal of the worms, and it is reported that pain disappears within a few hours.[137] Not surprisingly, given the current fashion of raw fish ingestion in the United States, cases of infestation have been reported, with some patients from California possibly setting a new American trend.[138]

Strongyloides stercoralis

Strongyloides infestation is endemic in certain parts of the United States.[139] It has been reported in a gastric biopsy of a patient with normal-appearing mucosa,[140] in a biopsy from a gastric ulcer,[141] and as a cause of emphysematous gastritis.[112]

Other Infestations

Endoscopic "capture" of hookworm has been documented,[142] *Schistosoma mansoni* was discovered at the edge of a gastric ulcer,[143] and *Cryptosporidium* has been seen in gastric biopsy sections from patients with AIDS.[144] It is not known whether *Cryptosporidium* produces gastritis.

Acknowledgments

I am indebted to Marilyn Weinstein for her indefatigable editorial assistance, to Klaus Lewin M.D. for stimulating clinico-pathological discussions, and to the UCLA GI Procedures Unit Staff for handling endoscopic biopsies with such care.

References

1. Sauerbruch T, Schreiber MA, Schüssler P, Permanetter W. Endoscopy in the diagnosis of gastritis. Diagnostic value of endoscopic criteria in relation to histological diagnosis. Endoscopy 1984; 16:101–4.
2. Nesland AA, Berstad A. Erosive prepyloric changes in persons with and without dyspepsia. Scand J Gastroenterol 1985; 20:222–8.
3. Jabbari M, Cherry R, Lough JO, et al. Gastric antral vascular ectasia: The watermelon stomach. Gastroenterology 1984; 87:1165–70.
4. Lee FI, Costello F, Flanagan N, Vasudev KS. Diffuse antral vascular ectasia. Gastrointest Endosc 1984; 30:87–90.
5. McCormack TT, Sims J, Eyre-Brook I, et al. Gastric lesions in portal hypertension: inflammatory gastritis or congestive gastropathy? Gut 1985; 26:1226–32.
6. Lucas CE, Sugawa C, Riddle J, et al. Natural history and surgical dilemma of "stress" gastric bleeding. Arch Surg 1971; 102:266–73.
7. Franzin G, Manfrini C, Musola R, et al. Chronic erosions of the stomach—A clinical, endoscopic and histological evaluation. Endoscopy 1984; 16:1–5.
8. Ito S, Lacy ER. Characteristics of ethanol-induced lesions in rat gastric mucosa. In: Allen A, et al, eds. Mechanisms of Mucosal Protection in the Upper Gastrointestinal Tract. New York: Raven Press 1984; 57–63.
9. Lambert R, Andre C, Moulinier B, Bugnon B. Diffuse varioliform gastritis. Digestion 1978; 17:159–67.
10. Stamm B, Heer M, Buhler H, Ammann R. Mucosal biopsy of vascular ectasia (angiodysplasia) of the large bowel detected during routine colonoscopic examination. Histopathology 1985; 9:639–46.
11. Wheeler MH, Smith PM, Cotton PB, et al. Abnormal blood vessels in the gastric antrum. A cause of upper gastrointestinal bleeding. Dig Dis Sci 1979; 24:155–8.
12. Marrone GC, Silen W. Pathogenesis, diagnosis and treatment of acute gastric mucosal lesions. Clin Gastroenterol 1984; 13:635–50.
13. Czaja AJ, McAlhany JC, Pruit BA Jr. Acute gastro-

14. Czaja AJ, McAlhany JC, Pruit BA Jr. Acute duodenitis and duodenal ulceration after burns. Clinical and pathological characteristics. JAMA 1975; 232:621–4.
15. Halloran LG, Zfass AM, Gayle WE, et al. Prevention of acute gastrointestinal complications after severe head injury: a controlled trial of cimetidine prophylaxis. Am J Surg 1980; 139:44–8.
16. Shepherd A, Harvey J, Jackson A, Colin-Jones DG. Recurrent retching with gastric mucosal prolapse. A proposed prolapse gastropathy syndrome. Dig Dis Sci 1984; 29:121–8.
17. Bown SG, Swain CP, Storey DW, et al. Endoscopic laser treatment of vascular anomalies of the upper gastrointestinal tract. Gut 1985; 26:1338–48.
18. Poelman JR, Hausman RH, Hoitsma HW. Endoscopy in lye burns of oesophagus and stomach. Endoscopy 1977; 9:172–7.
19. Cello JP, Fogel RP, Boland CR. Liquid caustic ingestion. Spectrum of injury. Arch Intern Med 1980; 140:501–4.
20. Loeb PM, Eisenstein AM. Caustic injury to the upper gastrointestinal tract. In: Sleisenger MH, Fordtran JS, eds. Gastrointestinal Disease: Pathophysiology, Diagnoses, Management. Ed 3. Philadelphia: WB Saunders 1983; 148–55.
21. Novak JM, Collins JT, Donowitz M, et al. Effects of radiation on the human gastrointestinal tract. J Clin Gastroenterol 1979; 1:9–39.
22. Palmer ED. Gastritis: a reevaluation. Medicine 1954; 33:199–290.
23. Gottfried EB, Korsten MA, Lieber CS: Alcohol-induced gastric and duodenal lesions in man. Am J Gastroenterol 1978; 70:587–92.
24. Lanza FL, Royer GL, Nelson RS, et al. Ethanol, aspirin, ibuprofen, and the gastroduodenal mucosa: An endoscopic assessment. Am J Gastroenterol 1985; 80:767–9.
25. Faintuch J, Shepard KV, Blackstone MD, Levin B. Acute gastro-duodenal mucosal injury due to hepatic arterial floxuridine chemotherapy. Gastrointest Endosc (Abstr) 1984; 30:135.
26. Bourdages R, Prentice RSA, Beck IT, et al. Atheromatous embolization to the stomach. An unusual cause of gastrointestinal bleeding. Am J Dig Dis 1976; 21:889–94.
27. Shepherd HA, Patel C, Bamforth J, Isaacson P. Upper gastrointestinal endoscopy in systemic vasculitis presenting as an acute abdomen. Endoscopy 1983; 15:307–11.
28. Hoare AM, Jones EL, Alexander-Williams J, Hawkins CF. Symptomatic significance of gastric mucosal changes after surgery for peptic ulcer. Gut 1977; 18:295–300.
29. Green PHR, Fevre DI, Barrett PJ, et al. Chronic erosive (verrucous) gastritis. Endoscopy 1977; 9:74–8.
30. Elta GH, Fawaz KA, Dayal Y, et al. Chronic erosive gastritis—a recently recognized disorder. Dig Dis Sci 1983; 28:7–12.
31. Weinstein WM. Gastritis. In: Sleisenger MH, Fordtran JS, eds. Gastrointestinal Disease: Pathology, Diagnosis, Management. Ed 3. Philadelphia: WB Saunders 1983; 559–78.
32. Terruzzi V, Minoli G, Butti GC, Rossini A. Gastric lipid islands in the gastric stump and in the non-operated stomach. Endoscopy 1980; 12:58–62.

33. Kimura K, Hiramoto T, Buncher CR. Gastric xanthelasma. Arch Pathol 1969; 87:110–7.

34. Domellof L, Eriksson S, Helander HF, Janunger KB. Lipid islands in the gastric mucosa after resection for benign ulcer disease. Gastroenterology 1977; 72:14–8.

35. Meshkinpour H, Orlando RA, Arguello JF, DeMicco MP. Significance of endoscopically visible blood vessels as an index of atrophic gastritis. Am J Gastroenterol 1979; 71:376–9.

36. Weinstein WM, Buch KL, Elashof J, et al. The histology of the stomach in symptomatic patients after gastric surgery: A model to assess selective patterns of gastric mucosal injury. Scand J Gastroenterol 1985; 20(Suppl 109):77–89.

37. Tatsuta M, Iishi H, Ichii M, et al. Chromoendoscopic observations on extension and development of fundal gastritis and intestinal metaplasia. Gastroenterology 1985; 88:70–4.

38. Kimura K. Chronological transition of the fundic-pyloric border determined by stepwise biopsy of the lesser and greater curvatures of the stomach. Gastroenterology 1972; 63:584–92.

39. Kreuning J, Bosman FT, Kuiper G, et al. Gastric and duodenal mucosa in 'healthy' individuals. J Clin Pathol 1978; 31:69–77.

40. Cheli R, Simon L, Aste H, et al. Atrophic gastritis and intestinal metaplasia in asymptomatic Hungarian and Italian populations. Endoscopy 1980; 12:105–8.

41. Siurala M, Varis K, Kekki M. New aspects on epidemiology, genetics, and dynamics of chronic gastritis. In: van der Reis L, ed. Frontiers of Gastrointestinal Research. Basel: S. Karger, 1980; 6:148–66.

42. Rösch W, Demling L, Elster K. Is chronic gastritis a reversible process? Follow-up study of gastritis by stepwise biopsy. Acta Hepatogastroenterol 1979; 22:252–5.

43. Ihamaki T, Kekki M, Sipponen P, Siurala M. The sequelae and course of chronic gastritis during a 30- to 34-year bioptic follow-up study. Scand J Gastroenterol 1985; 20:485–91.

44. Imai T, Murayama H. Time trend in the prevalence of intestinal metaplasia in Japan. Cancer 1983; 52:353–61.

45. Oi M, Oshida K, Sugimura S. The location of gastric ulcer. Gastroenterology 1959; 36:45–56.

46. Gear MWL, Truelove SC, Whitehead R. Gastric ulcer and gastritis. Gut 1971; 12:639–45.

47. Maaroos HI, Salupere V, Uibo R, et al. Seven-year follow-up study of chronic gastritis in gastric ulcer patients. Scand J Gastroenterol 1985; 20:198–204.

48. MacDonald WC. Correlation of mucosal histology and aspirin intake in chronic gastric ulcer. Gastroenterology 1973; 65:381–9.

49. Aukee S. Gastritis and acid secretion in patients with gastric ulcers and duodenal ulcers. Scand J Gastroenterol 1972; 7:567–74.

50. Kekki M, Sipponen P, Siurala M. Progression of antral and body gastritis in patients with active and healed duodenal ulcer and duodenitis. Scand J Gastroenterol 1984; 19:382–8.

51. Haenszel W, Correa P, Cuello C, et al. Gastric cancer in Colombia. II. Case-control epidemiologic study of precursor lesions. J Natl Cancer Inst 1976; 57:1021–35.

52. Imai T, Kubo T, Watanabe H. Chronic gastritis in Japanese with reference to high incidence of gastric carcinoma. J Natl Cancer Inst 1971; 47:179–95.

53. Stemmerman G, Haenszel W, Locke F. Epidemiologic pathology of gastric ulcer and gastric carcinoma among Japanese in Hawaii. J Natl Cancer Inst 1977; 58:13–9.

54. Sipponen P, Kekki M, Siurala M. Atrophic chronic gastritis and intestinal metaplasia in gastric carcinoma. Comparison with a representative population sample. Cancer 1983; 52:1062–8.

55. MacDonald WC. Clinical and pathologic features of adenocarcinoma of the gastric cardia. Cancer 1972; 29:724–32.

56. Antonioli DA, Goldman H. Changes in the location and type of gastric adenocarcinoma. Cancer 1982; 50:775–81.

57. Lewin KJ, Dowling F, Wright JP, Taylor KB. Gastric morphology and serum gastrin levels in pernicious anaemia. Gut 1976; 17:551–60.

58. Strickland RG, Mackay IR. A reappraisal of the nature and significance of chronic atrophic gastritis. Am J Dig Dis 1973; 18:426–40.

59. Mosbech J, Videbaek A. Mortality from and risk of gastric carcinoma among patients with pernicious anaemia. Br Med J 1950; 2:390–4.

60. Elsborg L, Mosbech J. Pernicious anaemia as a risk factor in gastric cancer. Acta Med Scand 1979; 206:315–8.

61. Elsborg L, Andersen D, Myhre-Jensen O, Bastrup-Madsen P. Gastric mucosal polyps in pernicious anaemia. Scand J Gastroenterol 1977; 12:49–52.

62. Stockbrugger RW, Menon GG, Beilby JOW, et al. Gastroscopic screening in 80 patients with pernicious anaemia. Gut 1983; 24:1141–7.

63. Borch K, Renvall H, Liedberg G. Gastric endocrine cell hyperplasia and carcinoid tumors in pernicious anemia. Gastroenterology 1985; 88:638–48.

64. Kekki M, Saukkonen M, Sipponen P, et al. Dynamics of chronic gastritis in the remnant after partial gastrectomy for duodenal ulcer. Scand J Gastroenterol 1980; 15:509–12.

65. Saukkonen M, Sipponen P, Varis K, Siurala M. Morphological and dynamic behavior of the gastric mucosa after partial gastrectomy with special reference to the gastroenterostomy area. Hepatogastroenterology 1980; 27:48–56.

66. Ramsey EJ, Carey KV, Peterson WL, et al. Epidemic gastritis with hypochlorhydria. Gastroenterology 1979; 76:1449–57.

67. Gledhill T, Leicester RJ, Addis B, et al. Epidemic hypochlorhydria. Br Med J 1985; 290:1383–6.

68. Marshall BJ, Warren JR. Unidentified curved bacilli in the stomach of patients with gastritis and peptic ulceration. Lancet 1984; 1:1311–5.

69. Steer HW. The gastro-duodenal epithelium in peptic ulceration. J Pathol 1985; 146:355–62.

70. Villako K, Ihamaki T, Tamm A, Tammur R. Upper abdominal complaints and gastritis. Ann Clin Res 1984; 16:192–4.

71. Cheli R, Perasso A, Giacosa A. Dyspepsia and chronic gastritis. Hepatogastroenterology 1983; 30:21–3.

72. Toukan AU, Kamal MF, Amr SS, et al. Gastroduodenal inflammation in patients with nonulcer dyspepsia. A controlled endoscopic and morphometric study. Dig Dis Sci 1985; 30:313–20.

73. Buch KL, Weinstein WM, Hill TA, et al. Sucralfate therapy in patients with symptoms of alkaline reflux gastritis. A randomized, double-blind study. Am J Med 1985; 79(Suppl 2C):49–54.

74. Sipponen P, Kekki M, Haapakoski J, et al. Gastric cancer risk in chronic atrophic gastritis: Statistical

calculations of cross-sectional data. Int J Cancer 1985; 35:173–7.

75. Schafer LW, Larson DE, Melton LJ, et al. The risk of gastric carcinoma after surgical treatment for benign ulcer disease. A population-based study in Olmsted County, Minnesota. N Engl J Med 1983; 309:1210–3.

76. Sonnenberg A. Endoscopic screening for gastric stump cancer—would it be beneficial? A hypothetical cohort study. Gastroenterology 1984; 87:489–95.

77. Stokkeland M, Schrumpf E, Serck Hanssen A, et al. Incidence of malignancies of the Billroth II operated stomach. A prospective follow-up. Scand J Gastroenterol 1981; 16(Suppl 67):169–71.

78. Offerhaus GJA, Huibregtse K, de Boer J, et al. The operated stomach: A premalignant condition? A prospective endoscopic follow-up study. Scand J Gastroenterol 1984; 19:521–4.

79. Scharschmidt BF. The natural history of hypertrophic gastropathy (Ménétrier's disease). Report of a case with 16 year follow-up and review of 120 cases from the literature. Am J Med 1977; 63:644–52.

80. Searcy RM, Malagelada J-R. Ménétrier's disease and idiopathic hypertrophic gastropathy. Ann Intern Med 1984; 100:565–70.

81. Chouraqui JP, Roy CC, Brochu P, et al. Ménétrier's disease in children: Report of a patient and review of sixteen other cases. Gastroenterology 1981; 80:1042–7.

82. Bjork JT, Geenen JE, Komorowski RA, Soergel KH. Ménétrier's disease diagnosed by electrosurgical snare biopsy. JAMA 1977; 238:1755–6.

83. Wood GM, Bates C, Brown RC, Losowsky MS. Intramucosal carcinoma of the gastric antrum complicating Ménétrier's disease. J Clin Pathol 1983; 36:1071–5.

84. Brooks AM, Isenberg J, Goldstein H. Giant thickening of the gastric mucosa with acid hypersecretion and protein-losing gastropathy. Gastroenterology 1970; 58:73–9.

85. Overholt BF, Jeffries GH. Hypertrophic, hypersecretory protein-losing gastropathy. Gastroenterology 1970; 58:80–7.

86. Daniel ES, Ludwig SL, Lewin KJ, et al. The Cronkhite-Canada syndrome. An analysis of clinical and pathologic features and therapy in 55 patients. Medicine 1982; 61:293–309.

87. Stamp GWH, Palmer K, Misiewicz JJ. Antral hypertrophic gastritis; a rare cause of iron deficiency. J Clin Pathol 1985; 38:390–2.

88. Ranchod M, Lewin KJ, Dorfman RF. Lymphoid hyperplasia of the gastrointestinal tract. A study of 26 cases and review of the literature. Am J Surg Pathol 1978; 2:383–400.

89. Brooks JJ, Enterline HT. Gastric pseudolymphoma. Its three subtypes and relation to lymphoma. Cancer 1983; 51:476–86.

90. Orr RK, Lininger JR, Lawrence W Jr. Gastric pseudolymphoma. A challenging clinical problem. Ann Surg 1984; 200:185–94.

91. Rubin LA, Little AH, Kolin A, Keystone EC. Lymphomatoid granulomatosis involving the gastrointestinal tract. Two case reports and a review of the literature. Gastroenterology 1983; 84:829–33.

92. Khan MH, Lam R, Tamoney HJ. Isolated granulomatous gastritis. Am J Gastroenterol 1979; 71:90–4.

93. Weinstock JV. Idiopathic isolated granulomatous gastritis. Spontaneous resolution without surgical intervention. Dig Dis Sci 1980; 25:233–5.

94. Hanada M, Takami M, Hirata K, Nakajima T. Hyalinoid giant cell gastritis. A unique gastric lesion associated with eosinophilic hyalinoid degeneration of smooth muscle. Acta Pathol Jpn 1985; 35:749–58.

95. Compton CC, Von Lichtenberg F. Necrotizing granulomatous gastritis and gastric perforation of unknown etiology: a first case report. J Clin Gastroenterol 1983; 5:59–65.

96. Rutgeerts P, Onette E, Vantrappen G, et al. Crohn's disease of the stomach and duodenum: a clinical study with emphasis on the value of the endoscopy and endoscopic biopsies. Endoscopy 1980; 12:288–94.

97. Danzi JT, Farmer RG, Sullivan BH Jr, Rankin GB. Endoscopic features of gastroduodenal Crohn's disease. Gastroenterology 1976; 70:9–13.

98. Schmitz-Moormann P, Malchow H, Pittner PM. Endoscopic and bioptic study of the upper gastrointestinal tract in Crohn's disease patients. Pathol Res Pract 1985; 179:377–87.

99. Klein NC, Hargrove RL, Sleisenger MH, Jeffries GH. Eosinophilic gastroenteritis. Medicine 1970; 49:299–319.

100. Cello JP. Eosinophilic gastroenteritis—a complex disease entity. Am J Med 1979; 67:1097–104.

101. Caldwell JH, Mekhjian HS, Hurtubise PE, Beman FM. Eosinophilic gastroenteritis with obstruction. Immunological studies of seven patients. Gastroenterology 1978; 74:825–9.

102. Leinbach GE, Rubin CE. Eosinophilic gastroenteritis: a simple reaction to food allergens? Gastroenterology 1970; 59:874–89.

103. Katz AJ, Goldman H, Grand R. Gastric mucosal biopsy in eosinophilic (allergic) gastroenteritis. Gastroenterology 1977; 73:705–9.

104. Abell MR, Limond RV, Blamey WE, Martel W. Allergic granulomatosis with massive gastric involvement. N Engl J Med 1970; 282:665–8.

105. Johnstone JM, Morson BC. Inflammatory fibroid polyp of the gastrointestinal tract. Histopathology 1978; 2:349–61.

106. Eugene C, Penalba C, Gompel H, et al. Le granulome eosinophile gastrique: intérét de la polypectomie endoscopique. A propos de deux observations. Sem Hop Paris 1983; 59:2249–50.

107. Palmer ED. Note on silent sarcoidosis of the gastric mucosa. J Lab Clin Med 1958; 15:231–4.

108. Bennington JL, Porus R, Ferguson B, Hannon G. Cytology of gastric sarcoid. Report of a case. Acta Cytol 1968; 12:30–6.

109. Konda J, Ruth M, Sassaris M, Hunter FM. Sarcoidosis of the stomach and rectum. Am J Gastroenterol 1980; 73:516–8.

110. Chinitz MA, Brandt LJ, Frank MS, et al. Symptomatic sarcoidosis of the stomach. Dig Dis Sci 1985; 30:682–8.

111. Miller AI, Smith B, Rogers AI. Phlegmonous gastritis. Gastroenterology 1975; 68:231–8.

112. Williford ME, Foster WL Jr, Halvorsen RA, Thompson WM. Emphysematous gastritis secondary to disseminated strongyloidiasis. Gastrointest Radiol 1982; 7:123–6.

113. Dutz W, Saidi F, Kohout E. Gastric anthrax with massive ascites. Gut 1970; 11:352–4.

114. Mittleman RE, Suarez RV. Phlegmonous gastritis

associated with the acquired immunodeficiency syndrome/preacquired immunodeficiency syndrome. Arch Pathol Lab Med 1985; 109:765–7.

115. Bron BA, Deyhle P, Pelloni S, et al. Phlegmonous gastritis diagnosed by endoscopic snare biopsy. Dig Dis Sci 1977; 22:729–33.

116. Lifton LJ, Schlossberg D. Phlegmonous gastritis after endoscopic polypectomy. Ann Intern Med 1982; 97:373–4.

117. Honnig D, Kuhn H, Stadelmann O, Botticher R. Phlegmonous gastritis after India ink marking. Endoscopy 1983; 15:266–9.

118. Novis BH, Bank S, Marks IN. Gastrointestinal and peritoneal tuberculosis. S Afr Med J 1973; 47:365–72.

119. Palmer KR, Patil DH, Basran GS, et al. Abdominal tuberculosis in urban Britain—a common disease. Gut 1985; 26:1296–305.

120. Butz WC, Watts JC, Rosales-Quintana S, Hicklin MD. Erosive gastritis as a manifestation of secondary syphilis. Am J Clin Pathol 1975; 63:895–900.

121. Reisman TN, Leverett FL, Hudson JR, Kalser MH. Syphilitic gastropathy. Am J Dig Dis 1975; 20:588–93.

122. Morin ME, Tan A. Diffuse enlargement of gastric folds as a manifestation of secondary syphilis. Am J Gastroenterol 1980; 74:170–2.

123. Eras P, Goldstein MJ, Sherlock P. Candida infection of the gastrointestinal tract. Medicine 1972; 51:367–79.

124. Cronan J, Burrell M, Trepeta R. Aphthoid ulcerations in gastric candidiasis. Radiology 1980; 134:607–11.

125. Minoli G, Terruzzi V, Butti G, et al. Gastric candidiasis: an endoscopic and histological study in 26 patients. Gastrointest Endosc 1982; 28:59–61.

126. Di Febo G, Miglioli M, Calo G, et al. Candida albicans infection of gastric ulcer. Frequency and correlation with medical treatment. Results of a multicenter study. Dig Dis Sci 1985; 30:178–81.

127. Orchard JL, Luparello F, Brunskill D. Malabsorption syndrome occurring in the course of disseminated histoplasmosis. Case report and review of gastrointestinal histoplasmosis. Am J Med 1979; 66:331–5.

128. Schulman A, Bornman P, Kaplan C, et al. Gastrointestinal mucormycosis. Gastrointest Radiol 1979; 4:385–8.

129. Berardi RS. Abdominal actinomycosis. Surg Gynecol Obstet 1979; 149:257–66.

130. Howiler W, Goldberg HI. Gastroesophageal involvement in herpes simplex. Gastroenterology 1976; 70:775–8.

131. Sperling HV, Reed WG. Herpetic gastritis. Dig Dis Sci 1977; 22:1033–4.

132. Buss DH, Scharyj M. Herpesvirus infection of the esophagus and other visceral organs in adults. Incidence and clinical significance. Am J Med 1979; 66:457–62.

133. McDonald GB, Sharma P, Hackman RC, et al. Esophageal infections in immunosuppressed patients after marrow transplantation. Gastroenterology 1985; 88:1111–7.

134. Strayer DS, Phillips GB, Barker KH, et al. Gastric cytomegalovirus infection in bone marrow transplant patients: an indication of generalized disease. Cancer 1981; 48:1478–83.

135. Franzin G, Musola R, Mencarelli R. Changes in the mucosa of the stomach and duodenum during immunosuppressive therapy after renal transplantation. Histopathology 1982; 6:439–49.

136. Balthazar EJ, Megibow AJ, Hulnick DH. Cytomegalovirus esophagitis and gastritis in AIDS. Am J Radiol 1985; 144:1201–4.

137. Sugimachi K, Inokuchi K, Ooiwa T, et al. Acute gastric anisakiasis. Analysis of 178 cases. JAMA 1985; 253:1012–3.

138. Kliks MM. Anisakiasis in the western United States: four new case reports from California. Am J Trop Med Hyg 1983; 32:526–32.

139. Milder JE, Walzer PD, Kilgore G, et al. Clinical features of Strongyloides stercoralis infection in an endemic area of the United States. Gastroenterology 1981; 80:1481–8.

140. Barr JR. Strongyloides stercoralis. Can Med Assoc J 1978; 118:933–5.

141. Scowden EB, Schaffner W, Stone WJ. Overwhelming strongyloidiasis. An unappreciated opportunistic infection. Medicine 1978; 57:527–44.

142. Dumont A, Seferian V, Barbier P. Endoscopic discovery and capture of Necator americanus in the stomach. Endoscopy 1983; 15:65–6.

143. Capdevielle P, Coignard A, Le Gal E, et al. Ulcere prepylorique et biharziose gastrique. Gastroenterol Clin Biol 1979; 3:153–6.

144. Pitlik SD, Fainstein V, Garza D, et al. Human cryptosporidiosis: spectrum of disease. Report of six cases and review of the literature. Arch Intern Med 1983; 143:2269–75.

Chapter 22

BENIGN AND MALIGNANT TUMORS OF THE STOMACH

DENNIS M. JENSEN, M.D.

MALIGNANT TUMORS OF THE STOMACH

Gastric Carcinoma

Clinical Synopsis

In the United States and Europe over 90% of patients with gastric carcinoma present with advanced malignancy, so that the diagnosis is usually made late in the course of the disease.[1, 2] Often, nonspecific upper gastrointestinal symptoms, such as nausea, anorexia, dyspepsia, and occasionally vomiting, have been present for several months. As the tumor increases in size, early satiety and abdominal pain become more common complaints and are often accompanied by substantial weight loss, gastrointestinal bleeding, obstruction, and/or perforation. Occasionally, patients have dysphagia or other symptoms or signs of local spread of the tumor.

Rarely, distant metastases and associated symptoms are the first manifestation of gastric cancer: a tender liver due to metastases, bone pain, bloody ascites, headache, or neurologic signs of metastases. Osteoarthropathy and cerebellar degeneration can occur as manifestations of gastric carcinoma. Acanthosis nigricans has also been associated with cancer of the stomach.[3] The clinical presentation of carcinoma of the gastric cardia can closely simulate achalasia.

The detection of gastric carcinoma in an early, asymptomatic stage occurs infrequently in the United States. In Japan, however, early gastric carcinoma is often detected by various screening methods, including endoscopy.

There are striking differences in the incidence rates for cancer of the stomach throughout the world.[4] Furthermore, mortality due to this malignancy has been declining in many, but not all, countries over the past several decades. This is probably not attributable to any significant improvement in therapy. In the United States, for example, the number of patients surviving 5 years after diagnosis has increased by only 2% to 5% over the past two decades.[5] Earlier diagnosis could be a factor in the declining mortality statistics in some countries.

Diagnosis

The diagnosis of gastric carcinoma is confirmed in most patients by upper gastrointestinal series rather than endoscopy in the United States. Since American patients often present with advanced carcinoma of the stomach, the upper gastrointestinal series usually reveals a large ulcerated mass (Figs. 22–1 and 22–2). In some cases the malignancy is so advanced that it is evident on a plain x-ray film of the abdomen (Figs. 22–3 and 22–4). In many other countries, and now more frequently in the United States, endoscopy is the primary diagnostic test.

Rarely, the clinical presentation of a patient will be that of a surgical emergency, the diagnosis of advanced gastric carcinoma being made at operation; cancer-related perforation and massive bleeding are two such circumstances. However, with the widespread use of endoscopy for diagnosis and treatment of upper gastrointestinal bleeding, it would now be rare for a patient to undergo surgery for gastrointestinal hemorrhage without preoperative endoscopy.

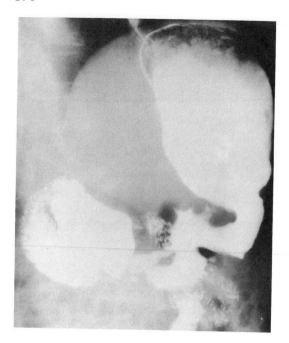

FIGURE 22–1. Upper gastrointestinal x-ray series of 68-year-old woman shows large, irregular, ulcerated antral mass. The patient had weight loss, upper gastrointestinal bleeding, and advanced gastric adenocarcinoma. (Courtesy of M. Weiner, M.D.)

FIGURE 22–2. 52-year-old man with Billroth II anastomosis and carcinoma in gastric remnant. Symptoms included abdominal pain and weight loss. There was evidence of partial obstruction on upper gastrointestinal x-ray series. Irregularity and scalloping along the inferior portion of the gastric remnant suggested carcinoma. Endoscopic biopsies revealed adenocarcinoma. The patient was not amenable to curative resection or palliative surgery. (Courtesy of B. Kadell, M.D.)

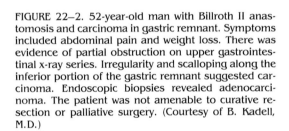

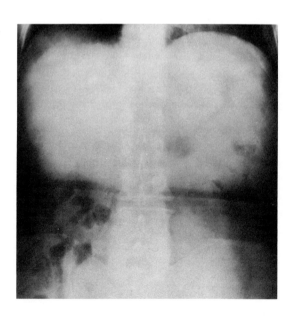

FIGURE 22–3. Plain x-ray film of abdomen showing compression of gastric profile suggesting malignant infiltration of stomach wall. This 64-year-old woman had weight loss, vague epigastric distress, and early satiety. (Courtesy of M. Weiner, M.D.)

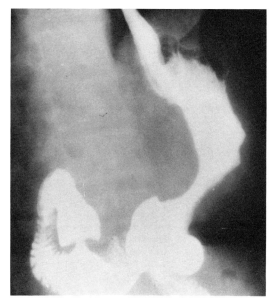

FIGURE 22–4. Upper gastrointestinal x-ray series on same patient as in Figure 22–3, showing carcinoma of the stomach. At endoscopy there were large gastric folds without mucosal ulceration and with lack of distensibility of the gastric body. Routine endoscopic biopsies were not diagnostic. Laparotomy with full-thickness biopsies confirmed the diagnosis of diffusely infiltrating, unresectable adenocarcinoma (linitis plastica) of the stomach. (Courtesy of M. Weiner, M.D.)

Endoscopy

Endoscopic confirmation of the diagnosis of gastric carcinoma has become common over the past decade. The location, size, extent, and macroscopic characteristics of the tumor can be established by standard endoscopic procedure. Endoscopic biopsies and cytologic studies characterize the carcinoma and aid in planning subsequent management. Even for gastric carcinoma diagnosed by upper gastrointestinal x-ray series, endoscopy is almost always performed for confirmation and biopsy, especially prior to laparotomy.

For a patient with gastrointestinal bleeding, endoscopy is almost always the first diagnostic test. Although biopsies should not be obtained from an actively bleeding carcinoma, brush cytology or biopsy of nearby or satellite lesions will often establish a tissue diagnosis. Occasionally, repeat endoscopy with routine biopsies can be diagnostic when bleeding has subsided. When initial endoscopic biopsies are not diagnostic, biopsy with a large ("jumbo") forceps (using an endoscope with a large-diameter accessory channel), or a snare-excision biopsy (using a double-chan-

nel endoscope) have been used to obtain larger specimens; this is rarely necessary if an adequate number of well placed biopsies have been obtained with standard diameter diagnostic endoscopes and their companion forceps.

Endoscopic Appearance

The gastric cancer classification suggested by Borrmann et al.[6] is useful in endoscopy for the description of these tumors. This classification refers to advanced gastric carcinoma. Although developed for characterization of the appearance of gross pathologic or surgical specimens, the classification easily lends itself to endoscopic description (Table 22–1).

Borrmann type I refers to a polypoid mass without a central ulceration. This polypoid cancer can be distinguished from a benign polyp because it is irregular, nodular, and does not have a smooth overlying mucosa. The surface of the resected mass consists of multiple tumor nodules (Plate 22–1). Biopsy of abnormal appearing mucosa over this polypoid mass or of the tumor nodules should confirm the diagnosis of gastric carcinoma over 90% of the time provided several biopsies are obtained.[7] Occasionally the mucosa over such a lesion will appear relatively normal. In such a case, large ("jumbo") forceps biopsies may be useful for detection of submucosally infiltrating carcinoma.

The Borrmann type II polypoid mass with a central ulceration is the most common endoscopic appearance of advanced gastric carcinoma. Because of the ulceration, such patients often have chronic gastrointestinal bleeding. Although the polypoid, mass-like features of such lesions are evident, central ulceration may be the predominant endoscopic feature. Typically, the ulceration has an irregular border, and the mucosal surface of the mass is obviously irregular and differs in appearance from that of surrounding nor-

TABLE 22–1. **Borrmann Macroscopic Classification of Advanced Gastric Cancer***

Type	Macroscopic Appearance
I	Polypoid mass
II	Polypoid mass with central ulceration
III	Infiltrating lesion with central ulceration
IV	Diffuse infiltrating lesion

*Adapted from: Borrmann R, Henke F, Lubarsch O. Handbuch der Speziellen pathologischen Anatomie und Histologie, Vol. 4. Berlin: Springer, 1926; 865.

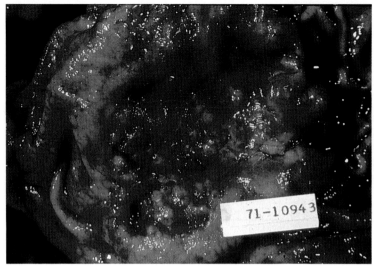

PLATE 22–1. Gross specimen of resected large gastric carcinoma is multiobulated, exophytic, and ulcerated. (Courtesy of K. Lewin, M.D.)

mal mucosa (Plates 22–2 and 22–3). Because of the exophytic nature of the mass, the endoscopic appearance of the associated ulceration should not be confused with that of a benign gastric ulcer. Forceps biopsies obtained via endoscopes with standard accessory channel diameters are usually positive.

The Borrmann type III macroscopically is an infiltrating lesion with central ulceration. This is the least common appearance endoscopically for advanced gastric carcinoma (Plates 22–4 and 22–5).

The Borrmann type IV lesion is a diffusely infiltrating carcinoma in a linitis plastica pattern. At endoscopy, there may be no break in the mucosa overlying large gastric folds (Plate 22–6). However, the involved region of the stomach may lack distensibility. Mucosal biopsy specimens may be negative for malignancy in such cases. For example, endoscopic biopsies were negative for carcinoma in the patient whose upper gastrointestinal x-ray series is shown in Figure 22–4. Large (jumbo) forceps biopsy or the snare-

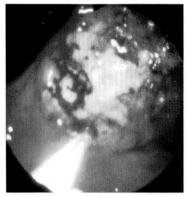
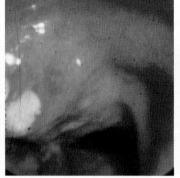
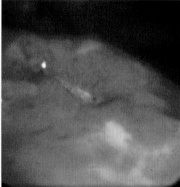

PLATE 22–2.   PLATE 22–3.   PLATE 22–4.

PLATE 22–2. Polypoid, ulcerated gastric carcinoma of body stomach (Borrmann type III). The yellow area is exudate on the base of the ulcerated mass. There is slight bleeding from the left side of the lesion. The biopsy forceps is evident in the 7 o'clock position. Biopsy specimens were positive for gastric adenocarcinoma. (Courtesy of M. Derezin, M.D.)

PLATE 22–3. Polypoid mass of the gastric body (Borrmann type II). Two superficial ulcers with exudate are seen on this large mass. The patient had upper gastrointestinal bleeding, anemia, and weight loss. Although cytologic studies done at endoscopy did not confirm malignancy, multiple biopsy specimens from the edge of the ulcerations revealed adenocarcinoma. (Courtesy of M. Derezin, M.D.)

PLATE 22–4. Ulcerated gastric carcinoma (Borrmann type III). At endoscopy a large submucosal mass and large gastric folds could be seen. One deep ulcer and several superficial ulcers are noted on a background of nodular mucosa and irregular folds. Tumor nodules have erupted through the mucosa in the ulcerated areas. Biopsies from the edge of the deep ulcer were positive for adenocarcinoma. Biopsies from the large folds in areas without mucosal ulceration were not diagnostic for the underlying carcinoma that in these areas had features of linitis plastica. (Courtesy of M. Derezin, M.D.)

excision technique for large particle biopsy may yield an endoscopic diagnosis in such cases in which the cancer is primarily submucosal.[8, 9] However, the snare-excision technique should be used with caution, if at all, when the mucosal surface is flat, and raised, nodular areas or enlarged folds are not clearly present.

Biopsy and Cytology

Both endoscopic biopsy and brush cytology may be used to establish a tissue diagnosis of gastric carcinoma. The role of each has been better defined in recent years. Depending on the gross morphologic characteristics of the lesion as described by the Borrmann classification, the use of cytology in addition to biopsy will increase the yield.

Multiple endoscopic biopsies obtained under direct visual control have a high yield when taken from ulcerated lesions that are suggestive of advanced gastric carcinoma. Biopsies from the edge of an ulcer and abnormal-appearing nodular mucosa are likely to yield a positive diagnosis for either polypoid or infiltrating cancers.[10, 11] Brush cytology in addition to biopsy may improve the yield, particularly in the case of the infiltrating type of lesion with central ulceration. Winawer et al.[11] found that multiple biopsies yielded a diagnosis in polypoid lesions with or without ulceration in 80% to 90% of cases. However, with routine mucosal biopsy of infiltrating, advanced gastric carcinoma, the yield was only 50% to 60% with multiple biopsies. The yield was 70% for infiltrating lesions with ulceration and increased to 80% when brush cytology was employed with mucosal biopsy. Others have reported that the yield for biopsy alone increases when more than six mucosal biopsies are taken;[12] dramatic increases in yield are described when 10 mucosal biopsies are taken from a gastric cancer.[7] Graham et al.[13] found that the first biopsy specimen yielded a correct diagnosis in 70% of gastric cancers. The yield increased to over 95% if four biopsies were obtained, and to over 98% with seven biopsy specimens.

With respect to positive diagnosis by endoscopic biopsy and/or brush cytology, infiltrating gastric carcinoma without ulceration is the most difficult; both brush cytology and routine mucosal biopsies may be nondiagnostic. Biopsies of the submucosa with either large (jumbo) biopsy forceps or snare-excision biopsy technique may be necessary to obtain a positive tissue diagnosis.[8, 9]

As will be noted throughout this chapter,

submucosal malignancies are a problem with respect to tissue diagnosis by endoscopy since in most cases the biopsy forceps used with current diagnostic endoscopes only sample the mucosa. In general, it is useful to search for and obtain biopsies in areas where the submucosal process has produced a break in the mucosa such as an erosion. If the mucosa is truly intact, a deeper biopsy that includes submucosal tissue is usually necessary for correct diagnosis. This may be obtained by using a larger forceps (sometimes referred to as a jumbo forceps) (Plate 22–7); an endoscope with a large diameter accessory channel is required, usually 3.5 mm or greater. Another approach is the so-called snare-excision biopsy or large-particle biopsy ("lift- and-cut technique"). This requires a double-channel endoscope (Plate 22–8). A polypectomy snare is passed through one channel and the snare loop is opened and placed on the region of mucosa to be sampled. A biopsy forceps is passed through the second accessory channel and a piece of mucosa within the perimeter of the loop is grasped and pulled upward from the mucosal surface but without pulling the forceps entirely away as would be the case with standard biopsy technique. The snare loop is closed around thickened mucosa and current (either coagulation or blended) is applied. The lift and cut technique entails some risk of perforation and should be used only when there is clearly defined thickening of the mucosa. Some endoscopists consider the large forceps technique to be satisfactory and to have less risk of perforation. There are, however, no comparative data for the two techniques. Occasionally, neither technique provides adequate tissue for diagnosis of submucosal disorders and laparotomy with full thickness gastric biopsy is required for histologic diagnosis.

Endoscopic biopsy techniques and the endoscopic appearance of benign gastric ulcers are discussed in Chapter 20.

Special Cases of Gastric Carcinoma

Early Gastric Carcinoma

Early gastric carcinoma refers to a special situation in which the carcinoma is confined to the mucosa or submucosa. This terminology is based upon a macroscopic classification of small gastric cancers found in Japan.[14] This lesion has a different natural history, prognosis, and therapy than most of the advanced gastric carcinoma seen in Europe

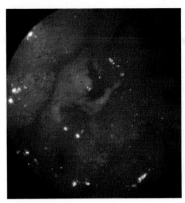 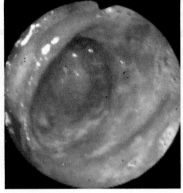 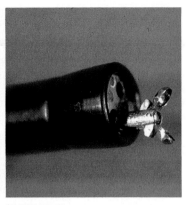

PLATE 22–5.   PLATE 22–6.   PLATE 22–7.

PLATE 22–5. Endoscopic view of gastric adenocarcinoma (Borrmann type III). Note central irregular ulcer crater with poorly defined margin and surrounding nodular, raised folds of the predominately submucosal tumor that produce a mass effect. (Courtesy of M.V. Sivak, Jr., M.D.)

PLATE 22–6. Endoscopic view of infiltrative adenocarcinoma of antrum (Borrmann type IV). The mucosal surface is erythematous and slightly nodular but there is no mass or ulceration. Antral contractile activity was absent. (Courtesy of M.V. Sivak, Jr., M.D.)

PLATE 22–7. Tip of therapeutic endoscope with large (jumbo) forceps extending from accessory channel.

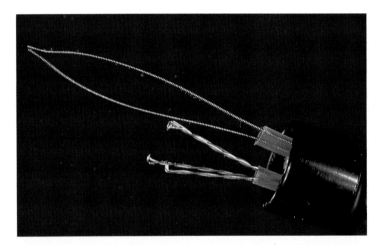

PLATE 22–8. Therapeutic two-channel endoscope with polyp grasper protruding from one channel and a standard monopolar electrocoagulation snare protruding from the other. This combination of accessories is useful for endoscopic polypectomy in the upper gastrointestinal tract and for obtaining large particle (lift-and-cut) biopsies.

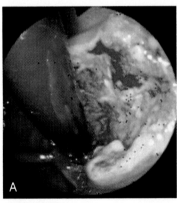 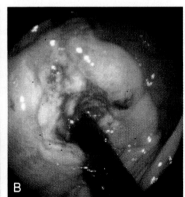 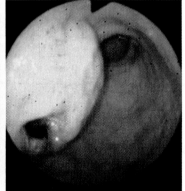

PLATE 22–9.   PLATE 22–10.

PLATE 22–9. A, Retroverted (turn-around) endoscopic view of gastric cardia showing ulcerated adenocarcinoma. B, Retroverted (turn-around) endoscopic view of gastric cardia, showing ulcerated, infiltrative adenocarcinoma. (Courtesy of M.V. Sivak, Jr., M.D.)

PLATE 22–10. Endoscopic view of large, ulcerated leiomyosarcoma on anterior wall of antrum (left). Pylorus is at upper right. (Courtesy of M.V. Sivak, Jr., M.D.)

TABLE 22–2. **Japanese Macroscopic Classification of Early Gastric Cancer**

Type	Name	Endoscopic Appearance
I	Protruded (polypoid)	Polypoid (sessile or pedunculated) Irregular contour Variable size
II	Superficial	
IIa	Elevated	Slightly elevated, plaque-like without inflamed mucosa
IIb	Flat	Flat Discolored mucosa
IIc	Depressed	Slight depression/irregular margin Clubbing or surrounding folds Intact areas of mucosa in depression Surface erosion possible
III	Evacuated (ulcerated)	Ulcer similar to benign gastric ulcer

and the United States. The diagnosis does not take into account lymph node spread.

Based primarily on extensive studies from Japan, the biologic behavior of early gastric carcinoma seems to differ from that found in the United States and Europe. It may begin as an ulcer, but this may spontaneously heal only to be followed by recurrence of the lesion.[15] The tumor has a slower growth rate and patients tend to survive longer, at least in Japan where early gastric cancer represents approximately 30% of the tumors detected by mass screening surveys.[16] It has been estimated that early gastric carcinoma represents only 4% to 7% of all gastric cancers detected in Europe and the United States. However, when early gastric carcinoma is found in non-Japanese patients, its biologic behavior appears to be similar to that described by the Japanese. Why the diagnosis is made less commonly in the United States and Europe than in Japan is uncertain. It probably relates to the use of mass screening for early detection and the high frequency of gastric carcinoma in Japan.

The macroscopic classification of early gastric carcinoma adopted by the Japan Gastroenterologic Endoscopic Society in 1962 is shown in Table 22–2 and Figure 22–5.[17] This classification and the corresponding endoscopic appearance are now used more commonly in Europe and the United States.[14, 18, 19] The results of some studies suggest that early gastric cancer is detected more often now in other countries, the increase in diagnosis being attributed to greater use of endoscopy.[18, 20–22]

The classification divides early gastric cancer into three main types and three subtypes based on macroscopic appearance at endoscopy and on gastrectomy specimens (Table 22–2).

The pure Type I early gastric carcinoma includes any sessile or pedunculated polyp. In comparison with benign gastric polyps, the contour of the polypoid or protruded early gastric carcinoma may be irregular; they are of variable size. Snare resection of the polyp is the best method to distinguish an early gastric carcinomatous polyp from a benign one. To obtain adequate tissue for histologic study, biopsies with a large (jumbo) forceps or a standard bayonet-type forceps are alternatives with small sessile polyps. (Plate 22–3).

The superficial type (Type II) of early gastric carcinoma is divided into three subtypes. Type IIa is slightly elevated, plaque-like, and well-circumscribed at endoscopy or

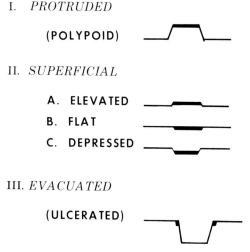

FIGURE 22–5. Schematic diagram of Japanese classification of early gastric carcinoma.

gastrectomy. When this type of lesion is found in pure form the surrounding mucosa is normal. Type IIa elevated lesions are raised by a few millimeters above the surrounding mucosa but have not formed into the polypoid Type I lesion. Multiple endoscopic biopsies with the jumbo biopsy forceps or the routine bayonet-type biopsy forceps should be considered for histologic diagnosis of this type of superficial gastric carcinoma.

Type IIb is a flat lesion with no abnormality visible macroscopically except discoloration of the mucosa. The mucosa may also be abnormal to palpation with the biopsy forceps, and as the mucosa is lifted with the forceps, tenting may not occur. Multiple biopsies of this type of lesion are indicated.

The Type IIc lesion is depressed slightly below the adjacent mucosa. Its margins may be irregular, and there may be clubbing of the surrounding folds. Areas of normal-appearing, intact mucosa may be present within the depression. Surface erosions within this depressed lesion can also be seen. The mucosa may be abnormal to palpation; tenting does not occur during biopsy. Multiple biopsies should be obtained for histologic diagnosis of this Type IIc lesion.

The Type III evacuated or ulcerated early gastric carcinoma is similar to a benign gastric ulcer. Endoscopic biopsy technique is comparable; 6 to 10 specimens depending on the size of the lesion should be obtained to distinguish Type II early gastric cancer from benign gastric ulcer. We often prefer to use the jumbo biopsy forceps for larger ulcers; the endoscopy technician checks each specimen for adequate size. The distinguishing features of benign gastric ulcers versus early gastric carcinoma are discussed in Chapter 20. In the United States approximately 3% of resected gastric specimens with benign-appearing gastric ulcers have carcinoma in part of the mucosa either adjacent to or at a distance from the ulcer.[23]

Because early gastric carcinoma does not always occur in pure form as one of the types or subtypes, combinations of types and subtypes may also occur. For example, an early gastric cancer of the ulcerated type (Type III) may be associated with surrounding focal mucosal discoloration (IIc) so that this combination would be classified as Type III plus IIc. At endoscopy or examination of a gross pathologic specimen, early gastric carcinoma is best described by employing combinations of the various types and subtypes of the Japanese classification. All possible combinations of the types listed in Table 22–2 have been described. The dominant macroscopic feature is listed first. For example, the commonest appearance of early gastric carcinoma described by Green et al.[18] was an ulcer with discolored or depressed margins. These early gastric cancers would, therefore, be classed as Type III plus IIc and Type IIb plus III.

Carcinoma of the Cardia Mimicking Achalasia

Carcinoma in the cardia of the stomach is best seen on turn-around (retroflexed, retroverted) examination of the proximal stomach (see Chapter 11) (Plate 22–9). Achalasia secondary to carcinoma of the cardia can mimic the manometric and clinical features of idiopathic achalasia.[18, 24] However, patients with achalasia secondary to carcinoma tend to be older and to have an abrupt onset of symptoms as well as other associated signs of carcinoma such as gastrointestinal blood loss, anemia, and pain. In the evaluation of all patients with achalasia, endoscopy with a turn-around examination of the fundus should be considered to rule out carcinoma. Some patients with carcinoma of the fundus mimicking achalasia will have intact mucosa rather than an ulcerated infiltrating mass of the type shown in Plate 22–9. Submucosal spread of tumor with involvement of the myenteric plexus of the esophagus accounts for the syndrome. This and the intact mucosa in many cases make this disorder difficult to diagnose short of surgery, even with meticulous endoscopic observation and biopsy technique.[25] Patients with achalasia secondary to carcinoma tend not to respond to pneumatic dilation.

Other Focal Malignant Gastric Tumors

Leiomyosarcoma

Leiomyosarcoma is a malignant tumor of smooth muscle origin. If the leiomyosarcoma increases in size, the patient may have nonspecific gastrointestinal symptoms and weight loss. Upper abdominal pain is common. Most patients are in the sixth or seventh decade of life.[26] Bleeding and anemia related to ulceration of the tumor are common symptoms. Patients with smaller lesions may be asymptomatic.

Except for larger size and evidence of local

extension or metastases, it is difficult to distinguish leiomyosarcoma from benign leiomyoma. Most leiomyomata are small and tend to remain asymptomatic. They may be discovered as an incidental radiographic or endoscopic finding. Leiomyosarcoma is usually detected as the tumor increases in size or causes some complication, e.g., gastrointestinal bleeding or symptoms from metastases (Figs. 22–6 and 22–7; Plate 22–10). Since much of the bulk of the tumor will be located beneath the mucosa, routine endoscopic biopsies are likely to be negative for malignancy. If the leiomyosarcoma is ulcerated, a large-particle (snare-excision) biopsy may reveal spindle cells with mitotic figures and irregular nuclei, features that are characteristic of leiomyosarcoma.[27, 28] However, pathologic differentiation of a benign leiomyoma from leiomyosarcoma may be difficult even when the entire specimen is available for study. Often the malignant nature of the lesion is inferred by its biologic behavior; invasion of adjacent organs, for example, indicates malignancy.

Kaposi's Sarcoma

Outside Africa, Kaposi's sarcoma of the stomach commonly occurs in patients with

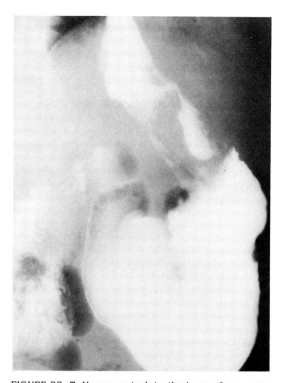

FIGURE 22–7. Upper gastrointestinal x-ray from same patient as in Plate 22–6, showing ulcerating leiomyosarcoma of the fundus of the stomach. Endoscopically, the appearance was that of an ulcerated submucosal tumor. Large-particle biopsy was interpreted as showing leiomyosarcoma, based on the presence of spindle cells with mitotic figures and irregular nuclei. (Courtesy of M. Weiner, M.D.)

acquired immunodeficiency syndrome (AIDS). Most of our patients with gastric Kaposi's sarcoma have had characteristic findings of cutaneous Kaposi's sarcoma. Gastrointestinal involvement in patients with AIDS and cutaneous Kaposi's sarcoma is common and may be diagnosed by either upper gastrointestinal endoscopy or colonoscopy.[29]

The usual appearance at endoscopy is a discrete, erythematous small-to-large nodule (Plate 22–11). Single or multiple lesions may be present in the stomach. Large nodules frequently have a reticulated white surface. A central umbilication or ulceration is common.

Because of the reddish color of the lesion of gastrointestinal Kaposi's sarcoma, profuse bleeding might be expected in response to endoscopic biopsy, but this has been uncommon in our experience. The histologic diagnosis can be difficult with routine mucosal biopsies because of the submucosal nature of

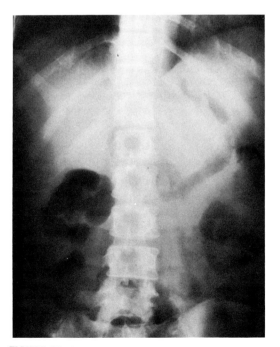

FIGURE 22–6. Upright plain abdominal x-ray of 40-year-old woman. The abnormal gastric shadow shows apparent compression of the lumen. (Courtesy of M. Weiner, M.D.)

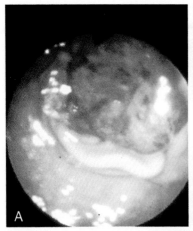
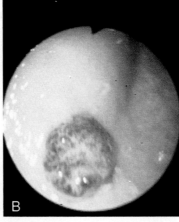

PLATE 22–11. A, Endoscopic view of gastric nodule of Kaposi's sarcoma in 30-year-old Caucasian man with nausea, weight loss, and fever. (Courtesy of M. Weinstein, M.D.) B, Endoscopic view of nodule of Kaposi's sarcoma in antrum of homosexual man with AIDS. (Courtesy of M.V. Sivak, Jr., M.D.)

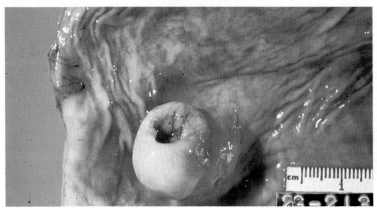
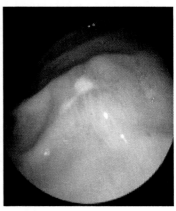

PLATE 22–12.   PLATE 22–13.

PLATE 22–12. Resected gastric specimen containing a leiomyoblastoma from same patient as in Figure 22-8. The endoscopic appearance would be similar. Despite metastases, this patient has done relatively well. (Courtesy of K. Lewin, M.D.)

PLATE 22–13. Endoscopic view of nodule of metastatic breast carcinoma in stomach. Note submucosal nature of lesion with central ulceration. Numerous such lesions were found in the stomach; biopsies were positive for carcinoma. (Courtesy of M.V. Sivak, Jr., M.D.)

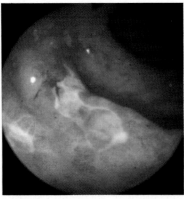
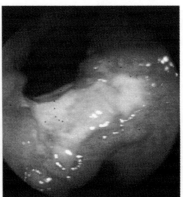
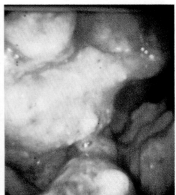

PLATE 22–14.   PLATE 22–15.   PLATE 22–16.

PLATE 22–14. Endoscopic view of infiltrative non-Hodgkin's lymphoma of stomach. There is distortion and ulceration of the mucosal surface. (Courtesy of M.V. Sivak, Jr., M.D.)

PLATE 22–15. Retroverted endoscopic view of angulus of stomach showing gastric ulcer that proved to be a non-Hodgkin's lymphoma. Note the irregular shape of the ulcer, poorly demarcatred margin, and nodularity in the surrounding mucosa. Proximal aspect of stomach is at top of the photograph, distal at bottom. (Courtesy of M.V. Sivak, Jr., M.D.)

PLATE 22–16. Endoscopic view of large gastric folds in body of stomach shown radiographically in Figure 22-11. The folds were rigid and somewhat friable. Jumbo forceps biopsy specimens revealed lymphoma. (Courtesy of M. Derezin, M.D.)

the lesions. Large biopsy specimens obtained with a large forceps or by snare excision may be necessary to confirm the diagnosis. The characteristic histologic appearance is of muscle-like spindle cells combined with increased vascular spaces containing endothelial cells.[29, 30]

Leiomyoblastoma

Leiomyoblastoma occurs rarely in the stomach as a submucosal malignancy of smooth-muscle origin (Fig. 22–8; Plate 22–12). This tumor is pathologically distinct from leiomyosarcoma; patients with this tumor tend to have a more benign course than those with leiomyosarcoma.[31] Unless these tumors ulcerate, cause complications such as gastrointestinal bleeding, or metastasize they may grow to a large size while remaining asymptomatic.

Metastatic Tumors to the Stomach

Metastasis to the stomach from nongastric primary carcinoma is rare but can cause symptoms or complications. Malignant melanoma, carcinoma of the breast, pancreatic carcinoma, carcinoma of the lung, and carcinoma of the colon metastasize to the gastric wall and can present as mucosal or submucosal lesions that are diagnosed by upper gastrointestinal radiography or endoscopy (Fig. 22–9). Clinically, patients with gastric

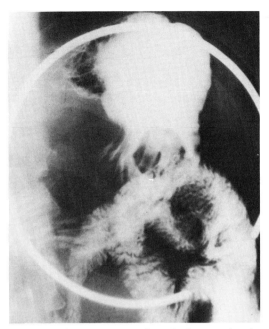

FIGURE 22–9. Upper gastrointestinal x-ray showing large, discrete polypoid mass in stomach of 52-year-old woman with breast cancer but without evidence of widespread metastatic disease. A submucosal lesion was found at endoscopy. Routine biopsies of the mucosa were not diagnostic. (Courtesy of B. Kadell, M.D.)

metastases may or may not have widespread metastatic disease. An upper gastrointestinal x-ray series or endoscopy may be obtained in these patients because of nonspecific symptoms or upper abdominal pain, gastrointestinal bleeding, or partial obstruction.

Carcinoma of the breast metastasizes to the gastric mucosa or submucosa. Common endoscopic or radiographic appearances are polypoid defects or ulcerations, umbilicated submucosal lesions (Plate 22–13), or infiltrating submucosal spread with thickened and enlarged gastric folds.[32] Routine mucosal biopsies may not be diagnostic. In such cases large-particle snare-excision or large-forceps biopsy or even laparotomy may be necessary to confirm the diagnosis of submucosal metastases.

Malignant melanoma metastasizes to the gut and characteristically presents as a "bull's eye" or target lesion on upper gastrointestinal x-rays (Fig. 22–10). At endoscopy, small metastases of malignant melanoma may be pigmented similar to the original cutaneous melanoma. Larger lesions often do not contain pigment. Although ulcerated metastases may be correctly diagnosed from routine mucosal biopsies, larger specimens may be necessary to confirm submucosal melanoma.[33, 34]

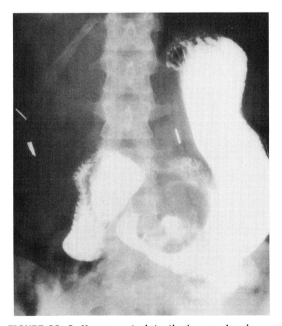

FIGURE 22–8. Upper gastrointestinal x-ray showing a large, ulcerated antral tumor that proved to be a leiomyoblastoma. (Courtesy of B. Kadell, M.D.)

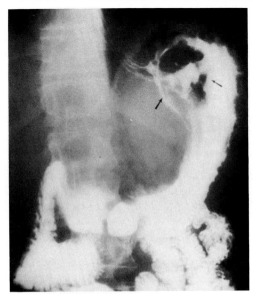

FIGURE 22–10. Upper gastrointestinal radiograph showing large, ulcerated mass (*arrows*) in the fundus of stomach. The patient had undergone resection of a cutaneous melanoma and presented with upper gastrointestinal bleeding. (Courtesy of M. Weiner, M.D.)

Gastric Lymphoma

Clinical Synopsis

Patients with gastric lymphoma usually have nonspecific symptoms such as upper abdominal pain, anorexia, nausea, vomiting, or weight loss that are indistinguishable from the symptoms of chronic ulcer disease or gastric adenocarcinoma. Complications such as gastrointestinal bleeding may be manifested by anemia, melena, and rarely hematemesis. Fever and loss of weight may also occur.[27, 35]

The stomach is the most common extranodal location for non-Hodgkin's lymphomas.[36] It is uncommon for the stomach to be the primary site of Hodgkin's disease.[35, 37] Disseminated lymphoma (Hodgkin's or non-Hodgkin's) can involve the stomach as well as other parts of the gastrointestinal tract. Clinically, patients with secondary gastrointestinal involvement are usually readily distinguishable from those with primary gastric lymphoma because of the advanced stage and extranodal disease.

Diagnosis

Lymphomas of the stomach may be primarily gastric, the only manifestation of extranodal disease, or they may involve the stomach secondarily as part of a generalized lymphoma involving several parts of the gastrointestinal tract. Although staging and treatment of primary gastric lymphoma differ from secondary gastric lymphoma, their radiographic and endoscopic appearances are similar.

On upper gastrointestinal x-rays or at endoscopy, lymphoma of the stomach may have several characteristic appearances. The most common is a diffuse infiltrative pattern of involvement of the gastric wall similar to the Borrmann type IV lesion of diffuse adenocarcinoma (Plate 22–14). The appearance may be that of single or multiple ulcers similar to the Borrmann III lesion of advanced adenocarcinoma (Plate 22–15). Lymphomatous ulcers are often deep and/or large. A polypoid mass with or without ulceration is another characteristic manifestation.

The diffuse infiltrative pattern of lymphomatous involvement of the stomach may produce abnormal gastric folds (Fig. 22–11). At endoscopy, such folds are characteristically large and the stomach does not distend in response to air insufflation. The large folds are thick and may appear gray (Plate 22–16). They may also be ulcerated, in which case routine mucosal biopsies taken from the edge

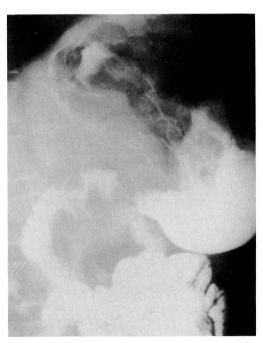

FIGURE 22–11. Upper gastrointestinal x-ray showing giant gastric folds that proved to be due to gastric lymphoma in 64-year-old man who presented with fever, weight loss, and early satiety. (Courtesy of M. Weiner, M.D.)

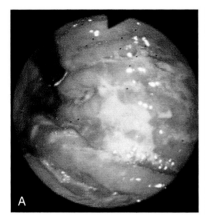 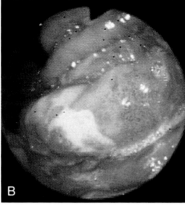

PLATE 22–17. *A,* Retroverted endoscopic view of enlarged, distorted, and ulcerated folds of gastric lymphoma. *B,* Closer view showing large, ulcerated fold with mottled surface. (Courtesy of M.V. Sivak, Jr., M.D.)

of the ulcer are often diagnostic of lymphoma (Plate 22–17). However, more commonly the submucosal nature of the lymphoma makes the diagnosis by routine forceps biopsy difficult. Larger specimens may be required for a positive tissue diagnosis[8, 9] (Plate 22–18).

Biopsy and Brush Cytology Yield

Despite the submucosal nature of a gastric lymphoma, routine endoscopic biopsies are positive in various series in from 70% to 87% of cases.[37, 38] Because of the problems of lymphoma typing, distinguishing primary from secondary involvement, and at times distinguishing pseudolymphoma from lymphoma, the mere finding of abnormal lymphocytes on biopsy or cytology may not be sufficient for specific diagnosis. When a specific diagnosis cannot be confirmed, a larger endoscopic biopsy specimen may be useful in conjunction with other staging techniques such as bone marrow biopsy, computed tomography (CT) of the abdomen, other directed biopsies (e.g., lymph node biopsy), and specific laboratory tests.

The Rappaport histologic classification of non-Hodgkin's lymphoma of the stomach is usually used.[39] On the basis of architecture, Rappaport has divided lymphomas into nodular and diffuse; then division on the basis of cell characteristics such as the presence of poorly differentiated or well-differentiated histiocytes, lymphocytes, or a mixed cell pattern (Plate 22–19). Unlike advanced adenocarcinoma of the stomach, gastric lymphoma often responds to radiotherapy and chemotherapy.

Pseudolymphoma

An intense lymphocyte infiltration may be present in the biopsies of benign-appearing lesions such as chronic gastric ulcers. The term pseudolymphoma is usually given to these findings, although the associated lymphocytic infiltrate is neither a malignant nor a benign tumor of the stomach. The true incidence of this lesion is unknown. It is probably more common than suspected and has probably been inadvertently included among true gastric lymphomas, an occurrence that may have resulted in some apparent improvement in survival statistics in some series of gastric lymphoma patients.[40]

The reported age range is wide, although most patients are middle-aged. Symptoms are

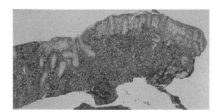

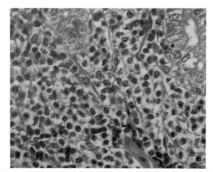

PLATE 22–18. Photomicrograph of specimen obtained by jumbo forceps biopsy from the same patient as in Figure 22-11 and Plate 22-16 *(top).* High-power magnification reveals gastric lymphoma *(bottom).* (Courtesy of W. Weinstein, M.D.)

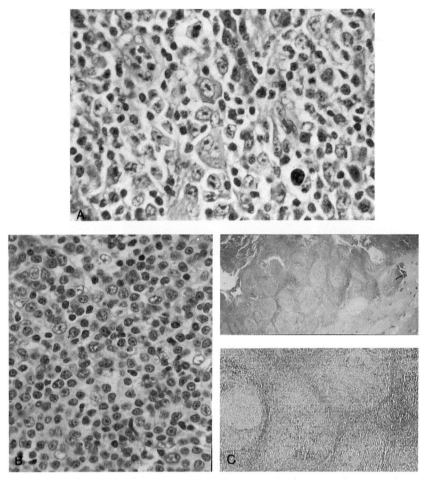

PLATE 22–19. *A,* Photomicrograph of high-power view of endoscopic biopsy specimen consistent with histiocytic lymphoma of the stomach. (Courtesy of K. Lewin, M.D.). *B,* Photomicrograph showing typical histology of nodular lymphoma of stomach. (Courtesy of K. Lewin, M.D.). *C,* Photomicrograph showing low-power view of gastric lymphoma of nodular type *(top).* High-power view shows cells to be well differentiated lymphocytes *(bottom).* (Courtesy of K. Lewin, M.D.)

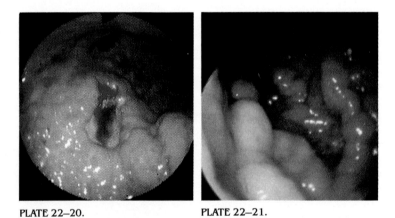

PLATE 22–20.   PLATE 22–21.

PLATE 22–20. Endoscopic view of enlarged, nodular gastric fold with surrounding nodularity and central ulcer in a patient with pseudolymphoma. Biopsies showed marked infiltration of the mucosa and submucosa by mature lymphocytes. Operative resection was performed; pathologic findings were consistent with pseudolymphoma. Patient was well at 2 years follow-up. (Courtesy of M.V. Sivak, Jr., M.D.)

PLATE 22–21. Endoscopic view of large gastric folds, extending from fundus into gastric body. Although no ulcers or erosions were seen, the stomach was poorly distensible in response to endoscopic air insufflation and these folds did not flatten.

entirely nonspecific. The radiographic and endoscopic appearances of pseudolymphoma of the stomach vary. Ulceration is a common feature. A well-demarcated crater may be the only finding, although ulceration is usually associated with a large mass and/or enlarged rugal folds (Plate 22–20). However, pseudolymphoma may also have predominantly infiltrative characteristics with multiple superficial ulcers and erosions. This variability in appearance parallels that of true gastric lymphoma.

Pseudolymphoma is often associated with evidence of prior peptic ulcer disease, and it has been suggested that it represents an exaggerated or unusual reaction to peptic ulceration in the stomach. However, similar lesions occur in other organs not subjected to the effects of acid or pepsin. Pseudolymphoma has also been regarded as a precursor of malignant lymphoma, but this is unlikely since a few patients have had extended periods of follow-up without evidence of malignant transformation.[41]

With the relatively small biopsy specimens obtained via standard diameter diagnostic endoscopes, the pattern of lymphocytic infiltration found in pseudolymphoma may be indistinguishable from a well-differentiated lymphocyte pattern characteristic of lymphoma. Large biopsy specimens or even surgical specimens may be necessary to distinguish pseudolymphoma from true lymphoma. Such biopsies may be indicated clinically, particularly with a slow-healing or non-healing chronic gastric ulcer whose initial biopsy specimens had many lymphocytes. The presence of lymphoid follicle formation with true germinal centers confirms the diagnosis of pseudolymphoma rather than lymphoma. In some cases, immunologic studies of biopsy specimens with monoclonal antibodies may be of assistance in differentiating pseudolymphoma from lymphoma.[42] Gastric lymphomas tend to have a monoclonal pattern of immunoglobulin.[43]

Differential Diagnosis of Large Gastric Folds

The significance of large gastric folds, discovered by either endoscopy or upper gastrointestinal series, is not a rare problem. Potentially serious conditions that require further study must be distinguished from benign disorders; various clinical and laboratory data are useful. However, certain endoscopic observations are of considerable value in this regard: whether the stomach distends and the rugal folds flatten in response to air insufflation, whether there are ulcerations, the appearance of the overlying mucosa be it normal or abnormal, and whether other lesions might be present and account for the finding of large folds such as gastric varices or polyps (Plate 22–21). The differential diagnosis of large gastric folds with intact mucosa is outlined in Table 22–3.

Many of the disorders listed in Table 22–3 may be predominantly submucosal. Therefore, it may be necessary to use the large forceps or lift-and-cut technique to obtain a specimen of adequate size and depth for histologic diagnosis (Fig. 22–12; Plate 22–22). These techniques should be used with caution and only in areas where the mucosa is clearly firm and thickened; biopsy of gastric varices, for example, is contraindicated (Fig. 22–13). Even with these special techniques the specimens obtained may be unsatisfactory, and occasionally laparotomy with full-thickness gastric biopsy is required.

Benign lesions that cause large gastric folds with intact mucosa are gastric varices, granulomatous disease, infections such as secondary syphilis, hypertrophic gastropathies, and Ménétrier's disease (Fig. 22–14; Plates 22–23 and 22–24). The histopathologic findings with the polyps of Ménétrier's disease are similar to those with hyperplastic polyps (see below). Other, rarer benign conditions may also have large gastric folds. Large rugal folds and diarrhea may also be characteristic of the Zollinger-Ellison syndrome (gastrinoma). A localized or metastatic pancreatic or duodenal tumor may be found in these patients.

TABLE 22–3. **Differential Diagnosis of Large Gastric Folds (Mucosa Intact)**

Malignancy Submucosal
  Metastatic carcinoma (breast, lung, etc.)
  Infiltrating adenocarcinoma (linitis plastica pattern)
  Leiomyosarcoma
  Lymphoma (primary or secondary)

Benign
  Gastric varices
  Granulomatous disease (e.g., tuberculosis, sarcoidosis)
  Secondary syphilis
  Hypertrophic gastropathy
  Ménétrier's disease

Other
  Zollinger-Ellison syndrome

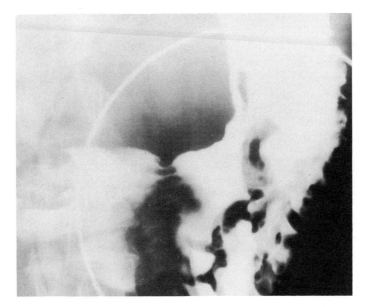

FIGURE 22–12. Upper gastrointestinal radiograph showing large gastric folds (hyperrugosity). This 24-year-old man was undergoing chronic hemodialysis. He had no gastrointestinal symptoms, and the x-ray study was obtained as he was being considered for cadaveric renal transplantation. Large gastric folds without ulceration or erosions were noted at endoscopy. These did not flatten with air insufflation although the stomach was distensible. (Courtesy of B. Kadell, M.D.)

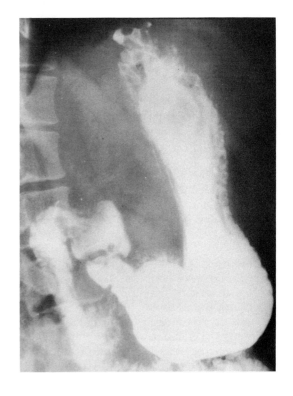

FIGURE 22–13. Upper gastrointestinal x-ray showing prominent folds of gastric fundus. Gastric fundal varices were suspected in this 38-year-old man with recurrent gastrointestinal bleeding. At endoscopy, gastric fundal varices were also suspected although esophageal varices were absent. The folds flattened somewhat with distention. No biopsies were obtained. Visceral angiography confirmed the presence of gastric varices, and liver biospy indicated cirrhosis. (Courtesy of M. Weiner, M.D.)

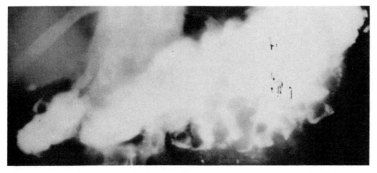

FIGURE 22–14. Upper gastrointestinal x-ray showing large folds in body of stomach suggestive of superimposed small polyps in 33-year-old man with weight loss, hypoalbuminemia, and severe protein wasting. The clinical and radiographic findings were consistent with Ménétrier's disease. After total gastrectomy there was significant improvement in the hypoalbuminemia. (Courtesy of B. Kadell, M.D.)

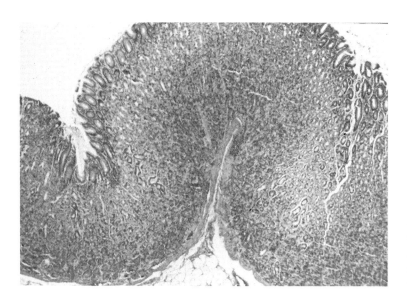

PLATE 22–22. Photomicrograph of large-particle biopsy from same patient as in Figure 22-12, showing hypertrophic gastritis without evidence of Menetrier's disease or lymphoma. (Courtesy of K. Lewin, M.D.)

PLATE 22–23. Gross surgical specimen of Menetrier's disease from same patient as in Figure 22-14. A similar appearance was evident at endoscopy. (Courtesy of K. Lewin, M.D.)

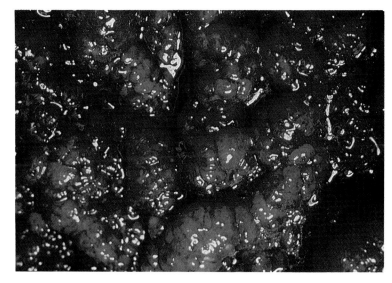

PLATE 22–24. Photomicrograph shows characteristic histopathology of Menetrier's disease in lower-power view. Mucosal and submucosal cystic and inflammatory changes are evident in one of the numerous polyps that carpeted the stomach. (Courtesy of K. Lewin, M.D.)

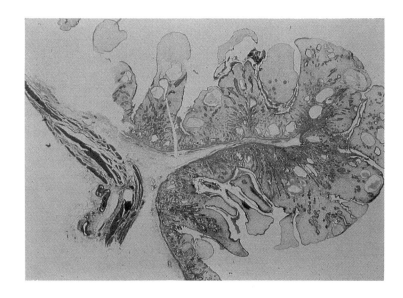

GASTRIC POLYPS

Single or Multiple Polyps

Clinical Synopsis

Gastric polyps are usually asymptomatic and are discovered incidentally on gastrointestinal radiographs or at endoscopy. However, occult or frank upper gastrointestinal bleeding may occur if one or more of the lesions become ulcerated or eroded. Rarely, prolapse of an antral polyp through the pylorus causes transient obstruction with gastric distention, nausea, and vomiting. Some patients with gastric polyps have nonspecific, chronic symptoms such as upper abdominal discomfort, nausea, and dyspepsia. Some patients who have polyps in the antrum may have presenting symptoms of partial obstruction, upper abdominal pain, nausea, or vomiting. When gastric polyposis is associated with gastric carcinoma, there may be weight loss and other signs or symptoms of gastric malignancy. Protein-losing enteropathy is evident with some polyposis syndromes, such as Cronkhite-Canada syndrome, but only rarely.[44]

Compared with the high frequency of colonic polyps in the United States and Europe, gastric polyps are uncommon. In autopsy series, the incidence of adenomatous polyps of the stomach is 0.4%.[45] The reported incidence in symptomatic patients in radiographic and endoscopic series is as high as 2%.[46] Multiple gastric polyps often occur in an individual patient; a polyposis syndrome should be considered if numerous polyps are found and other parts of the gut are involved (see below).

Diagnosis

In most cases, gastric polyps are demonstrated by gastrointestinal radiography or endoscopy. However, evidence of gastrointestinal blood loss may be the first clue to diagnosis; this may be manifested by laboratory findings alone, such as positive stool hemoccults and/or anemia. Since there is an association between atrophic gastritis and gastric polyp formation, achlorhydria may be documented by secretory testing and pernicious anemia by further laboratory testing.

The endoscopic and radiographic differential diagnosis of gastric polyps includes gastric carcinoma, pancreatic rest, metastatic tumor, submucosal tumors, foreign bodies, and hematomas. Endoscopy is especially useful to confirm the lesion as a discrete protru-

sion into the lumen of the stomach (see below); to characterize the size, location, number, and surface appearance; to obtain biopsies of the lesion itself or the often abnormal surrounding mucosa; and to perform polypectomy for histologic characterization of the polyp. Early gastric carcinoma, as defined by the Japanese classification (Table 22–2) can present as a polyp.

In this section, the (1) hyperplastic, (2) adenomatous, and (3) hamartomatous (juvenile) histologic types of gastric polyps will be discussed as individual lesions and within various polyp syndromes.

Endoscopy

Endoscopically, gastric polyps may be single or multiple; they appear as sessile, pedunculated, or occasionally multilobulated protuberances in the lumen of the stomach that do not disappear with maximal insufflation. Benign polyps are usually rounded, have a smooth surface, and may be pedunculated. However, they can also be ulcerated; the surface of the polyp may be erythematous, friable, and/or hemorrhagic. There may be associated changes in the surrounding mucosa, including evidence of atrophy, particularly in an abnormal stomach such as after gastric surgery (Plates 22–25 and 22–26). In patients with symptoms that suggest intermittent gastric obstruction, the obstructing behavior of the polyp may be noted at endoscopy (Figs. 22–15 and 22–16). Prolapse of an antral polyp through the pylorus can be observed at endoscopy (Plate 22–27). Although it is often difficult to attribute chronic nonspecific complaints to the presence of the polyp, some patients respond to polypectomy (Fig. 22–17; Plate 22–28).

Between 70% and 80% of polyps in the stomach are hyperplastic.[47, 48] Gastric hyperplastic polyps tend to be larger than their counterparts in the colon; usually they are less than 2 cm in diameter but may become larger (Fig. 22–18; Plate 22–29).

The hyperplastic polyp is the most common histologic type of gastric polyp encountered at endoscopy.[46, 49] Endoscopically, they are often solitary, smaller than 2 cm, and either pedunculated or sessile. They occur with equal frequency in the proximal stomach and antrum (Fig. 22–19). The method of endoscopic biopsy depends on the size and location of the polyp and whether it is pedunculated or sessile. For smaller polyps that are usually sessile, we prefer either a bayonet-

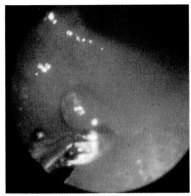
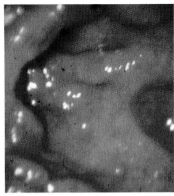
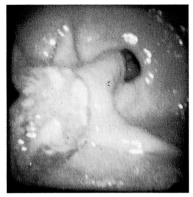

PLATE 22–25.   PLATE 22–26.   PLATE 22–27.

PLATE 22–25. Endoscopic view of an eroded antral polyp. The patient had hemoccult positive stools and dyspepsia. The polyp, too small for polypectomy, was removed with a large forceps and found to be an adenomatous polyp. Biopsies from the surrounding antral mucosa revealed atrophic changes without dysplasia.
PLATE 22–26. Endoscopic view of small, sessile, erythematous gastric polyps in gastric remnant 20 years after gastric resection with Billroth II anastomosis. The polyps proved to be adenomatous; severe atrophic changes were also found by biopsy in the gastric remnant. Endoscopic follow-up was initiated.
PLATE 22–27. Endoscopic photograph of pre-pyloric polyp prolapsing through pylorus. The patient had symptoms of partial obstruction. Endoscopic polypectomy revealed an adenomatous polyp; biopsies of the abnormal-appearing antral mucosa showed chronic atrophic gastritis. (Courtesy of M. Derezin, M.D.)

type forceps (spike within the forceps cups) or a large forceps (without coagulation). For larger polyps, either the large forceps or standard electrosurgical snare polypectomy are effective methods for obtaining adequate tissue for histologic characterization.

In the differential diagnosis of single gastric polyps, hematoma should be considered and can be seen either radiographically or endoscopically (Fig. 22–20).

Adenomatous polyps are the second most common type of gastric polyp. They occur with greater frequency in the antrum than in the proximal stomach and may be sessile or pedunculated (Fig. 22–21; Plate 22–30). The surface of the polyp is generally smooth and may have a reddish color in comparison to surrounding normal mucosa.

Unlike the colon, villous adenomas occur rarely in the stomach. In reported series, they tend to be large and frequently harbor malignant changes.[50, 51]

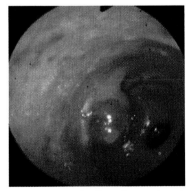

PLATE 22–28. Endoscopic view of the polyp shown in Figure 22-17. The polyp was removed by endoscopic polypectomy after biopsies were obtained of the surrounding mucosa. Histologically the polyp was an adenoma without malignant change. The patient's symptoms resolved after polypectomy.

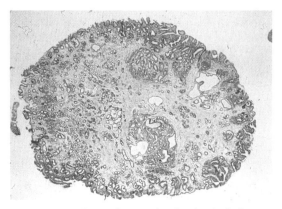

PLATE 22–29. Photomicrography showing typical histology for hyperplastic polyp of the stomach. There is elongation and branching of hyperplastic glands that are also dilated and show cystic changes. (Courtesy of K. Lewin, M.D.)

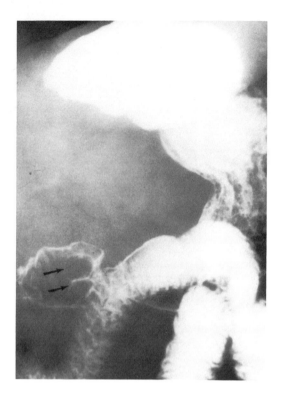

FIGURE 22–15. X-ray film showing prolapse of an antral polyp through the pylorus and into the duodenum (*arrows*). This 61-year-old patient had presenting symptoms of partial gastric outlet obstruction. (Courtesy of M. Weiner, M.D.)

FIGURE 22–16. Another x-ray film of same patient as in Figure 22–15, obtained during the same upper gastrointestinal x-ray series, that shows return of the polyp (*arrow*) to the antrum. The histologic diagnosis was benign antral polyp. (Courtesy of M. Weiner, M.D.)

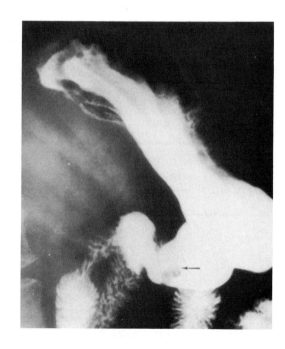

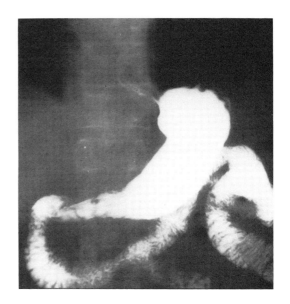

FIGURE 22–17. Upper gastrointestinal radiograph shows a smooth, round, pedunculated, benign-appearing antral polyp in an 81-year-old man with persistent dyspepsia and hemoccult-positive stool. (Courtesy of B. Kadell, M.D.)

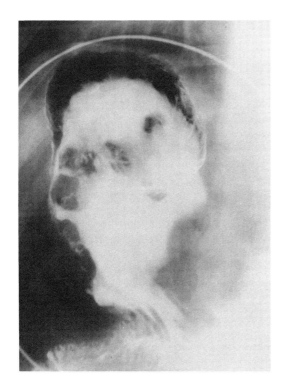

FIGURE 22–18. Gastrointestinal x-ray showing huge, multilobulated polyp in the body of stomach. The polyp, over 6 cm in diameter, caused early satiety, weight loss, upper abdominal pain, and chronic occult gastrointestinal bleeding. It was too large to remove endoscopically, although snare-excision biopsies revealed histologic findings of a hyperplastic polyp. Histologic examination of the resected lesion confirmed this diagnosis. (Courtesy of M. Weiner, M.D.)

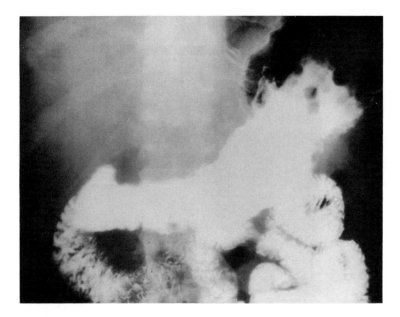

FIGURE 22–19. Upper gastrointestinal radiograph showing numerous, smooth polyps of varying size primarily in the fundus. Endoscopic polypectomy or biopsy would be indicated to determine histologic type and rule out coincident carcinoma. Although hyperplastic polyps are more common in the fundus, both hyperplastic and adenomatous polyps were found and endoscopic follow-up was planned. (Courtesy of B. Kadell, M.D.)

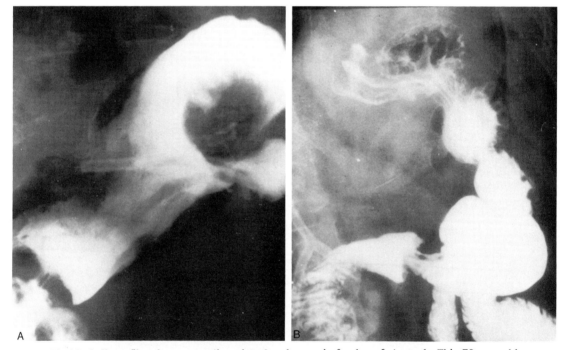

FIGURE 22–20. A, X-ray film shows smooth, submucosal mass in fundus of stomach. This 70-year-old woman had persistent nausea and vomiting postoperatively, for which a nasogastric tube had been placed. A coagulopathy was corrected. The lesion is a gastric hematoma. The patient's symptoms and the hematoma resolved gradually within one month. (Courtesy of B. Kadell, M.D.). B, X-ray film from same patient one month later, showing resolution of the fundal hematoma. (Courtesy of B. Kadell, M.D.)

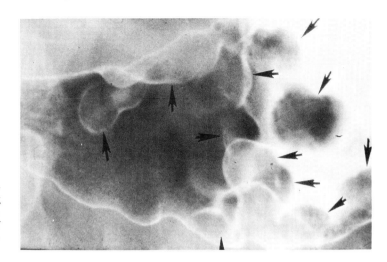

FIGURE 22–21. Double-contrast upper gastrointestinal x-ray showing multiple gastric polyps (*arrows*), some of which have an irregular shape. (Courtesy of W. Weinstein, M.D.)

Relation to Gastric Carcinoma

There are close morphologic and statistical relationships between gastric polyps, particularly adenomas, and gastric cancer. Gastric polyps are frequently found in association with gastric adenocarcinoma.[47, 48] Other mucosal abnormalities such as atrophic gastritis are frequently associated with gastric adenomas. The occurrence of a gastric adenoma is thought to place a patient at higher risk for the development of adenocarcinoma of the stomach.[47, 48, 52] Therefore, the presence of adenocarcinoma must be considered in the differential diagnosis and evaluation of patients with multiple benign polyps (Fig. 22–22).

Gastric hyperplastic polyps are not considered to be neoplastic; they do not undergo malignant degeneration. Although malignant change has been reported rarely in gastric hyperplastic polyps,[53] it is difficult to evaluate some reports because of differences in the terminology used to characterize polyps, and particularly because of the similarity in architecture between some hyperplastic polyps and adenomas. Adenomatous polyps, which are capable of malignant degeneration, can be found in patients who also have hyperplastic polyps. Also, hyperplastic polyps may occur in abnormal gastric mucosa (atrophic gastritis) that has an associated increased risk of adenocarcinoma.[46, 54]

It is well established that adenomatous polyps in the stomach may contain carcinoma, the frequency of carcinomatous change being dependent upon the size of the polyp.[47, 48, 55–57] For adenomatous polyps the chance of malignancy also depends upon the cell type and is greatest with villous adenomas. Carcinomatous degeneration has been found in 50% to 70% of specimens in some series.[50, 58]

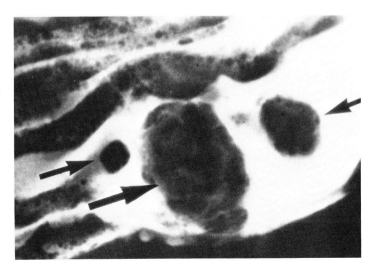

FIGURE 22–22. Upper gastrointestinal x-ray showing large gastric folds, two polyps (smaller arrows at left and right), and large, sessile gastric cancer (*larger arrow*) between the two polyps. Histologically, the two polyps proved to be adenomas. At endoscopy the mucosa surrounding the polyps and the carcinoma was markedly atrophic. The diagnoses were also confirmed at surgery. (Courtesy of W. Weinstein, M.D.)

Endoscopic biopsy alone may not reveal the extent or even the presence of carcinomatous change in a polyp, so that endoscopic or surgical polypectomy may be required for complete histologic characterization of a polyp, including the presence or absence of focal carcinoma.[49, 59]

There is less evidence that gastric adenomas are actual precursors of gastric carcinoma in comparison to the amount of data supporting the polyp–cancer sequence concept in the colon. Foci of cancer within gastric adenomas are usually small, superficial, and rarely invasive; metastasis from cancer within a gastric polyp is exceedingly rare.[60] Elsborg and Mosbech[61] reported a 4-year endoscopic follow-up study of 68 patients with pernicious anemia in which polyps were discovered in 25 patients; none were greater than 2 cm in diameter. Some polyps increased and others decreased in size during follow-up. Some polyps disappeared, and there was no observed transition of a polyp to carcinoma. Mizuno et al.[54] followed 118 patients with polyps. Four patients (3.4%) developed malignant polyps during endoscopic follow-up that ranged from 1.5 to 3.5 years. When strict histologic criteria were employed, there was only one specimen (0.9%) that harbored invasive cancer. Ming[62] concluded that the gastric adenoma is a precursor of gastric cancer, although the transition from polyp to cancer is probably an uncommon occurrence.

Management

The American Society for Gastrointestinal Endoscopy (ASGE) considers gastric polyps premalignant and has made several specific recommendations with respect to their management.[63] These are summarized as follows: If a polypoid defect is detected by upper gastrointestinal radiography or endoscopy, biopsy specimens should be taken, or the lesion should be removed, whether the patient is asymptomatic or has symptoms such as obstruction or bleeding due to the polyp(s). Endoscopic surveillance subsequent to polypectomy is dependent upon the histology, size, and number of polyps present at endoscopy. If the polyp is hyperplastic or hamartomatous (i.e., non-neoplastic), surveillance is unnecessary. Endoscopic follow-up is recommended, however, for adenomatous polyps. Any polyp larger than 2 cm should be removed by endoscopic polypectomy or surgical resection. If a polyp is less than 2 cm in diameter and it is solitary or there are only a few polyps, the polyp or polyps should be excised endoscopically and periodic follow-up endoscopy should be instituted. If polyp diameter is less than 2 cm, but there are multiple polyps, endoscopic polypectomy should be performed when feasible, and endoscopic follow-up is indicated. If endoscopic removal is not feasible, surgical excision should be considered.

The risks and complications of endoscopic polypectomy in the stomach are similar to those reported for colonoscopic polypectomy: hemorrhage, perforation, and delayed ulceration with slow healing at the polypectomy site. ReMine et al.[49] reported a 4% risk of hemorrhage that might require surgery. They routinely prescribed H_2 blockers or antacids after gastric polypectomy to induce healing of the ulceration that frequently occurs at the site of the polypectomy. Although some authors believe that the risk of gastroscopic polypectomy is greater than that for polypectomy in the colon, the risk of carcinoma in a polyp should be weighed against the potential risk of polypectomy. However, most authors believe that gastric polypectomy is a reasonably safe procedure. Should bleeding occur, endoscopic control is feasible using a variety of endoscopic hemostatic methods.[64]

Endoscopic Techniques for Diagnosis and Polypectomy

The previously described techniques of large-forceps biopsy and the lift-and-cut large-particle biopsy procedure are useful for biopsy or removal of gastric polyps of various sizes, configurations, and locations (Plates 22–7, 22–8, and 22–31). A two-channel endoscope is often preferred. For biopsy or polypectomy of small (less than 1 cm) sessile polyps and for biopsy of large folds, ulcers, or nodules, we often use the large (jumbo) biopsy forceps (Plate 22–7). This forceps is designed to cut rather than pinch off a tissue specimen, and it provides excellent tissue specimens for histologic assessment; it is used without cautery. The bayonet-type (spike) biopsy forceps is also useful for small polyps or nodules as well as for biopsy of the surrounding mucosa (Plate 22–31).

A two-channel endoscope facilitates polypectomy in the stomach as well as retrieval of the polyp (Plate 22–8). It is sometimes more difficult to retrieve a polyp from the stomach than one from the colon. Electrosurgery in the stomach often stimulates severe contractile activity. This can usually be

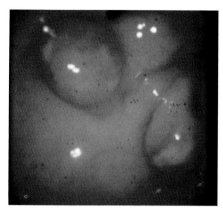
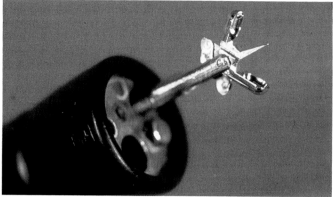

PLATE 22–30.   PLATE 22–31.

PLATE 22–30. Endoscopic view of polyps in same patient as in Figure 22-21. There were numerous sessile and pedunculated polyps, some with mucosal erosions. Several were removed by polypectomy; biopsies were obtained from others with the large forceps. Histologically, the polyps proved to be adenomas without carcinoma. After polypectomy, the patient was given a short course of H₂ blocker therapy. Serial endoscopic follow-up was planned.
PLATE 23–31. Tip of endoscope with standard bayonet-type (spike) forceps extending from accessory channel.

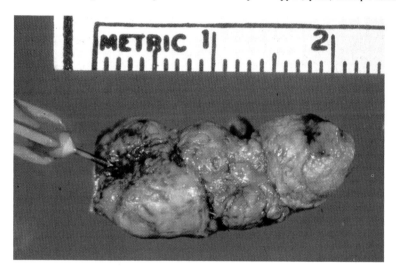

PLATE 22–32. Gastric polyp with needle in stalk after formalin fixation. Insertion of a 26-gauge needle in the stalk is useful for identification of the resected aspect of the polyp by the pathologist. (Courtesy of H. Weinstein, M.D.)

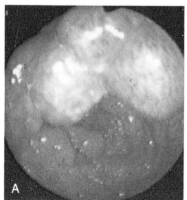
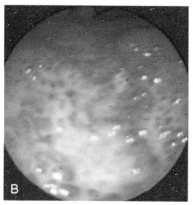
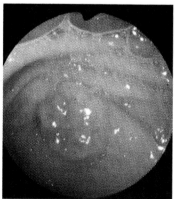

PLATE 22–33.   PLATE 22–34.

PLATE 22–33. Endoscopic views of antrum in 34-year-old Korean woman with Cronkhite-Canada syndrome. A, Large polyp with mottled, reticulated surface. B, Mottled mucosal surface with small polyps. (Courtesy of M.V. Sivak, Jr., M.D.)
PLATE 22–34. Endoscopic view of antral adenomatous polyp in a patient with familial polyposis coli. (Courtesy of M.V. Sivak, Jr., M.D.)

controlled pharmacologically by the intravenous administration of glucagon. Even large polyps can be retrieved either with the use of a polyp grasper or at times with this plus a polypectomy snare loop. Histologic examination of the polyp is facilitated by putting a 26-gauge needle in the stalk or line of resection immediately after retrieval of the specimen (Plate 22–32). This prevents the retraction of the stalk that occurs quickly after polypectomy, especially when the polyp is placed in a fixative. In the laboratory, the polyp is bisected through the stalk and each half is embedded for sectioning through the long axis.[65]

Polyposis Syndromes

The polyposis syndromes with gastric polyps are listed in Table 22–4.

Peutz-Jeghers and Cronkhite-Canada Syndromes

Histologically, the polyps of the Peutz-Jeghers syndrome are hamartomatous (juvenile). These polyps are nonmalignant and do not undergo carcinomatous change. Numerous gastric polyps are often present.

The Cronkhite-Canada syndrome is a noninherited, noncongenital disorder that occurs primarily in the sixth to seventh decade, although age range is 31 to 86 years in reported cases.[44, 66, 67] There is no definite sex predilection. Spontaneous remission has been reported,[66, 68] but the prognosis is generally poor with a mortality of 60%, most deaths occurring within 6 to 18 months.[69, 70] Numerous gastric polyps are usually present in the Cronkhite-Canada syndrome (Figs. 22–23 and 22–24). They are not adenomas or neoplastic and are considered not to be premalignant. The extragastric manifestations of the Cronkhite-Canada syndrome include generalized polyposis of the gastrointestinal tract, particularly the colon and small intestine, cutaneous hyperpigmentation, alopecia, and onychodystrophy.[67, 71]

On gross or endoscopic examination of either the stomach or the colon, multiple sessile polyps on a thickened mucosa are seen. The concentration of polyps within the stomach is usually heaviest in the antrum; they range from 0.5 to 1.5 cm in diameter and may have a mottled or reticulated surface pattern (Plate 22–33). Microscopically, there is intact surface epithelium, tortuous glands that are cystically dilated and filled with proteinaceous fluid, and edematous chronically inflamed lamina propria. Secondary acute inflammation may be superimposed.[44]

Familial Polyposis and Gardner's Syndrome

Patients with familial polyposis or Gardner's syndrome may have polyps in the upper gastrointestinal tract; these may be adenomatous polyps. Multiple polyps may be present in the stomach in either disorder. Gardner's syndrome is usually characterized by multiple colonic and small intestinal polyps, although gastric polyps occur rarely. Similarly, patients with familial polyposis have predominantly colonic polyps but rarely have gastric and small intestinal polyps.

The distribution of polyps in the upper gastrointestinal tract of patients with familial polyposis or Gardner's syndrome may have several patterns. Sivak and Jagelman[72] described fundic, duodenal, and fundic plus duodenal patterns. Other reports confirm a predilection for polyps to be located in the fundus.[73, 74] However, the distribution in 10 cases reported by Itai et al.[75] was random in the stomach. Watanabe et al.[76] found an antral distribution to be most common, with

TABLE 22–4. **Polyposis Syndromes with Gastric Polyps**

Syndrome	Polyp Type	Malignant Potential	Gastric Involvement	Extragastric Manifestations
Cronkhite-Canada	Hamartoma (juvenile)	No	Predominant	Generalized gastrointestinal polyposis Cutaneous hyperpigmentation Alopecia Onychodystrophy
Peutz-Jeghers	Hamartoma (juvenile)	No	Common	Mucocutaneous Generalized gastrointestinal polyposis
Gardner's	Adenoma	Yes	Rare	Colon polyposis Soft tissue and osseous abnormalities
Familial polyposis	Adenoma	Yes	Rare	Colon polyposis

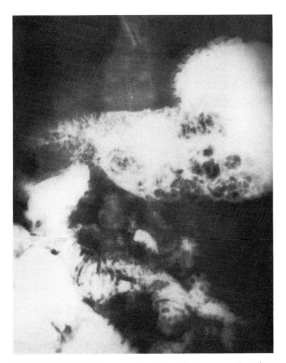

FIGURE 22–23. Upper gastrointestinal x-ray showing numerous polyps of stomach and small bowel of 50-year-old man with Cronkhite-Canada syndrome. The presenting symptoms were hypoalbuminemia, weight loss, alopecia, and dystrophic nails. (Courtesy of M. Weiner, M.D., and A. Schwabe, M.D.)

fundic polyposis being the second most common.

Gastric polyps may be either hyperplastic or adenomatous. Hyperplastic polyps appear to be more common.[73, 75, 77, 78] However, the pathologic type may also be related to the distribution of polyps within the stomach. In the series of 22 patients reported by Watanabe et al.,[76] polyps found in the antrum were more likely to be adenomas (Plate 22–34). Those in the fundus tended to be hyperplastic. Similar findings were reported by Ranzi et al.[74]

Endoscopically, fundic polyps are usually numerous, hemispheric, sessile, and orange-yellow and range from 2 to 7 mm in diameter[72] (Plates 22–35 and 22–36). Removal of larger adenomatous polyps when feasible is indicated. The need for endoscopic surveillance is not established, but most authors with experience with upper gastrointestinal polyposis in association with familial polyposis or Gardner's syndrome recommend some form of endoscopic surveillance that takes into account the number, size, and configuration of the gastric polyps.

OTHER MUCOSAL AND SUBMUCOSAL GASTRIC LESIONS

Clinical Synopsis

The lesions discussed in this section are the gastric leiomyoma, lipoma, angioma, and carcinoid. Ectopic pancreas in the stomach (pancreatic rest) is also a relatively common disorder that is discussed in Chapter 35. Some of these (leiomyoma, lipoma) are mainly submucosal, although they may involve the gastric mucosa by extension or ulceration. Most patients with submucosal lesions of this type will be asymptomatic or have nonspecific symptoms that prompt up-

FIGURE 22–24. Upper gastrointestinal x-ray showing numerous gastric polyps in a patient with Cronkhite-Canada syndrome. (Courtesy of M. Weiner, M.D.)

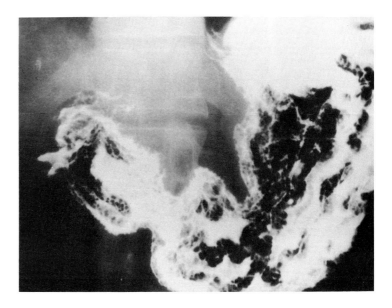

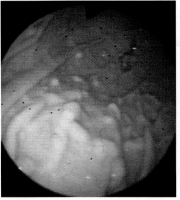 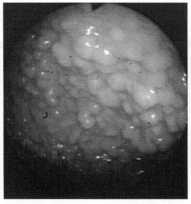 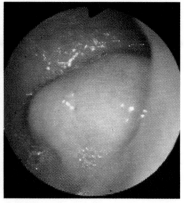

PLATE 22–35.   PLATE 22–36.   PLATE 22–37.

PLATE 22–35. Endoscopic view of hyperplastic polyps in body of stomach in patient with familial polyposis coli. (Courtesy of M. V. Sivak, Jr., M.D.)

PLATE 22–36. Endoscopic view of numerous small hyperplastic polyps in fundus of patient with familial polyposis coli. (Courtesy of M. V. Sivak, Jr., M.D.)

PLATE 22–37. Endoscopic view of submucosal mass in antrum. Note smooth surface of normal mucosa over the lesion. (Courtesy of M. V. Sivak, Jr., M.D.)

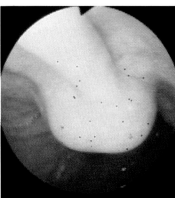 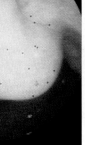 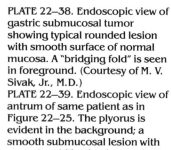

PLATE 22–38. Endoscopic view of gastric submucosal tumor showing typical rounded lesion with smooth surface of normal mucosa. A "bridging fold" is seen in foreground. (Courtesy of M. V. Sivak, Jr., M.D.)

PLATE 22–39. Endoscopic view of antrum of same patient as in Figure 22–25. The plyorus is evident in the background; a smooth submucosal lesion with central umbilication is seen in the foreground. The lesion was soft to palpation. A large forceps was used for histologic sampling. (Courtesy of W. Weinstein, M.D.)

PLATE 22–38.   PLATE 22–39.

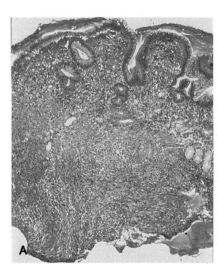 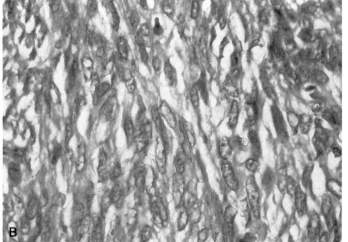

PLATE 22–40. A, Photomicrograph (low-power) of large forceps biopsy from same patient as in Figure 22–25 and Plate 22–39 shows lesion to be a leiomyoma. (Courtesy of W. Weinstein, M.D.). B, Photomicrograph (high-power) showing characteristic spindle-like muscle cells of a gastric leiomyoma. (Courtesy of W. Weinstein, M.D.)

per gastrointestinal x-ray study or endoscopy. Occasionally, patients with large submucosal lesions or ulcerated lesions will have more specific signs or symptoms such as gastrointestinal bleeding, anemia, or partial obstruction. A variant carcinoid syndrome is rarely reported with gastric carcinoid because most of these patients will not have liver metastases.[79–81]

Endoscopic Diagnosis and Technique

A submucosal tumor has a characteristic endoscopic appearance, although there are no features that distinguish one type of tumor from another. In general, submucosal tumors are rounded defects that project into the lumen of the stomach as a polypoid defect. Since the lesion is beneath the mucosa, the color and texture of the overlying surface mucosa are identical to that of the surrounding mucosa (Plate 22–37). The mucosa at the edges of the tumor may be pulled together to form one or more ridges ("bridging folds") that extend from the surrounding normal mucosa upward toward the summit of the tumor mound (Plate 22–38). The shape of the tumor may include a depression (umbilication), almost always at the apex of the lesion. Ulceration is another common endoscopic feature. An ulcerated submucosal lesion can occasionally be difficult to differentiate from a chronic gastric ulcer with surrounding edema and scarring.

If the submucosal tumor is ulcerated or found to be the source of upper gastrointestinal bleeding, endoscopic biopsy and surgical resection may be indicated. For such lesions, biopsy with standard or large-size forceps is recommended for histologic assessment. Since the lesion is for the most part submucosal, biopsy specimens may be nonrevealing unless in fact an error in endoscopic assessment led to misdiagnosis and the lesion is actually something other than a submucosal benign tumor, such as an adenomatous polyp. Thus endoscopic biopsy may either confirm the presence of the submucosal lesion or suggest another possibility. In some cases, biopsy specimens taken from the region of ulceration will suggest a more specific diagnosis. Surgical resection may be necessary for ulcerated lesions because these do not heal with medical therapy. Most submucosal lesions of this category, however, will be asymptomatic. Because it is often not pos-

sible to differentiate a benign from a malignant submucosal lesion with certainty, and because these lesions may grow and produce complications such as ulceration and bleeding, some endoscopists undertake periodic endoscopic follow-up, although the value of this approach has not been established.

Endoscopic treatment of bleeding gastric angioma is feasible and recommended instead of surgery.[82]

Removal of gastric carcinoid tumors is generally recommended because of the concern for malignancy. These tumors can be removed either endoscopically (using a forceps or by electrosurgical polypectomy) or surgically.

Gastric Leiomyoma

The most common benign gastric tumor is the leiomyoma. This arises from smooth muscle tissue in the submucosa and is usually found as an incidental lesion at endoscopy, upper gastrointestinal radiography, surgery, or autopsy in previously asymptomatic patients (Fig. 22–25; Plates 22–39 and 22–40). Gastrointestinal bleeding and upper abdominal pain are the most common symptoms. Surgical resection of gastric leiomyoma is curative and recurrences have not been reported.[83, 84]

Lipoma

Gastric lipomas are rare, submucosal soft tumors of various sizes. They are usually

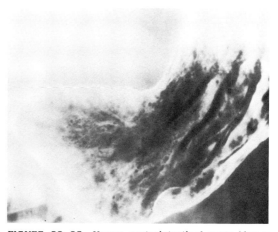

FIGURE 22–25. Upper gastrointestinal x-ray shows characteristic submucosal lesion with central umbilication in a 34-year-old patient with upper abdominal pain. (Courtesy of B. Kadell, M.D.)

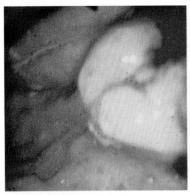
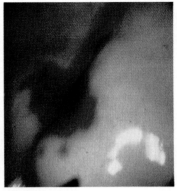
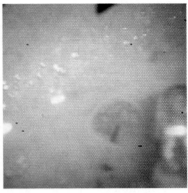

PLATE 22–41.   PLATE 22–42.   PLATE 22–43.

PLATE 22–41. Endoscopic appearance of an ulcerated lipoma of the stomach. The patient had symptons of early satiety and upper gastrointestinal bleeding. The soft submucosal ulcerated lesion was actively bleeding at endoscopy and was resected. The yellow color is characteristic.

PLATE 22–42. Endoscopic view of a large, umbilicated gastric angioma. The patient had upper gastrointestinal bleeding and iron-deficiency anemia that required transfusions. Selective visceral angiography did not show the lesion. Endoscopic biopsies were not obtained; endoscopic electrocoagulation was performed, following which the patient had no recurrence of upper gastrointestinal bleeding.

PLATE 22–43. Endoscopic view of 3 to 4 mm gastric carcinoid at left of open biopsy forceps in patient with gastric atrophy and achlorhydria. (Courtesy of M. V. Sivak, Jr., M.D.)

solitary and most often located in the distal stomach. Gastrointestinal bleeding is the most common symptom, although most lipomas are asymptomatic unless overlying gastric ulceration or erosion occurs.[85] A faint yellow hue beneath the mucosa may be detected at endoscopy (Plate 22–41). Lipomas may have several configurations including sessile, pedunculated, or multilobulated. Lipomas characteristically exude a yellow material when biopsies are obtained. If a lipoma is removed endoscopically by electrosurgical snare excision, it will float because of the low-density

fat. Significant bleeding may result after snare resection of part of a lipoma. In our experience, endoscopic hemostasis is less successful with bleeding due to excision of a lipoma than to bleeding after removal of other submucosal tumors.

Gastric Angioma

Large gastric angiomas commonly have a red mucosal component as well as a submucosal component (Plate 22–42). Endoscopic hemostatic methods have been used successfully in treating these lesions.[82] Because of the characteristic red, vascular appearance, it is not difficult to distinguish this lesion from the other mucosal or submucosal lesions described in this section. However, it may be necessary to wash such lesions to distinguish them from adherent blood.

Gastric Carcinoid

Gastric carcinoids are uncommon; they account for only a small percentage of carcinoid tumors occurring in the gastrointestinal tract. They may be an incidental finding at endoscopy, surgery, or autopsy. They may be multiple in the stomach.[86] Symptoms, when present, are nonspecific. There may be evidence of gastrointestinal blood loss, either as acute symptoms of hematemesis and/or melena, or in the form of chronic anemia.[87] There ap-

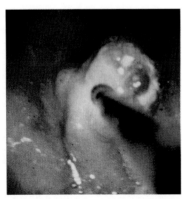

PLATE 22–44. Endoscopic biopsy of a polypoid mass that proved to be a gastric carcinoid.

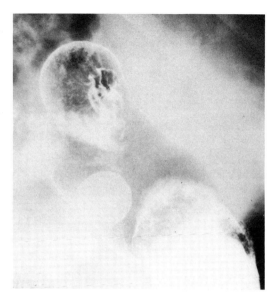

FIGURE 22–26. Upper gastrointestinal radiograph shows a large, sessile polypoid mass in a 45-year-old man. The lesion proved to be a gastric carcinoid on resection. (Courtesy of B. Kadell, M.D.)

pears to be an association of gastric carcinoid tumors with atrophic gastritis and achlorhydria[88, 89] (Plate 22–43). A syndrome that resembles the carcinoid syndrome associated with metastatic carcinoid of the small bowel has been described.[90, 91]

The first endoscopic description is probably that by Walley[92] in 1937. The endoscopic appearance varies. The lesions have been described as both polypoid (sessile and pedunculated) and submucosal.[46, 86, 93, 94] Characteristically, they resemble submucosal lesions and may have a central umbilication (Fig. 22–26). They may be located in either the antrum or the fundus of the stomach. If polypoid in configuration and at endoscopy they may be confused with gastric polyps[93] (Plate 22–44). Since gastric carcinoids originate in either the mucosa or the submucosa, endoscopic biopsy can be expected to suggest the diagnosis in a significant percentage of cases.

Gastric carcinoids may be malignant. Metastases have been present in about one third of cases reported, lymph nodes and/or the liver being the most common sites of spread. A carcinoid tumor cannot be termed malignant or benign on the basis of histologic appraisal alone. The occurrence of metastasis appears to be related to the size of the tumor.

Because of their malignant potential, either endoscopic or surgical resection of gastric carcinoids is recommended.[79, 80] Endoscopic

polypectomy may be undertaken for smaller submucosal or polypoid lesions. However, one report of angiography in a gastric carcinoid tumor suggests that these lesions may be highly vascular.[95] The risk of bleeding with endoscopic polypectomy could therefore be significant with larger lesions.

References

1. Adashek K, Sanger J, Longmire WP Jr. Cancer of the stomach: review of consecutive ten year intervals. Ann Surg 1979; 189:6–10.
2. Dupont JB Jr, Lee JR, Burton GR, Cohn I Jr. Adenocarcinoma of the stomach: Review of 1,497 cases. Cancer 1978; 41:941–7.
3. Brown J, Winkelmann RK. Acanthosis nigricans: A study of 90 cases. Medicine 1968; 47:33–51.
4. Coggon D, Acheson ED. The geography of cancer of the stomach. Br Med Bull 1984; 40:335–41.
5. Silverberg E. Cancer statistics, 1982. CA 1982; 32:15–31.
6. Borrmann R, Henke F, Lubarsch O. Handbuch der Speziellen Pathologischen Anatomie und Histologie, Vol. 4. Berlin: Springer, 1926; 865.
7. Dekker W, Tytgat GN. Diagnostic accuracy of fiber-endoscopy in the detection of upper intestinal malignancy: a follow-up analysis. Gastroenterology 1977; 73:710–4.
8. Bjork JT, Geenen JE, Soergel KH, et al. Endoscopic evaluation of large gastric folds: a comparison of biopsy techniques. Gastrointest Endosc 1977; 24:22–3.
9. Martin TR, Onstad GR, Silvis E, Vennes JA. Lift and cut biopsy technique for submucosal sampling. Gastrointest Endosc 1976; 23:29–30.
10. Hatfield ARW, Slavin G, Segal AW, Levi AJ. Importance of the site of endoscopic gastric biopsy in ulcerating lesions of the stomach. Gut 1975; 16:884–6.
11. Winawer SJ, Posner G, Lightdale CJ, et al. Endoscopic diagnosis of advanced gastric cancer: factors influencing yield. Gastroenterology 1975; 69:1183–7.
12. Sancho-Poch FJ, Bolanzo J, Ocana J, et al. An evaluation of gastric biopsy in the diagnosis of gastric cancer. Gastrointest Endosc 1978; 24:281–2.
13. Graham DY, Schwartz JT, Cain GD, Gyorkey F. Prospective evaluation of biopsy number in the diagnosis of esophageal and gastric carcinoma. Gastroenterology 1982; 82:228–31.
14. Morson BC. The Japanese classification of early gastric cancer. In: Yardley JH, Morson BC, Abell MR, eds. International Academy of Pathology Monograph. The Gastrointestinal Tract. Baltimore: Williams & Wilkins, 1977; 176–83.
15. Sakita T, Oguro Y, Takasu S, et al. Observations on the healing of ulcerations in early gastric cancer. The life cycle of the malignant ulcer. Gastroenterology 1971; 60:835–9.
16. Kawai K, Fernandez JMB, Seifert E, Murakami T. Proceedings of the symposium: Early Gastric Cancer, IVth World Congress of Digestive Endoscopy. Gastroenterologia Japonica, 1979; 14:266–91.
17. Murakami T, ed. Early Gastric Cancer. (Gann monograph on cancer research, No. 11) Baltimore: University Park Press, 1972; 301.

18. Green PHR, O'Toole KM, Weinberg LM, Goldfarb JP. Early gastric cancer. Gastroenterology 1981; 81:247–56.

19. Ito Y, Blackstone MO, Riddell RH, Kirsner JB. The endoscopic diagnosis of early gastric cancer. Gastrointest Endosc 1979; 25:96–101.

20. Paulino F, Roselli A. Early gastric cancer: report of twenty-five cases. Surgery 1979; 85:171–6.

21. Machado G, Davies JD, Tudway AJC, et al. Superficial carcinoma of the stomach. Br Med J 1976; 2:77–9.

22. Seifert E, Butke H, Gail K, et al. Diagnosis of early gastric cancer. Am J Gastroenterol 1979; 71:563–7.

23. Tedesco FJ, Best WR, Littman A, et al. Role of gastroscopy in gastric ulcer patients. Planning a prospective study. Gastroenterology 1977; 73:170–3.

24. Kolodny M, Schrader ZR, Rubin W, et al. Esophageal achalasia probably due to gastric carcinoma. Ann Intern Med 1968; 69:569–73.

25. Tucker HJ, Snape WJ Jr, Cohen S. Achalasia secondary to carcinoma: manometric and clinical features. Ann Intern Med 1978; 89:315–8.

26. Shiu MH, Farr GH, Papachristou DN, Hajdu SI. Myosarcomas of the stomach: natural history, prognostic factors and management. Cancer 1982; 49:177–87.

27. Bedikian AY, Khankhanian N, Valdivieso M, et al. Sarcoma of the stomach: clinicopathologic study of 43 cases. J Surg Ocol 1980; 13:121–7.

28. Cabre-Fiol V, Vilardell F, Sala-Clardera E, Perez Mota F. Preoperative cytological diagnosis of gastric leiomyosarcoma. Gastroenterology 1975; 68:563–6.

29. Derezin M, Lewin KJ, Groopman J, Weinstein WM. Gastrointestinal involvement with Kaposi's sarcoma in epidemic acquired immunodeficiency syndrome (AIDS). (Abstr) Gastrointest Endosc 1983; 29:178–9.

30. Friedman-Kien AE, Laubenstein LJ, Rubinstein P, et al. Disseminated Kaposi's sarcoma in homosexual men. Ann Intern Med 1982; 96:693–700.

31. Plantinga ERM, Mravunac M, Joosten HJM. Gastric leiomyoblastoma: three interesting cases. Acta Chir Scand 1979; 145:571–4.

32. Cormier WJ, Gaffey TA, Welch JM, et al. Linitis plastica caused by metastatic lobular carcinoma of the breast. Mayo Clin Proc 1980; 55:747–53.

33. Nelson RS, Lanza F. Malignant melanoma metastatic to the upper gastrointestinal tract. Gastrointest Endosc 1978; 24:156–8.

34. Menuck LS, Amberg JR. Metastatic disease involving the stomach. Am J Dig Dis 1975; 20:903–13.

35. Lewin KJ, Ranchod M, Dorfman RF. Lymphomas of the gastrointestinal tract. A study of 117 cases presenting with gastrointestinal disease. Cancer 1978; 42:693–707.

36. Freeman C, Berg W, Cutler SJ. Occurrence and prognosis of extranodal lymphomas. Cancer 1972; 29:252–60.

37 Nelson RS, Lanza FL. The endoscopic diagnosis of gastric lymphoma: gross characteristics and histology. Gastrointest Endosc 1974; 21:66–8.

38. Posner G, Lightdale CJ, Cooper M, et al. Reappraisal of endoscopic tissue diagnosis in secondary gastric lymphoma. Gastrointest Endosc 1975; 21:123–5.

39. Rappaport H. Tumors of the hematopoietic system. In: Atlas of Tumor Pathology, Section 3. Fasc 8, Washington DC: Armed Forces Institute of Pathology, 1966; 97–161.

40. Mattingly SS, Cibull ML, Ram MD, et al. Pseudolymphoma of the stomach. A diagnostic and therapeutic dilemma. Arch Surg 1981; 116:25–9.

41. Stroehlein JR, Weiland LH, Hoffman HN, Judd ES. Untreated gastric pseudolymphoma. Dig Dis 1977; 22:465–70.

42. Palestro G, Poggio E, Leonardo E, Coda R: Primary gastric lymphoid proliferations: immunological criteria to distinguish gastric lymphoma from reactive hyperplasia. Oncology 1977; 34:164–7.

43. Yamanaka N, Ishi Y, Koshiba H, et al. A study of surface markers in gastrointestinal lymphoma. Gastroenterology 1980; 79:673–7.

44. Daniel ES, Ludwig SL, Lewin KJ, et al. The Cronkhite-Canada syndrome: An analysis of clinical and pathologic features and therapy in 55 patients. Medicine 1982; 61:293–309.

45. Bentivegna S, Panagopoulos PG. Adenomatous gastric polyps (11 cases added to a previous report). Am J Gastroenterol 1965; 44:138–48.

46. Deyhle P. Results of endoscopic polypectomy in the gastrointestinal tract. Endoscopy 1980; (Suppl):35–46.

47. Ming SC, Goldman H. Gastric polyps: a histogenetic classification and its relation to carcinoma. Cancer 1965; 18:721–6.

48. Tomasulo J. Gastric polyps. Histologic types and their relationship to gastric carcinoma. Cancer 1971; 27:1346–55.

49. ReMine SG, Hughes RW Jr, Weiland LH. Endoscopic gastric polypectomies. Mayo Clin Proc 1981; 56:371–5.

50. Walk L. Villous tumor of the stomach: clinical review and report of two cases. Arch Intern Med 1951; 87:560–9.

51. Mark LK, Samter T. Villous adenomas of the stomach. Am J Gastroenterol 1975; 64:137–9.

52. Fabry TL, Frankel A, Waye JD. Gastric polyps. J Clin Gastroenterol 1982; 4:23–7.

53. Papp JP, Joseph JI. Adenocarcinoma occurring in a hyperplastic polyp. Removal by electrosurgical polypectomy. Gastrointest Endosc 1976; 23:38–9.

54. Mizuno H, Kobayashi S, Kasuguai T. Endoscopic follow-up of gastric polyps. Gastrointest Endosc 1975; 21:112–5.

55. Hay LJ. Surgical management of gastric polyps and adenomas. Surgery 1956; 39:114–9.

56. Huppler EG, Priestley JT, Morlock CG, Gage RP. Diagnosis and results of treatment in gastric polyps. Surg Gynecol Obstet 1960; 110:309–13.

57. Marshak RH, Feldman F. Gastric polyps. Am J Dig Dis 1965; 10:909–35.

58. Bremer EH, Battaile WF, Balle PH. Villous tumors of the upper gastrointestinal tract. Am J Gastroenterol 1968; 50:135–43.

59. Seifert E, Elster K. Endoskopische polypektomie am Magen. Indikation, Technik und Ergebnisse. Dtsch Med Wochenschr 1972; 97:1199–203.

60. Monaco AP, Roth SI, Castleman B, Welch CE. Adenomatous polyps of the stomach. A clinical and pathological study of 153 cases. Cancer 1962; 15:456–7.

61. Elsborg L, Mosbech J. Pernicious anaemia as a risk factor in gastric cancer. Acta Med Scand 1979; 206:315–8.

62. Ming S-C. The classification and significance of gastric polyps. Internat Acad Pathol Monogr 1977; 18:149–75.

63. American Society for Gastrointestinal Endoscopy guidelines for clinical application: "The role of endoscopy of the surveillance in premalignant condi-

tions of the upper gastrointestinal tract." ASGE, Manchester, MA, 1983.

64. Jensen DM. Endoscopic control of gastrointestinal bleeding. In: Berk JE, ed. Developments in Digestive Diseases. Philadelphia: Lea & Febiger, 1980; 1–27.

65. Weinstein WM, Hill TA. Gastrointestinal mucosal biopsy. In: Berk JE, ed. Bockus Gastroenterology. Ed. 4. Philadelphia: WB Saunders, 1985; 626–44.

66. Peart AG JR, Sivak MV Jr, Rankin GB, et al. Spontaneous improvement of Cronkhite-Canada syndrome in a postpartum female. Dig Dis Sci 1984; 29:470–4.

67. Johnson GK, Soergel KH, Hensley GT, et al. Cronkhite-Canada syndrome: gastrointestinal physiology and morphology. Gastroenterology 1972; 63:140–52.

68. Russell D McR, Bhathal PS, St. John DJB. Complete remission of Cronkhite-Canada syndrome. Gastroenterology 1983; 85:180–5.

69. Cotterill JA, Day JL, Hughes JP, et al. The Cronkhite-Canada syndrome. Postgrad Med J 1973; 49:268–73.

70. Jarnum S, Jensen H. Diffuse gastrointestinal polyposis with ectodermal changes. A case with severe malabsorption and enteric loss of plasma proteins and electrolytes. Gastroenterology 1966; 50:107–18.

71. Cronkhite LW Jr, Canada WJ. Generalized gastrointestinal polyposis; unusual syndrome of polyposis, pigmentation, alopecia, and onychotrophia. N Engl J Med 1955; 252:1011–5.

72. Sivak MV Jr, Jagelman DG. Upper gastrointestinal endoscopy in polyposis syndromes: familial polyposis coli and Gardner's syndrome. Gastrointest Endosc 1984; 30:102–4.

73. Denzler TB, Harned RK, Pergam CJ. Gastric polyps in familial polyposis coli. Radiology 1979; 130:63–6.

74. Ranzi T, Castagnone D, Velio P, et al. Gastric and duodenal polyps in familial polyposis coli. Gut 1981; 22:363–7.

75. Itai Y, Kogure T, Okuyama Y, Muto T. Radiographic features of gastric polyps in familial adenomatosis coli. Am J Roentgenol 1977; 128:73–6.

76. Watanabe H, Enjoji M, Yao T, Ohsato K. Gastric lesions in familial adenomatosis coli. Hum Pathol 1978; 9:269–83.

77. Utsunomiya J, Maki T, Iwama T, et al. Gastric lesions of familial polyposis coli. Cancer 1974; 34:745–54.

78. Ushio K, Sasagawa M, Doi H, et al. Lesions associated with familial polyposis coli: Studies of lesions of the stomach, duodenum, bones and teeth. Gastrointest Radiol 1976; 1:67–80.

79. Seifert E, Elster K. Carcinoids of the stomach: report of two cases. Am J Gastroenterol 1977; 68:372–8.

80. Feldman AJ, Weinberg M, Raess D, et al. Gastric carcinoid tumor. Its occurrence with ossification and diffuse argyophil-cell hyperplasia. Arch Surg 1981; 116:118–21.

81. Balthazar EJ, Megibow A, Bryk D, Cohen T. Gastric carcinoid tumors: radiographic features in eight cases. AJR 1982; 139:1123–7.

82. Jensen DM, Bown S. Gastrointestinal angioma; diagnosis and treatment with laser therapy and other endoscopic modalities, In: Fleischer D, Jensen D, Bright-Asare P, eds. Therapeutic Laser Endoscopy and Gastrointestinal Disease. Boston: Martinus Nijhoff, 1983, 151–60.

83. Morson BC, Dawson IP. Non-epithelial tumours. In: Morson BC, Dawson IP, eds. Gastrointestinal Pathology. Oxford: Blackwell Scientific Pub, 1979; 187–99.

84. Perrillo RP, Zuckerman GR, Shatz BA. Aberrant pancreas and leiomyoma of the stomach: indistinguishable radiologic and endoscopic features. Gastrointest Endosc 1977; 23:162–3.

85. Johnson DCI, DeGennaro VA, Pizzi WF, Nealon TF Jr. Gastric lipomas. A rare cause of massive upper gastrointestinal bleeding. Am J Gastroenterol 1981; 75:299–301.

86. Kornfeld HR, Sherlock P, Hertz R. Multiple carcinoid tumors of the stomach with endoscopic observations. Gastrointest Endosc 1971; 18:74–7.

87. Schoenfeld R, Cahan J, Dyer R. Gastric carcinoid tumor. An unusual case of hematemesis. Arch Intern Med 1959; 104:649–52.

88. Wilander E, Sundstrom C, Grimelius L. Pernicious anaemia in association with argyrophil (Sevier-Munger) gastric carcinoid. Scand J Haematol 1979; 23:415–20.

89. Harris AI, Greenberg H. Pernicious anemia and the development of carcinoid tumors of the stomach. JAMA 1978; 239:1160–1.

90. Christodoulopoulos JB, Klotz AP. Carcinoid syndrome with primary carcinoid tumor of the stomach. Gastroenterology 1961; 40:429–40.

91. Oates JA, Sjoerdsma A. A unique syndrome associated with secretion of 5-hydroxytryptophan by metastatic gastric carcinoids. Am J Med 1962; 32:333–42.

92. Walley GJ. A case of carcinoid tumor of the stomach. St. Bartholomew's Hosp J 1937; 44:141–2.

93. Gueller R, Haddad JK. Gastric carcinoids simulating benign polyps. Two cases diagnosed by endoscopic biopsy. Gastrointest Endosc 1975; 21:153–5.

94. DeLuca RF, Ferrer JP, Gambescia RA, Raskin JB. Gastric carcinoid endoscopically simulating leiomyoma. Case report and review of the literature. Am J Gastroenterol 1978; 70:163–6.

95. Andersen JB, Madsen B, Skjoldborg H. Angiography in a case of carcinoid tumour in the stomach. Br J Radiol 1971; 44:218–20.

Chapter 23

DISEASES OF THE DUODENUM

BERNARD M. SCHUMAN, M.D.

Diseases of the duodenum, other than bulbar peptic ulcer, are uncommon and may be overlooked at endoscopy. Moreover, the papilla—the most interesting duodenal structure—is ordinarily out of view or can be seen only tangentially with forward-viewing endoscopes and, thus, cannot be adequately studied. It is also unlikely that more than half of the linear extent of the duodenum is ever visualized by routine endoscopic examination, and what is confidently declared a normal duodenoscopy is in reality a normal semiduodenoscopy. The duodenum is not only a repository for peptic ulcer but may harbor a wide variety of diseases, both primary and secondary. Inflammatory, neoplastic or infectious disorders are readily identifiable endoscopically, and some may be definitively diagnosed by endoscopic biopsy.

INFLAMMATORY DISEASES

Crohn's Disease

Crohn's disease of the duodenum is uncommon, occurring in only 2% of patients with Crohn's disease.[1, 2] More than 200 cases have been reported,[1] most with involvement elsewhere in the digestive tract. Almost all patients with duodenal Crohn's disease have had epigastric pain as the major symptom. The diagnosis is usually made radiologically in the course of a small bowel series. Endoscopic study is done to confirm the diagnosis and to obtain biopsies for histologic study.

The endoscopic features of duodenal Crohn's disease were described in a study of 14 patients, 3 of whom had involvement of the duodenum alone.[3] The characteristic findings were not unlike those of Crohn's disease elsewhere in the intestine. The mucosal surface is granular and often nodular. Erosions and aphthoid ulcers are frequent,

but the long, deep linear ulcers with white base and narrow red margin are seen less often (Plate 23–1). The wall of the bowel lacks distensibility and contractions are not evident because of the stiffened folds. Indeed, mural inflammation commonly results in stenosis of the proximal duodenum that is sufficient to prevent passage of the endoscope (Plate 23–2).[2] By the time characteristic findings of Crohn's duodenitis are present, stenosis may already be a major feature. When there is associated gastric disease, which usually involves the antrum, duodenoscopy may be impossible because of antral and pyloric stenoses.

A rare complication of Crohn's duodenitis is the formation of a duodenoenterocutaneous fistula. Of 2 such cases, the fistula was identified by duodenoscopy in 1, although mucosal biopsies disclosed only nonspecific inflammation.[4] Endoscopic evaluation of duodenum involved with enterocolonic fistulas is essential to determine if the duodenal process is secondary to contiguous colonic granulomatous inflammation or a manifestation of primary Crohn's involvement. In 2 cases of coloduodenal fistulization, the duodenum was found at surgery to be involved only secondarily.[5]

Endoscopic duodenal biopsies in Crohn's disease have been disappointing for the most part. Nugent et al.[2] did not encounter any granulomas in endoscopic biopsies from the original 17 patients in their series, although these were found in 1 of 3 patients who had capsule biopsies. This suggests that a larger and perhaps deeper endoscopic biopsy will yield a higher percentage of granulomas. This was verified in their further experience (recounted in an addendum to their paper) with 8 additional patients with duodenal Crohn's disease, in 4 of whom granulomas were demonstrated by biopsy done, presum-

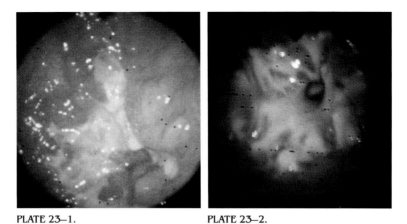

PLATE 23–1.   PLATE 23–2.

PLATE 23–1. Crohn's ulcer of duodenum. Narrowed duodenal lumen is in lower right of the field.
PLATE 23–2. Severe stricture of the descending duodenum in a patient with duodenal Crohn's disease. (Courtesy M.V. Sivak, Jr., M.D.)

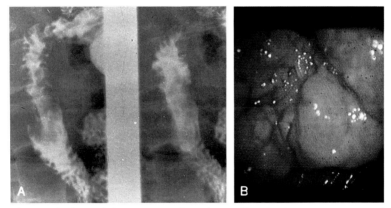

PLATE 23–3. A, Radiographic views of villous tumor of the descending duodenum. B, Endoscopic view of villous tumor. (Courtesy M.V. Sivak, Jr., M.D.)

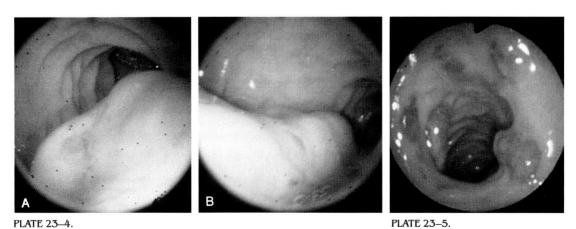

PLATE 23–4.   PLATE 23–5.

PLATE 23–4. Proximal (A) and distal (B) views of a large submucosal duodenal tumor that proved to be a leiomyoma at surgery. (Courtesy M.V. Sivak, Jr., M.D.)
PLATE 23–5. Circumscribed nodular form of Brunner's gland hyperplasia. (Courtesy M.V. Sivak, Jr., M.D.)

ably, with more modern endoscopes containing larger accessory channels.[2]

Eosinophilic Gastroenteritis

Marked eosinophilic infiltration of the wall of the stomach and small intestine is the hallmark of eosinophilic gastroenteritis. Patients with this uncommon disorder will often have a history of allergic disorders, and invariably marked peripheral eosinophilia is demonstrable.[6] Although the stomach is primarily involved, in one disease pattern there is multifocal involvement of the duodenum and jejunum in addition to the extensive submucosal infiltration of the antrum. Endoscopically the pattern of mucosal folds is accentuated and the mucosa hyperemic, but these findings are usually marked in the antrum and less obvious in the duodenum, where there may be only focal erythema and erosion.

Another pattern in adults, not distinguishable endoscopically from the first pattern although characterized by both mucosal and submucosal eosinophilic infiltration, lends itself more readily to definitive diagnosis by endoscopic biopsy, especially in the stomach but also in the duodenum and jejunum.[7] Dense collections of eosinophils—in effect eosinophilic microabscesses—can be found by microscopic study of biopsy material, although the absence of this finding does not exclude the disease. In fact, parasitic infection, radiation enteritis, lymphoma, and polyarteritis nodosa must be eliminated as diagnostic possibilities when biopsies show nonspecific inflammation.[6]

Pancreatitis

The question of whether alcohol has a noxious effect on duodenal mucosa remains unanswered. Lev et al.[8] could not correlate histologic change with alcohol consumption. However, in a group of alcoholic patients with chronic pancreatitis, endoscopic biopsy of the duodenal bulb showed an increased frequency of isolated duodenitis compared with patients with chronic alcoholism or liver cirrhosis alone.[9] Duodenal mucosal abnormalities appear to be associated with the inflammatory process of both acute and chronic pancreatitis, although mucosal alteration may not be evident endoscopically.

The inflammatory process may be progressive, so that actual stenosis of the second or third portion of the duodenum ensues. This finding on upper gastrointestinal series should not preclude endoscopic evaluation, even when stricturing is apparently severe, since duodenoscopy is nevertheless successful in most such cases.[10] However, this usually yields meager findings other than confirmation of the narrowed caliber, since in most cases the mucosa is intact and normal in appearance,[11] although occasionally there will be erythema and friability of the mucosa. Failure to identify the papilla is not unusual since it may be retracted and out of sight of the side-viewing duodenoscope.[12] Although the stenotic segment may be long, the stricture usually resolves as the contiguous inflammatory process subsides. A small percentage of patients will develop a fibrosing pancreaticoduodenitis and will ultimately require surgical bypass.[11] Considerable rigidity of the stenotic area may be appreciated by endoscopic palpation, but it cannot be assumed that mural fibrosis is the cause, because a similar abnormality may occur with a pseudocyst or pancreatic cancer. Before surgical intervention, duodenoscopy should be complemented by a thorough evaluation including ultrasonography, computed tomography, or endoscopic retrograde pancreatography.

INFECTIOUS DISEASES

Tuberculosis

Duodenal tuberculosis, when it is found in conjunction with ileocecal involvement, is frequently mistaken for Crohn's disease in the United States, where gastrointestinal tuberculosis is rare.[13] In Africa, Asia, and India, where intestinal tuberculosis is common,[14] duodenal tuberculosis is still infrequently encountered and constitutes only 3% of gastrointestinal tuberculosis. Since only 50% of patients with duodenal tuberculosis have involvement elsewhere in the digestive tract or other viscera, diagnosis is difficult, and laparotomy and surgical biopsy are necessary for histologic confirmation.

Duodenoscopy is undertaken to explain findings on upper gastrointestinal series of thickened folds, ulcerations, and stricture consistent with Crohn's disease, peptic ulcer, or neoplasm. In one report specifically related to duodenoscopic evaluation, the finding was a stricture 2 to 3 cm long, surrounded by hyperemic and granular mucosa.[14] Six endoscopic biopsies disclosed nonspecific chronic inflammation and fibrosis, but caseating granulomas were seen in subsequent surgical material. In another patient, marked bulbar duodenitis and a postbulbar stricture were found, but again biopsy specimens were not diagnostic and surgery was required to obtain histologic verification.[13] Pyloric obstruction may interfere with endoscopic evaluation of the duodenum.[15] Endoscopic biopsy was also disappointingly negative in the evaluation of an irregular ulcer 2 cm in widest diameter with a necrotic base in the distal transverse duodenum; again, surgical material from the duodenum contained granulomas in the submucosa and serosa.[16]

It is evident that duodenoscopic biopsy cannot provide the submucosal tissue in which the acid-fast bacilli proliferate. Whether the use of a larger biopsy forceps or special techniques such as snare biopsy will safely retrieve tissue deep enough for diagnosis remains to be seen, but in view of the rarity of duodenal tuberculosis in the United States such a study should be undertaken in an endemic area.

Parasites

Although in many countries the prevalence of parasitic infection is low, the endoscopist should consider the presence of parasitic infection, which is often amenable to therapy, when unexplained mucosal changes are encountered in the duodenum.

The endoscopist may rarely find a worm in the duodenum.[17] The worm should be removed with the biopsy forceps for specific identification. It is more likely that only the nonspecific duodenal mucosal inflammation that is a reaction to the parasite or its eggs will be seen, but the endoscopist should be alert to the possibility of a parasitosis, in order that aspiration of luminal fluid and mucosal biopsies may be appropriately performed.

Giardia lamblia is a protozoan of cosmopolitan distribution that is disseminated by contaminated water and fecal-oral spread. The diagnosis is ordinarily confirmed by finding the characteristic flagellate in diarrheal stool specimens. However, the prominence of upper gastrointestinal symptoms such as anorexia and nausea as well as loss of weight may initiate radiologic and endoscopic study of the stomach and duodenum. At duodenoscopy the valvulae conniventes may be thick-

ened although the mucosa itself may appear relatively normal.[18] In a patient with hypogammaglobulinemia, however, the mucosa may show numerous punctate nodules, a manifestation of lymphoid nodular hyperplasia. If giardiasis is suspected, the duodenal luminal contents should be aspirated to examine the fluid for the trophozoite. Endoscopic biopsy should yield a high degree of positive return, based on the excellent results achieved with capsule biopsy.[18] Giardiasis is not a condition that requires endoscopy for diagnosis, but if the opportunity arises incidentally during evaluation of a patient, it should not be lost.

Strongyloides stercoralis infests the duodenum and may cause a myriad of symptoms, the most common being epigastric pain. Upper gastrointestinal roentgenography may show minimal mucosal changes or, with severe involvement occurring in endemic areas or in immunosuppressed patients, thickened duodenal folds and mural rigidity.[19] These latter findings usually require endoscopy for definitive diagnosis, but the endoscopic appearance varies from "marked edema" in mild infections[20] to gross inflammatory hypertrophy of the mucosa, which in advanced disease nearly obliterates the lumen.[19] Strongyloidiasis must be suspected first if it is to be diagnosed endoscopically, because the diagnosis depends on aspiration of luminal mucus and juice, which will contain rhabditiform larvae of *S. stercoralis,* and on duodenal biopsy, which results in a high yield for the parasite buried in the mucosa.

A small luminal helminth such as hookworm may be aspirated via the suction channel of an endoscope into a trap, or it may be gently picked off the mucosa with a biopsy forceps.[17] Identification of any rhabditiform or filariform larvae obtained at biopsy, however, requires a parasitologist to differentiate hookworm from *S. stercoralis* and *Trichostrongylus* species.[20] The large helminth *Ascaris lumbricoides* presents no difficulty in recognition since its gross external features are characteristic. A heavy infection of *A. lumbricoides* may result in migration of the worm into the ampulla, from which it may be extracted if it is visible. Pancreatitis has been documented as a complication of ductal invasion by the roundworm.[21]

A bizarre encounter with a tapeworm in the duodenum led to extraction of the 250 cm worm with its head intact.[22] Because of increased immigration of people to the

United States from the Orient, the endoscopist should be prepared to recognize such trematodes as *Fasciola hepatica* and *Clonorchis sinensis*.[23]

TUMORS

Benign Neoplasms

The duodenum constitutes only 8% of the small bowel by length but harbors 10% to 20% of small bowel tumors.[24] Since only 3% to 6% of all gastrointestinal benign and malignant neoplasms originate in the small intestine, the actual number is relatively small. Moreover, only 50% of the benign tumors ever become symptomatic; the remainder are found incidentally at surgery, autopsy, or endoscopy.[25]

The diagnosis of duodenal tumors is usually first made in the course of an upper gastrointestinal series. The finding is unexpected if not incidental, but a duodenal defect does warrant further investigation.

The most direct approach for evaluation is duodenoscopy and biopsy. If the lesion appears pedunculate by radiographic study, the patient and duodenoscopist should be prepared for polypectomy in order to avoid an additional procedure. Selection of an endoscope for evaluation depends on the location and size of the tumor. A forward-viewing, small-diameter endoscope may permit the best view of bulbar tumors, but a lesion on the medial wall of the descending duodenum may be observed best by a side-viewing duodenoscope. When adequate biopsy specimens are essential, as in a large tumor, or when polypectomy is anticipated, a forward-viewing instrument with a large-caliber channel will allow adequate access to a lesion that is large enough to project into the lumen. On occasion, both forward- and side-viewing endoscopes are required for satisfactory study of the lesion.

In most instances routine upper gastrointestinal endoscopy probably does not include bowel beyond the second portion of the duodenum. To reach and examine a more distally located lesion identified on barium contrast study, endoscopy under fluoroscopy is preferable to be certain that the tip of the endoscope crosses the spine as it traverses the third portion of the duodenum.

Adenomas

Adenomas, the most common duodenal tumor, occur as single or multiple lesions and are usually pedunculate. Occult bleeding is the most frequent sign of an adenoma but, as in one of our cases,[24] massive hemorrhage may occur. Endoscopically the lesion projects into the lumen and may be a few millimeters to 50 mm in diameter.[26] The surface of the tumor is the same color as that of the surrounding mucosa, but it is usually lobulated, with particularly prominent lobules apparent in larger adenomas.

Adenomas of the duodenum can be classified histologically in the same manner as colonic adenomas. The tumor presumably progresses from one composed entirely of tubular glands to one that shows a florid or papillary glandular pattern. Thus, at one end of the spectrum is the tubular adenoma and at the other end the villous adenoma with a mixed tubulovillous type occupying an intermediate position. Large villous adenomas seem to have the same high degree of malignant potential as their colonic counterpart. For this reason pedunculate adenomas should be removed endoscopically. Those that are too large or cannot be removed endoscopically for other technical reasons should be removed by surgery.[27-33] Until 1975, of 41 reported cases of villous adenoma, 27% showed invasive malignant changes. Patients over age 50 with distal duodenal tumors larger than 4 cm are at particularly high risk for invasive cancer.[34]

Of our 10 cases of villous adenoma diagnosed by fiberoptic endoscopy,[35] we were impressed with the variable clinical presentation—bleeding in 5 cases, obstruction in 4, and jaundice in 2—as well as the variation in endoscopic appearance. The villous adenoma in the duodenum may be in the form of prominent folds or a verrucous encircling lesion (Plate 23–3); it is usually sessile, but 2 of our cases were pedunculate polyps. The pedunculate polyp should be removed in toto by duodenoscopic polypectomy and the specimen carefully studied for evidence of invasive cancer. The sessile lesion, which is usually shaggy and multilobulated, should be thoroughly studied by biopsy. Pancreaticoduodenectomy is in order only if an invasive cancer is identified; otherwise, a wide local excision is appropriate.[32] In a review of 44 cases of villous adenomas treated surgically, only 5 required pancreaticoduodenectomy, and 3 were amenable to endoscopic polypectomy alone.[36]

Leiomyoma

The leiomyoma is the most frequently occurring benign tumor in the small intestine and is found mainly in the jejunum.[37] Although least commonly found in the duodenum, the leiomyoma is, nevertheless, the second most prevalent neoplasm in the duodenum.[38]

Most leiomyomas arise from the muscularis propria and vary in size from a few millimeters to several centimeters.[25] Exoenteric tumors may become large enough to bleed or less commonly to produce obstruction and thus come to the attention of the endoscopist.[39]

Leiomyomas are submucosal tumors and offer no distinct mucosal feature that permits endoscopic diagnosis. The lesion bulges into the lumen as a round or ovoid sessile polyp with a smoothly tapering border (Plate 23–4); rarely it is pedunculate.[24] As the polyp enlarges, it may lead to pressure necrosis of the overlying mucosa and a resultant central ulceration. Bleeding from this ulcer usually leads to endoscopy, and this central hemorrhagic ulcer should arouse a suspicion of leiomyoma.

In our endoscopic series of 45 duodenal polyps, 19 biopsy specimens showed normal mucosa or mucosal inflammation.[24] It is likely that many small submucosal bulges generally ignored by the endoscopist are leiomyomas that probably originate in the muscularis mucosae.

Brunner's Gland Adenoma

Polyps that arise from Brunner's gland of the duodenum are rare lesions of the supra Vaterian duodenum and are most often found in the bulb. Although the adenoma is the most common form of Brunner's gland hyperplasia, there are diffuse nodular and circumscribed nodular forms (Plate 23–5) as well.[40] Because of the bulbar location and the propensity of these tumors to bleed or obstruct the lumen, the Brunner's gland adenoma, or brunneroma, is often mistaken as a manifestation of peptic ulcer disease.

The endoscopic picture may vary from multiple 2 to 3 mm nodules carpeting the mucosa of the proximal duodenum to a solitary polyp of a few millimeters to several centimeters in diameter. The diffuse nodular pattern accounts for the characteristic "Swiss cheese" radiographic appearance. Although Brunner's glands are submucosal, primarily below the muscularis mucosae, endoscopic biopsies are frequently diagnostic since hyperplasia results in extension of the glands into the mucosa.[24, 40, 41] Brunner's gland hyperplasia is not a premalignant lesion, and surgical excision is unnecessary unless tumor size becomes sufficient to cause obstruction by intermittent intussusception.[42]

Brunner's gland adenoma may bleed[43, 44] and require excision. If pedunculate, these polyps are best removed by endoscopic polypectomy (Plate 23–6); 3 cases of successful endoscopic removal have been described.[24, 43, 45] Some caveats should be observed with snare excision of a duodenal polyp. The papilla of Vater must be identified, so that if prominent or protuberant it is not inadvertently snared.[43] Excessive coagulation in the thin-walled duodenum increases the risk of perforation. Conversely, inadequate coagulation increases the danger of excessive bleeding from the richly vascular duodenum, which is bathed in acid-peptic juices.[46]

Lipoma

Lipomas are found three times more commonly in the small intestine than in the stomach but less than half as often as in the colon.[24] These submucosal tumors may become several centimeters in diameter and form a pseudopedicle as they enlarge. With a sessile lesion, a positive tissue diagnosis can be made by the so-called "drill" technique. This biopsy method involves taking several biopsies from the same site, so that underlying submucosal fat composing the lesion is retrieved.

The endoscopic appearance is similar to that of other submucosal duodenal tumors (Plate 23–7). However, the polypoid form lends itself to palpation with the blunt tip of the biopsy forceps, by means of which the soft nature of the tumor is appreciated and the characteristic "pillow" sign—a smooth indentation made by the forceps—is elicited. Intraluminal polypoid lipomas may intussuscept, producing intermittent obstruction; also, bleeding may occur as a result of superficial necrosis. When the lipoma is symptomatic, endoscopic polypectomy is feasible if a sufficiently developed pseudopedicle has formed.[23]

Neurofibroma

Solitary neurofibromas are usually found in the ileum. They occur in 15% of patients with von Recklinghausen's disease, with the most frequently involved intestinal segments being (in descending order) the jejunum, the ileum, and the duodenum.[37] In a review of 28 cases of neurogenic tumors of the small

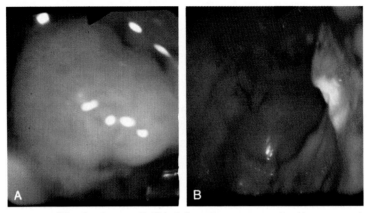

PLATE 23–6. *A,* Brunneroma of the duodenum. *B,* This 1.5 cm tumor was excised by snare polypectomy.

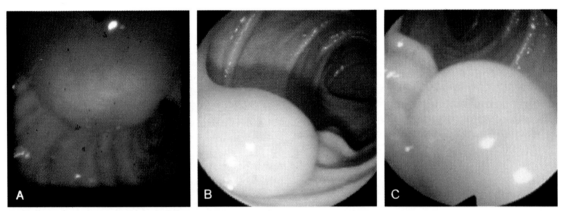

PLATE 23–7. *A,* Lipoma of the duodenum. This tumor was soft, indenting on pressure from the blunt forceps tip. Biopsy showed normal mucosa and the tumor was presumed to be a lipoma. *B* and *C.* Two views of a soft whitish, polypoid submucosal duodenal tumor presumed to be a lipoma. (*B, C* Courtesy M.V. Sivak, Jr., M.D.)

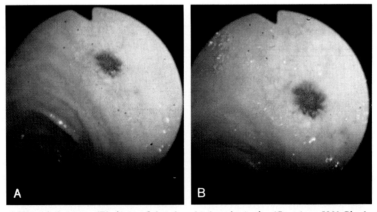

PLATE 23–8. Distant *(A)* and close-up *(B)* views of duodenal telangiectasia. (Courtesy M.V. Sivak, Jr., M.D.)

intestine reported since 1955, Sivak et al.[47] recorded 10 duodenal neoplasms, all of which had ulcerated and bled; 4 were neurofibromas, 2 neurofibromosarcomas, 2 paragangliomas, and 2 neuromas. In a patient with von Recklinghausen's disease, these workers performed endoscopic polypectomy of an ulcerated 2.5 cm round mass 4 cm beyond the papilla of Vater. The submucosal polyp was a neurilemoma.

In another patient with von Recklinghausen's disease, multiple submucosal elongated polypoid tumors were present in the pylorus and first and second portions of the duodenum.[48] Several of these tumors had a central umbilication similar to that seen with leiomyoma. The duodenal mucosa had a diffuse reticular brown pigmentation. Endoscopic biopsies of the polyps were consistent with diagnosis of a neurofibroma.

The duodenal neurogenic tumor is exceedingly rare. It is dangerous because of its propensity to bleed and to undergo malignant transformation. When solitary, it may be amenable to endoscopic polypectomy, but the upper gastrointestinal neurogenic tumor is usually one of several, and surgical resection is necessary.

Lymphangioma

Lymphatic cysts, or lymphangiomas, are rarely seen in the duodenum.[49-51] These lesions are located in the submucosa but give the mucosa a yellow color. The polypoid tumor is soft and can be removed by endoscopic polypectomy[50] or drained by means of multiple biopsies.[51]

Pancreatic Rest

Heterotopic pancreas may be found in the duodenum, more commonly in the bulb. These formations are usually noted incidentally at endoscopy as submucosal nodules with a central umbilication. Biopsy specimens infrequently contain pancreatic acini and ducts; therefore, diagnosis is essentially by endoscopic observation. Pancreatic rests have been responsible for duodenal obstruction, massive hemorrhage, and common bile duct obstruction,[52] but none of these major complications have as yet been reported as an endoscopic diagnosis. The pancreatic rest is also discussed in Chapter 35.

Telangiectasia

Telangiectasias may be seen in the duodenum either as solitary lesions or as part of the multiorgan involvement of Osler-Weber-Rendu disease. It would be unusual to see telangiectasias in the duodenum without also finding them in the stomach. Bleeding is a frequent complication and endoscopic evaluation provides definitive diagnosis. These lesions may be pale and not be readily visible if the patient is anemic. Patients should be re-examined after blood replacement if initial studies fail to explain the gastrointestinal hemorrhage. Telangiectasias have the characteristic raised central arteriolar bleb. Thin tendrils radiate outward from this central point (Plate 23-8). It would appear to be unusual to witness spontaneous bleeding from a gastrointestinal telangiectasia.

Telangiectasias can be eradicated by endoscopic electrocoagulation or photocoagulation, but this may not solve the problem of blood loss if there are more vascular lesions distally in the intestine.

Polyposis Syndromes

Adenomas of both stomach and duodenum occur with surprising frequency in patients with familial polyposis coli (FPC) and Gardner's syndrome (GS).[53, 54] In 49 patients with FPC or GS, endoscopy revealed duodenal adenomas in about one third; the adenomas were usually multiple, small, white, and located in the second portion of the duodenum.[53] Yao et al.[54] noted similar "minute-size adenomas" as well as larger lesions that ranged in size from 5 to 22 mm (Plate 23-9). In one of their cases biopsy specimens of a normal appearing papilla revealed an adenoma.[55] Using a side-viewing duodenoscope, this same group[55] studied the papilla in 24 patients with FPC and in 10 patients noted a granular to nodular surface that by biopsy proved to be a manifestation of adenomatous change.

Gastric and duodenal polyps are found in patients with GS, and in a review of the literature to 1976, 36 cases of gastric or small bowel (mostly duodenal) adenomas were collected.[56] In one case with only duodenal adenomas, superficial carcinoma was identified in a large adenoma.[56] Endoscopic removal of duodenal polyps, which proved to be adenomatous, was accomplished in another patient with GS, and severe dysplasia was evident on microscopic study of the adenomas.[57]

The exclusion of gastric and duodenal adenomas is sufficient reason to perform upper gastrointestinal endoscopy routinely on patients with FPC and GS. Since malignant

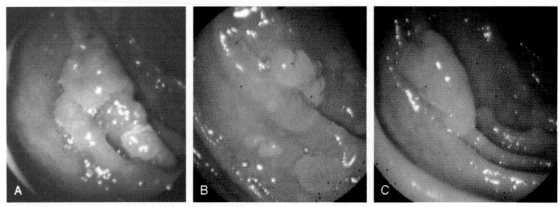

PLATE 23–9. Small, irregular-shaped sessile and semisessile polyps in patients with familial polyposis coli (A) and Gardner's syndrome *(B and C)*. (Courtesy M.V. Sivak, Jr., M.D.)

change has been demonstrated with duodenal adenomas, endoscopic polypectomy, when feasible, is appropriate for large polyps, and electrocoagulation or excision for smaller polyps. Adenomas of the papilla are a special problem; endoscopic follow-up with biopsy at intervals of 1 to 2 years to exclude dysplasia may be a reasonable approach.

Cronkhite-Canada syndrome is a rare disorder characterized by alopecia, skin pigmentation, nail atrophy, and diffuse gastrointestinal polyposis.[58] The polyps are an inflammatory type and contain mucous retention cysts; they are located mostly in the stomach and colon, but the small bowel, particularly the duodenum, may be affected. Small sessile polyps seen on endoscopy almost completely replace the mucosa, and biopsy reveals the characteristic retention cysts. These polyps have no malignant potential, and thus nothing more than correct identification is required. Spontaneous remission of the syndrome, with complete disappearance of the gastrointestinal polyps, has been reported.[58]

Hamartomatous polyps develop throughout the entire digestive tract in Peutz-Jeghers syndrome, an autosomal dominant disorder. The diagnosis is confirmed by the radiographic finding of multiple small bowel polyps, usually jejunal, in a patient with melanin spots on the lips, buccal mucosa, and the tips of the fingers and toes. Endoscopy is indicated in the unusual circumstance of bleeding localized to the duodenum or when duodenal intussusception from a large polyp is suspected. Endoscopic polypectomy may avoid surgical intervention. Microscopically the retrieved polyp will have the distinctive branching stalk of smooth muscle fibers that is thicker at the center of the polyp than at its periphery.[25]

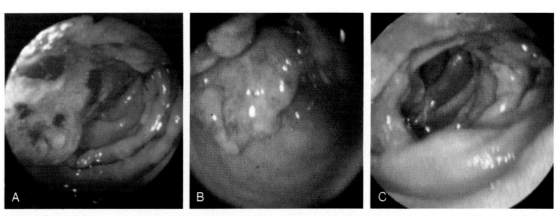

PLATE 23–10. Adenocarcinomas of the duodenum in three patients. The lesion seen in *A* was found in the patient with familial polyposis coli whose more proximal polyp is seen in Plate 23–9A. (Courtesy M.V. Sivak, Jr., M.D.)

Malignant Neoplasms

Adenocarcinoma

About 50% of all primary malignancies of the small intestine are adenocarcinomas.[59] Carcinomas of the duodenum account for only 0.35% of all gastrointestinal carcinomas, but relative to its length the duodenum harbors the largest number of cancers in the small bowel.[60] Duodenal carcinoma is usually classified according to its anatomic relationship to the ampulla of Vater. Since carcinoma of the bulb is very rare, supra-ampullary tumors are essentially found in the second portion of the duodenum and, in a study of 71 cases of duodenal carcinoma, these constituted 7% of cases[61]; infra-ampullary and periampullary tumors made up 56% and 32%, respectively. Discrete ampullary cancers are not always clearly separated from the periampullary group in many reports. For many authors[59, 62–64] the term "periampullary" has traditionally included ampullary adenocarcinoma. More often than not, it is impossible to decide, either endoscopically or at surgery, whether the cancer arose from duodenal mucosa and encroached on the papilla or vice versa. The other problem with classification of periampullary adenocarcinoma is the determination of the tissue origin, since the cancer may arise not only from contiguous duodenal mucosa but also from the distal bile and pancreatic duct, ampulla, and pancreas. The most accurate diagnosis of ampullary cancer is by gross pathologic and microscopic study of resected or autopsy specimens, although uncertainty may still persist in some cases.

Duodenoscopy has had an important impact on preoperative diagnosis of duodenal adenocarcinoma. In one series of 17 patients with adenocarcinoma of the duodenum, endoscopy provided a histologic diagnosis of cancer in 5 of the 7 cases in which it was performed.[59] In another series of 12 adenocarcinomas, 2 cases not diagnosed by radiographic study were confirmed by duodenoscopic biopsy.[60] The necessity for a complete examination of the entire duodenum in suspected cases was emphasized by Satake et al.[65]

The duodenoscopic appearance of adenocarcinoma is not specific and cannot be differentiated with confidence from leiomyosarcoma or lymphoma. The lesion is usually nodular and polypoid, but it may also be ulcerated or friable (Plate 23–10).[66] It is most often confined to the second or third portion of the duodenum, whereas lymphoma may be diffuse.[60] Because biopsies are generally easy to obtain, a tissue diagnosis can be made in most cases.[65] Walsh et al.[67] failed to obtain malignant tissue by endoscopic biopsy in 3 of 6 cases of adenocarcinoma of the ampulla of Vater, but the ampulla was considered abnormal visually in all 6 patients.

Leiomyosarcoma

In the small bowel, myogenic cancers are most common in the jejunum and least common in the duodenum (10%).[68] Compared to the entire duodenum, there are parallel percentages of leiomyoma (50%) and leiomyosarcoma (53%) in the descending portion of the duodenum.[69] At least one case has been followed from a 4 cm biopsy-proven leiomyoma to a 7 cm surgically excised leiomyosarcoma.[70] Thus, there is circumstantial evidence that the leiomyoma is the precursor of the leiomyosarcoma, suggesting that large leiomyomas should be excised even if found only incidentally. Until 1981, 123 cases of duodenal leiomyosarcoma were reported in a review of the literature.[71]

The endoscopic appearance will vary depending on the size of the tumor and whether it is intraluminal, intramural, or exoenteric. In one instance the endoscopist saw an umbilicated polypoid mass that was friable and bled profusely upon biopsy.[72] However, the tumor may be submucosal and develop a central ulceration as it enlarges (Plate 23–11).[69] The ulcerated form would presumably be the most common, since bleeding is the chief complaint in over half the cases.[25]

Endoscopic biopsy of duodenal leiomyosarcoma is not reliable or, more accurately, not interpretable as benign or malignant.[69, 72] Although large tumors are most often malignant, endoscopic biopsies are inadequate for a count of mitotic figures, upon which the diagnosis of malignancy rests. Indeed, at times the diagnosis of leiomyosarcoma must await the demonstration of metastases during the clinical course, since even the surgically excised tumor may not meet the pathologic criteria for cancer.[71]

Lymphoma

Although rare in the gastrointestinal tract of adults, lymphoma is the most common digestive tract tumor in children. Lymphoma occurs least frequently in the duodenum,

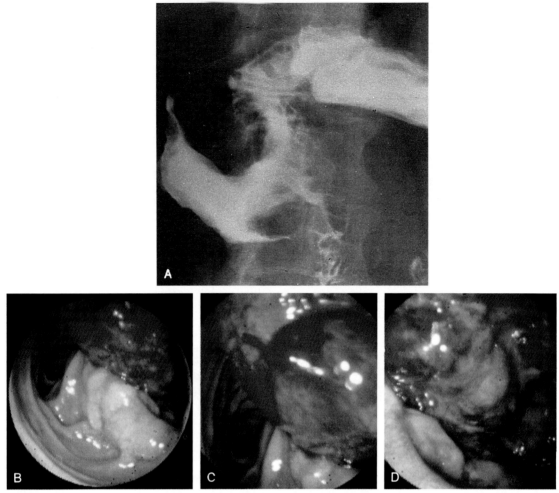

PLATE 23–11. A, X-ray showing ulcerated leiomyosarcoma of the duodenum, with a fistulous track. B, Endoscopic view with duodenum to the left of the field, the tumor in the center, and the fistula to the right. C, Closer view of the lesion, with duodenal lumen to the left. D, Close-up view of the lesion, with fistula to the right.

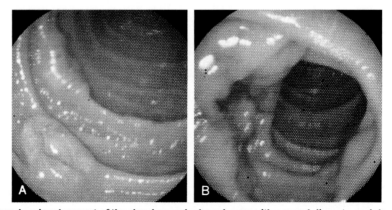

PLATE 23–12. A, Secondary involvement of the duodenum by lymphoma with several discrete nodules. B, More extensive and confluent involvement of the same area 2½ months later.

except in patients with immunoproliferative small intestinal disease (IPSID).[25]

The duodenum was involved in all of 6 cases of IPSID studied endoscopically.[73] The mucosa was thickened and covered by many sessile polyps of varying sizes. In one patient, scattered ulcers were seen, and in another a large ulcerative mass was found in the third portion of the duodenum (Plate 23–12). Unfortunately this report does not indicate whether endoscopic biopsies were diagnostic.

In another retrospective study,[74] in only 1 of 6 patients was primary malignant lymphoma diagnosed preoperatively. There were no characteristic endoscopic findings. Although duodenoscopic biopsy may provide a diagnosis of lymphoma, the differentiation into Hodgkin's and non-Hodgkin's types of lymphoma requires surgical biopsy.[74]

Lymphosarcoma of the duodenum has been described, but less than 75 cases have been collected since 1877.[75] Endoscopy in one patient showed a "fungating ulcerating lesion of the second portion of the duodenum."[75] The biopsy was originally interpreted as adenocarcinoma, but upon comparison with the surgical biopsy it was considered consistent with lymphosarcoma.

Metastases

Malignant invasion of the medial wall of the duodenum most likely originates in the pancreas, stomach, or biliary tree, but contiguous spread from the right kidney and the hepatic flexure of the colon either directly or via lymphatic channels may also occur.[25] Excluding the "obvious" carcinomas of the pancreas, stomach, and biliary tract, Veen et al.[76] collected 14 cases of duodenal metastases over a 10-year span: 5 from the colon; 2 from the kidney and pancreas, 2 from cutaneous melanoma; and 1 each from the uterus, esophagus, and gallbladder.

Pancreatic cancer compromising the duodenal lumen is a common development in patients who survive 10 months from presentation.[77] The usual endoscopic appearance is that of a soft polypoid tumor involving the second or third portion of the duodenum (Plate 23–13).[78, 79] Biopsies are almost always confirmatory of pancreatic cancer.

Cancer of the stomach only rarely spreads to the duodenum, perhaps because of the poor lymphatic connections between the two organs.[80] Lymphatic invasion by gastric cancer cells turned the color of the duodenal mucosa to white in one case,[80] but polypoid tumors surrounded by mucosa of a more normal color were also identified, biopsies from the latter yielding a histologic diagnosis (Plate 23–14).

Four cases of hypernephroma metastatic to the duodenum were discovered endoscopically because of the onset of upper gastrointestinal bleeding.[81] A nodular mass with ulceration was noted at duodenoscopy in 2 cases, a multilobulated smooth mass in 1 case, and a circumferential ulcer in another case (Plate 23–15). Biopsies in all cases were negative for malignancy, although cytologic findings were positive for malignant cells in one. The hypervascularity of the hypernephroma impedes retrieval of adequate biopsy material and contributes to the failure to obtain an appropriate pathologic diagnosis.[81]

Malignant melanoma metastasizes frequently to the stomach and duodenum. Bleeding or obstruction related to large ulcerated tumors warrants endoscopic examination. If pigmented, the duodenal tumor is recognized readily at endoscopy. The nodules vary in size and are usually ulcerated. Biopsy specimens are usually positive for melanoma.[82–84] The gastrointestinal metastasis may be the only one apparent, and endoscopic examination becomes an important evaluation since surgical resection may result in prolonged palliation.[82]

Metastases from carcinoma of the breast,[83] testis,[84] and ovary[84] have been identified at endoscopy.

Miscellaneous Malignant Tumors

An extramedullary plasmacytoma, a lesion usually associated with multiple myeloma, was identified in the first portion of the duodenum as a primary isolated tumor.[85] Endoscopic biopsy of this fungating mass was followed by severe hemorrhage that necessitated laparotomy.

Visceral involvement may occur in 10% of patients with Kaposi's sarcoma; the gastrointestinal tract is commonly affected, the majority of lesions being found in the stomach.[86] There may be duodenal extension of the maculopapular to polypoid tumor that takes on a dark red color as it enlarges. Lesions of 1 cm or greater may have a central umbilication of variable depth. Endoscopic biopsy is reliable for tissue diagnosis, this being essential for staging treatment of the disease.[86]

Carcinoid tumors of the gastrointestinal tract are found mainly in the appendix

(50%), and next most commonly in the small intestine (25%). The most frequent site in the small bowel is the distal 50 cm of ileum.[25] The duodenum is the second least common site, but duodenal carcinoids cause symptoms more often than do other types. Since foregut carcinoids exhibit an argyrophil reaction but not argentaffin staining, they rarely cause carcinoid syndrome. Endoscopically, they are typically small (less than 2 cm) submucosal lesions covered by normal mucosa that may have a yellow-orange tint.[24] Biopsies are usually diagnostic. Because carcinoid is considered a malignant lesion, surgical excision is mandatory, even for asymptomatic tumors.

Gastrinomas, of which two thirds are malignant, are most often localized to the pancreas, but the duodenal wall is a frequent extrapancreatic site. Because these tumors are small and submucosal, they are overlooked at endoscopy and may not become apparent until duodenoscopy is done after total gastrectomy.[87] The opportunity for preoperative biopsy diagnosis of a duodenal gastrinoma afforded by endoscopy should not be missed, since the surgical management will be governed by the endoscopic finding.[88-90] Indeed, Zollinger-Ellison syndrome has been "cured" by endoscopic polypectomy of a submucosal 3 to 4 mm tumor.[91]

MISCELLANEOUS DISEASE

Foreign Bodies

More than 99% of foreign bodies that enter the duodenum pass through the small intestine. The junction of the second and third portions of the duodenum is the first anatomic flexure at which the foreign body may become lodged.[92] Toothpicks account for 10% of intestinal perforations[92] and are particularly difficult to localize, since the wooden (now plastic as well) toothpick is not radiopaque. Toothpicks, however can be easily removed endoscopically from the duodenum with forceps, even if already perforating the wall (Plate 23–16).[93, 94]

Pins and needles have a high risk of perforation if retained in the duodenum, and immediate endoscopic extraction is indicated. A needle can be grasped with forceps and pulled safely into the accessory channel of the endoscope, but an open safety pin is best retrieved by putting the closed biopsy forceps through the loop. By opening the jaws of the forceps, the safety pin is captured and can

be pulled out with the endoscope.[95, 96] Use of an overtube with the endoscope also adds a margin of safety and may make the procedure technically easier.

A thermometer was extracted from the duodenum by placing a polypectomy snare around the neck of the thermometer.[97]

A duodenal bezoar was encountered between the second and third segments of the duodenum in a patient who had had a gastroduodenostomy. It was conjectured that narrowing of the flexure was a result of the surgery, although two diverticula were present in the area.[98] Duodenal bezoars are almost always associated with obstruction and have been reported in patients with duodenal web[99] and diaphragm.[100] Foreign bodies and their extraction by endoscopic methods are considered in detail in Chapter 14.

Diverticula, Diaphragms, and Stenosis

Duodenal diverticula are found during 10% to 20% of endoscopic examinations and, when juxtapapillary, are associated with an increased incidence of gallstones and pancreatitis (See Chapter 30).[101, 102] The diverticulum often encompasses the papilla at its superior border but, rarely, the papilla may be located entirely within the diverticulum. In one fifth of cases the diverticula are multiple and may, in a few cases, border either side of the papilla, giving a pantaloon effect.[103] Although diverticulitis with subsequent perforation has been recorded,[101] diverticula are not known to interfere with or complicate duodenoscopy.

An unusual variant of duodenal diverticula is the intraluminal duodenal diverticulum (IDD), a developmental abnormality resulting from the effect of peristaltic activity on a duodenal diaphragm.[104] The IDD has a diagnostic radiographic appearance, and duodenoscopy is invoked to evaluate the pouch for bleeding or inflammation and to localize the papilla.[105] A double aperture, one for the pouch and the other for the duodenal lumen, is better appreciated with the side-viewing duodenoscope.[106] However, only the pouch will be seen if it is circumferentially attached. Duodenoscopy may be useful for removal of impacted debris in the pouch or for dilation of the outflow ostium of the IDD.[107] Hajiro et al.,[108] using a polypectomy snare, endoscopically excised the tip of an IDD that had been inverted and thus provided an adequate opening in the center of the diverticulum.

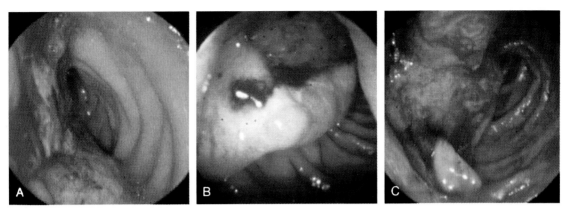

PLATE 23–13. *A,* Duodenal invasion by carcinoma of the pancreas. *B,* Ulcerated, bleeding carcinoma of the pancreas is visible in the medial wall of the duodenum. *C,* Cystadenocarcinoma of the pancreas, invading the duodenum. (Courtesy M.V. Sivak, Jr., M.D.)

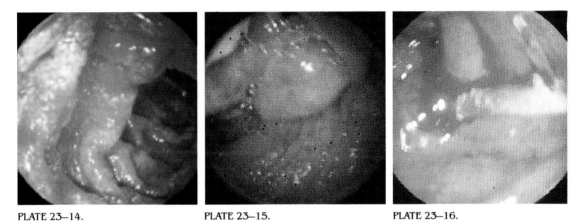

PLATE 23–14.   PLATE 23–15.   PLATE 23–16.

PLATE 23–14. Involvement of the duodenum by metastatic gastric adenocarcinoma. Note the very small, whitish nodules that cover much of the mucosal surface. Biopsy was positive for carcinoma. (Courtesy M.V. Sivak, Jr., M.D.)
PLATE 23–15. Hypernephroma metastatic to the duodenum. (Courtesy M.V. Sivak, Jr., M.D.)
PLATE 23–16. Toothpick in the duodenum. This toothpick was readily grasped and retrieved with the biopsy forceps.

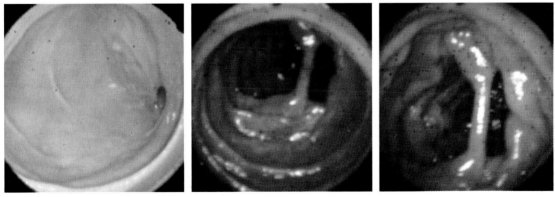

PLATE 23–17.   PLATE 23–18.

PLATE 23–17. Duodenal diaphragm in an elderly woman. Note the excentrically placed opening, about 6 or 7 mm in diameter, through the diaphragm. (Courtesy M.V. Sivak, Jr., M.D.)
PLATE 23–18. Duodenal diaphragm. This incomplete diaphragm was nonobstructing and so was not divided by endoscopic electrocoagulation.

This should become the technique of choice for obstructed IDD, replacing surgical duodenotomy and excision.

As of 1978, only 31 cases of duodenal diaphragm had been reported. Suarez and Bolden[99] reported endoscopic evaluation of a case in which they were unable to pass the gastroscope through the eccentrically positioned 10 mm aperture (Plate 23–17). A *form fruste* diaphragm was found by the author at duodenoscopy (Plate 23–18). Therapeutic intervention has been surgical in the past, but it is reasonable to anticipate that, in most cases, endoscopic dilation or incision will be used.

Congenital stenosis was identified endoscopically at the apex of the duodenal bulb, which had a circumferential cuffing of the mucosa "giving the appearance of a cervix."[109] The stenosis did not relax in response to intravenous glucagon. I have encountered a postsurgical, postbulbar stenosis that balloon dilation improved temporarily (Plate 23–19).

Varices

Duodenal varices may be found in patients with cirrhosis or with extrahepatic portal hypertension. In the latter, esophageal and gastric varices are often absent. Bleeding from duodenal varices can be severe and frequently is misinterpreted endoscopically as arising from duodenal ulcer.[110, 111] The varices are postbulbar and may not be suspected if the endoscopist has not already encountered esophageal varices.[112] When the source of active bleeding remains undiagnosed, the patient should undergo arteriography[113, 114] or hepatic portography,[110] which will demonstrate clearly, as a rule, the duodenal varices. On one occasion, however, arteriography was negative and a large, dilated, blue varix of the second portion of the duodenum was easily seen at duodenoscopy.[115]

The usual treatment of bleeding duodenal varices is portacaval shunt,[110] suture ligation,[112] or excision of the varix,[115] although Sauerbruch and colleagues[116] successfully performed sclerotherapy in a patient who had had a portacaval shunt and had bled from a duodenal varix.

Hemangiomatosis and Hematoma

Capillary hemangiomas of the duodenum are not rare, but cavernous hemangiomas are distinctly unusual. They are congenital and may develop in other organs, particularly the skin. Their endoscopic identification as a vascular lesion should not be difficult. A submucosal tumor with bridging folds and a lustrous slightly blue color is characteristic.[117] However, unless the entire duodenum is examined, even large hemangiomas will be missed, only to be demonstrated by angiography.[118]

Intraduodenal hematoma results primarily from blunt abdominal trauma, but anticoagulant therapy[119] and chronic pancreatitis[120] have also been incriminated. It has also been reported as a complication of endoscopic retrograde cholangiopancreatography (ERCP),[121] the hematoma forming in the peripapillary area as a result of accidental intramural injection of contrast material. With spontaneous intraduodenal hematoma associated with anticoagulant therapy, the duodenal lumen at duodenoscopy has been found to be concentrically narrowed by purple ecchymotic folds of varying thickness; "the duodenal bulb is never involved."[119] In one report of intraduodenal hematoma,[122] the fixed, thickened folds were misinterpreted as a secondary feature of pancreatic cancer by gastroduodenoscopy. In the other cases,[120, 121] only a purplish bleb was evident endoscopically.

Fistulas: Biliary-Duodenal, Duodenocolic, and Aortoduodenal

Cholecystoduodenal fistula is the most common type of biliary enteric fistula, but choledochoduodenal or cholecystoduodenocolic fistulas also occur. Most of these benign fistulas are caused by erosion of a large gallstone, but peptic ulcer may be responsible in a small number of cases. A stone larger than 2 cm may become impacted in the small bowel, usually the terminal ileum, and only rarely in the duodenum.[123] If impacted in the duodenum, the stone may be viewed endoscopically.[123] A stone impacted in the third portion of the duodenum was not found at fiberoptic duodenoscopy because the examination was terminated at the bulb.[124] I have seen one case in which attempts to trap the stone in a Dormia basket for withdrawal were unsuccessful (Plate 23–20). Disimpaction usually requires surgical duodenotomy.[125]

Duodenocolic fistulas usually represent erosion from carcinoma of the hepatic flexure of the colon but may also be caused by carcinoma of the gallbladder or duodenum.[126] Less frequently, benign conditions such as peptic ulcer disease, diverticulitis, and granulomatosis or ulcerative colitis may cause such fistulas. The diagnosis is most often confirmed by barium enema studies; upper gastrointestinal endoscopy ordinarily plays no role. Ergin et al.[127] observed endoscopically a necrotic mass with central ulceration in the duodenum in a patient with a fistulous communication between the second portion and the hepatic flexure; however, the communication had been documented by barium enema and upper gastrointestinal series prior to endoscopy. Nevertheless, endoscopic biopsy revealed adenocarcinoma.

About 80% of aortoenteric fistulas communicate with the duodenum. Because the third portion is relatively fixed retroperitonally between the abdominal aorta posteriorly and the mesenteric artery and vein anteriorly, it is subject to pressure necrosis from an infrarenal aneurysm (primary type of aortoenteric fistula) or from an aortic graft (secondary type).[128] An extensive review published in 1980 identified 186 patients with primary aortoenteric fistula.[129] The diagnosis of a secondary type aortoduodenal fistula can be made endoscopically if a bile-stained vascular prosthesis is recognized, a pulsatile mass appreciated, or arterial bleeding encountered in the second or third part of the duodenum.[130] Walsh and coworkers[67] and Perdue and associates[131] stressed the importance of recognition of the early signs of back pain, fever, and intermittent bleeding in alerting the physician to the possibility of impending aortoenteric hemorrhage; the first group noted that the Gallium scan and computed tomography were each positive in all of the 5 patients examined,[67] whereas endoscopy was diagnostic in only 3 of 8 cases reported by Perdue et al.[131] It is mandatory that endoscopy include examination of the third and fourth portions of the duodenum; otherwise the diagnosis of aortoduodenal fistula will not be made.[128] Some surgeons believe that upper gastrointestinal endoscopy is needed only to exclude another cause of hemorrhage in a patient with a known aortic prosthesis, and that visualization of the fistula should not even be attempted.[132] It is difficult, however, to discourage definitive diagnosis if the endoscopist sees blood in the distal duodenum.

Champion and coworkers[133] have insisted that endoscopy be repeated as often as necessary to establish the diagnosis of aortoduodenal fistula. However, significant upper gastrointestinal hemorrhage and the absence at endoscopy of other potential causes in a patient with an aortic graft can be reason enough for surgical exploration, since exsanguinating hemorrhage is a distinct possibility in patients with this condition. Since 1977, yearly reports of endoscopic diagnosis of aortoduodenal fistula have been published.[134–141] In some cases endoscopic diagnosis was made by recognition of the bile-stained graft (Plate 23–21),[133, 134, 137, 139] a late stage of pressure necrosis, but in most instances the lesion appeared as a smooth mass that was either ulcerated or pulsatile or both.[135–138, 140] The aortoenteric fistula is considered further in Chapter 24.

A "C" graft constructed for a mesocaval shunt for control of bleeding esophageal varices was seen protruding into the second portion of the duodenum by endoscopy; it is not only the aortic prosthesis that puts the patient at risk.[141]

Celiac Disease

Using the GIF-D3 panendoscope (Olympus Corp.), Stevens and McCarthy[142] concluded that endoscopic biopsy of the duodenal bulb excludes celiac disease if villi are present. Villi were recognizable endoscopically in 25 controls, but not in 11 untreated patients with celiac disease; spraying indigo carmine on the duodenal mucosa exaggerated the abnormal mosaic pattern for directed biopsy.[142] Reducing the focal distance of the GIF-D2 endoscope (Olympus Corp.) to 5 mm enhances the ability to discern villous atrophy and permits biopsy from definite sites of disease involvement.[143] Biopsies of the first and second part of the duodenum in 14 patients with celiac disease correlated well with proximal jejunal suction biopsies.[143] In another study, 27 patients with suspected celiac disease had duodenoscopic biopsies; 11 biopsies considered compatible with celiac disease were confirmed by suction jejunal biopsy, and 13 normal biopsies were also verified by subsequent suction biopsy.[144]

Biopsies taken with the smaller-sized forceps used with the thinner-caliber endoscopes are not as easy to interpret with respect to celiac disease. The mucosal abnormality in celiac disease, being patchy and variable, requires, moreover, several biopsies to ensure a reliable diagnosis, although it appears that the more severe changes are found twice as often in the duodenum as in the jejunum (Plate 23–22).[145]

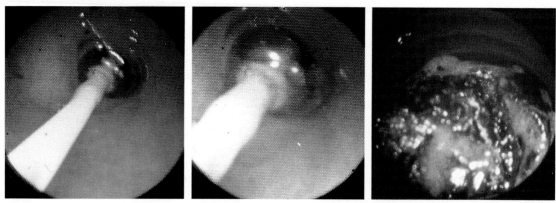

PLATE 23–19.   PLATE 23–20.

PLATE 23–19. *Left and Right,* Postsurgical, postbulbar stenosis. Balloon dilation was effective only temporarily.
PLATE 23–20. Gallstone impacted in descending duodenum. This stone could not be trapped in a Dormia basket.
(Courtesy of M. Ibrahim, M.D.)

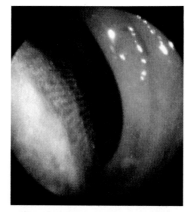

PLATE 23–21. Aortoduodenal fistula. The bile-stained, ribbed prosthesis is readily identifiable.

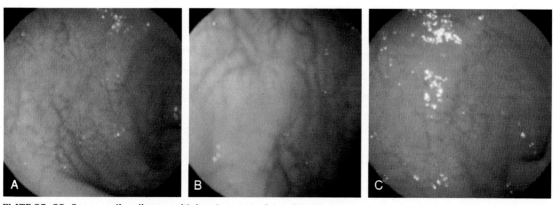

PLATE 23–22. Severe celiac disease with involvement of the distal duodenum. (Courtesy M.V. Sivak, Jr., M.D.)

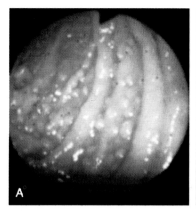
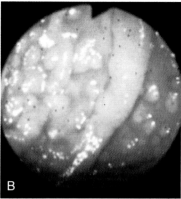

PLATE 23–23. A, Nodular lymphoid hyperplasia of duodenum in a patient with IgA deficiency. B, Close-up view of mucosal nodules. (Courtesy M.V. Sivak, Jr., M.D.)

Whipple's Disease

Duodenoscopic study of patients with untreated Whipple's disease reveals in most cases a typical pattern of thickened mucosa with discrete or confluent yellow-white granules between the folds.[146, 147] These pinhead-size projections actually represent distended villi. The mucosa was also friable[148] or had areas of petechial hemorrhage.[147] Biopsies correlated well with duodenoscopic findings, since the granular mucosa showed distended villi packed with PAS-positive macrophages, whereas the more normal appearing mucosa had slender villi and the PAS-positive macrophages were submucosal.[146, 147] After treatment, both duodenoscopic and histologic evaluation were essentially normal. A case can be made for duodenoscopic biopsy as the diagnostic method of choice, since duodenal and jejunal involvement by Whipple's disease may be patchy and the single biopsy obtained with the blind suction biopsy capsule may fail to retrieve tissue containing PAS-positive macrophages. At duodenoscopy, several biopsies of abnormal areas should result in a high percentage of positive findings.

Nodular Lymphoid Hyperplasia

Patients with acquired hypogammaglobulinemia may develop a nodular mucosal pattern of the small bowel. These nodules are the result of lymphoid hyperplasia which represents a response to deficiency or absence of IgA (Plate 23–23). Although they are seen predominantly in the jejunum or ileum, on one occasion these nodules were found endoscopically in the descending duodenum, where they appeared as 1 to 3 mm soft, polypoid excrescences covering the mucosa.[149] The biopsy specimens showed lymphoid hyperplasia, and aspirates from the duodenum revealed *Giardia lamblia*, a commonly associated infection.

Pseudomelanosis

Peculiar tiny black spots that have been seen in the duodenal mucosa in 7 patients were described in a series of papers.[150-154] It has been established by electron microscopy and electron probe x-ray analysis that these pigment granules are not melanin but iron sulfide.[154]

References

1. Frandsen PJ, Jarnum S, Malstrom J. Crohn's disease of the duodenum. Scand J Gastroenterol 1980; 15:683–8.
2. Nugent FW, Richmond M, Park SK. Crohn's disease of the duodenum. Gut 1977; 18:115–20.
3. Danzi JT, Farmer RG, Sullivan BH Jr, Rankin GB. Endoscopic features of gastroduodenal Crohn's disease. Gastroenterology 1976; 70:9–13.
4. Fitzgibbons TJ, Green G, Silberman H, et al. Management of Crohn's disease involving the duodenum, including duodenal cutaneous fistula. Arch Surg 1980; 115:1022–8.
5. Smith TR, Goldin RR. Radiographic and clinical sequelae of the duodenocolic anatomic relationship: two cases of Crohn's disease with fistulization to the duodenum. Dis Colon Rectum 1977; 20:257–62.
6. Greenberger N. Allergic disorders of the intestine and eosinophilic gastroenteritis. In: Sleisenger MH, Fordtran JS, eds. Gastrointestinal Disease: Pathophysiology, Diagnosis and Management. Philadelphia: WB Saunders, 1983:1069–76.
7. Robert F, Omura E, Durant JR. Mucosal eosinophilic gastroenteritis with systemic involvement. Am J Med 1977; 62:139–43.
8. Lev R, Thomas E, Parl FF, Pitchumoni CS. Pathological and histomorphometric study of the effects of alcohol on the human duodenum. Digestion 1980; 20:207–13.

9. Piubello W, Vantini I, Scuro LA, et al. Gastric secretion, gastroduodenal histological changes, and serum gastrin in chronic alcoholic pancreatitis. Am J Gastroenterol 1982; 77:105–10.
10. Makrauer FL, Antoniali DA, Banks PA. Duodenal stenosis in chronic pancreatitis. Clinicopathological correlation. Dig Dis Sci 1982; 27:525–32.
11. Bradley EL III, Clements JL Jr. Idiopathic duodenal obstruction: an unappreciated complication of pancreatitis. Ann Surg 1981; 193:638–48.
12. Grodsinsky G, Schuman BM, Black MA. Absence of pancreatic duct dilation in chronic pancreatitis. Arch Surg 1976; 112:444–9.
13. Black GA, Carsky EW. Duodenal tuberculosis. Am J Roentgenol 1978; 131:329–30.
14. Tandon RK, Pastakia B. Duodenal tuberculosis as seen by duodenoscopy. Am J Gastroenterol 1976; 66:483–6.
15. Tishler JM. Duodenal tuberculosis. Radiology 1979; 130:593–5.
16. Gleason T, Prinz RA, Kirsch EP, et al. Tuberculosis of the duodenum. Am J Gastroenterol 1979; 72:36–40.
17. Monroe LS. The endoscopic encounter with parasites. Gastrointest Endosc 1984; 30:113–4.
18. Brandborg LL, Owens R, Fogel R, et al. Giardiasis and traveler's diarrhea. Gastroenterology 1980; 78:1602–14.
19. Bone MF, Chesner IM, Oliver B, Asquith P. Endoscopic appearance of duodenitis due to strongyloidiasis. Gastrointest Endosc 1982; 28:190–1.
20. Peralta NR, Rodrigues MA. Strongyloides stercoralis larva in gastric and duodenal aspirates. Acta Cytol 1978; 22:61–3.
21. Winters C Jr, Chobanian SJ, Benjamin SB, et al. Endoscopic documentation of Ascaris-induced acute pancreatitis. Gastrointest Endosc 1984; 30:83–4.
22. Jager G, Voigtsberger P, Bohm S. Endoscopic removal of a tapeworm. Z Aerztl Fortbild 1978; 72:337.
23. Hauser SC, Bynum TE. Abnormalities on ERCP in a case of human fascioliasis. Gastrointest Endosc 1984; 30:80–2.
24. Reddy RR, Schuman BM, Priest RJ. Duodenal polyps: diagnosis and management. J Clin Gastroenterol 1981; 3:139–45.
25. Herbsman H, Wetstein L, Rosen Y, et al. Tumors of the small intestine. Curr Probl Surg 1980; 17:121–82.
26. Bar-Meir S, Hallack A, Baratz M. Endoscopic removal of a giant duodenal polyp. Endoscopy 1983; 15:29–30.
27. Dupas JL, Marti R, Caprou JP, Delamarre J. Villous adenoma of the duodenum. Endoscopic diagnosis and resection. Endoscopy 1977; 9:245–7.
28. Bunt TJ, Riley WJ. Villous adenoma of the duodenum. J Iowa Med Soc 1983; 73:52–4.
29. Bosseckert H. Villous tumors of the duodenum: a precancerous lesion? Praxis 1982; 71:903–6.
30. Widgren S. Does the polyp cancer sequence apply to the duodenum? Praxis 1982; 71:907–10.
31. Shead GV, Mathan M. Villoglandular adenoma of the duodenum. Aust NZ J Surg 1978; 48:193–5.
32. Cooperman M, Clausen KP, Hecht C, et al. Villous adenomas of the duodenum. Gastroenterology 1978; 74:1295–7.
33. Pollak EW, Crow J, Jacobs WH, Choctaw WT. Villous duodenal adenoma. A less aggressive approach. J Kans Med Soc 1981; 82:231–2.
34. Kutin ND, Ranson JH, Gouge TH, Localio SA. Villous tumors of the duodenum. Ann Surg 1975; 181:164–8.
35. Batra SK, Schuman BM, Reddy RR. The endoscopic variety of duodenal villous adenoma—an experience with ten cases. Endoscopy 1983; 15:89–92.
36. Delpy JC, Bruneton JN, Druillard J, Lecompte P. Non-vaterian duodenal adenomas: report of 24 cases and review of the literature. Gastrointest Radiol 1983; 8:135–41.
37. Wilson JM, Melvin DB, Gray G, Thorbjarnarson B. Benign small bowel tumors. Ann Surg 1975; 181:247–50.
38. Anderson JR, Ford MJ. Leiomyoma of the duodenum—an unusual presentation of a rare tumor. Postgrad Med J 1979; 55:218–20.
39. Morris SJ, Shifrin H, Feinberg A, Rogers AI. Duodenal leiomyoma as a cause of gastrointestinal hemorrhage. South Med J 1978; 71:470–3.
40. Farkas I, Patko A, Kovacs J, et al. The brunneroma, the adenomatous hyperplasia of the Brunner's glands. Gastroenterol Belg 1980; 43:179–86.
41. Maratka Z, Kocianova J, Kudrmann J, et al. Hyperplasia of Brunner's glands. Radiology, endoscopy, and biopsy findings in 11 cases of diffuse, nodular, and adenomatous form. Acta Hepatogastroenterol 1979; 26:64–9.
42. Maglinte DD, Mayes SL, Ng AC, Pickett RD. Brunner's gland adenoma: diagnostic considerations. J Clin Gastroenterol 1982; 4:127–31.
43. Appel MF, Bentlif PS. Endoscopic removal of bleeding Brunner gland adenoma. Arch Surg 1976; 111:301–2.
44. Barnhart GR, Maull KI. Brunner's gland adenomas: clinical presentation and surgical management. South Med J 1979; 72:1537–9.
45. Alper IA, Haubrich WS. Duodenoscopic removal of a Brunner's gland adenoma. Gastrointest Endosc 1973; 20:73.
46. Moulinier B, et al. Endoscopic removal of benign gastroduodenal tumors. Endoscopy 1975; 7:121–5.
47. Sivak MV Jr, Sullivan BH Jr, Farmer RG. Neurogenic tumors of the small intestine: review of the literature and report of a case with endoscopic removal. Gastroenterology 1975; 68:374–80.
48. Rutgeerts P, Hendricks H, Geboes K, et al. Involvement of the upper digestive tract by systemic neurofibromatosis. Gastrointest Endosc 1981; 27:22–5.
49. Sauerbruch T, Keiditsch E, Wotzka R, Kaess H. Lymphangioma of the duodenum. (Diagnosis by endoscopic resection.) Endoscopy 1977; 9:179–82.
50. Singer M, Busse R, Seib HJ, et al: Endoscopic polypectomy in the upper gastrointestinal tract. (Abstr) Endoscopy 1975; 7:216.
51. Gangl A, Polterauer P, Krepler R, Kumpan W. A further case of submucosal lymphangioma of the duodenum diagnosed during endoscopy. Endoscopy 1980; 12:188–90.
52. Laughlin EH, Keown ME, Jackson JE. Heterotopic pancreas obstructing the ampulla of Vater. Arch Surg 1983; 118:979–80.
53. Sivak MV Jr, Jagelman DG. Upper gastrointestinal endoscopy in polyposis syndromes: familial polyposis coli and Gardner's syndrome. Gastrointest Endosc 1984; 30:102–4.
54. Yao T, Ida M, Ohsato K, et al. Duodenal lesions in familial polyposis of the colon. Gastroenterology 1977; 73:1086–92.
55. Iida M, Yao T, Itoh H, et al. Endoscopic features

of adenoma of the duodenal papilla in familial polyposis of the colon. Gastrointest Endosc 1981; 27:6–8.

56. Schulman A. Gastric and small bowel polyps in Gardner's syndrome and familial polyposis coli. J Can Assoc Radiol 1976; 27:206–9.

57. Sweeney BF, Anderson DS. Endoscopic removal of duodenal polyp in a patient with Gardner's syndrome. Dig Dis Sci 1982; 27:557–60.

58. Russell DM, Bhathal PS, St. John DJ. Complete remission in Cronkhite-Canada syndrome. Gastroenterology 1983; 85:180–5.

59. Lillemoe K, Imbembo AL. Malignant neoplasms of the duodenum. Surg Gynecol Obstet 1980; 150:822–6.

60. Kerremans RP, Lerut J, Penninckx FM. Primary malignant duodenal tumors. Ann Surg 1979; 190:179–82.

61. Spira IA, Ghazi A, Wolff WI. Primary adenocarcinoma of the duodenum. Cancer 1977; 39:1721–6.

62. Blumgart LH. Duodenoscopy and endoscopic retrograde choledochopancreatography: present position in relation to periampullary and pancreatic cancer. J Surg Oncol 1975; 7:107–19.

63. Hall TJ, Blackstone MO, Cooper MJ, et al. Prospective evaluation of endoscopic retrograde cholangiopancreatography in the diagnosis of periampullary cancers. Ann Surg 1977; 187:313–7.

64. Langer B, Lipson R, McHattie JD, et al. Periampullary tumors: advances in diagnosis and surgical treatment. Can J Surg 1979; 22:34–7.

65. Satake K, Sowa M, Yamashita K, et al. Carcinoma of the duodenum: its preoperative diagnosis. Br J Surg 1975; 62:973–6.

66. Wald A, Milligan FD. The role of fiberoptic endoscopy in the diagnosis and management of duodenal neoplasms. Am J Dig Dis 1975; 20:499–505.

67. Walsh DB, Eckhauser FE, Cronewett JL, et al. Adenocarcinoma of the ampulla of Vater: diagnosis and treatment. Ann Surg 1982; 195:152–7.

68. Hauswald KR, Griffen WO. Smooth muscle tumors of the duodenum. Rev Surg 1977; 34:64–7.

69. Sato A, Hikosaka O, Koike Y, et al. Diagnostic and therapeutic considerations of myogenic tumors of the duodenum. Gastroenterol Jpn 1978; 13:65–71.

70. Wong J, Stephen MS, Ong GB, Lowenthal J. Leiomyosarcoma of the duodenum: a report of three cases. Aust NZ J Surg 1977; 47:793–8.

71. Barkan A, Wolloch Y, Dintsman M, Yeshurun D. Leiomyosarcoma of the duodenum. Two case reports and a literature review. Am J Proctol Gastroenterol Colon Rectal Surg 1981; 32:18–21, 28.

72. Yassinger S, Imperato TJ, Midgley R Jr, et al. Leiomyosarcoma of the duodenum. Gastrointest Endosc 1977; 24:38–40.

73. Helmy I. Endoscopic diagnosis of immunoproliferative small intestinal disease (IPSID). Endoscopy 1980; 12:114–6.

74. Kobler E, Buhler H, Fehr H, et al. Primary malignant lymphoma of the duodenum. Praxis 1982; 71:924–7.

75. Payson BA, Weingarten LA, Pollack J. Lymphosarcoma of the duodenum associated with carcinoma of the lung. Am J Gastroenterol 1979; 71:295–300.

76. Veen HF, Oscarson JE, Malt RA. Alien cancers of the duodenum. Surg Gynecol Obstet 1976; 143:39–42.

77. Bungay K, Dennistone S, Hunt PS. Duodenal ob-struction and carcinoma of the head of pancreas. Med J Aust 1980; 2:150–1.

78. Sharon P, Stalnikovicz R, Rachmilewitz D. Endoscopic diagnosis of duodenal neoplasms causing upper gastrointestinal bleeding. J Clin Gastroenterol 1982; 4:35–8.

79. Ashkenazi S, Sharom P, Levij IS, et al. Giant cell carcinoma of the pancreas: report of a case with upper gastrointestinal bleeding diagnosed by endoscopic brush cytology. Am J Gastroenterol 1978; 70:302–5.

80. Cronstedt JL, Kalczynski J, Jonsson NGE. Involvement of the duodenum by gastric carcinoma. Gastrointest Endosc 1982; 28:44–5.

81. Theodors A, Sivak MV Jr, Carey WD. Hypernephroma with metastasis to the duodenum: endoscopic features. Gastrointest Endosc 1980; 26:48–50.

82. Sivak MV Jr, Sullivan BH Jr. Endoscopic diagnosis of malignant melanoma metastatic to the duodenum. Gastrointest Endosc 1975; 22:36–8.

83. Coughlin GP, Bourne AJ, Grant AK. Endoscopic diagnosis of metastatic disease of the stomach and duodenum. Aust NZ J Med 1977; 7:52–5.

84. Lammli J, Buhler H, Bosseckert H, et al. Metastasen im duodenum. Praxis 1982; 71:1054–7.

85. Mannell A. Primary isolated extramedullary plasmacytoma of the duodenum. Aust NZ J Surg 1979; 49:577–80.

86. Ahmed N, Nelson RS, Goldstein HM, Sinkovics JG. Kaposi's sarcoma of the stomach and duodenum: endoscopic and roentgenologic correlations. Gastrointest Endosc 1975; 21:149–52.

87. Donovan DC, Dureza R, Jain U. Gastrinoma of duodenum. Diagnosis by endoscopy. NY State J Med 1979; 79:1766–8.

88. Woodtli W, Gemsenjager E, Heitz PU, et al. Endokrine Tumoren (APU Dome) des Duodenum—Eine kooperative Studie. Praxis 1982; 71:1045–53.

89. Hofmann JW, Fax PS, Wilson SD. Duodenal wall tumors and the Zollinger-Ellison syndrome. Surgical management. Arch Surg 1973; 107:334–9.

90. Wu WC, Kengis J, Whalen GE, et al. Endoscopic localization of a wall tumor in Zollinger-Ellison syndrome. Gastroenterology 1974; 66:1237–9.

91. Otten MH, Berkenhager JC, van Blankenstein M. Zollinger-Ellison syndrome treated by endoscopic removal of a duodenal gastrinoma. Neth J Med 1978; 21:248–51.

92. Wiest JW, Follette DM, Traverso LW. Toothpick perforation of the duodenum. West J Med 1980; 132:157–9.

93. Honaas TO, Shaffer EA. Endoscopic removal of a foreign body perforating the duodenum. Can Med Assoc J 1977; 116:164–9.

94. Schwartz JT, Graham DY. Toothpick perforation of the intestines. Ann Surg 1977; 185:64–6.

95. Thompson MH. Endoscopic removal of a duodenal foreign body. Br Med J 1975; 4:502–3.

96. Anderson FH. Removal of a safety pin from the duodenum with the fiberoptic endoscope. Am J Gastroenterol 1974; 61:301–3.

97. Kerlin P, Paull A. Removal of duodenal foreign body with endoscopic snare. Med J Aust 1978; 2:276–7.

98. Madura MJ, Naughton BJ, Craig RM. Duodenal bezoar: a case report and review of the literature. Gastrointest Endosc 1982; 28:26–8.

99. Suarez LA, Bolden EI. Congenital duodenal web in an adult. Curr Surg 1978; 35:366–9.

100. Turnbull A, Kussin S, Baines M. Radiographic and endoscopic features of a congenital duodenal diaphragm in an adult: a case report and review of the literature. Gastrointest Endosc 1980; 26:46–8.

101. Leinkram C, Roberts-Thomson IC, Kume GA. Juxtapapillary duodenal diverticula. Association with gallstones and pancreatitis. Med J Aust 1980; 1:209–10.

102. van der Spuy S. The relationship between juxtapapillary diverticula and biliary calculi. An endoscopic study. Endoscopy 1979; 11:197–202.

103. Cox CL. Perforated duodenal diverticulitis. South Med J 1980; 73:830.

104. Griffin M, Carey WD, Hermann R, Buonocore E. Recurrent acute pancreatitis and intussusception complicating an intraluminal duodenal diverticulum. Gastroenterology 1981; 81:345–8.

105. Wobser EC, Koischwitz D, Katz K, et al. Radiographical and endoscopical studies on two cases of intraluminal diverticulum of the duodenum. Endoscopy 1977; 8:101–5.

106. Karlsen S, Rosseland AR, Pytte R, Wilhelmsen T. Intraluminal duodenal diverticulum. Report of a case diagnosed by endoscopy. Endoscopy 1979; 11:267–71.

107. Karoll MP, Ghahremani GG, Port RB, Rosenberg JL. Diagnosis and management of intraluminal duodenal diverticulum. Dig Dis Sci 1983; 28:411–6.

108. Hajiro K, Yamamoto H, Matsui H, Yamamoto T. Endoscopic diagnosis and excision of intraluminal duodenal diverticulum. Gastrointest Endosc 1979; 25:151–4.

109. Halko M, Lo Presti PA, Ratel HD, et al. Congenital duodenal stenosis. Am J Gastroenterol 1978; 69:323–7.

110. Aagaard J, Burcharth F. Bleeding duodenal varices demonstrated by transhepatic portography: report of a case misinterpreted as bleeding duodenal ulcer. Acta Chir Scand 1980; 146:77–8.

111. Rappazzo JA, Kozarek RA, Altman M. Duodenal varices: endoscopic diagnosis of an unusual source of upper gastrointestinal hemorrhage. Gastrointest Endosc 1981; 27:227–8.

112. Kunert H, Ottenjann R. Endoscopy in bleeding duodenal varices: a rare cause of massive upper GI hemorrhage. Endoscopy 1977; 8:99–101.

113. Itzchak Y, Glickman MG. Duodenal varices in extrahepatic portal obstruction. Radiology 1977; 124:619–24.

114. Schoettle GP Jr, Davis WD Jr, Bowen JC. Duodenal varices: a rare cause of upper gastrointestinal hemorrhage. J La State Med Soc 1978; 130:7–10.

115. Richardson JD, McInnis WD, Pestana C. Duodenal varices. Am Surg 1976; 42:201–3.

116. Sauerbruch T, Weinzierl M, Dietrich HP, et al. Sclerotherapy of a bleeding duodenal varix. Endoscopy 1982; 14:187–9.

117. Ikeda K, Murayama H, Takano H, et al. Massive intestinal bleeding in hemangiomatosis of the duodenum. Endoscopy 1980; 12:306–10.

118. Sutton D, Murfitt J, Howarth F. Gastrointestinal bleeding from large angiomas. Clin Radiol 1981; 32:629–32.

119. Loison F, Patri B. Intramural hematoma of the duodenum with anticoagulants—role of endoscopy. Acta Endosc 1983; 13:225–7.

120. van Spreeuwel JP, van Garp LH, Bast TJ, Nadorp JH. Intramural hematoma of the duodenum in a patient with chronic pancreatitis. Endoscopy 1981; 13:246–8.

121. Patel R, Shaps J. Intramural duodenal hematoma—a complication of ERCP.. (letter) Gastrointest Endosc 1982; 28:218–9.

122. Freed JS, Roe G, Szuchmacher PH. Intramural duodenal hematoma mimicking carcinoma of the head of the pancreas. Mt Sinai J Med 1979; 46:564–7.

123. Ramanujam P, Shabeeb N, Silver JM. Unusual manifestations of gallstone migration into the gastrointestinal tract. South Med J 1983; 76:30–2.

124. Thorpe JA. Gallstone ileus. JR Coll Surg Edinb 1979; 24:299–300.

125. Argyropoulos GD, Velmachos G, Axenidis G. Gallstone perforation and obstruction of the duodenal bulb. Arch Surg 1979; 114:333–5.

126. Welch JP, Warshaw AL. Malignant duodenocolic fistulas. Am J Surg 1977; 133:658–61.

127. Ergin MA, Alfonso A, Auda SP, Waxman M. Primary carcinoma of the duodenum producing a malignant duodenocolic fistula. Dis Colon Rectum 1978; 21:408–12.

128. Gregson R, Craig O. Aorto-enteric fistulae: the role of radiology. Clin Radiol 1983; 34:65–72.

129. Steffes BC, O'Leary JP. Primary aortoduodenal fistulae: a case report and review of the literature. Am Surg 1980; 46:121–9.

130. Baker MS, Fisher JH, van der Reis L, et al. The endoscopic diagnosis of an aortoduodenal fistula. Arch Surg 1976; 111:304.

131. Perdue GD Jr, Smith RB III, Ansley JD, Constantino MJ. Impending aortoenteric hemorrhage: the effect of early recognition on improved outcome. Ann Surg 1980; 192:237–43.

132. Hill SL, Knott LH, Alexander RH. Recurrent aortoduodenal fistula: a lesson in management. Am Surgeon 1982; 48:137–40.

133. Champion MC, Sullivan SN, Watson WC. Aortoduodenal fistula: endoscopic diagnosis. Dig Dis Sci 1980; 25:811–2.

134. Brady PG. Aortoduodenal fistula. Role of endoscopy in diagnosis. Am J Gastroenterol 1978; 69:705–7.

135. Ott DJ, Kerr RM, Gelfand DW. Aortoduodenal fistula: an unusual endoscopic and radiographic appearance simulating leiomyoma. Gastrointest Endosc 1978; 24:296–8.

136. Brand EJ, Sivak MV Jr, Sullivan BH Jr. Aortoduodenal fistula: endoscopic diagnosis. Dig Dis Sci 1979; 24:940–4.

137. Puppala AR, Munasivamy M, Doshi AM, Steinheber FU. Endoscopic diagnosis of aortoduodenal fistula: complication of abdominal aortic by-pass grafts. Am J Gastroenterol 1980; 73:414–7.

138. Martin J, Cano N, Di-Costanzo J, Richiari JP. Aortoduodenal fistula: endoscopic diagnosis. Dig Dis Sci 1981; 26:956–7.

139. Banai J, Salfay G, Szeleczky M, Kun M. An uncommon endoscopic finding: bleeding secondary aortoenteric fistula. Endoscopy 1982; 14:185–6.

140. Baker HB, Baker MS, van der Reis L, Fisher JH. Endoscopy in the diagnosis of aortoduodenal fistula. Gastrointest Endosc 1977; 24:35–7.

141. Wexler RM, Falchuk KR, Horst DA, et al. Duodenal erosion of a mesocaval graft: an unusual complication of mesocaval shunt interposition surgery. Gastroenterology 1980; 79:729–30.

142. Stevens FM, McCarthy CF. The endoscopic dem-

onstration of coeliac disease. Endoscopy 1977; 8:177–80.

143. Gillberg R, Ahren C. Coeliac disease diagnosed by means of duodenoscopy and endoscopic duodenal biopsy. Scand J Gastroenterol 1977; 12:911–16.

144. Holdstock G, Eade OE, Isaacson P, Smith CL. Endoscopic duodenal biopsies in coeliac disease and duodenitis. Scand J Gastroenterol 1979; 14:717–20.

145. Scott BB, Losowsky MS. Patchiness and duodenal-jejunal variation of the mucosal abnormality in coeliac disease and dermatitis herpetiformis. Gut 1976; 17:984–92.

146. Volpicelli NA, Salyer WR, Milligan FD, et al. The endoscopic appearance of the duodenum in Whipple's disease. Johns Hopkins Med J 1976; 138:19–23.

147. Riemann JF, Rosch W. Synopsis of endoscopic and related morphological findings in Whipple's disease. Endoscopy 1978; 7:98–103.

148. Crane S, Schlippert W. Duodenoscopic findings in Whipple's disease. Gastrointest Endosc 1978; 24:248–9.

149. Feller ER, Weiser MM, Schapiro RH. Endoscopic visualization of nodular lymphoid hyperplasia. Gastrointest Endosc 1977; 24:37–8.

150. Bisordi WM, Kleinman MS. Melanosis duodeni. Gastrointest Endosc 1976; 23:37–8.

151. Breslaw L. Melanosis of the duodenal mucosa. Gastrointest Endosc 1980; 26:45–6.

152. Cowen ML, Humphries TJ. Pseudomelanosis of the duodenum. Endoscopic and histologic observations on a unique case of pigmentation in the duodenum. Gastrointest Endosc 1980; 26:107.

153. Ganju S, Adomavicius J, Salgia K, Steigman F. The endoscopic picture of melanosis in the duodenum. Gastrointest Endosc 1980; 26:44–5.

154. Yamase H, Norris M, Gillies C, et al. Pseudomelanosis duodeni: a clinicopathologic entity. Gastrointest Endosc 1985; 31:83–6.

Chapter 24

ENDOSCOPY IN THE POSTOPERATIVE UPPER GASTROINTESTINAL TRACT

MELODY J. O'CONNOR, M.D.
JOHN I. ALLEN, M.D.
JACK A. VENNES, M.D.

During 1983 11% of the patients who underwent endoscopy at the University of Minnesota had had gastrointestinal surgery. This percentage is similar to that in other major endoscopy centers[1] and emphasizes that endoscopists must understand not only normal anatomy but also the consequences of abdominal surgery and the pathologic lesions that may occur after surgery.

This chapter addresses the subject of endoscopy in patients who have undergone operations on the esophagus, stomach, duodenum, biliary tree, pancreas, and abdominal aorta. Basic surgical principles and the anatomic and physiologic consequences of commonly performed abdominal operations are described. Operative procedures are reviewed briefly, with exclusion of finer details. There are many variations in surgical approach, technique, and materials used; thus cooperation between the operating surgeon and endoscopist is essential.

INTRAOPERATIVE ENDOSCOPY

Upper gastrointestinal endoscopy is rarely required during surgery. The most frequent indication is bleeding that occurs distal to the ligament of Treitz.[2] Potential lesions include ulcers, tumors (leiomyoma and leiomyosarcoma), vascular malformations, and aortoduodenal fistulas in patients with abdominal aortic grafts.[3] Intraoperative endoscopy may identify small tumors, vascular abnormalities, and bleeding sites.

The entire small intestine may be visualized at operation with a 135 cm pediatric colonoscope. With the abdomen open, the small bowel can be gently and sequentially pleated, accordion-fashion, over the endoscope; this requires cooperation between the endoscopist and surgeon. The smooth muscle atony induced by anesthesia makes it difficult to advance the instrument, since the elastic bowel suspended on its mesentery tends to form a loop rather than permit advancement of the instrument tip. This is first noted along the greater curvature of the stomach. The surgeon may apply pressure to the greater curvature to aid advancement into the duodenum, and a relatively straight axis from esophagus to duodenum can also be maintained by periodic attention to this area. The tendency for the instrument to form a loop will also be noted in the jejunum. The best technique, therefore, is to allow the surgeon to present a short segment of bowel for endoscopic examination by holding a length of about 10 cm before the endoscope tip in as straight a configuration relative to the instrument tip as possible. After the endoscopist examines this section the surgeon gently pulls it over the insertion tube while the endoscopist advances the instrument a few centimeters.

During these maneuvers the bowel wall will be transilluminated by the endoscopic light. This makes small vascular lesions readily detectable by the surgeon (Plate 24–1). Since there is always a possibility that multiple lesions may be present, the location of each should be marked by a suture as it is encoun-

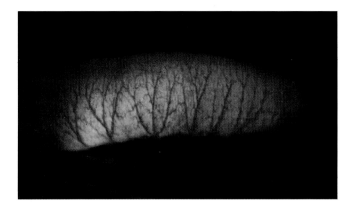

PLATE 24—1. Normal transilluminated bowel. Intraoperative endoscopy is performed to locate bleeding lesions of intestine beyond ligament of Treitz. The operating suite has been darkened and the bowel is transilluminated by the endoscope. Vascular lesions are readily demonstrated with this technique.

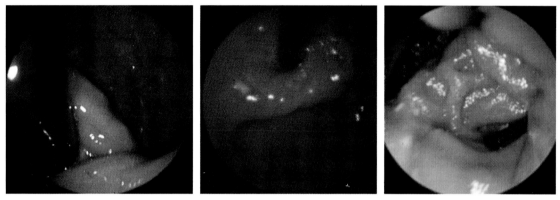

PLATE 24—2.   PLATE 24—3.   PLATE 24—4.

PLATE 24—2. Retroverted close-up view of 360 degree wrap of Nissen fundoplication. Note that the wrap spirals in a clockwise and posterior manner around endoscope.

PLATE 24—3. Retroflexed view of Nissen wrap from a distance. Fundus of stomach is in background.

PLATE 24—4. Esophagojejunostomy. Endoscope is positioned in distal esophagus looking into Roux-en-Y limb. Note dominant efferent limb which courses in straight caudad direction (left limb) and short blind limb of jejunum to right. This view is typical of an of esophageal-jejunal anastomosis (end to side respectively) of Roux-en-Y reconstruction (for both esophagojejunostomy and gastrojejunostomy) and should not be mistaken for a loop jejunostomy.

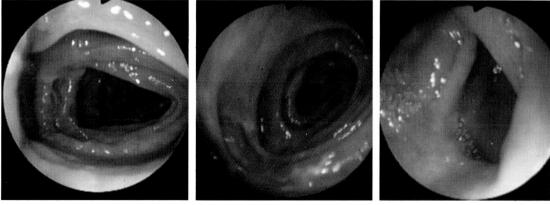

PLATE 24—5.   PLATE 24—6.   PLATE 24—7.

PLATE 24—5. Esophageal resection with colonic interposition. Endoscopic view from proximal anastomosis into lumen of interposed colonic segment.

PLATE 24—6. Esophageal resection with colonic interposition. Note transverse folds of interposed colonic segment and in the distance, distal colon anastomosis.

PLATE 24—7. Normal-appearing pyloroplasty with triangular, widely patent pylorus. Suture line of Heineke-Mickulicz incision is seen on anterior wall of pyloric channel left upper edge of photograph).

tered. As the instrument advances through the intestine, a certain amount of trauma will result to the mucosa. Small hemorrhages will often be noted on withdrawal, and these may be confused with small vascular lesions, especially as the former appear to the surgeon when transilluminated as dark areas. Therefore the endoscopic examination should be conducted as the instrument is being advanced, not during withdrawal.

Excessive air insufflation should be avoided, since this results in troublesome distention of the bowel. If the examination has been completed during insertion, much of the insufflated air can be aspirated on withdrawal. Prolonged postoperative ileus may occur as a result of intraoperative endoscopy. This can be avoided by close attention to detail and gentleness during the examination phase of the procedure, in addition to restricting air insufflation to the minimum necessary for proper examination.

POSTSURGICAL ENDOSCOPY OF THE ESOPHAGUS

This section summarizes the endoscopic techniques that ensure complete and accurate examination in patients who have undergone esophageal surgery. Three topics will be discussed: (1) antireflux procedures, (2) esophageal resection, and (3) esophageal replacement.

Antireflux Procedures

Surgical Techniques and Normal Endoscopic Appearance

Currently used antireflux operations include the Nissen fundoplication,[4-6] Belsey Mark IV repair,[7, 8] Hill repair,[9, 10] Collis repair,[11, 12] and placement of the Angelchik prosthesis.[13, 14]

The Nissen fundoplication, by far the most commonly used antireflux procedure, is performed by wrapping the gastric fundus 360 degrees around the distal esophagus (Figs. 24–1 and 24–2). This creates an intra-abdominal esophageal segment and a "flap-valve" mechanism at the gastroesophageal junction. The wrap is created with a 40 French (13 mm diameter) dilator in the esophagus to ensure a lumen diameter of at least 13 mm. The gastric fundus is sutured to the anterior serosal surface of the esophagus to prevent cephalad slippage of the stomach beneath the wrap. The Belsey Mark IV repair differs from the Nissen procedure in that the fundic wrap extends only 270 degrees around the distal esophagus, and the procedure is performed via a thoracotomy incision. Data from manometric studies suggest that both a mechanical and functional lower esophageal sphincter result with the Nissen and Belsey repairs.[15-19] Not only are resting lower esophageal sphincter pressures increased above preoperative levels, but there is appropriate elevation of sphincter pressure in response to cholinergic or pentagastrin stimulation.

The Hill and Collis repairs are rarely used and have a higher failure rate than the techniques described in the previous paragraph.[10, 12] Both anchor the cardia of the stomach posteriorly to the preaortic fascia and involve closure of the esophageal hiatus. The Angelchik prosthesis is a doughnut-shaped device designed to create an artificial sphincter mechanism at the distal esophagus. Experience with this device is limited, but early reports of dislodgement or disruption

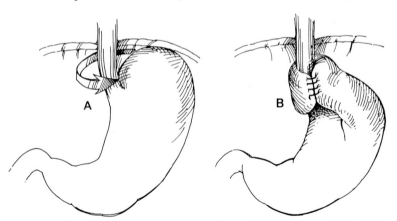

FIGURE 24–1. Nissen fundoplication, with 360-degree wrap of gastric fundus around intra-abdominal esophagus. Sutures fix wrap to anterior surface of esophagus to prevent intussusception of stomach underneath wrap ("slipped Nissen").

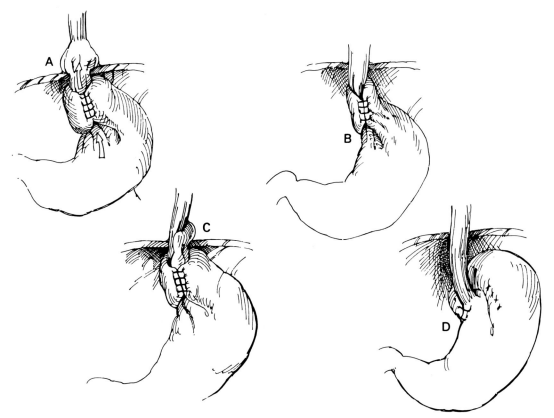

FIGURE 24–2. Complications of Nissen fundoplication. *A,* "Slipped Nissen"; *B,* tight wrap; *C,* paraesophageal hernia through wrap; *D,* disrupted Nissen fundoplication.

of the prosthesis suggest a high failure rate.[20–22]

Intact Nissen and Belsey repairs appear similar endoscopically. The esophageal mucosa should be normal, and the distal esophagus must be carefully examined for residual Barrett's epithelium. The gastroesophageal junction is narrowed and the normal angulation between the distal esophagus and the stomach lumen is lost. Normally there is no protrusion of gastric mucosa into the distal esophagus. The endoscope may be gently advanced through the lower sphincter, and the position of the sphincter at rest and its approximate diameter and length should be estimated.

A retroverted view of a Nissen (Plates 24–2 and 24–3) repair shows a thickened fold of stomach wall adjacent to the lumen of the fundus that spirals clockwise and posteriorly around the distal esophagus. The wrap should not be patulous around the endoscope. Redundant folds of mucosa should be flattened by air insufflation and carefully examined for paraesophageal herniation. Other than diminished gastric volume, the appearance of the stomach and duodenum is not altered.

Endoscopic Findings in Symptomatic Patients

Postoperative conditions that require prompt endoscopic evaluation include recurrence or persistence of reflux symptoms, dysphagia and odynophagia, "gas-bloat" syndrome, epigastric pain, and Barrett's esophagus. The overall success rate of antireflux operations is 85% to 90%[5, 6, 8] In studies reported in older literature, return of reflux symptoms was used to define recurrence; now manometry, pH monitoring, barium contrast studies, and radioisotope procedures more accurately define both recurrence and breakdown of the surgical repair.[8, 10, 15–18, 23]

Recurrence of reflux symptoms may result from a technically inadequate "loose" wrap or from postoperative disruption of the wrap (see Fig. 24–2D).[24–28] Endoscopically, a wide-open lumen at the gastroesophageal mucosal junction and mucosal changes consistent with reflux esophagitis suggest a disrupted wrap. A loose wrap may initially appear relatively intact but may be patulous when viewed by retroversion. Symptom relief in the early postoperative period followed by recurrence of similar complaints suggests an initially successful repair that has become disrupted. When there are recurrent symptoms of reflux, endoscopy is the appropriate procedure for diagnosis and may be followed by a trial of medical therapy, although reoperation may be necessary if symptoms are severe.

Dysphagia and odynophagia occur in patients with (1) an intact antireflux procedure plus an unrecognized motility disorder; (2) a "tight" Nissen; (3) persistent stricture; or (4) a "slipped" Nissen. Proper evaluation includes barium swallow under fluoroscopy, esophageal manometric studies and, when indicated, endoscopy.[24–28]

A motor disorder of the esophagus may coexist with significant reflux esophagitis and remain clinically silent. Dysmotility should be discovered before fundoplication. If dysphagia appears postoperatively, esophageal manometry is indicated, although barium swallow with fluoroscopy or cine esophagography are alternative or supplemental studies for the diagnosis of a motility disorder. Intractable symptoms may require take-down of the fundoplication, with further treatment being determined by the primary disorder.

A tight Nissen (see Fig. 24–2B) or a persistent stricture appear as a narrowing at the gastroesophageal junction with or without evidence of esophagitis and scarring. The occurrence of a tight Nissen is minimized by constructing the fundoplication around a dilator, limiting the length of the wrap to less than 4 cm, and avoiding an excessively tight closure of the diaphragmatic crura around the esophagus. Healing of a postoperative anastomotic leak can result in scarring around the distal esophagus, with resultant esophageal stricturing. Treatment for a tight Nissen or stricture begins with careful dilation under fluoroscopic guidance. Dilators larger than 13 mm (40 French) should not be used; otherwise the wrap may be disrupted. Persistent dysphagia may require resection and reconstruction of the esophagus by colonic interposition.

A slipped Nissen (see Fig. 24–2A) results from intussusception of the stomach body through the fundic wrap. This produces an "hourglass" deformity on barium swallow. Slippage occurs when the wrap is not adequately fixed to the esophagus during operation. Endoscopic examination reveals that the gastroesophageal junction is above the level of the diaphragm and the fundic wrap. Operative repair is necessary and dilation is not a therapeutic option.

The "gas-bloat" syndrome (postfundoplication syndrome) consists of early satiety, abdominal bloating, and weight loss and occurs in 10% to 40% of patients after a Nissen fundoplication.[24, 26, 27, 29] Usually it is a transient occurrence of uncertain etiology that resolves spontaneously. It may be caused by a tight fundic wrap or by gastric hypomobility resulting from intraoperative vagal nerve damage. The presence of a tight wrap or persistent stricture are recognizable endoscopically, and patients may respond dramatically to gentle dilation. Only 2% of patients with this syndrome have intractable symptoms requiring reoperation.[26, 29]

Epigastric pain after fundoplication may result from gastric ulcers[30] or a paraesophageal hernia[31] (see Fig. 24–2C). Ulceration may occur anywhere in the stomach. Initial therapy should be medical, but if ulceration is related to gastric stasis as a result of inadvertent vagotomy during fundoplication, a pyloroplasty may be required. Herniation of gastric fundus through an intact wrap occurs rarely after fundoplication and is diagnosed by barium swallow (Fig. 24–3) and endoscopy. The potential for strangulation necrosis of the incarcerated segment usually necessitates revision of the fundoplication.

Approximately 10% of patients with reflux esophagitis have Barrett's esophagus. The incidence of adenocarcinoma of the distal esophagus is higher in patients with Barrett's epithelium (8% to 26%) than in those with esophageal reflux but with otherwise normal distal esophageal mucosa.[32–36] This condition, which should be diagnosed endoscopically before fundoplication, is discussed in Chapters 17 and 18.

Whether antireflux surgery induces regression of Barrett's epithelium or whether surgery decreases the risk of cancer is not known.[32] Regression and even disappearance of the columnar lining of the distal esophagus after antireflux procedures have been reported.[37] Reports of adenocarcinoma of the distal esophagus after Nissen procedures suggest that the risk of cancer within Barrett's epithelium is not abolished by fundoplication.[38] Since both adenocarcinoma of the esophagus and Barrett's epithelium are relatively rare, clinical data on cancer risk and appropriate follow-up are insufficient and do

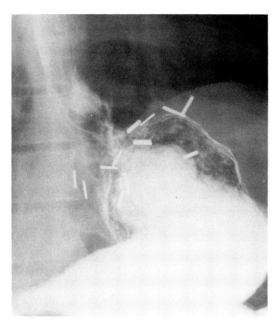

FIGURE 24–3. Paraesophageal hernia through Nissen fundoplication. Barium contrast study demonstrates intact Nissen fundoplication through which anterior gastric wall has herniated (underneath the Nissen wrap). Note diminished luminal diameter of distal esophagus. Metallic clips mark area of the wrap.

not permit firm conclusions. Current recommendations of the American Society for Gastrointestinal Endoscopy (ASGE) call for yearly endoscopic examination, with multiple biopsies and brushing for cytologic examination, in patients with Barrett's epithelium. This approach should also apply to patients who have undergone antireflux procedures. There is no established method of management in cases in which Barrett's epithelium has regressed or disappeared. The permanence or completeness of such apparently favorable changes is difficult to establish, and it is not certain that these therapeutic responses reduce the risk of cancer. Since more data on the course of treated Barrett's epithelium are needed, it would be prudent at this time to continue endoscopic surveillance regardless of apparent clinical and endoscopic responses.

Esophageal Resection

General Considerations

Esophageal resection is performed for carcinoma of the esophagus, gastroesophageal junction, or proximal stomach and for intractable strictures of the esophagus resulting from caustic substance ingestion or rarely severe reflux esophagitis. The type of disease (malignant vs. benign) and its location determine the extent of esophageal resection. The tendency for esophageal cancer to spread rapidly to lymphatics or adjacent vital structures (e.g., aorta and trachea) limits the number of patients in whom curative resection is possible.[39, 40]

If curative resection is undertaken, proximal margins of 10 cm are required to ensure removal of tumor, because of the tendency for submucosal spread (see Chapter 17). Palliative resection or bypass operation for extensive carcinoma of the esophagus may be indicated. The extent of esophagus resected dictates the method for restoration of gastrointestinal continuity: either primary reconstruction (esophagogastrostomy or esophagojejunostomy) or esophageal replacement. Esophageal resection, which frequently requires both abdominal and thoracic incisions, has significant morbidity and mortality. Early anastomotic leakage with sepsis and respiratory complications account for operative mortality (30 days) of 10% to 20%.[40] High early morbidity and a 5-year survival rate of 10% to 15% indicate that surgical therapy of esophageal cancer should be attempted only after careful preoperative evaluation.[41, 42]

Esophagogastrostomy

Esophagogastrostomy is the most commonly used method of reconstruction after resection of the middle or distal third of the esophagus for cancer (Fig. 24–4).[43, 44] The anastomosis may be hand-sewn or made with a stapling device. Resection with esophagogastrostomy is not performed for benign strictures because of severe postoperative reflux. Since resection of the distal esophagus includes resection of the vagi, concomitant pyloroplasty or pylorotomy is often performed.

There are few indications for endoscopy in the early postoperative period. When anastomotic leakage is suspected (pain, fever, leukocytosis, prolonged ileus, and pleural effusion) endoscopy is contraindicated until this diagnosis is eliminated radiographically.[45]

Late complications manifesting as pain or dysphagia after esophageal resection include alkaline reflux esophagitis, anastomotic stricture, and recurrence of carcinoma.[46–49] Alkaline or bile reflux results from the loss, inherent in the surgery, of normal esopha-

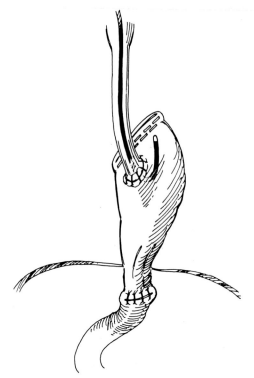

FIGURE 24–4. Proximal gastrectomy and esophago-gastrostomy. Resection of the proximal stomach and gastroesophageal junction included resection of the vagi; therefore, pyloroplasty is necessary to prevent gastric stasis. Position of the esophagogastric anastomosis is on anterior wall of the stomach, with small gastric pouch extending superiorly toward staple line.

geal and pyloric sphincters. Diagnosis is best confirmed by endoscopic examination, with biopsies when appropriate. Alkaline reflux esophagitis has the endoscopic appearance of bile-stained, edematous, friable mucosa, often with ulceration and localized hemorrhage in both the esophagus and gastric remnant. Medical therapy may be inadequate, and severely symptomatic patients may require complete gastrectomy and conversion to a Roux-Y esophagojejunostomy for diversion of duodenal secretions from the esophagus.[50, 51] Alkaline reflux esophagitis is discussed in Chapter 18.

Benign anastomotic strictures occur in 5% to 10% of patients with an esophagogastrostomy.[46–49] Most anastomotic strictures respond to pneumatic dilation with flexible Grundzig-type balloon-tipped catheters.[52] Endoscopic incision of densely fibrotic strictures that fail to respond to attempts at dilation by established methods has been reported, but experience with this technique is limited.[53, 54] When cancer recurs at the suture line, widespread recurrence or metastatic disease is probable. Endoscopic dilation may be palliative in some patients.[52] Recurrent anastomotic carcinoma frequently responds to laser therapy, as discussed in Chapter 9.

Esophagojejunostomy

Esophagojejunostomy is performed after total gastrectomy for cancer[55, 56] or for the Zollinger-Ellison syndrome (Fig. 24–5).[57] Free reflux of duodenal contents through the esophagojejunostomy into the distal esophagus may cause severe esophagitis and late development of a stricture.[58] Patients with symptoms that suggest bile reflux esophagitis should undergo endoscopy with biopsy to confirm the diagnosis and eliminate the diagnosis of cancer. If a loop esophagojejunostomy (Fig. 24–5A) is performed, a concomitant jejunojejunostomy is placed proximal to the esophagojejunostomy to allow duodenal juices to "bypass" the anastomosis. If a Roux-Y reconstruction (Fig. 24–5B) is performed, alkaline juices are diverted into the jejunum 40 cm distal to the anastomosis to minimize reflux esophagitis. Note that a Roux-Y jejunal limb is anastomosed to the distal esophagus in an end-to-side manner. This creates an efferent limb that courses directly in a caudal direction from the anastomosis plus a short afferent segment that ends blindly in an oversewn end (Plate 24–4). Knowledge of the surgical anatomy is critical to avoid mistaking the Roux-Y limb for a loop esophagojejunostomy, which in turn can lead to forceable attempts to intubate the blind limb.

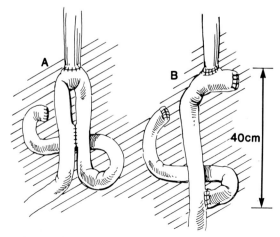

FIGURE 24–5. Total gastrectomy with esophagojejunostomy. A, Gastrectomy with loop esophagojejunostomy plus distal jejunojejunostomy. B, Gastrectomy with Roux-Y esophagojejunostomy; this variation emphasizes need to know surgical anatomy prior to endoscopy.

Esophageal Replacement

Resection of all or most of the esophagus for carcinoma or long corrosive strictures necessitates esophageal replacement. Skin tubes and jejunal grafts have been used for this purpose, but colonic interposition is preferred (Fig. 24–6).[59–61] The interposed segment may be intrathoracic, that is, in the position of the normal esophagus, substernal or subcutaneous.[62]

The normal endoscopic appearance of the interposed segment is similar to normal colon seen colonoscopically. The proximal anastomosis is easily traversed (Plate 24–5), whereupon a long, sometimes convoluted segment of colon is seen. The triangular configuration of the haustral folds of the transverse colon are usually apparent (Plate 24–6). The distal anastomosis may be widely patent and free reflux may be noted.

Stricture at the proximal anastomosis, the most frequent late occurring complication of colon interposition, is generally attributed to anastomotic leakage early in the postoperative course. Periodic pneumatic dilation with flexible Grundzig-type balloon catheters is effective therapy and reoperation is seldom

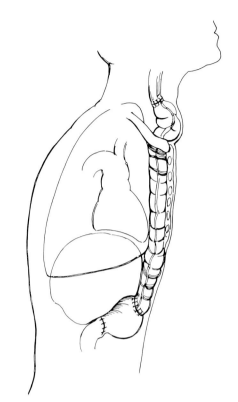

FIGURE 24–7. Colonic interposition. Protrusion of proximal segment of colon over clavicle produces mechanical obstruction and dysphagia.

required. A late developing stricture of the distal portion of the colonic segment due to reflux of gastric contents rarely occurs and must be evaluated endoscopically to exclude the possibility of recurrent tumor.

Redundancy of the colonic segment in its proximal portion may result in a mechanical obstruction to swallowing at the point where the colon passes underneath the clavicle (Fig. 24–7). Manual manipulation of the subcutaneous portion of the colon may facilitate passage of food under the bony prominence. This complication may not respond to dilation and resection of a small portion of interposed colon and reanastomosis to distal esophagus may be necessary.

POSTSURGICAL ENDOSCOPY OF THE STOMACH

Peptic Ulcer Surgery

General Considerations

Accurate endoscopic examination of patients after ulcer surgery requires knowledge of the procedures performed and the postsurgical anatomy. Surgical treatment for pep-

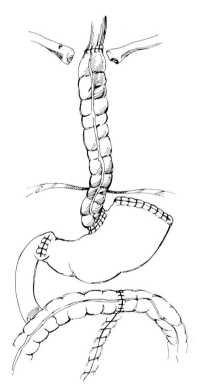

FIGURE 24–6. Esophageal resection. Esophagectomy, proximal gastrectomy, and reconstruction with colonic interposition.

tic ulcer disease is based on elimination of cholinergic and hormonal stimuli of acid secretion and reduction of parietal cell mass. Based on these principles, ulcer surgery involves truncal vagotomy with a drainage procedure or vagotomy with gastric resection.[63, 64] Highly selective vagotomy, an alternative to truncal vagotomy, eliminates vagal stimulation in the parietal cell mass, but maintains innervation of the antral pump mechanism. For this reason, drainage procedures are not necessary with highly selective therapy.

Ulcer surgery causes major alterations in gastric function, which usually result in no more than mild, transient symptoms. Therefore, postoperative complaints may be expected, such as mild diarrhea in the early postoperative period. The patient's complaints may also be due to a problem unrelated to the ulcer surgery—for example, unchanged chronic pain—or postoperative symptoms may indicate a pathologic process such as postgastrectomy obstruction or ulceration.[65] Clinical evaluation includes precise documentation of symptoms, careful physical examination, appropriate laboratory tests, and consideration of endoscopy. Although radiographic examination is occasionally helpful in certain situations, the accuracy of barium contrast studies is limited by the surgically altered anatomy and the rapid emptying of the stomach.[1, 66–70] False positive and false negative roentgenographic results are most common with respect to mucosal abnormalities. For these reasons endoscopy has become the primary diagnostic procedure to evaluate most complications after ulcer surgery.[1, 70–75]

Surgical Techniques and Normal Endoscopic Appearance

Close attention should be given to the specific notation of the following points during endoscopy in any patient who has undergone ulcer surgery: type of anastomosis (Billroth I or II); size of the gastric pouch; position and diameter of the gastrointestinal stoma; estimated quantity of bile refluxed into the gastric pouch and esophagus; degree and anatomic distribution of any inflammation; presence of retained food or secretions; any abnormal mucosal appearance suggesting intestinal metaplasia, cancer, or ulceration; intraluminal sutures or staples; and the presence or absence of antral motility.

Pyloroplasty and Gastroenterostomy

The drainage procedures used in patients who undergo truncal vagotomy without resection include pyloroplasty and gastroenterostomy. The Heineke-Mickulicz pyloroplasty[76, 77] (Fig. 24–8) involves a longitudinal incision through the muscular pylorus with approximation of the two ends of the surgical incision to form a suture line that is perpendicular to the original incision. This procedure disrupts the continuity of the pyloric sphincter mechanism and widens the gastric outlet. Gastroenterostomy drainage (Fig. 24–9) is accomplished by anastomosing proximal jejunum to the antrum or body in a dependent area along the greater curvature.

After pyloroplasty the appearance of the stomach is normal, with an identifiable antrum and a widely patent, somewhat distorted pylorus (Plate 24–7). Patients with active ulcer disease at the time of operation

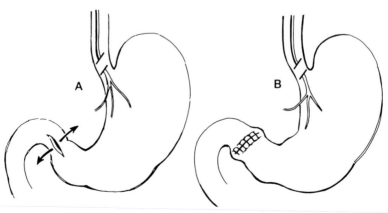

FIGURE 24–8. Truncal vagotomy and pyloroplasty.

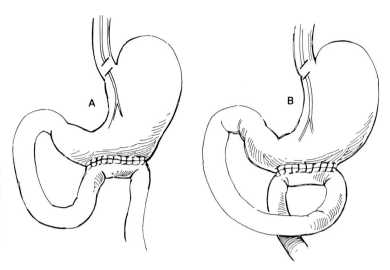

FIGURE 24–9. Truncal vagotomy and gastroenterostomy. *A,* Loop gastrojejunostomy with afferent limb (proximal jejunum) on patient's right and efferent limb (distal jejunum) on left. *B,* Loop gastrojejunostomy with afferent and efferent limbs reversed.

may have gastric outlet obstruction during the early postoperative period. On endoscopy, the pyloric channel may be edematous and difficult to intubate. By following the muscular folds of the antrum, gentle pressure can be exerted to traverse the pyloric channel and enter the duodenum. Prolonged nasogastric suction will usually resolve early postoperative outlet obstruction.

Endoscopy in a patient who has undergone a gastroenterostomy without resection requires specific knowledge of the surgical anatomy prior to intubation (Plate 24–8). The antrum and remaining pylorus must be identified, and a thorough examination must be made of the duodenum for residual or recurrent ulcers. In the early postoperative period, edema and friability may be present in the antrum and around the gastrointestinal stoma. The pylorus may be inflamed and difficult to intubate (Plate 24–9). The pylorus lies in a posterior-superior position relative to the stoma, the latter usually being located in a dependent position on the greater curvature of the stomach. The efferent limb is often identifiable by the ease with which it is entered. The afferent limb will contain bile.

Billroth I Anastomosis

The operative techniques in partial gastrectomy are similar for a Billroth I (gastroduodenostomy) and Billroth II (gastrojejunostomy) anastomosis.[77] The proximal stomach is transected at the antrum, and the duodenum is divided distal to the pyloric ring. The usual method of constructing a Billroth I anastomosis is the Hoffmeister technique in which the upper half of the gastric resection line beginning at the lesser curvature is closed and the lower half is used for anastomosis to the remaining duodenum (Fig. 24–10A).[77]

At endoscopy the size of the gastric pouch, the healed gastrotomy scar running longitudinally along the lesser curvature (Plate 24–10), and the stoma should be noted. Normally the stoma is widely patent, is in dependent position, and leads directly into duodenum (Plate 24–11). The presence of suture material, reflux of bile into the gastric pouch or esophagus, ulceration, or inflammation should be recorded and biopsies obtained if mucosal abnormalities are seen.

Billroth II Anastomosis

After gastric resection, a Billroth II anastomosis (Fig. 24–10B and C) is constructed using either the Hoffmeister or Polya technique to connect the distal stomach to a proximal loop of jejunum.[77] In the Polya technique the anastomosis is formed by using the entire width of the original transverse gastrostomy. With either the Hoffmeister or Polya technique, the two jejunal limbs may be separated by a wide distance or narrow raphe, depending on the width of the actual stoma (Fig. 24–11).

At endoscopy the area around the gastrointestinal stoma should be carefully inspected for sutures, staples, and ulcerations. An endoscopic description of the anatomic findings resulting from the surgery is essential. Complete examination of the anastomosis, particularly the jejunal side, may require gentle retroflexion of the endoscope within the stoma, a maneuver facilitated by use of small-diameter endoscopes with a 135-degree angle

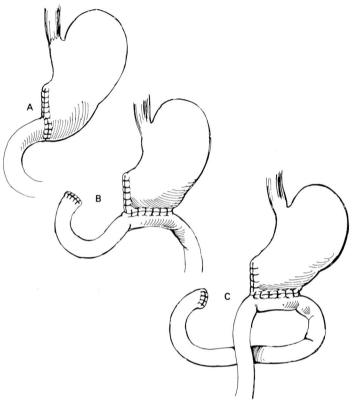

FIGURE 24–10. Antrectomy and gastroenterostomy (vagotomy not illustrated). *A,* Antrectomy with Billroth I gastroduodenostomy. *B,* Antrectomy with Billroth II loop gastrojejunostomy (afferent limb left, efferent limb right). *C,* Antrectomy with Billroth II loop gastrojejunostomy (afferent and efferent limbs reversed).

of view and tight bending radius (Plate 24–12). The efferent limb is dependent, is the most easily entered, and appears to continue in a straight caudad direction (Plate 24–13). The opening of the afferent limb is more difficult to enter, may be tucked behind a fold of the stoma, and may be situated to the left or right of the efferent limb depending on the method of surgical anastomosis. The afferent limb is identified by the presence of bile and the ampulla. With intubation to the proximal duodenum, the closure site may be examined and a biopsy obtained to diagnose retained antrum.[78]

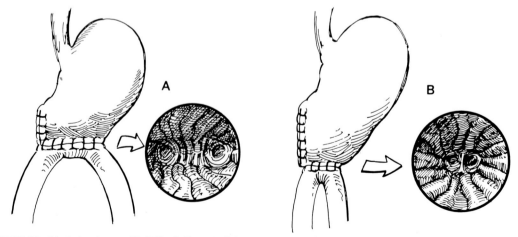

FIGURE 24–11. Antrectomy with Billroth II gastrojejunostomy. *A,* Wide anastomosis results in wide separation of jejunal limbs. *B,* Narrow anastomosis results in closely approximated limbs separated by narrow raphe.

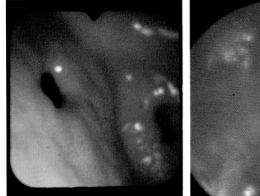 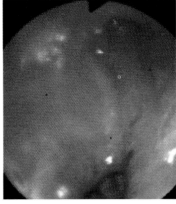 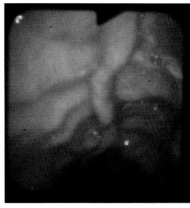

PLATE 24–8.   PLATE 24–9.   PLATE 24–10.

PLATE 24–8. Gastroenterostomy. Pylorus appears on right and gastroenterostomy stoma is to left (on anterior gastric wall); both are patent, with no inflammation. Antral mucosa is normal.

PLATE 24–9. Gastroenterostomy–seventh postoperative day. Pylorus (superior margin of photograph) is scarred and inflamed; surrounding antral mucosa is friable. Gastroenterostomy stoma is in dependent position on greater curvature (lower margin of photograph).

PLATE 24–10. Well-healed gastrotomy scar courses longitudinally along lesser curvature. (See Figure 24–6 for further illustration of location of gastrotomy scar).

Roux-Y Reconstruction

The Roux-Y gastrojejunostomy is primarily performed as a second operation when antrectomy and Billroth II (sometimes Billroth I) anastomosis results in symptomatic alkaline reflux.[46, 47, 50, 51, 79, 80] The operation involves division of the jejunum about 20 cm distal to the ligament of Treitz, anastomosis of the proximal end of the efferent jejunal limb to the gastric pouch, and a jejunojejunostomy (end-to-side) between the proximal intestinal limb and the distal jejunum 40 cm beyond the gastrojejunostomy. The distance between the gastric pouch and the jejunojejunostomy is a critical factor if bile reflux (too short) and recurrent ulceration (too long) are to be avoided.

Endoscopic examination of the gastric remnant after resection with Roux-Y anastomosis is the same as described for the Billroth II anastomosis. The gastrojejunostomy is a side-to-side anastomosis with a short blind limb

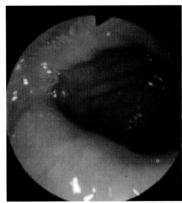 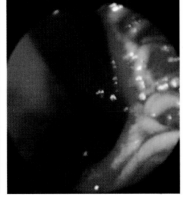 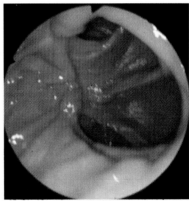

PLATE 24–11.   PLATE 24–12.   PLATE 24–13.

PLATE 24–11. Gastrectomy with Billroth I anastomosis. Normal appearing Billroth I stoma leads directly to duodenum.

PLATE 24–12. Jejunal side of Billroth II anastomosis. Endoscope is retroflexed in stoma of Billroth II anastomosis. Jejunal side of anastomosis may be inspected for inflammation or recurrent ulcers with this technique.

PLATE 24–13. Gastrectomy with Billroth II anastomosis (3 years post-resection), with jejunal limbs widely separated. Dominant limb (most easily entered) is usually efferent, whereas the afferent limb may be situated on either side of the efferent limb and is often tucked under a fold.

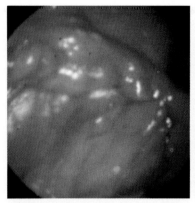 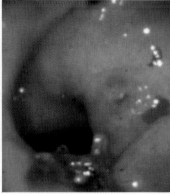 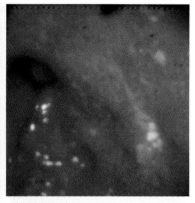

PLATE 24—14.   PLATE 24—15.   PLATE 24—16.

PLATE 24—14. Fresh 24 hr gastrotomy scar is not bleeding and is well secured. This area can be a source of postoperative bleeding and should be carefully examined if hemorrhage occurs in immediate postoperative period.

PLATE 24—15. Gastrectomy with Billroth I anastomosis. This is a fresh anastomosis with blood oozing from stoma where suture material is visible.

PLATE 24—16. Gastric erythema. Note intense erythema in gastric pouch after gastrectomy with Billroth I anastomosis. Erythema is most intense around stoma. Minimal gastritis was present histologically.

that must not be mistaken for a stenotic afferent jejunal limb (see Plate 24—4). The anastomosis should be examined for the presence of obstruction, inflammation, recurrent ulceration, dysplasia, and carcinoma.

Endoscopy in the Early Postoperative Period

Bleeding and obstruction are the two major complications in the early postgastrectomy period for which endoscopy may be requested.[81, 82] Endoscopy is usually indicated for significant bleeding, but early gastric outlet obstruction is often diagnosed radio-graphically, endoscopy being reserved for selected patients.

Although endoscopy in early postoperative patients is not technically difficult, care must exercised to avoid disruption of the fresh surgical anastomosis (Plate 24—14). A well-constructed anastomosis can withstand gentle endoscopic examination even immediately after surgery if minimal insufflation is used.[81–83] However, if an anastomotic leak is suspected, endoscopy is contraindicated; this diagnosis must be established roentgeno-graphically.

Endoscopic localization of the site of bleed-

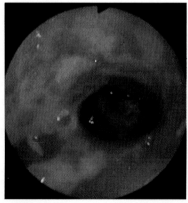 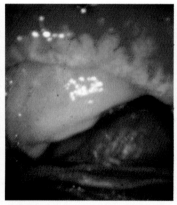 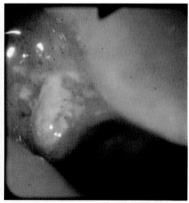

PLATE 24—17.   PLATE 24—18.   PLATE 24—19.

PLATE 24—17. Histologically proven severe gastritis seen diffusely throughout gastric pouch. Mucosa is friable and bile-stained.

PLATE 24—18. Intestinal metaplasia. Feathery white border of metaplastic intestinal epithelium can be seen on gastric side of Billroth II anastomosis. Intestinal metaplasia may also appear as white patches or larger white areas and should not be mistaken for cancer. Note eventration of efferent limb through stoma.

PLATE 24—19. Recurrent ulcer. Ulcer at stomal ring is flat and superficial and has adherent white pseudomembrane. Minimal gastritis was noted.

ing that occurs in the early postgastrectomy period is essential for diagnosis and appropriate choice of therapy. Minimal blood loss can occur as oozing at the anastomotic site; this is of little consequence. Significant postgastrectomy bleeding (more than 4 units of blood loss within 48 hours) may originate from operative suture lines, visible intraluminal sutures (Plate 24–15), active ulcer disease, erosions caused by a nasogastric tube, gastritis, or varices. Bleeding may be exacerbated by coagulopathy. Carefully performed endoscopy, with gentle washing and inspection of the anastomoses and remaining gastric pouch, will usually identify bleeding sites.

Outlet obstruction in the early postoperative period may be mechanical (tight anastomosis and edema) or functional (prolonged gastric atony or a nondependent stoma). It is suspected when attempts to discontinue postoperative nasogastric drainage fail or when drainage is excessive.[83] A barium contrast study is the initial diagnostic step for differentiation between mechanical and functional obstruction. Patients with prolonged gastric outlet obstruction or marked malnutrition preoperatively may require from weeks to months to regain normal gastric motility, especially after vagotomy. If mechanical obstruction is suspected, endoscopy is indicated to evaluate stomal size and position, to search for suture material that could compromise the lumen, or to diagnose severe inflammation and edema at the stoma. Rarely, intractable postoperative anastomotic obstruction may require reoperation.

Endoscopy in the Late Postoperative Period

The most common symptoms in the late postoperative period that prompt endoscopy are summarized in Table 24–1. About 80% of patients with postoperative complications require endoscopy within the first year after surgery.[1, 70] Since specific symptom patterns often suggest specific pathologic findings, the endoscopist should be familiar with the patient's symptoms, such as the pattern of pain and its relation to food or medications, the nature of vomitus (undigested food versus bilious secretions), and the duration and rate of bleeding.

Specific considerations having a bearing on endoscopy in postgastrectomy patients include the presence of duodenogastric bile/alkaline reflux, gastric mucosal changes, recurrent ulceration, mechanical obstruction,

TABLE 24–1. **Major Symptoms of Patients Referred for Endoscopy***

Symptom	Frequency (%)
Pain	51–66
Vomiting	41–48
Bleeding	14–39
Weight loss	33
Dumping	32
Anemia	18
Diarrhea	17
Early satiety or anorexia	12
Esophageal reflux	4–8

*Data collected from published reports[1, 70–75] and unpublished data from the authors' experience.

bleeding, and weight loss or malnutrition.[63–65, 77, 84, 85] Gastric carcinoma also is occasionally found in the postgastrectomy patient.

The following common endoscopic findings should not be considered pathologic. The usual angulation of the esophagogastric junction to the left may be lost. Although gastric mucosa may be normal with normal rugal folds, frequently the rugae are absent, there is mucosal pallor, and finely arborizing mucosal vessels are readily distinguished. Distensibility is normal, although maximum insufflation is difficult to maintain with an open stoma. On the gastric side of the stomal ring, small outpouchings, recesses, or nodules of granulation tissue are often noted. Portions of the stomach or jejunal limbs may be bound down or "tented" by postsurgical adhesions; these alter the normal course of the intestine, for which reason the endoscope should be advanced with caution and gentleness.

Duodenogastric Reflux

Terminology with respect to postoperative gastritis due to duodenogastric reflux is imprecise and confusing. Although postoperative gastritis is often referred to as bile gastritis, it is by no means certain that bile is the cause, or at least the exclusive etiologic factor. The term alkaline reflux gastritis is also used. Such terminology must not be mistakenly accepted as indicative of the pathophysiology of this poorly understood condition. For convenience, the term bile reflux will be used here. This subject is also considered in Chapter 21.

Duodenogastric reflux, manifested as bilious vomiting often with concurrent epigastric pain, may occur after all types of ulcer surgery.[47, 48, 79, 86–91] The pain of bile reflux differs from that of recurrent ulcer in that it is relieved by bilious vomiting. Bile reflux is normal in patients with incompetent or absent pyloric sphincters but is not clinically significant unless it produces symptoms.[92, 93] Endoscopy is useful for determining the cause of bilious vomiting and also the mucosal effects of duodenogastric reflux. In nearly all patients bile reflux causes the gastric mucosa to appear erythematous and friable[94, 95] (Plate 24–16), but in some patients—perhaps those with a greater degree of reflux—peristomal ulcers or esophageal inflammation occur. These patients require aggressive medical therapy; if this fails, a second operation (Roux-Y gastrojejunostomy) may be necessary to divert the normal duodenal juices from the stomach. Endoscopic evaluation of the effectiveness of medical therapy is mandatory in assessing healing and the need for reoperation.

Gastric Mucosal Changes

Important alterations of the gastric mucosa in the postgastrectomy patient include erythema, gastritis, intestinal metaplasia, dysplasia, and cancer.[1, 70, 75, 96–100] Dysplasia and cancer are discussed in a subsequent section.

Mucosal erythema develops in nearly all patients who undergo ulcer surgery; this cannot be quantified or correlated with clinical factors.[71, 72, 99–102] Although erythema is usually associated with bile staining (bile gastritis), gastritis cannot always be proved histologically. Erythema is usually most intense around the stoma; the mucosa can be extremely friable (see Plate 24–16). Erythema is abolished by biliary diversion surgery.[86, 88]

Histologic evidence of gastritis is found in 60% to 100% of patients who have undergone gastric resection for peptic ulcer disease[1, 71, 72, 90, 103] (Plate 24–17). There is no evidence that gastritis can be accurately quantitated or implicated in specific clinical symptoms.[1, 71, 72] In our experience, 75% to 80% of patients with Billroth II reconstruction after gastric resection will have histologically verifiable gastritis for prolonged periods that may extend to many years after surgery, regardless of clinical symptoms. In animal studies, gastritis has been induced by duodenogastric reflux,[104] but a similar relationship has not been demonstrated in man. Long-term sequelae of gastritis include mucosal atrophy and occasionally deficiency of intrinsic factor and hence a lack of vitamin B_{12}.[105, 106] Such gastritis is rarely the source of significant bleeding.

Intestinal metaplasia refers to the development of intestinal epithelium in gastric mucosa.[107, 100] The degree of intestinalization may be mild, with few intestinal elements, or severe, with formation of villi. Any cell type found in the intestine can also be found in metaplastic areas within the stomach. It is not known whether this lesion is heterotopic, that is, the result of misplacement of intestinal epithelium, or truly metaplastic, that is a transformation of gastric into intestinal epithelium.[108]

Some authors believe that intestinal metaplasia is a premalignant lesion, because of the frequent endoscopic finding of intestinal epithelium in association with carcinoma.[107–109] No long-term study in humans has prospectively followed metaplastic lesions to determine whether they degenerate into cancer. Animal experiments studying chemically induced intestinal metaplasia suggest that malignant degeneration does occur, but the extent to which these findings may be correlated with postgastrectomy metaplasia in humans is uncertain.[104]

The endoscopic appearance of intestinal metaplasia is distinctive (Plate 24–18). There is usually a superficial, flat, whitish, feathery edge of tissue beginning at or near the stoma that extends proximally into the gastric pouch. Occasionally lesions occur as white spots or islands in the peristomal area. Our policy for patients with intestinal metaplasia is annual or biannual endoscopic examinations with repeated biopsies.

Recurrent Ulcer

Recurrence rates after peptic ulcer surgery are as follows: vagotomy and pyloroplasty, 5% to 8%; vagotomy and antrectomy, 2% to 4%; highly selective vagotomy, 10% to 20%; and subtotal gastrectomy (without vagotomy) 20%.[63–65, 110–112] The presenting symptoms in 75% to 90% of patients with marginal ulcers include pain, and in over 50%, concurrent bleeding. Of all patients who present to the endoscopist with typical dyspeptic pain, 58% will have recurrent ulcers.[1, 70, 75] Unlike primary ulcer disease, which is characterized by intermittent and cyclical symptoms, recurrent ulcers after surgery tend to cause continuous symptoms that do not remit until effective therapy is instituted. Symptoms often persist despite medical therapy, and a second operation becomes necessary[113]—thus the need for timely re-evaluation of patients and accurate diagnosis of recurrent ulcer. Because radiographic examination of the postgastrectomy stomach is highly inaccurate,[1, 66, 70] endoscopy is the mandatory procedure of choice when ulcer recurrence is a consideration.

Peptic ulcers almost always occur on the stomal ring or the jejunal limb adjacent to the stoma; they rarely occur in gastric mucosa,[65, 114] although a recent report disputes this.[115] Several biopsies of gastric ulcers, especially in the absence of mechanical obstruction or bezoar, must be obtained to eliminate the possibility of carcinoma. Ulcers on the anastomotic ring are flat and linear in configuration with an overlying pseudomembrane (Plate 24–19). Stomal ulcers in jejunal mucosa are characteristically round and shallow (Plate 24–20). Stomal ulcers may be circumferential and may bleed easily on contact by the endoscope (Plate 24–21). Marked edema and consequent obstruction is unusual but does occur (Plate 24–22).

A recurrent ulcer requires careful investigation of its cause (Fig. 24–12), the most common being incomplete vagotomy.[65, 77, 113] The need for thorough endoscopy in a stomach that is clear of retained food or bezoar cannot be overstated; this includes careful inspection of remaining gastric mucosa for the cobblestoned appearance that suggests continued function or hypertrophy of acid-producing epithelium; estimation of stomal diameter; and investigation of the closed afferent limb for retained antrum.

Mechanical Obstruction

Gastric outlet obstruction that occurs late in the postoperative course is usually due to anastomotic stricture or recurrent ulceration with edema. Endoscopy is the examination of choice, with attention focused on the stomal area. The presence of a bezoar (Plate 24–23) or retained food may require lavage or a period of clear liquid intake before endoscopy will be successful.

Bleeding

The approach to management and therapy for hemorrhage in the postgastrectomy patient is similar to that used for bleeding in the nonsurgical patient.[116, 117] This is considered in detail in Chapter 6. Iced saline lavage or gastric hypothermia sometimes decreases the rate of bleeding.[118] If hemorrhage continues, emergency endoscopy is indicated, with a meticulous search for one or more of the following: esophageal varices, esophageal ulcers, esophagitis, Mallory-Weiss tears, gastritis, intraluminal sutures, and ulcers. Particular attention must be directed toward the jejunal side of the anastomosis, where stomal ulcers are most likely to occur. Gentle retroflexion of the endoscope within the stoma may reveal blind areas not readily seen when approaching the anastomosis in a forward-viewing direction (see Plate 24–12). Bleeding ulcers are sometimes refractory to medical therapy and may require surgical intervention.

Endoscopy may be performed in postgastrectomy patients with subclinical bleeding or anemia to search for recurrent ulcers, severe gastritis, or the rare gastric carcinoma. Anemia may develop in postgastrectomy patients from loss of blood, malabsorption of iron, or

FIGURE 24–12. Drawing illustrating conditions causing recurrent ulcers.

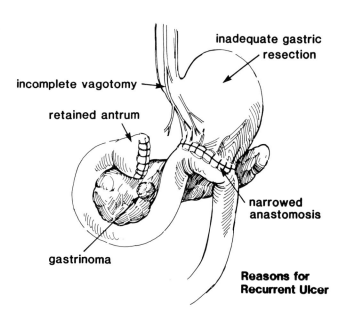

inadequate gastric resection

incomplete vagotomy

retained antrum

gastrinoma

narrowed anastomosis

Reasons for Recurrent Ulcer

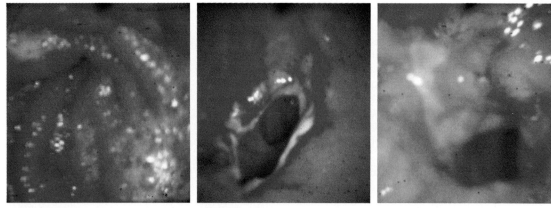

PLATE 24—20.   PLATE 24—21.   PLATE 24—22.

PLATE 24—20. Recurrent ulcer. Extreme close-up view of ulcer found in jejunal mucosa just beyond stoma in patient who had a gastrectomy and Billroth II anastomosis. Typically, ulcer is small and shallow.

PLATE 24—21. Recurrent ulcer surrounding stoma of Billroth II anastomosis. Ulcer was rather shallow but bled easily. Edema was not severe enough to cause outlet obstruction in this patient. Note visible suture in inferior edge (6 o'clock position) of stoma.

PLATE 24—22. Ulceration and outlet obstruction. Deep ulceration and intense inflammation is present in patient with Billroth II anastomosis, who presented with outlet obstruction.

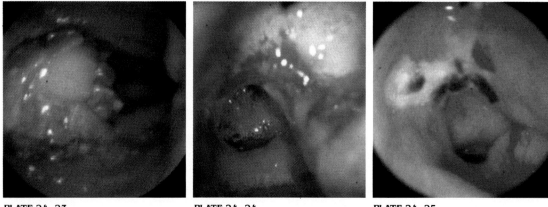

PLATE 24—23.   PLATE 24—24.   PLATE 24—25.

PLATE 24—23. Moderate size gastric pouch with erythema and phytobezoar. Patient had narrowed anastomosis which required surgical supervision.

PLATE 24—24. Malignant ulcer. Deep, irregular gastric ulcer is visible in patient who had undergone gastrectomy with Billroth I anastomosis. Biopsies revealed adenocarcinoma.

PLATE 24—25. Suture ulcer. Suture material is visible within ulcer bed. Endoscopic removal of the suture resulted in healing of ulcer.

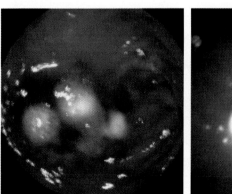

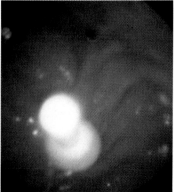

PLATE 24—26. Large gastric pouch and stenotic stoma in patient who had undergone gastric bypass. Three pills are seen adjacent to pinhole-sized stoma. Surgical revision with reduction of pouch size was necessary.

PLATE 24—27. Feeding gastronomy tube within stomach lumen. Typically these enter stomach at antral-fundic junction. Pylorus seen in distance.

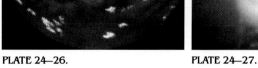

PLATE 24—26.   PLATE 24—27.

intrinsic factor deficiency.[65] Recurrent ulcer is suspect in the anemic patient with dyspeptic pain. Even in the absence of this type of pain, recurrent ulceration, gastritis, or other causes of blood loss, including colonic lesions, must be eliminated before assuming anemia is due to iron or intrinsic factor deficiency.[1, 70–72]

Malnutrition and Weight Loss

Weight loss and malnutrition are sometimes indications for endoscopy in the postgastrectomy patient, although the examination is usually not helpful except to rule out bleeding lesions, as discussed above. The incidence of gastric remnant cancer is small, but it is necessary to exclude this lesion from consideration when there has been significant loss of weight.

Cancer

In 1922 Balfour[119] reported the case of a patient who developed adenocarcinoma in the gastric remnant after ulcer surgery for non-neoplastic disease. Subsequently, several investigators reported an increased incidence of so-called gastric "stump" cancer, compared with nonoperated controls, and advocated routine endoscopic screening with biopsy for all patients beginning 10 to 15 years after operation.[120–126]

The range of histologic changes in the gastric mucosa of postgastrectomy patients includes chronic atrophic gastritis, intestinal metaplasia, gastric gland dilation (cystic dilation, or cystification), papillary and glandular hyperplasia, and adenomatous transformation.[98–100, 127] The severity of these histologic changes may be related to the amount of duodenogastric reflux; animal studies suggest that the frequency of gastric remnant cancer correlates quantitatively with bile reflux.[104]

Although the results of retrospective studies suggest an increased risk for gastric cancer among postgastrectomy patients, the results of other retrospective studies[128–131] and several population-based studies[132–134] do not support this conclusion. The ASGE does not advocate routine screening of asymptomatic postgastrectomy patients. Decision analysis methods suggest that in the United States, where the incidence of gastric cancer is low, minimal if any benefit would result from routine screening.[135] Based on currently available data, endoscopy with multiple biopsies[8–12] of abnormal appearing mucosa[136–138] and recurrent gastric ulcers is indicated in postgastrectomy patients only if new or recurrent symptoms develop. If gastric ulcers are found, biopsy for evidence of carcinoma is indicated (Plate 24–24).

Other Problems

Other problems that may prompt endoscopy include retained sutures, postgastrectomy dumping syndrome, afferent loop syndrome, symptoms suggesting esophageal reflux, and dysphagia.

Nonabsorbable suture material or *staples* may appear on the luminal surface of the gastric mucosa. These can cause pain, ulceration, and bleeding.[139] At endoscopy sutures are usually found within ulcers in the region of the anastomosis or at the gastrotomy closure (Plate 24–25). Symptoms may be relieved and bleeding may cease after removal of suture material. When sutures are noted during endoscopy, a gentle attempt at removal should be made even in the absence of ulceration.

The dumping syndrome is usually a transient problem in the postgastrectomy patient and is alleviated by appropriate dietary manipulation. Endoscopic examination rarely is helpful in defining the problem or directing therapy.

The afferent loop syndrome, now considered extremely rare, results from a narrowed afferent loop outlet.[72] Postprandial accumulation of pancreatic and biliary secretions within the limb causes pain and nausea; these symptoms are relieved when the secretions suddenly enter the stomach and induce bilious vomiting. Experimental studies using balloon occlusion of the afferent loop or radionucleotide imaging of biliary secretions have failed to demonstrate an association between symptoms and a dysfunctional afferent loop.[65, 140] Endoscopy assists in evaluating the patency of afferent and efferent limbs and in defining other more probable causes of postgastrectomy pain such as recurrent ulcer.

Symptoms referable to the esophagus are common after ulcer surgery. Usually symptoms of *reflux* and *dysphagia* are transient and related to physiologic adaptation to vagotomy. If dysphagia continues beyond the immediate postoperative period, endoscopy should be performed to rule out severe reflux esophagitis or stricture, both of which are manageable by conventional means.

ERCP in the Postgastrectomy Patient

ERCP is a commonly available and accurate procedure to image the biliary and pancreatic ducts.[141, 142] Patients who have undergone ulcer surgery often present unique problems to the endoscopist attempting ERCP or endoscopic sphincterotomy. Although esophageal surgery, pyloroplasty, or gastrectomy with Billroth I anastomosis do not ordinarily add to the technical difficulty in cannulation of the ampulla, ERCP after gastrectomy and Billroth II anastomosis can be extremely difficult.[143–145] A Roux-Y anastomosis virtually precludes successful cannulation.

In patients who have undergone gastric resection with Billroth II drainage, it is often difficult to locate the afferent limb with a side-viewing endoscope. For this reason an end-viewing endoscope may be used to establish the position of the afferent limb and the ampulla of Vater and to attempt cannulation. (This technique is discussed in Chapter 25.) The length of the afferent loop is rarely the reason for failure of ERCP. Since the courses from the stomach of the afferent and efferent limbs of a loop jejunostomy vary (see Fig. 24–10), the position of the endoscope should be confirmed fluoroscopically before concluding that the length of the afferent limb makes ERCP impossible. The success rate of ERCP after gastrectomy and Billroth II anastomosis is approximately 50% and often entails a long and arduous procedure.

Cancer Operations

The extent of resection for gastric carcinoma depends on tumor size and location.[63, 64, 77] Proximal gastric carcinomas are usually treated by esophagogastrectomy with anastomosis of the remaining esophagus to stomach or with colonic interposition if esophageal involvement is extensive (see Figs. 24–4 and 24–6).[77, 146, 147] Carcinoma of the midstomach is treated by total or near-total gastrectomy (see Fig. 24–4),[56, 77] whereas distal cancer is treated by distal gastrectomy with gastrojejunostomy (see Fig. 24–10).[77, 148, 149] Billroth II (gastrojejunostomy) anastomosis is most often used rather than Billroth I (gastroduodenostomy) to avoid obstruction of the anastomosis after resection if the tumor should recur in the duodenum.

Postoperative problems usually relate to recurrence of carcinoma at the site of anastomosis. The presenting features may be upper gastrointestinal bleeding, abdominal pain, or obstruction. Endoscopic examination of the remaining gastric pouch and stoma should be performed for evidence of recurrent carcinoma. We routinely obtain biopsies in the area of the stoma in patients with gastric cancer even when there is no visible evidence of recurrent tumor. Obstructing carcinoma at the anastomosis occasionally can be treated by Grundzig-type balloon dilation, although the risk of bleeding or perforation is significant.

Weight Reduction (Bariatric) Surgery

The complications and decreased life expectancy of patients with morbid obesity may warrant operative intervention. Although jejunoileal bypass is no longer done because of severe postoperative metabolic problems,[150, 151] gastric bypass or gastroplasty is currently used for weight reduction.[152, 153] These procedures reduce the size of the gastric pouch and gastric outlet, thereby limiting caloric intake.

Three commonly performed gastric bypass procedures are illustrated in Figure 24–13. Endoscopic evaluation after gastric bypass should include estimations of pouch size and stomal diameter in addition to examination for mucosal abnormalities such as gastritis or ulcer. Examination of the bypassed segment is difficult but may be accomplished using a pediatric colonoscope in patients in whom drainage is carried out via a loop gastrojejunostomy.

Postoperative problems that require both radiographic and endoscopic investigations include failure of weight reduction, stomal obstruction, and upper gastrointestinal bleeding.[154] Failure to lose weight may be due to staple line disruption, gastric pouch dilation, stomal dilation, and dietary indiscretion.[155] A large gastric pouch or a large diameter anastomosis require reoperation with replacement of the staple line or reduction in pouch size. Stomal obstruction results in frequent emesis and regurgitation (Plate 24–26) and is sometimes amenable to dilation with Grundzig-type balloons.[156, 157] The incidence of stomal ulceration, which produces pain and bleeding, is less than 2%.[158] Stomal ulceration in association with a small gastric pouch usually responds to medical therapy; ulceration associated with a large pouch may require pouch revision and vagotomy. Symptomatic bleeding from the bypassed stomach and duodenum rarely occurs (0.3%).[159]

Gastrostomy Tubes

Gastrostomy tubes are used for enteric feeding or, less frequently, for gastric de-

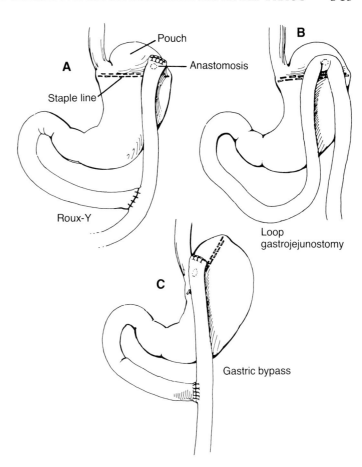

FIGURE 24–13. Gastric bypass operations. *A,* 85% Gastric bypass with horizontal double row of staples and Roux-Y gastrojejunostomy. *B,* Gastric bypass with loop gastrojejunostomy. *C,* 85% Bypass with diagonal row staples and a Roux-Y gastrojejunostomy (in direct line with distal esophagus).

compression. Either Foley catheters with large balloons or Malinckrodt catheters are placed in the dependent portion of the stomach near the fundic-antral junction on the greater curvature (Plate 24–27). The catheter is pulled toward the skin and sutured to approximate the stomach wall and the abdominal peritoneal surface.[77]

Patients with gastrostomy tubes undergo endoscopy primarily for bleeding or obstruction. The technique of endoscopy is not difficult, although the anatomy of the stomach is somewhat distorted by the gastrostomy tube. The usual method of following rugal folds to the antrum may not be helpful because of the tension produced by the gastrostomy tube on the stomach wall. Endoscopy can be performed immediately after placement of the tube if care is taken to minimize air insufflation. Maturation of the tube tract requires about 6 weeks, at which time endoscopy can be performed through the fistula using a small endoscope.

ENDOSCOPY AFTER CHOLEDOCHOENTEROSTOMY

Choledochoenterostomy is used for permanent decompression of a biliary tree obstructed by stones or cancer.[77, 160] This involves anastomosis of the common bile duct to the posterior superior aspect of the duodenal bulb (Fig. 24–14A). Choledochojejunostomy, used when duodenal abnormalities or cancer preclude duodenal anastomosis, may be either a loop choledochojejunostomy or a Roux-Y (Fig. 24–14B and C).

Complications of choledochoenterostomy include cholangitis, biliary obstruction, and "sump" syndrome.[160, 161] Each is related to stomal stenosis or obstruction, which requires endoscopy with cholangiography for diagnosis.[160–164] A choledochoduodenostomy is located in the duodenum immediately beyond the pylorus on the superior aspect of the bulb. At endoscopy, which is facilitated by a side-viewing instrument, this normally ap-

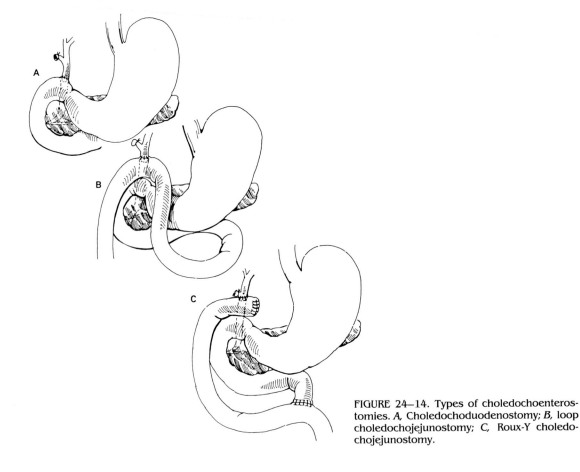

FIGURE 24–14. Types of choledochoenterostomies. A, Choledochoduodenostomy; B, loop choledochojejunostomy; C, Roux-Y choledochojejunostomy.

pears as a patent, round anastomosis approximately 1 cm in diameter (Plate 24–28). A choledochojejunostomy can be examined with a pediatric colonoscope, although even this endoscope may not be long enough to reach the anastomosis. Cholangiography of the proximal biliary tract is performed using a balloon-tipped catheter to occlude the anastomosis and permit adequate filling of the biliary system with a contrast agent (Fig. 24–15A). Injection of contrast agent at the ampulla will demonstrate the anatomy of the distal blind segment of the common duct (Fig. 24–15B). If stones or debris are shown in the distal common bile duct, as occurs in the "sump" syndrome, endoscopic sphincterotomy may be beneficial (Fig. 24–16). Since recurrent cholangitis, biliary obstruction, and the sump syndrome are probably related to stricture of the choledochoduodenostomy, endoscopic dilation of a strictured anastomosis with removal of debris may be curative.[165]

ENDOSCOPY AFTER PANCREATIC OPERATION

Chronic Pancreatitis

Surgery for chronic pancreatitis involves resection of portions of the pancreas and pancreatic duct drainage.[77, 166–169] The most commonly performed procedures are the Puestow-Gillesby[170] and the DuVall[171] (Fig. 24–17). Symptomatic relief after surgical therapy can be expected in 75% of patients if rigid indications for operation are imposed.

The Puestow-Gillesby procedure is used to treat patients with long, dilated segments of the main pancreatic duct and involves incision of the entire length of the duct with drainage by means of a side-to-side anastomosis of a jejunal limb to the gland (see Fig. 24–17). Chronic pancreatitis involving the body or tail of the gland can be treated by resection of the tail and end-to-end anastomosis of the pancreatic duct to a Roux-Y limb (DuVall procedure) (see Fig. 24–17B).

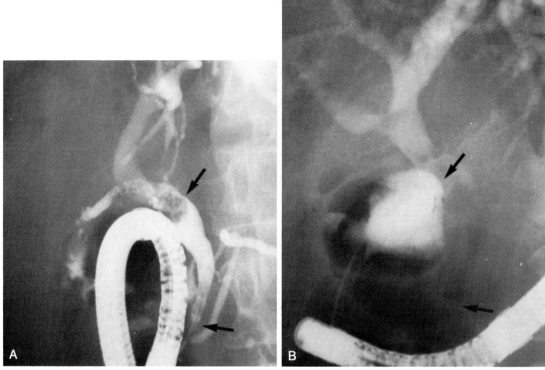

FIGURE 24–15. Injection of contrast material. *A,* Injection of contrast material into common bile duct via papilla (*arrow at bottom*) demonstrates free flow through choledochoduodenostomy and into proximal biliary radicals. A stone is visible within common bile duct at level of anastomosis (*arrow at top*). *B,* Contrast material is injected into proximal biliary radicals after placement of occlusive balloon through choledochoduodenostomy (*arrow at top*). Air outlines distal common duct and portion of pancreatic duct (*arrow at bottom*).

FIGURE 24–16. "Sump" syndrome. Position of stoma is superior-posterior on wall of duodenal bulb just distal to pyloric sphincter. Stones and debris are shown accumulating in distal blind end of common bile duct ("sump" syndrome).

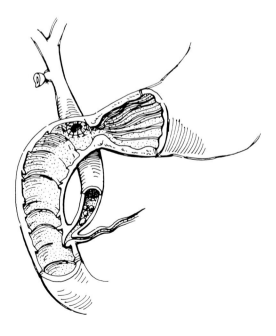

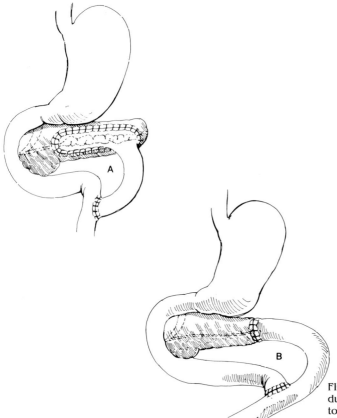

FIGURE 24–17. Pancreatic drainage procedures. *A*, Longitudinal pancreaticojejunostomy with Roux-Y reconstruction (Puestow-Gillesby procedure). *B*, End-to-end pancreatojejunostomy (DuVall procedure).

Preoperative ERCP is mandatory when considering surgical therapy, because this outlines the specific anatomic features and therefore aids in planning the surgical approach.[172] Endoscopy should be considered postoperatively when symptoms recur after a pain-free period. Postoperative retrograde pancreatography will define ductal anatomy and establish the patency of an anastomosis, or the lack thereof, although anastomotic patency does not always correlate with the presence or absence of symptoms (Fig. 24–18).

Pancreatic Pseudocysts

Surgical procedures for internal drainage of pseudocysts include cystgastrostomy (Fig. 24–19) and cystjejunostomy.[77] For cystgastrostomy, an incision is made via an anterior gastrotomy through the posterior wall of the stomach into the pseudocyst cavity located directly posterior and adherent to the stom-

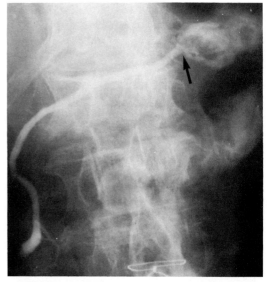

FIGURE 24–18. ERCP of DuVall Procedure. Pancreatography after DuVall end-to-end pancreaticojejunostomy shows patent proximal pancreatic duct with free flow of contrast material into jejunal limb (*arrow*).

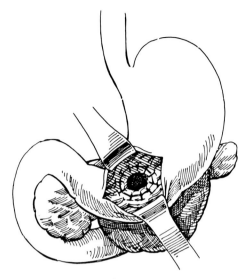

FIGURE 24–19. Pancreatic pseudocystgastrostomy. Illustration of operative appearance of cystgastrostomy performed via anterior gastrotomy.

ach wall. The cystgastrostomy is oversewn circumferentially to insure hemostasis of the highly vascular gastric wall.

After this type of surgery endoscopy will demonstrate the anterior gastrotomy suture line (Plate 24–29) and the entrance to the cyst cavity, which is usually on the posterior gastric wall. Pseudocysts rapidly collapse after drainage; thus endoscopy in the later postoperative period will fail to demonstrate the cyst anastomosis. A 7-day-old cystgastrostomy is shown in Plate 24–30.

Endoscopy is indicated for postoperative upper gastrointestinal bleeding. Early onset bleeding after operation may originate from the margin of the cystgastrostomy, the gastrotomy suture line, the interior of the cyst, or from sources unrelated to the procedure. Sometimes angiography is required to localize bleeding sites.

Whipple Operations

Less than 10% of patients with pancreatic cancer have tumors that are resectable for cure. The surgical procedures are distal pancreatectomy for lesions in the tail and pancreatoduodenectomy (Whipple procedure) for lesions of the head and periampullary region (Fig. 24–20).[77] The Whipple operation involves resection of the pancreatic head, distal common bile duct, and duodenum along with adjacent node-bearing tissue.[173] A

gastrojejunostomy, choledochojejunostomy and pancreatojejunostomy are performed to reconstitute intestinal continuity and biliary and pancreatic drainage. The endoscopic appearance of the stomach is identical to that of a gastric resection with Billroth II anastomosis performed for ulcer disease. Endoscopy is occasionally performed for recurrent biliary obstruction or pancreatitis to determine the patency of the biliary and pancreatic anastomoses. A pediatric colonoscope is recommended. Considerable skill and patience are required for this type of complex endoscopic examination.

ENDOSCOPY AFTER VASCULAR SURGERY

Graft-enteric fistulas occur in 1% to 4% of patients treated for abdominal aortic aneurysms.[174, 175] Mortality rates of 100% in unoperated patients and 50% to 75% in surgically treated patients warrant an aggressive search for this lesion in patients with intraabdominal grafts who present with gastrointestinal bleeding.[174–176] Successful management depends on early, accurate diagnosis.[176] Aortoenteric fistula is considered in Chapter 23.

Graft-enteric fistulas result in part from mechanical forces between the proximal suture line of the graft and the overlying third portion of the duodenum.[174] A second important pathogenetic component is probably subclinical infection of the graft.[174] Initially patients with this disorder usually have a small to moderate amount of upper gastrointestinal bleeding which often stops spontaneously (the "herald bleed"). Concomitant ulcers are often present and should not be cause for a relaxed diagnostic evaluation. Barium contrast studies, computed tomography, and angiography may fail to diagnose the fistula, especially in the absence of active bleeding.[174–176]

Every patient with an abdominal aortic graft and upper gastrointestinal bleeding requires emergency endoscopy to the ligament of Treitz[177–180] (Fig. 24–21). We recommend a 135 cm length pediatric colonoscope for this purpose. Because bleeding from a graft fistula always recurs and is potentially lethal, rapid diagnosis is essential. At endoscopy one or more of the following may be found: absence of any bleeding source, extrinsic compression of the third portion of the duodenum, bleeding in the distal duodenum, superficial erosions of the distal duodenum,

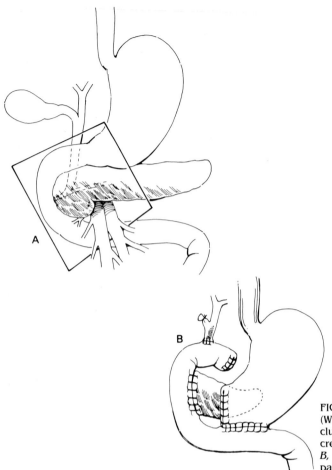

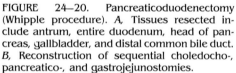

FIGURE 24–20. Pancreaticoduodenectomy (Whipple procedure). A, Tissues resected include antrum, entire duodenum, head of pancreas, gallbladder, and distal common bile duct. B, Reconstruction of sequential choledocho-, pancreatico-, and gastrojejunostomies.

FIGURE 24–21. Aorto-graft duodenal fistula. Fistula from proximal aortic graft suture line into fourth portion of the duodenum near ligament of Treitz. Pediatric colonoscope is needed to provide sufficient length for endoscopic examination.

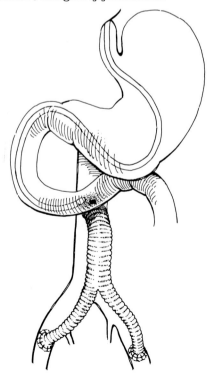

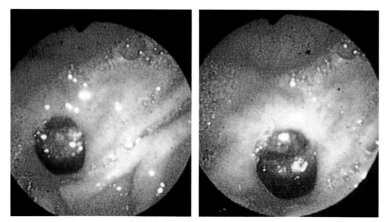

PLATE 24–28. Choledochoduodenostomy viewed with side-viewing endoscope. Stoma is located in duodenal bulb just byond pylorus. Diameter of stoma is approximately 1 cm. (Photograph courtesy of Dr. J. Segal.)

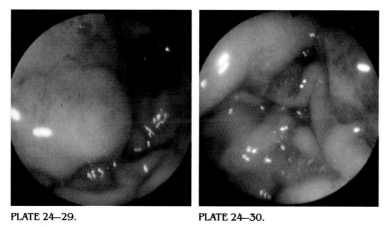

PLATE 24–29.   PLATE 24–30.

PLATE 24–29. Pseudocystgastrostomy. Gastrotomy scar can be seen on anterior side of stomach with cystgastrostomy just below and to right.
PLATE 24–30. Pseudocystgastrostomy. Stoma is still visible in this 7-day old cystgastrostomy. Usually cyst rapidly collapses after decompression and stoma disappears.

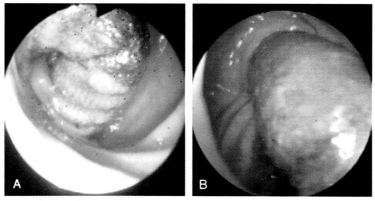

PLATE 24–31. Aorto-enteric graft fistula. Dacron graft material is visible in lumen of fourth part of duodenum viewed with pediatric colonoscope. (Courtesy of M. V. Sivak, Jr., M.D.)

and graft material protruding into the lumen of the duodenum (Plate 24–31).

Extreme care must be taken not to dislodge clot or impacted graft material; otherwise massive hemorrhage may occur. Endoscopic findings suggesting a graft-enteric fistula should prompt emergency operative exploration for confirmation and treatment. Some authors advocate endoscopy in the operating suite just prior to anesthesia induction to minimize delay in definitive management and avoid massive bleeding.[179] Our policy is to consider each patient individually, but always to err on the side of aggressive surgical intervention should a question concerning therapy arise. Every patient with upper gastrointestinal bleeding should be questioned specifically about prior intra-abdominal vascular surgery.

References

1. Hirschowitz BI, Luketic GC. Endoscopy in the postgastrectomy patient: An analysis of 580 patients. Gastrointest Endosc 1971; 18:27–30.
2. Shinya H, McSherry C. Endoscopy of the small bowel. Surg Clin North Am 1982; 62:821–4.
3. Brand EJ, Sivak MV Jr, Sullivan BH Jr. Aortoduodenal fistula: Endoscopic diagnosis. Dig Dis Sci 1979; 24:940–4.
4. Nissen R. Gastropexy and "fundoplication" in surgical treatment of hiatal hernia. Am J Dig Dis 1961; 6:954–61.
5. Skinner DB, Belsey RH. Surgical management of esophageal reflux and hiatus hernia: Long-term results with 1,030 patients. J Thorac Cardiovasc Surg 1967; 53:33–54.
6. Negre JB, Markkula HT, Keyrilainen O, Matikainen M. Nissen fundoplication: Results at 10 year follow-up. Am J Surg 1983; 146:635–8.
7. Baue AE, Belsey RH. The treatment of sliding hiatus hernia and reflux esophagitis by the Mark IV technique. Surgery 1967; 62:396–406.
8. Demeester TR, Johnson LF, Kent AH. Evaluation of current operations for the prevention of gastroesophageal reflux. Ann Surg 1974; 180:511–25.
9. Hill LD. An effective operation for hiatal hernia: An eight year appraisal. Ann Surg 1967; 166:681–92.
10. Woodward ER. Surgical treatment of reflux peptic esophagitis. Am Surgeon 1982; 48:647–51.
11. Collis JL, Kelly TD, Wiley AM. Anatomy of the crura of the diaphragm and the surgery of hiatus hernia. Thorax 1954; 9:175–89.
12. Henderson RD, Marryatt G. Total fundoplication gastroplasty: Long-term follow-up in 500 patients. J Thorac Cardiovasc Surg 1983; 85:81–7.
13. Angelchik J-P, Cohen R. A new surgical procedure for the treatment of gastroesophageal reflux and hiatal hernia. Surg Gynecol Obstet 1979; 148:246–8.
14. Starling JR, Reichelderfer MO, Pellett JR, Belzer FO. Treatment of symptomatic gastroesophageal reflux using the Angelchik prosthesis. Ann Surg 1982; 195:686–91.
15. Lipshutz WH, Eckert RJ, Gaskins RD, et al. Normal lower-esophageal reflux. N Engl J Med 1974; 291:1107–10.
16. Higgs RH, Castell DO, Farrell RL. Evaluation of the effect of fundoplication on the incompetent lower esophageal sphincter. Surg Gynecol Obstet 1975; 141:571–5.
17. Bowes KL, Sarna SK. Effect of fundoplication on the lower esophageal sphincter. Can J Surg 1975; 18:328–33.
18. Hallgrimsson JG, Linnet H, Jonasson H, et al. Postoperative evaluation after correction of oesophageal hiatus hernia. Scand J Thorac Cardiovasc Surg 1976; 10:257–61.
19. Noble HGS, Christie DL, Cahill JL. Follow-up studies on patients undergoing Nissen fundoplication utilizing intraoperative manometry. J Pediatr Surg 1982; 17:490–3.
20. Lackey C, Potts J. Penetration into the stomach: A complication of the antireflux prosthesis. JAMA 1982; 248:350.
21. Condon RE. More misadventures with the esophageal collar. Surgery 1983; 93:477–8.
22. Lilly MP, Slafsky F, Thompson WR. Intraluminal erosion and migration of the Angelchik antireflux prosthesis. Arch Surg 1984; 119:849–53.
23. Behar J, Sheahan DG, Biancani P, et al. Medical and surgical management of reflux esophagitis. A 38-month report on a prospective clinical trial. N Engl J Med 1975; 293:263–8.
24. Leonardi HK, Ellis FH Jr. Complications of the Nissen fundoplication. Surg Clin North Am 1983; 63:1155–65.
25. Henderson RD. Nissen hiatal hernia repair: Problems of recurrence and continued symptoms. Ann Thorac Surg 1979; 28:587–93.
26. Hill LD, Ilves R, Stevenson JK, Pearson JM. Reoperation for disruption and recurrence after Nissen fundoplication. Arch Surg 1979; 114:542–8.
27. Leonardi HK, Crozier RE, Ellis FH Jr. Reoperation for complications of the Nissen fundoplication. J Thorac Cardiovasc Surg 1981; 81:50–6.
28. Boesby S, Sorensen HR, Madsen T, Wallin L. Failures after surgical treatment of patients with hiatus hernia and reflux symptoms: A pathophysiological study. Scand J Gastroenterol 1982; 17:219–24.
29. Hocking MP, Maher JW, Woodward ER. Definitive surgical therapy for incapacitating "gas-bloat" syndrome. Am Surgeon 1982; 48:131–3.
30. Herrington JL Jr, Meacham PW, Hunter RM. Gastric ulceration after fundic wrapping: Vagal nerve entrapment, a possible causative factor. Ann Surg 1982; 195:574–81.
31. Festen C. Paraesophageal hernia: A major complication of Nissen's fundoplication. J Pediatr Surg 1981; 16:496–9.
32. Sjogren RW Jr, Johnson LF. Barrett's esophagus: A review. Am J Med 1983; 74:313–21.
33. Naef AP, Savary M, Ozzello L. Columnar-lined lower esophagus: An acquired lesion with malignant predisposition. J Thorac Cardiovasc Surg 1975; 70:826–35.
34. Radigan LR, Glover JL, Shipley FE, Shoemaker RE. Barrett esophagus. Arch Surg 1977; 112:486–91.
35. Haggitt RC, Tryzelaar J, Ellis FH, Colcher H. Adenocarcinoma complicating columnar epithelium-lined (Barrett's) esophagus. Am J Clin Pathol 1978; 70:1–5.

36. Skinner DB, Walther BC, Riddell RH, et al. Barrett's esophagus: Comparison of benign and malignant cases. Ann Surg 1983; 198:554–66.
37. Brand DL, Ylvisaker JT, Gelfand M, Pope CE II. Regression of columnar esophageal (Barrett's) epithelium after anti-reflux surgery. N Engl J Med 1980; 302:844–8.
38. Hamilton SR, Hutcheon DF, Ravich WJ, et al. Adenocarcinoma in Barrett's esophagus after elimination of gastroesophageal reflux. Gastroenterology 1984; 86:356–60.
39. Postlethwait RW, Sealy WC. Surgery of the Esophagus. New York: Appleton-Century-Crofts, 1979.
40. Cukingnan RA, Carey JS. Carcinoma of the esophagus. Ann Thorac Surg 1978; 26:274–86.
41. Le-Tian X, Zhen-Fu S, Ze-Jian L, Lian-Hun W. Surgical treatment of carcinoma of the esophagus and cardiac portion of the stomach in 850 patients. Ann Thorac Surg 1983; 35:542–7.
42. Postlethwait RW. Complications and deaths after operations for esophageal carcinoma. J Thorac Cardiovasc Surg 1983; 85:827–31.
43. Gunnlaugsson GH, Wychulis AR, Roland C, Ellis FH Jr. Analysis of the records of 1,657 patients with carcinoma of the esophagus and cardia of the stomach. Surg Gynecol Obstet 1970; 130:997–1005.
44. Hopkins RA, Alexander JC, Postlethwait RW. Stapled esophagogastric anastomosis. Am J Surg 1984; 147:283–7.
45. Ancona E, Bardini R, Nosadini A, et al. Esophagogastric anastomotic leakage. Int Surg 1982; 67:143–5.
46. Anderson HN. Postoperative alkaline reflux gastritis and esophagitis. Am Surg 1977; 43:670–7.
47. Herrington JL Jr, Sawyers JL, Whitehead WA. Surgical management of reflux gastritis. Ann Surg 1974; 180:526–37.
48. Nath BJ, Warshaw AL. Alkaline reflux gastritis and esophagitis. Ann Rev Med 1984; 35:383–96.
49. Payne WS. Surgical treatment of reflux esophagitis and stricture associated with permanent incompetence of the cardia. Mayo Clin Proc 1970; 45:553–62.
50. Herrington JL Jr, Mody B. Total duodenal diversion for treatment of reflux esophagitis uncontrolled by repeated antireflux procedures. Ann Surg 1976; 183:636–44.
51. Payne WS. Prevention and treatment of biliary-pancreatic reflux esophagitis: The role of long-limb Roux-Y. Surg Clin North Am 1983; 63:851–8.
52. Keshishian JM, Smyth NPD, Maxwell DD, Chua M. Dilation of difficult strictures of the esophagus. Surg Gynecol Obstet 1984; 158:81–5.
53. Thorsen G, Rosseland AR. Endoscopic incision of postoperative stenoses in the upper gastrointestinal tract. Gastrointest Endosc 1983; 29:26–9.
54. Weiss W, Hold H, Neumayr A, Schuller J. Endoscopic treatment of stenosized anastomosis after gastrectomy. Endoscopy 1977; 9:242–4.
55. Inberg MV, Heinonen R, Rantakokko V, Viikari SJ. Surgical treatment of gastric carcinoma: A regional study of 2,590 patients over a 27-year period. Arch Surg 1975; 110:703–7.
56. Shiu MH, Papacristou DN, Kosloff C, Eliopoulos G. Selection of operative procedure for adenocarcinoma of the midstomach. Ann Surg 1980; 192:730–7.
57. Jensen RT, Gardner JD, Raufman J-P, et al. Zollinger-Ellison syndrome: Current concepts and management. Ann Intern Med 1983; 98:59–75.
58. Morrow D, Passaro ER Jr. Alkaline reflux esophagitis after total gastrectomy. Am J Surg 1976; 132:287–91.
59. May IA, Samson PC. Esophageal reconstruction and replacements. Ann Thorac Surg 1969; 7:249–77.
60. Mansour KA, Hansen HA II, Hersh T, et al. Colon interposition for advanced nonmalignant esophageal stricture: Experience with 40 patients. Ann Thorac Surg 1981; 32:584–91.
61. Hankins JR, Cole FN, McLaughlin JS. Colon interposition for benign esophageal disease: Experience with 23 patients. Ann Thorac Surg 1984; 37:192–6.
62. Postlethwait RW, Sealy WC, Dillon ML, Young WG. Colon interposition for esophageal substitution. Ann Thorac Surg 1971; 12:89–109.
63. Sabiston DC Jr, ed. Davis-Christopher Textbook of Surgery. Ed 12. Philadelphia: W. B. Saunders, 1981.
64. Schwartz SI, Shires GT, Spencer FC, Storer EH, eds. Principles of Surgery. Ed 4. New York: McGraw-Hill, 1984.
65. Sleisenger MH, Fordtran JS. Gastrointestinal Disease. Ed 3. Philadelphia: W. B. Saunders, 1983.
66. Martin TR, Vennes JA, Silvis SE, et al. A comparison of upper gastrointestinal endoscopy and radiology. J Clin Gastroenterol 1980; 2:21–5.
67. Knutson CO, Max MH, Ahmad W, Polk HC Jr. Should flexible fiberoptic endoscopy replace barium contrast study of the upper gastrointestinal tract? Surgery 1978; 84:609–15.
68. Max MH, West B, Knutson CO. Evaluation of postoperative gastroduodenal symptoms: Endoscopy or upper gastrointestinal roentgenography? Surgery 1979; 86:578–82.
69. Gohel VK, Laufer I. Double-contrast examination of the postoperative stomach. Radiology 1978; 129:601–7.
70. Cotton PB, Rosenberg MT, Axon ATR, et al. Diagnostic yield of fibre-optic endoscopy in the operated stomach. Br J Surg 1973; 60:629–32.
71. Bowden TA Jr, Hooks VH III, Mansberger AR Jr. The stomach after surgery: an endoscopic perspective. Ann Surg 1983; 197:637–44.
72. Koelz HR, Gewertz BL. The stomach. Part I: Vagotomy. Clin Gastroenterol 1979; 8:305–21.
73. Alexander-Williams J, Hoare AM. The stomach. Part II: Partial gastric resection. Clin Gastroenterol 1979; 8:321–53.
74. Spainhour JB, Webster PD. Endoscopy in the evaluation of patients following gastrectomy. Arch Intern Med 1974; 134:52–5.
75. Donahue PE, Nyhus LM. Surgeon-endoscopists and the assessment of postoperative patients. South Med J 1982; 75:1570–5.
76. Hayden WF, Read RC. A comparative study of Heineke-Mikulcz and Finney pyloroplasty. Am J Surg 1968; 116:755–9.
77. Maingot R, ed. Abdominal Operations. Ed 7. New York: Appleton-Century-Crofts, 1980.
78. Sakai P, Filho UL, Cabrera PAI, et al. Fiberoptic endoscopy in the diagnosis of retained gastric antrum. Endoscopy 1983; 15:246–8.
79. de Langen ZJ, Slooff MJM, Jansen W. The surgical treatment of postgastrectomy reflux gastritis. Surg Gynecol Obstet 1984; 158:322–6.
80. Powell DC, Bivins BA, Bell RM, Griffen WO Jr.

Technical complications of Roux-en-Y gastrojejunostomy. Arch Surg 1983; 118:922–5.

81. Waldmann D, Ruckauer K, Salm R. Early postoperative endoscopy of the operated intestine. Endoscopy 1981; 13:108–12.

82. Manegold BC. Early postoperative endoscopy in the operated stomach. Endoscopy 1981; 13:104–7.

83. Waye JD. Surgical problems with the postoperative stomach: A technique for meaningful endoscopic evaluation. Mt Sinai J Med 1976; 43:291–3.

84. Clark CG. Medical complications of gastric surgery for peptic ulcer. Compr Ther 1981; 7:26–32.

85. Reber HA, Way LW. Surgical treatment of late postgastrectomy syndrome. Am J Surg 1975; 129:71–7.

86. Davidson ED, Hersh T. The surgical treatment of bile reflux gastritis: A study of 59 patients. Ann Surg 1980; 192:175–8.

87. Ritchie WP Jr. Alkaline reflux gastritis: An objective assessment of its diagnosis and treatment. Ann Surg 1980; 192:288–98.

88. Fiore AC, Malangoni MA, Broadie TA, et al. Surgical management of alkaline reflux gastritis. Arch Surg 1982; 117:689–94.

89. Boren CH, Way LW. Alkaline reflux gastritis: A re-evaluation. Am J Surg 1980; 140:40–6.

90. Van Heerden JA, Phillips SF, Adson MA, McIlrath CC. Postoperative reflux gastritis. Am J Surg 1975; 129:82–8.

91. Berardi RS, Siroospour D, Ruiz R, et al. Alkaline reflux gastritis: A study in forty postoperative duodenal ulcer patients. Am J Surg 1976; 132:552–7.

92. Hoare AM, Keighley MRB, Starkey B, Alexander-Williams J. Measurement of bile acids in fasting gastric aspirates: An objective test for bile reflux after gastric surgery. Gut 1978; 19:166–9.

93. Keighley MRB, Asquith P, Edwards JAC, Alexander-Williams J. The importance of an innervated and intact antrum and pylorus in preventing postoperative duodenogastric reflux and gastritis. Br J Surg 1975; 62:845–9.

94. Keighley MRB, Asquith P, Alexander-Williams J. Duodenogastric reflux: A cause of gastric mucosal hyperaemia and symptoms after operations for peptic ulceration. Gut 1975; 16:28–32.

95. Mosimann F, Burri B, Diserens H, et al. Enterogastric reflux; experimental and clinical study. Scand J Gastroenterol 1981; 16(Suppl 67):149–52.

96. Geboes K, Rutgeerts P, Broeckaert L, et al. Histologic appearance of endoscopic gastric mucosal biopsies 10–20 years after partial gastrectomy. Ann Surg 1980; 192:179–82.

97. Domellof L, Eriksson S, Janunger K-G. Carcinoma and possible precancerous changes of the gastric stump after Billroth II resection. Gastroenterology 1977; 73:462–8.

98. Johnston DH. A biopsy study of the gastric mucosa in postoperative patients with and without marginal ulcer. Am J Gastroenterol 1966; 46:103–18.

99. Burbige EJ, French SW, Tarder G, Belber JP. Correlation between gross appearance and histologic findings in the postoperative stomach. Gastrointest Endosc 1979; 25:3–5.

100. Stempien SJ, Dagradi AE, Tan DTD. Endoscopic aspects of the gastric mucosa ten years or more after vagotomy-pyloroplasty. Gastrointest Endosc 1971; 18:21–2.

101. Lees F, Grandjean LC. The gastric and jejunal mucosae in healthy patients with partial gastrectomy. Arch Intern Med 1958; 101:943–51.

102. Hoare AM, Jones EL, Alexander-Williams J, Hawkins CF. Symptomatic significance of gastric mucosal changes after surgery for peptic ulcer. Gut 1977; 18:295–300.

103. Savage A, Jones S. Histological appearances of the gastric mucosa 15–27 years after partial gastrectomy. J Clin Pathol 1979; 32:179–86.

104. Langhans P, Heger RA, Hohenstein J, Bunte H. Gastric carcinoma after gastric surgery—an experimental study. Hepatogastroenterology 1981; 28:34–7.

105. Siurala M, Lehtola J, Ihamaki T. Atrophic gastritis and its sequelae: Results of 19–23 years' follow-up examinations. Scand J Gastroenterol 1974; 9:441–6.

106. Kliems G, Paquet KJ, Lindstaedt H, Miederer S. Atrophic gastritis after Billroth I gastrectomy. Endoscopy 1979; 11:127–30.

107. Reynolds KW, Johnson AG, Fox B. Is intestinal metaplasia of the gastric mucosa a premalignant lesion? Clin Oncol 1975; 1:101–9.

108. Korn ER. Intestinal metaplasia of the gastric mucosa: Endoscopic recognition and review of the literature. Am J Gastroenterol 1974; 61:270–4.

109. Morson BC. Carcinoma arising from areas of intestinal metaplasia in gastric mucosa. Br J Cancer 1955; 9:377–85.

110. Siim C, Lublin HKF, Jensen H-E. Selective gastric vagotomy and drainage for duodenal ulcer: a 10–13 year follow-up study. Ann Surg 1981; 194:687–91.

111. Welch CE, Malt RA. Medical progress. Abdominal surgery. N Engl J Med 1983; 308:624–32; 685–95; 753–60.

112. Grossman MI (Moderator). Peptic ulcer: New therapies, new diseases. Ann Intern Med 1981; 95:609–27.

113. Thompson BW, Read RC. Secondary operations for duodenal ulcer. Am J Surg 1977; 134:758–62.

114. Stabile BE, Passaro E Jr. Recurrent peptic ulcer. Gastroenterology 1976; 70:124–35.

115. Sharaiha ZK, Smith JL, Cain GD, et al. Recurrent ulcers after gastric surgery: Endoscopic localization to gastric mucosa. Am J Gastroenterol 1983; 78:269–71.

116. Yajko RD, Norton LW, Eiseman B. Current management of upper gastrointestinal bleeding. Ann Surg 1975; 181:474–80.

117. Larson DE, Farnell MB. Upper gastrointestinal hemorrhage. Mayo Clin Proc 1983; 58:371–87.

118. Himal HS, Watson WW, Jones CW, MacLean LD. The management of bleeding acute gastric erosions: The role of gastric hypothermia. Br J Surg 1975; 62:221–3.

119. Balfour DC. Factors influencing the life expectancy of patients operated on for gastric ulcer. Ann Surg 1922; 76:405–8.

120. Eberlein TJ, Lorenzo FV, Webster MW. Gastric carcinoma following operation for peptic ulcer disease. Ann Surg 1978; 187:251–6.

121. Kobayashi S, Prolla JC, Kirsner JB. Late gastric carcinoma developing after surgery for benign conditions. Endoscopic and histologic studies of the anastomosis and diagnostic problems. Am J Dig Dis 1970; 15:905–12.

122. Domellof L, Janunger KG. The risk for gastric carcinoma after partial gastrectomy. Am J Surg 1977; 134:581–4.

123. Klarfeld J, Resnick G. Gastric remnant carcinoma. Cancer 1979; 44:1129–33.

124. Osnes M, Lotveit T, Myren J, Serck-Hanssen A. Early gastric carcinoma in patients with a Billroth II partial gastrectomy. Endoscopy 1977; 9:45–9.

125. Totten J, Burns HJG, Kay AW. Time of onset of carcinoma of the stomach following surgical treatment of duodenal ulcer. Surg Gynecol Obstet 1983; 157:431–3.

126. Orlando R III, Welch JP. Carcinoma of the stomach after gastric operation. Am J Surg 1981; 141:487–91.

127. Mortensen NJMcC, Thomas WEG, Jones SM. Endoscopic screening for premalignant changes 25 years after gastrectomy: Results of a five-year prospective study. Br J Surg 1984; 71:363–7.

128. Kivilaakso E, Hakkiluoto A, Kalima TV, Sipponen P. Relative risk of stump cancer following partial gastrectomy. Br J Surg 1977; 64:336–8.

129. DeJode LR. Gastric carcinoma following gastroenterostomy and partial gastrectomy. Br J Surg 1961; 48:512–4.

130. Liavaag K. Cancer development in gastric stump after partial gastrectomy for peptic ulcer. Ann Surg 1962; 155:103–6.

131. Dougherty SH, Foster CA, Eisenberg MM. Stomach cancer following gastric surgery for benign disease. Arch Surg 1982; 117:294–7.

132. Logan RFA, Langman MJS. Screening for gastric cancer after gastric surgery. Lancet 1983; 2:667–70.

133. Schafer LW, Larson DE, Melton LJ III, et al. The risk of gastric carcinoma after surgical treatment for benign ulcer disease: A population-based study in Olmsted County, Minnesota. N Engl J Med 1983; 309:1210–3.

134. Ross AHM, Smith MA, Anderson JR, Small WP. Late mortality after surgery for peptic ulcer. N Engl J Med 1982; 307:519–22.

135. Sonnenberg A. Endoscopic screening for gastric stump cancer: Would it be beneficial? A hypothetical cohort study. Gastroenterology 1984; 87:489–95.

136. Graham DY, Schwartz JT, Cain GD, Gyorkey F. Prospective evaluation of biopsy number in the diagnosis of esophageal and gastric carcinoma. Gastroenterology 1982; 82:228–31.

137. Winawer SJ. Tissue diagnosis in upper gastrointestinal malignancy (Editorial). Gastroenterology 1982; 82:379–82.

138. Green PHR, O'Toole KM, Weinberg LM, Goldfarb JP. Early gastric cancer. Gastroenterology 1981; 81:247–56.

139. Bono JA. Upper gastrointestinal fiberoptic endoscopy reveals the silk suture-line ulcer. Am Surg 1978; 44:282–5.

140. Sivelli R, Farinon AM, Sianesi M, et al. Technetium-99m HIDA hepatobiliary scanning in evaluation of afferent loop syndrome. Am J Surg 1984; 148:262–5.

141. Vennes JA. Applications of endoscopy to the visualization of biliary and pancreatic ducts. Minnesota Med 1973; 56:843–6.

142. Geenen JE, Vennes JA, Silvis SE. Résumé of a seminar on endoscopic retrograde sphincterotomy (ERS). Gastrointest Endosc 1981; 27:31–8.

143. Thon H-J, Loffler A, Buess G, Gheorghiu T. Is ERCP a reasonable diagnostic method for excluding pancreatic and hepatobiliary disease in patients with a Billroth II resection? Endoscopy 1983; 15:93–5.

144. Rosseland AR, Osnes M, Kruse A. Endoscopic sphincterotomy (EST) in patients with Billroth II gastrectomy. Endoscopy 1981; 13:19–24.

145. Safrany L, Neuhaus B, Portocarrero G, Krause S. Endoscopic sphincterotomy in patients with Billroth II gastrectomy. Endoscopy 1980; 12:16–22.

146. Papchristou DN, Fortner JG. Adenocarcinoma of the gastric cardia: The choice of gastrectomy. Ann Surg 1980; 192:58–64.

147. Zacho A, Cederqvist C, Fischerman K. Surgical treatment of gastric malignancies: A twenty-year series comprising mainly far advanced and high-seated tumors. Ann Surg 1974; 179:94–101.

148. Cady B, Ramsden DA, Stein A, Haggitt RC. Gastric cancer. Contemporary aspects. Am J Surg 1977; 133:423–9.

149. Dupont JB Jr, Lee JR, Burton GR, Cohn I Jr. Adenocarcinoma of the stomach: Review of 1,497 cases. Cancer 1978; 41:941–7.

150. Nachlas MM, Crawford DT, Pearl JM. Current status of jejunoileal bypass in the treatment of morbid obesity. Surg Gynecol Obstet 1980; 150:256–70.

151. Hocking MP, Duerson MC, O'Leary JP, Woodward ER. Jejunoileal bypass for morbid obesity: Late follow-up in 100 cases. N Engl J Med 1983; 308:995–9.

152. Halverson JD, Zuckerman GR, Koehler RE, et al. Gastric bypass for morbid obesity: A medical-surgical assessment. Ann Surg 1981; 194:152–60.

153. Thompson WR, Amaral JF, Caldwell MD, et al. Complications and weight loss in 150 consecutive gastric exclusion patients: A clinical review. Am J Surg 1983; 146:602–12.

154. Halverson JD, Koehler RE. Assessment of patients with failed gastric operations for morbid obesity. Am J Surg 1983; 145:357–63.

155. Ellison EC, Martin EW Jr, Laschinger J, et al. Prevention of early failure of stapled gastric partitions in treatment of morbid obesity. Arch Surg 1980; 115:528–33.

156. Wolper JC, Messmer JM, Turner MA, Sugerman HJ. Endoscopic dilation of late stomal stenosis. Arch Surg 1984; 119:836–7.

157. Paulk SC. Formal dilation after gastric partitioning. Surg Gynecol Obstet 1983; 156:502–4.

158. Printen KJ, Scott D, Mason EE. Stomal ulcers after gastric bypass. Arch Surg 1980; 115:525–7.

159. Printen KJ, LeFavre J, Alden J. Bleeding from the bypassed stomach following gastric bypass. Surg Gynecol Obstet 1983; 156:65–6.

160. Madden JL, Chun JY, Kandalaft S, Parekh M. Choledochoduodenostomy: an unjustly maligned surgical procedure? Am J Surg 1970; 119:45–54.

161. McSherry CK, Fischer MG. Common bile duct stones and biliary-intestinal anastomoses. Surg Gynecol Obstet 1981; 153:669–76.

162. Akiyama H, Ikezawa H, Kameya S, et al. Unexpected problems of external choledochoduodenostomy: Fiberscopic examination in 15 patients. Am J Surg 1980; 140:660–5.

163. Siegel JH. Duodenoscopic sphincterotomy in the treatment of the "sump" syndrome. Dig Dis Sci 1981; 26:922–8.

164. Barkin JS, Silvis S, Greenwald R. Endoscopic therapy of the "sump" syndrome. Dig Dis Sci 1980; 25:597–601.

165. Teplick SK, Wolferth CC Jr, Hayes MF Jr, Amrom G. Balloon dilatation of benign postsurgical biliary-enteric anastomotic strictures. Gastrointest Radiol 1982; 7:307–10.

166. Traverso LW, Tompkins RK, Urrea PT, Longmire WP Jr. Surgical treatment of chronic pancreatitis: Twenty-two years' experience. Ann Surg 1979; 190:312–9.

167. Potts JR III, Moody FG. Surgical therapy for chronic pancreatitis: Selecting the appropriate approach. Am J Surg 1981; 142:654–9.

168. Bolman RM III. Surgical management of chronic relapsing pancreatitis. Ann Surg 1981; 193:125–31.

169. Cooperman AM. Chronic pancreatitis. Surg Clin North Am 1981; 61:71–83.

170. Puestow CB, Gillesby WJ. Retrograde surgical drainage of pancreas for chronic relapsing pancreatitis. AMA Arch Surg 1958; 76:898–907.

171. DuVall MK Jr. Caudal pancreatico-jejunostomy for chronic relapsing pancreatitis. Ann Surg 1954; 140:775–85.

172. Kugelberg CH, Wehlin L, Arnesjo B, Tylen U. Endoscopic pancreatography in evaluating results of pancreaticojejunostomy. Gut 1976; 17:267–72.

173. Whipple AO, Parsons WB, Mullins CR. Treatment of carcinoma of the ampulla of Vater. Ann Surg 1935; 102:763–79.

174. Connolly JE, Kwaan JH, McCart PM, et al. Aortoenteric fistula. Ann Surg 1981; 194:402–12.

175. Champion MC, Sullivan SN, Coles JC, et al. Aortoenteric fistula: Incidence, presentation, recognition, and management. Ann Surg 1982; 195:314–7.

176. Perdue GD Jr, Smith RB III, Ansley JD, Costantino MJ. Impending aortoenteric hemorrhage: The effect of early recognition on improved outcome. Ann Surg 1980; 192:237–43.

177. Mir-Madjlessi SH, Sullivan BH Jr, Farmer RG, Beven EG. Endoscopic diagnosis of aortoduodenal fistula. Gastrointest Endosc 1973; 19:187–8.

178. Baker MS, Fisher JH, van der Reis L, Baker BH. The endoscopic diagnosis of an aortoduodenal fistula. Arch Surg 1976; 111:304.

179. Kleinman LH, Towne JB, Bernhard VM. A diagnostic and therapeutic approach to aortoenteric fistulas: Clinical experience with twenty patients. Surgery 1979; 86:868–80.

180. Martin J, Cano N, Di-Costanzo J, Richierei JP. Aortoduodenal fistula: Endoscopic diagnosis. (Letter) Dig Dis Sci 1981; 26:956–7.

Section III

PANCREAS AND BILIARY TRACT: ERCP

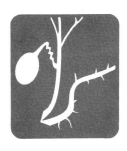

Chapter 25

TECHNIQUE OF ERCP

JACK A. VENNES, M.D.

The pancreas and biliary tree are no longer considered remote areas, as they were in the late 1960's and early 1970's when endoscopic retrograde cholangiopancreatography (ERCP) was introduced. Precise diagnosis is now the rule, and the location and etiology of many abnormalities can be determined with a high degree of accuracy.[1,2]

Present-day economic considerations increasingly favor early use of the most definitive diagnostic and therapeutic measures available. In many cases we now have the ability to select a single test that provides sufficient primary diagnostic detail for sound management choices. The diagnostic test may also be part of a subsequent clinical step, such as ultrasound or computed tomography (CT) with guided needle aspiration cytology, percutaneous transhepatic cholangiography (PTC) with placement of an endoprosthesis across a stricture, or ERCP with endoscopic sphincterotomy.

During the past decade of increasing diagnostic accuracy much has been learned about disease processes. Accurate diagnostic conclusions based on ERCP depend on precise radiographic recording of the normal and abnormal details of one or both ductal systems.[3] To accomplish this efficiently and safely requires attention to technical details, some of which are included in this chapter. Insertion of the cannula into one or the other duct is important, but only a beginning.

ERCP is a sophisticated technique that can be mastered by the trained endoscopist with a reasonable commitment of training time. Guided personal experience greatly facilitates learning; however, specific written instructions on ERCP technique can be useful, particularly if they can be referred to repeatedly as training progresses. There are often several methods for doing things properly; the method described here is only one of these.

Before beginning, some basic requirements for success should be considered: facilities, equipment, personnel, patients, and patience. An x-ray examining room equipped with a high-resolution fluoroscopic monitor and spot film device is required. A radiographic tube with a small focal spot (0.3–0.6 mm) and a large-milliamperage generator produces sharply detailed x-ray images with short exposure times.

ERCP is a two-component procedure—endoscopic and radiologic. The latter consists of high-quality radiographic technique as well as interpretation of results. A team approach with a radiologist is crucial to the initial success with respect to both components. During the initial development of an ERCP routine, it is important to work with one interested radiologist to gradually combine the endoscopic and radiographic techniques into a smooth disciplined routine. With skill, experience, and teamwork, detailed information will be available from only a few well-positioned, coned x-rays; thus there will be less radiation exposure to the patient and the endoscope fiber bundle. After the procedure routine is well established and as the endoscopist gains experience, the presence of a radiologist is usually unnecessary, except in unusual cases.

A trained gastrointestinal assistant is an important team member in ERCP because the procedure frequently takes longer than routine upper and lower gastrointestinal endoscopic procedures and requires the complete attention of the endoscopist, and because patients may require more sedation. For these reasons another experienced observer, and preferably two, should be available to monitor the patient's vital functions, response to medications, and the many items of equipment that may be required during the procedure.

It is advisable to determine early whether the number of patients for whom ERCP is indicated will provide sufficient experience for development and maintenance of proficiency. When skillfully performed, the results of ERCP are accurate and informative; the therapeutic extension of ERCP, endoscopic sphincterotomy, is a major advance. However, when performed with only modest success ERCP is another expensive road to diagnostic equivocation. Moreover, it is frustrating to the endoscopist, the referring physician, and the patient when the desired clinical information is unclear or unavailable despite a lengthy attempt at the procedure.

ERCP can be rewarding or discouraging for the endoscopist. The time required for training varies greatly from person to person, but a certain period of practice with patients is necessary. It is clearly best that this be done with the guidance of an experienced endoscopist who has the ability and patience to teach the procedure. The final prerequisites for learning the procedure are patience and close attention to detail.

ENDOSCOPIC EQUIPMENT FOR ERCP

Side-viewing instruments 120 cm in working length are routinely used for ERCP. Forward-viewing instruments are used only for cannulating the papilla after Billroth II anastomosis. Newer side-viewing instruments greatly improve the efficiency of ERCP because they have a wider angle of view and greater maneuverability. Some have a larger

accessory channel which is useful for therapeutic procedures, but the principal advantage of the larger channel is that it permits aspiration of duodenal contents while a cannula is within the channel (Fig. 25–1). The larger channel accepts the standard 1.6 mm diameter Teflon ERCP cannula which is used with the smaller channel endoscopes. In at least one instrument the axis of the visual field has been angled 15 degrees in a proximal or retrograde direction relative to the axis of the insertion tube. When the tip of this endoscope is deflected to observe the papilla, the additional retroflexion of the visual field provides a more "tucked under" view and facilitates the cephalically directed approach often needed for cholangiography (Fig. 25–2).

Standard commercially available cannulas generally function well, but they should have an indwelling stylus wire long enough to stiffen the section of the cannula that remains outside the duodenoscope during cannulation. This permits a firm finger grip and authoritative advancement of the cannula without crimping. Tapered tip cannulas should be available and may be used successfully when attempts with a standard cannula have failed (Fig. 25–3). Occasionally, cannulation of the minor or accessory papilla is required, and usually this is only possible with use of a cannula with a long tapering tip.

PREPARATION FOR ERCP

If the patient is informed and confident, there is a greater likelihood that the ERCP will be well tolerated, expeditious, and suc-

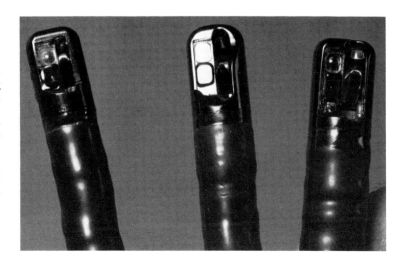

FIGURE 25–1. Side-viewing endoscopes are available with channels and elevators of varying sizes. *Left,* Older instrument with a 2.0 mm diameter channel. *Center,* A modern instrument with wide angle of view has a 2.8 mm diameter channel. *Right,* A "treatment" endoscope has a channel diameter of 4.2 mm. Outer measurements of diameters of distal segments are 10, 12, and 12 mm, respectively.

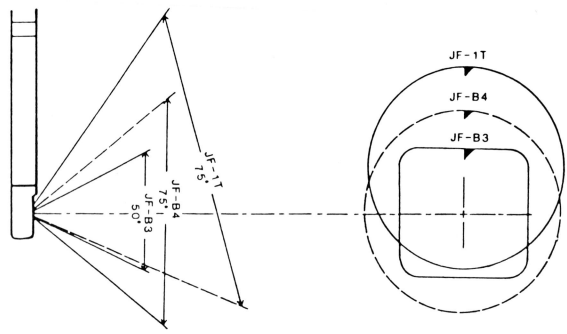

FIGURE 25–2. In this diagram, relative fields of view of three endoscopes are superimposed. Tilting the image retrograde, as shown, frequently permits a more "tucked under" position for viewing the papilla. (Courtesy of H. Ichikawa, Olympus Corp.)

cessful. The risks and indications should be discussed before the actual procedure is undertaken. ERCP can be performed with safety as an outpatient procedure in reasonably healthy patients. Smooth muscle activity

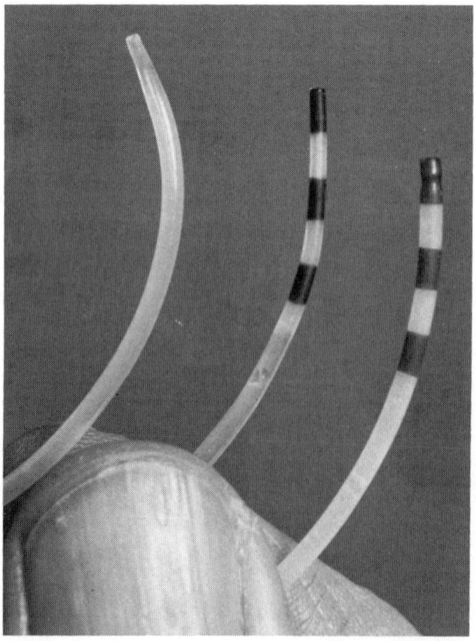

FIGURE 25–3. Standard 1.6-mm Teflon cannulas may be variably tapered at the tip to facilitate ductal entry.

of the duodenum and perhaps of the papilla is related to the emotional state and awareness of the patient. Smooth muscle relaxation is important and is accomplished in large measure by the reassurance of prior discussion, an atmosphere of quiet unhurried competence in the x-ray room, and appropriate medication.

If an obstructing lesion is thought to be present and surgical management is tentatively planned, it should be clearly explained to the patient that, to preclude sepsis, ERCP is being done the day of, or at most a day prior to, surgery. The patient should be informed before the procedure that hospitalization may be necessary in the event of possible sepsis or pancreatitis. In our experience pancreatitis is unlikely and hospitalization for observation is unnecessary if the patient does not experience pain during the procedure or within 2 hours afterward.

The fasting patient lies comfortably on a padded x-ray table. A scout film of the upper abdomen is taken to evaluate any soft tissue densities and to ensure correct radiographic technique. Residual barium in the colon from previous radiographic studies can present a problem (as can oral contrast agent from a recent CT), but satisfactory studies can usually be obtained without interference from overlying contrast material. Medications, prepared in advance for use, are administered through an intravenous line, preferably in the right arm or hand. When the patient is prone or in a left lateral position, the right extremity is preferred for administration of drugs. Opiates such as alphaprodine (Nisentil) or diazepam or both are administered slowly to preclude idiosyncratic reactions or respiratory depression in sensitive (usually elderly) patients. Atropine (0.6 mg) or its equivalent will usually control duodenal motility and will provide some relaxation of ampullary smooth muscle. Glucagon (0.2 mg) can be be given as often as needed during the procedure and provides a 15 to 20 minute period of duodenal atony after each dose. Small amounts of a topical anesthetic are usually used for pharyngeal anesthesia to increase the comfort of the patient. Premedication should be unhurried and precise. Within wide limits, the correct amount of drug administered is that amount the patient requires for comfort. This amount is less if the patient is relaxed and the endoscopist is gentle. Equipment and drugs for cardiopulmonary resuscitation and other emergencies must be available and, as for any procedure that requires premedication, the endoscopist and gastrointestinal assistants must be familiar with and practice the resuscitation techniques and procedures.

Final preparation includes checking the mechanical functions, illumination, and image systems of the endoscopic equipment. ERCP differs from other procedures in at least three respects. First, the mechanism for elevation of the cannula is unique to side-viewing instruments, and this function should be checked before each procedure. Second, vertical and lateral flexion to the maximum limits of the endoscope are frequently required for successful cannulation. If much of this flexion is lost as a result of wear and tear and stretching of the deflection cables, the ease or success of the procedure is compromised.

The third unique characteristic of ERCP is the potential for bacterial infection. Any bacterial contamination of semiclosed spaces must be scrupulously avoided. Unlike all other fiberoptic gastrointestinal endoscopic procedures, there is a potential for septic events, especially cholangitis or formation of a pancreatic abscess.[4] To avoid infection, several additional safeguards are mandatory. Endoscopes should be disinfected after each use; the side-viewing instrument should be soaked in glutaraldehyde and rinsed again just prior to the procedure if the endoscope has been stored.[5] Water bottles and tubing should be disinfected or gas-sterilized after each day's use, and a clean, disinfected, dried bottle and tubing should be used each day. The air-water channel of the instrument should be cleaned and disinfected as part of total care. Since water-loving organisms such as *Pseudomonas* are most frequently responsible for ERCP-related sepsis, it is important that their growth in stored endoscopes is prevented by air-drying the channels prior to storage. For the same reason sterile water should be used in wash bottles to avoid the possibility of *Pseudomonas* contamination from tap water. If all these measures are used in conjunction with the clinical safeguards of appropriate antibiotic usage and timely surgery for relief of obstruction, the complication of exogenously introduced sepsis is virtually eliminated.

BEGINNING THE PROCEDURE

With the patient in the left lateral position, the side-viewing endoscope is gently introduced. It will be easier to turn the patient to the prone position later if the left arm is placed behind the patient before beginning. With the deflection controls unbraked (unlocked) and running free, the endoscope usually traverses the esophagus blindly. If there is resistance to advancement of the instrument, or if some information about the esophagus is desired, gentle downward deflection affords a variably adequate view (especially during withdrawal upon completion of the procedure). The endoscopist should have an appreciation of the usual resistance offered by the cricopharyngeus muscle and the esophagogastric junction, based on prior experience with forward-viewing endoscopes. If there is any question that the resistance to gentle passage of side-viewing instruments is unusual or abnormal, the instrument should be withdrawn and a forward-viewing instrument substituted to investigate the problem.

As the stomach is entered, insufflation will result in a view of gastric mucosa, usually of the proximal lesser curvature. A convention is used for radial orientation of a side-viewing instrument in which 12 o'clock becomes the reference point when the valve projections on the control surface of the endoscope point vertically. Rotating clockwise 90 degrees results in a 3 o'clock position, and so on (Fig. 25–4). As the control head is turned with the wrist, the endoscope tip responds with rotation. If the endoscopist performs the procedure in the standing position, simply turning slightly to the left or right will result in rotation of the tip of the instrument. Grasping and rotating the insertion tube with the right hand, as may be done in colonoscopy, is unnecessary. As the stomach is entered without deflection of the instrument tip, with the control section in the 12 o'clock orientation, and with the patient in the left lateral position, the endoscopic view shows the proximal lesser curvature. The image may be

"redded out," that is, the tip may be on or very close to the mucosa. Rotating counterclockwise, with downward deflection, will usually result in an image of the lumen. From this point, upward deflection to a neutral or slightly upward position in conjunction with advancement of the insertion tube and clockwise rotation will produce a smooth spiraling motion downward into the antrum. Upon entering the stomach, downward deflection may place the instrument tip in the gastric pool. As with end-viewing instruments, it is well to aspirate once and then reinsufflate and proceed, but repetitive time-consuming aspiration and insufflation should be

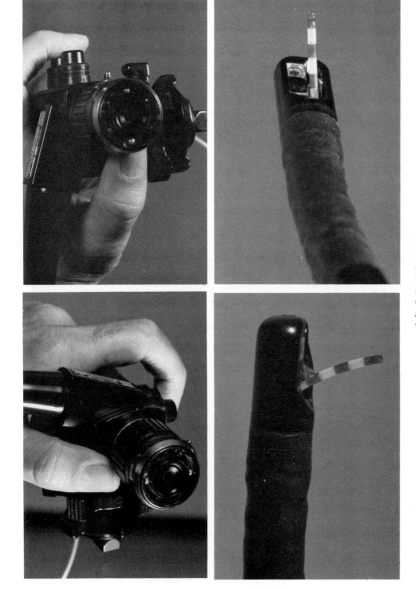

FIGURE 25–4. Endoscope controls and tip at 12 o'clock (*top*) and 3 o'clock (*bottom*) positions. The 12 o'clock view in the stomach is directed to the lesser curvature. In the duodenum of a prone patient, the 12 o'clock view is of the medial wall.

avoided. Stomachs with a cascade configuration can be confusing and appear to have no outlet; it may be necessary to rotate the endoscope to 9 o'clock to get across the spine and out of the pouch, moving clockwise into the antrum.

Depending on clinical considerations, it may be advisable to study the stomach and duodenum on the way to the papilla. When familiar with the side-viewing endoscope, this can be accomplished expeditiously and may be routinely added to each examination. Retroflexion of the side-viewing instrument tends to occur easily in the stomach. Downward deflection of the endoscope tip will usually afford a tubular view of the body of the stomach. In the neutral tip position one is frequently looking at a wall of the stomach; the 12 o'clock position faces the lesser curvature, 3 o'clock the posterior wall, and so on (Fig. 25–4). As with all gastrointestinal endoscopy procedures the image may become obscure; when lost, one should back up, withdraw a bit, insufflate, and look for landmarks.

ENTERING THE DUODENUM

Proceeding from the antrum into the bulb is usually easily accomplished if a few rules are observed. With side-viewing endoscopes, the tip will next advance to the area just disappearing from view at 6 o'clock. As the pylorus is approached with controls in neutral or down-deflected slightly, the pyloric ring sinks into the "setting sun" position. With continued slow advancement and slight upward deflection of the instrument tip as the pyloric ring disappears, the mucosa will suddenly rush by and the next view will be the typical villous mucosa of the duodenal bulb. There are many variations on this usual theme. Hypermotility may require pharmacologic control. As the pylorus is approached it may move laterally from the 6 o'clock position in the field of view. This is managed by locking the lateral flexion control after using it to rotate the pylorus in the visual field to its "proper" 6 o'clock position and then proceeding as usual. In a horizontal stomach the approach to the pylorus will be oblique rather than *en face;* the endoscope will enter the duodenum with the tip in the neutral position, and upward deflection (tip elevation) is not required. The mucosa of the duodenal bulb has a distinctive villous appearance when viewed up close. The superior

aspect and anterior and posterior walls of the bulb can be examined quickly and easily. Some of the floor or inferior aspect of the bulb is usually evident as the endoscope is withdrawn and rotated toward 3 o'clock.

In planning an easy exit from the bulb, recall that it is usually oriented in a somewhat cephalad direction. If the endoscope tip is therefore deflected slightly downward and withdrawn toward the pylorus, the entire length of the bulb will be seen. The apical fold (superior duodenal angle) is usually visible and the entire bulb will be seen to angle upward (cephalad) and turn in a rather straight posterior direction (posterior being more or less to the right with the patient in the left lateral position). Therefore, the endoscope tip should be vertically (upward) deflected to a slight degree, the control section rotated clockwise to 3 o'clock (posteriorly), and the endoscope gently advanced. The view of the lumen is usually lost during this maneuver and mucosa is seen to slide across the visual field. Further rotation to 6 o'clock and slight lateral deflection to the right usually results in a new view of duodenal mucosal folds (plicae). The operator then does whatever is necessary with the controls to safely achieve a tubular view of the lumen ("always pursue lumen" applies here as in the rest of endoscopy). Parenthetically, it is possible to over-organize the maneuvers through the bulb. Leaving the bulb may be as simple as downward deflection in the 12 o'clock position, with some lateral deflection as needed. Remembering that the bulb turns generally in a posterior direction (that is, 3 to 6 o'clock) one can cast about gently using both deflection controls to find and follow the lumen to the descending duodenum. Whichever method is used, a little blind mucosal "slide-by" frequently occurs and, therefore, gentleness is required along with a constant tactile appreciation of the degree of resistance encountered, since obstructing lesions can be overlooked visually with side-viewing instruments. If the endoscope tip does not advance smoothly, partial withdrawal may uncoil the insertion tube in the stomach so that the tip moves easily into the distal duodenum. As soon as the descending duodenum is entered, the patient should be turned to a prone position. This is equivalent to further rotation of the instrument in a clockwise direction (except that in this case the patient is rotated), which facilitates a tubular view of the duodenum that can be maintained with minimal insufflation and also affords the best position for later imaging of both ductal systems with contrast medium.

VIEWING THE PAPILLA

As the descending duodenum is entered and the patient is turned to a prone position, the control section of the endoscope is oriented to the 12 o'clock position. The papilla will frequently be sighted as the tubular view of the lumen unfolds, but it may be lost again as the patient is turned. Assume that the endoscope tip has advanced to the mid-descending duodenum and the papilla is located somewhat proximal to this point; the medial wall of the duodenum will now be viewed directly. A slow, steady withdrawal of the endoscope with scanning of the posteromedial wall from 10 to 2 o'clock in the visual field should be initiated. Clues to the location of the papilla include (1) a vertical fold running perpendicularly across and often disrupting the transverse duodenal folds and (2) a trickle of bile on the mucosa. Following either in a proximal direction will lead to the major papilla. If there is peristaltic activity it should be controlled with intravenous glucagon, because a relatively immobile duodenum is necessary for early discovery of the papilla. With wide-angle endoscopes the papilla is usually found without difficulty. Most often it has a round pink or red face with papillary folds, concentric rings, or a central dimple.

One reason for failure to locate the papilla is premature termination of the proximally moving search pattern. There is a tendency for the novice to avoid withdrawal to the bulb because of a largely unfounded concern about falling back into the antrum: that is, that the instrument can only be reinserted to the descending duodenum with difficulty. The descending duodenum often courses posteriorly, then caudad; the fold at this turn may be mistaken for the bulb and the search may be stopped just short of the papilla.

Another luminal bulge proceeds *cephalad* from the papilla as a broader band that typically merges with the duodenal wall after crossing one or two duodenal folds. This is the *intramural segment* of the distal common bile duct seen as it obliquely traverses the duodenal wall. Its length varies, and this is important to endoscopic sphincterotomy in that the intramural segment defines the an-atomic limits of a safe incision. The longitudinal axis of the intramural segment is also of importance in the success of ERCP, because the cannula must be precisely aligned with this axis for bile duct cannulation. The intramural segment may not be apparent initially if the folds that cross the papilla are prominent. These are referred to as hooded folds. The redder color of the papilla may be the main clue in the initial search for the papilla, since the papillary bulge or mound may be obscured by overlying folds (duodenal plicae). When the tip of the papilla is discovered, the hooded folds may be laid back, using the cannula as a probe, to reveal the entire structure.

APPROACHING THE PAPILLA

Positioning the papillary surface in the field of view is the single most important component of a successful procedure. Seen up close and directly *en face*, the orifice(s) is usually evident and is cannulated with most authority and success from a precisely angulated vantage point. Attempts at cannulation at some distance from the papilla are often haphazard, permissive, and unsuccessful. The detail of the papillary structure must be visualized, approach angles and points of contact must be precise, and cannula advancement should be forceful and smoothly coordinated for consistent success.

Cannulation is at times easily accomplished by trial and error, but typically a series of sequential maneuvers works best. With the deflection controls in neutral and at 12 o'-clock, the patient prone, and the endoscope usually in a partially advanced or greater curve position, the medial wall of the descending duodenum will be in view. The term *greater curve position* refers to placement of the insertion tube along the greater curvature of the stomach so that a loop is formed within the stomach (Fig. 25–5). The papilla will first be sighted in the left of the visual field facing obliquely somewhere to the right and caudad (Fig. 25–6). The deflection controls are braked (partially locked) and the cannula, which has already been filled with contrast medium, should be passed just far enough into the field of view so that its axis and trajectory are evident. The endoscope should then be rotated counterclockwise with the left hand, which will center the papilla in the visual field. Next, right lateral deflection of the instrument tip (that is, clockwise motion

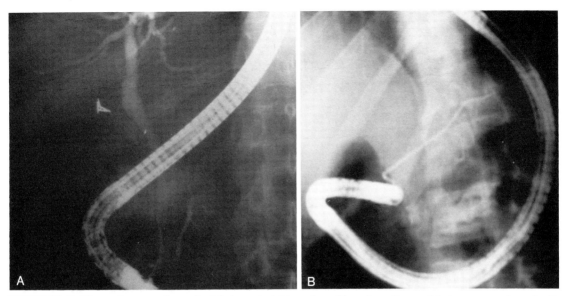

FIGURE 25–5. The endoscope shown in *A* is in a straightened position along the gastric lesser curvature. In *B*, the endoscope is advanced to a greater curvature (loop) position. Optimal cannulating positions frequently lie somewhere between. The papilla typically appears on the left side of the endoscopic view in the advanced position and on the right side in the straightened position.

of the outermost deflection knob) will result in rotation of the axis of the papilla so that it is approximately in line with the anticipated vector of the cannula (see Fig. 25–6). The endoscope tip should be moved close to the papilla by a variable combination of upward (vertical) flexion and advancement and withdrawal of the insertion tube. At this point only small, fine motions will be needed to precisely align the cannula with the presumed axis of the ampulla.

There are several important variations of these standard maneuvers. Cannulation of the common duct frequently requires that the papilla be approached from right to left, since the duct follows this course on entering the duodenal wall (Fig. 25–7). This right-to-left orientation is usually easier to achieve if the endoscope is slowly withdrawn to a straightened lesser curvature position. In the lesser curvature position, the insertion tube follows a relatively straight course along the lesser curvature of the stomach from cardia to descending duodenum. The maneuver to this position is sometimes referred to as the "straightening maneuver." When the instru-

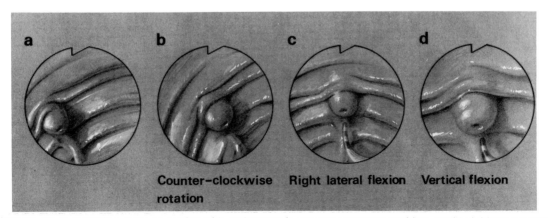

FIGURE 25–6. Squaring away on papilla with endoscope in greater curvature position. Papilla initially appears on left, pointing down and to right (*a*); papilla is centered by rotating endoscope, in a counter-clockwise direction toward it (*b*); next, axes of papilla and cannula are (roughly) aligned with right lateral flexion (*c*); papilla is then brought up close by advancing and withdrawing the endoscope and by vertical flexion (*d*). Fine tuning can now begin.

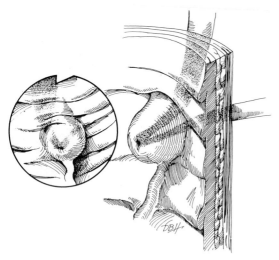

FIGURE 25–7. Shaded areas outline courses of biliary system and pancreatic duct. Bile duct pursues immediately cephalad course, often with a lateral "jog" in its intrapapillary terminus. Pancreatic duct typically does not course immediately upward and, in the lateral plane, moves straight or to the right.

ment is in this configuration, the length of insertion tube within the patient is typically only 60 to 70 cm (see Fig. 25–5). The lesser curvature position contrasts with the looped greater curvature position. Both positions as well as intermediate ones can be appreciated fluoroscopically. The straightening maneuver is accomplished with controls braked, full right lateral deflection, and slow steady withdrawal of the insertion tube, frequently with the addition of clockwise rotation by the left hand and wrist. The image of the papilla will move from the left to the right side of the visual field, and an oblique, right-to-left, close-up position is usually possible.

To review, the standard maneuvers for squaring the papilla in the visual field when in the greater curvature position include counterclockwise rotation of the endoscope combined with right lateral deflection. In the straightened position, clockwise rotation and left lateral deflection are often most useful. If these maneuvers are initially memorized and then practiced, they will in time begin to make sense and will become reflexive.

The initial position achieved in the duodenum may be the straightened one, and it may be unnecessary to change this instrument configuration; that is, initial entry to the descending duodenum may have resulted in immediate identification of the papilla in the right of the visual field without much deflection of the instrument tip and certainly not in a fully developed greater curvature position.

Another frequent variation of the usual configuration of the papilla is the caudal orientation (Fig. 25–8). This may occur as a normal variant and is often associated with a prominent intramural bile duct segment proximal to the papilla. Impacted stones in the distal common duct produce the most marked examples of this variant in which the papilla is large and bulging as well as oriented caudally. Cannulation of the downward deflected papilla requires that the endoscope be positioned distal (below) the papilla, and then turned back up (upward tip deflection) in a "tucked-under" position (Fig. 25–9). Actually, this is a good position with most papillas for entry into the common duct because the duct has an immediate cephalad course in the papilla. The tucked-under position thus orients the cannula in this cephalically directed plane (Fig. 25–10).

The rather structured lock-step maneuvers described above are useful but insufficient by themselves. These standard maneuvers are highly interrelated and varied, and some hours of practice time are always necessary to refine hand-eye coordination.

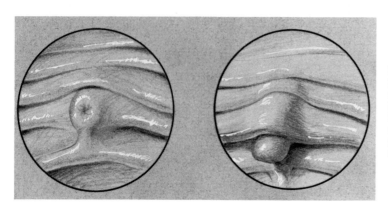

FIGURE 25–8. Two basic papilla positions. *Left,* papilla face looks directly out into duodenum; *right,* papilla is directed caudad. The orifice is directed down also, and successful cannulation requires lifting papilla with a cannula or flexing endoscope tip up under papilla.

FIGURE 25–9. Standard endoscope positions. *Left,* Instrument is straightened along the
lesser curvature of the stomach.
Center, A good working position
is frequently between extremes,
as in this drawing. *Right,*
Greater curvature, or extended,
position, is depicted. The
"tucked-under" position for
viewing the papilla, as also illustrated on the right, is usually
obtained in intermediate endoscope positions.

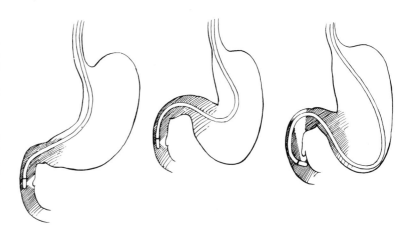

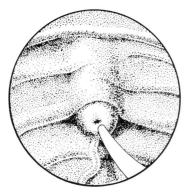

FIGURE 25–10. "Tucked-under" view of Vaterian segment. Intramural bile duct courses cephalad from
papilla. Advancing cannula easily follows cephalad
course of the duct in this endoscope position.

When the papilla has been identified and
brought into the closest possible position, it
is tempting to attack immediately, cannula at
the ready. Not quite yet. The locking mechanism for the deflection controls should be
used to brake (partially lock) both controls,
if this has not been already done. The papilla
should be observed carefully for evidence of
a duct orifice, or even the presence of two
orifices. With the patient fully medicated and
duodenal atony complete, it is often desirable
to watch for two minutes. Whether the papillary surface is smooth or papillomatous, an
opening may become evident as a transiently
appearing minute black hole. Lacking this,
the orifice may be evident as a punctate
depression, a small cluster of fine papillomatous fronds, or a spot that is redder than
the rest of the papillary tip. If the face of the
papilla is round, the orifice is usually in the
middle, especially if there appear to be concentric rings. Occasionally a tissue flap or
"trap door" overlies the orifice(s) and must
be lifted aside with the cannula tip.

A second orifice is present in less than 10%
of patients, and the best opportunity for this
discovery is by initial close observation before
the papilla is traumatized with the cannula.
If the two orifices lie in a vertical plane in
the visual field, the cephalad opening always
belongs to the biliary tree. If the two orifices
lie on a horizontal plane, the left (or posterior) orifice is in continuity with the biliary
tract. An imaginary but useful concept is
demonstrated in this regard in Figure 25–11.

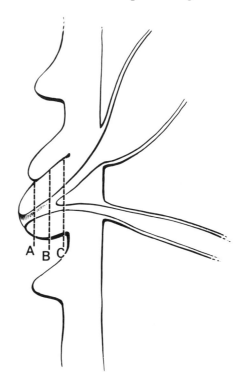

FIGURE 25–11. Three possibilities are conceptually
related in this drawing. If the ductal junction protrudes
successively toward the duodenal lumen, or as one
"slices" the papilla, the following relationships can be
seen: a short common channel (usual) (*A*), a long
common channel (*B*), or separate orifices (*C*).

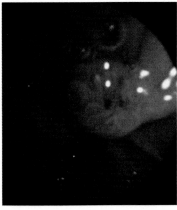

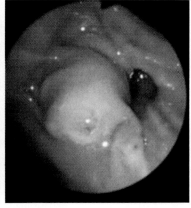

PLATE 25–1. Papilla of Vater with two separate orifices. Common duct drains via the cephalad orifice. A juxta-ampullary diverticulum is present posteriorly.

PLATE 25–2. Normal papilla viewed from below in "tucked under" position. Bulge coursing cephalad from papillary orifice is made by common duct segment that traverses the duodenal wall. Juxta-ampullary diverticulum is evident on the right (anterior).

PLATE 25–1.   PLATE 25–2.

If the combined ductal systems are imagined to protrude successively toward the duodenum, or if one figuratively "slices" the papilla, any of three relationships may be seen, namely a long common channel, a short common channel (the usual circumstance), and separate orifices. In the last-named instance the common duct lies in a cephalad position or to the left of the pancreatic duct orifice as it follows its normal course. The two orifices may be obvious and separated by 2 mm or less (Plate 25–1). Rarely a second small black hole can be seen on the rim of a main or larger opening. Time is saved and the probability of a successful result increases if these observations are made before cannulation is attempted.

The details of the now precisely mapped papilla should be memorized. Edema or friability may occur early in the course of attempted cannulation in some patients and obscure fine papillary detail; thus the opportunity to make these necessary observations is lost. At some point it is also desirable to briefly move the tip of the instrument away from the papilla to gain an impression of the apparent course of the common duct in the intramural ridge proximal to the papillary opening.

Next, with the tip of the cannula (filled with contrast medium) positioned at the periphery of the visual field, the controls braked, the patient prone, and the duodenum at rest, the papilla is brought as close as possible to the instrument tip. The axis of the cannula and of the desired duct are now aligned by a series of fine tuning micromaneuvers. The coordinated movements described earlier may now be repeated in miniature. If the papilla lies in the left of the visual field with the instrument in greater curvature position, the required small moves

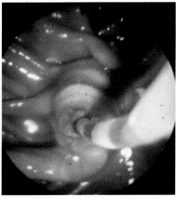

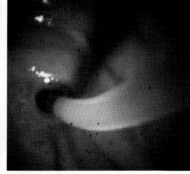

PLATE 25–3. Cannulation of biliary duct. The papilla is viewed from below; hence the cannula is oriented somewhat cephalad. The cannula tip is elevated as it enters the orifice, rising over the septum, and initially angled slightly from right to left.

PLATE 25–4. Cannulation of pancreatic duct. The papilla is best approached directly without cephalad orientation. In the lateral plane, the cannula is directed straight in or from left to right.

PLATE 25–3.   PLATE 25–4.

for alignment will be some combination of counterclockwise rotation and right lateral tip deflection (see Fig. 25–6). Conversely, the moves will be clockwise rotation and left lateral tip deflection if the endoscope is pulled up to the straightened lesser curvature position and the papilla is therefore in the right side of the visual field. In either configuration an optimal close approach is also the result of advancement or withdrawal of the insertion tube plus vertical tip deflection. The common duct tends to course to the left and immediately cephalad in the endoscopic view, whereas the pancreatic duct tends to travel straight through the papilla and to the right (see Fig. 25–7). If respiratory motion is a problem, alignment and cannulation must be timed with the phases of respiration or the motion can be reduced by turning the patient from the prone to right oblique position. "Cheap shots" should not be taken by lunging with the cannula at a papillary target which is moving or not in position; this will not succeed, it is a waste of time, and the trauma of futile attempts may obscure important details.

The cannula and duct should be aligned before cannulation. Precise location of the cannula tip is primarily a left-hand function which utilizes slight rotatory movements of the endoscope (left wrist or turning the whole body) and elevation of the cannula as needed. The left thumb controls the cannula elevator of the endoscope. The cannula is advanced smoothly but with authority by the right hand as the tip is precisely directed with the left. As the cannula tip engages the papillary orifice, it should be held firmly in position by pressure on the cannula and elevator.

At this point one of several things occur. The cannula may pass freely into a duct, in which case it is most probably in the bile duct but may be in a long, straight cephalad-directed section of the pancreatic system. Injection of a minimal amount of contrast agent under fluoroscopic control will identify the location. Frequently, the cannula traverses the soft folds of the papilla, but stops after advancing 3 to 10 mm. The tip should be held in place firmly but gently while making small corrections in the trajectory of the cannula with the cannula elevator and the vertical and lateral deflection controls. It is helpful to imagine that the cannula tip is seeking its way through more fronds and blind passages into the main channel. A more directive approach with orientation of the

catheter in specific directions may be of use later in the procedure, but at this stage firm but not forceful advancement of the cannula tip may cause it to slide into a free position in the ampulla or one of the ducts. If this is not successful, the lateral deflection control can be used to alter the axis of the cannula somewhat while the tip is firmly within the orifice of the papilla. If this does not succeed in moving the cannula into a free position, the vertical axis should be changed by advancing or withdrawing the cannula. (In making these minor changes in either the horizontal or vertical axis or both, the cannula should nevertheless remain pointed in the general direction of the duct to be opacified first.) When free in either duct, the cannula may remain stationary with about 1 to 2 cm of its length within the duct, or it may move further into the duct for a variable distance. Most commercially available cannulas are marked at the distal end to help estimate the length of the cannula that has been inserted into the ampulla. Generally the spacing of the marks is at 3 mm intervals.

If the cannula tip seems to be impacted and does not respond to the gentle but firm maneuvers described above, a small amount of contrast material can be injected under fluoroscopic control. The cannula may already be in direct contact with the duct, either impacted at the furthest possible point or angulated against the wall of the duct; if this is the case, the desired x-ray study may be obtainable from this impacted position. During such an injection the cannula may move unassisted to a free position. This may be helpful if the impacted cannula happens to be in a common channel, as filling of both ducts will result. This provides an immediate reference as to the position of both ducts. However, simultaneous filling to complete opacification of both ducts should be avoided if possible because of the potential for over-filling the pancreatic duct, which has a much smaller capacity for contrast than the biliary system. Overfilling may predispose to pancreatitis. Another minor problem with injection of contrast agent when the cannula is impacted is that contrast medium refluxes into the duodenum and collects within the duodenal bulb or stomach of the prone patient, in which locations it often overlies parts the pancreas and biliary system and thus obscures radiographic detail. When injecting from an impacted position, one duct (not necessarily the desired one) may be opacified, but not the other system. Then the cannula should be withdrawn slightly, because the wedged tip may have resulted in a coaption of the opposite walls of the duct as a result of stretching and the general deformity of the anatomic structures produced by the wedged cannula. If so, withdrawal and reinjection may result in ductal opacification.

When the cannula has been placed precisely, it may initially pass freely into a duct. It may be held up after entry for 5 to 10 mm, and then after further manipulation it may move further inward into an unrestricted position, or it may remain impacted. The various maneuvers described above may result in a successful procedure.

PROBLEMS IN APPROACHING THE PAPILLA

A squared-away, *en face* position close to the papilla is occasionally difficult to achieve despite application of the usual maneuvers and principles. Prior gastric or duodenal surgery may be the problem if the duodenum is fixed in position or if its normal course is altered. The papilla may be "relocated" to a position nearer the bulb or in a further posterior position, particularly after a Billroth I anastomosis. Such changes in position of the papilla present some difficulty but are usually manageable.

Another cause for such difficulty is a malfunctioning endoscope. The maximum degree of deflection of the distal bending segment of the endoscope is frequently required for successful studies. With heavy usage the control wires may stretch, and this reduces the deflection capability of the instrument. Although this is uncommon in newer model endoscopes, it may nevertheless occur gradually and not be detected unless the instrument is tested periodically to be certain that deflection of the distal tip meets the manufacturer's specifications.

A third reason for an inability to approach the papilla closely is failure to use all available insertion levels of the endoscope. Most endoscopists are familiar with the fully inserted or greater curvature position *(vide supra)*, and many will withdraw the instrument to what they consider a straightened or lesser curvature position. However, the normal postbulbar duodenum frequently courses posteriorly from the bulb and then turns in a caudad direction. When proceeding from a deeply inserted greater curvature configuration, this

junction between the caudally directed and horizontal sections will be viewed up close. If this point is mistaken for the bulb, the examiner may stop the straightening maneuver without ever achieving a full lesser curvature straightened position or without examining the horizontal segment that may contain the papilla.

Unusual anatomic relationships may require maneuvers other than the customary ones. It may be useful to attempt to approach the papilla after returning the patient to the left lateral position. It may be advantagous not to suppress duodenal motility, when it reappears, with further doses of glucagon, because the motion of the duodenal wall may bring the papilla close enough for cannulation. Generally this must be timed to the motility phases or respiratory motion and requires skill and practice. In some cases the papilla may be brought closer to the instrument tip by simply deflating the duodenum.

As a last resort, cannulation across a greater than ideal distance can be attempted. A previously unused cannula can sometimes be used to correct problems encountered in approaching the papilla. A new cannula will remain relatively straight at the distal tip before it assumes a curved shape by repeated usage. This may be useful if it is necessary to attempt cannulation at a distance. On occasion, a cannula will veer off course as it is advanced toward the papilla. This can occur when the cannula has acquired a spiral shape in addition to the usual curve at the distal end. This can sometimes be corrected during the procedure by moving the cannula repeatedly in and out of the accessory channel with the cannula elevator in a half-raised position.

Finally, the situation may arise where it is possible to approach the papilla closely enough for cannulation, but the axis of the cannula stubbornly remains unaligned with the presumed duct axis. This means that the cannula only approaches the axis of the ampulla in a tangential fashion. While this may seem to be the only alternative, such tangential passes usually do not work. In addition to other measures already discussed, an "impaling" technique may be appropriate. The cannula is advanced so that the tip engages the orifice. Then the cannula tip is held at the orifice of the papilla using the elevator, the deflection controls are locked, and the cannula is swung into proper alignment by smoothly rotating the insertion tube or using the lateral deflection controls or both. Generally some trial and error is required to determine the best sequence of maneuvers to bring the cannula into an alignment that is calculated to be in line with the axis of the ampulla.

PROBLEMS IN DUCTAL FILLING

Injection of contrast medium may not fill either duct despite a close *en face* position with the catheter impacted. There are several possible explanations for this. Most frequently, the orifice has not been precisely identified. Rarely a large minor papilla (the accessory duct of Santorini) may be mistaken for the major papilla (the duct of Wirsung) which may be only a few centimeters distal in position, perhaps hidden by a bend or duodenal fold. It is also possible that the ducts may take an unusual course through the Vaterian segment (papilla and duodenal wall). Various aspects of this small but complex anatomic area are discussed in Chapters 27 and 33.

There are several obvious solutions to the problem of non-filling. The papilla should be re-examined unhurriedly at close range for evidence of an orifice that was overlooked at initial inspection. The more distal aspect of the duodenum should be examined to be certain that the major papilla has not escaped notice. Inexperience may lead to attempts at cannulation of all manner of folds and depressions that are not in reality the papilla. When certain of the correct anatomic structure, and when the above measures including those for realigning the axis of the catheter have failed, a tapered tip cannula should be used. When the papilla appears papillomatous or protruded with no obvious orifice, success is often a matter of patient, systematic probing for the proper orifice and axis from multiple directions, including those which are seemingly tangential in alignment. This is not necessarily traumatic, although care must be exercised in the use of this type of cannula. When advanced forcefully, especially after a long unsuccessful attempt at cannulation and opacification, intramural injection of contrast medium may appear as a gray bulbous swelling. While this is worrisome in appearance, intramural injection has not to my knowledge led to morbid events. However, an event such as this indicates that it is time (or past time) to stop. When a procedure is unsuccessful, a point is reached at which the patient's tolerance will soon be exceeded and the endoscopist becomes too fatigued to be effective. Dogged persistence beyond this point does not increase skill or success.

FILLING THE DESIRED DUCT

ERCP is a useful procedure only if either ductal system can be visualized with predictability so that precise diagnostic information can be acquired in the majority of cases. Failure to obtain a cholangiogram when management decisions depend heavily on knowledge of the details of biliary anatomy is an extremely vexing problem.

An understanding of the anatomy of the Vaterian segment is necessary for resolution of this problem. For the purpose of this discussion, consider that the papilla has been approached closely and is in a squared-away, *en face* position in the visual field of the endoscope. In general the pancreatic duct courses through the duodenal wall without much, if any, cephalad orientation. In the lateral plane (as observed endoscopically) the course of the duct is to the right (medial) of the papilla. The common bile duct usually follows an immediate cephalad course in the vertical plain, even within its intrapapillary portion (see Fig. 25–7). In the lateral plane, however, the bile duct frequently turns to the left (posteriorly) for a short intrapapillary distance before turning back in line with the vertical axis of the duodenum. This short, initial posterior swing does occur, although the intraduodenal bile duct imprint running proximal to the papilla in parallel with the vertical duodenal axis seemingly belies its existence.

The other anatomic correlate to keep firmly in mind is the variable presence of a common channel. It is most useful to assume that a short common channel exists, beyond which there is a septum dividing the two ductal systems (Fig. 25–12). In order to unify the concept of an initial leftward (posterior) turn in the course of the bile duct with the concept of a common channel that is shortly in its course divided by a septum that defines the two ducts, it is useful to visualize the septum as being *functionally* rotated toward a vertical position relative to the long axis of the duodenum.

With these anatomic concepts in mind, the biliary tree can be cannulated with about the same frequency as the pancreatic system. This requires a tight vertical orientation of

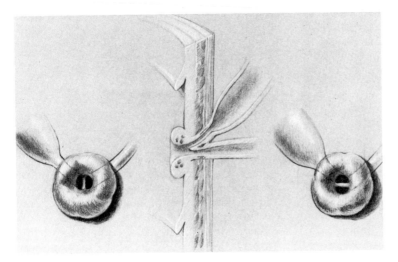

FIGURE 25–12. Center, sagittal section showing usual short channel. Beyond it is a septum dividing the two ductal systems shown on right. The need to raise the cannula along the roof of the channel in order to enter the bile duct is evident in the diagram at the right. It is helpful to combine this with the frequent initial leftward course of the common duct, which *conceptually* rotates the septum toward vertical as seen on the diagram to the left. The relationships are exaggerated for emphasis in this figure. The usual vertical course of the bile duct, once it is outside of the duodenum, is shown in center of the figure.

the cannula tip, and frequently this must be combined with an initial right-to-left course through the distal intrapapillary portion. This can be visualized by imagining a clock face over the *en face* papilla centered on the ampullary orifice. The proscribed right-to-left course now proceeds from some point in the quadrant between 3 and 6 toward the quadrant demarcated by 9 and 12 on the clock face. The tight vertical orientation must be applied to the cannula tip just as it enters the papilla so as to lift it over the nearby septum. Once the cannula is "trapped" on the pancreatic side of the septum, no maneuver will succeed in biliary visualization.

Successful vertical orientation of the cannula depends on two more factors. First, it must be determined whether the endoscope tip is above, at, or below the level of the papilla in the duodenum (Fig. 25–13). The papilla is easy to identify with modern instruments with wide-angle visual fields, but the position of the tip of the instrument relative to the level of the papilla may not be apparent by reference to the visual field alone. A close

orientation to the papilla is possible by vertical flexion of the instrument tip, but if this is done from an instrument tip position that is proximal to the level of the papilla, vertical flexion of the cannula for bile duct entry is not possible. The appearance of the transverse duodenal folds is often a clue to the position of the instrument tip relative to the papilla (see Fig. 25–13). If the pancreatic duct has been opacified, the position of the tip can be determined fluoroscopically. The bile duct can sometimes be entered from a position at the level of the papilla by pulling the cannula and hence the papilla upward with the elevator as the cannula tip enters the orifice. This will orient the cannula in a cephalad or vertical direction in the general direction of the bile duct. However, this is not always effective, and the obvious choice of position for vertical catheter deflection is that distal to the papilla, from which position the instrument tip can be deflected upward to approach the papilla closely in a vertical or cephalad orientation, which almost looks retrograde along the course of the descend-

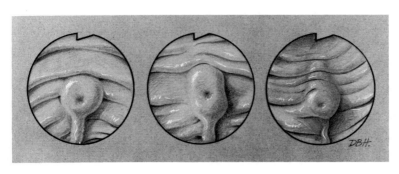

FIGURE 25–13. Appearance of papilla from three endoscopic vantage points. *Left to right*, endoscope is positioned above, opposite, and below papilla. Direction of the plicae longitudinalis in endoscopic field identifies each position. For example, plicae appear concave downward when viewed from above the papilla, as depicted in the drawing on the left.

ing duodenum. This is sometimes referred to as the tucked-under position. (Plates 25–2 and 25–3).

A related factor of importance is the direction the papilla takes as it enters the duodenum. This may be perpendicular to the duodenal wall or it may be directed downward or distally into the duodenum (see Fig. 25–8). A variable degree of downward direction is the usual situation with most normal papillas. This caudad orientation becomes extreme when a stone is impacted in the intramural duct, pushing the papilla outward and downward.

With all these anatomic considerations in mind, free cannulation of the biliary tree is often straightforward. If the endoscope tip is stationed opposite the papilla, the cannula tip is lifted strongly with the left thumb on the elevator just as it disappears into an orifice. If the endoscope tip is tucked under (that is, advanced beyond the papilla and then vertically flexed to a close position), it is often simply a matter of threading the cannula along the visible axis of the intramural segment (see Fig. 25–10) as though it were crawling up under duodenal mucosa. To this vertical or cephalad trajectory of the cannula tip, a short, initial right-to-left course may be added in a coordinated fashion as the catheter is advanced (see Fig. 25–7). This is accomplished by rotating the papilla face slightly to the left in the endoscopic view, usually by means of lateral deflection of the tip, so that the cannula tip not only will follow a cephalad course but also will sweep slightly right to left across the papillary surface (see Fig. 25–7).

To summarize: From a position opposite the papilla, the cannula tip, and thus the papilla itself, can be forcefully lifted as the cannula is advanced to enter the duct above the septum. From a tucked-under position, the cannula is already pointed in a cephalad direction. Entry into the bile duct from either of these positions frequently requires the addition of a short coordinated move to the left before moving straight up the axis of the intramural portion of the bile duct.

These are standard maneuvers which are important for consistent cannulation of the bile duct, but unfortunately they are not always sufficient. Therefore other strategies are necessary for consistent cholangiography. If the pancreatic duct is cannulated initially and identified by partial filling with 1 to 2 ml of contrast agent, it may be possible to enter the common duct by withdrawing the cannula until all but the distal 3 to 4 mm remains in the duct. Then, with the deflection controls braked, the cannula tip can be moved cephalad and to the left by means of rotation of the insertion tube or use of the deflection controls or both. If a significant common channel is present, this maneuver may permit re-advancement of the cannula into the biliary system. The endoscope position can be changed, proceeding to a more or less tucked-under position. The best tucked-under orientation is often found when the instrument configuration in the stomach is midway between the fully advanced greater curvature and fully straightened lesser curvature instrument configurations in combination with acute vertical deflection of the instrument tip. Other positions should be tried in a systematic fashion. This can include a nearly perpendicular catheter entry, a cephalad orientation (but to the right rather than left), an exaggeration of the standard right-to-left directedness so that the catheter is nearly tangential in its approach. A tapered cannula may be used. This may be helpful in separating the two ducts if the common channel is very short or nonexistent. A change in the patient's position to an oblique or lateral one will change the position of the papilla relative to the tip of the instrument. This type of minor alteration may be sufficient for successful cannulation. Previous maneuvers can be repeated from a position very near the papilla for authoritative cannula control. A careful search should be made for a minute second orifice to the left or cephalad to the identified one. It is important to be certain that the accessory papilla has not been mistaken for the major papilla.

If the systematic approach using all these maneuvers fails, then it is best to stop and attempt the procedure again in a few days if this is still warranted by the clinical circumstances. About half the time such repeat attempts are successful, perhaps because of greater familiarity with and consideration of the technical aspects of the problem. Furthermore, the edema and inflammation resulting from the initial attempts will have subsided. However, further procedures beyond a second attempt are unlikely to succeed. Note also that failure to cannulate either or both ductal systems is not reliable evidence for a ductal abnormality or papillary stenosis.

Usually the pancreatic system is readily

entered by approaching the papilla in a straight perpendicular direction with the cannula or from left to right in the lateral plane (left to right on the imaginary clock face) (Plate 25–4). Generally a position close to the papilla works best. However, a tucked-under position is undesirable for pancreatography. The tucked-under position can be changed to a more optimal one by withdrawing the insertion tube slightly or advancing to a full greater curvature position.

RADIOLOGIC CONSIDERATIONS

It is a good rule to fill the clinically relevant duct with contrast agent first, if this is feasible; then, filling the opposite system will not interfere with either entry or radiographic visualization of the ductal system in question. It is possible that a duct filled with contrast medium will at times keep the walls of the contiguous duct coapted and thus interfere with cannulation and opacification. Therefore, the initial part of the study period when conditions are optimal should concentrate on the ductal system of major clinical interest. If the clinical question concerns the bile duct, approaching this duct first will reduce the possibility of pancreatitis. This is often the prime reason for attempting cannulation of the biliary system first. It is likely, based on studies in animals, that acute ERCP-induced pancreatitis is in part a function of ductal filling pressure and duration of ductal filling.[6] During attempted cholangiography it is not unusual to enter the pancreatic duct repeatedly and to confirm this position each time by contrast injection. This may leave the pancreatic duct filled with contrast agent to a variable degree for an appreciable period of time. If the pancreatic duct is filled completely with contrast medium initially and this is followed by repeated unsuccessful attempts at cannulation of the biliary system, inadvertent overfilling of the already opacified pancreatic ductal system may occur.

Fluoroscopic confirmation of cannula position is frequently necessary during ERCP. This can be done by injecting a small amount of contrast agent. It is also accomplished by noting cannula position relative to the distal portions of a duct(s) already outlined by contrast medium. For example, when the cannula slips into the bile duct, this is evident fluoroscopically if the cannula position is obviously separate from the contrast agent–filled pancreatic duct. Alternately, the cannula may be seen fluoroscopically as being still within an already opacified duct. In this case, further injection of contrast medium to confirm the position of the catheter is not necessary. This is useful in avoiding overfilling of an already opacified pancreatic duct when trying to cannulate the biliary system.

Modern fiberoptic endoscopes are not impervious to radiation damage to fiber bundles. It is essential to minimize radiation to the endoscope as well as to the patient and personnel. This can be done by frequent use of coning shutters, by restricting the number of spot films to the minimum necessary for complete demonstration of the ductal system, and by withdrawing the endoscope into the antrum out of the radiation field when taking multiple spot films. Fluoroscopy time can be minimized by use of brief interrupted views to check instrument and cannula positions and to monitor opacification of the ducts. All these measures require a disciplined intention to reduce radiation. They then require periodic re-attention, as they tend to be forgotten, especially in the early stages of training in the procedure. Judicious use of x-rays is an important component in the skillful performance of ERCP.

SPECIAL CIRCUMSTANCES

Prior gastroduodenal surgery is a special problem for the endoscopist, as mentioned above. The patient who has had a subtotal gastrectomy and Billroth II gastrojejunostomy presents the greatest challenge.[7, 8] The first problem is to identify and enter the afferent loop, this being accomplished best with a forward-viewing endoscope. The next problem is to traverse the afferent loop safely and successfully. This will be a highly variable distance which depends on the prerogative of the surgeon. Next, the papilla must be located, and this too is best done with a small-caliber forward-viewing endoscope. The final problem is to identify and cannulate the orifices; at this point a side-viewing instrument might be preferable.

All things considered, it is usually best to begin with a small-diameter forward-viewing endoscope when the patient has had a Billroth II gastrojejunostomy. The afferent loop may be located in the visual field to the right or left of the efferent loop. Its lumen is frequently less evident and may be tucked into a corner. Afferent loop secretions are usually bile-tinged, and this observation is sometimes helpful in separating the two possible channels. The lumen of the efferent loop is likely to be more evident and will proceed in a straight caudad direction as seen endoscopically or fluoroscopically. Once the afferent loop is entered it is necessary to gently negotiate the various abrupt turns. This may require techniques that are more familiar in colonoscopy with frequent withdrawal and straightening of the insertion tube as loops form. The afferent loop may be fixed in position as a result of fibrous adhesions, in which case the difficulty may be increased. Although the length of the afferent loop varies to a considerable degree, the closed end and the nearby papilla can usually be reached.

It should be kept in mind that the anatomic relationships in the Vaterian segment and papilla still hold. Since the bile duct will course in a cephalad direction roughly parallel to the long axis of the duodenum, it is often easier to cannulate the bile duct than the pancreatic duct, which encounters the duodenal wall at an almost perpendicular angle. One of the problems with the use of a forward-viewing instrument for cannulation is that most such instruments do not have a capability for direction of the cannula. Although some forward-viewing instruments do have an elevator mechanism, the range of movement possible with this is limited. Thus it is necessary to aim the cannula by deflecting the tip of the endoscope. Therefore, a small-caliber endoscope with a very maneuverable tip and a tight-bending radius will function best. Unfortunately, even with the most maneuverable instruments, the range of possible approaches to the papilla is still limited because the papilla must be kept in view during cannulation. Frequently it is only possible to change the axis of the cannula after inserting it into the orifice, and this may compromise the endoscopic view of the papilla. If cannulation of one or both relevant ducts fails, the process should be repeated with the side-viewing duodenoscope. Here the major problem may be entry into the afferent loop. Its position at the gastrojejunal stoma as noted during use of the forward-viewing endoscope should be kept in mind for placing the second instrument in the afferent loop. Changes in the patient's position and fluoroscopic monitoring may be helpful.

In patients with pancreas divisum (see Chapter 35) the main pancreatic drainage is via the minor papilla and accessory duct of Santorini. Pancreatography requires cannulation of this small accessory or minor papilla. It is usually identified slightly to the right of, and about 2 to 4 cm proximal to, the endoscopically viewed major papilla. A careful close up visual inspection is essential so that the usually tiny orifice may be located if possible. Sometimes this orifice can be identified as a small, black, pinpoint hole that opens and closes. The tip of the catheter must be placed exactly at this point. It is crucial that the catheter be aligned precisely and to know exactly where to place the cannula tip. The area around the orifice of the minor papilla becomes traumatized very quickly, and the edema, inflammatory reaction, and slight bleeding thus induced quickly obscure the structure; thus only one or two good passes can be expected before this sequence of events begins. Therefore, two elements in successful cannulation are the time taken to position the instrument tip properly and inspection of the structure in an effort to locate the orifice. Locating the orifice requires maximal endoscopic illumination and an endoscope with excellent resolution. It may be necessary to remove the lecturescope to maximize observing conditions. It is usually necessary to try every manner of instrument configuration until the most *en face* position can be achieved, but frequently the fully inserted greater curvature position is useful. Finally, the accessory papilla is so small and its orifice so tiny that a tapered fine-tip catheter is mandatory for cannulation.

CONCLUSION

At all levels of experience it is well to step back occasionally and review what is being done. The following "Do's and Don'ts" are repeated here for occasional review.

Optimally prepare the patient and his smooth muscle. Insist on complete duodenal atony, because this facilitates discovery and cannulation of the papilla. Selective cannulation is usually (not always) more successful with the patient in the prone position. This position is also best for capturing radiographic details. Attempted cannulation at a great distance from the papilla is a major cause of failure. A prerequisite for success is the ability to bring the papilla into a close-up *en face* position for detailed inspection and cannulation; thus the ability to maneuver the instrument is of major importance. Often the novice adopts one instrument configuration as the only one possible. Frequently this is because of fear that further maneuvering will result in loss of view of the papilla or that the instrument tip will fall back into the antrum, and that either event may result in failure. However, it is necessary to become comfortable with frequent changes in instrument configuration, from the full greater curvature to the full lesser curvature straightened position as well as the numerous positions between these extremes.

The ability to concentrate is mandatory. The papilla should always be studied carefully for clues to the location of the ampullary orifice(s) before attempting cannulation. Patience is also mandatory. Tentative passes with the cannula before careful study and alignment of the papilla usually result in failure.

It is necessary to develop a sense of the probable axis and direction of both ducts and to be able to align the cannula in every direction without limit in both the vertical and lateral planes. Repetition of maneuvers and approaches that do not work is pointless. Always change something! This may be as simple as changing the patient's position to an oblique or lateral one or switching to a tapered catheter. Prolonged procedures that become an endurance test for patient and endoscopist alike are usually unsuccessful. A second procedure several days later, if clinically warranted, has a greater chance of success.

A high level of hand/eye coordination is required. Although various maneuvers have been described here in a sequential fashion, it is in reality necessary to perform many of these simultaneously in a smooth, coordinated manner. Practice with the cannula in the instrument to learn pinpoint positioning by means of the elevator is useful.

A commonly unrecognized cause of failure is a malfunctioning endoscope. Since maximum possible deflection may be required for cannulation, the instrument must meet the manufacturer's specifications.

Successful ERCP requires more skill and hand/eye coordination than most endoscopic

procedures, but the learning process can be facilitated by attention to specific details. Early in this process there is considerable random or vaguely directed motion without knowing why something worked or whether it will apply to the next patient. However, specific maneuvers and an understanding of certain anatomic points will evolve gradually from this experience. The general pattern of this process has been outlined in this chapter; nevertheless it is impossible to put into writing a complete description of such a complex procedure. Hopefully, this description will guide one's thinking and shorten the learning process, but it cannot address every nuance or account for every contingency. Thus it is not possible to learn ERCP from a book. As stated, individual guidance by an experienced endoscopist in the actual "hands-on" performance of the procedure is clearly the best method. Finally, ERCP can only be judged successful when it results in radiographs that contain all necessary diagnostic information.

References

1. Matzen P, Haubek A, Holst-Christensen J, et al. Accuracy of direct cholangiography by endoscopic or transhepatic route in jaundice: A prospective study. Gastroenterology 1981; 81:237–41.
2. Cotton PB. Progress report: ERCP. Gut 1977; 18:316–41.
3. Vennes JA, Bond JH. Approach to the jaundice patient. (Editorial) Gastroenterology 1983; 84:1615–8.
4. Bilbao MK, Dotter CT, Lee TG, Katon RM. Complications of endoscopic retrograde cholangiopancreatography (ERCP). A study of 10,000 cases. Gastroenterology 1976; 70:314–20.
5. Gerding DN, Peterson LR, Vennes JA. Cleaning and disinfection of fiberoptic endoscopes: Evaluation of glutaraldehyde exposure time and forced-air drying. Gastroenterology 1982; 83:613–8.
6. Olson RC, Vennes JA, Silvis SE. Pancreatitis secondary to endoscopic retrograde cholangiopancreatography. (Abstr) Gastrointest Endosc 1976; 22:232.
7. Katon RM, Bilbao MK, Parent JA, Smith FW. Endoscopic retrograde cholangiopancreatography in patients with gastrectomy and gastrojejunostomy (Billroth II): A case for the forward look. Gastrointest Endosc 1975; 21:164–5.
8. Safrany L. Endoscopy and retrograde cholangiopancreatography after Billroth II operation. Endoscopy 1972; 4:198–202.

Chapter 26

INDICATIONS, CONTRAINDICATIONS, AND COMPLICATIONS OF ERCP

D. ROY FERGUSON, M.D.
MICHAEL V. SIVAK, JR., M.D.

OVERVIEW

Endoscopic cannulation of the papilla of Vater by McCune et al.[1] in 1968 introduced a remarkable period of nonoperative visualization of the biliary and pancreatic ducts. This procedure evolved rapidly over the past decade as therapeutic maneuvers were added to the basic technique of endoscopic retrograde cholangiopancreatography (ERCP). During this time extraordinary progress occurred in other investigative techniques that provided means for study of the biliary system and pancreas such as ultrasonography, computed tomography (CT), and percutaneous transhepatic cholangiography (PTC). These and other highly technical methods of investigation are readily available and it therefore becomes incumbent upon the physician to select the test or tests that will provide accurate and clinically pertinent information at the least cost and with the greatest safety and comfort for the patient. The endoscopist must not only have a thorough knowledge of the indications and complications of ERCP but must also recognize that all these available tests have a comparative value and limitations relative to a specific diagnostic problem. It is therefore relevant to consider not only the indications for ERCP in the following sections but also to compare ERCP with other diagnostic modalities.

INDICATIONS FOR ERCP
Biliary Tract Disease

Jaundiced patients can be accurately separated into the broad diagnostic categories of nonobstructive hepatic parenchymal disease and obstructive biliary tract disease on clinical grounds alone in about 90% of cases.[2, 3] Ideally, any additional test must provide further specific information on the exact nature of a biliary or pancreatic disorder. When biliary obstruction is suspected, for example, diagnostic studies must define the location and nature of the obstruction and suggest a specific diagnosis. Often no single test meets all these specifications.

The evaluation of jaundiced patients was one of the earliest applications of ERCP. Ultrasonography, CT, and PTC can be alternatives to ERCP. Intravenous cholangiography, although fairly specific, is insensitive and is seldom employed in the investigation of jaundice.

Ultrasonography and CT

Ultrasonography is at least 90% accurate in differentiating between biliary obstruction and hepatocellular disease.[4] The sine qua non of obstruction is ductular dilation. Berk et al.[5] have stated that an ultrasonographic bile duct diameter in excess of 5 mm justifies cholangiography. However, some increase in the bile duct diameter is said to occur normally in older individuals.[6, 7] There are other complicating factors. For example, there are obstructive disorders in which the bile ducts are not dilated, such as sclerosing cholangitis. If the obstruction is of recent onset, there may be no ultrasonographic evidence if the bile ducts are not yet dilated.[8]

CT is also highly accurate in defining biliary obstruction, and depends also on the

581

presence of dilated bile ducts for diagnosis. The comparative accuracy for CT and ultrasonography was found by Goldberg et al.[9] to be 87% and 91%, respectively. Matzen et al.[2] compared the ability of ultrasonography, CT, and cholescintigraphy to define bile duct patency in 56 patients. There were no significant trends that favored ultrasonography over CT. Morris et al.[10] in a study of a small number of patients with cholestatic jaundice, found that both CT and ultrasonography detected dilated ducts in the majority of cases, but that CT was superior for determining cause.

Biliary dilation may be present in the absence of obstruction after cholecystectomy. A variety of studies suggest that compensatory physiologic dilation of the extrahepatic bile ducts does not occur after cholecystectomy.[11, 12] Graham et al.[11] found no increase in diameter in 77 asymptomatic patients who underwent preoperative and follow-up ultrasonography from 4 to 16 months post-cholecystectomy. The results of these studies suggest that if the diameter of the extrahepatic system is normal before removal of the gallbladder, it will remain so after surgery. This applies also if surgical exploration of the bile duct was performed. If the bile ducts are dilated preoperatively, they will remain dilated or in a few cases return to normal diameter after surgery. It has been suggested that this relates to the integrity of ductular elastic fibers that may be damaged as a result of intermittent long-standing obstruction. However, small undetected stones may account for persistent postoperative dilation. If an increasing diameter of the extrahepatic ducts is demonstrated after cholecystectomy, obstruction is probably present. If the patient is asymptomatic, the process may be low-grade or intermittent, as by stone or perhaps papillary dysfunction.

Although ultrasonography is reasonably accurate in defining the level of obstruction, it is significantly less reliable with regard to the cause of obstruction. In a report by Dewbury et al.[13] ultrasonography correctly defined the presence or absence of obstruction in 97% of cases, but it was diagnostic in only 58%.

Ultrasonography has a significant technical failure rate, particularly in patients who have undergone surgery or in those with gaseous distention of the intestine. Prior surgery also limits CT, but excess gas usually does not present any difficulty. Both CT and ultrasonography, although highly accurate in classifying hepatobiliary disorders as obstructive or nonobstructive, often do not provide additional information on the nature of the obstruction. Problems encountered by ultrasonography with respect to biliary dilation after cholecystectomy and obstruction in the absence of dilation also apply to CT.

Ultrasonography is particularly prone to error in choledocholithiasis, especially after cholecystectomy. Stones may be present without ductular dilation.[14] Cronan et al.,[15] in a prospective study of 87 patients with proven bile duct stones, found that choledocholithiasis was confirmed by ultrasonography in only 13%. About two thirds of the patients had dilated ducts, and in 20% of these a calculus was demonstrated. In the remaining one third without dilation, none of the stones were visualized. In a study of 90 patients by Gross et al.,[16] the sensitivity of ultrasonography for the detection of stones was 25% overall. It was slightly higher if the ducts were dilated. CT can detect calculi as small as 2 mm in vitro if they are calcified, but non-calcified stones are difficult to identify with certainty unless 4 to 5 mm in diameter.[17]

There are no known complications of diagnostic ultrasonography or CT. The one theoretical disadvantage of CT is radiation exposure. Actual dosages are poorly described in the literature, especially from the viewpoint of the non-radiologist physician who orders the examination. McCullough and Payne[18] reported that in most clinical situations CT radiation exposure ranges from 2 to 10 rads per study, but that much larger doses are possible with improvements in the imaging capabilities of CT scanners.

PTC and ERCP

Success Rates

The fine-needle (Chiba) method has replaced earlier percutaneous cholangiography techniques because it is technically easier, has a greater success rate, and has fewer complications. There are definite differences for percutaneous opacification of the biliary system with dilated versus non-dilated ducts. With dilated bile ducts, opacification success is reported to be 100%.[19–22] With non-dilated ducts, however, the success rate ranges from 25%[23] to 95%.[20] A survey of the literature is given in Table 26–1. The overall success rate for visualization of dilated bile ducts based on the reports summarized in this table is 97.4%, and that for non-dilated ducts is

TABLE 26–1. **Fine-needle Transhepatic Cholangiography Success Rates**

		Success Rate (%)	
Author	**N***	*Dilated*	*Non-dilated*
Okuda et al.[24]	314	91	67.5
Shirakabe et al.[25]	687	96	85
Redeker et al.[19]	40	100	60
Elias et al.[23]	60	95	25
Pereiras et al.[20]	129	100	95.6
Goldstein et al.[21]	35	100	53
Jain et al.[26]	80	94.4	50
Ariyama et al.[27]	885	99	85
Kocher and Mousseau[28]	90	97.6	68
Choi et al.[22]	78	100	68
Mueller et al.[29]	450	99	74

*N = total number of patients (i.e., obstructed and non-obstructed).

60.3%. Harbin et al.,[30] in a survey of 2,006 cholangiographic studies from 31 centers, found a success rate of 97.8% with dilated ducts and 70.2% with nondilated ducts. Success increased 4% to 5% if more than six passes were performed. Kreek and Balint[31] reported a survey of fine-needle cholangiography from 21 centers. Diagnostic information was obtained in 89% of examinations. However, if the bile ducts were not dilated, opacification was successful in only 50%. If obstruction was due to malignancy, the failure rate was only 4%; if due to sclerosing cholangitis 20% of examinations failed, and if there was choledocholithiasis 10% failed.

In a survey of more than 10,000 ERCP procedures, Bilbao et al.[32] found the overall success rate for visualizing the biliary tree to be 70%. There was a significant difference in the success rate for experienced endoscopists (200 or more procedures) versus inexperienced endoscopists (25 or less procedures): 85% vs. 38%, respectively.

Comparative Studies

Frederic et al.[4] in a prospective study compared the results of ultrasonography and ERCP in hepatobiliary disease. They found that for lesions of the common bile duct and ampulla, ultrasonography led to a correct and specific diagnosis in 33 of 92 cases (36%), whereas ERCP led to the correct specific diagnosis in 90 of 92 cases (98%). Of particular note is that ultrasonography failed for technical reasons in 17 of 92 examinations and produced false-negative results in 42 of 92 cases. ERCP failed in one case and yielded a false-negative result in another. Ultrasonography was more accurate than ERCP with respect to focal hepatic disease, and both

were more than 80% accurate in the recognition of diffuse liver disease. Correct diagnoses of gallbladder lesions were approximately the same, with ERCP having the higher failure rate.

PTC and ERCP are comparable in that the biliary tree is visualized radiographically after a radiopaque contrast medium is injected into the bile ducts. The specificity for both procedures is high. Elias et al.[23] reported the results of an early study comparing PTC with ERCP in 60 patients; overall success rates for ERCP and PTC were 65% and 50% respectively. With extrahepatic obstruction, PTC was successful in 95%, but with nonobstructed bile ducts the success rate was only 25%. In a randomized trial of 21 postcholecystectomy patients with jaundice, Ertan et al.[33] found that the results with ERCP were satisfactory in 75% of patients and that PTC produced a satisfactory outcome in 100% of cases. Satake et al.[34] compared ERCP and PTC with regard to localization of the obstruction and correct diagnosis in 187 patients with obstructive jaundice. ERCP localized the obstruction in 90% and provided the correct diagnosis in 55%; PTC localized the obstruction in 82% and gave a correct diagnosis in 37%. Matzen et al.[35] also reported a randomized study in 52 jaundiced patients. Opacification was achieved by ERCP in 85%, and by PTC in 84%. ERCP was diagnostic in 89%, and PTC diagnostic in 68%. The difference was not statistically significant. ERCP yielded significantly more cholangiograms, however, in patients with lower bilirubin values, while PTC resulted in significantly more cholangiograms if the ducts were dilated.

From the foregoing it is clear that the success rate for visualization of the biliary system for PTC is higher than that for ERCP if the bile ducts are dilated. The success rate for ERCP is higher if the ducts are not dilated.

It is difficult to estimate which procedure is more comfortable for patients. Pain occurs in a significant number of those undergoing PTC, as a result of irritation of the capsule of the liver. Therefore, patients frequently are sedated and are given analgesics. There are no studies with regard to the time required for each procedure. In expert hands, ERCP can be accomplished in about 20 minutes. PTC is probably about the same. PTC requires less skill and experience than ERCP. The cost for ERCP in the United States is higher at present than that for PTC.[36]

Complications

The overall complication rate for ERCP in a survey of 10,000 procedures reported by Bilbao et al.[32] was 3%; that for experienced endoscopists was 3%. However, the complication rate for inexperienced physicians was 7% if unsuccessful, and 15% if successful. In a survey of over 400 members of the A/S/G/E, the complication rate for ERCP was 2.16%.[37] Specific complications are discussed in a following section.

The complication rates for percutaneous fine-needle cholangiography procedures cited in Table 26–1 are shown in Table 26–2. The composite complication rate for these 11 reports is 3.8%. It is difficult to separate major from minor complications in many of these studies. Furthermore, the complication rate for opacification of obstructed ducts by PTC is probably higher than that for non-obstructed ducts. A major complication occurred in 10.2% of the cases reported in the survey by Kreek and Balint,[31] and in 3.4% of the cases surveyed by Harbin et al.[30] The reason(s) for the discrepancy between the complication rate in these two surveys is unclear. Mueller et al.[38] have suggested that the higher rate in the report by Kreek and Balint may be due to inexperience. However, Harbin et al.[30] found no relationship between experience and complications. The majority of procedures were in fact performed by individuals with experience with 25 or less procedures. In this series, the success rate increased 4% to 5% if the number of attempts at opacification of the biliary system was not limited. But the authors found no increase in complications with unrestricted passes. This was also confirmed by Ariyama et al.[27]

TABLE 26–2. Fine-needle Transhepatic Cholangiography Complication Rate

Author	Complication Rate (%)
Okuda et al.[24]	8*
Shirakabe et al.[25]	0.29†
Redeker et al.[19]	5
Elias et al.[23]	5
Pereiras et al.[20]	3.1
Goldstein et al.[21]	0
Jain et al.[26]	5
Ariyama et al.[27]	0.2†
	8.4*
Kocher and Mousseau[28]	2.2
Choi et al.[22]	0
Mueller et al.[29]	4.8

*Includes major and minor complications.
†Major complications only.

The most common serious complications of PTC are sepsis, bile leakage with bile peritonitis, and intraperitoneal hemorrhage. Less common are hemobilia, endotoxic shock, and bile pulmonary embolism.[39, 40] Other, usually minor problems include fever, subcapsular hematoma, pneumothorax, contrast reactions, vasovagal reactions, and hypotension.

Bile leakage was discovered in 1.45% of patients undergoing PTC in the survey by Harbin et al.[30] This is probably an underestimate. Juler et al.[41] found bile in the peritoneal cavity at operation or autopsy in 40% of patients. The average amount present was 200 ml. Although bile leakage may be common, bile peritonitis requiring prompt surgical intervention is relatively rare.

Intraperitoneal hemorrhage occurs in less than 0.5% of PTC studies.[30] Subcapsular hematomas occurred in 12% in the survey by Harbin et al.[30] of over 2000 procedures. Hemobilia was not reported. An intrahepatic arteriovenous fistula was discovered incidentally in only one patient. As with bile leakage, however, vascular lesions occur more often than suspected. Hoevels and Nilsson[42] performed angiography in 83 patients from 1 to 70 days after PTC (average 13 days). Intrahepatic vascular lesions discovered in 27 patients included aneurysms, hematoma, and arterioportal and arteriohepatic venous fistulas. As with bile leakage, the great majority of these remain clinically silent.

Sepsis is a potential problem for both ERCP and PTC in that most patients with biliary obstruction have infected bile. Cholangitis as a contraindication to ERCP, and sepsis as a complication of ERCP are discussed in following sections.

Comparison of Complications of ERCP and PTC

Septicemia occurred in 2 patients in the PTC group and 1 patient studied by ERCP in the trial of Elias et al.[23] In the trial of ERCP versus PTC reported by Satake et al.[34] complications occurred in 7.9% of patients undergoing ERCP, the most serious being sepsis. The mortality in the ERCP group was 2.9%. Complications occurred in 9.2% of those patients who had PTC; mortality was 1.5%. A severe complication occurred in 3.8% of the patients undergoing PTC. External drainage was instituted during PTC in most cases.

Some untoward sequelae, such as sepsis, occur with both ERCP and PTC, whereas other complications are unique to one procedure or the other. For practical purposes, the overall complication rates for both investigations are approximately equal. That for PTC ranges from 2% to 8%[27] and is similar to the range for ERCP, which is 2% to 7%.[32, 37] Most PTC-related complications occur in the setting of biliary obstruction, and in this situation the incidence is probably higher, since inclusion of normal studies of nonobstructed ducts in reported series tends to decrease the calculated complication rate in many series. Some authors regard the experience of the examiner as important with respect to PTC complications;[38] others do not.[30] The level of the endoscopist's skill and experience does play a role in ERCP complications.[32]

Contraindications

Associated medical conditions and technical problems can also be significant factors with respect to success and potential complications. In some situations, these determine the choice of cholangiographic procedure.

There are relatively few contraindications to PTC. Severe coagulopathy contraindicates PTC but not ERCP. A prolonged prothrombin time as occurs in a variety of diseases is a relative contraindication to PTC, but this often can be corrected prior to the procedure. Septic cholangitis is also a contraindication, unless biliary drainage is also to be performed. The prognosis for such patients if left untreated is poor, and biliary drainage is a therapeutic option although the complication rate will be high. Kadir et al.[43] performed percutaneous biliary drainage in 18 patients with biliary sepsis due to acute obstructive cholangitis. Septic shock occurred in 3 patients and sepsis without hypotension in 2. The mortality was 17% after the procedure, which the authors felt was substantially lower than that anticipated for operative decompression. PTC is also more difficult and perhaps has a higher complication rate in patients with ascites.

The relatively few contraindications to ERCP are discussed in a following section. Acute pancreatitis is a relative contraindication, as is septic cholangitis. However, ERCP with endoscopic sphincterotomy has been undertaken in such circumstances as a therapeutic measure. Prior operative procedures such as a partial gastrectomy with Billroth II or Roux-Y anastomosis will reduce the success rate for ERCP or render it technically impossible. With regard to successful visualization, PTC probably has an advantage over ERCP when the patient has undergone a Billroth II procedure, regardless of the presence or absence of duct dilation.

Approach to the Jaundiced Patient

Based on the reports cited above, some general rules can be promulgated for the approach to the problem of jaundice. The clinical assessment of the patient remains the fundamental starting point. Ultrasonography or CT should be the first step in "visualization" of the biliary system. In a study concerned with the differentiation of obstructive from nonobstructive jaundice, O'Connor et al.[44] compared sensitivity, specificity, and overall accuracy for clinical assessment, ultrasonography, CT, and nuclear biliary scans. Sensitivities were 95%, 55%, 63%, and 41%, respectively; specificities were 76%, 93%, 93%, and 88%, respectively. The overall accuracy was 84% for clinical evaluation, 78% for ultrasonography, 81% for CT, and 68% for the biliary scan. These results generally agree with those of other studies.

Generally, clinical evaluation and noninvasive imaging studies yield a reasonably accurate appraisal of the disease. In this simplified scheme, the role of cholangiography in the evaluation of cholestatic jaundice is one of delineating the final diagnosis.[36] However, when biliary obstruction is the working clinical diagnosis, the choice of further diagnostic and/or therapeutic procedures can still be complex.

The ironic fact is that greater technical ability has actually increased and not lessened the physician's burden of judgment. Clinical assessment may be at odds with the results of noninvasive imaging procedures, in which case cholangiography for diagnosis may become more imperative. If biliary obstruction is the apparent problem, PTC is preferable to ERCP, as a general rule, if dilated intrahepatic biliary ducts have been demonstrated by CT or ultrasonography. However, specific clinical situations alter the approach to the individual patient to such a degree that this rule often becomes moot.

Ultrasonography or CT guided aspiration biopsy may confirm a diagnosis of carcinoma in the region of the head of the pancreas. In this circumstance, ERCP or PTC, by way of insertion of an endoprosthesis, is entirely therapeutic. If ampullary carcinoma is suspected, ERCP with biopsy is the diagnostic and sometimes therapeutic procedure of choice. When chronic pancreatitis is the main possibility and operative intervention is under consideration, ERCP will provide additional information on the status of the pancreatic duct that may be of value in planning surgery. There are compelling reasons to consider ERCP with possible endoscopic sphincterotomy and stone extraction as the sole diagnostic and therapeutic procedure when clinical assessment indicates choledocholithiasis. Thus, it is clinical assessment of the individual patient that most often guides the selection of further diagnostic and therapeutic procedures.

There are two broad indications for ERCP in obstructive jaundice: (1) delineation of the site and nature of the obstruction and (2) therapeutic intervention. Interventional methods include endoscopic sphincterotomy, extraction of gallstones, placement of an endoprosthesis or nasobiliary drain, and dilation of strictures of the biliary system. Over the past decade many centers with extensive experience in ERCP noted a gradual transition in the role of ERCP from one that was exclusively diagnostic to that of therapeutic intervention in at least half of the patients undergoing the procedure. These therapeutic modalities are discussed in following chapters.

ERCP in Specific Disorders of the Bile Ducts

Two primary conditions that affect the liver and are difficult to differentiate clinically are sclerosing cholangitis and primary biliary cirrhosis. Primary biliary cirrhosis usually occurs in middle-aged women; sclerosing cholangitis also occurs in this age group. In most studies of bile duct visualization by PTC, sclerosing cholangitis has the highest failure rate and is the single most difficult diagnosis. In some series, failure to visualize the bile ducts after more than six passes with the Chiba needle has been considered as prima-facie evidence of sclerosing cholangitis. This is, however, far less satisfactory than cholangiographic demonstration, which can be virtually diagnostic in most cases. CT and ultrasonography which depend on the presence of dilated ducts for diagnosis are likewise unsatisfactory and cannot differentiate the thickened ducts of sclerosing cholangitis from normal tissue. Because of these limiting factors for other investigative procedures, ERCP is the procedure of choice when the clinical setting is appropriate for sclerosing

cholangitis.[45] Suspicious clinical circumstances include a cholestatic syndrome without other obvious cause or a cholestatic syndrome in a patient with inflammatory bowel disease, particularly ulcerative colitis. ERCP methods of stricture dilation and endoprosthesis placement have also been suggested as therapy for dominant strictures in sclerosing cholangitis. ERCP also provides a means of monitoring medical, endoscopic, or surgical therapy. Sclerosing cholangitis, including the cholangiographic appearance of the ducts, is discussed in Chapters 31 and 32.

Carcinoma of the extrahepatic bile duct is another cause of obstructive jaundice that may be difficult to differentiate from choledocholithiasis in its early stages in patients with a prior cholecystectomy. When this question can not be resolved clinically and by reference to CT and ultrasonographic findings, ERCP with potential bile duct stone extraction is the procedure of choice. If an ampullary tumor is also considered in the differential diagnosis, as might be the case, for example, if there is evidence of gastrointestinal blood loss, then ERCP with biopsy and collection of material for cytologic examination becomes the favored procedure.

Although ultrasonography and CT are effective in defining mass lesions in the liver and in the head of the pancreas, they are considerably less satisfactory for recognition of intraluminal bile duct stones. ERCP is clearly the procedure of choice when there is a question of choledocholithiasis in a patient who has undergone cholecystectomy, since the biliary system can be cleared of stones by endoscopic methods in most cases. Endoscopic sphincterotomy and extraction of bile duct stones is also indicated in patients with intact gallbladders who are not candidates for surgery.

ERCP has also been suggested as a preoperative procedure in patients with chronic cholecystitis and cholelithiasis, especially those with persistent jaundice, as a substitute for operative cholangiography and/or common bile duct exploration. Choledocholithiasis, if found, can be managed by endoscopic sphincterotomy and stone extraction. The rationale for this is that ERCP provides a cholangiogram that is technically superior to operative cholangiography; that preoperative ERCP shortens the surgical procedure, especially when common duct exploration is expected to be difficult; that it defines associated abnormalities of importance to the surgeon such as a common duct stricture or papillary stenosis; and that it can define certain concomitant diseases, if they are present, such as peptic ulcer. This use of preoperative ERCP has not been studied prospectively and should be considered a theoretic indication at this time.

A number of pancreatic disorders may produce secondary biliary obstruction. This problem is discussed in a following section.

ERCP can have a secondary role in trauma and hemobilia. Although hemobilia is primarily an angiographic diagnosis, it may also be recognized at endoscopy. The classic triad of right upper quadrant pain, jaundice, and gastrointestinal tract bleeding should alert the endoscopist to this possibility. Calculus disease of the biliary tree, amenable to ERCP intervention, may also cause hemobilia. This, however, is rare, and accounts for hemobilia in only 13% of cases.

Pancreatic Diseases

CT and Ultrasonography

Prospective and retrospective studies have shown that the sensitivity and specificity of ultrasonography in the detection of pancreatic disease is in the range of 80% to 90%.[46] With regard to pancreatic carcinoma, Taylor et al.[47] reported a sensitivity and specificity of 94% and 99%, respectively. The failure rate for visualization of the pancreas was 10%. Pollock and Taylor[48] reported adequate visualization in 87% in a study of 112 patients with suspected cancer, and a sensitivity and specificity of 94% and 96%, respectively. There is thus some reason to question the need for additional studies such as ERCP in the diagnosis of pancreatic causes of obstruction. However, inclusion criteria that strongly favored the diagnosis of carcinoma and access to clinical information considerably decreased the value of these studies.

Hessel et al.[49] undertook a prospective study of the ability of CT and ultrasonography to differentiate between pancreatic disease and a normal pancreas. The sensitivity and specificity of CT were about 90%, whereas ultrasonography had a sensitivity of about 69% and a specificity of 82%. The technical failure rate for ultrasonography was high, 44 of 279 examinations being unsatisfactory. In another study, the overall diagnostic accuracy for CT was 84% in pancreatic disease; that for ultrasonography was 64%.[50] This calculation included 20% of the ultra-

sonography examinations that were unsuccessful. If these were eliminated the success rate for the two examinations was about equal. The overall sensitivity for CT and ultrasonography in another study of 81 patients with suspected pancreatic disease was 76.2% and 57.1% respectively, while the specificity was 98% for CT and 86.1% for ultrasonography.[51]

Cotton et al.[52] reported a comparison trial of gray-scale ultrasonography and retrograde pancreatography in patients with no pancreatic disease as well as patients with a variety of pancreatic disorders. The failure rate was 7.2% for ultrasonography and 5.8% for ERCP. Overall, the comparison between the two was about equal, although ultrasonography was slightly superior when the pancreas ultimately proved to be normal; there was a slight advantage for ERCP in the diagnosis of cancer. The authors recommended a combination of the two techniques as providing the best comprehensive approach to diagnosis.

A retrospective as well as prospective study of the relative efficiency and predictive value of ultrasonography and retrograde pancreatography by Gowland et al.[53] in 1981 found the specificity for ultrasonography and pancreatography to be 90% and 65%, respectively; the sensitivity was 55% and 80%, respectively. Twenty-five per cent of the ultrasonography procedures and 11% of the pancreatographic studies were unsatisfactory. The low specificity of pancreatography was thought to be due to its unreliability in minimal degrees of chronic pancreatitis, whereas the low sensitivity for ultrasonography was said to result from difficulty with recognition of chronic pancreatitis in the absence of acute inflammatory changes.

ERCP

Chronic Pancreatitis

Traditionally, the diagnosis of chronic pancreatitis depended upon the presence of chronic abdominal pain, a history of recurrent bouts of pancreatitis, elevation of serum amylase and/or lipase, demonstration of calcification in the region of the pancreas on plain x-rays of the abdomen, and/or the development of pseudocysts. Given this former lack of investigative procedures, the best assessment of the presence or degree of chronic pancreatitis was observation, operative pancreatography, and palpation at the time of surgery. Since chronic pancreatitis produces radiographic abnormalities in the main pancreatic duct and its branches, its presence is detectable by ERCP. CT and ultrasonography can also detect the presence of chronic pancreatitis, and as with other clinical problems the comparative accuracy and specificity must be considered for these several methods of studying the pancreas.

High-resolution CT can detect dilated pancreatic ducts, but usually the diagnosis of chronic pancreatitis by CT is based on the presence of calcification and atrophy of the gland and the presence of pseudocysts. The most favorable aspect of ultrasonography and CT in the diagnosis of chronic pancreatitis is specificity. When chronic pancreatitis is unequivocally demonstrated by either imaging technique, a close correlation will be found with the results of other studies including ERCP, and positive diagnostic accuracy (specificity) approaches 100%.[51]

Earlier studies that compare the value of ultrasonography and ERCP in chronic pancreatitis reflect author preference. In a prospective study, however, Swobodnik et al.[51] found that ERCP was more sensitive and more specific in the diagnosis of chronic pancreatitis than either ultrasonography or CT. The most recent studies indicate that sensitivity is about equal with respect to the diagnosis of chronic pancreatitis.

When the diagnosis of chronic pancreatitis cannot be confirmed by CT and ultrasonography, ERCP yields a small percentage increase in the rate of positive diagnosis. Available data suggest that ERCP should be reserved for clinical problems in which the results of CT and ultrasonography are inconclusive, and for delineation of the pancreatic ducts prior to surgery.[54, 55] ERCP is part of the standard preoperative planning for pancreatic surgery in many institutions. Preoperative knowledge of pancreatic anatomy may result in a change in the type of surgery or it may alter the expectations of the surgical procedure. For example, pancreatico-pleural fistulas have been discovered in association with pseudocysts; in one case this abnormality was treated nonsurgically by radiation after diagnosis by ERCP.[56]

The diagnosis of chronic pancreatitis, whether by ERCP, CT, ultrasonography, or another modality, does not determine the necessity of surgical intervention. This decision must be based upon clinical assessment of the patient and the results of various tests and procedures. However, when surgery becomes a consideration, ERCP provides the best means for delineating pancreatic ductal pathology including the presence of strictures, ductal filling defects, ductal continuity with pseudocysts, main pancreatic duct disruption, and anomalous pancreatic anatomy. ERCP has also demonstrated that the changes of chronic pancreatitis are by no means uniform throughout the gland in all patients. The surgical decision for pancreatic drainage rather than amputation often depends on the demonstration of a dilated duct or the presence of obstruction within the head of the gland or at the sphincter of Oddi.

Comparisons of pancreatic secretory testing and ERCP have provided uncertain results. A study by Valentini et al.[57] compared secretin, cholecystokinin, and pancreatozymin (S-CCK-Pz) stimulation with ERCP in 124 patients, 65 of whom had proven chronic pancreatitis and 59 suspected pancreatitis. In those with established chronic pancreatitis, pancreatography was abnormal in 85% and S-CCK-Pz stimulation was abnormal in 78.5%. In the 59 cases of suspected chronic pancreatitis, pathologic ductal changes were found in 12%, and 40.7% had abnormal S-CCK-Pz stimulation tests. Since these data pertain to suspected cases interpretation is difficult. It is possible that retrograde pancreatography in conjunction with pancreatic stimulation may provide more information than either study performed alone, but different authors arrive at different conclusions with regard to this question.

The role of ERCP in chronic pancreatitis, including its relation to other methods of investigation, is discussed in Chapters 36 and 37.

Pseudocyst of the Pancreas

CT and ultrasonography are the initial procedures of choice for detection of a pseudocyst. Although the presence of a pseudocyst presents a special hazard for ERCP, this need not be a contraindication to the procedure. Certain important information can only be obtained by pancreatography. For example, continuity between the pancreatic duct and a pseudocyst has important implications for surgical management.[58] The approach to management of the pseudocyst that is in continuity with the main pancreatic duct may differ from that of the isolated lesion with regard to its expected resolution and to surgical drainage.[58] In some cases internal surgical drainage might be deferred if continuity can be demonstrated. As a general rule, ERCP in the presence of a pseudocyst should be performed in anticipation of surgery. Pseudocyst of the pancreas is discussed in Chapter 38.

Acute Pancreatitis

Traditionally, ERCP has had virtually no role in acute pancreatitis. More recently a few authors have advocated the procedure in this disorder. For example, Gebhardt et al.[59] found ERCP to be of value in hemorrhagic pancreatitis. When the cause of recurrent pancreatitis is not known, ERCP may assist in delineating biliary tract related disease from other causes such as alcoholism. A number of reports indicate that ERCP and endoscopic sphincterotomy should be considered in known or suspected gallstone-induced acute pancreatitis. For example, Safrany and Cotton[60] reported the use of endoscopic sphincterotomy as a first-treatment method in 22 patients severely ill with acute pancreatitis and jaundice or cholestasis. The use of ERCP and sphincterotomy in acute pancreatitis is considered further in several of the following chapters.

Pancreatic Trauma

When epigastric pain radiates to the left side in association with gastrointestinal bleeding, the possibility of pancreatic duct hemorrhage must be considered, especially if there is a history of trauma or a pseudocyst is present. Blood clots in the pancreatic duct can be defined by ERCP, and several authors have demonstrated the ERCP findings; some have proposed endoscopic sphincterotomy for relief of the pain associated with ductal obstruction by clots.[61-63] The role of ERCP in pancreatic duct hemorrhage is potentially greater than in hemobilia. Documentation of a pseudocyst in the presence of bleeding may indicate surgery; ERCP may delineate possible methods of drainage.[64]

Pancreatic trauma is a rare indication for ERCP. Safrany's[65] experience of 6000 ERCP procedures over a 10-year period included only 56 cases of traumatic lesions of the biliary tree and pancreas. Eleven patients had alterations of the pancreatic ductal system after blunt trauma, and in 7 of these there was complete rupture of the main pancreatic duct where it crosses the spine. Of the other four patients, cyst formation was found in three and a fistula was discovered in the fourth. Before 1980 it was thought that ERCP might cause further harm in pancreatic trauma; however, other more recent reports confirm the value of retrograde pan-

creatography for demonstration and localization of disruption of the main pancreatic duct after blunt trauma. Linos et al.[66] reported an incidence of pseudocysts in association with blunt abdominal trauma perhaps as high as 30%. They argued that the demonstration of main pancreatic duct disruption is an indication for surgical drainage. Comparison data on the value of ERCP, ultrasonography, and CT in pancreatic trauma are currently not available. ERCP in pancreatic trauma is discussed in Chapter 38.

Carcinoma of the Pancreas

The diagnosis of pancreatic cancer remains problematic. Hessel et al.[49] found that the sensitivity of CT and ultrasonography was 84% and 56%, respectively, in the detection of carcinoma in 279 patients. Swobodnik et al.[51] found that ERCP was more sensitive for carcinoma than CT or ultrasonography, but the specificity with respect to malignancy was about equal for ERCP and CT. Moss et al.[67] compared CT and ERCP in 61 patients with suspected pancreatic carcinoma. The accuracy of ERCP was 62%, with a false-negative rate of 8% and a failure rate of 30%. If only successful ERCP studies were considered, accuracy was 88%. CT yielded a correct diagnosis in 76% with false-positive, false-negative, and indeterminate results in 5%, 13%, and 6%, respectively. When CT and ERCP were in agreement diagnostic accuracy was 93%, i.e., greater than either study alone.

Savarino et al.[68] reviewed all these diagnostic modalities to determine whether their use had resulted in an increase in the detection of pancreatic cancer at a resectable stage. They concluded that these tests produced no increase in the rate of resectability although diagnosis was accurate and reliable. None of these modalities have been employed prospectively in the screening of asymptomatic patients for pancreatic cancer because this would be expensive and impractical. Furthermore, there are no sufficiently reliable factors that could be used to define an at-risk population. Despite these uncertainties, it is nevertheless likely that none of the currently available modalities are sufficiently sensitive and specific in the detection of small pancreatic carcinomas in an early stage.

The clinical question of pancreatic carcinoma is not resolved by CT or ultrasonography in some cases. Frick et al.[69] assessed the value of ERCP in patients with suspected carcinoma who had indeterminate CT results. ERCP proved helpful in 25 of 26 patients studied and was considered a suitable second imaging modality for pancreatic neoplasm.

One of the major difficulties in ERCP diagnosis is the differentiation of pancreatic carcinoma from chronic pancreatitis. Frick et al.[70] reported that ERCP was 90% accurate in differentiating benign from malignant pancreatic disease in 71 patients. However, in patients with concomitant chronic pancreatitis and carcinoma, ERCP results were inaccurate and differentiation was virtually impossible. This differential diagnosis may also be a formidable problem for CT and ultrasonography, although fine-needle biopsy of the pancreas under the guidance of either imaging method enhances diagnostic specificity.

Freeny et al.[71] proposed the use of percutaneous fine needle pancreatic biopsy during ERCP. Since the safety of CT-guided aspiration biopsy has been established, ERCP-guided biopsy would seem to be a reasonable alternative in high-grade obstructing lesions of the main pancreatic duct. In the study by Freeny et al.,[71] a positive diagnosis of adenocarcinoma was obtained for 13 of 14 patients who underwent the procedure. However, the reported experience with this technique is not extensive. ERCP in pancreatic carcinoma is discussed in Chapter 39.

ERCP with endoscopic biopsy is the procedure of choice in cancer of the ampulla of Vater, but it also has similar potential advantages in periampullary cancer. A positive diagnosis of carcinoma within the distal common bile duct or in the immediate retropapillary area may sometimes be obtained by brushing cytology. Cancer in the head of the pancreas may also invade through the duodenal wall, so that a tissue diagnosis may be obtained by endoscopic biopsy. In such circumstances, ERCP is the procedure of choice.

Pancreatic Disorders Causing Biliary Obstruction

Pseudocysts can impinge upon the biliary tract, and there is ample documentation of distal common bile duct abnormalities secondary to pseudocysts, particularly in the head of the pancreas.[72] Carcinoma of the pancreas may produce the so-called "double duct sign" in which a neoplasm within the head of the pancreas obstructs both the common bile and pancreatic ducts.[73] The double duct sign was thought to be relatively specific for carcinoma of the head of the pancreas, but the results of more recent work suggest

that it may also occur in chronic pancreatitis.[74] Ralls et al.[75] questioned the value of pancreatographic findings such as the double duct, which they found in association with chronic pancreatitis as well as carcinoma. Despite certain limitations, ERCP better delineates pancreatic ductal abnormalities than other radiologic procedures, and at present it is probably the best procedure available short of laparotomy for differentiating intrinsic biliary tract disease from secondary biliary tract involvement by pancreatic disease.

Miscellaneous Indications

Miscellaneous indications for ERCP include selective cannulation of the pancreatic or bile duct for aspiration or stimulation studies of either bile or pancreatic duct secretions ("pure juice biochemistry").[76] This is discussed in Chapter 37.

Diseases of the duodenal papilla remain a diagnostic dilemma. Certain disorders such as dysfunction of the sphincter of Oddi are poorly defined, although duodenoscopic measurement of papillary function by manometric methods provides a relatively new avenue of investigation. The treatment of papillary dysfunction is controversial but may include endoscopic sphincterotomy. When sphincter of Oddi dysfunction is considered, carcinoma of the papilla of Vater and small bile duct stones must also be included in the differential diagnosis and ERCP is indicated. The sphincter of Oddi is considered in Chapter 33.

Pancreas divisum is an interesting anomaly that may be more common than previously suspected. Whether or not this plays a role in some cases of recurrent acute pancreatitis and chronic pancreatitis remains controversial. Pancreas divisum is discussed in Chapter 35.

Abdominal Pain

One of the more problematic indications for ERCP is evaluation of abdominal pain. When this is a particularly difficult diagnostic problem, and the results of less invasive studies are consistently negative or inconclusive, ERCP is often considered. The overall value of this is difficult to ascertain, and there have been few reports that address this question.

Bull et al.[77] reported that of 806 ERCP examinations, 140 had been requested for patients who had undiagnosed upper abdominal pain, 70 of whom had not undergone biliary surgery. In the group that had not undergone surgery, at least one duct was opacified in 59 patients (84%). ERCP was diagnostic in 7 patients (10%), but in 3 of these the diagnosis was peptic ulcer disease. Four had pancreatic disease. There was a 25% incidence of psychiatric disorders in the group with abdominal pain unexplained by any tests. There was also about a 10% incidence in which ERCP was not helpful and in which symptoms proved to be due to underlying organic causes. Of the 70 patients who had had biliary surgery, 45 were found to have other abnormal test results. Of the remaining 25 patients, the results of ERCP were similar to those in the group who had not undergone surgery. Ruddell et al.[78] studied 140 patients who had not undergone biliary surgery. An ERCP diagnosis was achieved in 24%, including 25 patients with abnormal pancreatograms and one with pancreatic carcinoma. However, significant alcohol abuse was detected in the history of a number of the patients in this report.

Whether ERCP should be considered a final step in evaluation of unexplained abdominal pain remains in question; if the procedure is performed, a low yield should be anticipated. In some cases further careful attention to the clinical history, physical examination, and laboratory tests will lead to a more specific diagnosis. ERCP is an alternative to laparotomy in particularly difficult cases, as the morbidity and mortality are significantly less.

CONTRAINDICATIONS

The only truly absolute contraindication to ERCP is refusal of the patient to undergo endoscopy or the patient's inability to cooperate during the procedure for whatever reason. Even in the latter circumstance, ERCP can be performed under general anesthesia when the study is considered essential to management. By and large, a contraindication to a procedure is a logical conclusion based on clinical assessment and the results of other tests and studies. Accordingly, most contraindications are relative and vary to the degree that the results of the procedure are of importance. The degree of risk must always be balanced against the potential benefit. In some clinical situations risk may outweigh any potential benefit. Acute myo-

cardial infarction, for example, is a strong contraindication to ERCP, and it is difficult to conceive a situation in which ERCP would be required during the unstable phases of acute myocardial infarction. In some cases only certain aspects of a procedure are contraindicated. For example, respiratory failure precludes the use of sedative drugs, and severe uncorrectable coagulopathy restricts the use of endoscopic sphincterotomy.

Certain structural abnormalities of the upper gastrointestinal tract may increase the risk of the procedure or render it technically difficult or impossible. Passage of the side-viewing duodenoscope into the esophagus is a "blind" maneuver. Hence patients with an unrecognized esophageal stricture or large diverticulum are at risk for esophageal perforation. Esophageal dilation might precede ERCP. The endoscope might be passed under fluoroscopy to avoid entering a diverticulum, although this structural abnormality remains a relatively strong contraindication. A large paraesophageal hiatal hernia also represents a special hazard, especially if it is not recognized before attempting to maneuver the duodenoscope to the duodenum. Pyloric stenosis or gastric outlet obstruction may restrict entry into the duodenum; marked degrees of obstruction can be considered a contraindication.

Cholangitis has been considered a contraindication, based primarily on studies in patients with obstructive jaundice and fever.[79] Cholangitis and biliary obstruction are usually coexistent conditions. Pretreatment with antibiotics and endoscopic relief of obstruction have made this a relative contraindication.

Acute pancreatitis and pancreatic pseudocyst have also been considered contraindications to ERCP. However, Safrany and Cotton[60] have advocated the use of endoscopic sphincterotomy for acute gallstone-induced pancreatitis. It does not appear that the morbidity or mortality with this approach is excessive, but available data on the results are limited at present. Pseudocyst of the pancreas is considered a relative contraindication to ERCP, since opacification and filling with contrast medium, especially if excessive, may convert the cavity to a pancreatic abscess. The latter has a markedly higher morbidity and mortality than pseudocyst alone. ERCP should not be considered for diagnosis alone since CT and ultrasonography are noninvasive methods of accurate diagnosis. Therefore, the role of ERCP in pseudocyst is limited. ERCP should be performed only when certain specific types of information are being sought that will have a significant bearing on management, especially surgical management. As a general rule, ERCP in the presence of a pseudocyst should be performed only as a preoperative procedure so that adequate surgical drainage of the pseudocyst within a short span of time is assured. The special problems that are encountered when ERCP is performed in the presence of a pseudocyst are discussed in Chapter 38.

It is the experience of most endoscopists that patients who have had reactions to iodinated contrast medium in other radiologic procedures do not have similar difficulty when this type of medium is used for ERCP. However, it is clear that the contrast agent is absorbed during the procedure. Renal excretion, for example, has been documented.[80] When this question remains of concern, some endoscopists pretreat patients with an antihistamine drug or an antihistamine and corticosteroids. The efficacy of this practice is not established.

The presence of hepatitis B infection in a patient undergoing ERCP is also thought to be a contraindication, albeit a weak one. The question of transmission of hepatitis B virus (HBV) at endoscopy has been considered in relation to various procedures, but it is especially important with cannulation of the bile duct, since this structure may potentially harbor a high concentration of HBV. The contraindication lies in the risk to the operator and subsequent patients in whom the endoscopic instruments will be used. Risks to the endoscopist and endoscopy assistants can be minimized by adequate protection such as the use of gloves, care in handling aspirated secretions and bile, and vaccination against HBV. Retrospective studies have not identified any significant problem with HBV transmission by means of endoscopic equipment and procedures. A recent prospective study demonstrated a lack of transmission for all types of endoscopy.[81] The issue of HBV transmission is also discussed in Chapter 12.

Technically difficult procedures also become more hazardous for patients if the endoscopist does not recognize his or her limitations or that the procedure is actually impossible. The survey of the 10,000 ERCP procedures by Bilbao et al.[32] confirms that failure and complication rates are highest for the inexperienced physician.

COMPLICATIONS

Complication Rate

The complication rate in most reported series varies from 2% to 7%, with death occurring as a result of the procedure in 0.001% to 0.8% of patients. Brandes et al.[82] reported an overall complication rate of 5%, with untoward events being equally divided between pancreatitis and complications related to infection. In the extensive review of Bilbao et al.,[32] the overall complication rate was 3%; the rate was significantly greater for inexperienced physicians. The survey of 400 members of the American Society for Gastrointestinal Endoscopy quoted the complication rate as 2.2%.[37] Most fatalities were related to sepsis or bacterial infections, and from this perspective they are the most serious hazards. Zimmon et al.[83] found an overall complication rate of 5% in a retrospective study of 300 procedures in 278 patients.

The ASGE survey reported the risk of instrument perforation at some site in the upper gastrointestinal tract as 0.3 cases per thousand.[37] Of these, esophageal perforation occurred in a few patients. The perforation rate associated with endoscopic sphincterotomy is substantially higher than that for routine diagnostic ERCP. The complications of endoscopic sphincterotomy are discussed in Chapter 29.

Endoscopic Complications

Certain potential complications are common to all upper gastrointestinal endoscopic procedures. These are discussed in Chapter 12. Aspiration to some extent is a function of the depth of sedation, age of the patient, and co-morbid states. With adequate precautions this should be a minor problem. Drug reactions, a more common problem, may be manifestations of an allergic reaction or oversedation leading to respiratory and/or cardiac arrest. The incidence of this has been estimated to be 0.1% to 0.6%. Vagally mediated reactions also occur.[84]

Sepsis

The leading and most serious complication of ERCP is sepsis. In prospective studies the incidence of bacteremia was as high as 14%, although in other studies this was negligible.[85-88] Helm[89] noted 38 clinical episodes of septicemia after 4359 endoscopic bile duct interventions, including a variety of therapeutic maneuvers in 34 patients, an incidence of 0.87%. Thirteen patients with septicemia died, sepsis being the direct cause of death in 6 patients. The risk of sepsis is related in part to the underlying disease. Disorders that result in stasis, particularly in the bile ducts, are known to result in bacterial colonization. However, organisms may also be introduced into either ductal system by the ERCP procedure.

There is ample evidence that contamination of the cannula, duodenoscope, or the water bottle of the endoscopic light source can cause infection.[90–92] *Pseudomonas aeruginosa* is a particularly common contaminating organism.[91, 93] Other enterobacteriaceae, *Staphylococcus epidermidis*, and other organisms have also been incriminated. There are numerous documented cases of septicemia in which organisms found in the patient's blood had the same serotype as organisms cultured from the duodenoscope, water bottle, and/or endoscopic accessories such as the cannula.[92, 93] Thorough cleaning of the equipment reduces the incidence of *Pseudomonas* infection.

Although careful disinfection and drying of endoscopic equipment minimizes the risk of nosocomial infection, these measures do not alter the potential for sepsis following instrumentation of an infected ductal system.[94] Biliary infection represents a potential complication with respect to all forms of biliary manipulation. In the survey by Bilbao et al.,[32] 90% of the cases of septic cholangitis occurred in patients with obstructed bile ducts; all of the fatal cases also occurred in this group. Since sepsis clearly can occur, endocarditis is also a possibility in susceptible patients. Reviews of bacterial endocarditis have not specifically implicated gastrointestinal procedures, but the degree of risk in susceptible patients has not been established.[95] Fluid samples aspirated from an obstructed system or at the papilla of Vater usually contain bacteria that are the same as those found in blood cultures from patients with post-ERCP sepsis.[88]

Most patients with obstructing choledocholithiasis have infected bile. The incidence is somewhat lower if obstruction is caused by malignancy.[96, 97] Helm[89] obtained bile samples for culture immediately after catheterization of the bile duct at ERCP in 142 patients. *Escherichia coli* was the most common bacterium isolated (63% of cultures), followed by *Pseudomonas* species.

In man and experimental animals the transfer of biliary contents to the circulation during cholangiography is directly related to pressure increases during injection.[98] Animal experiments suggest that lymphatics play a major role in septicemia after intrabiliary manipulation.[99, 100] Pathways have been demonstrated in experimental animals by which particulate substances may gain access to the systemic circulation through the parenchyma of either the liver or the pancreas.[101–103]

Methods for minimizing or eliminating the problem of sepsis related to instrumentation of an obstructed and infected bile duct include use of antibiotic-containing contrast medium, prophylactic use of antibiotics, and early and adequate drainage.[104]

The stability and antibacterial activity of the aminoglycoside antibiotics tobramycin and gentamicin were studied in vitro in a mixture of bile and a radiographic contrast agent by Jendrzejewski et al.[105] Although the results of this study showed that the antibacterial activity of these agents was not altered by an environment that simulated ERCP, they did not establish the efficacy of including antibiotics in the contrast. Generally, the value of adding antibiotics to the contrast agent is discounted.

Dutta et al.,[106] in a prospective evaluation of the risk of bacteremia and the role of antibiotics in ERCP in 51 patients, found the incidence of bacteremia to be minimal. Opacification of at least one ductal system was achieved in 42 patients (84%); an abnormal ductal system was demonstrated in 17 cases. *Streptococcus pneumoniae* was cultured from a patient's blood after opacification of a pancreatic duct with multiple strictures. Although the incidence of bacteremia was only 2% overall in this study, the incidence in patients with an abnormal ductal system was considerably higher (i.e., 1 of 17 cases). Dutta et al.[106] advocated that antibiotics be administered only after procedures that demonstrated biliary abnormalities. In an accompanying editorial, McMahon and Gorelick[107] pointed out that the questions raised were of more significance than the findings of this study. Although it was reassuring that sepsis following ERCP occurred in 1% to 2% of cases in this study (significantly less than the reported 14%), a specific approach to the treatment of post-ERCP sepsis has not been established, and the role for antibiotics before and/or after the procedure remains undefined.

Parenteral antibiotics normally excreted in bile do not attain high concentration if the biliary system is obstructed.[108] However, adequate blood levels of an appropriate antibiotic will reduce the incidence of septicemia.[109] About two thirds of the organisms present in bile infected as a result of obstruction will be gram-negative, and about two thirds of patients will have more than one organism.[97] Sudden endotoxic shock in the absence of evidence of sepsis may also occur after manipulation as gram-negative organisms are forced into the circulation. This event is probably not preventable even if serum antibiotic concentration is high.

Antibiotic prophylaxis is indicated in all cases of biliary obstruction where manipulation of the bile duct is planned. It is also indicated when ductal obstruction is likely to be present and the patient's condition is such that sepsis would be poorly tolerated (e.g., elderly patients) or life-threatening. It should also be used when the potential consequences of sepsis would be serious, as for example in patients with prosthetic devices. Antibiotic prophylaxis is most effective if the drug(s) is given in advance of the procedure, allowing enough time to achieve an adequate blood level at the time of the procedure. However, attempts at sterilization of the bile ducts prior to intervention are time-consuming and ineffective. It is our practice to administer parenteral antibiotics about 1 to 2 hours before ERCP when there is a reasonable possibility that biliary obstruction will be present. When this proves to be the case, antibiotics are continued for about 12 hours after the procedure. The antibiotic(s) of choice has not been established. Generally, this includes an aminoglycoside and cephalosporin. With respect to ERCP, the efficacy of this practice has not been verified in controlled trials, but it is justified and indicated based on data derived from non-endoscopic studies of bacterial colonization and sepsis associated with obstructed bile ducts.

One of the best methods of dealing with an infected closed space such as an obstructed bile duct is to establish adequate drainage as quickly as possible. Prior to the development of endoscopic sphincterotomy, this required either surgical or percutaneous drainage procedure. However, this can now be achieved by endoscopic methods at the time of diagnostic cholangiography. Endoscopic sphincterotomy with extraction of bile duct stones is an effective drainage procedure. A biliary endoprosthesis or a nasobiliary tube can also be placed endoscopically in many cases of biliary obstruction so that adequate drainage occurs.

Pancreatic sepsis is a rare but serious complication that has a high mortality and extensive morbidity. A major risk is that a pseudocyst will be converted into an abscess following injection of contrast material contaminated by bacteria from the gastrointestinal tract or from the endoscope and/or its accessories. In the survey by Bilbao et al.[32] there was a very low incidence of pancreatic sepsis, but 20% of the patients with this complication died. Hershey et al.[110] studied the concentrations of systemically administered ampicillin, gentamicin, and clindamycin in the pancreatic juice of 12 patients, 10 of whom had pancreatic disease. The levels of ampicillin and gentamicin found were considered ineffective; there were detectable levels of clindamycin. However, there is no evidence that prophylactically administered antibiotics will prevent pancreatic sepsis. Complications of ERCP in pancreatic pseudocyst are discussed in Chapter 38.

Acute Pancreatitis

The reported incidence of acute pancreatitis in early reports of ERCP series ranges from 1% to 17%.[111–115] It occurred after 1% of the 10,000 procedures composing the survey of Bilbao et al.;[32] pancreatitis occurred after 51 of 3884 procedures in the survey of Nebel et al.[37] In most cases pancreatitis is mild and self-limiting, but there have been rare fatalities as a result of this complication.[115, 116]

ERCP-induced pancreatitis appears to be related to the number of injections of contrast medium into the pancreatic duct, the volume of contrast used, and perhaps the injection pressure.[117] Ruppin et al.[115] reported a decline from 7.4% to 1.3% in the incidence of acute pancreatitis as a result of careful monitoring of contrast volume, avoiding acinar opacification, and the use of tetracycline; the value of the latter is doubtful. Control of injection pressure by means of a manometer is said to decrease the level of postprocedure hyperamylasemia as well as the incidence of acute pancreatitis.[118] However, this method has not been adopted widely; most endoscopists rely on fluoroscopic control during opacification of the pancreatic duct. Galvan and Klotz[119] suggested that pancreatitis may occur more often in patients who have had acute episodes in the past. In the survey of Bilbao et al.,[32] 66% of the patients who developed post-ERCP pancreatitis had prior episodes. However, data on this point are limited.

Serum amylase elevation, sometimes to extremely high levels, occurs after ERCP in 50% to 60% of cases.[120] Post-ERCP hyperamylasemia is generally accepted as not having any significance, and routine post-ERCP serum amylase determinations have no value. Therefore, there must be clinical evidence of acute pancreatitis in addition to elevated serum amylase levels before considering that a complication has occurred.

Miscellaneous Complications

A variety of complications may result from endoscopic therapeutic measures involving the bile and pancreatic ducts. These are usually related to endoscopic sphincterotomy and related maneuvers and include perforation and hemorrhage. These complications are discussed in Chapter 29.

Study of the urine specimens of patients who have undergone routine ERCP procedures indicates that an appreciable amount of contrast medium may be excreted by the kidneys.[79] In the study by Sable et al.,[121] absorption was documented after instillation into the duodenum alone, but the amount of contrast medium excreted was less than that found after pancreatic or bile duct injections. The implications of these results are not clear. Perhaps urinary excretion is related to excessive volumes of contrast medium and/or high injection pressure, but this is not certain. Sable et al.[121] have suggested that allergic reactions to iodinated contrast materials are possible, but this complication appears to be extremely rare.

Radiation dosages in patients undergoing ERCP are comparable to that for other standard radiographic procedures.[122, 123]

References

1. McCune WS, Shorb PE, Moscovitz H. Endoscopic cannulation of the ampulla of vater: a preliminary report. Ann Surg 1968; 167:952–6.
2. Matzen P, Malchow-Møller A, Brun B, et al. Ultrasonography, computed tomography, and cholescintigraphy in suspected obstructive jaundice—a prospective comparative study. Gastroenterology 1983; 84:1492–7.
3. Schenker S, Balint J, Schiff L. Differential diagnosis of jaundice: Report of a prospective study of 61 proved cases. Am J Dig Dis 1962; 12:449–63.
4. Frederic N, Deltenre M, d'Hondt M, et al. Comparative study of ultrasound and ERCP in the diagnosis of hepatic, biliary, and pancreatic diseases: A prospective study based on a continuous series of 424 patients. Eur J Radiol 1983; 3:208–11.
5. Berk RN, Cooperberg PL, Gold RP, et al. Radiography of the bile ducts. A symposium on the use of new modalities for diagnosis and treatment. Radiology 1982; 145:1–9.
6. Lasser RB, Silvis SE, Vennes JA. The normal cholangiogram. Am J Dig Dis 1978; 23:586–90.
7. Mahour GH, Wakim KG, Ferris DO. The common bile duct in man: its diameter and circumference. Ann Surg 1967; 165:415–9.
8. Lapis JL, Orlando RC, Mittelstaedt A, et al. Ultrasonography in the diagnosis of obstructive jaundice. Ann Intern Med 1978; 89:61–3.
9. Goldberg HI, Filly RA, Korobkin M, et al. Capability of CT body scanning and ultrasonography to demonstrate the status of the biliary ductal system in patients with jaundice. Radiology 1978; 129:731–7.
10. Morris AI, Fawcitt RA, Wood R, et al. Computed tomography, ultrasound, and cholestatic jaundice. Gut 1978; 19:685–8.
11. Graham MF, Cooperberg PL, Cohen MM, et al. Ultrasonographic screening of the common hepatic duct in symptomatic patients after cholecystectomy. Radiology 1981; 138:137–9.
12. Mueller PR, Ferrucci JT Jr, Simeone JF, et al. Postcholecystectomy bile duct dilation: myth or reality? AJR 1981; 136:355–8.
13. Dewbury KC, Joseph AEA, Hayes S, Murray C. Ultrasound in the evaluation and diagnosis of jaundice. Br J Radiol 1979; 52:276–80.
14. Greenwald RA, Pereiras R Jr, Morris SJ, Schiff ER. Jaundice, choledocholithiasis, and a nondilated common duct. JAMA 1978; 240:1983–4.
15. Cronan JJ, Mueller PR, Simeone JF, et al. Prospective diagnosis of choledocholithiasis. Radiology 1983; 146:467–9.
16. Gross BH, Harter LD, Gore RM, et al. Ultrasonic evaluation of common bile duct stones: prospective comparison with endoscopic retrograde cholangiopancreatography. Radiology 1983; 146:471–4.
17. Moss AA, Filly RA, Way LW. In vitro investigation of gallstones with computed tomography. J Comput Assist Tomogr 1980; 4:827–31.
18. McCullough EC, Payne JT. Patient dosage in computed tomography. Radiology 1978; 129:457–63.
19. Redeker AG, Karvountzis GG, Rickman RH, et al. Percutaneous transhepatic cholangiography. An improved technique. JAMA 1975; 231:386–7.
20. Pereiras R Jr, Chiprut RO, Greenwald RA, et al. Percutaneous transhepatic cholangiography with the "skinny" needle. A rapid, simple, and accurate method in the diagnosis of cholestasis. Ann Intern Med 1977; 86:562–8.
21. Goldstein LI, Sample WF, Kadell BM, et al. Grayscale ultrasonography and thin-needle cholangiography. Evaluation in the jaundiced patient. JAMA 1977; 238:1041–4.
22. Choi SH, Pralzer FA Jr, Park HC. Percutaneous transhepatic cholangiography with thin needle: recent update. J Med 1981; 12:147–58.
23. Elias E, Hamlyn AN, Jain S, et al. A randomized trial of percutaneous transhepatic cholangiography

with the Chiba needle versus endoscopic retrograde cholangiography for bile duct visualization
in jaundice. Gastroenterology 1976; 71:439–43.

24. Okuda K, Tanikawa K, Emura T, et al. Nonsurgical, percutaneous transhepatic cholangiography—Diagnostic significance in medical problems
of the liver. Dig Dis 1974; 19:21–36.

25. Shirakabe H, Ariyama J, Kurosawa K, et al. Experience with a new technique for percutaneous
transhepatic cholangiography. (Abstr) Gastroenterology 1975; 68:909.

26. Jain S, Long RG, Scott J, et al. Percutaneous
transhepatic cholangiography using the "Chiba"
needle—80 cases. Br J Radiol 1977; 50:175–80.

27. Ariyama J, Shirakabe H, Ohashi, et al. Experience
with percutaneous transhepatic cholangiography
using the Japanese needle. Gastrointest Radiol
1978; 2:359–65.

28. Kocher R, Mousseau R. Percutaneous transhepatic
cholangiography with the Chiba needle. Am J
Gastroenterol 1979; 71:39–44.

29. Mueller PR, Harbin WP, Ferrucci JT Jr, et al. Fine-
needle transhepatic cholangiography: reflections
after 450 cases. AJR 1981; 136:85–90.

30. Harbin WP, Mueller PR, Ferrucci JT, Jr. Transhepatic cholangiography: complications and use
patterns of the fine-needle technique. A multi-
institutional survey. Radiology 1980; 135:15–22.

31. Kreek MJ, Balint JA. "Skinny needle" cholangiography—results of a pilot study of a voluntary
prospective method for gathering risk data on new
procedures. Gastroenterology 1980; 78:598–604.

32. Bilbao MK, Dotter CT, Lee TG, et al. Complications of endoscopic retrograde cholangiopancreatography (ERCP). A study of 10,000 cases. Gastroenterology 1976; 70:314–20.

33. Ertan A, Kandilci U, Danisoglu V, et al. A comparison of percutaneous transhepatic cholangiography and endoscopic retrograde cholangiopancreatography in postcholecystectomy jaundice. J
Clin Gastroenterol 1981; 3:67–72.

34. Satake K, Cho K, Tatsumi S, et al. Evaluation of
cholangiographic procedures in diagnosis of obstructive jaundice. Am Surg 1981; 47:387–92.

35. Matzen P, Malchow-Moller A, Lejerstofte J, et al.
Endoscopic retrograde cholangiopancreatography
and transhepatic cholangiography in patients with
suspected obstructive jaundice. A randomized
study. Scand J Gastroenterol 1982; 17:731–5.

36. Scharschmidt BF, Goldberg HI, Schmid R. Current
concepts in diagnosis: Approach to the patient with
cholestatic jaundice. N Engl J Med 1983; 308:
1515–9.

37. Nebel OT, Silvis SE, Rogers BHG, et al. Complications associated with retrograde cholangiopancreatography. Results of the 1974 ASGE survey.
Gastrointest Endosc 1975; 22:34–6.

38. Mueller PR, vanSonnenberg E, Simeone JF. Fine-
needle transhepatic cholangiography. Indications
and usefulness. Ann Intern Med 1982; 97:567–72.

39. Armellin GM, Smith RC, Faithfull GR. Pulmonary
bile emboli following percutaneous cholangiography and biliary drainage. Pathology 1981; 13:615–
8.

40. Peven DR, Yokoo H. Bile pulmonary embolism:
report of a case and a review of the literature. Am
J Gastroenterol 1983; 78:830–4.

41. Juler GL, Conroy RM, Fuelleman RW. Bile leakage
following percutaneous transhepatic cholangiog-

raphy with the Chiba needle. Arch Surg 1977;
112:954–8.

42. Hoevels J, Nilsson U. Intrahepatic vascular lesions
following nonsurgical percutaneous transhepatic
bile duct intubation. Gastrointest Radiol 1980;
5:127–35.

43. Kadir S, Baassiri A, Barth KH, et al. Percutaneous
biliary drainage in the management of biliary sepsis. AJR 1982; 138:25–9.

44. O'Connor KW, Snodgrass PJ, Swonder JE, et al. A
blinded prospective study comparing four current
noninvasive approaches in the differential diagnosis of medical versus surgical jaundice. Gastroenterology 1983; 84:1498–1504.

45. MacCarty RL, LaRusso NF, Wiesner RH, et al.
Primary sclerosing cholangitis: findings on cholangiography and pancreatography. Radiology 1983;
149:39–44.

46. Lawson TL. Sensitivity of pancreatic ultrasonography in the detection of pancreatic disease. Radiology 1978; 128:733–6.

47. Taylor KJW, Buchin PJ, Viscomi GN, Rosenfield
AT. Ultrasonographic scanning of the pancreas.
Prospective study of clinical results. Radiology
1981; 138:211–3.

48. Pollock D, Taylor KJW. Ultrasound scanning in
patients with clinical suspicion of pancreatic cancer:
a retrospective study. Radiology 1981; 47:1662–5.

49. Hessel SJ, Siegelman SS, McNeil BJ, et al. A
prospective evaluation of computed tomography
and ultrasound of the pancreas. Radiology 1982;
143:129–33.

50. Husband JE, Meire HB, Krell L. Comparison of
ultrasound and computer-assisted tomography in
pancreatic diagnosis. Br J Radiol 1977; 50:855–62.

51. Swobodnik W, Meyer W, Brecht-Kraus D, et al.
Ultrasound, computed tomography and endoscopic retrograde cholangiopancreatography in the
morphologic diagnosis of pancreatic disease. Klin
Wochenschr 1983; 61:291–6.

52. Cotton PB, Lees WR, Vallon AG, et al. Gray-scale
ultrasonography and endoscopic pancreatography
in pancreatic diagnosis. Radiology 1980; 134:453–
9.

53. Gowland M, Warwick F, Kalantzis N, Braganza J.
Relative efficiency and predictive value of ultrasonography and endoscopic retrograde pancreatography in diagnosis of pancreatic disease. Lancet
1981; II:190–3.

54. Grodinsky C, Schumann B, Brush BE. Endoscopic
retrograde pancreatic duct cannulation (ERCP) as
an aid to pancreatic surgery. Bull Soc Int Chir
1975; 34:605–10.

55. Cooperman AM, Sivak MV, Sullivan BH Jr, et al.
Endoscopic pancreatography: its value in preoperative and postoperative assessment of pancreatic
disease. Am J Surg 1975; 129:38–43.

56. Greenwald RA, Deluca RF, Raskin JB. Pancreaticpleural fistula: demonstration by endoscopic retrograde cholangiopancreatography (ERCP) and successful treatment with radiation therapy. Dig Dis
Sci 1979; 24:240–4.

57. Valentini M, Cavallini G, Vantini I, et al. A comparative evaluation of endoscopic retrograde cholangiopancreatography and the secretin-cholecys-
tokinin test in the diagnosis of chronic pancreatitis:
a multicentre study in 124 patients. Endoscopy
1981; 13:64–7.

58. Martin EW Jr, Catalano P, Cooperman M, et al.

Surgical decision-making in the treatment of pancreatic pseudocysts. Internal versus external drainage. Am J Surg 1979; 138:821–4.

59. Gebhardt CH, Riemann JF, Lux G. The importance of ERCP for the surgical tactic in haemorrhagic necrotizing pancreatitis (preliminary report). Endoscopy 1983; 15:55–8.

60. Safrany L, Cotton PB. A preliminary report: Urgent duodenoscopic sphincterotomy for acute gallstone pancreatitis. Surgery 1981; 89:424–8.

61. Carr-Locke DL, Westwood CA. Endoscopy and endoscopic retrograde cholangiopancreatography findings in traumatic liver injury and hemobilia. Am J Gastroenterol 1980; 73:162–4.

62. McDougal EG, Mandel SR. Traumatic hemobilia. Successful nonoperative treatment in two cases. Am Surg 1984; 50:169–72.

63. Jensen AR, Matzen P. Hemobilia with jaundice: treatment by endoscopic papillotomy. Am J Gastroenterol 1982; 77:162–3.

64. Struyven J, Cremer M, Pirson P, et al. Posttraumatic bilhemia: diagnosis and catheter therapy. AJR 1982; 138:746–7.

65. Safrany L. (from Course Syllabus). ERCP: diagnostic and therapeutic aspects. Cleveland Clinic Foundation, Cleveland, Ohio, March 1984.

66. Linos DA, King RM, Mucha P Jr, et al. Blunt pancreatic trauma. Minn Med 1983; 66:153–60.

67. Moss AA, Federle M, Shapiro HA, et al. The combined use of computed tomography and endoscopic retrograde cholangiopancreatography in the assessment of suspected pancreatic neoplasm: a blind clinical evaluation. Radiology 1980; 134:159–63.

68. Savarino V, Mansi C, Bistolfi L, et al. Failure of new diagnostic aids in improving detection of pancreatic cancer at a resectable stage. Dig Dis Sci 1983; 28:1078–82.

69. Frick MP, Feinberg SB, Goodale RL. The value of endoscopic retrograde cholangiopancreatography in patients with suspected carcinoma of the pancreas and indeterminate computed tomographic results. Surg Gynecol Obstet 1982; 155:177–82.

70. Frick MP, O'Leary JF, Walker HC Jr, et al. Accuracy of endoscopic retrograde cholangiopancreatography (ERCP) in differentiating benign and malignant pancreatic disease. Gastrointest Radiol 1982; 7:241–4.

71. Freeny PC, Kidd R, Ball TJ. ERCP-guided percutaneous fine-needle pancreatic biopsy. West J Med 1980; 132:283–7.

72. Siegel JH, Sable RA, Ho R, et al. Abnormalities of the bile duct associated with chronic pancreatitis. Am J Gastroenterol 1979; 72:259–66.

73. Freeny PC, Bilbao MK, Katon RM. "Blind" evaluation of endoscopic retrograde cholangiopancreatography (ERCP) in the diagnosis of pancreatic carcinoma: the "double duct" and other signs. Radiology 1976; 119:271–4.

74. Plumley TF, Rohrmann CA, Freeny PC, et al. Double duct sign: Reassessed significance in ERCP. AJR 1982; 138:31–5.

75. Ralls PW, Halls J, Renner I, Juttner H. Endoscopic retrograde cholangiopancreatography (ERC) in pancreatic disease. A reassessment of the specificity of ductal abnormalities in differentiating benign from malignant disease. Radiology 1980; 134:347–52.

76. Cotton PB. Progress report. ERCP. Gut 1977; 18:316–41.

77. Bull J, Keeling PW, Thompson RP. Endoscopic retrograde cholangiopancreatography for unexplained upper abdominal pain. Br Med J 1980; 280:764.

78. Ruddell WSJ, Lintott DJ, Axon ATR. The diagnostic yield of ERCP in the investigation of unexplained abdominal pain. Br J Surg 1983; 70:74–5.

79. Thurnherr M, Bruhlmann WF, Krejs GI, et al. Fulminant cholangitis and septicemia after endoscopic retrograde cholangiography (ERC) in two patients with obstructive jaundice. Am J Dig Dis 1976; 21:477–81.

80. Weizel A, Gelhaus-Klamant U. Renal excretion of contrast medium after endoscopic retrograde investigations. Endoscopy 1978; 10:30–2.

81. Villa E, Pasquinelli C, Rigo G, et al. Gastrointestinal endoscopy and HBV infection: no evidence for a causal relationship. A prospective controlled study. Gastrointest Endosc 1984; 30:15–7.

82. Brandes JW, Scheffer B, Lorenz-Meyer H, et al. ERCP: Complications and prophylaxis—a controlled study. Endoscopy 1981; 13:27–30.

83. Zimmon DS, Falkenstein DB, Riccobono C, et al. Complications of endoscopic retrograde cholangiopancreatography. Analysis of 300 consecutive cases. Gastroenterology 1975; 69:303–9.

84. Goncalves D. Endoscopic procedures hazard—vagovagal syncope with heart standstill due to ERCP. Arq Gastroenterol 1979; 16:200–2.

85. Geenen JE. ERCP and the problem of sepsis. In: Sivak MV Jr, Levin B, eds. Selected papers from the Cleveland Clinic Course. "ERCP: diagnostic and therapeutic aspects—an international symposium", March 19–21, 1981. Gastrointest Endosc 1982; 28:197–209.

86. Stray N, Midtvedt T, Valnes K. Endoscopy-related bacteremia. Scand J Gastroenterol 1978; 13:345–7.

87. Siegel JH, Berger SA, Sable RA, et al. Low incidence of bacteremia following endoscopic retrograde cholangiopancreatography (ERCP). Am J Gastroenterol 1979; 71:465–8.

88. Parker HW, Geenen JE, Bjork JT, Stewart ET. A prospective analysis of fever and bacteremia following ERCP. Gastrointest Endosc 1979; 25:102–3.

89. Helm EB. Direct choledochography and related diagnostic methods. Part 3: ERCP and biliary infections. Clin Gastroenterol 1983; 12:115–23.

90. Schousboe M, Carter A, Sheppard PS. Endoscopic retrograde cholangio-pancreatography: related nosocomial infections. NZ Med J 1980; 92:275–7.

91. Low DE, Micflikier AB, Kennedy JK, et al. Infectious complications of endoscopic retrograde cholangiopancreatography. Arch Intern Med 1980; 140:1076–7.

92. Doherty DE, Falko JM, Lefkovitz N, et al. Pseudomonas aeruginosa sepsis following retrograde cholangiopancreatography (ERCP). Dig Dis Sci 1982; 27:169–70.

93. Elson CO, Hattori K, Blackstone MO. Polymicrobial sepsis following endoscopic retrograde cholangiopancreatography. Gastroenterology 1975; 69:507–10.

94. O'Connor HJ, Axon ATR. Gastrointestinal endoscopy: infection and disinfection. Gut 1983; 24:1067–77.

95. Shorvon PJ, Eykyn SJ, Cotton PB. Gastrointestinal instrumentation, bacteraemia, and endocarditis. Gut 1983; 24:1078–93.

96. Keighley MRB, Lister DM, Jacobs SI, et al. Hazards of surgical treatment due to microorganisms in the bile. Surgery 1974; 75:578–83.

97. Keighley MRB. Micro-organisms in the bile. A preventable cause of sepsis after biliary surgery. Ann R Coll Surg Engl 1977; 59:328–34.

98. Hultborn A, Jacobsson B, Rosengren B. Cholangiovenous reflux during cholangiography. An experimental and clinical study. Acta Chir Scand 1962; 123:111–4.

99. Huang T, Bass JA, Williams RD. The significance of biliary pressure in cholangitis. Arch Surg 1969; 98:629–32.

100. Jacobsson B, Kjellander J, Rosengren B. Cholangiovenous reflux. An experimental study. Acta Chir Scand 1962; 123:316–21.

101. Bockman DE. Route of flow and micropathology resulting from retrograde intrabiliary injection of India ink and ferritin in experimental animals. A combined light- and electron-microscopic study. Gastroenterology 1974; 67:324–32.

102. Waldron RL II, Luse SA, Wollowick HE, Seaman WB. Demonstration of a retrograde pancreatic pathway: correlation of roentgenographic and electron microscopic studies. AJR 1971; 111:695–9.

103. Bockman DE, Schiller WR, Anderson MC. Route of retrograde flow in the exocrine pancreas during ductal hypertension. Arch Surg 1971; 103:321–9.

104. Collen MJ, Hanan MR, Maher JA, et al. Modification of endoscopic retrograde cholangiopancreatography (ERCP) septic complications by the addition of an antibiotic to the contrast media. Am J Gastroenterol 1980; 74:493–6.

105. Jendrzejewski JW, McAnally T, Jones SR, Katon RM. Antibiotics and ERCP: In vitro activity of aminoglycosides when added to iodinated contrast agents. Gastroenterology 1980; 78:745–8.

106. Dutta SK, Cox M, Williams RB, et al. Prospective evaluation of the risk of bacteremia and the role of antibiotics in ERCP. J Clin Gastroenterol 1983; 5:325–9.

107. McMahon LF Jr, Gorelick FS. ERCP and bacteremia. J Clin Gastroenterol 1983; 5:358–9.

108. Keighley MRB, Baddeley RM, Burdon DW, et al. A controlled trial of parenteral prophylactic gentamicin therapy in biliary surgery. Br J Surg 1975; 62:275–9.

109. Keighley MRB, Drysdale RB, Quoraishi AH, et al. Antibiotics in biliary disease: the relative importance of antibiotic concentrations in the bile and serum. Gut 1976; 17:495–500.

110. Hershey SD, Sugawa C, Cushing R, et al. The value of prophylactic antibiotic therapy during endoscopic retrograde cholangiopancreatography. Surg Gynecol Obstet 1982; 155:801–3.

111. Blackwood W, Vennes J, Silvis S. Post endoscopy pancreatitis and hyperamylasemia. Gastrointest Endosc 1973; 20:56–8.

112. Cotton PB. Cannulation of the papilla of Vater by endoscopy and retrograde cholangiopancreatography (ERCP) Gut 1972; 13:1014–25.

113. Kasugai T, Kuno N, Aoki I, et al. Fiberduodenoscopy: analysis of 353 examinations. Gastrointest Endosc 1971; 18:9–16.

114. Kasugai T, Kuno N, Kobayashi S, Hattoni K. Endoscopic pancreatocholangiography. I. The normal endoscopic pancreatocholangiogram. Gastroenterology 1972; 63:217–26.

115. Ruppin H, Amon R, Ett W, et al. Acute pancreatitis after endoscopic/radiological pancreaticography (ERP). Endoscopy 1974; 6:94–8.

116. Ammann RW, Deyhle P, Butikofer E. Fatal necrotizing pancreatitis after peroral cholangiopancreatography. Gastroenterology 1973; 64:320–3.

117. Hamilton I, Lintott DJ, Rothwell J, et al. Acute pancreatitis following endoscopic retrograde cholangiopancreatography. Clin Radiol 1983; 34:543–6.

118. Kasugai T, Kuno N, Kizu M. Manometric endoscopic retrograde pancreatocholangiography. Technique, significance, and evaluation. Dig Dis Sci 1974; 19:485–502.

119. Galvan A, Klotz AP. Is transduodenal pancreatography ever contraindicated? A case report of provoked pancreatitis and pseudocyst. Gastrointest Endosc 1973; 20:28–30.

120. Skude G, Wehlin L, Maruyama T, Ariyama J. Hyperamylasaemia after duodenoscopy and retrograde cholangiopancreatography. Gut 1976; 17:127–32.

121. Sable RA, Rosenthal WS, Siegel J, et al. Absorption of contrast medium during ERCP. Dig Dis Sci 1983; 28:801–6.

122. Peters PE, Katz G, Safrany L, Weitemeyer R. Radiation exposure in patients undergoing endoscopic retrograde cholangiopancreatography and endoscopic papillotomy. Gastrointest Radiol 1978; 3:353–5.

123. Cohen G, Brodmerkel GJ Jr, Lynn S. Absorbed doses to patients and personnel from endoscopic retrograde cholangiopancreatographic (ERCP) examinations. Radiology 1979; 130:773–5.

Chapter 27

ANATOMY AND EMBRYOLOGY OF THE BILIARY TRACT AND PANCREAS

BERNARD H. HAND*, M.S., F.R.C.S.

It has been rightly said that variation in the biliary tree is rampant and even that such variation is constant. It is estimated that less than 50% of subjects possess so-called normal anatomy when considering vascular variation,[1] whereas ductal variations are less common and occur in about 13% of cases.[2] The word anomalous has been used to describe the differences, which implies abnormality; but these must surely be regarded as normal variations distinct from true congenital abnormalities. Bearing in mind that the liver, biliary tract, and pancreas develop close to each other from small buddings of the gut tube, these variations must be expected. With the advent of preoperative x-rays, endoscopic retrograde cholangiopancreatography (ERCP), ultrasound, computed tomography, and arteriography, a more realistic appreciation has become possible than was obtained from earlier postmortem studies.

EMBRYOLOGY

The liver, biliary tract, and pancreas develop from diverticula, or cylinders, which appear at the junction of foregut and midgut as early as the nineteenth somite embryo, on or about the twenty-fifth day, although some anatomists put this a little earlier. These endodermal buds produce the epithelium and secretory cells, whereas the musculature, connective tissue, and blood vessels develop from the splanchnic mesoderm and the septum transversum, the latter being invaded by a plexus of vessels derived from the vitelline and umbilical veins.

The diverticulum for the liver and biliary tract is the first of the buds to be seen, this at the beginning of the fourth week projecting into the ventral mesentery. A further bulge develops, resulting in its division into a larger cranial portion, destined to become the liver and bile ducts, and a smaller caudal portion that will produce the gallbladder and cystic duct. The cranial portion divides into two solid cords, ultimately to produce the right and left hepatic ducts. These cords push into the adjacent septum transversum and anastomose round clusters of mesenchyme cells which form small blood vessels. In turn these blood vessels become confluent with the vitelline and umbilical veins and eventually produce the liver sinusoids.

Major blood vessels appear in the liver by the thirty-second day, namely the right and left umbilical veins, the transverse portal sinus, and the hepatic part of the inferior vena cava; later the right umbilical vein atrophies. In utero, the blood is shunted from the left umbilical vein directly into the inferior vena cava via the ductus venosus. At birth this atrophies and remains as the ligamentum venosum.

The septum transversum becomes one of the main sites for hematopoiesis until near full term. It also produces the Kupffer cells, the liver capsule, and all the ligaments that suspend the liver, as well as the central tendon of the diaphragm.

The hepatic cords eventually acquire a lumen and with the rapid growth of the liver parenchyma, far in excess of other tissues,

---

*Deceased.

599

the gallbladder, cystic duct, and bile ducts increase in size and length. Ultimately the liver is about 10% of total body weight, whereas at birth this proportion falls to 5%. Bile is secreted beginning at the fourth or fifth month.

The pancreas develops from two diverticula of the duodenal endoderm when the embryo is about 30 days old (Fig. 27–1). The first to appear lies dorsal and slightly cranial to the hepatic diverticulum and grows out into the dorsal mesentery to the left of the vitelline veins, reaching eventually as far as the developing spleen. The ventral bud, paired initially, arises a little later in the angle below the hepatic diverticulum. The left bud of the pair atrophies.

As the common bile duct bud elongates and the ventral bud extends away from the duodenum, it appears that the ventral bud is actually a branch of the common bile duct. Soon the duodenum rotates 90 degrees on its long axis, and there is a more rapid growth of the left side of the duodenum. This converts the original ventral surface into the right side and brings the ventral pancreas into the mesoduodenum in a position in front of the bile duct and caudal to the dorsal pancreas. The left vitelline vein, destined to become the portal vein, thus lies behind the dorsal pancreas and in front of the ventral pancreas (viewing from anterior to posterior). After this rotation the mesoduodenum fuses with the posterior peritoneum to make most of the duodenum and the whole pancreas except the tail retroperitoneal structures.

At about six to seven weeks the two lobes fuse into a single organ. The ventral pancreas becomes the uncinate lobe and the lower part of the head, while the dorsal pancreas forms the rest of the head, neck, body, and tail.

The duct systems of these two portions usually fuse in the head, the duodenal entry of the dorsal duct (Santorini) being cranial

and dorsal to that of the ventral duct (Wirsung). The former frequently seals completely so that all pancreatic juice flows via the ventral duct. The ventral duct may drain directly into the duodenum or acquire a common opening with the bile duct. Occasionally the two ducts do not fuse, and therefore their respective parts of the pancreas drain separately into the duodenum. Least commonly of all, the ventral duct obliterates and all drainage takes place through the dorsal duct. These variations should be expected, since any one may be the normal mode in higher mammalian species.

Within the now-formed gland the major pancreatic ducts lengthen into the surrounding mesenchyme, and by sprouting and subsequent canalization the collecting ducts and acini are produced by the twelfth week. At about the tenth week cells bud off from the pancreatic endoderm, become disconnected from the duct system, and are destined to differentiate into the endocrine cells. By the fourth month secretory granules appear in the exocrine pancreas.

GENERAL ANATOMIC DESCRIPTION

Liver

The liver is the largest of the viscera and fills most of the abdominal cavity enclosed between the diaphragm and ribs. It normally weighs about 1500 gm, about one fortieth of total body weight. The anterosuperior, posterior, and right lateral surfaces are in curved continuity and are referred to as the diaphragmatic surface. Classically the liver is divided into a larger right and a smaller left lobe by the falciform ligament, which contains the ligamentum teres as the obliterated left umbilical vein (Fig. 27–2).

The under, or visceral, surface is further divided into two additional smaller lobes by four vertical fissures and one transverse fis-

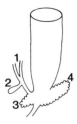 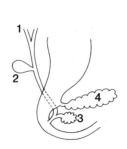 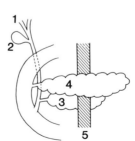

FIGURE 27–1. Embryologic development of the pancreas. 1, bile ducts; 2, gallbladder; 3, ventral bud; 4, dorsal bud; 5, superior mesenteric and portal veins.

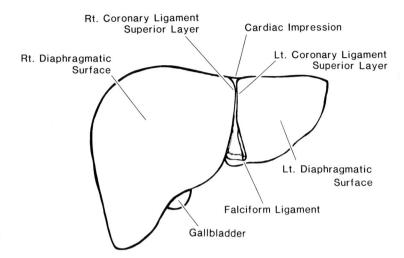

FIGURE 27–2. Diaphragmatic surface of the liver.

sure. The latter is the porta hepatis, which provides entry of vessels and bile ducts into the liver. Anterior to this and lying between the ligamentum teres and the gallbladder fossa is the quadrate lobe, whereas posterior to it and lying between the inferior vena cava and the ligamentum venosum lies the caudate lobe and its caudate process, which bridges into the right lobe (Fig. 27–3).

This standard description of the liver lobes is no longer acceptable for clinical purposes. From studies of human liver corrosion casts and x-rays, a segmental division has been demonstrated. This is based on the distribution of the intrahepatic bile ducts and associated branches of the hepatic artery and portal vein, which closely follow one another to the finest branches. There are no cross connections between segments that are sufficient in size to maintain an area in which the ducts or arteries have been occluded. Furthermore, although these segments are easily discernible in the casts, they have no anatomical landmarks that can be seen on the surface of the liver or within its substance.[3–9]

Extensive research has shown that the right and left lobes are demarcated by a line, not quite sagittal in section, that runs from the gallbladder fossa to the left of the inferior vena cava. The quadrate lobe and most of the caudate lobe, with the exception of the caudate process, therefore lie within the left lobe.

These two main lobes have been further subdivided into segments. There have been

FIGURE 27–3. Visceral surface of the liver and its relations.

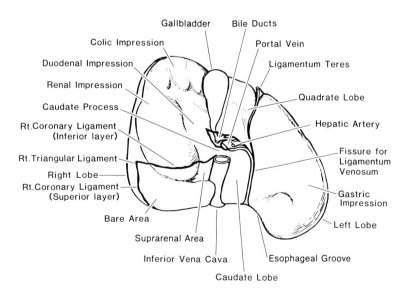

some slight differences in nomenclature, but it is now generally accepted that the right lobe is divided into anterior inferior, anterior superior, posterior inferior, and posterior superior segments; the left lobe is divided into medial superior, medial inferior, lateral superior, and lateral inferior segments; subsegmental ducts are also described (Figs. 27–4 and 27–5). A branch of the anterior inferior segment of the right lobe lies close to the surface under the gallbladder fossa, and this has been named the subvesical duct.

The caudate process drains into the right hepatic duct, and sometimes the right side of the caudate lobe does so also. Most of the caudate lobe usually drains into the left hepatic duct. The quadrate lobe drains into the left hepatic duct.

It must be further appreciated that the hepatic veins do not follow the same segmental drainage but pass in an oblique posterior direction to reach the inferior vena cava and therefore cross these segments.

As might be anticipated there is some variation in the segmental and subsegmental ducts. Aberrant drainage of subsegmental ducts within the right lobe occurs in 20% of cases; the anterior and posterior segmental ducts do not join to form a right hepatic duct in 28%; the posterior segmental duct joins the left hepatic duct in 22%; and in 6% the right anterior segmental duct joins the left hepatic duct.

The medial and lateral segmental ducts of the left lobe unite to form a left hepatic duct

in 67% of cases; in 25%, the medial segmental duct drains into the lateral inferior duct. Other variations are much less common (Fig. 27–6). These and even more minor variations, which are really of significance only in hepatic surgery, may be found in the literature.[10]

The liver is suspended from the diaphragm and the anterior abdominal wall by ligaments. The anterior falciform ligament divides, proceeding over the superior surface of the liver, into right and left coronary ligaments. These are oriented to the left and right on the superior surface. The width of each coronary ligament narrows as their anterior and posterior layers come closer together toward their farthest attachment to the left and right, the terminal edges being called the left and right triangular ligaments. The liver is also held by the inferior vena cava which passes in a groove posteriorly. It is covered by peritoneum, except on these ligaments and a small bare area in contact with the diaphragm to the right of the inferior vena cava, which is skirted by the separated layers of right coronary ligament. Beneath the peritoneum lies a thin connective tissue covering, known as Glisson's capsule.

From the visceral surface the lesser omentum extends downward from the porta hepatis and the fossa for the ligamentum venosum to attachments to the lesser curvature of the stomach and the first part of the duodenum. The bile ducts, portal vein, and hepatic arteries are found within the free

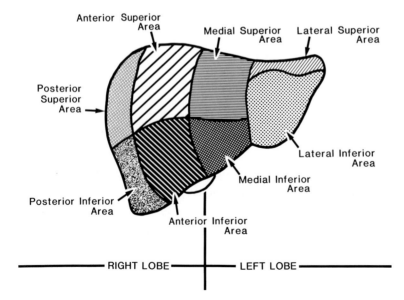

FIGURE 27–4. Segmental pattern of intrahepatic ducts: diaphragmatic surface.

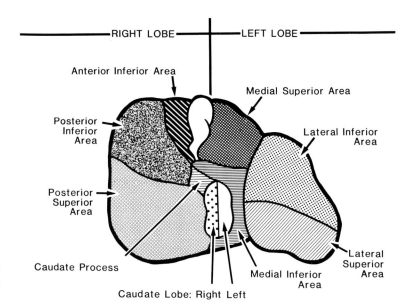

FIGURE 27–5. Segmental pattern of the intrahepatic ducts: visceral surface.

edge of the lesser omentum. They therefore lie anterior to the foramen of Winslow which leads from the main peritoneal cavity into the lesser sac.

The first three surfaces (vida supra) of the liver are in contact with the diaphragm and the anterior abdominal wall. The visceral surface on the left is related to the esophagus and the lesser curvature of the stomach; to the right, it is in contact with the right kidney, the right suprarenal gland, the hepatic flexure, the pylorus, and the duodenum.

Hepatic Ducts

The right and left hepatic ducts join just outside the porta hepatis to form the common hepatic duct, which has a diameter sim-

FIGURE 27–6. Variations of the segmental intrahepatic ducts. A–C, Variations related to the right lobe; D–J, variations related to the left lobe. ASD, anterior segmental duct; PSD, posterior segmental duct; RHD, right hepatic duct; LHD, left hepatic duct; CHD, common hepatic duct; LS, lateral segmental duct; MS, medial segmental duct; LSA, lateral superior area duct; LIA, lateral inferior area duct. (*Adapted from* Linder RM, Cady B. Hepatic resection. Surg Clin North Am 1980; 60:349–67. Reproduced with permission.)

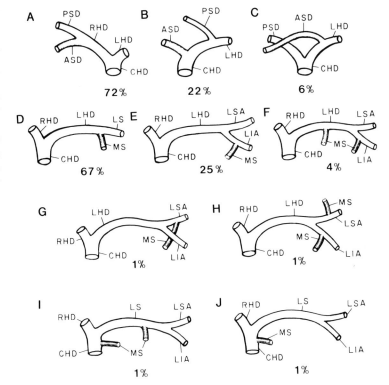

ilar to that of the common bile duct. Although on average the common hepatic duct is 2.5 to 3.5 cm in length, the union of the left and right ducts may be lower, and they have even been reported as opening separately into the duodenum.[11] This, combined with the variable site of entry of the cystic duct, determines the lengths of the common bile and common hepatic ducts. The common hepatic duct passes down the free edge of the lesser omentum with the hepatic artery or with one of its two main branches, the artery lying to the left of the bile duct and the portal vein lying behind. The cystic artery usually crosses the common hepatic duct posteriorly, but in 25% of cases it passes anterior to the duct. Also, in 15% of cases the right hepatic artery lies anterior to the duct.[1, 11, 12]

Gallbladder

The gallbladder, with a capacity of about 50 ml, is a pear-shaped sac lying in a fossa on the right visceral surface of the liver lateral to the quadrate lobe and separated from the caudate lobe by the structures leading to the porta hepatis. It is covered by peritoneum to a variable extent and may even be on a mesentery.[13, 14]

The gallbladder is composed of a columnar epithelium thrown into folds, giving it a honeycombed appearance, outside of which lies a fibromuscular layer mainly longitudinal in direction. There are mucous glands, but the neck of the gallbladder contains goblet cells. The gallbladder consists of a fundus which may or may not project beyond the liver to come in contact with anterior abdominal wall at the level of the ninth costal cartilage.[15, 16] Posteriorly the gallbladder is in contact with the transverse colon. With the normal tilt of the liver the body passes upward, backward, and to the left and narrows to form the neck. A dilatation here, called Hartmann's pouch, is a pathologic and not an anatomic entity. The body is in contact with the liver superiorly, into which it may be embedded to a variable extent and with the duodenum and transverse colon below; the neck narrows into the cystic duct.

Cystic Duct

The cystic duct, usually 3 to 4 cm long, runs backward and to the left in a series of S-shaped bends to join the common hepatic duct, thereby forming the common bile duct.

It contains the valves of Heister, which have a splinting effect.

Common Bile Duct

This duct continues downward and slightly to the left in the free edge of the lesser omentum, with the hepatic artery proper on its left and the portal vein behind. It passes behind the first part of the duodenum, where now the gastroduodenal artery lies to its left and the retroduodenal artery lies in front. It then passes into a groove in the head of the pancreas and runs to the right in front of the inferior vena cava. Its entry into the pancreas is recognized radiologically as the apex of a curve or even a sharp angle, and here the common bile duct may narrow slightly. Behind the pancreas it is approached by the pancreatic duct, and the two ducts become enveloped in a common muscular and connective tissue sheath and pass together through the choledochal window in the duodenal muscle to open on the major papilla about 8 to 10 cm from the pylorus.

In about 15% of cases there is no pancreatic tissue behind the common bile duct as it lies in the pancreatic groove. In the remaining 85% of cases, it is partly or wholly covered by pancreatic tissue. Even if the duct is completely covered there is a dissectable plane between the two organs.[17–19] It may lie quite close to the duodenum, or it may be as much as 2 mm away. In this region it is usually crossed by the superior pancreatoduodenal vessels. Measurements of the diameter have been made radiologically, on postmortem specimens, at intravenous or operative cholangiography and by ultrasonography. In comparing these, magnification factors must be taken into account. Table 27–1 shows some reported series.[20–28] It is generally accepted that the upper normal limit is 10 mm, or at most 12 mm, measured radiologically. This measurement is taken conventionally at point of entry of the duct into the pancreas. The normal appearance of the bile duct by ERCP is discussed in Chapter 28.

Choledochoduodenal Area

Although the existence of a sphincter at the lower end of the common bile duct was postulated by Glisson in 1659,[29] researches into the anatomy of the choledochoduodenal area actually began in the 19th century, when

*Reproduced by courtesy of the Editor of the British Journal of Hospital Medicine.
†Diameter in mm on entry into the pancreas measured on x-ray films.

TABLE 27–1. Measurements of the Internal Diameter of the Normal Common Bile Duct*

Authors	Date	Diameter†
Partington and Sachs[20]	1951	5–11
Poppel and Jacobson[21]	1953	4–6
Sullens and Sexton[22]	1955	Up to 7
Cole and Harridge[23]	1956	Up to 15
Wise and O'Brien[24]	1956	3–15
Hutchinson and Blake[25]	1957	Up to 8
LeQuesne et al.[26]	1959	Up to 10
Mahour et al.[28]	1967	4–12

the existence of a sphincter mechanism at the lower end of the common bile duct appears to have been established.[30, 31]

Early in the 20th century further studies were carried out, mainly to determine the etiology of pancreatitis.[32, 33] Later, the microscopic appearance of this area was extensively investigated, and the more important works have been reviewed and acknowledged.[34–36] Unfortunately, the initial researches tended to confuse the issue as to the extent of the musculature and as to whether the sphincter muscle was a functional entity separate from the duodenal muscle.

Let us consider first the functional independence: In the early part of this century several authorities believed that the sphincter was only partly responsible for control of the flow of bile.[37–39] A little later it was considered to be fully independent of the duodenal muscle.[40–42] In more recent times, with the advent of the image intensifier, it was concluded that the sphincter was fully independent.[43–46] Subsequent electromyographic studies have confirmed this.[47]

Consider next the anatomic studies: Comprehensive study of fetal sections established the existence of a sphincter that was anatomically separate from the duodenal wall and involved both the common bile duct and the pancreatic duct. Initially it was thought that the sphincter around the pancreatic duct was incomplete and that the common channel was not encompassed by the sphincter.[48, 49] Later studies on adult tissue, however, showed that the sphincter encircled the pancreatic duct and the common channel.[50]

It was not appreciated until the 1950's, when cholangiography was being more widely practiced, that radiologically the com-

mon bile duct becomes abruptly narrowed as it approaches the duodenum.[20, 21, 34, 51–55]

Even with these extensive investigations, no clear picture emerged of the relationship between the macroscopic, microscopic, and radiologic appearances of the choledochoduodenal area. A study of autopsy material, using cholangiography and pancreatography, followed by the preparation of ductal casts and subsequent dissection of the specimens, made it possible to correlate the configuration of the cast with the gross anatomy and the radiologic appearance. By microscopic study of these specimens it was possible to correlate the sphincter mechanism with the radiologic appearance.[34, 35]

This work demonstrated that the terminal narrowing of the common bile duct, not detectable on its external surface, was due to the marked increase of muscle fibers in the wall. This produced an abrupt reduction in the width of the lumen that correlated to a radiologically recognizable notch. The notch was found to lie some 2 mm proximal to the duodenal wall and corresponded to the upper edge of the superior choledochal sphincter. The muscular narrow-lumened portion of the common bile duct, referred to as the thickened segment, varies in length from 11 mm to 27 mm, the average being 16 mm. The length of the intraduodenal part of the thickened segment is thus 2 mm less, i.e., 9 mm to 25 mm (Fig. 27–7).

Based on these findings, it was suggested that the previous subdivision of the common bile duct into four portions—supraduodenal, retroduodenal, retropancreatic and intraduodenal—should be abandoned in favor of only two portions: namely, an upper, longer, wide-lumened, thin-walled portion and a lower, shorter, narrow-lumened, thick-walled portion demarcated by a notch. This division relates not only to the radiologic appearance, but also to microscopic appearance and function. The upper part is merely a conduit composed of mucosa and a lot of elastic and connective tissue, but very little muscle, the latter having a predominantly longitudinal orientation. In this section numerous mucous glands can be seen opening as depressed pores. The second lower part of the common bile duct is the sphincteric mechanism.

The pancreatic duct, lying posteriorly or posteromedially, approaches the common bile duct just above the level of the notch. Here the two ducts become surrounded by a common muscular sheath but remain sepa-

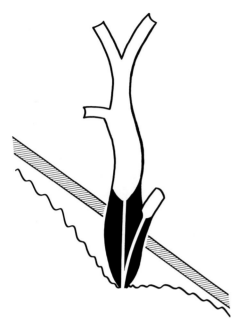

FIGURE 27–7. Diagrammatic representation of the common bile duct, showing a notch that divides it into two distinct parts: an upper, wide-lumened, thin-walled portion and a lower, narrow-lumened, thick-walled portion. The lower portion is seen to lie mainly in the submucous layer of the duodenum. (*From:* Hand BH. An anatomical study of the choledochoduodenal area. Br J Surg 1963; 50:486–94. Reproduced with permission.)

the pancreatic drainage passes via the duct of Santorini.[34, 35] Tradition refers to the common channel as the ampulla of Vater,[58] but recent studies fail to demonstrate any dilation in this region.[27, 34, 35, 57] The length of the common channel has been reported as measuring between 1 mm and 17 mm, the majority being between 2 mm and 7 mm long.[35]

The orifice of the major papilla is round or slit-like and between 2 and 5 mm in diameter. Sometimes minute fronds of mucosa prolapse through the orifice. These are called valvules and arise from the common channel mucosa; they contain a central core of muscle that permits lengthening and shortening.[59]

Pancreas

The pancreas, which is 12 to 25 cm in length and weighs 70 to 100 gm depending on the sex, lies retroperitoneally on the posterior abdominal wall and possesses an ill-defined connective tissue capsule. It is prismatic in cross section and therefore has three borders—superior, inferior, and anterior.

The pancreas is divided anatomically into head, neck, body, and tail. Its form is hook-

rated by a muscular septum.[35, 56, 57] This muscular sheath is predominantly circular in configuration and surrounds both the common bile duct and pancreatic duct separately and also passes across the septum between them in a figure-of-8 fashion. This muscle extends to the apex of the papilla and therefore envelops the common channel when present or surrounds both ducts individually if there are separate openings. An outer layer of the longitudinal muscle is present and is thought to produce shortening and lengthening and thus erection of the papilla.

In the submucous layer of the duodenum, the two ducts may fuse by a gradual thinning and breakdown of the septum to form a common channel or pancreatobiliary canal (Fig. 27–8). Alternatively the two ducts may open separately on the major papilla (Fig. 27–9). A great deal of work has been done on the frequency of these two modes of entry and the length of the common channel. Based on a comprehensive review of the literature involving some 3000 specimens, it would appear that some 85% have a common channel and 13% have separate openings; in 2% the duct of Wirsung is not patent and all

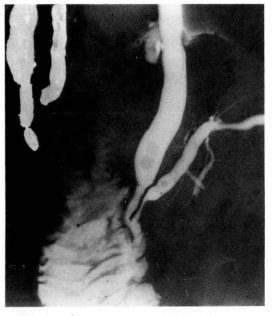

FIGURE 27–8. Autopsy cast and cholangiogram showing a well-marked notch on the common bile duct. The narrow-lumened portion, called the thickened segment, and the common channel are well known. The pancreatic duct has a similar appearance. (*From:* Hand BH. An anatomical study of the choledocho-duodenal area. Br J Surg 1963; 50:486–94. Reprinted with permission.)

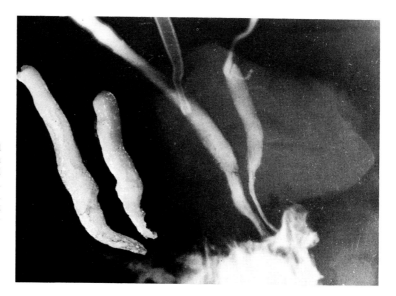

FIGURE 27–9. Autopsy cast and cholangiogram of specimen with separate openings of the bile and pancreatic ducts into the duodenal lumen. The notch of the common bile duct is not prominent, but that of the pancreatic duct is well defined. (*From*: Hand BH. An anatomical study of the choledochoduodenal area. Br J Surg 1963; 50: 486–94. Reproduced with permission.)

like, the "hook" being the head and the body, and the "handle" being the tail. It is pale yellow and has a slightly lobulated surface. In the past the pancreas was regarded as a fixed structure, but computed tomography indicates that some movement occurs during respiration, with the tail being more mobile.

Anatomically the pancreas passes from right to left, usually in a cephalad direction; the shape of the gland has been described as oblique (36% of cases), sigmoid (19%), transverse (3%), horseshoe (8%), L-shaped (33%), and inverted (11%).[60, 61] Where it crosses the spine and aorta there is a forward bulge, and it is here that the pancreas is vulnerable to injury as a result of blunt abdominal trauma. Its relationship to the spine is variable. Whereas the head may be as low as the first sacral and the tail as high as the tenth thoracic vertebra, usually the whole gland lies between first lumbar and twelfth thoracic vertebrae.

The mean thickness of the pancreas is 2.3 cm in the head, 1.9 cm in the neck, 2 cm in the body, and 1.5 cm in the tail; the mean width is 4.4 cm, 3.4 cm, 3.5 cm, and 3 cm at these respective anatomic divisions. This indicates that its vertical dimension is twice that of the anteroposterior direction.

The head lies within the duodenal loop and is overlapped by it superiorly but overlaps it elsewhere. In 98% of patients it lies between twelfth thoracic and second lumbar vertebrae.[62] It lies in front of the common bile duct, the medial edge of the right kidney and its vessels, the inferior vena cava, the right gonadal vein, the end of the left renal vein, and the right crus of the diaphragm.

The hepatic artery lies at the upper border of the head, whereas the transverse colon, part of the greater omentum, and the root of the transverse mesocolon lie anteriorly. In the lower part of the head lies the uncinate process, which extends to the left behind the superior mesenteric vein, separating it from the aorta behind.

The neck, which is more triangular in shape than the head and is slightly constricted, lies approximately level with the pylorus and the gastroduodenal artery. It is in front of the superior mesenteric vein, the beginning of the portal vein, and the cysterna chyli. The celiac artery hooks over its top edge. The body passes obliquely upward, slightly backward, and to the left across the spine at levels that vary between twelfth thoracic and second lumbar vertebrae, in front of the superior mesenteric artery, the aorta, the left suprarenal gland and the left kidney and its vessels, and finally the left crus. The splenic vein runs behind its upper border and may be partly embedded in its substance; the splenic artery lies above, running a tortuous course. The inferior mesenteric vein passes posteriorly to join the splenic vein. The transverse mesocolon is attached to its inferior edge. Anteriorly it forms the stomach bed, separated by the lesser sac. The left end of the body is related to the duodenojejunal junction and the splenic flexure.

The tail moves away from the posterior abdominal wall to enter the lienorenal ligament with its splenic vessels, and it usually reaches the hilum of the spleen. It normally lies at the level of the twelfth thoracic or first lumbar vertebra, but may be as low as the second lumbar and as high as the eleventh thoracic vertebrae.

Pancreatic Ducts

The main pancreatic duct begins at the tail and runs in an undulant fashion through the gland nearer to its upper edge and posterior surface and receives its branches at right angles in a herringbone pattern. At the point of junction of the ducts of Santorini and Wirsung, frequently there is a slight constriction or a loop segment may be present. Occasionally the main duct becomes bifurcate in the body or begins as the confluens of several small ducts in the tail. The length of the pancreatic duct varies between 16.4 cm and 24.2 cm.[62] As it approaches the duodenum it turns sharply downward and slightly backward and to the right. This segment may have a slightly wider diameter relative to the other portions of the duct and may appear somewhat dilated. In the head, the herringbone pattern of main pancreatic duct branches is not so obvious, although several branches are found. In particular it receives a branch from the uncinate lobe. Close to the duodenal wall it comes to lie alongside the common bile duct and, just outside the duodenal muscle, it becomes enveloped with it in a common muscle sheath. A notch identical to that occurring on the common bile duct also occurs at the same level on the pancreatic duct, so that the lowest part of the pancreatic duct is markedly narrowed relative to the diameter of the adjacent segment of the duct (see Fig. 27–8).[35] The main pancreatic duct, or duct of Wirsung, drains directly into the duodenum in approximately 13% of cases; in 2%, the duct is not patent, whereas in the remaining 85% it forms a common channel with the common bile duct before duodenal entry. The course of the main pancreatic duct has been reported at ERCP as ascending in 48.5% of cases, horizontal in 26.5%, sigmoid in 16.2%, and descending in 8.8%.[63]

The normal range of diameter of the main pancreatic duct is 3 to 7 mm in the head, the usual diameter being between 4 and 5 mm. Narrowing occurs in its terminal portion, which is about 2 mm in diameter. The diameter in the body ranges from 2.5 to 5 mm, with most ducts being between 3 and 3.5 mm, and from 1.5 to 3 mm in the tail, with 2 to 2.5 mm being the usual dimension. Maximum normal diameters for the head, body,

and tail have been quoted as 6.5 mm, 5 mm, and 3 mm, respectively,[64] but higher measurements have been reported.[65] There is evidence that, with increasing age, the diameter of the duct increases and the level of the papilla is lower in the body.[60] This was not confirmed in similar reports on the site of the papilla, the course and the caliber of duct, and so forth.[66] The radiologic features of the retrograde pancreatogram are discussed in Chapter 28.

Papillae

The major papilla is a smooth elevation that usually lies in the second part of the duodenum on the posterior or posteromedial wall. A transverse mucosal fold may obscure the papilla, but a characteristic longitudinal fold extends distally from its lower edge— the plica longitudinalis. The major papilla usually lies about 8 cm from the pylorus, but some authors have found it to be as close as 5 cm or as far away as 14 cm, which means that it can be located at any point from the junction of the first and second parts of the duodenum to within the third part.[15, 21, 67] One author[68] reports that 74% of papillae were found in the second part of the duodenum, 18% at the junction of the second and third parts, and 8% in the third part. Thus, both vertical and horizontal levels of the papilla in relation to the spine are variable, the structure lying between the first lumbar and the second sacral vertebrae; however, 90% lie between the second and third lumbar vertebrae in a vertical direction; and 49% are to the right of the spine, 46% are over the spine, and about 5% are to the left side of the spine in the horizontal plane.[60]

The external appearance of the major papilla has been described as flat, papillary, or hemispherical.[69] Whereas hemispherical would appear to be the commonest form, other shapes such as unformed, swollen, villous, cone-shaped, nipple-shaped, and sharply pointed have been described.[70] There appears to be considerable variation in size. The average is about 1 cm in diameter but a diameter as large as 3 cm has also been reported.[21]

The duct of Santorini lies anterior and cranial to the main duct and drains the anterosuperior part of the gland. It passes anterior to the common bile duct and enters the duodenum on the minor papilla. The duct usually widens just proximal to the orifice (Fig. 27–10). The minor papilla lies either ventral to or level with the major papilla in a transverse plane and either proximal to or level with it in a vertical plane, but it is never found dorsal or distal to the major papilla.

The minor papilla lies on a transverse mucosal fold which may be bifurcate. Its distance from the major papilla is usually 1.0 to 3.5 cm, its size variable, and in dissected specimens it is nearly always identifiable. It may be as large as or even larger than the major papilla, but surprisingly its size bears no direct relationship to patency. The minor papilla may be too small to be identified endoscopically, or even if it is large enough to be identified, its orifice may be too narrow to permit cannulation. Details of its incidence and microscopic structure were reported long ago.[19]

In microscopic anatomic studies, minute accessory pancreatic ducts have been found entering the common bile duct in its intrapancreatic and intraduodenal portions and also entering the duodenum directly.[71]

ANOMALIES AND CONGENITAL ABNORMALITIES

Liver

Biliary atresia, as the name suggests, was originally thought to be due to a failure of

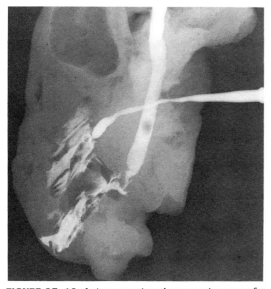

FIGURE 27–10. Autopsy cast and pancreatogram of a specimen in which the duct of Wirsung could not be found. The duct of Santorini can be seen to drain into the duodenum. There is marked dilation before entry. The minor papilla is outlined by a halo of contrast. The common bile duct is well notched, but the thickened segment is short. (*From:* Hand BH. An anatomical study of the choledochoduodenal area. Br J Surg 1963; 50:486–94. Reproduced with permission.)

cannulization involving variable amounts of the intrahepatic and extrahepatic duct systems. Although its cause is still unknown, it is now considered an infective or ischemic condition and not truly a congenital abnormality and therefore will not be considered further in this section.

Cystic disease affecting the liver is not rare.[72, 73] In the polycystic form it appears to be associated with renal cysts in 50% of cases. Solitary cysts may also occur. None of these mucus-containing cysts communicates with the bile ducts. Rarely, cystic disease is associated with hepatic fibrosis.[74] A rare diffuse dilation of the intrahepatic ducts has been recorded.[75]

Right, Left, and Common Hepatic Ducts

It has been stated that the right and left hepatic ducts may fuse within the liver. This has rightly been denied, and it is now established that fusion takes place 7 to 15 mm below the hilum.[10, 16] The left hepatic duct follows a more oblique course and is therefore longer. In some cases major tributaries of the right, but not the left, hepatic duct may also be outside the liver, specifically the right anterior and right posterior segmental ducts. In other cases the right anterior and right posterior segmental ducts may join the left hepatic duct as a confluence. Less commonly the right posterior segmental duct joins the left hepatic duct. In these last two examples no true right hepatic duct exists (Fig. 27–11). Rarely the right and left hepatic ducts fuse far down in the free edge of the lesser omentum, in which case the cystic duct is more liable to join the right hepatic duct. Naturally, when the cystic duct joins a confluence, as it does in about 2% of cases, there is no common hepatic duct. These variations have been well documented.[27, 76, 77] The right hepatic duct has been reported as draining into the gallbladder, into the cystic duct, and directly into the duodenum.[78, 79]

With the recognition of the segmental structure of the liver, the term accessory bile duct is no longer tenable. These ducts are not additional in any sense, but merely ducts draining a specific part of the liver which run an aberrant extrahepatic course. A wide range of incidence has been reported, with this aberrant finding occurring in up to 28% of cases. Differences in incidence are related to the method of demonstration. Many of these ducts are quite small, they may possibly

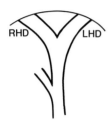
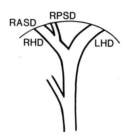

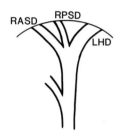
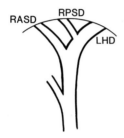

FIGURE 27–11. Modes of junction of the hepatic ducts. The upper two drawings show the findings of 75% of cases in which a true right hepatic duct is formed. In the lower two drawings, no true right hepatic duct is present, either because the three ducts join as a confluence (*left*) or the right posterior segmental duct joins the left hepatic duct (*right*). RHD, right hepatic duct; LHD, left hepatic duct; RASD, right anterior segmental duct; RPSD, right posterior segmental duct.

TABLE 27–2. **Incidence and Mode of Entry of So-called Accessory Hepatic Ducts***

Author	Date	Meth	N	% AD	RHD	CHD	CD/CHD	CD	GB	CBD	Anast
Flint[11]	1923	Dis	200	15	9	9	10				1
Lurje[15]	1937	Dis	194	11		10	4	5			3
Michels[1]	1951	Dis	200	18	7	20				2	
Moosman and Coller[80]	1951	Dis	250	16	5	15	5	5	3	1	6
Hayes et al.[82]	1958	Op	400	18				6	59	5	2
Dowdy et al.[27]	1962	Dis	100	15			12		3		
Grant[81]	1962	Dis	95	7		4		2			1

*Reproduced by courtesy of the Editor of the British Journal of Hospital Medicine.

Meth = method of detection; N = number of specimens; % AD = percentage with accessory ducts; RHD = right hepatic duct; CHD = common hepatic duct; CD/CHD = junction of cystic duct and common hepatic duct; CD = cystic duct; GB = gallbladder; CBD = common bile duct; Anast = anastomosing or double ducts; Dis = dissection; Op = operative.

result from infection, and they are of no clinical significance. They have been reported as draining into the right hepatic duct, common hepatic duct, cystic duct, gallbladder, and common bile duct. Some reported series are listed in Table 27–2. Few of these would be demonstrated either radiologically or at operation. The most important variation, from an operative point of view, is an aberrant right segmental hepatic duct which joins the common hepatic duct low down in 16% of cases.[1, 2, 4, 5, 11, 15, 16, 27, 80–82]

GALLBLADDER

Unlike in other higher mammals, especially the cat, in humans congenital abnormalities of the gallbladder are rare.[83, 84] However, Phrygian cap deformity, or folded fundus, is seen in 18% of cholecystograms.[85] Diverticulum of the gallbladder, which may occur anywhere on the wall, is rare,[86] and must be distinguished, together with hourglass constriction, from an inflammatory condition known as cholecystitis glandularis proliferans.[87]

Bilobed gallbladder and a multiseptate form have been reported and usually look normal on the external surface.[88] Very rarely the gallbladder may be rudimentary or absent without being part of congenital biliary atresia. Absence is usually associated with other congenital abnormalities, and over 150 cases have been reported.[89–93]

Double gallbladder may be expected in 1 in 3000 to 4000 cases.[94] It may be associated with two separately opening cystic ducts, one of which may join the right hepatic duct, or the two ducts may join in a "Y" fashion before entry. (Fig. 27–12) There is some question as to whether this condition is related to an increased incidence of gallstone formation.[95–97]

Ectopic positions of the gallbladder may occur. The gallbladder may lie intrahepatically, a condition which must be distinguished from absence, or it may lie under the left lobe of the liver without transposition, where its cystic duct may drain into the left hepatic duct. This has been recorded as being accompanied by a normal right-sided gallbladder. The gallbladder has also been found retrodisplaced onto the inferior and posterior part of the liver and also lying transversely, in which case both hepatic ducts may drain into it.

Cystic Duct

The cystic duct is extremely variable in length and course, as well as its site and mode of termination. It has been reported as absent,[98] but it is likely that this is most often the result of pathologic processes. Although it normally joins the common bile duct, it may join the right hepatic duct, an aberrant right segmental duct, the confluence of the right and left hepatic ducts, or even the left hepatic duct. Its length depends upon its site of junction with the common hepatic duct, which may be high and close to the origin of the common hepatic duct or low and close to the entry of the common bile duct into the duodenum.

Its mode of entry has been described as angular, long and short, parallel, and spiral. In the last two types the cystic duct may be separated from the common duct by loose connective tissue, or they may be fused in a nondissectable plane. In these two types the site of entry will be nearer to the duodenal terminus of the bile duct, lying retroduodenally or even intrapancreatically, in which case it could be as long as 6 cm. In spiral entry, the cystic duct usually passes posterior to the common hepatic duct, but it may pass anteriorly, and a double spiral has been reported.[16, 27, 80, 99] These variations and their approximate incidence, based on a review of the literature, are depicted schematically in Figure 27–13.

Common Bile Duct

Anomalies of the common bile duct are rare. Both absence[100] and duplication[101] are reported. Drainage into the stomach and double entry into the duodenum have been described, but there is some suspicion that these were the result of pathologic processes.[102]

Choledochal cyst, which is uncommon, is encountered more often in the Orient and takes various forms. The widely accepted classification[103] into types 1, 2, and 3 is shown in Figure 27–14. These types are discussed further in Chapter 31 from the clinical and radiographic viewpoints. The capacity of the cyst may vary from a few milliliters to 8 liters. When intrahepatic cystic dilations were recognized, types 4 and 5 were added to the classification.[104–106] All of these cysts are part of, or communicate with, the bile ducts and

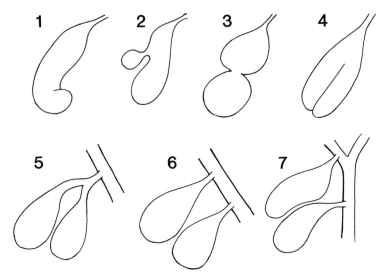

FIGURE 27–12. Congenital variations of the gallbladder. 1, Phrygian cap deformity; 2, diverticulum; 3, hourglass; 4, septum; 5, double gallbladder with single cystic duct; 6, double gallbladder with two cystic ducts draining into the common bile duct; 7, double gallbladder with two cystic ducts, one of which drains into the right hepatic duct.

FIGURE 27–13. Modes of entry of the cystic duct and approximate percentage of incidence as obtained from a review of the literature. POST, posterior; ANT, anterior.

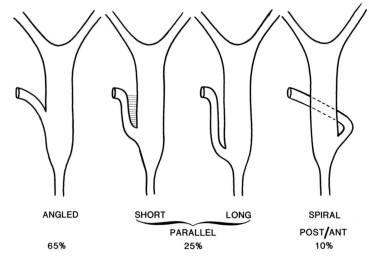

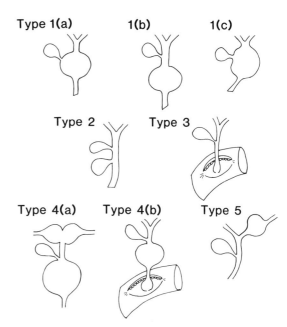

FIGURE 27–14. Types of choledochal cysts.

are not associated with polycystic disease, nor are they visible on the surface of the liver.

The intrahepatic variety has been divided into two groups: (1) a simple type with a tendency to stone formation and subsequent sepsis, now known as Caroli's disease,[107] and (2) a type associated with periportal fibrosis, which develops into cirrhosis and portal hypertension.

Pancreas

Anomalies of the pancreas are also discussed in Chapter 35, with emphasis on endoscopic, radiologic, and clinical aspects.

Arrested development resulting in absence of the pancreas, failure of formation of either dorsal or ventral buds, and failure of the two buds to fuse are exceedingly rare and are associated with other major congenital abnormalities that are usually incompatible with life. Pancreatic hypoplasia is also known to occur. This familial condition, known as the Shwachman-Diamond syndrome, is associated with hematologic disorders.

Inherited cystic fibrosis affecting the pancreas and lungs is a functional and not an anatomic abnormality. True cysts of the pancreas are not uncommon. They are usually unilocular and associated with cystic disease of the liver and kidneys. They contain serous fluid and are not connected with the pancreatic duct system.

A bifid tail of the pancreas, each limb having its own duct, has been described, as has suspension of the pancreas on a short mesentery from the posterior abdominal wall.

Ectopic Pancreas

Ectopic pancreatic tissue has been found in postmortem studies; when a specific search was made, an incidence of over 13% was recorded. These islands may be as small as 1 mm or as large as 5 cm in diameter. They may be multiple and may be located almost anywhere in the abdomen. About 80% are found in the stomach or duodenum, but they have also been found in the spleen, in the gallbladder and bile ducts, and in the midgut loop to its apex in a Meckel's diverticulum.[108]

It is not clear whether these islands arise from displaced bud tissue (which would seem likely, since a high proportion are close to the area where the buds develop), or whether the gut epithelium spontaneously produces them heterotopically.

Annular Pancreas

Annular pancreas is uncommon, and it is difficult to assess its incidence. One authority has reported 3 cases in 7000 autopsies[109]; another found only 1 adult case in 20,000 autopsies.[110] It may present soon after birth or later in life or may be found incidentally at postmortem examination.

Early presentation usually occurs within the first few days of life and appears to be associated with duodenal stenosis or atresia in over 40% of cases.[111] It is frequently associated with other congenital abnormalities such as esophageal atresia, imperforate anus, congenital heart disease, malrotation of the gut, and Down's syndrome. Annular pancreas causes no more than 1% of neonatal intestinal obstructions and less than 5% of duodenal obstructions.[112, 113] The site of the annular pancreas in 85% of cases is in the second part of the duodenum. It has a variable relationship to the papilla of Vater, but is usually proximal to it, even though bile can frequently be aspirated. Its site has also been reported in the first and third parts of the duodenum. Radiologically the dilated duodenum proximal to the narrowing and the duodenal bulb produce a "double bubble" appearance. The pancreatic tissue is usually embedded in the duodenal muscle and has its own duct.[114] These two facts render local excision or division highly undesirable.

When presenting later in life, the symptoms are similar to those of peptic ulcer, and patients usually have duodenal obstruction. Peptic ulcer has been documented in a third of the cases. Acute pancreatitis and jaundice have also been reported.[115–119] Duodenal obstruction produced by kinking due to general visceroptosis has been suggested as the explanation for the presentation in later life.

It has been postulated that annular pancreas is derived embryologically from persistence of the left part of the ventral bud, or alternatively that it is due to fixation of a portion of the right part of the ventral bud to the duodenal wall before rotation occurs. It has also been suggested that it is merely a major variety of ectopic pancreas.[120]

Pancreas Divisum

Greater attention has been given to the anatomy of the pancreatic duct as a result of increasing use of endoscopic pancreatography. Although referred to earlier in this chapter, pancreas divisum requires elaboration in the light of reports that patients with chronic pancreatitis appear to have a higher incidence of this anomaly than occurs in the general population.[121]

There is still some confusion over nomenclature. Some authors refer to the ducts as those of Wirsung and Santorini, whereas others refer to them as the main and accessory pancreatic ducts, respectively. If the main drainage occurs via the duct of Santorini and the minor papilla, clearly it is nonsense to refer to the former as an accessory duct. It is better, therefore, to use classic terminology when referring to the ducts, particularly in relation to their embryologic development.

The dorsal pancreas—that is, the tail, body, neck, and the upper anterior part of the head—relates to the duct of Santorini; the rest of the head relates to the duct of Wirsung. In humans these two ducts most often fuse in the head and varying degrees of drainage take place through both ducts, although most often the greater part occurs via the duct of Wirsung. In some cases in which fusion of the ducts has occurred, the duct of Santorini ends blindly in the duodenal wall. Occasionally fusion of the two ducts does not occur. Least common of all is obliteration of the duct of Wirsung in its terminal portion. There are, therefore, five possible drainage patterns (Fig. 27–15).

The early researches into pancreatic anatomy, which were based on autopsy material, were attempts to explain the occurrence of acute pancreatitis when a stone became im-

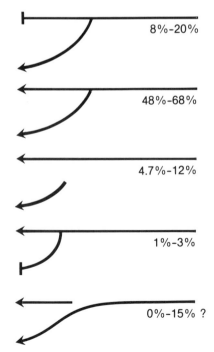

FIGURE 27–15. Pancreatic duct drainage pattern. Does type 5 (*bottom*) exist?

pacted in the lower common bile duct and obstructed the duct of Wirsung.[32, 33]

Notable among these studies was one in which the orifice of the major papilla was obstructed by a fine suture in 200 autopsy specimens and pancreatograms were performed. The duct of Wirsung was shown to be the sole or main pancreatic outlet in 91% of cases. The duct of Santorini was found in 50% of cases but was the sole or main outlet in only 9%, usually without communication with the duct of Wirsung. In 2.5% of cases the duct of Santorini was the sole outlet, since the terminal part of the duct of Wirsung was obliterated. From these figures it was calculated that the duct of Santorini could substitute for the duct of Wirsung in 21% of cases and relieve the obstruction in 12%. In 10% of cases it could not relieve the obstruction at all, and it ended blindly in 8%.[122, 123]

In another investigation, injection of air under water, dye injections, and dissections showed that the duct of Santorini was always present, communicated with the duct of Wirsung in 89% of cases, and drained into the duodenum in 73% of cases. Although this was not actually mentioned, presumably the duct of Santorini merely drained part of the head and drained separately into the duodenum in 11% of cases. In 4% the duct of Santorini was larger than the duct of Wirsung.[124]

In a study using bismuth or barium gelatin injections, it was found that the duct of Santorini was present in 68% of cases but ended blindly in 13%, whereas in 4% it proved to be the main drainage route of the pancreas.[65]

Another study using dye injections and pancreatograms showed that fusion between the ducts of Santorini and Wirsung occurred in 57.5% of cases and drainage occurred via both papillae; in 35% the duct of Santorini was blind and in 7.5% the ducts did not fuse. It was concluded in this report that in over 50% of cases the duct of Santorini could decompress the duct of Wirsung.[67]

Since these autopsy studies were carried out by different techniques and the statistics were reported in different ways, unfortunately it is not possible to obtain an accurate idea of the relative incidence of the five patterns of drainage (see Fig. 27–15). Indeed most authors do not specifically mention type 5, although by subtraction of their figures it must be presumed to exist. However, the percentages shown in Figure 27–15 are an attempt to rationalize the figures quoted

here, together with others that have been reported.

In a review of the literature on the incidence of pancreas divisum, an analysis of the findings in 750 autopsy specimens gave figures ranging from 4.7% to 14%, whereas the incidence was reported as being between 0.3% and 5.8% in over 9000 ERCP studies.[121] This latter work, of course, was carried out in patients with symptoms who were thought to have a normal pancreas. No ERCP studies have been carried out on normal volunteers. Earlier autopsy work was not designed to study pancreas divisum specifically, but it would not be difficult to carry out further duct studies with this in view.

Acknowledgements

I am deeply indebted to Mrs. Janice Henney, M.A., A.L.A. and the staff of the Ipswich Medical Library; to Mr. Philip Dove and the staff of the Medical Illustration Department of the Ipswich Hospital; and to Mrs. Diane Robertson, who typed the manuscript.

References

1. Michels NA. The hepatic, cystic and retroduodenal arteries and their relations to the biliary ducts. Ann Surg 1951; 133:503–24.
2. Benson EA, Page RE. A practical reappraisal of the anatomy of the extrahepatic bile ducts and arteries. Br J Surg 1976; 63:853–60.
3. Hjortsjo CH. Topography of the intrahepatic duct systems. Acta Anat (Basel) 1951; 11:599–615.
4. Healey JE Jr, Schroy PC. Anatomy of biliary ducts within the human liver; analysis of prevailing pattern of branchings and major variants of biliary ducts. AMA Arch Surg 1953; 66:599–616.
5. Hobsley M. Intra-hepatic anatomy: A surgical evaluation. Br J Surg 1958; 45:635–44.
6. Goldsmith NA, Woodburne RT. Surgical anatomy pertaining to liver resection. Surg Gynecol Obstet 1957; 105:310–8.
7. Gupta CD, Mittal VK, Gupta SC. Intrahepatic pattern of biliary ducts and their major variations. Indian J Med Res 1975; 63:1130–7.
8. Couinaud C. Etudes des voies biliares intra-hepatiques. J Chir (Paris) 1954; 70:310–28.
9. Chevrell JP, Duchene P, Salama A, Flament JB. Anatomical bases of intrahepatic biliodigestive anastomoses. Anat Clin 1980; 2:159–67.
10. Linder RM, Cady B. Hepatic resection. Surg Clin North Am 1980; 60:349–67.
11. Flint ER. Abnormalities of the right hepatic cystic and gastroduodenal arteries and of bile ducts. Br J Surg 1923; 10:509–19.
12. Daseler EH, Anson BJ, Hambley WC, Reimann AF. Cystic artery and constituents of the hepatic pedicle. Study of 500 specimens. Surg Gynecol Obstet 1947; 85:47–63.

13. Carter R, Thompson RJ Jr, Brennan LP. Volvulus of the gallbladder. Surg Gynecol Obstet 1963; 116:105–8.
14. Ashby BS. Acute and recurrent torsion of the gallbladder. Br J Surg 1965; 52:182–4.
15. Lurje A. Topography of extrahepatic biliary passages with reference to dangers of surgical technique. Ann Surg 1937; 105:161–8.
16. Johnston EV, Anson BJ. Variations in the formation and vascular relationship of the bile ducts. Surg Gynecol Obstet 1952; 94:669–86.
17. Lytle WJ. The common bile duct groove in the pancreas. Br J Surg 1959; 47:209–12.
18. Smanio T. Varying relations of common bile duct with posterior face of pancreatic tissue in Negroes and white persons. J Int Coll Surg 1954; 22:150–73.
19. Baldwin WM. The pancreatic ducts in man together with a study of the microscopic structure of the minor duodenal papilla. Anat Rec 1911; 5:197–228.
20. Partington PF, Sachs MD. Monographs in Surgery. New York: Nelson, 1951.
21. Poppel MH, Jacobson NG. Roentgen aspects of papilla of Vater. Am J Dig Dis 1956; 1:49–58.
22. Sullens WE, Sexton GA. Indications for use of operative cholangiography. Ann Surg 1955; 141:499–503.
23. Cole WH, Harridge WH. Symposium on diagnosis in general surgery; diagnostic use of cholangiography in biliary tract disease. Surg Clin North Am 1956; 36:149–59.
24. Wise RE, O'Brien RG. Interpretation of the intravenous cholangiogram. JAMA 1956; 160:819–27.
25. Hutchinson WB, Blake T. Operative cholangiography. Surgery 1957; 41:605–12.
26. Lequesne LP, Whiteside CG, Hand BH. The common bile duct after cholecystectomy. Br Med J 1959; 1:329–32.
27. Dowdy GS Jr, Waldron GW, Brown WG. Surgical anatomy of the pancreaticobiliary ductal system. Observations. Arch Surg 1962; 84:229–46.
28. Mahour GH, Wakin KG, Ferris DO. The common bile duct in man, its diameter and circumference. Ann Surg 1967; 165:415–419.
29. Glisson F. Anatomia Hepatis. London, 1659.
30. Oddi R. Sphincteric fibres around the termination of the common bile duct. Arch ital Biol 1887; 8:317–22.
31. Hendrickson WF. A study of the musculature of the entire extrahepatic biliary system including that of the duodenal portion of the common bile duct and sphincter. Johns Hopkins Hosp Bull 1898; 9:221–32.
32. Opie EL. The aetiology of acute haemorrhagic pancreatitis. Johns Hopkins Hosp Bull 1901; 12:182–8.
33. Opie EL. The anatomy of the pancreas. Johns Hopkins Hosp Bull 1903; 14:229–32.
34. Hand BH. M.S. thesis, University of London, 1958.
35. Hand BH. An anatomical study of the choledochoduodenal junction. Br J Surg 1963; 50:486–94.
36. Hand BH. Anatomy and function of the extrahepatic biliary system. Rev Gastroenterol 1973; 2:3–29.
37. Buget GE. The regulation of the flow of bile. Am J Physiol 1925; 74:583–9.
38. Elman R, McMaster PD. The physiological variations in resistance to bile flow to the intestine. J Exp Med 1926; 44:151–71.
39. Potter JG, Mann FC. Pressure changes in the biliary tract. Am J Med Sci 1926; 171:202–17.
40. Lueth HC. Studies on the flow of bile into the duodenum and the existence of a Sphincter of Oddi. Am J Physiol 1931; 99:237–52.
41. Bergh GS, Layne JA. A demonstration of the independent contraction of the sphincter of the common bile duct in human subjects. Am J Physiol 1940; 128:690–4.
42. Long H. Observations on choledochoduodenal mechanisms and their bearing on physiology and pathology of biliary tract. Br J Surg 1942; 29:422–37.
43. Smith JL, Walters RL, Beal JM. A study of choledochal sphincter action. Gastroenterology 1952; 20:129–37.
44. Caroli J, Porcher P, Pequignot G, Delattre M. Contribution of cineradiography to the study of function of the human biliary tract. Am J Dig Dis 1960; 5:677–96.
45. Daniels BT, McGlone FB, Job H, Sawyer RB. Changing concepts of common bile duct anatomy and physiology. JAMA 1961; 178:394–7.
46. Nebesar RA, Pollard TJ, Potsaid MS. Cinecholangiography; some physiological observations. Radiology 1966; 86:475–9.
47. Ono K, Watanabe N, Suzuki K, et al. Bile flow mechanism in man. Arch Surg 1968; 96:869–74.
48. Schwegler RA Jr, Boyden EA. Development of pars intestinalis of the common bile duct in the human fetus with special reference to origin of ampulla of Vater and sphincter of Oddi: composition of musculus proprius. Anat Rec 1937; 68:193–219.
49. Kreilcamp BL, Boyden EA. Variability in composition of sphincter of Oddi, possible factor in pathologic physiology of biliary tract. Anat Rec 1940; 76:486–97.
50. Boyden EA. Anatomy of the choledochoduodenal junction in man. Surg Gynecol Obstet 1957; 104:641–52.
51. Sterling JA. Termination of common bile duct. Rev Gastroenterol 1949; 16:821–45.
52. Sterling JA, Friedmann RS, Ravel VP, Sollis-Cohen L. Analysis of postoperative cholangiograms. Surg Gynecol Obstet 1949; 89:292–8.
53. Hicken NF, McAllister AT, Coll DW. Residual choledochal stones, etiology and complications. AMA Arch Surg 1954; 68:643–56.
54. Wapshaw H. Radiographic and other studies of the biliary and pancreatic ducts. Br J Surg 1955; 43:132–41.
55. Kantor HG, Evans JA, Glenn F. Cholangiography: a critical analysis. AMA Arch Surg 1955; 70:237–52.
56. Hughes ESR, Kernutt RH. Terminal portions of the common bile duct and pancreatic duct of Wirsung. Aust NZ J Surg 1954; 23:223–35.
57. Kune GA. Surgical anatomy of the common bile duct. Arch Surg 1964; 89:995–1004.
58. Vater A. Novum bilis diverticulum. Hallers disputationum. Anatomicarum Selectarum Gottingae 1748; 3:259–73.
59. Kirk J. Observations on the histology of choledochoduodenal junction and papilla duodeni with particular reference to ampulla of Vater and sphincter of Oddi. J Anat Lond 1944; 78:118–20.
60. Kreel L, Sandin B. Changes in pancreatic morphology associated with aging. Gut 1973; 14:962–70.

61. Kreel L, Sandin B, Slavin G. Pancreatic morphology. A combined radiological and pathological study. Clin Radiol 1973; 24:154–61.
62. Classen M, Hellwig H, Rosch W. Anatomy of the pancreatic duct, a duodenoscopic-radiological study. Endoscopy 1973; 5:14–7.
63. Kasugai T, Kuno N, Kobayashi S, Hattori K. Endoscopic pancreatocholangiography. The normal endoscopic pancreatocholangiogram. Gastroenterology 1972; 63:217–26.
64. Cotton PB. The normal endoscopic pancreaticogram. Endoscopy 1974; 6:65–70.
65. Birnstingl M. A study of pancreatography. Br J Surg 1959; 47:128–39.
66. Varley PF, Rohrmann CA Jr, Silvis SE, Vennes JA. The normal endoscopic pancreaticogram. Radiology 1976; 118:295–300.
67. Dawson W, Langman J. An anatomical-radiological study of the pancreatic duct in man. Anat Rec 1961; 139:59–68.
68. Schwartz A, Birnbaum D. Roentgenologic study of the topography of the choledocho-duodenal junction. Am J Roentgenol 1962; 87:772–6.
69. Oi J, Takemoto T, Kondo T. Fibreduodenoscopy: Direct observations on the Papilla of Vater. Endoscopy 1969; 1:101–3.
70. Phillip J, Koch H, Classen M. Variations and anomalies of the Papilla of Vater, pancreas and biliary duct system. Endoscopy 1974; 6:70–7.
71. Cross KR. Accessory pancreatic ducts; special reference to the intrapancreatic portion of the common bile duct. Arch Pathol 1956; 61:434–40.
72. Melnick PJ. Polycystic liver. Analysis of 70 cases. Arch Pathol 1955; 59:162–72.
73. Rashed A, May RE, Williamson RC. The management of large congenital liver cysts. Postgrad Med J 1982; 58:536–41.
74. Kerr DN, Harrison CV, Sherlock S, Walker RM. Congenital hepatic fibrosis. Q J Med 1961; 30:91–117.
75. Foulk WT. Congenital malformations of the intrahepatic tree in the adult. Gastroenterology 1970; 58:253–6.
76. Kune GA. The influence of structure and function in the surgery of the biliary tract. Ann R Coll Surg Engl 1970; 47:78–91.
77. Balasegaram M. Hepatic surgery: present and future. Ann R Coll Surg Engl 1970; 47:139–58.
78. Paul M. An important anomaly of the right hepatic duct and its bearing on the operation of cholecystectomy. Br J Surg 1948; 35:383–5.
79. Rabinovitz J, Rabinovitch P, Zisk HJ. Rare anomalies of the extrahepatic bile ducts. Ann Surg 1956; 144:93–8.
80. Moosman DA, Coller FA. Prevention of traumatic injury to the bile ducts. Study of structures of the cystohepatic angle encountered in cholecystectomy and supraduodenal choledochostomy. Am J Surg 1951; 82:132–43.
81. Grant JCB. Atlas of Anatomy. Ed 5. Baltimore: Williams & Wilkins, 1962.
82. Hayes MA, Goldenberg IS, Bishop CC. The developmental basis for bile duct anomalies. Surg Gynecol Obstet 1958; 107:447–56.
83. Gross RE. Congenital anomalies of the gall bladder; review of 148 cases with a report of a double gall bladder. Arch Surg 1936; 32:131–62.
84. Lockwood BC. Congenital abnormalities of the gall bladder. JAMA 1948; 136:678–9.
85. Boyden EA. "Phrygian cap" in cholecystography: congenital anomaly of the gallbladder. Am J Roentgenol 1935; 33:589–602.
86. Weisel W, Walters W. Diverticulosis of the gallbladder. Proc Staff Meet. Mayo Clin 1941; 16:753–7.
87. Lequeene LP, Ranger I. Cholecystitis glandularis proliferans. Br J Surg 1957; 44:447–58.
88. Hobby JA. Bilobed gall bladder. Br J Surg 1970; 57:870–2.
89. Latimer EO, Mendez FL Jr, Hage WJ. Congenital absence of the gallbladder. Ann Surg 1947; 126:229–42.
90. Mouzas G, Wilson AK. Congenital absence of the gall-bladder with stone in the common bile-duct. Lancet 1953; 1:628–9.
91. Gerwig WH Jr, Countryman LK, Gomez AC. Congenital absence of gallbladder and cystic duct. Report of six cases. Ann Surg 1961; 153:113–25.
92. Rogers AI. Congenital absence of gall bladder with choledocholithiasis. Gastroenterology 1965; 48:524–9.
93. Ferris DO, Glazer IM. Congenital absence of gall bladder. Arch Surg 1965; 91:359–61.
94. Boyden EA. Accessory gall-bladder, embryological and comparative study of aberrant biliary vesicles occurring in man and domestic animals. Am J Anat 1926; 38:177–231.
95. Stolkind E. Double gall bladder: a report of a case and a review of 38 cases. Br J Surg 1940; 27:760–6.
96. Corcoran DB, Wallace KK. Congenital anomalies of the gall bladder. Am Surg 1954; 20:709–25.
97. Harlaftis N, Gray SW, Skandalakis JE. Multiple gallbladders. Surg Gynecol Obstet 1977; 145:928–34.
98. Adam Y, Metcalf W. Absence of cystic duct: a case report, the embryology and a review of the literature. Ann Surg 1966; 164:1056–8.
99. Hess N. Surgery of the Biliary Passages and Pancreas. New York: van Nostrand, 1965; 241–301.
100. Markle GB. Agenesis of the common bile duct. Arch Surg 1981; 116:350–2.
101. Swartley WB, Weeder SD. Choledochus cyst with double common bile duct. Ann Surg 1940; 141:499–503.
102. Quintana EV, Labat R. Ectopic drainage of the common bile duct. Ann Surg 1974; 180:119–23.
103. Alonso-Lez A, Rever WB, Pessagno DJ. Congenital choledochal cyst. Int Abstr Surg 1959; 108:1–30.
104. Longmire WP Jr, Mandiola SA, Gordon HE. Congenital cystic disease of the liver and biliary system. Ann Surg 1971; 174:711–26.
105. Watts DR, Lorenzo GA, Beal JM. Congenital dilatation of the intrahepatic biliary ducts. Arch Surg 1974; 108:592–8.
106. Todani T, Watanabe Y, Narusue M, et al. Congenital bile duct cysts. Classification; operative procedures and review of thirty-seven cases including cancer arising from choledochal cyst. Am J Surg 1977; 134:263–9.
107. Caroli J. Diseases of the intrahepatic ducts. Clin Gastroenterol 1973; 2:147–61.
108. Feldman M, Weinberg T. Aberrant pancreas: a cause of duodenal syndrome. JAMA 1952; 148:893–8.
109. Stofer BE. Annular pancreas: tabulation of recent literature and report of a case. Am J Med Sci 1944; 207:430–5.

110. Havitch MM, Wood SA Jr. Annular pancreas. Ann Surg 1950; 132:1116–27.
111. Whelan TJ Jr, Hamilton GB. Annular pancreas. Ann Surg 1957; 146:252–62.
112. Hays DM, Greaney EM Jr, Hill JT. Annular pancreas as a cause of acute neonatal duodenal obstruction. Ann Surg 1961; 153:103–12.
113. Ravitch MM. The pancreas in infants and children. Surg Clin North Am 1975; 55:377–85.
114. Heyman RL, Whelan TJ Jr. Annular pancreas: demonstration of the annular duct on cholangiography. Ann Surg 1967; 165:470–2.
115. Lloyd-Jones W, Mountain JC, Warren KW. Annular pancreas in the adult. Ann Surg 1972; 176:163–70.
116. Swynnerton BF, Tanner NC. Annular pancreas. Br Med J 1953; 1:1028–9.
117. McGregor AMC, Green BJ, Stein MA. Symptomatic annular pancreas in the adult. Br J Surg 1969; 56:713–5.
118. Huebner GD, Reed PA. Annular pancreas. Am J Surg 1962; 104:869–73.
119. Anderson JR, Wapshaw H. Annular pancreas. Br J Surg 1951; 39:43–9.
120. O'Rahilly R, Muller F. A model of the pancreas to illustrate development. Acta Anat 1978; 100:380–5.
121. Cotton PB. Congenital anomaly of pancreas divisum can cause obstructive pain and pancreatitis. Gut 1980; 21:105–14.
122. Millbourn E. Calibre and appearance of the pancreatic ducts and relevant clinical problems. A roentgenographic and anatomical study. Acta Chir Scand 1960; 118:286–303.
123. Millbourn E. On excretory ducts of pancreas in man, with special relations to each other, to the common bile duct and to duodenum. Radiological and anatomical study. Acta Anat 1950; 9:1–34.
124. Rienhoff WR, Pickerell KL. Pancreatitis: an anatomical study of the pancreatic and extrahepatic systems. Arch Surg 1945; 51:205–19.

Chapter 28

THE NORMAL RETROGRADE PANCREATOGRAM AND CHOLANGIOGRAM

MICHAEL V. SIVAK, JR., M.D.

Postmortem radiographic contrast study of the biliary system was reported in 1921,[1] and percutaneous cholangiography was introduced into clinical practice by Huard and Do-Xuan-Hop in 1937,[2] although the procedure was not practiced widely until after the report of Carter and Saypol.[3]

The main pancreatic duct was described in 1642 by Wirsung; 100 years later Santorini defined the accessory pancreatic duct. There are numerous subsequent descriptions of pancreatic anatomy, some dealing with the morphology of the ductal system. These had little clinical relevance, however, until the development of intraoperative pancreatography in the early 1950's by Doubilet and Mulholland.[4] With the introduction of this technique, the fine points of pancreatic ductal anatomy assumed greater clinical importance. Furthermore, operative pancreatography demonstrated the feasibility and safety of radiographic contrast study of the pancreatic duct, although the clinical application of this method was restricted by the need for a laparotomy.

Because of earlier availability of radiologic techniques for visualization of the bile ducts, familiarity with the radiographic anatomy of the biliary system became common whereas pancreatography remained relatively obscure. The inception in 1968 of endoscopic retrograde cannulation of the ampulla of Vater resulted in detailed radiographs of the entire pancreatobiliary system; thus a greater knowledge of the roentgenographic anatomy of these structures became of paramount importance to endoscopists.

Knowledge of the essential features of the embryologic development of the pancreas contributes to an understanding of pancreatobiliary ductal anatomy. Pancreatic embryology is presented in Chapter 27.

THE NORMAL RETROGRADE PANCREATOGRAM

The endoscopic retrograde pancreatogram is a representation of a limited portion of the anatomy of the pancreas, since only the main pancreatic duct and its branches are demonstrated and the bulk of the parenchyma is not visualized. The pancreatic ducts have been studied by different methods including standard dissection, casts of the ductal system, and postmortem radiographs in cadavers, or after removal of the gland. The results of each are not strictly comparable with respect to the dimensions of the ductal system.

The Radiographic Configuration and Location of the Main Pancreatic Duct

The general "shape" of the main pancreatic duct demonstrated by retrograde pancreatography is angulated or "pistol shaped" (Fig. 28–1). An abrupt bend, or genu, sometimes greater than 90 degrees, is characteristically found to the right of the spine. This frequently corresponds to the point of embryologic fusion of the dorsal and ventral ducts. If the accessory pancreatic duct is opacified by retrograde contrast injection, its junction with the main pancreatic duct is usually found near this bend (Fig. 28–2).

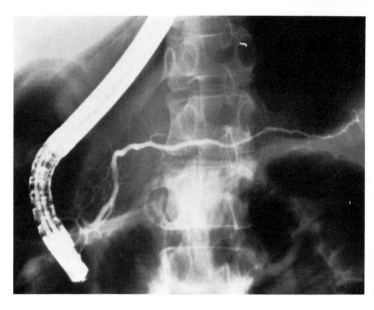

FIGURE 28–1. Normal pistol-shaped retrograde pancreatogram demonstrates the characteristic angulation or genu.

However, this angulation in the course of the duct need not be present.

The main pancreatic duct often follows a generally cephalad course within the retroperitoneum proceeding from the medial duodenal wall upwards and to the left. In one autopsy series the position of the main pancreatic duct in the head remained within 5 mm of the common bile duct over a mean duct length of 3.9 cm in 68% of the specimens studied.[5] However, this ascending course was found by Kasugai et al.[6] in only

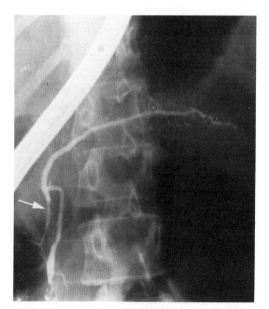

FIGURE 28–2. Normal retrograde pancreatogram demonstrates accessory duct (arrow) and pattern of main pancreatic duct branches in the tail.

48.5% of patients. The mean incline (measured from a line perpendicular to the spine) was 74, 19 and 21 degrees for the main pancreatic duct in the head, body, and tail, respectively.[7] The course of the main duct may be approximately parallel to the spine in the head of the gland, a relatively constant relationship, while it tends to be horizontal in the body.[8, 9] The greatest variation in course is usually found in the tail of the pancreas. Varley et al.[10] found that the origin of the pancreatic duct at the papilla of Vater was separated from the spine by a mean of 22.8 mm (± 10.0 mm); the maximum value found for this distance was 49.0 mm.

Retrograde pancreatograms most often present the ductal anatomy in an anterior-posterior view of the gland that offers no three-dimensional perspective. The course of the duct is actually not flat within the retroperitoneal space. Rather, it is U-shaped by virtue of lying over the spine (Fig. 28–3). The main pancreatic duct in the body may be several centimeters anterior to the ductal sections in the head and tail. This also means that slight rotation of the patient from the prone position to an oblique one will markedly alter the radiographic "shape" of the main duct. The anterior-posterior separation of the main duct from the spine was determined by Varley et al.[10] to be 56.7 mm (± 17.4 mm); the wide range of normal (7.9 to 96.1 mm) for this measurement negates its value for determination of pathologic displacement of the gland.

Radiographically, the entire main pancreatic duct is usually located within the span

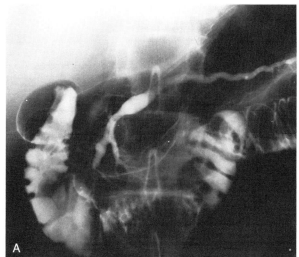
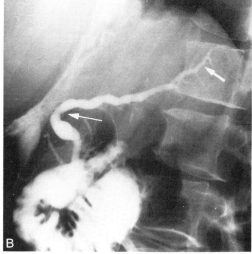
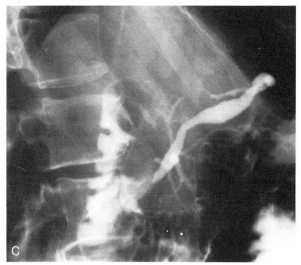

FIGURE 28–3. *A,* Anteroposterior retrograde pancreatogram. *B,* Left lateral view of pancreatogram demonstrates U-shaped configuration. Note position of midportion of ductal system in body of pancreas posterior to contrast-filled stomach (*long thin arrow*) and posterior position of pancreatic tail relative to position of pancreatic body (*short arrow*). *C,* Right lateral view of duct in head of pancreas. Note posterior position of duct in head of gland relative to that of duct in body.

of the twelfth thoracic to second lumbar vertebrae when viewed with the patient in a perfectly prone position. There is, however, a large variation in normal location.

Classifications of the radiographic "shape" as well as course and position of the main pancreatic duct have been proposed by many investigators. However, its configuration and location are so highly variable that assessment of these characteristics is of limited practical value.[9]

Radiographic Characteristics of the Pancreatic Ductal System

General Appearance

The main pancreatic duct has a smooth or somewhat undulating contour and progressively decreases in caliber proceeding from its duodenal terminus to the tail of the gland.* Minor variations in width are usually present, although the variations in caliber from point to point along the course of the duct are only slight and never abrupt.

---

*Editor's note: The terms proximal and distal as applied to the main pancreatic duct usually engender an argument. Using a strict dictionary definition, the term proximal refers to a structure nearest an anatomic reference point. If the papilla is taken as a reference point, the main duct in the head of the pancreas becomes proximal in position. However, a functional sense is often added. With regard to the biliary system, for example, the intrahepatic ducts are designated as proximal and the common bile duct as distal to reflect the direction of bile flow. It is more complicated to apply this reasoning to the pancreas since pancreatic juice enters the main duct along its entire course, but using this logic the main pancreatic duct nearest the duodenum becomes distal, that in the tail proximal.

Normal Narrowing of the Main Pancreatic Duct

Narrowing of the roentgenographic outline of the main pancreatic duct may occur normally in two locations. The first is near the genu in proximity to the junction with the accessory pancreatic duct. Birnstingl[11] found this relative stenosis to be present in 3% of cases in an autopsy study but found no associated histologic abnormality (Fig. 28–4). He attributed this finding to anatomic "folding" of the duct at the junction of the head and body. Berman et al.[12] also found this narrowing in a postmortem study using vinyl acetate and latex casts of the ductal system, and it has been noted in other autopsy and roentgenographic studies[13, 14] and operative pancreatograms as well.[15]

The second normal narrowing of the main pancreatic duct occurs within the body of the gland where the main duct overlies the superior mesenteric vessels. Berman et al.[12] found this narrowing to be consistently present, and distortion of the pancreatographic anatomy by the superior mesenteric vessels has been noted in other postmortem studies.[16] Although narrowing has been noted at this location in ERCP series,[14] it is not described in most pancreatographic studies or in other postmortem investigations.

Good quality pancreatograms with complete opacification of the pancreatic ductal system often demonstrate the terminus of the main duct at the duodenal wall and ampulla of Vater (Fig. 28–5). The diameter of the duct decreases as it encounters these structures. Kasugai et al.[6] were able to measure ductal length and diameter within these areas on a few retrograde pancreatograms. The section of the main pancreatic duct in the head of the gland immediately adjacent to the duodenal wall and papilla may also appear widened in a fusiform fashion. This is also a normal finding and does not indicate obstruction to flow at the ampulla of Vater. This appearance has been attributed to the decrease in diameter of the ductal system as it passes through the duodenal wall and papilla.[17]

Main Pancreatic Duct Branches

In the body and tail of the pancreas, branching of the main pancreatic duct occurs in an orderly fashion. Branches join the main duct at right angles, and usually alternate points of attachment with adjacent ducts on the opposite side of the main duct (Fig. 28–6). The branches in the mid-body are said to be fewer in number.[9] In contrast, the branching pattern in the pancreatic head is more disorderly and reflects the extensive embryologic transposition of the ventral anlagen.

With good technique, it is usually possible to opacify safely the first and some second order main pancreatic duct branches during retrograde pancreatography. Ishibashi and Matsubara[18] in their study of 33 cadaveric pancreases, found the mean number of main pancreatic duct first order branches to be 56, with a range of 52 to 66. The number of main pancreatic duct branches is thought by some investigators to decrease with increasing age of the patient, although this was not found by Ishibashi and Matsubara.

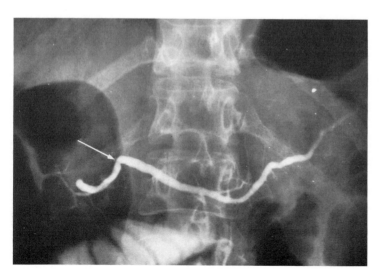

FIGURE 28–4. Retrograde pancreatogram shows slight narrowing (arrow) of the main duct at the genu. (From: Sivak MV Jr, Sullivan BH Jr. Endoscopic retrograde pancreatography. Analysis of the normal pancreatogram. Am J Dig Dis 1976; 21:263–9. Reprinted with permission of the Plenum Publishing Corporation.)

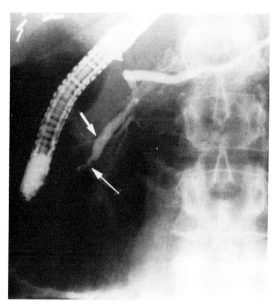

FIGURE 28–5. Retrograde pancreatogram shows narrowing of duct in region of duodenal wall and papilla (*long thin arrow*) with "fusiform" widening of the main duct in its retropapillary portion (*short arrow*). Main duct branch to the uncinate process is also present.

When demonstrated by retrograde contrast injection, the branch ducts taper smoothly and gradually, proceeding from the main duct. Marked variations in caliber, especially a wider peripheral diameter relative to that near the point of origin, are usually considered pathologic, especially in younger patients. This contrasts, however, with the necropsy study of Kreel and Sandin,[19] in which cystic changes and other irregularities of the branch ducts were found, especially in

older and apparently normal subjects. Similar distortions were found in association with increasing age in the necropsy study by Ishibashi and Matsubara.[18] It is unclear why these alterations in the main pancreatic duct branches are recognized in postmortem studies but not noted in endoscopic investigations. It appears that cystic dilation, tortuosity, and narrowing of branch ducts are not due to postmortem changes in the pancreas. Microscopic study of the abnormal areas generally reveals some evidence of mild fibrosis, but no inflammatory cells. It is possible that the postmortem radiographs are of better quality than those obtained in vivo, or that distortion is caused by postmortem methods of investigation. It is more likely, however, that minor degrees of cystic change, tortuosity, and narrowing of the main pancreatic duct branches may be a normal accompaniment of aging. As discussed in Chapter 36, this radiographic appearance may also be interpreted as evidence of minimal pancreatitis. It is possible that some similar cases were excluded from endoscopic series as being examples of a mild degree of pancreatitis. This problem is not considered or is unrecognized in endoscopic investigations, and some latitude within the normal range may be allowable with respect to the radiographic appearance of the main pancreatic duct branches in elderly patients.

Other than the accessory pancreatic duct, the only relatively consistent branch is a large unpaired one in the head of the gland that is directed inferiorly to the uncinate process of the pancreas (Fig. 28–7). Birnstingl[11] credited Cordier with the first description in 1952 of this branch. It has been noted by numer-

FIGURE 28–6. Normal retrograde pancreatogram demonstrates normal branching pattern in body and tail. Note orderly arrangement of branches.

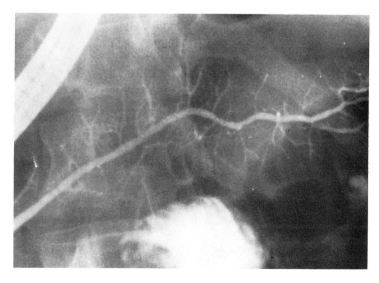

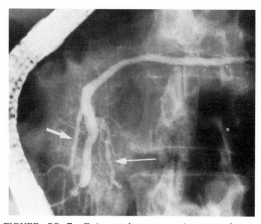

FIGURE 28–7. Retrograde pancreatogram demonstrates large unpaired main pancreatic duct branch to uncinate process of pancreas (*long thin arrow*). Note accessory duct also (*short arrow*). (From Sivak MV Jr, Sullivan BH Jr. Endoscopic retrograde pancreatography. Analysis of the normal pancreatogram. Am J Dig Dis 1976; 21:263–9. Reprinted with permission of the Plenum Publishing Corporation.)

ous investigators in both operative and endoscopic pancreatographic studies.[6, 20] In the endoscopic study of Sivak and Sullivan[14] it was found in 55.5% of pancreatograms; in the autopsy study by Rienhoff and Pickrell[21] it was noted in 61% of cases. This branch to the uncinate process may be quite long, and there are instances reported of its termination in a third papilla in the third portion of the duodenum.[21]

Accessory Pancreatic Duct

Opacification of the accessory pancreatic duct by retrograde pancreatography is unpredictable. In the report by Sivak and Sullivan[14] it was found in only 14% of pancreatograms. Kasugai et al.[6] noted the accessory duct in 32.4% of normal pancreatograms; Roberts-Thompson[22] in 40%; Varley et al.[10] in 62%. The accessory duct is found, however, in most specimens studied by postmortem methods. Rienhoff and Pickrell[21] noted it in 100% of autopsy specimens; Birnstingl[11] in 68%, although it was patent in 55.3%. The accessory pancreatic duct may not communicate with the main duct. In a postmortem study by Hand[17] the two ducts communicated in 88% of specimens; Rienhoff and Pickrell[21] found a communication in 89%.

Generally, visualization or lack of filling at retrograde pancreatography is not a reliable indicator of accessory duct patency, nor does caliber relate to functional status. Occasionally, careful observation at the time of retro-

grade injection at the main papilla may reveal flow of contrast into the duodenum via the accessory duct and papilla, but it is unusual to observe this.

Dimensions of the Main Pancreatic Duct

The dimensions of the main pancreatic duct have been obtained in a number of ways. Roentgenograms have been made by contrast injection into the duct in cadavers[13]; they have also been obtained after the pancreas has been removed from cadavers and placed flat on an x-ray cassette.[11] Differences in radiologic technique undoubtedly produce variations in the ductal measurements. In the postmortem study by Kreel and Sandin,[19] the length of the main duct was determined by contrast radiography in cadavers and after the pancreases were removed. The dimensions obtained by the two techniques differed by 1 to 2 cm, the measurements made with the pancreas in situ being the lesser in most cases. Another method utilizes injection casts of the ductal system. The latter technique, probably the most accurate, also produces a three-dimensional representation of the ductal system, although postmortem tissue changes may cause discrepancies from the true normal features.

Measurements may also be obtained from endoscopic retrograde pancreatograms with the aid of calipers and a magnifying lens. The length of the main pancreatic duct can be approximated with an instrument designed for measurement of distance on road maps. Although opacification of progressively finer branches of the ductal system and ultimately the pancreatic acini is a function of the injected volume of contrast material, the radiographic ductal diameters probably do not change appreciably in response to fluctuations or differences in injection pressure. Different radiologic techniques produce variations from one study to another. In particular, it is necessary to correct for the magnification that occurs in making the x-rays. The magnification factor associated with the usual ERCP procedure with the patient prone on the x-ray table is about 10% to 20%. This may be estimated by comparing the known diameter of the tip of the duodenoscope with its apparent diameter on the x-ray films. Since the position of the pancreas is not completely flat within the retroperitoneum, the use of a correction factor will be more accurate with measurements in the

TABLE 28–1. **Radiographic Dimensions of the Pancreatic Duct by Retrograde Pancreatography**

Author(s)	No.	Head	Body	Tail	Length	Range
Ogoshi et al.[23]	25	3.4	2.9	2.0	—	—
Classen et al.[7]	48	4.8	3.5	2.4	20.1	16.4–24.2
Kasugai et al.[6]	68	3.5	2.7	1.7	16.2	±2.5
Cotton[9]	57	3.3	2.5	—	14.5	9.5–18
Seifert*	28	4.0	3.0	2.3	18.6	17–21
Okuda et al.[24]	20	3.9	3.4	2.1	15.7	—
Sivak and Sullivan[14]	35	3.2	2.3	1.2	15.4	12.2–19
Moshal and Engelbrecht[25]	27	3.7	2.7	1.7	16.3	—
Varley et al.[10]	102	3.1	2.0	0.9	16.9	10.7–22.3
Roberts-Thompson[22]	30	3.1	2.4	1.4	—	—

*Seifert's data quoted by Cotton.[9]

head of the pancreas than in the body and the tail. The reported dimensions of the pancreatic duct are corrected for magnification in some ERCP reports of normal pancreatographic anatomy,[9, 10, 14, 23] but not in others.[7]

Despite the technical limitations of the various methods, an approximation of the normal dimensions of the pancreatic ductal system can be obtained by collective reference to published reports. The dimensions obtained by in vivo endoscopic studies are shown in Table 28–1, and those from postmortem investigations in Table 28–2. Howard and Short[15] found 4 mm to be the upper limit of normal for the diameter of the main duct by intraoperative pancreatography. Cotton[9] accepts 6 mm as the upper limit of normal for ductal diameter by retrograde pancreatography. Birnstingl,[11] in an autopsy-roentgenographic study of 150 pancreases, found that the diameter of the duct in the head of the gland ranged from 1.8 to 9.2 mm, and recommended that diameters up to 8 mm be considered normal unless there is other evidence of pancreatic disease. As a general rule, the dimensions found in autopsy studies are somewhat greater than those obtained from retrograde pancreatograms. The greatest variability in duct diameter occurs in the head of the pancreas.

In some postmortem studies, the diameter of the main pancreatic duct has been found to be greater in specimens from older than from younger individuals.[18, 26] The findings from two such studies are tabulated in Table 28–3. Kreel and Sandin[19] in studying 120 necropsy cases found that the width of the main pancreatic duct increased by about 8% with each decade of increase in age of the subjects. The lengths of the main duct when separated according to age category did not differ significantly in this study. Kasugai et al.[6] found a tendency for the diameter of the main duct on retrograde pancreatograms to be greater in older age groups, but this increase was not statistically significant. Other studies of retrograde pancreatograms fail to demonstrate a relation between age of the patient and ductal diameter.[9, 14, 22]

There have been attempts to relate ductal dimensions to sex and body habitus. Cotton[9] found the main duct to be significantly longer in men than in women in a review of retrograde pancreatographic data from several sources. Others have not found any relation between main pancreatic duct length and sex.[6, 14, 22] Milbourn[26] did not find any correlation between length and sex in a postmortem study. No difference in ductal diameter with respect to sex was found in the necropsy study by MacCarty et al.[27] Sivak and Sullivan[14] attempted to correlate the length of the main pancreatic duct with body surface area, but no relation was found.

The length of the main pancreatic duct visualized by retrograde pancreatography may be reduced by virtually any disease that

TABLE 28–2. **Dimensions of the Main Pancreatic Duct in Postmortem Studies**

Author(s)	No.	Head	Body	Tail	Length
Hand[17]	50	3.0–4.0	—	—	—
Birnsting[11]	150	4.1	—	—	—
Trapnell et al.[13]	45	4.0	2.0	1.0	—
Milbourn[26]	146	4.4	2.1	—	—

TABLE 28–3. **Dimensions of the Main Pancreatic Duct by Age in Postmortem Studies**

Author(s)	Age	Head	Body	Tail	Length
Kreel and Sandin[19]	<50	3.2	2.4	1.4	17.0
	50–59	4.3	3.5	1.8	19.0
	60–69	5.0	3.5	2.0	19.6
	70–79	4.6	3.5	2.1	19.8
	80–	5.3	4.0	2.1	19.4
MacCarty et al.[27]	31–50	3.3			
	51–70	3.5			
	71–90	4.6			

affects the pancreas. In particular, pancreatic carcinoma (which usually originates within the ductal system) may produce the radiographic pattern of ductal obstruction. When this occurs in the head or body, there is little difficulty with recognizing an abnormal pancreatogram. However, obstruction nearer to or within the tail of the pancreas may be more problematic; it is more difficult to be certain that some portion of the main duct remains unopacified.

It would be desirable from the standpoint of diagnosis to be able to categorize pancreatograms as normal or abnormal by obtaining measurements of the pancreatic duct from x-rays. Unfortunately, this is not possible in practice. For example, there is relatively close agreement among the various reports cited in Table 28–1 with respect to the mean length of the main duct. This is approximately 16 to 17 cm. However, the range for the normal length of the main duct, as noted in Table 28–1, is too great for determination of ductal length to be of value in the diagnosis of obstructing carcinoma in the tail of the pancreas. The normal roentgenographic length of the main duct is never less than 9 cm in any report. A relatively short duct may still be within normal limits, although a duct with a length of less then 9 cm will usually be pathologic.

The diameter of the main duct is also altered by certain diseases, for example chronic pancreatitis. For practical purposes, the values 3 to 4 mm, 2 to 3 mm and 1 to 2 mm (corrected for magnification) may be used as normal diameters for the main duct in the head, body and tail, respectively. However, a diameter of up to 6 mm in the head, 5 mm in the body and 3 mm in the tail of the pancreas can be normal.[9] By measurement alone, this upper limit of normal probably overlaps the dimensions of the duct in chronic pancreatitis.

NORMAL RETROGRADE CHOLANGIOGRAM

The subdivisions and terminology applied to the radiographic anatomy of the biliary system are the same as those used for surgical and gross anatomic description. Gross anatomic features of the bile ducts are discussed in Chapter 27. The many normal variations in the biliary ducts and anomalies are also discussed in Chapter 27. There are relatively few reports of the normal radiographic anatomy of the biliary system as demonstrated by retrograde cholangiography. Upon cannulation of the bile duct it is usually possible to demonstrate the common bile duct, cystic duct, common hepatic duct, and at least some parts of the right and left hepatic ducts and intrahepatic system. Certain technical problems with opacification and radiographic demonstration of the gallbladder and intrahepatic ducts are discussed in Chapter 32.

Radiographic Characteristics of the Biliary System

General Appearance

The radiographic appearance of the biliary ducts is similar to a leafless tree. Branching into progressively smaller tributaries occurs within the liver, whereas the extrahepatic ducts are without branches. The length, course, and origin of the cystic duct are highly variable. The origin may be in a very distal location on the medial aspect of the bile duct where it is in close relation to the pancreas. When in this position the cystic duct may be confused momentarily with the common duct during the initial injection of contrast agent.

When viewed from anterior to posterior, the bile duct is usually aligned in an inferior-superior direction parallel to the spine. However, it may be angulated in the elderly or its course may be distorted as a result of prior surgery. The point of contact with the superior margin of the pancreas is sometimes marked roentgenographically by a slight curve or bend toward the left. Viewed laterally, the course of the duct is directed somewhat anteriorly (Fig. 28–8).

For practical purposes, the extrahepatic bile ducts have no muscular component except at the most distal aspect of the common duct. The muscular component of the distal common duct can produce an abrupt narrowing in the radiographic contour of the duct; this may be noted as occurring within a few millimeters of the duodenal wall itself. This narrowing may be abrupt in some cases and has been described as a "notch" by Hand.[17] The ERCP cannula may also distort and exaggerate the normal radiographic anatomy of the distal bile duct (Fig. 28–9). A radiographic shelflike deformity of the bile duct just above the papilla can be misinterpreted as a constricting lesion. This can often be resolved by removing the cannula after opacification of the duct and observing the choledochoduodenal area with sequential x-ray views over the course of time (Fig. 28–10). As pharmacologically induced duodenal atony wanes, the outline of the distal muscular portion of the bile duct and choledochoduodenal area will change in appearance as the bile duct empties.

There are no normal points of narrowing within the biliary system with the exception of that which occurs in the region of the choledochoduodenal junction as described above.

Dimensions of the Biliary System

There are only a few reports of the dimensions of the bile ducts by retrograde cholangiography. Belsito et al.[28] determined that measurements of the bile ducts on ERCP x-rays exceeded corresponding determinations from intravenous cholangiogram x-rays in almost all instances, the average difference being about 3 mm. There are no reports comparing radiographic dimensions taken from retrograde cholangiograms with ones from percutaneous transhepatic cholangiograms.

As with pancreatography, variations in technique will produce different values with respect to measurement of the width of the bile duct at any given point. O'Dwyer et al.,[29] for example, measured the mean maximum diameter of the common hepatic and common bile ducts on radiographs taken in both the supine and prone positions in 12 patients. The width of the common hepatic duct with patients supine and prone was 10.1 mm (±0.9) and 11.0 mm (±1.0), respectively. The diameter of the common duct, supine and prone, was 13.0 (±1.1) and 11.6 mm

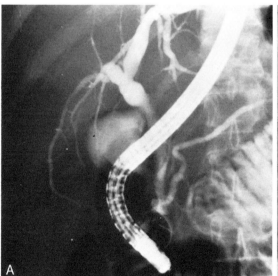
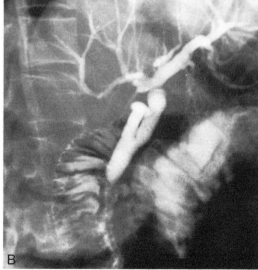

FIGURE 28–8. Retrograde pancreatocholangiogram of patient who has had cholecystectomy. *A,* Anteroposterior view demonstrates relatively straight course of extrahepatic bile duct that is approximately parallel to the spine except for slight medial angulation of common hepatic duct. *B,* Anteriorly directed plane of extrahepatic system is demonstrated by lateral view.

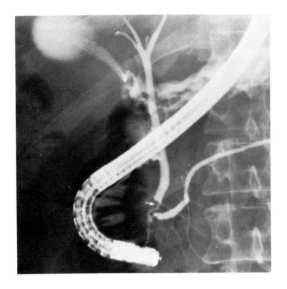

FIGURE 28–9. Notching of distal common duct (*arrow*) in choledochoduodenal area. Appearance suggests constricting lesion. Note that bile duct is not dilated. Impaction of cannula may alter appearance.

(±1.0), respectively. Measurements from retrograde cholangiogram x-rays must be corrected for magnification. Usually this is done by comparing the known diameter of the tip of the endoscope with its apparent diameter on the x-ray films. O'Dwyer et al.[29] found that the average magnification of the common bile and common hepatic ducts was about 23%. However, there was a marked variation from one patient to the next; the magnification factor ranged from about 8% to almost 50%. Since such a marked degree of magnification is possible, all retrograde cholangiograms should be corrected for magnification before considering the possibility of dilation of the biliary system.

The normal dimensions for the bile ducts from retrograde cholangiographic studies in

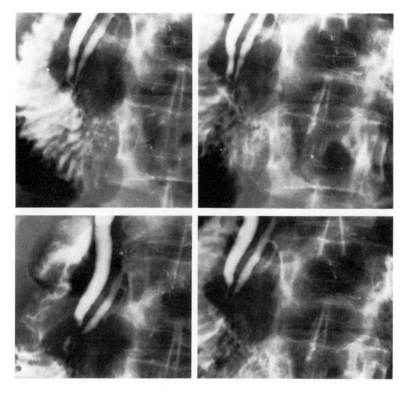

FIGURE 28–10. X-rays taken several minutes apart (arranged in sequence from left to right, top to bottom) demonstrate change in radiographic configuration of bile duct in choledochoduodenal area. View at lower left suggests constricting lesion, but appearance is normal on earlier views.

TABLE 28-4. **Normal Bile Duct Diameters by Retrograde Cholangiography***

Author(s)	No.	CBD	CHD	LHD	RHD
O'Dwyer et al.[29]	30	6.1	6.1		
Hamilton et al.[30]	50	6.5(p) 4.5(i)	6.0	4.5	4.5
Lasser et al.[31]	49	4.9(p) 4.3(i)	4.6		

*Mean maximum values in mm corrected for magnification. No., number of subjects; CBD, common bile duct; CHD, common hepatic duct; LHD, left hepatic duct; RHD, right hepatic duct; (p), prepancreatic; (i), intrapancreatic.

several reports are summarized in Table 28-4. The range for the reported normal diameters in Table 28-4 is given in Table 28-5. Hamilton et al.[30] also give mean values for three generations of intrahepatic ducts after the bifurcation into the left and right hepatic ducts; these are 2.5 mm (1.5-4.5), 2 mm (1-3), 1 mm (1-2). These authors also found that the diameters of the ducts of the left and right intrahepatic system did not differ significantly.

Lasser et al.[31] found that the diameters of the prepancreatic portion of the common bile duct and the common hepatic duct (but not the intrapancreatic portion of the common duct) were significantly greater in older than in younger individuals. This conclusion is supported by data from other investigators.[32, 33] However, O'Dwyer et al.[29] found no correlation between diameter and age; this view has also been supported by data from other investigators.[34] Extrahepatic duct diameters are also not influenced by the presence of parenchymal liver disease.[31]

It is not possible to determine that an abnormality of the biliary system is present or absent by simply measuring the caliber of the ducts. O'Dwyer et al.[29] determined bile duct diameters in 14 patients who had had cholecystectomies and found that the mean maximum diameters of the common bile and

common hepatic ducts were significantly greater than the corresponding values in normal patients. However, the measured duct diameter was beyond the upper limit of the normal range in only 2 of the 14 patients. These same authors also measured duct diameters in 46 patients with biliary obstruction. The mean maximum diameters were again significantly greater than the normal values, but for 25 patients they were still within the range of normal for the common duct, and for 13 patients they were within the range of normal for the common hepatic duct. Hamilton et al.[30] performed a similar study and also found that the degree of overlap between the measurements in normal ducts, postcholecystectomy ducts without obstruction, and obstructed ducts was so marked that abnormality of the ductal system could not be established by reference to ductal diameters alone.

It is usual to think of the biliary system as tapering in diameter from proximal to distal. This is true of the intrahepatic ducts, but the extrahepatic system is relatively uniform in diameter. However, Lasser et al.[31] found that while the diameter of the extrahepatic biliary segments did not vary by more than 1 to 2 mm, a given segment was wider in about one third of cases. This was most often the prepancreatic portion of the duct, followed

TABLE 28-5. **Range of Normal Bile Duct Diameters by Retrograde Cholangiography***

Author(s)	No.	CBD	CHD	LHD	RHD
O'Dwyer et al.[29]	30	3.5-10	3.5-13.3		
Hamilton et al.[30]	50	3-13(p) 3-10(i)	3-13	2.5-9	2.5-8.5
Lasser et al.[31]	49	2.3-8.5(p) 2.3-6.9(i)	2.1-9.2		

*In mm, corrected for magnification. No., number of subjects; CBD, common bile duct; CHD, common hepatic duct; LHD, left hepatic duct; RHD, right hepatic duct; (p), prepancreatic; (i), intrapancreatic.

closely by the common hepatic duct, and less frequently by the intrapancreatic section.

Editor's note: References 35 to 37 are also of interest in relation to the normal radiographic features of the biliary tree and pancreas as demonstrated by ERCP.

References

1. Burckhardt H, Muller W. Versuche über die Punction der Gallenblase und ihre Rontgendarstellung. Dtsch Z Chir 1921; 162:168–97.
2. Huard P, Do-Xuan-Hop. La ponction transhepatique des canaux biliares. Bull Soc Med Chir 1 Indochine 1937; 15:1090–1100.
3. Carter RF, Saypol GM. Transabdominal cholangiography. JAMA 1952; 148:253–5.
4. Doubilet H, Mulholland JH. Intubation of the pancreatic duct in the human. Proc Soc Exp Biol Med 1951; 76:113–44.
5. Dawson PM, Allen-Mersh TG. The anatomical relationship between the retropancreatic part of the bile duct and the main pancreatic duct. Ann R Coll Surg Engl 1983; 65:188–90.
6. Kasugai T, Kuno N, Kobayashi S, Hattori K. Endoscopic pancreatocholangiography. I. The normal endoscopic pancreatocholangiogram. Gastroenterology 1972; 63:217–26.
7. Classen M, Hellwig H, Rosch W. Anatomy of the pancreatic duct. A duodenoscopic-radiological study. Endoscopy 1973; 5:14–7.
8. Porter A, Warren G. The morphology of the main pancreatic duct at E.R.C.P. as a guide to its demonstration by ultrasound. Australas Radiol 1982; 26:149–55.
9. Cotton PB. The normal endoscopic pancreatogram. Endoscopy 1974; 6:65–70.
10. Varley PF, Rohrmann CA Jr, Silvis SE, Vennes JA. The normal endoscopic pancreatogram. Radiology 1976; 118:295–300.
11. Birnstingl M. A study of pancreatography. Br J Surg 1959; 47:128–39.
12. Berman LG, Prior JT, Abramow SM, Ziegler DD. A study of the pancreatic duct system in man by the use of vinyl acetate casts of 143 postmortem preparations. Surg Gynecol Obstet 1960; 110:391–403.
13. Trapnell JE, Howard JM, Brewster J. Transduodenal pancreatography; an improved technique. Surgery 1966; 60:1112–9.
14. Sivak MV Jr, Sullivan BH Jr. Endoscopic retrograde pancreatography. Analysis of the normal pancreatogram. Dig Dis 1976; 21:263–9.
15. Howard JM, Short WF. An evaluation of pancreatography in suspected pancreatic disease. Surg Gynecol Obstet 1969; 129:319–24.
16. Kreel L, Sandin B, Slavin G. Pancreatic morphology. A combined radiological and pathological study. Clin Radiol 1973; 24:154–61.
17. Hand BH. An anatomical study of the choledochoduodenal area. Br J Surg 1963; 50:486–94.
18. Ishibashi T, Matsubara O. Studies on the retrograde pancreatography in autopsy specimens. Bull Tokyo Med Dent Univ 1977; 24:43–51.
19. Kreel L, Sandin B. Changes in pancreatic morphology associated with aging. Gut 1973; 14:962–70.
20. Newman HF, Weinberg SB, Newman EB, Northup JD. The papilla of Vater and distal portions of the common bile duct and duct of Wirsung. Surg Gynecol Obstet 1958; 106:687–94.
21. Rienhoff WF Jr, Pickrell KL. Pancreatitis; an anatomic study of the pancreatic and extrahepatic biliary systems. Arch Surg 1945; 51:205–19.
22. Roberts-Thompson IC. Endoscopic retrograde pancreatography. Analysis of the normal pancreatogram, and changes which are associated with chronic pancreatitis and pancreatic cancer. Med J Aust 1977; 2:793–6.
23. Ogoshi K, Niwa M, Hara Y, Nebel OT. Endoscopic pancreatocholangiography in the evaluation of pancreatic and biliary disease. Gastroenterology 1973; 64:210–16.
24. Okuda K, Someya N, Goto A, et al. Endoscopic pancreatocholangiography; a preliminary report on technique and diagnostic significance. Am J Roentgenol Radium Ther Nucl Med 1973; 117:437–45.
25. Moshal MG, Engelbrecht H. Technique and results of endoscopic retrograde pancreaticocholangiography. A preliminary report on 140 patients. S Afr Med J 1975; 49:218–24.
26. Milbourn E. Calibre and appearance of the pancreatic ducts and relevant clinical problems. A roentgenographic and anatomical study. Acta Chir Scand 1960; 118:286–303.
27. MacCarty RL, Stephens DH, Brown AL Jr, Carlson HC. Retrograde pancreatography in autopsy specimens. Am J Roentgenol Radium Ther Nucl Med 1975; 123:359–66.
28. Belsito AA, Marta JB, Cramer GG, Dickinson PB. Measurement of biliary tract size and drainage time. Comparison of endoscopic and intravenous cholangiography. Radiology 1977; 122:65–9.
29. O'Dwyer JA, Pemberton J, Thompson RPH. Measurement of the endoscopic retrograde cholangiogram. Dig Dis Sci 1981; 26:561–4.
30. Hamilton I, Ruddell WSJ, Mitchell CJ, et al. Endoscopic retrograde cholangiograms of the normal and postcholecystectomy biliary tree. Br J Surg 1982; 69:343–5.
31. Lasser RB, Silvis SE, Vennes JA. The normal cholangiogram. Dig Dis 1978; 23:586–90.
32. Faris I, Thomson JPS, Grundy DJ, LeQuesne LP. Operative cholangiography: A reappraisal based on a review of 400 cholangiograms. Br J Surg 1975; 62:966–72.
33. Mahour GH, Wakim KG, Ferris DO. The common bile duct in man: Its diameter and circumference. Ann Surg 1967; 165:415–9.
34. Sachs MD. Routine cholangiography, operative and postoperative. Radiol Clin North Am 1966; 4:547–70.
35. Chang VH, Cunningham JJ, Fromkes JJ. Sonographic measurement of the extrahepatic bile duct before and after retrograde cholangiography. AJR 1985; 144:753–5.
36. Freise J, Gebel M, Kleine P, Weyand C. The diameter of the common bile duct determined by ultrasound and ERCP is not necessarily comparable. Ann Radiol (Paris) 1985; 28:5–8.
37. Schmitz-Moormann P, Himmelmann GW, Brandes JW, et al. Comparative radiological and morphological study of human pancreas. Pancreatitis-like changes in postmortem ductograms and their morphological pattern. Possible implication for ERCP. Gut 1985; 26:406–14.

Chapter 29

ENDOSCOPIC PAPILLOTOMY

MEINHARD CLASSEN, M.D.

Not many years after Langenbuch performed the first cholecystectomy, McBurney introduced surgical sphincterotomy. Seventy-five years later, the first endoscopic papillotomies of the papilla of Vater were carried out simultaneously in Japan and in Germany, and shortly thereafter successful endoscopic papillotomy (EPT) procedures were reported in the United States by Zimmon et al.[1] and by Geenen.[2] EPT* is now an established therapeutic procedure for various disorders of the papilla of Vater, the biliary tract, and the pancreas. In the past 10 years it has, in fact, become an indispensable procedure of choice for many of these disorders. A reasonable estimate of the total number of papillotomies that were performed throughout the world in 1985 is 50,000 to 60,000.

The number of EPT applications has greatly increased since its introduction because of various technical extensions of the procedure. EPT not only widens the normal or, in some cases, the abnormally constricted opening of the bile and pancreatic ducts, but it also facilitates access to both duct systems for further endoscopic treatment procedures such as biliary decompression by means of nasobiliary tubes, insertion of an endoprosthesis, pneumatic dilation of ductal stenoses, or local irradiation of inoperable tumors by implantation of a radioactive source such as an iridium wire. Stones in the bile duct and in the pancreatic duct can be extracted with balloon catheters or Dormia baskets; chemical, mechanical, and hydraulic methods are used to reduce the size of stones too large to be extracted by the usual means.

INDICATIONS FOR EPT

With the development of EPT in recent years there has been a shift in the pattern of endoscopic retrograde cholangiopancreatography (ERCP) procedures. Although ERCP was used exclusively for diagnosis between 1970 and 1974, this indication has been supplanted to a significant degree by EPT and related procedures. Since 1979 there has been a continuing increase in the number of therapeutic procedures so that in many centers these now account for as much as 60% of the indications for ERCP. A further shift in the reasons for EPT itself is also occurring; whereas choledocholithiasis had hitherto been the indication for EPT in 80% of cases, endoscopic management of bile duct stenoses by insertion of a biliary endoprosthesis has become increasingly common.

The indications for surgical sphincterotomy at the papilla of Vater were standardized by surgeons and pathologists years ago and still apply to EPT. However, the range of indications has broadened so that the spectrum now includes virtually all causes of obstruction of the biliary system as well as occlusion of the pancreatic ducts in some situations such as a stone near the papilla (Table 29–1).

Choledocholithiasis is an indication for sphincterotomy and stone extraction. In my view, this indication should be restricted to patients over age 50 in whom the surgical risk is high. The reason is that at present the long-term effects of EPT and its attendant loss of sphincter function are largely unknown. At the moment it is considered important to retain an intact sphincter, al-

---

*Editor's note: The term endoscopic papillotomy is preferred in many parts of continental Europe and some parts of Asia; the procedure is usually designated endoscopic sphincterotomy by most endoscopists in North America and England and in other areas of the Orient. For practical purposes these terms are interchangeable.

TABLE 29–1. **General Indications for
Endoscopic Papillotomy**

Papillary stenosis
Choledocholithiasis
Acute biliary pancreatitis
Suppurative cholangitis
To facilitate endoscopic therapy in bile duct
Pancreatolithiasis

though it is possible that this reservation may be discarded in the future if emerging data prove that loss of the sphincter of Oddi does not adversely affect the composition of bile and that loss of the barrier function of the sphincter against bacterial infection from the intestine has no significance, or that sphincterotomy reduces the frequency of recurrent bile duct stones.

The presence or absence of the gallbladder is irrelevant when the indication for EPT is emergency decompression of the bile duct. In this instance, removal of a stone obstructing the bile duct is of primary clinical importance and substantially improves the condition of the patient. Whether cholecystectomy is necessary after EPT is a controversial issue. This cannot be resolved until long-term prospective data are available on the course of patients who have undergone EPT but not removal of the gallbladder.

Foreign material, such as vegetable matter and debris, and parasites may occasionally be found in the biliary ducts. EPT with endoscopic extraction has been performed in many instances. The so-called "sump syndrome" is a recognized complication, albeit rare, of side-to-side choledochoduodenostomy or choledochojejunostomy when the distal non-functioning portion of the common bile duct becomes a sump or well in which lithogenic bile, gastrointestinal contents, and debris accumulate. This may produce obstruction of the enterobiliary anastomosis that can result in cholestasis and cholangitis. A variety of endoscopic maneuvers including EPT have been utilized in the non-surgical management of the sump syndrome.

Papillary stenosis is a long established indication for papillotomy. This includes not only benign stenosis of a short, circumscribed type, but also obstructing papillary carcinoma. An association between the congenital anomaly of pancreas divisum and recurrent episodes of pancreatitis has been proposed (see Chapter 35). Although this question has not been resolved, one of the possible explanations for such an association is that the minor papilla may be anatomically and/or functionally inadequate to handle secretion from the larger portion of the pancreatic parenchyma. Despite uncertainties concerning the relation between pancreas divisum and recurrent pancreatitis, EPT of the minor papilla has been performed in patients with this anomaly. However, the procedure is extremely difficult, and the complication rate and the clinical benefit have not been established.

EPT has been performed to remove concrements from the main pancreatic duct in patients with chronic pancreatitis and to facilitate placement of an endoprosthesis in main pancreatic duct stenoses near the papilla.[3, 4] However, only a small number of cases have been reported, so that abnormalities of the main pancreatic duct are not established indications for EPT at this time.

Acute obstructive cholangitis is also an indication for EPT and EPT-related maneuvers such as stone extraction, nasobiliary drainage, and insertion of a biliary endoprosthesis. The technical approach will differ according to the cause of obstruction. The most common causes are choledocholithiasis and malignancy.

TECHNIQUES AND METHODS

Equipment

In principle, all duodenoscopes with lateral optics are suitable for EPT. Over the years, however, improvements in the instrument have substantially increased its capabilities, including an increase in the viewing angle, increases in the range and tightness of the deflection angle of the instrument tip, and increases in the diameter of the accessory channel. The most recent models have instrument channels to 4.2 mm diameter; these are particularly suitable for implantation of an endoprosthesis.

The Erlangen-type papillotome is now in general use (Plate 29–1). The basic construction of this device is as follows: the outer Teflon catheter contains a thin steel wire that exits the catheter about 3 cm before its distal end and reenters the catheter about 3 mm from its tip. Tension applied to the wire produces a bowing effect in the catheter, the wire forming the bowstring. When the device

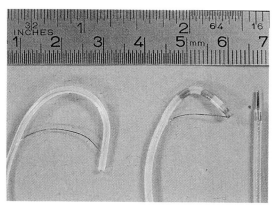

PLATE 29–1. *Left to right:* Standard papillitome (Erlangen model of Classen and Demling), minipapillotome, and needle-knife (Mori knife).

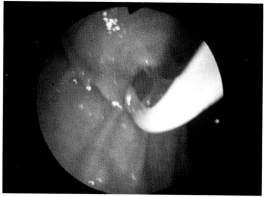

PLATE 29–3. Endoscopic view of papillotome in correct position in bile duct with proper tension applied to the wire. The roof of the papilla "rides" on the tensed wire. The cutting procedure can be initiated in this position.

has been properly placed in the papilla and bile duct, the exposed wire functions as a knife when high-frequency electrosurgical current is applied. The tip of the catheter, which has no wire, serves as a pathfinder during cannulation of the bile duct. There are numerous variations of this basic papil-

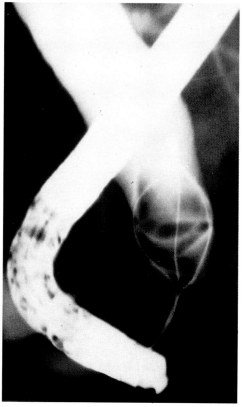

PLATE 29–2. Dormia basket introduced into bile duct. A stone has been captured in the Dormia basket.

lotome. One modification is to shorten the length of the exposed portion of the wire to 15 or 20 mm. This papillotome (Plate 29–1) is useful for making short incisions ("mini-cutting") and for "precutting"; the latter technique is used when deep cannulation and standard placement of the papillotome cannot be achieved. A special piercing knife or "needle-knife" papillotome (Olympus Optical Co) is also available (Plate 29–1). This instrument consists simply of a catheter and wire; the end of the wire can be extended 2 or 3 mm from the distal tip of the catheter. The needle-knife can be used to puncture and incise the roof of the duodenal papilla, a procedure termed fistulotomy.

Most commercially available high-frequency electrosurgical generators with cutting and coagulation modes are suitable for EPT. The machine should have a "rapid-start" function that helps to initiate the incision.[5] The output of an electrosurgical generator can fluctuate according to the electrical resistance it encounters. Machines with the "rapid-start" function have electronic circuitry that provides an initial high-power current for a fraction of a second to ensure that the electrosurgical incision will begin whatever electrical resistance is encountered (see Chapter 7 for a discussion of the principles of electrosurgery). If a machine without this capability is used, the onset of cutting may be delayed and unnecessary heating of the papillary area may occur.

Dormia baskets (Fig. 29–1 and Plate 29–2) and balloon catheters (Fig. 29–2) are used to extract stones from the bile duct. Additional

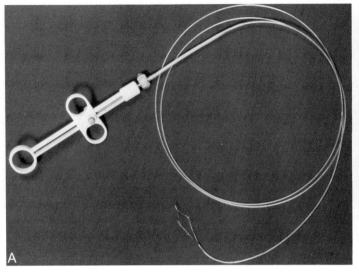

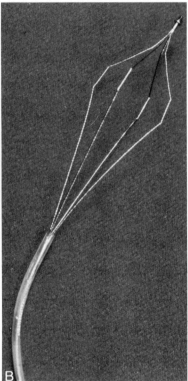

FIGURE 29–1. *A,* Dormia basket catheter. *B,* Close-up of Dormia basket.

instruments for lithotripsy and litholysis are described in the Methods section.

Preparation

As with every invasive procedure, the patient, and when appropriate his relatives, must be informed beforehand of the goal(s) and nature of the procedure, the premedication required, the risks and potential complications, and, when appropriate, the alternatives to endoscopic treatment. Because serious complications may occur, the endoscopist must have the close cooperation of an experienced abdominal surgeon. A coagulation profile should be obtained, and any coagulopathy should be corrected prior to the procedure.

Although hemorrhage is a recognized and potentially life-threatening complication of EPT, units of blood are cross matched before the procedure only in isolated instances. Endoscopic Doppler ultrasonography has been used to locate the retroduodenal artery in the wall of the duodenum along with any aberrant branches of this vessel in the region of the papilla.[6, 7] This technique helps the endoscopist to avoid arterial vessels as the EPT incision is made and is thought to reduce the risk of life-threatening hemorrhage.

We administer antibiotic prophylaxis prior to the procedure only in isolated instances, although there are differences of opinion on the need for these measures (see Chapter 26 for a discussion of the complications of ERCP).

Methods

Endoscopic Papillotomy

Except for minor modifications, the technique of EPT has remained virtually unchanged since it was first described. Following endoscopic retrograde cholangiography (ERC), the papillotome is introduced into the bile duct (Plate 29–3) while its position at the papilla and within the duct is monitored endoscopically and fluoroscopically (Plate 29–4). If there is any doubt whether or not the papillotome has been placed in the bile duct, a small amount of contrast medium can be instilled through the papillotome for confirmation. The proximal aspect or roof of the papilla should "ride" up and down on the cutting wire of the papillotome when tension is exerted on the wire because this assures that the cut will correspond to the course of the bile duct and that the tension on the wire is not excessive. About one third of the length of the tensed cutting wire should be visible outside the papilla. This ensures that the cutting process will be controlled and that cutting will proceed by increments (Plate 29–5). If the papillotome is introduced too deeply into the bile duct, the cut cannot be controlled, and an abrupt incision of excessive length may occur with the attendant danger of perforation and/or hemorrhage.

The correct length of the incision varies. Usually this will be about 10 to 15 mm when the papilla itself is normal. With short pulses of current, the roof of the papilla is incised as far as the point at which it enters the wall of the duodenum. In most cases this transition point can be readily seen endoscopically (Plate 29–5). Dilation of the distal aspect of the bile duct may produce a bulge in the duodenal wall proximal to the papilla. When observable, this bile duct infundibulum usually defines the course of the bile duct endoscopically. If, however, the papilla is small

and flat and the bile duct is not dilated, it may be more difficult to determine the length to which the cut can be made safely. The position of the bile duct in relation to the duodenal wall as observed fluoroscopically is also of assistance in gauging the length of the incision. If the duct lies close beneath the wall and is dilated, a relatively long cut can be made safely as a general rule. If the duct is not dilated and for the most part is positioned some distance from the duodenal wall on fluoroscopy, then the length of the incision must be reduced and there is less margin for error.

In up to 10% of cases, a small incision (precut, minicut) must be made first so that the standard papillotome can be selectively introduced into the bile duct to a sufficient depth. The modified version of the papillotome with a shorter exposed cutting wire section is first introduced as far as possible into the papilla. Then the roof of the papilla

FIGURE 29–2. *A,* Balloon catheter (American Edwards Co) for extraction of bile duct stones. *B,* Fully inflated 1-cm diameter balloon of balloon extraction catheter.

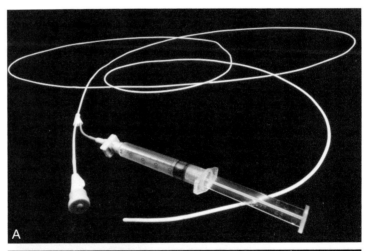

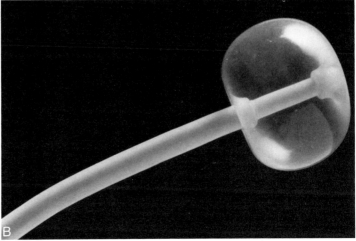

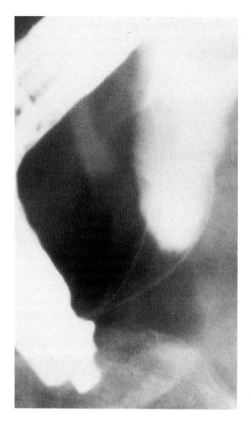

PLATE 29–4. Radiographic view of papillotome correctly introduced into the bile duct; one-third of the length of the exposed wire is in the duodenum and outside the bile duct.

PLATE 29–5. Endoscopic view of the EPT procedure. *Left:* Papillotomy is half complete. *Right:* Papillotomy complete.

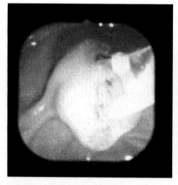
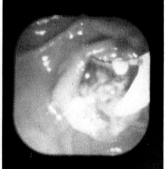

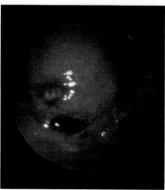
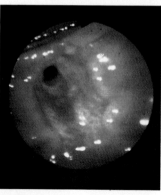

PLATE 29–6. Endoscopic view of papilla in biliary pancreatitis. The papilla is distended and inflamed. Two ulcers due to pressure from the stone are seen in the orifice and the roof of the papilla. The surface of an intrapapillary stone can be seen in the ulcerated areas.

PLATE 29–7. Endoscopic view of papilla post-EPT. A healed, irritation-free orifice is seen with free communication between the bile duct and the duodenum.

PLATE 29–6.   PLATE 29–7.

is incised as far as possible. If, as a result, the bile-colored mucosa of the biliary duct can be seen, the precut papillotome can be exchanged for the standard one, whereupon selective cannulation of the duct is usually successful or can be accomplished at a second session a few days later. We frequently use the needle-knife as another method of mini-cutting. The papilla is incised from its meatus along its roof in the direction of the bile duct. The papilla must be opened cautiously, using small incisions. When the ampulla is reached, the papillotomy is completed using the standard papillotome. These precut maneuvers require considerable expertise and experience if a satisfactory degree of safety is to be maintained. EPT with the use of a laser has also been reported.[8]

Another endoscopic technique for incision into the common bile duct is endoscopic fistulotomy (choledochoduodenostomy).[9, 10] This method is sometimes suitable when there is obstruction at the papilla of Vater. It is necessary that the distal bile duct produce a prominent impression on the wall of the duodenum that can be seen endoscopically proximal to the papilla. The prominence of this intramural segment is usually the result of dilation of the distal bile duct proximal to the point of obstruction. This dilated segment is also a necessary factor if the procedure is to be accomplished safely. Furthermore, it is advisable to inject contrast medium into the bile duct to demonstrate dilation and proximity of the bile duct to the wall of the duodenum. If these prerequisites are present, the intramural segment is simply punctured using an electrosurgical device such as a needle-knife. Depending on the anatomic circumstances in the individual case, the incision can be lengthened using a standard or precut papillotome. As with the precut techniques, endoscopic choledochoduodenostomy should be undertaken only by the most expert endoscopists.

In contrast to previous opinion, there is no increased risk of perforation in patients with juxtapapillary diverticula. Usually a diverticulum does not present any particular technical difficulty. Occasionally, the papilla will be entirely within a diverticulum and cannulation may be difficult or impossible. Even if the papillotome is placed in the bile duct, the anatomy may make it difficult to control the incision. If the papilla is at the distal margin of a shallow diverticulum there may be a ridge-like structure that bisects the diverticulum from distal to proximal to terminate at the papilla. This is usually the bile duct. EPT may actually be easier in this case since the course of the bile duct is clearly visible and the duct is close to the duodenal lumen.

The papilla is occasionally difficult to find in patients who have undergone Billroth II operations. Moreover, once it is located, the papillotome frequently cannot be properly placed for cutting. Even the use of an endoscope with forward viewing optics does not always resolve this problem. Some new papillotomes that are variations of the Erlangen type are designed for use in patients who have had Billroth II operations.[11] These devices are thought to reduce the risk of injury to the pancreas.

Endoscopic Treatment of Gallstones

Most gallstones are discharged spontaneously from the bile duct after EPT.[12] Nevertheless, it is advisable to extract as many calculi as possible using a Dormia basket or balloon catheter. Before papillotomy the size of the stone should be estimated and related to the possible length of the incision. On occasion, extraction will not be successful until some days have passed, and the edema produced by the papillotomy has regressed. If a stone is larger than the papillotomy incision, distal impaction of the stone followed by septic cholangitis may occur either spontaneously or during attempts to remove the stone endoscopically. Spontaneous stone impaction can be prevented by insertion of a nasobiliary tube.[13] The EPT incision can often be extended, but this should not be done before 1 week has elapsed. EPT results in hypervascularization of the papilla that increases the risk of hemorrhage if an attempt is made to extend the incision shortly after the first procedure.[14] If the stone has already become impacted during attempted extraction with a Dormia basket, then a nasobiliary tube is advanced beyond the entrapped basket into the bile duct to ensure outflow of bile. Another attempt at extraction after a few days is frequently successful. Otherwise, surgical removal of the stone is necessary. Lithotripsy or chemical litholysis can reduce the size of some stones that are unsuitable for extraction because of their large size or because of limits on the maximum possible length of the incision. Once such stones are rendered smaller by dissolution or fracturing, the fragments can usually be removed by Dormia basket or balloon catheter extraction.

Electrohydraulic and mechanical methods are available for lithotripsy. In mechanical lithotripsy, the stone is captured in an appropriate Dormia basket and is then broken by forcefully closing the basket. This requires that the basket be made of particularly strong wires. When the stone is trapped, the endoscope is removed from the patient. This requires that the handle or proximal mechanism of the basket be removed by cutting the wire. The outer Teflon sheath of the Dormia basket catheter is also removed so that only the wire remains. The basket now remains around the stone in the bile duct, and the opposite end of the wire exits via the patient's mouth. A flexible metal rod is then passed over the wire and is advanced to the basket and stone under fluoroscopic guidance (Fig. 29–3). Once the rod is in proper position the Dormia basket wire is attached to a knurled-wheel drive (Fig. 29–3). This allows the operator to forcefully close the basket by winding the wire onto the cylinder of the lithotripsy device. Essentially, the wire is pulled into the flexible metal rod; as the basket is pulled into the rod it is forced to close. This causes the stone to disintegrate into several pieces.[15] Even stones that are trapped in a Dormia basket at the papilla of Vater can be crushed in this manner.[16] Occasionally, it has been possible to introduce a mechanical lithotriptor into the bile duct to crush a stone without previous EPT. Fragments must then be extracted through the intact papilla.[17]

Experience with the electrohydraulic lithotripsy probe is limited.[18, 19] This method employs an electrode device that is placed in the bile duct near the stone to be broken. A high-voltage electrical discharge from the electrode produces a steep high-pressure hydraulic wave in a fluid medium that fractures the stone.[20] Electrohydraulic lithotripsy should be considered investigational at the present time. Other methods of crushing stones in the bile duct such as water jet cutting,[21] ultrasound,[22] and lasers are in preclinical stages of development.

Bile salt solutions have been used for the chemical dissolution of cholesterol stones in the bile duct. However, 40% of recurrent stones after cholecystectomy are calcium bilirubinate and not cholesterol stones. Because of this chemical composition, our group has investigated the alternating infusion of bile acid–EDTA and glycerol monoctanoate solutions.[23]

Our general approach to endoscopic management of choledocholithiasis can be seen in our results from a 1-year period that are representative of our overall experience (Table 29–2). In approximately 12% of cases some technical problem with stone extraction is encountered. In many of these cases the nasobiliary drainage tube is used to prevent impaction of the stone and in some cases for chemical litholysis. With these additional techniques the success rate for clearing the bile duct of stones increases to about 96%. Calculous disease of the extrahepatic bile ducts is discussed in detail in Chapter 30.

The methods of biliary drainage, endo-

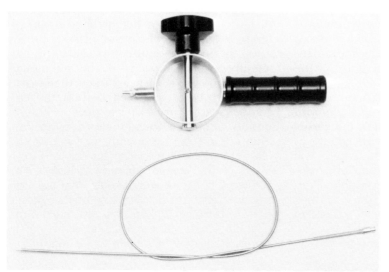

FIGURE 29–3. Mechanical lithotriptor with flexible wire sheath to contain Dormia basket wire.

TABLE 29–2. **Methods of Bile Duct Stone Extraction after EPT: 1-Year Experience at University Hospital, Frankfurt/Main***

Procedure	No. Patients	%
EPT		
Immediate extraction	89	63.2
Extraction at follow-up	19	13.5
Spontaneous passage	15	10.6
EPT + Nasobiliary Tube		
Extraction at follow-up	5	3.6
Reincision with extraction	2	1.4
Direct litholysis	4	2.8
Lithotripsy	1	0.7
EPT, Extraction Not Possible		
Palliative insertion of prosthesis	2	1.4
Surgery	4	2.8
Total	141†	100.0

*1/1/82 to 12/31/82.
†Indication was choledocholithiasis in 141 (56.2%) of 251 patients referred for EPT.

scopic dilation of biliary strictures, and local irradiation of inoperable malignancies of the bile duct are reported elsewhere (see Chapter 31).

RESULTS

Success Rates

Success rates for EPT, as determined by surveys of endoscopists, are reported from several countries (Table 29–3).[24–28] These reports pertain mainly to experience through the end of the 1970's. Choledocholithiasis was the indication for EPT in the majority of cases. Success rates for EPT from some single centers or individuals reporting 250 or more procedures are shown in Table 29–4.

Safrany et al.[36] reported successful EPT in 25 of 35 patients who had had a Billroth II gastrectomy. A complication occurred in each of two patients. The authors described the technical difficulties of the procedure and suggested that the complication rate might be higher than that associated with EPT in patients who had not undergone surgery. EPT was successful in 13 of 18 patients with prior gastrectomy and Billroth II procedures reported by Rosseland et al.[37] Forbes and Cotton[38] were successful in 8 of 10 such cases, and they emphasized the difficulty of ERCP and EPT after Billroth II procedures. Although results improved with experience, Forbes and Cotton recommended alternative diagnostic and therapeutic techniques whenever possible in these patients.

Russell et al.[39] attempted endoscopic enlargement of the orifice of the accessory pancreatic duct papilla in 12 patients with pancreas divisum. This was successful in only 5 cases, and only one of these patients had a good clinical result. The response to surgical sphincteroplasty in 7 patients was somewhat better, although 1 patient died postoperatively. The clinical result was also more sat-

TABLE 29–3. **Surveys of EPT Success Rates, Complications, and Mortality During the 1970's**

Country and reference	W. Germany (26)	Japan (24)	Italy (27)	England (25)	USA (28)
No. centers	9	25	8	14	21
Year reported	1978	1979	1979	1981	1981
No. patients	955	468	239	679	1250
Success (%)	92.1	96.5	81	87	89
Complications (%)	7.3	8.5	6.7	8.5	8.7
Mortality (%)	1.7	0.4	0.5	1.0	1.2

TABLE 29–4. **EPT Success Rates, Morbidity, and Mortality in Series of 250 or More Procedures**

Author (Ref)	No. Procedures	Success (%)	Morbidity (%)	Mortality (%)
Viceconte et al. (29)	296	86.1	7.0	0.8
Leese et al. (30)	394	98.0	10.4	0.8
Safrany (31)	265	92.0	10.0	1.2
Koch et al. (32)	267	95.0	7.1	0.8
Siegel (33)	267	96.6	5.0	0.77
Escourrou et al. (34)	443	92.0	7.0	1.5
Wurbs (35)	808	94–99*	7.3	1.4

*Varies with experience.

isfactory in patients with recurrent acute pancreatitis than in those with chronic pain.

Choledocholithiasis

EPT is successful in 98% of cases. A second session is necessary for 8% and a third session for 0.5% of patients. With respect to clearing the bile duct of stones, the success rate for groups working in Great Britain, Japan, and Germany is about 85%. Failure can be accounted for by factors such as anatomic abnormalities of the duodenum, prior surgery such as Billroth II resection, abnormalities of the papilla such as extreme stenosis, and prior biliary surgery. In addition, the large stone still presents a technical problem. However, gallstones are impossible to extract, as a rule, only if they are too large, are in the intrahepatic ducts, or are located above a biliary stricture (see Chapter 34 for endoscopic approaches to intrahepatic duct stones). It is virtually always possible to extract stones with a diameter less than 10 mm; the difficulties increase with stones above 15 mm in diameter, although every experienced endoscopist has encountered spontaneous discharge of concrements larger than 25 mm.[40] Notwithstanding this, attempted extraction of stones wider than 15 mm in diameter can be difficult, and success is less predictable.

Chemical litholysis offers the prospect of dissolution or reduction in size of large stones by a relatively less invasive and less traumatic means. Leuschner et al.[23] reviewed the experience up to about 1982 with chemical dissolution (litholysis) of stones in the bile duct. They concluded that the overall success rate was about 50% and that side effects occurred in the majority of patients. We have studied alternating infusions of bile acid–EDTA (BA-EDTA) and glycerol monoctanoate (GMOC).[23] During the period of study, most stones (87%) were extracted by EPT and the usual methods. Surgery was required in 4.2% of the cases. Chemical litholysis was undertaken in 17 patients (8.8%). In 8 of these cases (47%) this resulted in dissolution of the stones or reduction in size with subsequent extraction. Nausea and diarrhea occurred in 60% of the patients. Histologic examination of the gallbladders of patients subjected to operation showed acute ulceration and mild chronic inflammation. Better results are reported by another group,[41] but at the onset of treatment the stones were smaller in this series than in ours. Preliminary work with butyl ether would seem to indicate that the search for an appropriate agent for chemical litholysis of common bile duct stones still continues.

Foreign Bodies

A foreign body in the bile duct is a rarity. Following choledochoduodenostomy, retention of foodstuff in the biliary tract, particularly in the distal stump, may occur (sump syndrome, cholangiophytiasis). EPT and endoscopic methods are effective in eliminating this condition.[42–45]

Parasites in the bile duct or pancreatic duct (e.g., *Ascaris lumbricoides* and *Fasciola hepatica*) are rare in Western countries. They may cause obstructive jaundice or pancreatitis and should be extracted with a Dormia basket following EPT.[46,47]

Biliary Pancreatitis

The passage of a stone through the papilla of Vater with temporary blockade of the outflow of secretions from the pancreas is the most frequent cause of acute pancreatitis.[48] Persistence of the stone in the papilla or the discharge of many stones in a short time may lead to life-threatening pancreatitis with its attendant complications. Biliary pancreatitis is also discussed in Chapter 30.

The identification of the cause of biliary pancreatitis is usually more difficult than the treatment. A biliary origin may be assumed when there is a history of gallstones and when alcohol abuse can be eliminated as a cause. The specificity of abdominal ultrasonography is 68% for the detection of stones in the gallbladder associated with pancreatitis.[49] ERC, which until recently was regarded as contraindicated in acute pancreatitis, is reasonably risk-free when the pancreatic duct system is carefully opacified.[49] In most cases, the appearance of the papilla of Vater at duodenoscopy is characteristic (Plate 29–6).

In 1978, we collected data on 58 patients with pancreatitis and bile duct stones who had been successfully treated with EPT and, when appropriate, by stone extraction.[50] Since then, several other studies with successful results have been reported.[51, 52]

Safrany and Cotton[51] performed EPT in 11 patients with acute gallstone-related pancreatitis. In 6 of these patients the stone was impacted at the papilla, and in 1 patient a stone was present in the pancreatic duct. The condition of all patients improved promptly after EPT except in 1 case of a pancreatic pseudocyst. Van der Spuy[52] reported a favorable experience in 10 cases of acute pancreatitis due to bile duct stones.

It appears that after endoscopic treatment gallstone induced–pancreatitis recurs infrequently. It can be concluded that EPT is a genuine alternative to surgery for acute biliary pancreatitis due to bile duct stones.

Obstruction of the Papilla of Vater

Benign Papillary Stenosis

Benign papillary stenosis is a logical indication for EPT. There is a wide range in the reported incidence of benign papillary stenoses in endoscopic series, varying from 0.04% to 28.4%; the incidence in postmortem studies ranges from 0.04% to 0.12%.[53] Papillary stenosis was diagnosed 363 times (2.7%) in 13,300 diagnostic ERCP examinations at five gastroenterologic centers in the Federal Republic of Germany. Calculous disease of the bile ducts occurred as an associated pathologic finding in 61% and was considered to

be the most important associated or causative factor. Papillary stenosis was regarded as the result of surgical manipulation at the papilla of Vater in 7%, as due to papillary carcinoma in 14%, and as related to a juxtapapillary diverticulum in 1%.

According to the collected statistics reported by Seifert et al.[54] in 1982, circumscribed short papillary stenosis is the indication for papillotomy in 10.6% of all cases. EPT may be technically difficult in true papillary stenosis. It may be difficult to place the standard papillotome properly, and the fibrotic papilla may resist electrosurgical cutting. Moreover, recurrent stenosis after EPT for papillary stenosis is much more common (11.5% of cases) than after EPT for other indications. In addition, the complication and mortality rates for EPT in papillary stenosis without choledocholithiasis are higher than with EPT for other indications.

Neoplastic Papillary Obstruction

Benign papillary tumors are rare, being found in 1.5% of our patients who underwent papillotomy. However, the frequency of this diagnosis may increase as endoscopic methods become more widespread.

Papillary carcinoma is the third most common tumor causing obstructive jaundice (9% to 13% of cases), after carcinoma of the head of the pancreas and of the bile duct. However, it must be given special emphasis among tumors that obstruct the bile duct since it is often resectable, with a low operative mortality and a favorable survival of about 2 years on average.

Malignant papillary tumors are difficult to diagnose even with available endoscopic methods, including biopsy. Inability to obtain an adequate specimen (or specimens) for pathologic study is a significant problem. From the pathologic standpoint, the difficulties associated with the histologic diagnosis of papillary carcinoma derive from the juxtaposition of benign and malignant elements that is typical of this tumor. Thus, benign hyperplasia and adenomas may be found in association with carcinoma. Although a large particle biopsy by means of an electrosurgical snare wire improves diagnosis, in our experience it is more important to open the papilla by EPT and then obtain a large number of specimens from all exposed areas in the inner aspect. In 55 cases of periampullary carcinoma reported by Bourgeois et al.,[55] the diagnosis was confirmed histologically by biopsy of the papilla before EPT in only 50%

of the cases. When biopsy specimens were obtained after EPT, the diagnosis was confirmed in all cases. These authors also obtained biopsy specimens within 48 hours of EPT in 22 cases of benign biliary tract disease and found cellular atypism in these specimens.

In advanced cases, carcinoma of the papilla of Vater may be obvious endoscopically as an exophytic growth in the duodenum. Biopsy specimens from such a lesion will usually be positive. However, the diagnosis of small tumors originating from inside the ampulla (ampullomas) is particularly difficult. The duodenal aspect of the papilla of Vater may be normal or enlarged. Careful fluoroscopic study of the emptying of contrast medium from the bile duct and pancreatic duct may show defective, irregular filling of the ampulla. A small ampullary tumor, in addition to passage of small stones, should be considered in the differential diagnosis of every case of papillary obstruction.

EPT has both diagnostic and therapeutic roles in the management of carcinoma of the papilla of Vater. EPT is frequently necessary for accurate diagnosis by biopsy when the tumor is small and confined within the papilla. It has not been shown that preoperative EPT with biliary decompression improves operative results in terms of morbidity and mortality. However, EPT in patients with papillary carcinoma gains time for both patient and physician during which the operability of the tumor and the surgical risk for the patient can be determined. The patient can be prepared for surgery by correcting abnormalities such as coagulation defects and protein deficiency. If the operation is contraindicated or the tumor is unresectable, EPT with or without implantation of an endoprosthesis will improve the quality of the patient's remaining life. Recurrent stenosis occurs in about one-half of patients but can be eliminated by repeat EPT with or without implantation of a biliary endoprosthesis.

Acute Obstructive Cholangitis

We undertook a retrospective study of the efficacy of endoscopic treatment of 112 patients with acute obstructive cholangitis. Sixty-one patients had benign obstruction; the causes were gallstones in 51 patients and benign stenoses in 10 patients. Malignancy was the cause of obstruction in the remaining 51 patients, and in these cases cholangitis

occurred following endoscopic manipulation of the bile duct ("postendoscopic cholangitis"). The relatively high percentage of patients with "postendoscopic cholangitis" and malignant obstruction of the bile duct emphasizes the importance of carefully cleansing and disinfecting the endoscopic equipment.

Cholangitis was eliminated in all patients in whom the obstruction to bile flow was eliminated by EPT and, when appropriate, the EPT-related maneuvers of stone extraction, drainage by nasobiliary tube and/or endoprosthesis, and litholysis. All these patients survived. The endoscopic procedure failed in 7 patients. Five patients died, 4 of whom were in the group in whom endoscopic extraction was unsuccessful. The clinical condition of these patients deteriorated after endoscopic treatment failed and was complicated by shock and kidney failure to such an extent that surgical intervention could not be considered. Changes in laboratory values after successful endoscopic decompression of the bile ducts in patients with choledocholithiasis are shown (Fig. 29–4).

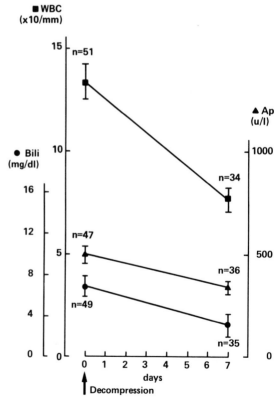

FIGURE 29–4. Changes in serum bilirubin, serum alkaline phosphatase, and leukocyte count after EPT in 51 patients with acute obstructive cholangitis due to choledocholithiasis.

TABLE 29–5. Endoscopic Methods of Treatment for Acute Obstructive Cholangitis Due to Malignant Bile Duct Obstruction

Treatment	No. Patients
Endoscopic papillotomy	2
Nasobiliary drainage	13
Bilioduodenal prosthesis	10
Nasobiliary drainage, subsequent prosthesis	22
Endoscopic drainage, examination technically impossible	3
Death before endoscopic examination	1
Total	51

the common bile duct. The procedure was successful in 88%, and complete clearing of stones from the bile duct was achieved in 91.7% of the cases of successful EPT. Major complications occurred in 7.5%, about one-half of which required surgery. More than 85% of the patients were over age 60, and over one-third had other significant illnesses. The mortality was 1.5%. This compared favorably with an operative mortality of 7% in a similar group of patients who underwent surgical sphincteroplasty. Five of 109 patients without residual stones after EPT developed mild to moderate symptoms of cholangitis during follow-up from 6 months to 6 years (mean 2.3 years).

The 51 patients with acute cholangitis due to malignant obstruction of the bile duct were treated by EPT and related maneuvers, as shown in Table 29–5. One patient with malignant obstruction died before EPT could be attempted. Endoscopic management was unsuccessful in 14 patients, all of whom died. Six of the remaining patients with effective biliary drainage established by EPT died in the hospital, a mortality rate of 16%. Two of these 6 patients died as a result of cholangitis; 3 died as a result of the primary disease while still hospitalized, and 1 died after elective surgery, presumably as a result of the primary disease.

Analysis of this small group of patients clearly demonstrates that the need to eliminate restrictions to the outflow of bile must have absolute priority in the endoscopic treatment of patients with biliary obstruction. Ninety percent of cases of acute obstructive cholangitis due to stones can be treated successfully by endoscopy. The mortality rate for endoscopic treatment appears to be markedly lower than that for surgical treatment.[56] This point is developed more fully in Chapter 30. It is also possible to manage about three-fourths of patients with acute cholangitis due to malignant obstruction of the bile duct by endoscopic means. Although the hospital mortality for patients is still high even if the treatment is successful, many deaths are due to the underlying malignancy. Furthermore, mortality is virtually 100% if the treatment fails.

Acute suppurative cholangitis is more common in Asia than in other parts of the world. Lam[57] attempted EPT in 134 patients with this condition, most of whom had stones in

Long-Term Results

EPT was introduced more than 10 years ago. Despite this, there have been few careful follow-up studies of sizable groups of patients.

In 1980, we undertook follow-up studies on 51 patients by endoscopic, radiologic, manometric, and laboratory methods; an additional 66 patients received questionnaires. The mean time lapse after EPT was 21.6 months. Ninety percent of the patients were symptom-free; one-third had minor changes in laboratory values that could be explained by other disorders, such as excessive consumption of alcohol. The biliary-duodenal pressure gradient had been completely abolished in 75% of the patients; duodenobiliary reflux of contrast medium was detected in 25% and aerobilia in 65%. None of the patients had signs of cholangitis or any detectable adverse sequelae.[58]

In 1982, Seifert et al.[54] reported results of a study of 9041 patients who had undergone EPT in 25 centers in the Federal Republic of Germany. Follow-up investigations in the form of ERCP, percutaneous transhepatic cholangiography, or intravenous cholangiography were obtained in 1050 of these patients. Recurrent bile duct stones were found in 5.77%; post-EPT stenosis occurred in 3.4%. Most of the patients were symptom-free (93.55%); symptoms were unchanged in 4.9% and worse in 1.63% of patients.

An interesting observation reported by Seifert et al.[54] was that recurrent stenosis occurred in 11.5% of patients who underwent EPT for papillary stenosis versus a post-EPT stenosis rate of only 2.9% in patients in whom the indication was choledocholithiasis. Stones recurred in about 5.9% of patients who had had choledocholithiasis, but none were found in those who underwent EPT for papillary stenosis. Recurrent stone formation is not necessarily related to the presence of a stricture and may occur even when the orifice produced by EPT is widely patent (Plate 29–7). It would appear that abnormalities in the composition of bile still have an important role in the pathogenesis of these stones.

There is a difference of opinion on the importance of the intact gallbladder as a risk factor following EPT. The results of several investigations with catamnestic data with follow-up to 7 years post-EPT have been published.[34, 59–63]

Hagenmüller et al.[59] and Escourrou et al.[34] have grouped patients in their series according to those who retained and those who did not retain gallbladders. The mean age of patients who did not undergo cholecystectomy was 75 years in both studies, 10 years more than the mean age of the patients in each study who had had cholecystectomy before EPT. The long-range survival of this older group of patients did not seem to be adversely affected by the intact gallbladder (Table 29–6). However, 4% to 15% of patients had long-term biliary complications.

In the series reported by Escourrou et al.,[34] EPT was performed in 234 patients with intact gallbladders because of advanced age or poor condition for surgery. Late complications occurred in 16 patients (12%) who retained gallbladders after EPT. Follow-up in 130 patients ranged from 6 to 66 months (mean, 22 months). In 8 patients acute cholecystitis developed from 1 to 9 months (mean, 4 months) after EPT; 7 of these underwent cholecystectomy.

EPT was performed by Neoptolemos et al.[61] in 100 patients with intact gallbladders. Fifty-nine were considered unsuitable for operation. Five of these patients eventually required surgery, 3 because of technical failure

and 2 because of empyema of the gallbladder. One patient in this group died after a large stone could not be extracted. Follow-up ranged from 4 to 50 months, and during this time 16 patients died, although only 1 death was attributable to sepsis related to cholecystitis. One patient underwent cholecystectomy because of persistent pain. In a second group of 38 patients, the EPT procedure preceded cholecystectomy. Choledochotomy was avoided in 29 of these patients. In a third group of 3 patients, EPT was performed after emergency cholecystostomy. No further surgery was required in these cases.

Cotton and Vallon[62] attempted EPT in 71 elderly patients with intact gallbladders with acute presenting symptoms due to bile duct stones. The procedure was successful in 70 patients, and the duct was cleared of stones in 61 patients (86%). Two patients underwent cholecystectomy for acute cholecystitis within 1 week of the endoscopic procedure. One patient with a retained stone who was considered a poor operative candidate died 6 weeks after EPT. Eleven patients underwent elective cholecystectomy. Follow-up (mean, 19 months) was obtained in 44 of 48 patients (mean age, 75 years) who did not undergo cholecystectomy. Five of these patients required cholecystectomy because of persistent pain, but neither cholangitis nor jaundice developed in this group. The authors recommended EPT for all patients who were acutely ill because of bile duct stones regardless of whether or not the gallbladder was present. Although longer follow-up was thought necessary to determine the indications for cholecystectomy subsequent to EPT, they also recommended that indefinite postponement of cholecystectomy be considered after successful endoscopic treatment of choledocholithiasis in elderly and poor surgical risk patients.

In the series of Solhaug et al.,[63] EPT was

TABLE 29–6. **Mortality in Patients Not Undergoing Cholecystectomy after EPT**

Author (Ref)	No. Patients	Cause of Death	
		Biliary (%)	*Non-Biliary (%)*
Escourrou et al. (34)	226	0	28 (12)
Hagenmüller et al. (59)	68	1 (1.5)	14 (21)
Riemann et al. (60)	206	4 (2.0)	38 (18)
Total	500	5 (1.0)	80 (16)

TABLE 29–7. **Mortality for Elective Cholecystectomy After EPT**

Author (Ref)	Total No. Patients	Elective Cholecystectomy After EPT (%)	Fatalities
Cotton et al. (64)	44	9 (20)	0
Cremer et al. (65)	496	20 (4)	0
Hagenmüller et al. (59)	68	5 (7)	0
Riemann et al. (60)	184	24 (13)	0
Tulassay et al. (66)	74	38 (51)	0
Total	866	96 (11)	0

performed in 22 patients who had not undergone cholecystectomy and in whom the risk of operation was considered prohibitive. In each of the 5 patients who required cholecystectomy subsequent to EPT, obstruction of the cystic duct had been demonstrated by cholangiography at the time of the EPT.

The results of Escourrou et al.[34] and of our group show that patients without a gallbladder have fewer long-term complications after EPT than patients with the gallbladder in situ. In more than 50% of the patients with gallbladders, the complication is related to the gallbladder itself. Surgery is usually necessary in these patients, whereas long-term biliary complications in patients without gallbladders can be managed endoscopically in most cases. For this reason, we are continuing elective cholecystectomy following endoscopic treatment of bile duct problems whenever the risk of surgery seems acceptable.

The mortality resulting from biliary complications that occur in patients with intact gallbladders after EPT is about 1% (Table 29–6).[34, 59, 60] This low mortality has been adduced as a reason against elective cholecystectomy after EPT. However, among almost 900 cases of elective cholecystectomy after EPT, there were no fatalities (Table 29–7).[59, 60, 64–66] It is possible that this is a chance result, but it strengthens our recommendation of elective cholecystectomy after EPT when the risk is acceptable.

COMPLICATIONS

The overall complication rate for EPT as determined in large surveys ranges from 6.5% to 8.7%; the mortality rate ranges from zero to 1.3%. The most frequent complications are hemorrhage, pancreatitis, cholangitis, and perforation of the duodenal wall. Perforations and hemorrhages usually become manifest within 12 to 24 hours, whereas pancreatitis and cholangitis may appear later. In the series of 71 patients over age 70 who underwent EPT for choledocholithiasis reported by Mee et al.,[67] a complication occurred in 9 patients (13%), although there were no deaths.

The length of the EPT incision is related to the risk of hemorrhage. The mean diameter of the vessels in the papillary arterial plexus is about 0.98 mm; the mean diameter of vessels in the roof (proximal aspect) of the papilla is only about 0.43 mm. However, in about 4% of cases the retroduodenal artery is in the region of the papillotomy. Thus, severe hemorrhage may occur in a minority of patients undergoing EPT procedures.

Operation is necessary to control bleeding in only about 11% of cases of hemorrhage following EPT. Endoscopic tamponade of the incision using special balloon catheters has been performed to control hemorrhage in a few patients with some success.[68] It is a reasonable expectation that EPT-related hemorrhage can be avoided by use of endoscopic Doppler ultrasonography, a procedure not yet widely available. It is possible to measure reasonably intense arterial signals within the wall of the duodenum. Thus, at present the best way to avoid hemorrhage is to restrict the length of the incision to the visible roof of the papilla.

Goodall[69] found evidence of post-EPT bleeding in 21 of 194 patients who underwent 235 EPT procedures. However, bleeding was occult in 7 cases. Six of the 14 patients with overt bleeding required operation, and 2 patients died as a result of hemorrhage. There was an increased risk of bleeding with repeated procedures. The author did not indicate the time interval between the first and the subsequent EPT procedures, and whether the bleeding could be related to excessive length of the incision or the hypervascularity that occurs at the papillotomy site after EPT was not stated. In almost all cases, bleeding began within 24 hours of EPT, although in 2 patients without evidence of bleeding during EPT, the onset of bleeding was delayed for 5 days.

Perforations may occur even when the length of the incision is properly restricted to the roof of the papilla. This may be accounted for in part by anatomic variations in the distal retropapillary aspect of the papilla, although the degree to which such variations are of importance is not certain and can be determined only by a careful prospective study. After every EPT incision, the choledochoduodenal junction should be checked radiographically for leakage. Extravasation of contrast medium and/or air into the retroperitoneum confirms the presence of a perforation.

Detection of a perforation does not necessarily mean that surgery must be performed immediately. Byrne et al.[70] encountered 5 perforations in approximately 500 procedures. They found that most patients responded satisfactorily to conservative management provided that biliary drainage was adequate. Evidence of perforation is usually present on plain x-rays of the abdomen as free air in the retroperitoneal space that sometimes outlines retroperitoneal structures such as the kidney. Many perforations heal spontaneously with or without nasobiliary drainage. If operation is not performed immediately upon detection of the perforation, the patient must be monitored clinically at close intervals, and if there are any signs of deterioration such as increasing pain, abdominal tenderness, or fever, surgery should be performed immediately. As a general rule, we recommend early surgery, since complications of the perforation such as retroperitoneal abscess increase surgical risk and morbidity.

The bile ducts in patients with choledocholithiasis harbor bacteria in almost all cases. If biliary blockage is not eliminated or is worsened by endoscopic intervention, cholangitis may occur. This may result if the stone(s) becomes impacted because the incision is too short to allow removal or passage of the stone or the stone is too large. Inser-

tion of a nasobiliary tube will greatly reduce the likelihood of impaction and cholangitis, and the tube can be used for drainage.

Pancreatitis is thought to result from too many inadvertent injections into the pancreatic duct during attempts at placement of the papillotome into the bile duct, direct trauma to the pancreatic duct with the papillotome by repeated or forceful cannulation, and excessive use of coagulation current during the EPT with resultant occlusion of the mouth of the pancreatic duct because of edema or direct tissue damage.

As a rule, these complications can be avoided if careful attention is given to 2 important principles: (1) the position of the papillotome in the bile duct should be checked carefully before starting the incision and (2) drainage of bile must be ensured following the EPT. Strict adherence to these principles has reduced the EPT-related complication rate in our patients from 7.4% to 4.8%; the necessity for surgical treatment has been reduced by one-third. Hemorrhage requiring surgery now occurs in only 0.5% of patients, and the EPT-related mortality has fallen to 0.7%. With the use of a nasobiliary tube, stone impaction and cholangitis have declined from 4.7% to 2.0%. The statistics collected from many countries by Machado[71] show a similar trend; the complication rate has decreased from 7.5% to 4.5% since 1980, and the mortality has fallen from 1.0% to 0.6%.

Gallstone ileus may occur after EPT for large stones in the bile duct. In the case reported by Halter et al.,[72] a 3.5-cm diameter calculus lodged in the jejunum about 50 cm distal to the ligament of Treitz 3 days after EPT, at which time stone extraction from the bile duct was unsuccessful. The stone was removed at laparotomy 9 days after the endoscopic procedure.

Death after EPT is probably caused in most cases by the underlying disorder, such as recurrent cholangitis and sepsis, rather than as a direct consequence of the endoscopic papillotomy (Table 29–8).

The complications and mortality following EPT are higher in patients with benign papillary stenosis (without choledocholithiasis) than in other patients. In fact, the mortality rate is about twice that in patients with choledocholithiasis without papillary stenosis (Table 29–8). The complication rate of EPT for papillary tumors is 5.3%. This rate and a

TABLE 29–8. **EPT Mortality**[54]

Indication	No. Patients	No. Deaths	Mortality (%)
Choledocholithiasis	7582	77	1.02
Papillary stenosis (without choledocholithiasis)	813	18	2.21
Papillary tumor	187	1	0.53
Total	8582	96	1.12

mortality rate of 0.5% are lower than those for EPT in patients with choledocholithiasis and papillary stenosis.

FUNCTIONAL CONSEQUENCES OF EPT

Changes in Bile Composition

The composition of the bile is influenced by changes in the anatomy of the extrahepatic biliary system. Cholecystectomy leads to a decrease in bile acid pool size, especially in patients with a large pool size preoperatively.[73] At the same time, the fractional turnover of primary bile acids increases, and there is a rise in the proportion of secondary bile acids in the bile.

EPT may accentuate the effects of cholecystectomy or induce changes that resemble those associated with cholecystectomy in patients who have retained their gallbladders. Sauerbruch et al.[74] studied the effect of EPT on bile acid pool and lipid composition in 3 patients with gallbladders and 7 patients who had undergone cholecystectomy. Determinations were made within several days and at several months after EPT. Total bile acid pool size was markedly reduced by EPT in patients with gallbladders, whereas there was no significant change in pool size in those without gallbladders.

We have found that cholesterol saturation of bile obtained from the bile duct decreases after EPT in patients with intact gallbladders.[75] However, Sauerbruch et al.[74] found no increase in the degree of cholesterol saturation in hepatic bile after EPT in patients with intact gallbladders.

Stellaard et al.[76] studied the effect of EPT on bile acid composition and cholesterol saturation of bile in 13 women who had undergone cholecystectomy at least 9 months before the endoscopic procedure. Twelve women who had had cholecystectomy and

did not undergo EPT comprised a control group. The EPT group exhibited a significantly higher percentage of chenodeoxycholic acid in bile, but no difference in the proportion of cholic acid. The percentages of the secondary bile acids were also lower in the EPT group, but the differences were not statistically significant. The biliary lipid composition in the EPT group did not differ from that in controls, so that the cholesterol saturation index in the patients undergoing EPT was similar to that of the control patients. The authors suggested that the changes demonstrated in bile composition would not be deleterious to the biliary or gastrointestinal systems. The significance of these findings remains unclear.

The normal diurnal fluctuations in biliary lipid concentrations are unchanged after cholecystectomy or EPT.

Manometric Investigations

The duodenobiliary pressure gradient is normally 8 mm Hg.[77] This is abolished in 80% of patients and reduced to 1 to 5 mm Hg in 20% of patients after EPT for bile duct stones in which the incision produced is relatively long. When the EPT incision is shorter, such as in minor papillotomies for the purpose of endoprosthesis insertion, the duodenobiliary pressure gradient usually remains unchanged or is reduced to an insignificant degree. In 11 patients who underwent this type of EPT and had manometry before and after the procedure, the pressure difference was eliminated in only 3 cases. Thus, this more selective type of papillotomy probably leaves remnants of the sphincter mechanism substantially intact. These observations have been confirmed by Staritz et al.[78]

Geenen et al.[12] studied the length of the incision after EPT using the papillotome itself and an inflated Fogarty balloon for reference. At 12 and 24 months after EPT, the duodenobiliary pressure gradient and the basal sphincter of Oddi pressure had been virtually abolished, and the amplitude of the phasic sphincter of Oddi contractions had decreased significantly. However, an increase in the amplitude of the phasic contractions was found 24 months after EPT to the point that the difference between the determinations at 24 months and the baseline determinations before EPT no longer reached statistical significance. Over the long term, the size of the papillary opening (length of the incision) decreased from 11.6 ± 0.8 mm to 7.5 ± 0.7 mm after 1 year and to 6.5 ± 0.7 mm after 2 years. These morphologic and manometric investigations confirm that the papillary orifice widened by EPT remains open to a significant degree for at least 2 years.

An intact sphincter of Oddi is probably an important barrier to spread of bacteria from the intestines. In 39 patients undergoing follow-up several months to some years after EPT, we found that there was considerable bacterial colonization in bile aspirated selectively from the bile duct (Table 29–9). However, none of these patients had symptoms or biochemical evidence of cholangitis. For this reason, we regard bacteriocholia as innocuous as long as bile flow remains unhindered.

Gregg et al.[79] studied the bacterial content of bile before and after either EPT or surgical sphincteroplasty in 45 patients with sphincter

TABLE 29–9. **Bacteria Strains in the Bile Duct Following EPT in 39 Patients***

Strain of Bacteria	No. Patients in Whom Strain Was Detected
E. coli	34
Klebsiella sp.	7
Enterobacter sp.	3
Proteus sp.	13
Providencia	1
Pseudomonas sp.	6
Enterococci	18
Streptococcus sp.	1
Staphylococcus aureus hemolytica	2
Candida sp.	1

*Cultures of bile obtained by endoscopic retrograde aspiration.

of Oddi stenosis. In all cases the bile was sterile prior to the procedure. Bile recultured 6 to 36 months after EPT contained bacteria in 70% of cases. However, there was no associated clinical evidence of cholangitis. More than one type of bacteria was found in most patients, and the majority were enteric organisms.

Greenfield et al.[80] studied 25 patients after EPT (mean, 36 months) for choledocholithiasis. Although symptomatic improvement occurred in all and there were no cases clinically of acute cholangitis, 20% of the patients had experienced mild episodes of abdominal pain, and a similar number had elevated serum gamma glutamyl transpeptidase activity as great as 3 times the normal level. In about half the patients, air in the biliary system was shown radiographically. In these patients, liver biopsy revealed mild portal tract fibrosis and inflammation. There was a statistical correlation between episodes of mild upper abdominal pain and air in the biliary system radiographically, which the authors accepted as evidence of biliary reflux of gastrointestinal contents. The long-term significance of observations such as these is unclear.

Alternatives to EPT

Although it is clear that EPT can result in changes in the physiology of the gastrointestinal tract, it is not certain to what degree these are of importance. There are thus some reservations about EPT in relatively young individuals in whom normal life expectancy would allow adequate time for any adverse effect to arise as a result of these alterations in anatomy and physiology. Because of this, other approaches to endoscopic therapy that produce a more physiologic result are being attempted. The most important indication for endoscopic opening of the papilla of Vater and the sphincter of Oddi is choledocholithiasis. Recently, Staritz et al.[81] have shown that the extraction of small stones from the bile duct may be possible following pharmacologic dilation of the sphincter of Oddi using glycerol trinitrate. The extraction of 32 bile duct stones 6 to 12 mm in diameter from 21 patients was attempted after administration of 1.2 to 3.6 mg of glycerol trinitrate. Thirty stones were extracted without difficulty. The remaining two stones were reduced in size by endoscopic mechanical lithotripsy and were then extracted. Subsequent manometric investigations showed that papillary function was retained.

This same group of investigators proposed balloon dilation of the papilla of Vater, using a special banana-shaped balloon 4 cm in length and 1.5 cm in diameter as an alternative to EPT.[82] This method also appears to be suitable for the removal of smaller stones from the bile duct.

Editor's note: References 83 and 84 are recent reports pertaining to endoscopic sphincterotomy.

References

1. Zimmon DS, Falkenstein DB, Kessler RE. Endoscopic papillotomy for choledocholithiasis. N Engl J Med 1975; 293:1181–2.
2. Geenen JE. Endoscopic papillotomy. In: Demling L, Classen M, eds. Endoscopic Sphincterotomy of the Papilla of Vater. Stuttgart: Thieme Verlag, Seite 1978: 81–2.
3. Schneider MU, Lux G. Floating pancreatic duct concrements in chronic pancreatitis. Pain relief by endoscopic removal. Endoscopy 1985; 17:8–10.
4. Fuji T, Amano H, Harima K, et al. Pancreatic sphincterotomy and pancreatic endoprosthesis. Endoscopy 1985; 17:69–72.
5. Hagenmüller F, Roos E. Electrosurgical aspects of endoscopic papillotomy. In: Endoscopic Papillotomy (EPT)—Now Ten Years Old. Heidelberg: Springer Verlag, in press.
6. Silverstein FE, Deltenre M, Tytgat G, et al. An endoscopic Doppler probe: preliminary clinical evaluation. Ultrasound Med Biol 1985; 11:347–53.
7. Martin RW, Gilbert DA, Silverstein FE, et al. An endoscopic Doppler probe for assessing intestinal vasculature. Ultrasound Med Biol 1985; 11:61–9.
8. Sander R, Poesl H. Endoscopic papillotomy with the Nd YAG laser. Endoscopy 1985; 17:115–6.
9. Osnes M: Endoscopic choledochoduodenostomy for common bile duct obstructions. Lancet 1979; 1:1059–60.
10. Schapira L, Khawaja FI. Endoscopic fistulo sphincterotomy: an alternative method of sphincterotomy using a new sphincterotome. Endoscopy 1982; 14:58–60.
11. Cremer M, Gulbis A, Toussaint J, et al. Techniques of endoscopic papillotomy. In: Delmont J, ed. The Sphincter of Oddi. Basel: Karger Verlag, 1977.
12. Geenen JE, Toouli J, Hogan WJ, et al. Endoscopic sphincterotomy: follow up evaluation of effects on the sphincter of Oddi. Gastroenterology 1984; 87:754–8.
13. Wurbs D, Phillip J, Classen M. Experiences with the long-standing nasobiliary tube in biliary diseases. Endoscopy 1980; 12:219–23.
14. Stolte M, Wiessner V, Rösch W. Todesursachen nach endoskopischer Papillotomie. Z Gastroenterol 1982; 20:452–8.
15. Riemann JF, Seuberth K, Demling L. Clinical application of a new mechanical lithotripter for smashing common bile duct stones. Endoscopy 1982; 14:226–30.
16. Frimberger E, Weingart J, Kühner W, et al. Einge-
klemmter Papillenstein: mechanische Lithotripsie moglichkeit. Dtsch Med Wochenschr 1983; 108:38.
17. Riemann JF, Seuberth K, Demling L. Mechanical lithotripsy through the intact papilla of Vater. Endoscopy 1983; 15:111–3.
18. Frimberger E, Kühner W, Weingart J, et al. Eine neue Methode der elektrohydraulischen Cholelithotripsie (Lithoklasie). Dtsch Med Wochenschr 1982; 107:213–5.
19. Tanaka M, Yoshimoto H, Ikeda S, et al. Two approaches for electrohydraulic lithotripsy in the common bile duct. Surgery 1985; 98:313–8.
20. Martin EC, Wolff M, Neff RA, et al. Use of the electrohydraulic lithotriptor in the biliary tree in dogs. Radiology 1981; 139:215–7.
21. Jessen K, Phillip J, Classen M. Endoscopic jet cutting—A new method for stone destruction in the common bile duct. 6th International Symposium on Jet-cutting Technology. BH RA Fluid Engineering, Cranfield, Bedford MK 43 OAJ, England, 1982; 39.
22. Demling L, Ermert H, Riemann JF, et al. Lithotripsy in the common bile duct using ultrasound. Preliminary in vitro experiments. Endoscopy 1984; 16:226–8.
23. Leuschner U, Baumgärtel H, Klempa J. Chemical treatment of choledocholithiasis. In: Classen M, Geenen J, Kawi K, eds. Non-Surgical Biliary Drainage. Berlin, Heidelberg: Springer Verlag, 1984; 81–5.
24. Nakajima M, Kizu M, Akasaka Y, Kawai K. Five years experience of endoscopic sphincterotomy in Japan: a collective study from 25 centres. Endoscopy 1979; 11:138–41.
25. Cotton PB, Vallon AG. British experience with duodenoscopic sphincterotomy for removal of bile duct stones. Br J Surg 1981; 68:373–5.
26. Seifert E. Endoscopic papillotomy and removal of gallstones. Am J Gastroenterol 1978; 69:154–9.
27. Montori A, Viceconte G, Viceconte GW, et al. ERCP and EPT: Italian experience. Endoscopy 1979; 2:142–5.
28. Geenen JE, Vennes JA, Silvis SE. Resumé of a seminar on endoscopic retrograde sphincterotomy (ERS). Gastrointest Endosc 1981; 27:31–8.
29. Viceconte G, Viceconte GW, Pietropaolo V, Montori A. Endoscopic sphincterotomy: indications and results. Br J Surg 1981; 68:376–80.
30. Leese T, Neoptolemos JP, Carr-Locke DL. Successes, failures, early complications and their management following endoscopic sphincterotomy: results in 394 consecutive patients from a single centre. Br J Surg 1985; 72:215–9.
31. Safrany L. Duodenoscopic sphincterotomy and gallstone removal. Gastroenterology 1977; 72:338–43.
32. Koch H, Rösch W, Schaffner O, et al. Endoscopic papillotomy. Gastroenterology 1977; 73:1393–6.
33. Siegel JH. Endoscopic papillotomy in the treatment of biliary tract disease. 258 procedures and results. Dig Dis Sci 1981; 26:1057–64.
34. Escourrou J, Cordova JA, Lazorthes F, et al. Early and late complications after endoscopic sphincterotomy for biliary lithiasis with and without the gallbladder 'in situ.' Gut 1984; 25:598–602.
35. Wurbs D. Endoscopic papillotomy. Scand J Gastroenterol 1982 (Suppl); 77:107–15.
36. Safrany L, Neuhaus B, Portocarrero G, Krause S. Endoscopic sphincterotomy in patients with Billroth II gastrectomy. Endoscopy 1980; 12:16–22.
37. Rosseland AR, Osnes M, Kruse A. Endoscopic

sphincterotomy (EST) in patients with Billroth II gastrectomy. Endoscopy 1981; 13:19–24.

38. Forbes A, Cotton PB. ERCP and sphincterotomy after Billroth II gastrectomy. Gut 1984; 25:971–4.

39. Russell RC, Wong NW, Cotton PB. Accessory sphincterotomy (endoscopic and surgical) in patients with pancreas divisum. Br J Surg 1984; 71:954–7.

40. Weizel A, Stiehl A, Raedsch R. Passage of a large bilirubin stone through a narrow papillotomy. Endoscopy 1980; 12:191–3.

41. Swobodnik W, Wechsler JG, Kluppelberg U, et al. Auflosung von Rezidivsteinen im Choledochus durch modifizierte Spulbehandlung über eine nasobiliare Verweilsonde. Dtsch Med Wochenschr 1984; 109:1232–6.

42. Siegel JH. Biliary bezoar: The sump syndrome and choledochoenterostomy. Endoscopy 1982; 14:238–40.

43. Baker AR, Neoptolemos JP, Carr-Locke DL, et al. Sump syndrome following choledochoduodenostomy and its endoscopic treatment. Br J Surg 1985; 72:433–5.

44. Siegel JH. Duodenoscopic sphincterotomy in the treatment of the "sump syndrome." Dig Dis Sci 1981; 26:922–8.

45. Tanaka M, Ikeda S, Yoshimoto H. Endoscopic sphincterotomy for the treatment of biliary sump syndrome. Surgery 1983; 93:264–7.

46. Phillip J, Classen M. Endoskopische Eingriffe an Papilla Vateri und Gallenwegen. In: Bilio-pankreatischer Chirurgie im Druck.

47. Houang MT, Franklin A, Arozena X. *Ascaris lumbricoides* detected in common bile duct following routine cholecystectomy and common bile duct sphincterotomy. Br J Radiol 1980; 53:804–5.

48. Acosta JM, Ledgesma CL. Gallstone migration as a cause of acute pancreatitis. N Engl J Med 1984; 190:484.

49. Lux G, Riemann JF, Demling L. Biliare Pankreatitis—Diagnostische und therapeutische Moglichkeiten durch ERCP und endoskopische Papillotomie. Z Gastroenterol 1984; 22:246–56.

50. Classen M, Ossenberg FW, Wurbs D, Hagenmüller F. Pancreatitis—an indication for endoscopic papillotomy? Endoscopy 1978; 10:223.

51. Safrany L, Cotton PB. A preliminary report: urgent duodenoscopic sphincterotomy for acute gallstone pancreatitis. Surgery 1981; 89:424–8.

52. van der Spuy S. Endoscopic sphincterotomy in the management of gallstone pancreatitis. Endoscopy 1981; 13:25–6.

53. Classen M, Leuschner U, Schreiber HW. Papilla stenosis and common duct calculi. Clin Gastroenterol 1983; 12:203–29.

54. Seifert E, Gail K, Weismüller J. Langzeitresultate nach endoskopischer Sphinkterotomie. Dtsch Med Wochenschr 1982; 107:610–4.

55. Bourgeois N, Dunham F, Verhest A, Cremer M. Endoscopic biopsies of the papilla of Vater at the time of endoscopic sphincterotomy: difficulties in interpretation. Gastrointest Endosc 1984; 30:163–6.

56. O'Connor MJ, Schwartz ML, McQuarrie DG, Sumner HW. Acute bacterial cholangitis; an analysis of clinical manifestations. Arch Surg 1982; 117:437–41.

57. Lam SK. A study of endoscopic sphincterotomy in recurrent pyogenic cholangitis. Br J Surg 1984; 71:262–6.

58. Burmeister W, Wurbs D, Hagenmüller F, Classen M. Langzeituntersuchungen nach endoskopischer Papillotomie. Z Gastroenterol 1980; 18:527–31.

59. Hagenmüller F, Wurbs D, Classen M. Long-term complications after endoscopic papillotomy (EPT) in patients with gallbladder in situ. (Abstr) Endoscopy 1973; 4:283–4.

60. Riemann JF, Gierth K, Lux G, et al. Die belassene Steingallenblase—ein Risikofaktor nach endoskopischer Papillotomie? Z Gastroenterol 1984; 22:188–93.

61. Neoptolemos JP, Carr-Locke DL, Fraser I, Fossard DP. The management of common bile duct calculi by endoscopic sphincterotomy in patients with gallbladders in situ. Br J Surg 1984; 71:69–71.

62. Cotton PB, Vallon AG. Duodenoscopic sphincterotomy for removal of bile duct stones in patients with gallbladders. Surgery 1982; 91:628–30.

63. Solhaug JH, Fokstuen O, Rosseland A, et al. Endoscopic papillotomy in patients with gallbladder in situ. Acta Chir Scand 1984; 150:475–8.

64. Cotton PB, Vallon AG. Duodenoscopic sphincterotomy in patients with gallbladders. (Abstr) Gastrointest Endosc 1981; 27:120.

65. Cremer M, Toussaint J, Dunham F, Jeanmart J. Endoscopic sphincterotomy (ES) with gallbladder in situ. (Abstr) Gastrointest Endosc 1981; 27:141.

66. Tulassay Z, Papp J. Endoskopische Sphinkterotomie bei Patienten mit Gallenblase in situ. Z Gastroenterol 1983; 27:492.

67. Mee AS, Vallon AG, Croker JR, Cotton PB. Nonoperative removal of bile duct stones by duodenoscopic sphincterotomy in the elderly. Br Med J [Clin Res] 1981; 283:521–3.

68. Staritz M, Ewe K, Goerg K, et al. Endoscopic balloon tamponade for conservative management of severe hemorrhage following endoscopic sphincterotomy. Z Gastroenterol 1984; 22:644–6.

69. Goodall RJ. Bleeding after endoscopic sphincterotomy. Ann Roy Coll Surg Engl 1985; 67:87–8.

70. Byrne P, Leung JW, Cotton PB. Retroperitoneal perforation during duodenoscopic sphincterotomy. Radiology 1984; 150:383–4.

71. Machado G. Acute complications of EPT in endoscopic papillotomy. In: Endoscopic Papillotomy EPT—Now Ten Years Old. International Symposium Erlangen, June, 1983.

72. Halter F, Bangerter U, Gigon JP, Pusterla C. Gallstone ileus after endoscopic sphincterotomy. Endoscopy 1981; 13:88–9.

73. Paumgartner G, Sauerbruch T. Secretion, composition and flow of bile. Clin Gastroenterol 1983; 12:3–23.

74. Sauerbruch T, Stellaard F, Paumgartner G. Effect of endoscopic sphincterotomy on bile acid pool size and bile lipid composition in man. Digestion 1983; 27:87–92.

75. Classen M, Kurtz W, Hagenmüller F. The gallbladder after endoscopic papillotomy. In: Trends in Hepatology. Lancaster: MTP, 1985.

76. Stellaard F, Sauerbruch T, Brunholzl C, et al. Bile acid pattern and cholesterol saturation of bile after cholecystectomy and endoscopic sphincterotomy. Digestion 1983; 26:153–8.

77. Rösch W, Koch H, Demling L. Manometric studies during ERCP and endoscopic papillotomy. Endoscopy 1977; 8:30–3.

78. Staritz M, Schmidt HD, Meyer zum Buschenfelde KH. Einflub der Cholecystektomie auf die Funktion

der Papilla Vateri: Eine prä- und postoperative endoskopisch manometrische Studie. (Abstr) Z Gastroenterol 1983; 21:423.

79. Gregg JA, DeGirolami P, Carr-Locke DL. Effects of sphincteroplasty and endoscopic sphincterotomy on the bacteriologic characteristics of the common bile duct. Am J Surg 1985; 149:668–71.

80. Greenfield C, Cleland P, Dick R, et al. Biliary sequelae of endoscopic sphincterotomy. Postgrad Med J 1985; 61:213–5.

81. Staritz J, Poralla T, Dormeyer HH, Meyer zum Buschenfelde KH. Endoscopic removal of common bile duct stones through the intact papilla after medical sphincter dilation. Gastroenterology 1985; 88:1807–11.

82. Staritz M, Ewe K, Meyer zum Buschenfelde KH. Endoscopic papillary dilation (EPD) for the treatment of common bile duct stones and papillary stenosis. Endoscopy 1983; 15:197–8.

83. Staritz M, Ewe K, Meyer zum Buschenfelde KH. Investigation of the sphincter of Oddi before, immediately after and six weeks after endoscopic papillotomy. Endoscopy 1986; 18:14–6.

84. Osnes M, Rosseland AR, Aabakken L. Endoscopic retrograde cholangiography and endoscopic papillotomy in patients with a previous Billroth-II resection. Gut 1986; 27:1193–8.

Chapter 30

CALCULUS DISEASE OF THE BILE DUCTS

DIETMAR F. W. WURBS, M.D.

During the past ten years diagnosis and therapy of calculi in the gallbladder and bile ducts have undergone profound and in some respects revolutionary changes. Ultrasonography has become the method of choice for demonstration of stones of the gallbladder.[1, 2] However, the diagnostic approach with respect to the bile ducts is more complex; ultrasonography can demonstrate the level of obstruction,[3] but identification of the cause is often impossible. This is particularly true for stones in the preampullary portion of the common bile duct. The conventional intravenous cholangiogram is error-prone with incorrect conclusions in as many as 40% of examinations, even with technically adequate procedures in non-jaundiced patients. The usefulness of this procedure is therefore in question.[4, 5]

A complete and detailed cholangiogram is a necessity in cholestasis to decide if operative therapy is indicated. Cholangiograms may be made either by percutaneous transhepatic cholangiography (PTC) or by endoscopic retrograde cholangiography (ERC). Both are effective, but in a sense ERC is performed via a natural route and therefore is less invasive than PTC. The technique of PTC is less difficult to master, and PTC is less expensive than ERC in many areas of the world. However, in experienced hands ERC may be performed in a short time, with little patient discomfort and with a success rate of about 80% to 90%. Endoscopic retrograde cholangiopancreatography (ERCP) also provides information about the papilla of Vater, duodenum, and pancreas. Furthermore, therapeutic manipulations are added to diagnostic ERC in up to 60% of procedures, eliminating the need for surgery in the majority of cases.[6]

Both PTC and ERCP have potential complications, and the mortality rate with both methods is about 0.1%.[7-10] Satisfactory results using either method depend on the skill and experience of the operator. Because many complications are related to bile stasis, the operator must be able to decompress the biliary system, either by percutaneous transhepatic drainage (PTD) or by endoscopic papillotomy (EPT) and drainage by nasobiliary tube or insertion of a biliary stent (also called a biliary endoprosthesis). A comprehensive analysis of the choice of diagnostic and non-surgical therapeutic measures for biliary tract disease is given in Chapter 26.

TECHNIQUE OF ERCP IN STONE DISEASE

The technique of ERCP is described in Chapter 25 and elsewhere.[11] Some special problems may arise in the course of this procedure, such as a juxtapapillary diverticulum, which may make cannulation of the papilla more difficult. Normally a 60% concentration of water-soluble contrast medium will produce excellent radiographs; however, with dilated bile ducts small stones may be obscured by this high concentration of radiopaque material. Therefore, a 30% concentration is preferable when choledocholithiasis is suspected. X-ray films made early during injection of contrast medium are helpful, as are delayed films at 30 minutes after ERCP. Normally, the procedure is done with the patient in a semi-prone position with the right side raised slightly from the x-ray table. In this position, the x-ray penetration distance through the body is shortest and does not encounter the spine. A nearly equal dis-

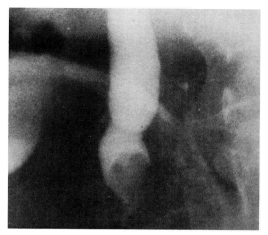

FIGURE 30–1. Round filling defect in the ampulla was initially interpreted as a stone. After endoscopic papillotomy (EPT), a polypoid carcinoma protruded into the duodenum.

THE PAPILLA AND PERIPAPILLARY FINDINGS IN STONE DISEASE

The most impressive endoscopic finding is a stone impacted in the ampulla of Vater. It may be visible in the meatus of the papilla (Plate 30–1) or, even if it is not visible, the stone may cause the whole papilla to protrude into the duodenum to an extreme degree (Plate 30–2). Redness around the meatus indicates inflammation, sometimes referred to as "papillitis." An enlarged papillary meatus with a red and fissured margin together with recent and usually severe colic may be interpreted as evidence of passage of a stone(s) (Plate 30–3). In such cases selective cannulation of the common bile duct is not difficult.

The incidence of duodenal diverticula increases with age. Usually they are located on the medial wall of the descending duodenum close to the papilla (Plate 30–4). Duodenoscopy with ERCP permits accurate localization, definition of their relation to the papilla, and correct diagnosis of associated bile duct stones[13–15] (Figs. 30–5 and 30–6). Lotveit and associates[14] reported on ERCP studies of pa-

tribution of contrast medium in the biliary tree can be attained by turning the patient to the supine or upright position. Only filling defects that are mobile and completely surrounded by contrast can be classified as stones. Tumors (Fig. 30–1), cysts (Fig. 30–2), and even normal papillas[12] (Fig. 30–3) can mimic stones. Conversely, a stone may mimic a tumor (Fig. 30–4).

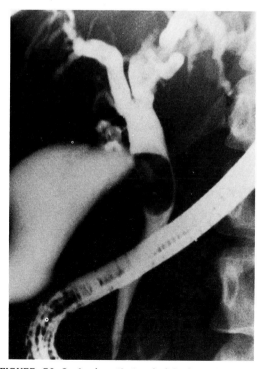

FIGURE 30–2. Lesion that mimicked a stone was shown at operation to be a bile duct cyst.

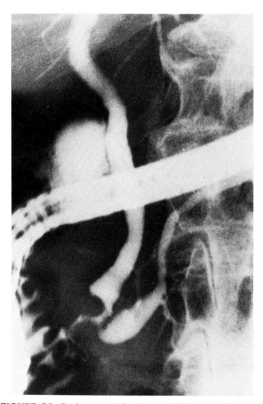

FIGURE 30–3. Asymmetric shape of the ampulla was initially interpreted as an impacted stone in the ampulla.

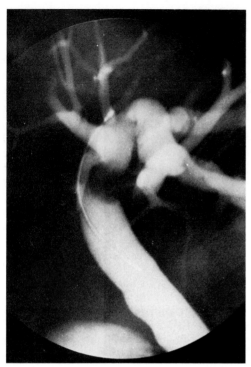

FIGURE 30–4. Stone simulates a tumor at the confluence of the hepatic ducts. The stone completely obstructs the right hepatic duct.

a causal relationship between duodenal diverticula and gallstone disease. Although the relationship of diverticula to the pathogenesis of biliary calculi is speculative, it has been suggested that the diverticulum causes stasis by impeding the flow of bile into the duodenum. In a study of a small number of patients, there were no significant differences in common bile duct pressure in relation to the presence or absence of diverticula.[16] Phasic activity and peak sphincter of Oddi pressure were similar in both groups.

Beta-glucuronidase is produced by bacteria—especially by *Escherichia coli*. This enzyme splits conjugated bilirubin, which in turn combines with calcium to form insoluble calcium bilirubinate.[17] There is a very high incidence (70% to 92%) of *E. coli* colonization of the bile ducts in association with papillary or peripapillary diverticula. In contrast, there is a lower incidence (45%) when diverticula are located at some distance from the papilla.[18] In about two thirds of cases there is a high incidence of pigment stones in gallbladders of patients with juxtapapillary diverticula.[19] There is also some evidence that beta-glucuronidase in the bile ducts may be the

tients in whom symptoms of biliary tract or pancreatic disease developed after cholecystectomy and who were asymptomatic for intervals of two years or more. The incidence of recurrent calculi in patients with diverticula was 87.5%; without diverticula the incidence was 39.1%. Studies such as this indicate

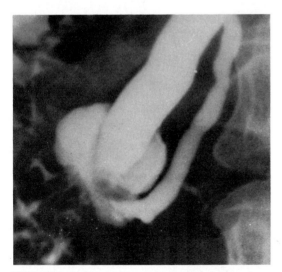

FIGURE 30–5. Retrograde cholangiogram in the same case as in Plate 30–4 demonstrating diverticulum surrounding the distal end of the bile duct.

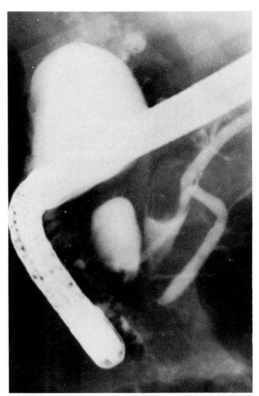

FIGURE 30–6. Normal pancreatic duct. Common bile duct with 10 × 20 mm stone and a diverticulum between bile duct and duodenum.

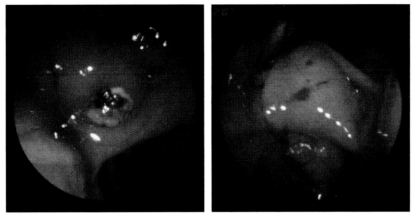

PLATE 30–1.   PLATE 30–2.

PLATE 30–1. A large stone (17 mm) has impacted in the ampulla causing recurrent acute pancreatitis.
PLATE 30–2. This large, prominent papilla harbors a 20 mm stone. Meatus of the papilla is directed caudally and cannot be seen. On the protruding papilla there is a second opening–probably a spontaneous perforation due to the presence of the stone.

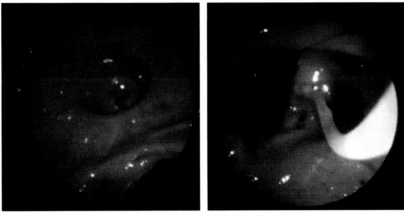

PLATE 30–3.   PLATE 30–4.

PLATE 30–3. Papilla is atypically located in a diverticulum. Meatus is large and red as a result of passage of a stone.
PLATE 30–4. Two large juxtapapillary diverticula. The papilla is usually located at the brim of the diverticulum in a dorsocaudal or ventrocaudal position. Here the diverticulum surrounds the papilla.

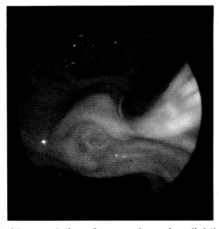

PLATE 30–5. Normal papilla (arrow) with cannulation of a second opening slightly cephalad to the papilla. Surgery with "bougienage of the papilla" had been performed previously.

result of a metabolic defect in the liver,[20] although this finding is controversial and lacks confirmatory data. Normally there is a metabolic pathway from glucuronic acid to glucaro-1,4-lactone, which is excreted in bile and which inhibits beta-glucuronidase. It has been suggested that this pathway prevents stone formation,[21] but this has not been established.

Another interesting finding of duodenoscopy and ERCP is the choledochoduodenal fistula (Plate 30–5; see also Plate 30–2). Typically the fistulas are located in the roof of the papilla or a little cephalad to this in the infundibular portion of the bile duct. This has been explained as the result of spontaneous stone-induced perforation;[22] however, similar fistulas were found in 18 of 36 patients after surgical sphincterotomy and after surgery during which the distal bile duct was probed blindly.[23] In my experience this fistula was discovered in 26 of 3000 patients undergoing ERCP; 5 patients with fistulas had no prior surgery, and operative reports were available in 16 of the remaining 21 patients. In all of these patients, probing in

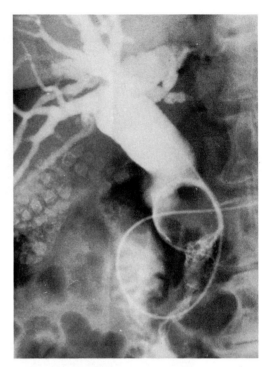

FIGURE 30–8. Multiple calculi in gallbladder. Contrast does not enter the gallbladder, and therefore cystic duct occlusion can be inferred. A large stone can be seen in the bile duct. This 83-year-old patient had right upper quadrant colicky pain about 50 years ago, a symptom-free interval of more than 40 years, and recurrent episodes of mild jaundice during the last 4 years. Now she has acute suppurative cholangitis, and a nasobiliary tube has been inserted to decompress the biliary tree.

a blind fashion or somewhat forceful passage of dilators "through the papilla" because of suspected stenosis had been carried out. It therefore seems probable that these fistulas represent unintended perforations in a significant number of cases (unpublished data). Endoscopic fistulotomy has been suggested as treatment of these fistulas.[24] Therapeutic intervention is probably necessary only if there are stones in the bile duct. In my series this was the case in 11 of the 26 patients.

STONES IN THE BILIARY TRACT: TYPICAL AND ATYPICAL FINDINGS

The most common finding is the small or medium-sized mobile stone up to 15 mm diameter in normal caliber or slightly dilated bile ducts. If the ducts are dilated, as many as 50 or more stones may be present (Fig. 30–7). These may be cholesterol stones. It has been suggested that the dilated bile duct to some extent assumes the function of the

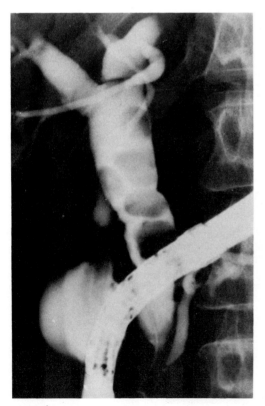

FIGURE 30–7. Multiple stones in common bile duct proved on analysis to be cholesterol stones.

gallbladder when this has been resected or is not functioning.[25] Patients with very large bile duct stones may have a long history with mild symptoms and long asymptomatic intervals (Fig. 30–8).

Hundreds of intrahepatic stones are sometimes found in Caroli's disease or after bile duct surgery. These stones, dilated ducts, and in some cases a relative or real stenosis can be demonstrated by ERC (Fig. 30–9). Jaundiced patients who have had biliary surgery, especially for calculus disease, are always highly suspect for recurrent stones. Bile duct stricture, with and without associated stones, must also be considered, since this is a frequent occurrence (Fig. 30–10). Even a patent choledochoduodenal anastomosis may be complicated by recurrence of stones (Figs. 30–11 and 30–12). In many cases in which there has been prior surgery, endoscopy with stone extraction is preferable to re-operation.

The Mirizzi syndrome consists of a triad of cystic duct stone, chronic cholecystitis with shrinkage of the gallbladder, and benign ste-

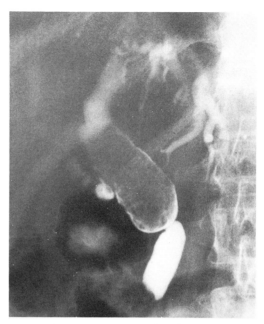

FIGURE 30–10. Large stone in bile duct above a stricture. Cholecystectomy and choledochotomy had been performed. Endoscopic removal is not possible.

nosis of the hepatic duct which may also lead to cholestasis and often cholangitis. Direct cholangiography typically demonstrates an asymmetric stenosis with a smooth configuration, an appearance that can usually be interpreted as due to compression (Fig. 30–13). Occasionally, however, interpretation of the findings may be difficult and the correct diagnosis may be made only at operation (Fig. 30–14).

Sometimes there may be more than one reason for a patient to be jaundiced; for example, a stone and carcinoma may both be present (Fig. 30–15), or a long cystic duct may harbor stones (Fig. 30–16).

The incidence of bile duct stones in patients who undergo operation for acute or chronic cholecystitis is 9% to 10%.[26] Residual or recurrent stones after cholecystectomy performed without duct exploration occur in 1% to 4% of patients.[27] The frequency of retained or recurrent stones after removal of bile duct stones at operation is 10%.[26] About 20% of patients who have undergone reoperation for bile duct stones will develop choledocholithiasis again.[28]

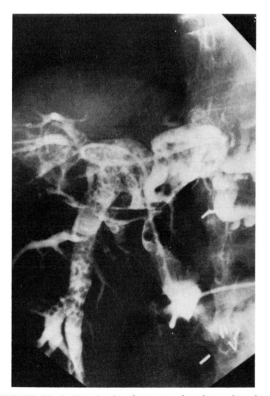

FIGURE 30–9. Hundreds of stones of various sizes in dilated intrahepatic bile ducts. There is free reflux of the radiographic contrast into the duodenum. Three choledochotomies were performed in this patient; after each operation, the number of stones increased. A nasobiliary tube has been inserted. An attempt at stone dissolution was unsuccessful.

GALLSTONE PANCREATITIS

One of the most common causes of acute pancreatitis is migration of bile duct stones through the papilla (see Plate 30–1). Delivery

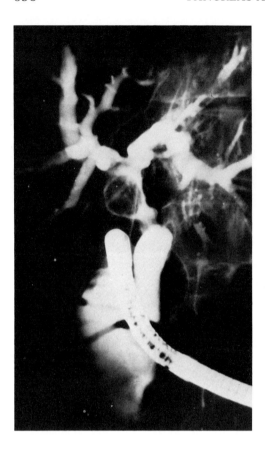

FIGURE 30–11. Recurrent stone after choledocho-duodenostomy. Bile duct is cannulated through the small-diameter anastomosis. Relative to the diameter of the stone, stenosis of the bile duct is narrow below the position of the stone in the bile duct. This stone and others that later recurred were composed of soft material and were extracted endoscopically.

FIGURE 30–12. This 93-year-old patient has had a Billroth II procedure, cholecystectomy, and choledochoduodenostomy. Cannulation and retrograde opacification through the anastomosis demonstrates complete filling of the bile duct with stones. The stones were soft, yellow material and thus extractable.

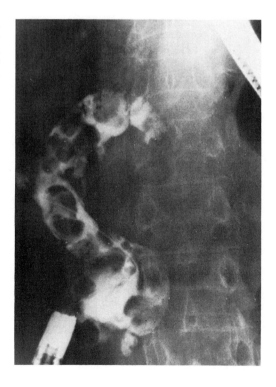

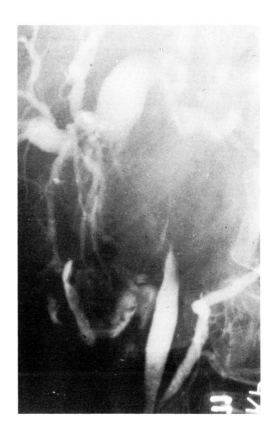

FIGURE 30–13. Mirizzi syndrome. A 7 cm × 3 cm stone compresses the common bile duct.

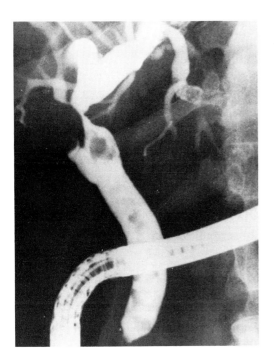

FIGURE 30–14. Mirizzi syndrome. Bile duct contains multiple stones. The bow-shaped impression at the bifurcation directed from the patient's right is caused by a stone. Preoperatively, a tumor was suspected.

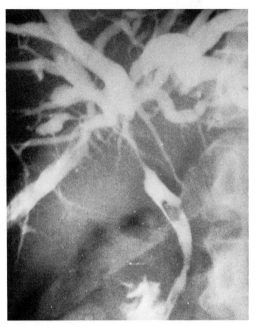

FIGURE 30–15. Stone and carcinoma of the bile duct with prestenotic dilation of the intrahepatic ducts.

of stones into the duodenum is accompanied by relief of symptoms and rapid decrease in serum amylase and bilirubin values. In the great majority of patients with known gallstones, calculi are found in the stool within 10 days after an attack.[29] Gallstone pancreatitis is a self-limiting disease with a benign natural course, for the most part. However, some patients develop severe and life-threatening pancreatitis because of persistent ampullary obstruction by a stone. Others will have recurrent severe pancreatitis because of repeated passage of stones. Therefore, surgery to remove the stone from the papilla and/or to resect the gallbladder which is acting as the stone reservoir is generally accepted. However, the timing of surgical intervention following the onset of pancreatitis is controversial. Acosta et al.[30] reported that results are most favorable if surgery is performed within 6 to 48 (average 28) hours. Others report that the most satisfactory outcome occurs when surgery is delayed for 5 to 7 days.[31, 32] Delayed surgery carries the risk of further episodes of pancreatitis.[31, 32] The earlier the operation the more often stones are found in the ampulla.[30, 31] The incidence of stone impaction at the papilla is increased in patients who have undergone surgery for gallstone pancreatitis and who sustain a further episode of biliary pancreatitis.[33]

Endoscopic techniques have profoundly altered the therapeutic approach to gallstone disease of the bile ducts. The first endoscopic extraction of a papillary stone performed by enlarging the papillary opening with a biopsy forcep was reported in 1974.[34] The systematic use of EPT in the management of gallstone pancreatitis was reported in 1978.[35] A survey in 1979 resulted in reports of 58 successful procedures with no fatalities.[36] Stones have even been extracted from the main pancreatic duct[37, 38] (Fig. 30–17). Duodenoscopy and EPT on an emergency basis for acute gallstone pancreatitis is now widely practiced by experienced endoscopists.[37, 39] The procedure is not contraindicated or limited by severity of the pancreatitis, age of the patient, or accompanying diseases. Improvement in the patient's general clinical condition and in laboratory parameters is prompt and sometimes dramatic.

CHOLEDOCHOLITHIASIS AND CHOLANGITIS

Cholangitis is often associated with choledocholithiasis. Its pathogenesis relates to the presence of bacteria in an obstructed duct. Bacterial colonization of bile is more frequent with obstruction caused by stones as opposed to tumor.[40] Additional predisposing factors may be the duration of time during which the obstruction has been present, number of episodes of colic, and age of the patient.[41] With repeated operations on the bile ducts,

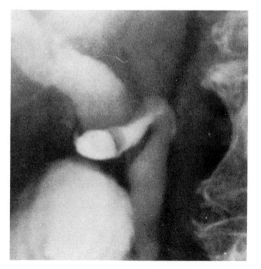

FIGURE 30–16. Long cystic duct with stone; whether it is residual or recurrent is not known.

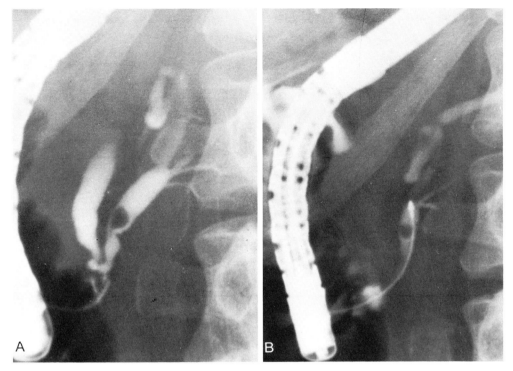

FIGURE 30–17. Endoscopic retrograde cholangiopancreatography (ERCP) was done because of recurrent acute pancreatitis. A, Simultaneous opacification of both pancreatic and bile ducts through a common channel. There is a 2–3 mm stone in the pancreatic duct. Stones of the same size were present in the gallbladder (not illustrated). B, Dormia basket is introduced into the pancreatic duct to extract the stone, which proved to be of yellow material.

bacterial colonization approaches 100% of cases.[40, 42, 43] It is mandatory that these facts be kept in mind when performing diagnostic or therapeutic procedures on the bile ducts. ERCP, PTC, and even T-tube cholangiography have septic complications that range from uncomplicated bacteremia to fatal endotoxic shock.[7, 43–45] It is possible that bacterial spreading during PTC results from iatrogenic biliovenous fistulas, but bacterial propagation may also occur with retrograde cannulation.[7, 45] It appears that an important factor, especially with respect to life-threatening endotoxic shock, is the pressure increase that occurs in an obstructed and infected duct. It is well established that the occurrence of cholangiovenous bile reflux depends on the degree to which intraductal pressure is increased.[46–48] The critical pressure level is 30–40 mm H_2O,[47, 48] and this is easily exceeded with every method of direct cholangiography.

From these data it must be assumed that infection of the bile ducts is probable in cases of biliary obstruction, especially if caused by calculi. ERCP must be performed by cau-tiously injecting only as much contrast medium as is necessary to determine the cause of obstruction. Antibiotic prophylaxis is recommended for all types of direct cholangiography when obstruction is likely to be present. This has been done by addition of aminoglycoside antibiotics, which are not antagonized by iodinated agents or bile, to the contrast agent[49] or by systematic administration of beta-lactamantibiotics, which achieve high serum levels, are excreted into bile, and are not antagonized by bile.[50–52] Selection of antibiotics should be based on the expected or identified bacterial contaminants of the ducts. These will be mainly *E. coli* and *Klebsiella*, *Enterobacter*, and *Pseudomonas* species. If bacteremia or sepsis occurs, it is not unusual to culture several different organisms from the blood. The spectrum of bacteria in the bile ducts as determined by ERC studies differs from that found in samples collected at surgery.[45] Endoscopes are notorious for harboring *Pseudomonas aeruginosa*. This species is a more significant problem in patients with tumors than in those with calculus disease.[45] It should be emphasized that biliary

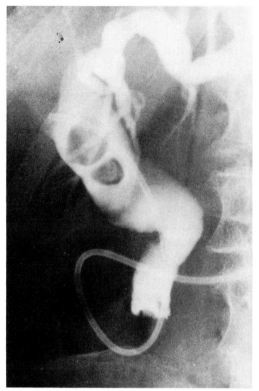

FIGURE 30–18. Nasobiliary tube. Stones have been mobilized from the prepapillary bile duct and pushed upward in the duct. Solvents have been perfused through the tube, and both stones have lacunae as signs of beginning dissolution.

excretion, including excretion of antibiotics into bile, is reduced when there is obstruction and stasis,[50, 52] and therefore antibiotic sterilization of obstructed bile ducts is impossible.[53] Although systemic antibiotic administration will reduce the incidence of septic

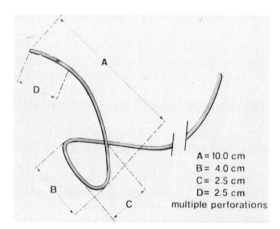

FIGURE 30–19. Diagram shows distal position of Wurbs-type nasobiliary tube.

A = 10.0 cm
B = 4.0 cm
C = 2.5 cm
D = 2.5 cm
multiple perforations

complications, it is logical that free bile flow must be established immediately after the cause of obstruction is determined. In the past this has been possible only by surgery. However, during the past 10 years temporary or definitive endoscopic therapy has become established as an effective approach. This includes EPT with stone extraction,[54] biliary stenting using an indwelling prosthesis, and the use of nasobiliary tubes for drainage, decompression,[55, 56] and dissolution of stones[57, 58] (Figs. 30–18 and 30–19).

ACUTE OBSTRUCTIVE SUPPURATIVE CHOLANGITIS

Acute obstructive suppurative cholangitis is the most dangerous form of bacterial cholangitis. In nearly all cases it is caused by common duct stones, and almost all patients will die if treated conservatively. Immediate mechanical decompression is mandatory.

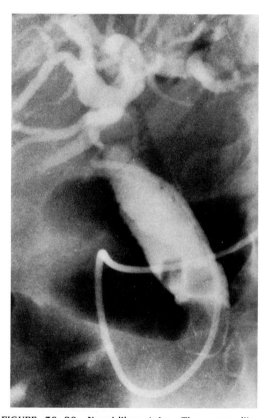

FIGURE 30–20. Nasobiliary tube. The prepapillary stone has not been mobilized. There is no free reflux of contrast medium around the stone and tube into the duodenum and decompression is incomplete. Slight suction on the nasobiliary tube will evacuate the bile tree.

This principle was formulated by Rogers in 1903,[59] and it has proved valid over many years.[60]

Endoscopists became more familiar with acute cholangitis with the introduction of EPT. During the early development of EPT, cholangitis was a serious problem, especially suppurative cholangitis associated with stone impaction after the procedure. The mortality rate was 16% during this period.[61] However, the problem has been largely resolved by the development and endoscopic use of nasobiliary drainage tubes which may be left in the bile ducts for long periods of time[55, 56] (Figs. 30–18 and 30–20). Endoscopic insertion of a nasobiliary tube fulfills the requirements for decompression by mobilizing the impacted stone, preventing reimpaction, and ensuring free flow of bile into the duodenum. If there is concern that bile flow around the nasobiliary tube and into the duodenum is inadequate, suction can be applied to the tube to drain the ducts externally. In my early experience the nasobiliary tube was used to treat septic complications arising from EPT that otherwise would have required urgent surgery. However, I now use nasobiliary drainage in all cases of acute obstructive suppurative cholangitis, including those patients who present with this condition, with satisfactory results in comparison with surgical or other non-surgical methods of management. In a collected series (Table 30–1) the mortality rate with non-surgical management was 100%. This was reduced to one third of patients by surgical intervention. The mortality rate for patients undergoing endoscopic decompression by means of nasobiliary tube insertion was 23%. Although there are difficulties with the use of collected data which are not quite comparable, this type of analysis indicates a favorable trend that supports the logical basis for the endoscopic management of acute suppurative cholangitis in association with biliary obstruction.

The endoscopic method of decompression of the bile ducts via the upper gastrointestinal tract and papilla of Vater is physiologic in its approach. Only a small papillotomy incision is required for introduction of the nasobiliary tube. Endoscopic decompression may be performed in virtually any patient, and the use of sedation can be minimized by an experienced endoscopist. General anesthesia is not required and the procedure can be performed by an experienced endoscopist even if there are additional problems of a serious nature such as shock, fever, mental confusion, defects in blood clotting, advanced age, or other disease.

In contrast, only 88 of 110 patients in the collected surgical series underwent operation (Table 30–1).[60, 62–69] These severely ill patients are less likely to tolerate the trauma of general anesthesia and laparotomy. The 22 non-operable patients died. This underscores the fact that immediate biliary decompression in acute suppurative obstructive cholangitis is the only effective treatment. PTD is also an effective method of decompression.[70, 71]

TABLE 30–1. **Acute Suppurative Cholangitis: Comparison of Surgical and Endoscopic Therapy**

	Patient Mortality			Mean age (years)
	Whole Group	*Operated Group*	*Non-operated Group*	
Surgical Decompression				
Reynolds and Dargan (1959)[60]	2/5	1/4	1/1	67.5
Glenn and Moody (1961)[62]	3/8	0/5	3/3	53.7
Ostermiller et al. (1965)[63]	6/8	6/8	0/0	68.3
Wadell (1966)[64]	3/6	0/3	3/3	67.3
Haupert et al. (1967)[65]	7/15	4/12	3/3	70–70
Dow and Lindenauer (1969)[66]	6/10	4/8	2/2	65
Hinchey and Couper (1969)[67]	8/24	6/22	2/2	60–70
Andrew and Johnson (1970)[68]	8/14	4/10	4/4	NA*
Welch and Donaldson (1976)[69]	8/20	4/16	4/4	72
Total	51/110	29/88	22/22	
Per cent	46%	33%	100%	
Endoscopic Decompression				
Wurbs (1983)	5/22	5/22	0/0	79
Per cent	23%	23%	—	

*Not available.

After an interval of satisfactory endoscopic decompression, further treatment of choledocholithiasis may be endoscopic or surgical. When the clinical situation is stable, the papillotomy can be enlarged if necessary and stones removed from the bile duct by basket or balloon extraction in most cases, although special problems may be encountered, such as excessively large stones. In addition to these simple methods for stone extraction, endoscopic therapy includes electrohydraulic lithotripsy,[72] mechanical crushing of stones (mechanical lithotripsy),[73] and chemical dissolution of stones[57, 58] (Table 30–2).

STONE DISSOLUTION

All solvents that can be perfused through T-tubes can also be given through nasobiliary drainage tubes. In recent years alpha-1-glycero-monooctanoin has been studied to the greatest extent.[74] This agent is theoretically most effective for stones composed mainly of cholesterol. However, it has been recognized postoperatively that the chemical composition of residual stones differs from that of stones that recur in the bile ducts after a long period of time. The former likely contains large amounts of cholesterol, whereas the latter usually has many components, including calcium bilirubinate and an organic matrix. Better results using monooctanoin perfusion can be expected with predominantly cholesterol stones detected in the early postoperative period. For stones present in the ducts for long periods of time, the sequential use of several different solvents has been proposed.[58] Complete dissolution or reduction of the stone to an extractable size is reported to occur in about two thirds of patients.[56] Intrahepatic stones can also be treated[57] (see Fig. 30–9).

Before the dissolution procedure is begun, it must be established radiographically that there is free reflux of perfused fluid from the ducts into the duodenum. If not, cholangitis will be induced. If it is suspected that pressure is rising in the duct, the perfusion must be stopped, and the nasobiliary tube used to drain the duct externally. Aliquots of bile may also be taken from the tube for culture.

There are some drawbacks to stone dissolution. Complete dissolution may require perfusion for more than 1 to 2 weeks. An adequate rate of flow must be maintained and this may not be tolerated by all patients. Side effects include abdominal cramps and diarrhea. However, it is often not necessary to completely dissolve the calculi. The solvent may reduce the size of the stone or soften it to the point that endoscopic extraction is possible.

MANAGEMENT OF CHOLEDOCHOLITHIASIS

In 1976 Berk and Kaplan[26] stated, "It is entirely possible that as more endoscopists become skilled in their [EPT] performance, these procedures may well assume the status of standard methods for removing low-lying stones from the common bile duct." Endoscopic papillotomy with stone extraction has been performed for 13 years and there are now enough data available to test this prophecy. However, there are caveats. It is impossible to compare the basically different surgical and endoscopic methods of stone removal with respect to all possible circumstances. Further, comparisons must be based on reports that have usually been published some years apart. Collected statistics from numerous investigators and centers where the procedures are performed in great numbers are most reliable. Pooled data are often obtained by questionnaire with the knowledge that success may be overstated, and risks and complications may be underestimated. In collected series, the diverse results of different investigators make interpretation of the composite data more difficult. Although there are reservations inherent in this method, and prospective comparative controlled studies are more desirable in princi-

TABLE 30–2. **Acute Obstructive Suppurative Cholangitis: Therapy after Nasobiliary Drainage***

Type of Therapy	No. Patients
Endoscopic Therapy	
Spontaneous delivery/extraction	10
Stone dissolution	3
Surgery	2
No Treatment	
Died before treatment	5
Unresolved†	2
Total	22

*Author's series.

†Not extractable or dissolvable; surgery impossible. One patient had pigtail drain.

TABLE 30–3. **Mortality: Biliary Surgery**

Type of Surgery		References
Cholecystectomy		
Chronic Cholecystitis	*Acute Cholecystitis*	
1.50% (*n* = 24,415)	3.50% (*n* = 4206)	75
1.02% (*n* = 3885)	3.15% (*n* = 564)	76
0.18% <60 years	0.39% <60 years	
3.00% >60 years	4.85% >60 years	
1.30% (*n* = 4327)		77
0.40% <60 years		
4.00% >60 years		
Cholecystectomy and Choledochotomy		
4.26% (*n* = 844)		76
1.66% <60 years		
6.19% >60 years		
5.30% (*n* = 1358)		77
2.40% <60 years		
12.80% >60 years		
47.68% (emergency surgery)		
Reoperation for Retained Stones		
3%–4%		78, 79
Transduodenal Sphincterotomy		
4.3% (*n* = 13,225)		84*

*Collected data.

ple, these are the only data available. It is probable that a controlled study comparing stone extraction using EPT with surgical removal of stones will not be undertaken given the established success with the endoscopic procedure.

Data on mortality rates for endoscopic therapy of choledocholithiasis compare favorably with those for operative therapy (Tables 30–3, 30–4, and 30–5). The surgical mortality rate for choledocholithotomy alone is not precisely known, but it is probably similar to that for cholecystectomy with choledochotomy and to reoperation for retained stones. The surgical mortality rate in acute obstructive suppurative cholangitis is about 46% (see Table 30–1).

The late complications of common bile duct surgery include stricture, papillary stenosis, and retention of suture material or clips in the bile duct. The incidence is not known. In a minimum of 0.3% to 0.7% of patients, retained, overlooked, or forgotten calculi are discovered by postoperative T-tube cholangiography.[28, 77] The usual reported frequency is 1% to 4%.[27] Reoperation has been mandatory treatment for these stones. However, about 10% to 26% will pass spontaneously, and therefore reoperation should be delayed for 4 to 6 weeks.[28] After a second operation residual stones are found by postoperative cholangiography in about 20% of patients.[28] Endoscopic therapy or extraction through the T-tube channel are alternatives to operation.[80–82]

Patients who have had calculi removed from the common bile duct at cholecystectomy seem more likely to develop recurrent calculi months or years later than those who did not have choledocholithiasis at a primary operation. However, confirmatory data for this impression are lacking.[25]

The success rate for the initial attempt at EPT and stone extraction is reduced 6% to

TABLE 30–4. **Mortality: Biliary Surgery for Gallstone-Induced Pancreatitis**

Overall	Early	Delayed	Late	Reference
11.0% (132)*	2% (46)	16% (86)	7% (14)	30
2.3% (172)	12% (24)	0% (134)		31
5.3% (114)	31% (17)	2% (98)		32

*Number of patients in parentheses.

TABLE 30–5. **Mortality: Endoscopic Treatment of Gallstones in Bile Duct**

	Mortality (%)	No. of Patients	Reference
Choledocholithiasis	1.10	1,989	61*
(including	0.87†	20,000	80*
cholestasis and	1.30	1,060‡	Author
cholangitis)			
Acute obstructive suppurative cholangitis	23	22	56
Biliary pancreatitis	0	58	36*
	18	11	37

*Collected data.
†Varied with level of experience from 0.3% to 5.1%.
‡Mean age, 68 years.

9% by the presence of stones that cannot be removed. The exact risks entailed in further endoscopic maneuvers to remove these retained calculi are not known. The new technique of mechanical destruction, referred to as mechanical lithotripsy, will decrease the number of instances in which all stones cannot be cleared from the bile duct.[73] In this technique, a strong basket is closed with considerable force to shatter any stone trapped within the basket (Fig. 30–21). Beginning in 1983 I found that with the use of this type of device, failure to remove all stones occurred in 1.3% of those patients in whom EPT was successful (unpublished data) (Table 30–6). Nevertheless, a certain percentage of stones will remain unextractable by endoscopic methods because of large size or intrahepatic position (see Figs. 30–9 and 30–10) or because it is impossible to reach the papilla, as in some patients with periampullary diverticulum or who have had previous surgery such as a Billroth II resection.

Endoscopic papillotomy has not been performed long enough to permit follow-up for extended periods of time. In one report[83] 51 patients underwent follow-up evaluation including ERCP at a mean of 21.6 months after EPT. None had papillary stenosis, recurrent stones, or cholangitis, although massive bacterial colonization of the bile ducts with colony counts of 10^5 to 10^8 viable organisms per milliliter was present in nearly all cases. This report agrees with findings after surgical sphincterotomy in which duodenobiliary reflux was found to be common but without adverse consequences.[84] In one collective series ($n = 954$) recurrent stones were found in 6% of patients who had undergone EPT and stone extraction.[85] Normally such stones

are soft and can be extracted easily. The lithogenicity of bile is known to fluctuate according to a circadian pattern, and this is retained after EPT.[86] There is no increase in the degree to which bile is saturated with cholesterol after EPT.[87]

A dilated bile duct after EPT seems to predispose to recurrent stones; this has been described in patients who have undergone surgery.[88] Stenosis of the papilla of Vater occurred after EPT in 2.3% of patients.[85]

Another theoretical problem that remains unresolved is the potential for carcinoma of the colon as a result of changes in bile acid metabolism, such as occurs after cholecystectomy,[89, 90] with resultant accelerated turnover in the enterohepatic circulation of the bile acid pool and a consequent increase in secondary bile acids. It has been shown that after EPT in patients who have undergone cholecystectomy there is no further augmentation in the turnover of bile acids.[91] However, epidemiologic studies of this question are not available because EPT therapy is too recent.

Another problem after EPT and successful clearance of stones from the bile duct is the effect on the intact gallbladder. Follow-up of patients with intact gallbladders after EPT has disclosed that complications may occur that require further surgery.[83, 92] It is not known whether the incidence of gallbladder complications changes after EPT. Up to the present it has seemed rational to perform elective cholecystectomy in low-risk patients with gallbladder stones whose bile ducts have been cleared of stones by endoscopic techniques. However, if the cystic duct is patent after EPT, and the gallbladder is without stones, there may be no reason to perform cholecystectomy.[93]

When comparing the results of surgical and endoscopic treatment, it must be remembered that the endoscopically treated patients are older (mean age 68 years for all patients[91] and 79 years for those with suppurative cho-

TABLE 30–6. **Stone Extraction After EPT*: 1983**

EPT and stone extraction	197
Mechanical lithotripsy	23
Extraction unsuccessful	1
Extraction not attempted	2
Total No. Patients	223

*In patients in whom extraction was unsuccessful at initial EPT.

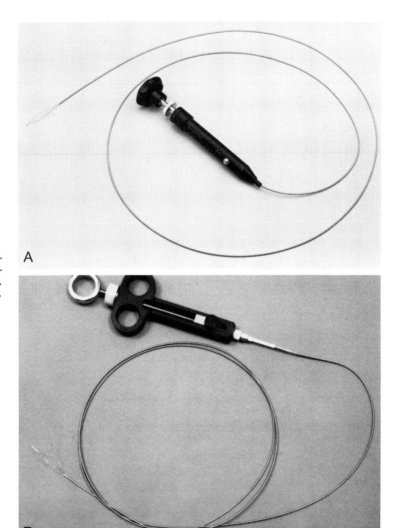

FIGURE 30–21. Two types of mechanical lithotriptor. A, Manufactured by American Endoscopy, Inc. B, Manufactured by Wilson-Cook, Inc.

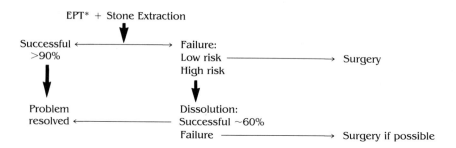

*EPT: Endoscopic papillotomy.

FIGURE 30–22. Suggested approach to treatment of cholodocholithiasis with history of previous cholocystectomy.

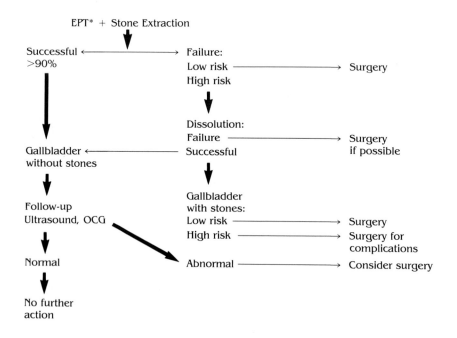

*EPT: Endoscopic papillotomy.

FIGURE 30–23. Suggested approach to treatment of cholodocholithiasis with no history of previous surgery.

TABLE 30–7. **Surgical vs. Endoscopic Treatment of Bile Duct Stones: Comparison of Mortality Rates**

Common Duct Stone—Gallbladder Resected		
Age	*Choledocholithotomy*	*EPT/Stone Extraction*
<60 years	~2%	~1.2%*
>60 years	~9%	~1.2%
Common Duct Stone—Gallbladder in Situ		
Age	*Choledocholithotomy plus Cholecystectomy*	*EPT/Stone Extraction plus Cholecystectomy*
<60 years	~2%	~1.5%*
>60 years	~9%	~2.5%
Acute Obstructive Suppurative Cholangitis		
Surgery		*Endoscopic Decompression plus Subsequent Stone Removal*
46%		23%
Gallstone-Induced Pancreatitis		
Surgery		*Endoscopy*
6%†		3%

*No exact data available; probably less.
†Substantial variation.

langitis; see Table 30–1), and that endoscopic series invariably include patients who are considered to be high operative risks. Potential long-term complications for older patients are less relevant. Conversely, potential complications that are related to the length of time elapsed after EPT may be a more significant factor for younger patients, and in this respect additional data on long-term complications are needed.

An overview of the mortality inherent in different approaches to treatment of bile duct stones in different clinical situations is given in Table 30–7. These estimates are based on a review of the literature and collected series rather than data with strict scientific validity.

The aim of surgical and endoscopic approaches to choledocholithiasis is the same: to cure as many patients as possible of bile stones with the lowest possible risk. Endoscopy is safer and the convalescent period after the procedure is minimal; however, not all stones can be removed and problems with the gallbladder cannot be resolved. Surgery has a higher risk and requires a prolonged recovery period, but bile duct problems and gallbladder disease can be treated by one operation. In some situations it is possible to combine the two methods to minimize risk. Indeed EPT can be used to remove remaining or recurrent stones or to relieve papillary stenosis following surgery, thereby shortening operative time. Conversely, surgery can

follow EPT in cases in which large stones are not extractable by endoscopy and when resection of the gallbladder is necessary for removal of stones. Suggested approaches to choledocholithiasis are outlined in Figures 30–22 and 30–23.

For the elderly or severely ill patient, endoscopic treatment of choledocholithiasis now is generally accepted as the treatment of choice without respect to presence or absence of the gallbladder. The issue of correct treatment for younger patients and for those clearly able to withstand surgery is more controversial: should the less traumatic, less hazardous, less invasive, and less expensive endoscopic method of therapy be withheld from younger patients because of a fear of long-term, as yet unknown, complications? In point of fact, many endoscopists offer EPT with stone extraction as the treatment of choice when bile duct stones are suspected in patients who have undergone cholecystectomy, regardless of age.

References

1. Cooperberg PL, Burhenne HJ. Real-time ultrasonography. Diagnostic technique of choice in a calculous gallbladder disease. N Engl J Med 1980; 302:1277–9.
2. Hessler PC, Hill DS, Deforie FM, Rocco AF. High accuracy sonographic recognition of gallstones. AJR 1981; 136:517–20.
3. Rettenmaier G. Sonografischer Oberbauchstatus. Aussagefähigkeit und Indikationen der Ultraschall-

Schnittbilduntersuchung des Oberbauchs. Internist 1976; 17:549–64.

4. Goodman MW, Ansel HJ, Vennes JA, et al. Is intravenous cholangiography still useful? Gastroenterology 1980; 79:642–5.

5. Osnes M, Grondseth K, Larsen S, et al. Comparison of endoscopic retrograde and intravenous cholangiography in diagnosis of biliary calculi. Lancet 1978; II:230.

6. Wurbs D, Classen M. Bedeutung der endoskopisch-retrograden Cholangio-Pankreatographie fur die Differenzierung der Cholestase. Dtsch med Wochenschr 1976; 101:291–3.

7. Bilbao MK, Dotter CT, Lee TG, Katon RM. Complications of endoscopic retrograde cholangiopancreatography (ERCP). Gastroenterology 1976; 70:314–20.

8. Harbin WP, Mueller PR, Ferrucci JT Jr. Transhepatic cholangiography: Complications and use patterns of the fine-needle technique. Radiology 1980; 135:15–22.

9. Kreek MJ, Balint JA. "Skinny Needle" cholangiography—results of a pilot study of a voluntary prospective method for gathering risk data on new procedures. Gastroenterology 1980; 78:598–604.

10. Nebel OT, Silvis SE, Rogers G, et al. Complications associated with endoscopic retrograde cholangiopancreatography: results of 1974 A.S.G.E. survey. Gastrointest Endosc 1975; 22:34–6.

11. Classen M, Wurbs D, Mairose UB. Duodenoskopie, retrograde Cholangio-Pankreatographie. In: Ottenjann R, Classen M, eds. Gastroenterologische Endoskopie, Lehrbuch und Atlas. Stuttgart: Enke, 1979.

12. Beneventano TC, Schein CJ. The pseudocalculous sign in cholangiography. Arch Surg 1969; 98:731–3.

13. Hoffman L, Weiss W, Classen M. Untersuchungen zum juxtapapillaren Duodenaldivertikel. Inn Med 1978; 5:22–6.

14. Lotveit T, Osnes M, Larsen S. Recurrent biliary calculi. Duodenal diverticula as a predisposing factor. Ann Surg 1982; 196:30–2.

15. van der Spuy S. The relationship between juxtapapillary diverticula and biliary calculi. An endoscopic study. Endoscopy 1979; 11:197–202.

16. Funch-Jensen P, Csendes A, Kruse A, Oster MJ. Common bile duct pressure and Oddi sphincter pressure in patients with common bile duct stones with and without juxta-ampullar diverticula of the duodenum. Scand J Gastroenterol 1979; 14:253–5.

17. Maki T. Pathogenesis of calcium bilirubinate gallstone: role of E. Coli, beta-glucoronidase and coagulation by inorganic ions, polyelectrolytes and agitation. Ann Surg 1966; 164:90–100.

18. Eggert A, Kirschner H, Teichmann W. Bakteriologische Befunde bei Patienten mit Cholelithiasis und Duodenaldivertikeln. Chirurg 1979; 50:441–4.

19. Lotveit T. The composition of biliary calculi in patients with juxtapapillary duodenal diverticula. Scand J Gastroenterol 1982; 17:653–6.

20. Tritapepe R, DiPadova C, Rovagnati P. Are pigmented gallstones caused by a "metabolic" liver defect? Br Med J 1980; 280:832.

21. Yamaguchi I, Sato T, Matsushiro T, Sato H. Quantitative determination of D-glucaric acid in bile in relation to inhibitory effect of bile on bacterial beta-glucuronidase. Tohoku J Exp Med 1965; 87:123–32.

22. Ikeda S, Okada Y. Classification of choledocho-

duodenal fistula diagnosed by duodenal fiberscopy and etiological significance. Gastroenterology 1975; 69:130–7.

23. Soehendra N. Endoskopische und radiologische Kontroll-untersuchungen nach transduodenaler Papillotomie. Langenbecks Arch Chir 1976; 341:39–49.

24. Urakami Y, Kishi S. Endoscopic fistulotomy (EFT) for parapapillary choledochoduodenal fistula. Endoscopy 1979; 10:289–94.

25. Glenn F. Postcholecystectomy choledocholithiasis. Surg Gynecol Obstet 1972; 134:249–52.

26. Berk JE, Kaplan AA. Choledocholithiasis. In: Bockus HS, ed. Gastroenterology. Vol. III. Philadelphia: W. B. Saunders, 1976; 843.

27. Girard RM, Legros G. Retained and recurrent bile duct stones. Surgical or nonsurgical removal? Ann Surg 1981; 193:150–4.

28. Way LW. Retained common duct stones. Surg Clin North Am 1973; 53:1139–47.

29. Acosta JM, Ledesma CL. Gallstone migration as a cause of acute pancreatitis. N Engl J Med 1974; 290:484–7.

30. Acosta JM, Rossi R, Galli OMR, et al. Early surgery for acute gallstone pancreatitis: evaluation of a systematic approach. Surgery 1978; 83:367–70.

31. Kelly TR. Gallstone pancreatitis: The timing of surgery. Surgery 1980; 88:345–50.

32. Tondelli P, Stutz K, Harder F, et al. Acute gallstone pancreatitis: best timing for biliary surgery. Br J Surg 1982; 69:709–10.

33. Kelly TR, Swaney PE. Gallstone pancreatitis: The second time around. Surgery 1982; 92:571–5.

34. Treske U, Schroeder U. Endoskopische Entfernung eines Konkrementes aus der Vaterschen Papille. In: Lindner H, ed. Fortschritte der gastroenterologischen Endoskopie Bd. 5. Baden-Baden, Koln, New York: Witzstrock, 1974; 117.

35. Classen M, Ossenberg FW, Wurbs D, et al. Pancreatitis—an indication for endoscopic papillotomy? Endoscopy 1978; 10:223.

36. Classen M, Ossenberg FW. Indications for endoscopic papillotomy. In: Classen M, et al., eds. The Papilla Vateri and Its Diseases. Baden-Baden, Koln, New York: Witzstrock 1979; 143.

37. Safrany L, Cotton PB. A preliminary report: Urgent duodenoscopic sphincterotomy for acute gallstone pancreatitis. Surgery 1981; 89:424–8.

38. Wurbs D. Gallensteinextraktion aus dem Ductus Wirsungianus. In: Henning H, ed. Fortschritte der gastroenterologischen Endoskopie Bd. 10. Baden-Baden, Koln, New York: Witzstrock, 1979; 182.

39. Koch H, Lux G. Results of endoscopic papillotomy. In: Demling L, ed. Endoscopic Papillotomy Now 10 Years Old. International Symposium, Heidelberg: Springer (in press 1985).

40. Scott AJ. Bacteria and disease of the biliary tract. Gut 1971; 12:487–92.

41. Gross E. Bakteriologische und histologische Untersuchungen an Leber und Gallenwegen vor und nach Eingriffen am Sphinkterapparat. Med Welt 1977; 28:1024–6.

42. Eggert A, Wittmann DH, Schroder HJ, Schimmel G. Die Bedeutung intraoperativer bakterieller Befunde bei Gallenblasen-und Gallenwegsoperationen. Munch med Wochenschr 1977; 119:955–8.

43. Keighley MRB, Wilson G, Kelly JP. Fatal endotoxic shock of biliary tract origin complicating transhepatic cholangiography. Br Med J 1973; 3:147–8.

44. Blumgart LH, Cotton PB, Burwood R, et al. Endos-

copy and retrograde choledochopancreatography in the diagnosis of the jaundiced patient. Lancet 1972; 2:1269–73.

45. Helm EB, Hagenmuller F, Stille W. Septikamie nach endoskopischen Eingriffen am Gallengangs-system. Munch med Wochenschr 1983; 125:210–2.

46. Huang T, Bass JA, Williams RD. The significance of biliary pressure in cholangitis. Arch Surg 1969; 98:629–32.

47. Jacobsson B, Kjellander J, Rosengren B. Cholangiovenous reflux. An experimental study. Acta Chir Scand 1962; 123:316–21.

48. Williams RD, Fish JC, Williams DD. The significance of biliary pressure. Arch Surg 1967; 95:374–9.

49. Jendrzejewski JW, McAnally T, Jones SR, Katon RM. Antibiotics and ERCP: In vitro activity of aminoglycosides when added to iodinated contrast agents. Gastroenterology 1980; 78:745–8.

50. Helm EB, Wurbs D, Gundlach H, et al. Keimelimination und Konzentrationsbestimmungen unter Mezlocillin in der Galle bei Gallenwegsinfektionen. Dtsch med Wochenschr 1981; 106:1087–90.

51. Helm EB, Wurbs D, Haag R, et al. Elimination of bacteria in biliary tract infections during ceftizoxime therapy. Infection 1982; 10:67–70.

52. Wurbs D, Fock R, Bulow B. Bacteria elimination from bile by cefotiam. In: Spitzy KH, Karrer K, eds. Proceedings of the 13th International Congress of Chemotherapy. Vienna: H. Egermann, 1983.

53. Williams R. The management of ascending cholangitis. I. Bacteriology and choice of antibiotic. Proc R Soc Med 1969; 62:243–4.

54. Classen M, Demling L. Endoskopische Sphinkterotomie der Papilla Vateri und Steinextraktion aus dem Ductus choledochus. Dtsch Med Wochenschr 1974; 99:496–7.

55. Wurbs D, Classen M. Transpapillary long-standing tube for hepatobiliary drainage. Endoscopy 1977; 9:192–3.

56. Wurbs D. Endoscopic papillotomy. Scand J Gastroenterol, Suppl 1982; 77:107–15.

57. Leuschner U, Wurbs D, Landgraf H. Dissolution of biliary duct stones with mono-octanoin. (Letter) Lancet 1979; 2:103–4.

58. Leuschner U, Wurbs D, Baumgartel H, et al. Alternating treatment of common bile duct stones with a modified glyceryl-1-monooctanoate preparation and a bile acid–EDTA solution by nasobiliary tube. Scand J Gastroenterol 1981; 16:497–503.

59. Rogers L. Biliary abscesses of the liver with operation. Br Med J 1903; 2:706.

60. Reynolds BM, Dargan EL. Acute obstructive cholangitis: a distinct clinical syndrome. Ann Surg 1959; 150:299–303.

61. Cremer M. Complications of endoscopic sphincterotomy. In: Classen M, et al., eds. The Papilla Vateri and Its Diseases. Baden-Baden, Koln, New York: Witzstrock, 1979; 134.

62. Glenn F, Moody FG. Acute obstructive suppurative cholangitis. Surg Gynecol Obstet 1961; 113:265–73.

63. Ostermiller W Jr, Thompson RJ Jr, Carter R, Hinshaw DB. Acute obstructive cholangitis. Arch Surg 1965; 90:392–5.

64. Wadell GF. Acute obstructive cholangitis. Scot Med J 1966; 11:137–42.

65. Haupert AP, Carey LC, Evans WE, Ellison HE. Acute suppurative cholangitis. Experience with 15 consecutive cases. Arch Surg 1967; 94:460–8.

66. Dow RW, Lindenauer SM. Acute obstructive suppurative cholangitis. Ann Surg 1969; 169:272–6.

67. Hinchey EJ, Couper CE. Acute obstructive suppurative cholangitis. Am J Surg 1969; 117:62–8.

68. Andrew DJ, Johnson SE. Acute suppurative cholangitis, a medical and surgical emergency. Am J Gastroenterol 1970; 54:141–54.

69. Welch JP, Donaldson GA. The urgency of diagnosis and surgical treatment of acute suppurative cholangitis. Am J Surg 1976; 131:527–32.

70. Ferrucci JT Jr, Mueller PR, Harbin WP. Percutaneous transhepatic biliary drainage. Technique, results, and applications. Radiology 1980; 135:1–13.

71. Nakayama T, Ikeda A, Okuda K. Percutaneous transhepatic drainage of the biliary tract. Gastroenterology 1978; 74:554–9.

72. Koch H, Stolte M, Walz V. Endoscopic lithotripsy in the common bile duct. Endoscopy 1977; 9:95–8.

73. Frimberger E, Weingart J, Kuhner W, Ottenjann R. Eingeklemmter Papillenstein: mechanische Lithotripsie moglich. Dtsch med Wochenschr 1983; 108:38.

74. Thistle JL, Carlson GL, Hofmann AF, et al. Monooctanoin, a dissolution agent for retained cholesterol bile duct stones: Physical properties and clinical application. Gastroenterology 1980; 78:1016–22.

75. American College of Surgeons, Ohio Chapter; 28,621 Cholecystectomies in Ohio. Results of a survey in Ohio Hospitals by the Gallbladder Survey Committee. Am J Surg 1970; 119:714–7.

76. Chigot JP. Le risque operatoire dans la lithiase biliare. A propos de 5433 interventions. Sem Hop Paris 1981; 57:1311–9.

77. Spohn K, Fux HD, Muller-Kluge M, et al. Gallenwegserkrankungen—Chirurgische Therapie und intraoperative Diagnostik. Therapiewoche 1975; 25:1033–47.

78. Hess W. Nachoperationen an den Gallenwegen. Stuttgart: Enke, 1977.

79. Way LW, Motson RW. Dissolution of retained common duct stones. Adv Surg 1976; 10:99–119.

80. Machado G. Acute complications of endoscopic papillotomy. In: Demling L, ed. Endoscopic papillotomy Now 10 Years Old. International Symposium, Heidelberg: Springer 1985 (in press).

81. Burhenne HJ. Complications of nonoperative extraction of retained common duct stones. Am J Surg 1976; 131:260–2.

82. Mazzariello RM. A fourteen-year experience with nonoperative instrument extraction of retained bile duct stones. World J Surg 1978; 2:447–55.

83. Burmeister W, Wurbs D, Hagenmuller F, Classen M. Langzeituntersuchungen nach endoskopischer Papillotomie (EPT). Z Gastroenterol 1980; 10:527–31.

84. Bohmig HJ, Zeidler G, Tuchmann A. Sphincterotomy for benign papillary stenosis. In: Classen M, et al., eds. The Papilla Vateri and Its Diseases. Baden-Baden, Koln, New York: Witzstrock 1979; 103.

85. Seifert E, Gail K, Weismuller J. Langzeitresultate nach endoskopischer Sphinkterotomie. Dtsch med Wochenschr 1982; 107:610–4.

86. Kurtz W, Leuschner U, Schneider S, et al. Diurnal rhythm of biliary lithogenicity persists after cholecystectomy and papillotomy. (Abstr) Gastroenterology 1982; 82:1107.

87. Sauerbruch T, Stellard F, Paumgartner G. Effect of endoscopic sphincterotomy on bile acid pool size and bile lipid composition in man. Digestion 1983; 27:87.

88. Nagase M, Setoyama M, Hikasa Y. Recurrent common duct stones, with special reference to primary common duct stones. Gastroenterol Jpn 1978; 13:290–6.

89. Linos DA, Beard CM, O'Fallon WM, et al. Cholecystectomy and carcinoma of the colon. Lancet 1981; 2:379–81.

90. Peters H, Keimes AM. Die Cholezystektomie als pradisponierender Faktor in der Genese des Kolorektalen Karzinoms? Dtsch Med Wochenschr 1979; 104:1581–3.

91. Stellaard F, Sauerbruch T, Brunholzl C, et al. Bile acid pattern and cholesterol saturation of bile after cholecystectomy and endoscopic sphincterotomy. Digestion 1983; 26:153–8.

92. Cotton PB, Vallon AG. Duodenoscopic sphincterotomy for removal of bile duct stones in patients with gallbladders. Surgery 1982; 91:628–30.

93. Gracie WA, Ransohoff DF. The natural history of silent gallstones. The innocent gallstone is not a myth. N Engl J Med 1982; 307:798–800.

Chapter 31

STENOSIS AND DILATION OF THE BILIARY AND PANCREATIC DUCTS

DAVID ZIMMON, M.D.

Dilation and stenosis are descriptive terms given to alterations of a duct system identified by visual, mechanical, or radiologic methods. There are assumed relationships between such findings and pathophysiologic changes as well as symptoms, although objective proof may be difficult to achieve. Relief of symptoms and normalization of biochemical parameters after intervention are considered indicative of diagnostic accuracy and therapeutic efficacy. However, placebo response, failed follow-up, and misjudgment must also be considered.

In addition to being descriptive, the terms dilation and stenosis are also relative. A segment of a duct is stenotic only in relation to another ductal segment that is considered to be normal. Ductal dimensions can be compared with a statistical norm, but objective standards are based on inexact techniques of measurement. Furthermore, there may be many variations from the norm according to sex, age, body habitus, and a variety of other factors. Although the relative meaning of these terms is unimportant when dilation and/or stenosis is extreme, it may be difficult or impossible to distinguish normal from abnormal with minor changes in ductal caliber.

Alterations in the radiographic features of the pancreatic duct associated with aging and those of chronic pancreatitis provide an example of the difficulties in differentiating abnormal from normal ductal dimensions.[1] The main pancreatic duct diameter increases and cystic changes occur in the main duct branches with advancing age, changes that are also indicative of chronic pancreatitis in young individuals.[2] As with all organs, pancreatic function (secretion) diminishes with age. The decision to consider changes such as these either pathologic or physiologic may be problematic.

The pancreatographic pattern of chronic pancreatitis includes segments of ductal dilation alternating with stenoses. Here also it is difficult to know the pathophysiologic sequence of events. This radiographic appearance could derive from episodes of obstruction that result in focal dilation in which narrowed sections may actually be segments that are simply less dilated because of periductal fibrosis. The contrary, generally accepted explanation is that dilation follows atrophy and fibrosis of the pancreas rather than obstruction,[3] but proof is lacking. Therefore, various methods of decompression, both surgical and endoscopic, are offered by those who consider obstruction the primary pathogenetic mechanism, resulting in remarkable but short-term clinical success in a few highly selected patients.[4]

Similar problems may be encountered with biliary tract disease. There is great variation in normal bile duct diameter.[5] Except in its distal sphincteric segment, the bile duct wall has essentially no muscular component. Once widened, the duct usually remains so. In sclerosing cholangitis, the extreme example of biliary stenosis, focal stenosis of a remarkable degree and extent may occur in the intrahepatic and extrahepatic biliary tree with relatively little or no apparent functional abnormality. It becomes difficult to define radiographically those areas of intrahepatic and/or extrahepatic stenosis or dilation that

673

may be contributing to the limitation of bile flow and/or the persistence of infection.

This discussion illustrates the problems encountered in compiling useful and valid information in a field in which currently available publications are few, often anecdotal, and enthusiastic and consist of reports on highly selected patients with limited follow-up. Despite these difficulties, endoscopic approaches to the biliary tract and pancreatic duct offer opportunities for diagnosis and therapy of various disorders that produce pancreatic or biliary dilation and/or stenosis.

ENDOSCOPIC METHODS OF BILIARY AND PANCREATIC DECOMPRESSION

Techniques

The basic technique of endoscopic biliary and pancreatic drainage is relatively simple. A wire guide, inserted through the accessory channel of the duodenoscope, is advanced through the orifice of the duodenal papilla or sphincterotomy opening and inserted through the stricture using fluoroscopic guidance. The stent* is then pushed along the wire guide by means of a tube of the same diameter until the distal and proximal ends of the prosthesis are positioned above and below the stricture, respectively. The tube used to push the stent into position should be a color different from the stent so that the abutment of the stent and pushing tube can be distinguished endoscopically. Once the stent is in position the wire guide is withdrawn, causing the pushing tube to disengage from the stent and leaving the latter in place.

This technique is satisfactory for placement of stents up to 7-French† diameter. Insertion of larger diameter stents requires additional maneuvers. The inner diameter of a 10-French or greater diameter stent is large relative to the diameter of the wire guide. Since the stent does not fit snugly over the wire, it cannot be pushed into position with a simple pushing tube, as this will cause the stent to bend and buckle. Therefore, an inner catheter is first passed over the wire guide and through the stricture. The large-diameter stent, which fits snugly over the inner catheter, is then advanced into position over

---

*The term endoprosthesis is used by some authors in preference to "stent."

†1-French is approximately 0.33 mm.

the combination wire–inner catheter guide system using a pushing tube (Plate 31–1).

One of the basic principles of endoscopic stent insertion is to keep the end of the duodenoscope close to the orifice of the duodenal papilla or sphincterotomy opening. If this is not done, the wire guide, sometimes along with the pushing tube and stent, may loop into the duodenal lumen, which may retract the wire guide from the duct. The stent cannot be withdrawn along the wire guide, and once it has been advanced beyond the end of the duodenoscope and into the duodenal lumen, it cannot be retracted into the duodenoscope even if it remains on the wire guide.

The technique of nasobiliary drainage is almost the same as stent insertion, except that a single long catheter is left in the duct. The nasobiliary drainage tube is also advanced along the previously positioned wire guide. Once the distal end of the drainage tube is positioned in the duct, the endoscope is withdrawn while the drainage tube is slowly advanced through the instrument channel so that the length of insertion tube withdrawn is matched by advancement of an approximately equal length of the nasobiliary tube. With careful fluoroscopic monitoring the endoscope can be removed completely, leaving the nasobiliary tube in place. The tube is then rerouted through the posterior pharynx and out one of the patient's nostrils with the aid of a second somewhat larger tube that is passed via the nostril and brought out through the patient's mouth.

Stents

There are some basic, largely unresolved problems with regard to the shape and size of stents as well as the type of material used to make the stent. Some endoscopists prefer to use relatively large-diameter stents (10-French and greater) (Fig. 31–1). This is done to obviate clogging or at least postpone the onset of occlusion. There are two basic shapes: the straight or slightly curved stent that usually has two side flaps to anchor it in place and the pigtail stent (either single or double) (Fig. 31–2). There are no comparison trials to indicate which, if any, of these devices is superior in any respect. Another approach to increasing overall stent diameter is to insert a bundle of stents of smaller diameter. It would seem that some of these issues could be resolved by controlled com-

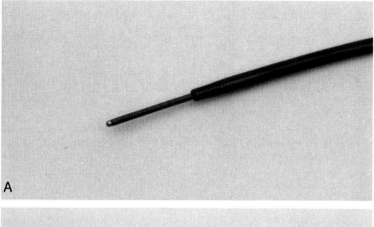

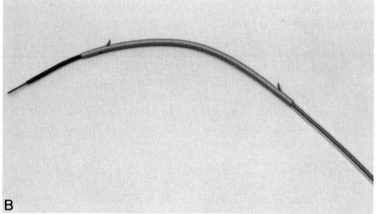

PLATE 31–1. *A,* Wire guide (green) and inner catheter (brown) used for insertion of 10-French stent (Wilson-Cook Medical). Note the tapered tip of the inner catheter. *B,* 10-French stent (blue) with pushing tube placed over wire guide and inner catheter.

parison trials. However, great differences from patient to patient with regard to anatomy, pathology, rate of disease progression, presence or absence of a gallbladder, and many other factors make such comparisons difficult.

Although a single 5-French stent with a 1-mm lumen will accommodate total bile flow, we prefer to place at least two 5-French stents, since one may become occluded. The space between two stents serves also as an additional pathway for bile flow. Currently, the use of a large diameter single stent (8- to 10-French) has no advantage compared with placement of a group of smaller stents. The lumen of two 5-French stents is equivalent to the lumen of a single 9-French tube; three 5-French stents are equivalent to a single 12-French tube. Experience has shown that 8.3-French percutaneous stents with a lumen diameter of 2 mm usually function 3 to 5 months and that this functional longevity is not increased by increases in stent diameter. Our experience with cancer palliation suggests that erosion with bleeding is a common

cause of stent obstruction. This is not obviated by a stent with a larger lumen and must be managed by frequently changing stents as the disease progresses. In this circumstance, extraluminal bile flow may be more satisfactory with a cluster of 5-French stents than with a single large-lumen stent.

Stents of 5-French diameter easily deform to fit irregular or angled stenoses. We have not observed proximal or distal bile duct or duodenal erosions when several such stents are used together. For removal, a cluster of stents can be grasped with a snare-loop or basket and withdrawn en masse. However, this may be more difficult if the stricture is extremely tight, in which case the stents can be removed and replaced one by one. The use of multiple 5-French stents has a further advantage in that a special endoscope with a large operating channel is not required. The standard duodenoscope with its smaller accessory channel is generally easier to manipulate than the larger channel special duodenoscopes needed for insertion of a large-diameter stent, and this can be used to

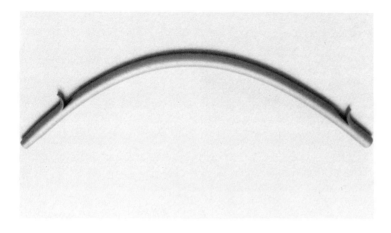

FIGURE 31–1. 10-French stent slightly curved with anchoring side flaps (Wilson-Look, Inc).

advantage when the duodenal lumen is narrowed and deformed by a malignant process, particularly carcinoma of the pancreas.

BILE DUCT DILATION

Bile duct dilation is common and often unassociated with disease. Unfortunately, absolute criteria for bile duct diameter are lacking, although by consensus a diameter greater than 10 to 11 mm is usually abnormal.[6] However, bile ducts of this diameter are often present in asymptomatic patients with no evidence of biliary dysfunction. Bile duct diameter is influenced by many factors, including duct wall compliance, bile flow, sphincter function, the availability of a gallbladder or fistula as an alternative runoff, and technique of measurement. Bile duct dilation in the absence of symptoms is most commonly found in patients who have had a cholecystectomy. Hepatic cirrhosis is also commonly associated with a dilated bile duct and gallbladder.

Hamilton et al.[7] measured the diameter of the extrahepatic and intrahepatic bile ducts on retrograde cholangiograms from 50 normal patients and 109 post-cholecystectomy patients. There was no evidence of obstruction on 70 of the post-cholecystectomy cholangiograms, although evidence of obstruction, either a stone or a stricture, was found in the other 39. Compared with measurements of bile ducts on cholangiograms of normal patients, bile duct diameter was greater at all points on post-cholecystectomy cholangiograms. Diameters were even greater on the cholangiograms that also had evidence of an obstructing lesion. However, the overlap in the dimensions for the three groups was so marked that measurement alone could not be used to assign patients to groups with and without obstruction.

A confounding problem, especially in symptomatic patients with post-cholecystectomy dilation of the extrahepatic bile ducts, is the limitations of radiologic techniques in identifying stones within the duct. Direct cholangiography is the favored method; we prefer endoscopic retrograde cholangiopan-

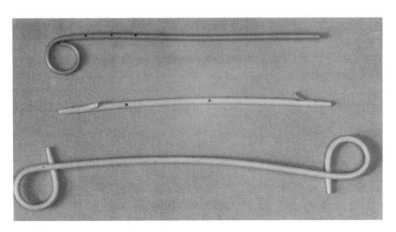

FIGURE 31–2. Three basic stent designs: 5-French, single pigtail (*top*), 5-French straight (*middle*) (American Endoscopy, Inc), 5-French double pigtail (*bottom*) (American Endoscopy, Inc).

creatography (ERCP) to percutaneous transhepatic cholangiography (PTC) because of greater safety of the former technique. Even with direct cholangiography problems abound, including false-negative examinations because of the inability to detect small (3 to 4 mm) stones in a dilated duct.

The nature of the disease process itself may foil radiologic diagnosis. Recurrent calculi from the gallbladder, cystic duct stump, or left hepatic duct may cause symptoms during distal impaction and later passage and yet leave no residual evidence of their presence. In gallstone pancreatitis ERCP may identify a common channel, and a normal study renders other causes of pancreatitis less likely, but the offending stone often has passed. Diagnosis of dysfunction of the duodenal papilla with intermittent biliary obstruction is also difficult.

CYSTIC DISORDERS OF THE BILE DUCTS

In 1959 Alonso-Lej et al.[8] classified cystic disorders of the biliary system into three types. Type I cysts, the most common, are dilations of the extrahepatic biliary system, usually the common duct (Fig. 31–3). The Type II lesion is a diverticulum of the common bile duct and is extremely rare. A Type III cyst is a dilation of the segment of the common duct within the muscular portion of the duodenal wall and is also termed a cho-

ledochocele. A Type III cyst often bulges, sometimes intermittently, into the duodenal lumen as a round smooth defect associated with the papilla of Vater (Plate 31–2). Several investigators classify Caroli's disease, a variant of intrahepatic and extrahepatic biliary cystic dilation, as a Type IV lesion.[9–11] Solitary hepatic cysts have also been reported in a few patients and have been classified as Type V.[12] Other more elaborate classifications of cystic disorders of the biliary system have been proposed that reflect the numerous variations of the appended basic classification of Alonso-Lej.[13]

Choledochal Cyst

A choledochal cyst is an uncommon biliary tract malformation thought to be congenital in origin. It is more common in Orientals and women.[12, 14] The incidence in Caucasians is estimated at less than 1 in 200,000.[15]

Although this defect most commonly produces symptoms in the young, over 20% of patients are older than 40 years of age.[16] The clinical features of choledochal cyst include abdominal pain, right upper quadrant mass, and jaundice. However, this classic clinical triad is found in only about 40% of patients.[16] Even in patients with typical findings, choledochal cyst is seldom considered unless there is a high index of suspicion. Although it is more likely to be suspected in Oriental pa-

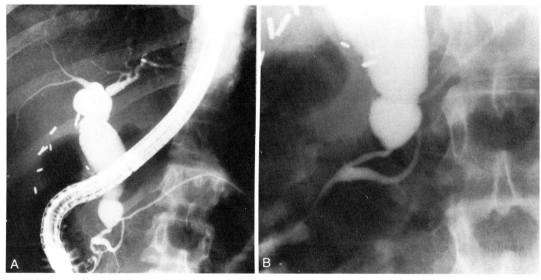

FIGURE 31–3. *A,* Type I biliary cyst (choledochal cyst). *B,* Close view of anomalous junction of bile and pancreatic ducts. Note long common channel. (From: Thatcher BS, Sivak MV, Hermann RE, Esselstyn CB: ERCP in evaluation and diagnosis of choledochal cysts: report of five cases. Gastrointest Endosc 1986; 32:27–31, with permission.)

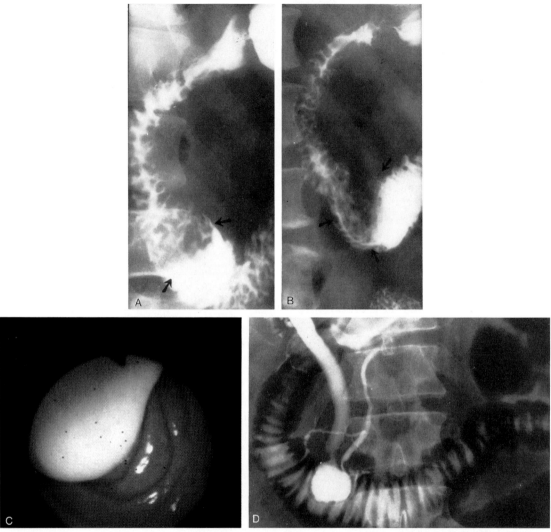

PLATE 31–2. *A* and *B,* Upper gastrointestinal x-ray films showing smooth, round filling defect *(arrows)* in descending duodenum that changes shape with motion of the duodenum. *C,* Endoscopic view showing smooth, round defect in the region of the duodenal papilla. *D,* Pancreatocholangiogram made by retrograde injection after cannulation of a pinpoint opening on the surface of the lesion showing Type III biliary cyst (choledochocele). (Photographs courtesy M.V. Sivak, Jr., M.D.)

tients, in a recent report all but 1 of 5 patients were Caucasians.[17]

The intrahepatic bile ducts may or may not be dilated in association with a choledochal cyst. Associated intrahepatic duct dilation was estimated by Todani et al.[18] to be present in approximately 30% of cases. However, there is considerable variation, with the reported incidence ranging from about 3% to 66% of cases.[16, 19] This may reflect differences in patient populations. Associated intrahepatic ductal dilation is uncommon in pediatric patients in the United States, and Todani et al.[18] have pointed out that intra-

hepatic ductal dilation is unusual before the age of 10 years.

The pathogenesis of choledochal cyst is uncertain. Babbitt[20] suggested an anomalous connection between the pancreatic and biliary ductal systems as the primary factor (Fig. 31–3). The essential feature of this anomaly is that the bile duct joins the pancreatic duct at some distance from the ampulla so that a long common channel conducts bile and pancreatic secretions to the duodenum. When the length of the common channel external to the duodenal wall is greater than 0.6 cm, this variant is said to be present.[21] This finding, plus the absence of a functional distal bile duct sphincter, is thought to promote reflux of pancreatic juice into the bile ducts with resultant inflammation and stricturing of the bile duct at the pancreaticobiliary ductal junction. It is suggested that high-grade stenosis results in cystic dilation of the extrahepatic bile ducts and that low-grade stenosis leads to cylindrical dilation.[14] In two reports by different groups of Japanese investigators, a total of 53 of 61 patients had this anomalous connection.[14, 21] All 5 patients in the report of Thatcher et al.[17] had this finding. Although the ductal segment between the pancreaticobiliary junction and the duodenum is referred to as a common channel, the exact anatomic nature of this segment is uncertain. Loss of the septum between the bile and pancreatic ducts as they approach the duodenal papilla results in the ordinary variety of pancreaticobiliary common channel. This segment may be relatively long in normal individuals, in which case retrograde injection of contrast medium via the papilla may produce simultaneous opacification of both ductal systems. However, in patients with choledochal cyst, the common ductal segment is inordinately long, and it is thought that this segment is actually a portion of the main pancreatic duct

Miyano et al.[22] performed an end-to-side biliary-pancreatic ductal anastomosis in 40 dogs as an experimental animal model of this anomalous union of the bile and pancreatic ducts. During follow-up for as long as 1 year, fusiform dilation of the bile duct occurred in all animals and was maximum at 1 week after surgery. Reflux of pancreatic juice into the biliary system was demonstrated in every animal, although stricturing of the anastomosis appeared to be a more important factor in the development of biliary dilation. The only significant morphologic change in the wall of the bile duct was epithelial hyperplasia. Chronic pancreatitis developed in one dog at 16 months after operation.

The anomalous connection between the bile duct and pancreatic duct appears to be unusual in other disorders of the bile ducts. Muller et al.[23] reviewed the cholangiographic anatomy of the choledochopancreatic ductal junction in 20 patients with primary sclerosing cholangitis. An abnormally long (> 15 mm) common channel was present in 2 cases (10%).

Abnormalities of the pancreatic duct have also been reported in patients with this anom-

alous pancreaticobiliary junction. In one series of 9 patients, pancreatography in 6 cases demonstrated an abnormal duct in 5, with marked dilation of the main pancreatic duct upstream from the anomalous connection being the most common finding.[24]

With the widespread use of biliary imaging techniques, the number of reported cases of this anomaly is increasing, and more than 80% of these are being diagnosed preoperatively.[25] Although ultrasonography, computed tomography (CT), and radionuclide scanning are advocated as useful in diagnosis,[26–31] these tests do not delineate anatomic relationships or the anomalous junction. In a few cases, PTC has been of value.[21, 32] However, ERCP is the procedure of choice for diagnosis.[14, 15, 17, 21] In addition to delineating anatomic features, ERCP will also demonstrate the presence of cystolithiasis and assist in operative planning.

The complications of choledochal cyst include intracystic formation of calculi, biliary obstruction, carcinoma, and perforation. The last of these is a rare complication usually associated with trauma.

The incidence of bile duct carcinoma is increased in association with choledochal cyst and is estimated at 2% to 5% versus 0.012% to 0.40% for the general population.[33] Flanigan[34] found adenocarcinoma to be the most common type and the posterior cyst wall to be the most frequent site. Approximately one-third of patients with cystolithiasis had biliary carcinoma. Kimura et al.[35] found an association between the anomalous pancreaticobiliary ductal union and gallbladder carcinoma. Carcinoma in association with choledochal cyst has an early age of onset. Even after excision of the cyst, cancer has been reported as developing within the intrahepatic ducts or at the anastomotic site.[36, 37]

There is no effective medical therapy for choledochal cyst.[11, 38] Cyst rupture with secondary peritonitis, cholangitis, and hepatic cirrhosis with secondary complications are common causes of death. The anomalous junction of the biliary and pancreatic ductal systems has certain technical implications with regard to endoscopic management. These probably contraindicate endoscopic sphincterotomy and prohibit endoscopic access to the biliary system for stone extraction in virtually all cases. Surgery is the recommended therapy, although the best operative approach is debated.[21] The two primary options are cyst excision with a drainage procedure or internal drainage alone, although excision of the Type I cyst is currently recommended if technically feasible.[25, 39]

Biliary Diverticulum

Biliary diverticulum is the least common of the cystic disorders of the bile duct. Farkas et al.[40] found only 24 cases in a review of the literature and reported 2 additional cases. The age range of patients is wide. The lesions are usually solitary but can be multiple. Most often they occur in the distal portion of the bile duct. An intrahepatic biliary diverticulum is extremely rare. Generally the lesion is small and discovered incidentally. However, patients may complain of right upper quadrant pain and tenderness, and jaundice and a palpable mass may occur. Occasionally a biliary diverticulum may harbor stones.

Choledochocele

Choledochocele is an unusual disorder that is the subject of sporadic case reports. It occurs equally in men and women; the age range is wide, with the mean occurring in the fourth decade.

The majority of patients have symptoms, chiefly epigastric pain, nausea, and vomiting. Some authors believe that choledochocele predisposes to the formation of stones, even though calculi were not present in the majority of cases reported. Scholz et al.[41] found 5 patients with choledocholithiasis or stones within the cyst itself in a review of 16 cases. A sixth patient had cholecystolithiasis. These authors suggested that the prevalence of stone disease among the cases reviewed indicated a predisposition for stone formation. Pancreatitis is reported to occur in association with choledochocele.[42-45] Calculi were found within the choledochocele in the case of pancreatitis reported by Jensen.[42] Reflux of contrast medium from the choledochocele into the pancreatic duct was noted in the case reported by Goldberg et al.[45] Choledochocele may cause obstructive jaundice.[46] Carcinoma arising within the cyst has also been reported.[47]

Several anatomic variations of choledochocele have been described.[48] In one type the pancreatic and bile ducts empty into a cystic cavity that communicates via a small pinpoint opening with the duodenum. In a second type the bile duct enters the duodenum in a relatively normal fashion, except that there is an intraduodenal sac-like herniation of the duct a few millimeters prior to its termination.

Several theories of pathogenesis have been proposed. Choledochocele may result from an inflammatory obstruction in the region of the ampulla. Another theory proposes a congenital duodenal duplication at the ampulla. Another possibility is that choledochocele is actually a congenital diverticulum of the common bile duct. Herniation of the bile duct in the region between the sphincter of Oddi and the choledochal sphincter has also been suggested as being due to an asynchronous or spastic contraction pattern in these sphincters.

Differential diagnosis includes duodenal duplication cyst, intraluminal duodenal diverticulum,[49] and a variety of benign and malignant tumors of the duodenal papilla. Although CT findings are said to be characteristic,[50, 51] the best method to determine the nature of the lesion is duodenoscopy with ERCP.

Choledochocele can be treated by endoscopic sphincterotomy. This must be guided by careful study of pancreatic and biliary ductal anatomy prior to making the incision. Drainage of a choledochocele by endoscopic sphincterotomy has been accomplished in a small number of patients.[52-54] Further evaluation of this approach is required.

Caroli's Disease

Focal cystic dilation of the intrahepatic bile ducts, also known as Caroli's disease, is probably an inherited disorder. It occurs most often in childhood, but may appear during early adult life. There are several forms, and the disorder may occur in association with hepatic fibrosis. The dilated, cystic segments of the biliary tree may contain debris, stones, and purulent material. The most frequent symptom is recurrent episodes of fever, with pain and jaundice being less common. There appears to be an increased incidence of cholangiocarcinoma in association with Caroli's disease.[33, 55]

A variety of methods, including ultrasonography, CT, and ERCP, are available for diagnosis.[56-58] Since bacterial cholangitis is a recognized complication of Caroli's disease, invasive procedures such as ERCP should be performed cautiously and probably with antibiotic prophylaxis.

ENDOSCOPIC DECOMPRESSION AS A THERAPEUTIC TRIAL

Despite the problems inherent in the diagnosis of symptomatic stenosis and/or dilation of the biliary or pancreatic ducts, the demonstration of these findings usually raises the issue of mechanical decompression. In the past, enthusiasm for this was limited by the pain, expense, morbidity, and mortality associated with transabdominal surgery, especially when an examination of the duodenal papilla, as well as the biliary and pancreatic sphincters, was necessary.[59]

When the indications for surgical or endoscopic therapy for symptoms related to stenosis with or without dilation of a ductal system are not clearly defined, a trial of temporary duct decompression by endoscopic insertion of a nasobiliary or nasopancreatic drain or a biliary or pancreatic duct stent may give some indication of the result to expect with a more permanent drainage procedure, either surgical or endoscopic.

A 5-French stent (outer diameter 1.6 mm) may be placed in either the biliary or the pancreatic duct without prior endoscopic sphincterotomy in most patients. Ductal systems of minute diameter sometimes found in normal persons (more often in women) may, however, present a problem. Such a finding is not abnormal nor necessarily a cause of symptoms, but insertion of a 5-French nasobiliary drain or stent into a duct of very small diameter could conceivably cause pancreatitis or inflammatory stenosis. Pain occasionally follows introduction of a 5-French stent or drain. When a nasobiliary or nasopancreatic drain is inserted, there is the option of immediate removal without the necessity of a second endoscopic procedure. If a drain with a duodenal side hole (0.025 inch) is used, decompression without external drainage is achieved. A nasobiliary drain without a duodenal side hole assures decompression by means of external (gravity) drainage and provides a means of injecting contrast medium. In some cases, this may reproduce a patient's pain.

If a stent is used for temporary decompression, its position can be determined at intervals with serial abdominal films. In some patients with pain presumed to be of pancreatic origin, a short 5-French stent without a pigtail can be placed in the pancreatic duct. This will usually fall out of the duct in a few days. If pain recurs after the stent has left the duct, the presumption of pain arising from pancreatic duct obstruction is confirmed and appropriate long-term decompression can be performed.

Although a trial of mechanical decompression may be helpful in deciding the efficacy of a more permanent drainage procedure, frequently neither relief of symptoms nor recurrence of pain after the stent has left the duct is clear-cut. There may be no change in biochemical parameters of obstruction such as a decrease in serum alkaline phosphatase or amylase levels, and it becomes difficult to judge the efficacy of the therapeutic trial of stent placement (Fig. 31–4).

STENOSIS OF THE DUODENAL PAPILLA

Stenosis of the anatomically and physiologically complex duodenal papilla is an insidious process usually associated with inflammatory biliary or pancreatic disease. When there is no obvious evidence of an associated disorder of the bile duct or pancreas, and in all older patients, neoplasia must be excluded by adequate and sometimes repeated biopsy. Endoscopic stent placement or balloon dilation is precluded by the necessity of eliminating neoplasia as the cause of stenosis of the duodenal papilla. With inflammatory stenosis of the biliary sphincter, adequate drainage of the dilated proximal biliary tree requires endoscopic sphincterotomy to obliterate the pressure gradient between the bile duct and the duodenum.

Dysfunction of the duodenal papilla with absent or minimal evidence of pathologic changes in the papilla itself may also be a cause of biliary and/or pancreatic duct obstruction. Sometimes termed biliary dyskinesia, this syndrome is poorly defined and difficult to diagnose. This disorder is discussed further in Chapter 33.

TECHNIQUE OF PROXIMAL BILIARY DRAINAGE

Not too many years ago PTC and percutaneous transhepatic biliary drainage were procedures of choice in biliary obstruction because of the limited ability to inject contrast medium proximal to an obstruction via an endoscopic approach. However, the techniques of deep bile duct cannulation or balloon cholangiography can usually be used to force contrast medium through obstructed segments. Balloon cholangiography requires insertion of a balloon catheter of the type

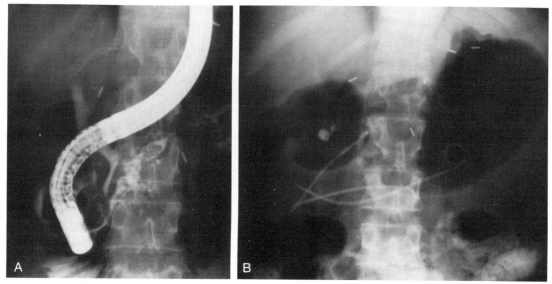

FIGURE 31–4. A, Retrograde pancreatocholangiogram demonstrating distorted, encased distal common bile duct and irregularly dilated pancreatic duct with numerous filling defects in a patient with chronic alcoholic pancreatitis and pain and fever after distal pancreaticojejunostomy. The lateral pancreaticojejunostomy is stenosed, although contrast medium enters the jejunum during high pressure injection after passing the catheter through the distal area of stenosis. B, Both ducts drained after placement of a short 5-French pigtail pancreatic duct stent. Two stents that could not be placed successfully are in the transverse part of the duodenum and will pass per rectum. There was resolution of pain and fever following pancreatic duct stent placement that confirmed the radiologic impression of pancreaticojejunostomy stenosis and obstruction of the pancreatic duct near the duodenum.

used to extract stones into the bile duct distal to the stricture, inflation of the balloon within the duct, and injection of contrast medium. When these methods fail a soft tip wire guide inserted through a catheter or nasobiliary drain that has been used to cannulate the distal bile duct can often be passed through the stenosis. The cannulating catheter or a nasobiliary drain with a tapered tip is then forced through the stenosis. The wire guide is withdrawn, and after a sample of bile is obtained for culture, contrast medium is injected to visualize the proximal ducts. Gravity drainage via the nasobiliary tube is then begun. This is often an appropriate point to interrupt the sequence of steps in endoscopic management since the endoscopist and patient will be fatigued, abdominal distention with stimulation of peristalsis due to air insufflation may be developing, and prolonged sedation as well as increasing doses of antiperistaltic drugs may be necessary in order to proceed.

Delayed lateral and supine films or fractional contrast medium injection via the nasobiliary tube with delayed films after drainage may be necessary to visualize important anatomic details not appreciated on films obtained during the endoscopic phase of the procedure.

When drainage is adequate, bile volumes of 600 to 800 ml per day can be anticipated, and a decline in serum bilirubin levels should be demonstrable within 48 hours. Clinical improvement in the patient's condition and sense of well-being should also occur within this space of time. Upon demonstration of a salutary response to nasobiliary drainage, stents may be placed endoscopically. If cholestasis does not continue to resolve after stent placement, the problem is probably mechanical if the response to nasobiliary drainage was satisfactory.

When it is difficult to separate obstructive cholestasis from liver failure as causes of jaundice, a poor response to nasobiliary drainage obviates endoscopic stent placement since hepatic failure, whether due to cirrhosis or to parenchymal replacement by metastases, is a primary component of the jaundice. It is important to identify such patients immediately by a trial of nasobiliary drainage since life expectancy will be short and further efforts at biliary decompression will be costly, lack benefit, and may monopolize valuable time remaining to the patient.

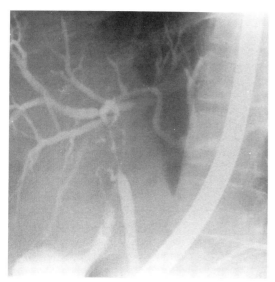

FIGURE 31–5. Retrograde cholangiogram showing long, narrow stricture of common hepatic duct that proved to be a carcinoma. Note the absence of intrahepatic duct dilation. The patient was not jaundiced at the time of this study. (Courtesy of M. V. Sivak, Jr., M.D.)

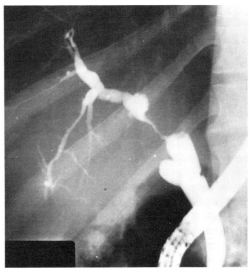

FIGURE 31–7. Retrograde cholangiogram of carcinoma at the bifurcation of the bile duct. The left hepatic duct is completely obstructed. There is a long, narrow stricture of the right hepatic duct with right intrahepatic duct dilation. (Courtesy of M. V. Sivak, Jr., M.D.)

NEOPLASTIC BILE DUCT OBSTRUCTION

Diagnosis

Nichols et al.[60] reviewed the cholangiographic findings in 82 patients with biopsy proven bile duct carcinoma. The most common morphologic type (75.6%) was a focal stenosis of the duct (Figs. 31–5 to 31–7). This

may completely obstruct the retrograde flow of contrast medium during ERCP and produce a cholangiographic picture of complete ductal obstruction (Figs. 31–8 and 31–9). Polypoid and diffuse sclerosing types were less common and occurred with about equal frequency (Fig. 31–10). The prognosis was best with the polypoid type and worst with the diffuse sclerosing variety. Survival was

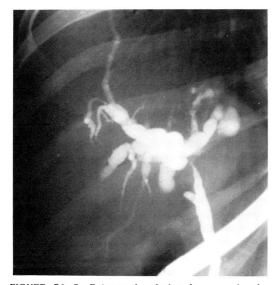

FIGURE 31–6. Retrograde cholangiogram showing carcinomatous stricture at the bifurcation of the bile duct with intrahepatic duct dilation. (Courtesy of M. V. Sivak, Jr., M.D.)

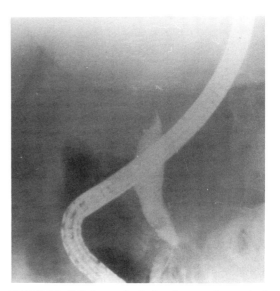

FIGURE 31–8. Retrograde cholangiogram demonstrating tapering complete obstruction of the bile duct due to carcinoma and a calculus in the distal common bile duct. (Courtesy of M. V. Sivak, Jr., M.D.)

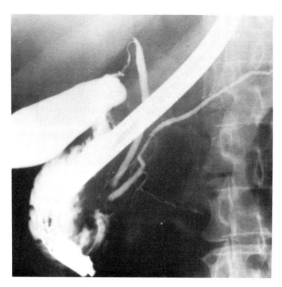

FIGURE 31–9. Complete obstruction of the common hepatic duct due to cholangiocarcinoma demonstrated by retrograde pancreatocholangiography. (Courtesy of M. V. Sivak, Jr., M.D.)

longer and surgical cure more likely when the tumor was limited to the distal extrahepatic bile duct. However, the neoplasm involved the intrahepatic or proximal extrahepatic ducts in 84% of cases. Operative resection was difficult or impossible for tumors in this location.

Cytologic methods have been employed to increase the accuracy of endoscopic diagnosis of both pancreatic and bile duct carcinoma. With bile duct carcinoma, however, the number of positive cytologic specimens obtained has usually been small. Roberts-Thomson and Hobbs[61] obtained cytologic specimens by duct aspiration in 17 patients with pancreatic carcinoma and 10 patients with bile duct cancer. Although a positive specimen was obtained in 60% of the pancreatic lesions, only 20% of the bile duct specimens were positive for carcinoma.

Primary extranodal non-Hodgkin's lymphoma is reported as arising in the bile duct in association with a clinical picture that initially resembled primary sclerosing cholangitis.[62] However, this is a rare occurrence, and in most cases biliary obstruction caused by lymphoma is due to compression of the bile ducts by enlarged lymph nodes in the porta hepatis.[63] Many other malignant neoplasms may metastasize to the porta hepatis and produce bile duct compression and obstruction (Figs. 31–11 to 31–13).

Neoplastic obstruction of the distal bile duct commonly arises from pancreatic adenocarcinoma that may be identified by scanning techniques or endoscopic retrograde pancreatography. The operative salvage of diagnosed pancreatic cancer is nil, and in most cases only palliation can be considered.[64] Pancreatic cancer is discussed in Chapter 39. Surgery is a consideration with other periampullary neoplasms because the high operative mortality (20%) and morbidity are balanced by a 30% 5-year survival for patients in whom resection is performed for cure.[65]

The first issue is to determine if any therapy (endoscopic, percutaneous, or operative) can benefit the individual patient with bile duct cancer. More than 30% of these patients die within 30 days of diagnosis with or without successful relief of bile duct obstruction and jaundice.[66] Prompt determination that no treatment will be effective in the deeply jaundiced, often aged patient is invaluable and avoids fruitless and expensive therapeutic maneuvers in cases in which death is imminent. Frequently, such a determination can be made without harm to the patient by temporary nasobiliary drainage (Fig. 31–14).

Endoscopic Therapy

The approach to bile duct obstruction is determined by the site of obstruction and the clinical manifestations.

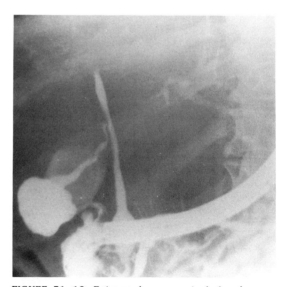

FIGURE 31–10. Retrograde pancreatocholangiogram demonstrating diffuse narrowing of the common bile duct, cystic duct, and common hepatic duct with obstruction at the bifurcation due to a diffuse sclerosing carcinoma of the bile duct. (Courtesy of M. V. Sivak, Jr., M.D.)

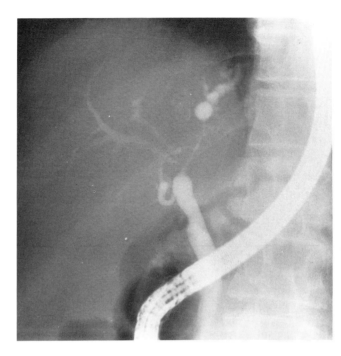

FIGURE 31–11. Retrograde cholangiogram showing stricturing of the left hepatic duct and only partial filling of the right hepatic ductal system in a patient with metastatic adenocarcinoma to the porta hepatis. (Courtesy of M. V. Sivak, Jr., M.D.)

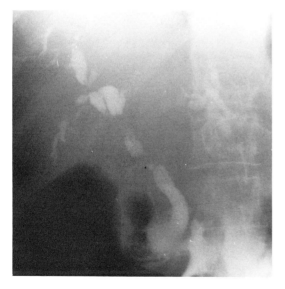

FIGURE 31–12. Retrograde cholangiogram showing multiple strictures of the proximal extrahepatic and intrahepatic bile ducts due to metastatic breast carcinoma. (Courtesy of M. V. Sivak, Jr., M.D.)

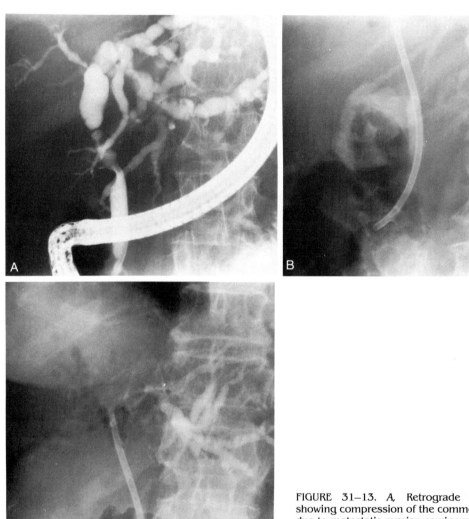

FIGURE 31–13. A, Retrograde cholangiogram showing compression of the common hepatic duct due to metastatic ovarian carcinoma. B and C, 10-French straight stent placed in duct for decompression. (Courtesy of M. V. Sivak, Jr., M.D.)

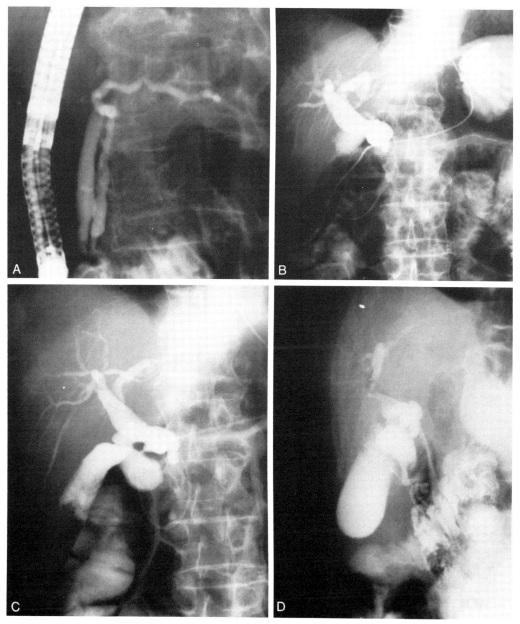

FIGURE 31–14. *A,* Retrograde pancreatocholangiogram in a jaundiced 83-year-old man with several serious diseases shows a normal pancreatic duct and obstruction of the proximal common bile duct. *B,* Opacification of the proximal biliary system and gallbladder via a 5-French nasobiliary drain inserted above the stenosis. This demonstrates a typical neoplastic bile duct lesion, dilation of the intrahepatic ducts, and distention of the gallbladder that contains a large quantity of biliary mud. Contrast medium outlines the gallbladder wall to the left of the nasobiliary drain, which is looped in the duodenum. *C,* Cholangiogram via a nasobiliary tube after 24 hours of decompression demonstrates reduction in diameter of the intrahepatic duct as well as decompression of the gallbladder that is 50% filled with contrast medium and still contains a large quantity of biliary mud. *D,* Cholangiogram after another 24 hours of decompression demonstrates complete filling of the gallbladder. The nasobiliary drain has been replaced with three 5-French, 7-cm double pigtail stents. This oblique view shows rapid emptying of the intrahepatic biliary tree through the stents. An endoscopic biopsy was positive for adenocarcinoma.

Obstruction of the Distal Bile Duct and/or Duodenal Papilla

Obstruction of the intraduodenal bile duct segment is typical of a terminal bile duct neoplasm or carcinoma of the duodenal papilla without proximal infiltration. Dilation of the bile duct proximal to the tumor often produces a soft, endoscopically visible bulge in the duodenal wall above the papilla. Palpation of this bulge with a catheter or biopsy forceps helps to confirm the impression of bile duct dilation. If a cholangiogram is obtained, compression of this dilated bile duct infundibulum may be observed fluoroscopically during palpation. With this type of lesion a 2- to 3-mm electrosurgical incision can be made into the bile duct infundibulum proximal to the obstructing tumor[67] (see Chapter 29). Then we often place one or two 5-French, 4-cm long, double pigtail stents through the incision to assure continued drainage and to prevent closure of the choledochoduodenostomy as a result of neoplastic infiltration. If a cholangiogram could not be obtained prior to incision of the infundibulum, the bile duct can be cannulated through the infundibulotomy for cholangiography or nasobiliary drainage. This technique of infundibulotomy avoids the risk of bleeding associated with incision of the terminal bile duct tumor itself and the difficulty of inserting stents through the obstructed distal biliary and papillary segments. A concerted effort should be made to obtain a pancreatogram before performing the infundibulotomy to determine if the tumor is pancreatic in origin.

In patients who remain jaundiced, technical failure of the procedure in providing decompression can be determined only by quantitating bile flow. In the seriously ill patient to be managed endoscopically, nasobiliary drainage offers a method for measuring technical success that may be combined with sphincterotomy or placement of stent(s) if feasible. The nasobiliary tube can be removed when cholangitis resolves, bile flow is assured, and cholestasis is subsiding. With removal of the nasobiliary tube a second or third 5-French stent may be placed in the space formerly occupied in the incised opening by the drainage tube.

Obstruction of the Middle Extrahepatic Bile Duct

The endoscopic approach to decompression of a bile duct obstruction due to a neoplastic stricture of the mid-portion of the extrahepatic bile duct is facilitated by the relatively normal distal segment. However, irritability and edema in the region of the duodenal papilla due to neoplastic infiltration, pancreatitis, or operative trauma may make selective bile duct cannulation difficult. A sphincterotomy incision of limited length simplifies initial and subsequent access to the bile duct and obviates the rare complication of pancreatitis as well as pancreatic pain that may occur following stent placement. The simplest sequence of maneuvers is opacification followed by insertion of a 5-French stent or nasobiliary drain. Then a second 5-French stent may be placed through the lesion. Alternatively, two successive stents or a stent and a nasobiliary drain may be inserted after sphincterotomy.

If it is only possible to place a nasobiliary drain alone or a single stent during an initial attempt at endoscopic decompression, the procedure can be completed at a second sitting, by which time a somewhat widened channel through the obstruction will have been established by the indwelling stent or drain. This facilitates selective bile duct cannulation. Endoscopic sphincterotomy can then be performed so that bile duct access is no longer problematic.

Once drainage is established by a stent in neoplastic obstruction of the bile duct, it cannot be discontinued. Even when stents have been present 3 to 6 months and there is a well-defined channel, the proximal biliary ducts drain poorly if the stents are removed. Based on extensive experience with 8.3-French percutaneous stents (2-mm lumen), we prefer to use two 5-French endoscopic stents, each having a 1-mm lumen, and may use three 5-French stents in patients when tumor debris or hemobilia produces intermittent occlusion of the lumen or when a gallbladder is present, as there is a requirement for high peak flow rates in the latter case (Fig. 31–14).

Obstruction of the Left and/or Right Hepatic Ducts

For mechanical reasons, malignant stenosis of the proximal bile ducts presents difficult technical problems for endoscopic management. Because such lesions are at a distance from the tip of the endoscope, the endoscopist has relatively less mechanical control in maneuvering wire guides and stents through the stenosis. When both the left and right hepatic ducts are involved, endoscopic decompression of both sides can be a formidable problem. Torque-stable catheters and soft-tipped wire guides with a movable core may resolve some of the technical problems.

When a lesion approaches or involves the hepatic bifurcation, an attempt should be made to stent both the left and right systems (Fig. 31–15). Drainage via a percutaneous approach can be used for one or the other ductal system when unfavorable anatomy results in technical failure. However, for short-term palliation of a patient with a disseminated malignancy a concerted effort at establishing endoscopic drainage is indicated, since the morbidity and mortality associated with two (left and right hepatic duct) percutaneous stents are substantial (Fig. 31–16).

BENIGN BILE DUCT STENOSIS

Benign stenosis of the bile duct involves diverse problems of varying severity and course. The majority of such lesions occur after abdominal surgery and include bile duct

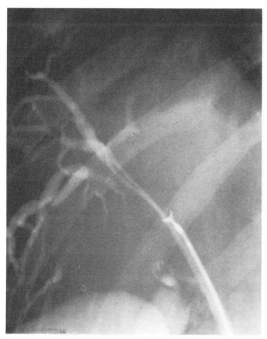

FIGURE 31–15. Retrograde cholangiogram in a 68-year-old man with jaundice. Prior ERCP demonstrated proximal common hepatic duct obstruction. After 24 hours of drainage with a 5-French nasobiliary drain and an endoscopic sphincterotomy, two 5-French, 10-cm double pigtail stents were placed above the obstruction; one stent is in the left hepatic duct, the other in the anterior division of the right hepatic duct. Following stent placement a 2.4-mm biopsy forcep was used to obtain a biopsy of the tumor and confirmed the diagnosis of adenocarcinoma.

stricture following cholecystectomy or sphincteroplasty (Figs. 31–17 to 31–19). Bile duct injury occurs during approximately 1 of every 200 cholecystectomies. Narrowing of the bile duct may develop very slowly so that symptoms of obstruction may appear at a relatively long time after surgery. The longest interval we have observed between inadvertent bile duct injury and the appearance of jaundice and cholangitis is 9 years. An interval of 29 years has been recorded.[68]

Endoscopic Management

Dilation of bile duct stenoses is technically feasible, if often difficult, and may provide long-term relief. Endoscopic as well as percutaneous dilation of biliary strictures has a morbidity and mortality that are less than those following transabdominal surgery, and the procedure can be repeated if stenosis recurs.[69] In some cases a combined percutaneous and endoscopic approach is required.

Experience with dilation of benign biliary strictures is limited. Furthermore, the technical problems encountered in each patient are unique, and anatomic distortion resulting from the surgery as well as distortion secondary to inflammation must be taken into account.

The first principle of management is to begin treatment as soon as signs or symptoms point to the presence of a postoperative stricture. Most postoperative bile duct stenoses are short (1 to 3 mm in length) (Fig. 31–20). When a postoperative biliary stricture limits bile flow, the diameter of the lumen in the narrow segment is usually minute. Often, a 0.035-inch diameter soft-tipped wire guide cannot be passed through the stenosis. With a percutaneous approach in such cases a further attempt can be made to pass small-diameter wire guides and catheters after an interval of drainage, decompression, and antibiotic therapy. These options are not available with the endoscopic approach, since the stenosis must first be passed to achieve proximal decompression.

However, if a 0.035-inch wire guide can be passed through the stenosis endoscopically, dilation is possible. We rarely proceed beyond insertion of a 5-French nasobiliary drainage tube at the first procedure. This initiates drainage and decompression and also provides a specimen for bacterial culture of the bile. Specific antibiotic therapy based upon culture results with antibiotic sensitivi-

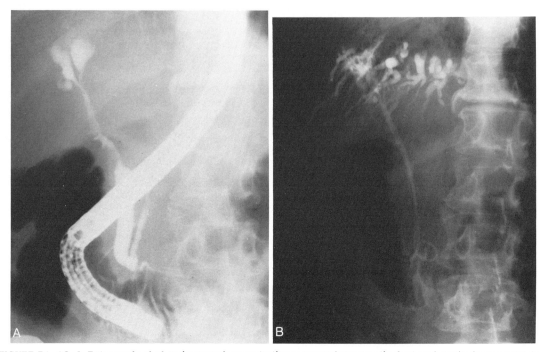

FIGURE 31–16. A, Retrograde cholangiogram demonstrating a normal pancreatic duct and extrinsic compression of the proximal common bile duct and entire hepatic duct in a jaundiced 66-year-old women with metastatic small cell carcinoma of the lung. B, Cholangiogram showing a 5-French, 7-cm double pigtail stent in the left hepatic duct and a 5-French, 10-cm double pigtail stent in the right hepatic duct that were placed after endoscopic sphincterotomy.

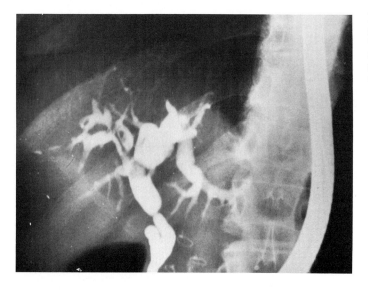

FIGURE 31–17. Retrograde cholangiogram showing postoperative stricture of the common hepatic duct with dilation of the ducts proximal to the stricture along with an intraductal calculus. (Courtesy of M. V. Sivak, Jr., M.D.)

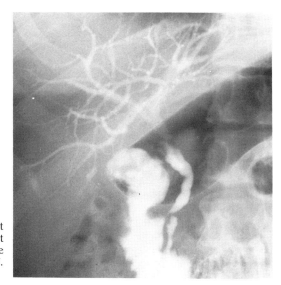

FIGURE 31–18. Retrograde cholangiogram in a patient with a choledochoduodenostomy. There is a stricture at the anastomosis and also a stricture just distal to the anastomosis in the common bile duct. (Courtesy of M. V. Sivak, Jr., M.D.)

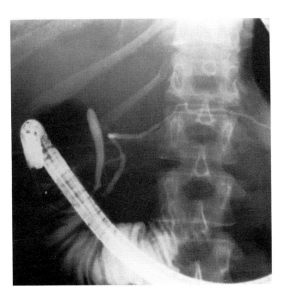

FIGURE 31–19. Retrograde pancreatocholangiogram demonstrating complete obstruction of the bile duct due to operative trauma. Note deep cannulation with placement of the catheter tip at the point of obstruction in an effort to opacify the bile duct proximal to the obstruction. (Courtesy of M. V. Sivak, Jr., M.D.)

FIGURE 31–20. Retrograde pancreatocholangiogram of short, very narrow postoperative stricture of the common bile duct. (Courtesy of M. V. Sivak, Jr., M.D.)

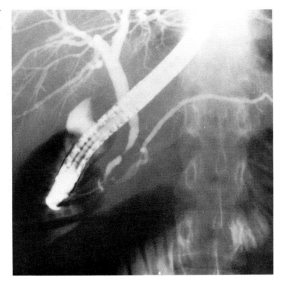

ties is extremely important. Unfortunately, a culture of the bile is often obtained only after the patient has received several antibiotics empirically.

The effectiveness of the nasobiliary drainage can be monitored by measuring bile flow and by serial cholangiography. The latter also provides a valuable demonstration of biliary anatomy that may identify additional lesions or problems such as stones or other anatomic or postsurgical variations of the bile ducts. Leakage of bile from the duct or collections of bile, often infected, outside the bile duct may be found. Prolonged drainage is often required for resolution of these problems.[70] The chronically infected biliary tree always contains cellular debris and commonly bile pigment stones. This material obstructs stents and drains, preventing decompression and resolution of cholangitis. With the use of a nasobiliary drain the duct system can be irrigated and drainage maintained. Abscesses may also resolve, since large amounts of pigment or pus will pass through a 5-French nasobiliary tube by gravity drainage. Serial cholangiography is invaluable for defining anatomy, following resolution of an abscess, and identifying stones that will not spontaneously fragment and pass.

Placement of a nasobiliary drain at the initial ERCP procedure eliminates the necessity of performing definitive cholangiography at the outset of endoscopic management. Excess contrast medium within the obstructed biliary tree increases intraductal pressure and forces bacteria and endotoxin into the adjacent hepatic sinusoids. This may cause fever, hypotension, and even septic shock. When hyperosmolar contrast medium remains in the bile duct, water continues to enter the biliary system to achieve isotonicity. This forces infected bile out of the biliary tree unless there is adequate drainage. The density of contrast medium required for adequate radiographic visualization often prevents fluoroscopic visualization of the wire guide and drain or pigtail portion of a stent. This, combined with inadequate radiographs and the limited time available for study of pathologic anatomy, may lead to errors in catheter placement or failed placement.

Balloon Dilation

Nonsurgical percutaneous balloon dilation of proximal postsurgical biliary stenoses was first described by Molnar and Stockum.[71] At that time, traversing and dilating these markedly narrowed, very firm strictures was a remarkable technical accomplishment. This technique reduced cholestasis and cholangitis in addition to providing a clear cholangiographic definition of the pathologic anatomy. In addition to removing stones from the bile duct, Molnar and Stockum also proposed this method as a definitive and curative procedure. Unfortunately, long-term follow-up of patients who have undergone this procedure has not been provided.

Although the simple concept of balloon dilation of sphincters and/or stenotic ductal segments is appealing, repeated procedures with forceful balloon dilation of stenotic bile ducts and enterobiliary anastomoses are usually required to maintain patency. When such a lesion is dilated via a percutaneous approach, a waist is often observed in the radiographic outline of the balloon at the level of the stenosis. High pressures of 6 to 8 atmospheres are required to eliminate this waist. The stenosis often reappears when the balloon is deflated, and on reinflation the narrow segment persists. This phenomenon probably relates to the inherent elasticity of the circumferential fibrosis and inflammation. Forceful dilation causes pain. This may indicate the presence of active inflammation surrounding the duct even in the absence of fistulas and periductal collections of bile. Rupture of the bile duct or perforation is a serious complication since leakage of infected bile produces a virulent infection and provokes intense fibrosis (Fig. 31–21). Aspiration of bile via the percutaneous route after balloon dilation often reveals hemorrhage, which can be severe. Blood clots within the duct after balloon dilation may occlude indwelling stents and the intrahepatic ducts themselves, with exacerbation of pain and cholangitis. For these reasons, dilation and irrigation are performed on a gradual, daily basis when using the percutaneous approach.[71]

An occasional patient may respond temporarily to balloon dilation. In the absence of circumferential fibrosis a single forceful dilation might be sufficient to establish a lumen, provided progressive inflammation and fibrosis do not occur. The stenotic bile duct segments of sclerosing cholangitis may also be a special case (Fig. 31–21).

Short-term follow-up of patients who have undergone balloon dilation of biliary strictures produces deceptive results, since gradual contraction of the scar takes place over a number of years. However, these endoscopic

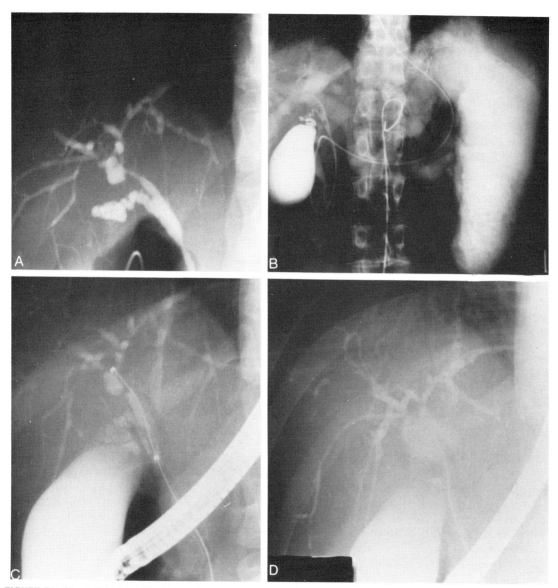

FIGURE 31–21. A, Intrahepatic cholangiogram performed via a 5-French nasobiliary drain in the distal common hepatic duct in a 43-year-old man with ulcerative colitis, fluctuating jaundice, fever, and abdominal pain. The drain, placed during a previous procedure, passes through a distal common hepatic duct stenosis into a short, dilated segment. The numerous stenoses of the intrahepatic ducts are typical of sclerosing cholangitis. B, Arteriogram demonstrates massive splenomegaly with dilated portal vein and collateral vessels. Varices were noted endoscopically. The nasobiliary drain is in good position proximal to the stricture. Nondrainage of the gallbladder is due to occlusion of narrow distal common bile duct by the nasobiliary drain. C, Inflation of 7-French catheter with a 4-mm dilating balloon that has been passed through the stenosis. D, Cholangiogram made after balloon dilation by means of a nasobiliary drain. The drain was inserted over a 0.035-inch soft-tip wire guide that passed easily through the dilated segment and into the right hepatic duct. Cholangiogram demonstrates extravasation of contrast medium, indicating partial hepatic duct rupture. After 24 hours of decompression, the drain was removed without untoward sequelae and with a satisfactory clinical response lasting for over 1 year.

techniques may be applied with such small risk in comparison with surgical correction of postoperative and inflammatory bile duct stenoses, and the results of therapy can be followed with such accuracy, that techniques for dilation of benign bile duct strictures merit investigative trials of therapy as an alternative to operative management.[72, 73]

It seems unlikely that sphincter of Oddi dysfunction would be improved by traumatic balloon dilation of the sphincter, but data are limited.[64]

Dilation Using Biliary Stents

Incremental dilation using biliary stents increasing from 5-French to 8.3-French avoids the problems of forceful balloon dilation and probably requires fewer percutaneous procedures. This technique can also be used endoscopically, or a number of 5-French stents may be placed serially. Since the lumen (1-mm diameter) of a single 5-French stent is adequate to carry the total daily output of 800 ml of bile, the interval between subsequent insertion of additional stents may be several weeks, and endoscopic placement of successive stents may be done on an outpatient basis. Ideally the stenotic segment should be dilated to a diameter slightly less than the lumen of the adjacent uninjured bile duct. This is often 7 to 9 mm and may require 5-French stents with an aggregate outside dimension of 25-French (8 mm) (Fig. 31–22).

Once a satisfactory number of stents have been inserted, they should be left in place for at least 1 year to allow complete maturation of the inflammatory scar tissue. Otherwise, rapid contraction of the actively forming scar will occur. Probably this process of healing and fibroblast (myofibroblast) contraction accounts for many of the problems and failures of forceful balloon dilation.

SCLEROSING CHOLANGITIS

Classification

Sclerosing cholangitis is classified as either a primary or a secondary disorder. Secondary sclerosing cholangitis implies an etiology, the two most commonly recognized causes being biliary infection and choledocholithiasis. Primary sclerosing cholangitis (PSC) can on rare occasion exist as a solitary entity. However, it is frequently, perhaps most often, associated with some other process or disease. Some of the known associated conditions are listed in

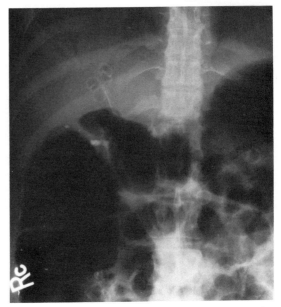

FIGURE 31–22. Plain x-ray film of the abdomen of a 34-year-old woman who had a distal bile duct stenosis following cholecystectomy and sphincteroplasty complicated by a duodenal leak. Residual barium is present in the right midabdomen. The distal bile duct stenosis was progressively dilated by the serial insertion of 5-French, 4-cm double pigtail stents. The four stents visualized in the bile duct represent an aggregate diameter of 8 mm. The stents were maintained in place for 1 year and then removed. At 2-year follow-up the patient is asymptomatic and has normal liver function.

Table 31–1. Inclusion of some disorders in this table is based on a few case reports.

Associated Disorders

There is a strong, but poorly understood, association between PSC and idiopathic inflammatory bowel disease (IBD), especially ulcerative colitis but also Crohn's disease. Between 1% and 3% of patients with IBD will have PSC, but about 50% of patients with

TABLE 31–1. **Disorders Known to be Associated with Sclerosing Cholangitis**

Retroperitoneal fibrosis
Riedel's thyroiditis
Thyrotoxicosis
Mediastinal fibrosis
Chronic pancreatitis
Sicca complex (with chronic pancreatitis)
Pseudotumor (orbit)
Peyronie's disease
Rheumatoid arthritis
Hypertrophic osteoarthropathy
Renal tubular acidosis
Vitiligo
Weber-Christian disease
Histiocytosis X

PSC will have IBD.[74] Schrumpf et al.[75] found that 14% of 336 patients with ulcerative colitis had evidence of hepatobiliary disease, and retrograde cholangiography demonstrated PSC in 19 of 39 cases. In a similar investigation by Tobias et al.,[76] evidence of hepatobiliary disease (i.e., persistent elevation of serum alkaline phosphatase greater than twice normal) was present in 9 of 250 patients with ulcerative colitis and in 3 of 164 patients with Crohn's disease; PSC was demonstrated in 3% of these IBD patients.

Clinical and Laboratory Features

The clinical presentation of PSC may be chronic biliary obstruction, hepatic cirrhosis with portal hypertension, or abnormal biochemical parameters of liver function in a patient with no symptoms of biliary tract disease. There is a definite male predominance, an interesting fact given the slight female predominance for ulcerative colitis. Although the age range is wide, PSC usually appears during middle age. PSC has been reported in children and infants.[77–79] When associated with IBD, it may be diagnosed many years after onset of the bowel disease and may even appear after colectomy for ulcerative colitis. PSC may rarely precede the appearance of IBD.[80] In almost all patients with IBD and PSC the clinical evolution of the two diseases is not parallel. For example, a flare in the colonic process is not usually associated with rapid worsening of the biliary disease. Because of early diagnosis by cholangiography, the course of PSC is known to be more prolonged than once thought.[81] However, PSC slowly progresses to biliary cirrhosis and death.

Prior to the use of direct cholangiography, particularly ERCP, the criteria for diagnosis of PSC were absence of biliary calculi, no prior biliary surgery, an operative cholangiogram that demonstrated typical findings, operative biopsy of the bile duct disclosing a fibrotic process without evidence of carcinoma, and relatively long follow-up to exclude carcinoma.[82] The greater use of retrograde cholangiography and the recognition that liver biopsy findings may be misleading in ulcerative colitis–associated hepatobiliary disease (vide infra) have changed the clinical profile of the patients with PSC in reported series such that a higher percentage will be asymptomatic and will have undergone ERCP on the basis of abnormal biochemical parameters of liver function.[83] Typical cholangiographic findings are often the major

criterion for diagnosis of PSC; remote cholecystectomy does not exclude the diagnosis. The only difficulty with this approach is the occasional case of sclerosing cholangiocarcinoma (vide infra).

Etiology

Speculation concerning the pathogenesis of PSC includes (1) damage as a result of portal bacteremia or other infectious processes,[84, 85] (2) absorption of toxins in patients with IBD, (3) generalized fibrotic disorder,[86–88] (4) autoimmune disease,[89] (5) hereditary factors, (6) drugs, and (7) viral infection.[90] A clinicopathologic picture of sclerosing cholangitis has been described in patients with histiocytosis X.[91] An increase in HLA-B8 in patients with PSC and ulcerative colitis is of interest since there are no increased frequencies for HLA antigens in patients with only ulcerative colitis.[92, 93] HLA-B8 is known to be associated with diseases that have a component of immunologic dysfunction. PSC has been described in association with reticulum cell sarcoma and in immune deficiency states.[77, 94]

Liver Biopsy

A variety of hepatobiliary disorders occur in association with IBD, including fatty infiltration of the liver, chronic active hepatitis, "cryptogenic cirrhosis," cholangiocarcinoma (with ulcerative colitis), and calculi (with Crohn's disease). In the past, many patients were classified as having "pericholangitis" on the basis of liver histology alone without the benefit of cholangiography.

Liver biopsy has merit in the classification of hepatobiliary disorders associated with IBD, but histologic findings alone are unreliable and can be misleading. Chapman et al.[95] retrospectively reviewed liver biopsy findings in 29 patients with PSC. Although all patients had a mixed portal inflammatory infiltrate and bile duct proliferation was demonstrated in the majority, evidence of cholestasis was present in a minority. In the study of Ludwig et al.[96] there were no characteristic histologic changes in liver biopsy specimens in 15% to 20% of patients with PSC. Barbatis et al.[97] studied liver biopsies from 16 patients with radiographically proven PSC and found that PSC could be diagnosed on the basis of established histologic criteria in only half the cases. However, these authors maintained that by reference to more specific findings PSC could be diagnosed by histologic criteria alone in the majority of the biopsy specimens in the series of 16 patients.

Many authorities have proposed that the term "pericholangitis" be abandoned, and there is an emerging concept of a spectrum of hepatobiliary disorders that occurs in association with IBD. Blackstone and Nemchausky[98] described intrahepatic cholangiographic abnormalities in patients with ulcerative colitis who had evidence of "pericholangitis." The intrahepatic ducts were abnormal in 8 patients, and in 2 of these the extrahepatic ducts were also abnormal. The authors suggested that the intrahepatic cholangiograms may commonly be abnormal in asymptomatic or mildly symptomatic patients with "pericholangitis." Ludwig et al.[96] have proposed that hepatic parenchymal findings in patients with PSC and in some patients with ulcerative colitis be referred to as "chronic nonsuppurative obliterative cholangitis," and that PSC be considered as either "small duct" or "large duct," i.e., predominantly intrahepatic or extrahepatic. Galambos and Brooks[99] described 4 patients with a cholestatic syndrome intermediate between primary biliary cirrhosis (PBC) and sclerosing cholangitis. These patients did not have antimitochondrial antibodies or elevated IgM levels and 3 of the 4 were men. The characteristic cholangiographic findings of sclerosing cholangitis were absent in the extrahepatic ducts and the immediate tributaries of the left and right hepatic ducts. However, cholangiograms demonstrated rapid attenuation and narrowing of the smaller intrahepatic bile ducts.

ERCP

Cholangiography has become more essential in the differential diagnosis of IBD-associated hepatobiliary disease.

Radiographic Findings. The characteristic radiographic findings in PSC include stenosis, ectasia, obstruction, sacculation, diffuse narrowing, and mural irregularity (Figs. 31–23 and 31–24). These may occur in the intrahepatic ducts, the extrahepatic biliary system, or both. There are slight differences in reported series with regard to the pattern of involvement, i.e., intrahepatic only, extrahepatic only, or a combined pattern. In 20 cases reported by Rohrmann et al.[100] the intrahepatic ducts were abnormal in all patients, whereas the extrahepatic ducts were abnormal in 15. In the series of 86 cases reported by MacCarty et al.[101] only the intrahepatic ducts and proximal extrahepatic system were involved in 20% of patients. In practice, it may be difficult to distinguish

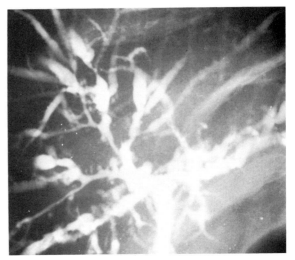

FIGURE 31–23. Retrograde cholangiogram demonstrating sclerosing cholangitis of the intrahepatic ducts. Short segmental stenoses alternate with areas of normal caliber or dilation to produce a beaded appearance. In dilated segments the ductal wall is also irregular. (Courtesy of M. V. Sivak, Jr., M.D.)

exclusive intrahepatic or extrahepatic involvement. Furthermore, there are no data on the detection of early, mild disease by cholangiography.

The most important intrahepatic ductal radiographic features found by Rohrmann

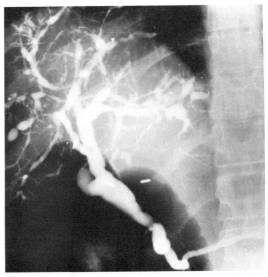

FIGURE 31–24. Retrograde cholangiogram showing predominantly intrahepatic duct sclerosing cholangitis. The main cholangiographic findings are multiple ductal strictures along with dilated segments. (From: Ferguson DR. Cholestasis syndromes. In: Farmer RG, Achkar E, Fleshler B, eds. Clinical Gastroenterology. New York: Raven Press, 1983: 517–30, with permission.)

et al.[100] were diminished arborization, stenosis, and ectasia. Severe obliterative changes occurred in a few patients. The principal cholangiographic finding within the left and right hepatic ducts was stenosis, with mural irregularity and ectasia being less frequent. However, mural irregularities were frequent in the common hepatic and common bile ducts. Marginal outpouchings or diverticula were found in about half of the cases (Fig. 31–25). Stenotic areas were less common than in the intrahepatic portion, as were ectasia and obstruction. Rohrmann et al.[100] also suggested that saccular diverticula of the extrahepatic ducts occurred exclusively in patients with IBD-associated PSC, but this is disputed.[101]

The most common radiographic feature in the study by MacCarty et al.[101] was multifocal stricturing of both the extrahepatic (Figs. 31–23 and 31–24) and the intrahepatic ducts. Strictures were usually not more than 1 to 2 cm in length and alternated with either normal or minimally dilated segments to produce a "beading" pattern. "Band-like" strictures measuring 1 to 2 mm in length were seen in 21% of patients, chiefly in the extrahepatic ducts. Confluent stricturing with long connected segments was thought to indicate advanced disease. Mural irregularity was noted in 44% of patients, and as in the series by Rohrmann et al.,[100] this was more often

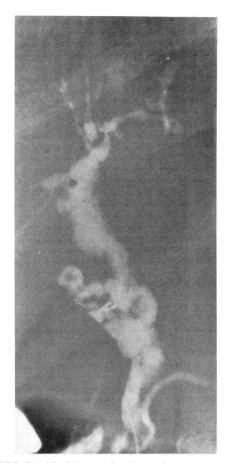

FIGURE 31–26. Retrograde cholangiogram showing irregular extrahepatic duct with mural irregularities due to sclerosing cholangitis. (Reprinted from Sclerosing cholangitis. By Sivak, M. V., Jr. From Scand J Gastroenterol 1983; 18(Suppl 88):18–23. By permission of Norwegian University Press (Universitetsforlaget AS), Oslo.

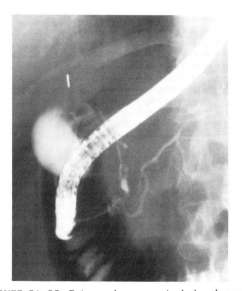

FIGURE 31–25. Retrograde pancreatocholangiogram of a patient with severe sclerosing cholangitis. There is limited opacification of the biliary system, but filling of the distal portion demonstrates diverticulum-like pockets. (Courtesy of M. V. Sivak, Jr., M.D.)

found in the extrahepatic ducts (Fig. 31–26). The cystic duct was abnormal in a few patients in each of these series.[100, 101]

The retrograde pancreatogram may also be abnormal in patients with PSC. MacCarty et al.[101] found pancreatographic abnormalities in 8% of patients. These were characterized as various degrees of stricturing. Epstein et al.[102] found abnormal pancreatograms in 3 of 20 patients with PSC. In this retrospective study, pancreatic duct abnormalities were also found in 43% of 35 patients with PBC. Palmer et al.[103] studied retrograde pancreatograms in a group of patients with cholestasis. There were 13 patients with PSC, 15 patients with proximal cholangiocarcinoma, and 13 normal individuals. Pancreatograms were reviewed and graded as to degree of abnormality by two independent observers without knowledge of the diagnosis. Results of pancreatography were abnormal in 77% of patients with PSC and in 60% of patients with cholangiocarcinoma. Irregularity of the main pancreatic duct branches was the main finding, although in 5 patients with PSC and 2 with cholangiocarcinoma the main pancreatic duct was markedly irregular.

Differential Diagnosis

Several disorders resemble PSC cholangiographically: PBC, cirrhosis from any cause, cholangiocarcinoma, and postoperative stricturing.

Summerfield et al.[104] studied 23 patients with PBC by endoscopic retrograde cholangiography. The intrahepatic ducts were irregular in caliber and tortuous in 7 cases. Although 39% of the patients had gallstones, the authors attributed the intrahepatic cholangiographic abnormalities to the concomitant histologically proven cirrhosis that was present in all cases.

Rohrmann et al.[105] have suggested that there are distinguishing intrahepatic cholangiographic features for these several diseases. In a study of 107 patients with a variety of liver diseases they found that cirrhosis was characterized by stenosis, diminished arborization, tortuosity, and approximation of the intrahepatic ducts.

Falkenstein et al.,[106] in a postmortem study of 30 patients, found that generalized crowding of the hepatic ducts plus a "zigzagging and corkscrewing" course of the finer radicles was characteristic of cirrhosis. Infiltrative disorders produced straightening and elongation of the radicles plus spreading apart of the bile ducts in association with hepatomegaly. These findings occurred with alcoholic hepatitis, diffuse hepatic carcinomatosis, and myeloproliferative disorders. With metastatic tumors, which frequently compress bile ducts, some patients had a distinctive pattern of segmental narrowing with peripheral dilation.

The single most reliable differential point between PSC and PBC (i.e., cirrhosis associated with PBC) or cirrhosis is the absence of extrahepatic duct involvement in the latter two disorders.

Although it is usually not difficult to differentiate postoperative stricturing from PSC, cholangiocarcinoma presents a greater problem. MacCarty et al.[101] compared cholangiograms of 86 patients with PSC with those of 82 patients with primary bile duct carcinoma. Although in most instances carcinoma

presented a focal stricture, in about 10% of cases there was diffuse stricturing of the biliary system. This diffuse radiographic pattern of carcinoma probably cannot be distinguished cholangiographically from PSC, although band-like strictures and diverticula were not found in any case of carcinoma, and these features appeared to be characteristic of PSC.[101]

The difficult differential diagnosis of PSC and carcinoma is compounded by the possibility that cholangiocarcinoma may occur in long-standing PSC.[107–109] Wee et al.[108] reported 8 cases of cholangiocarcinoma in association with chronic ulcerative colitis. Five of these patients had PSC involving the larger bile ducts; 3 patients had so-called "small-duct" PSC or "pericholangitis." The cancers were extrahepatic in origin in 5 and intrahepatic in 2 patients, and the neoplasm affected both the gallbladder and the liver in 1 patient. In support of a PSC-associated predisposition to neoplasia, the authors noted the presence of carcinoma in situ in areas of fibrous cholangitis, multicentric origin of malignancy, tumor-free segments of the bile duct involved by PSC at a distance from malignant tumors, and documented long-standing inflammatory hepatobiliary disease prior to the discovery of carcinoma in some cases. Although the reported cases of bile duct cancer in association with PSC are increasing, the data in support of an increased incidence of cholangiocarcinoma in patients with PSC are limited.

MacCarty et al.[107] compared cholangiograms from patients with PSC alone and those of 13 patients with PSC plus biopsy or autopsy proven cholangiocarcinoma. Marked dilation of the bile duct or a segment of the duct was noted in all cases of cholangiocarcinoma with PSC, but this finding also occurred in about one-fourth of the patients with PSC alone. The radiographic appearance of a polypoid mass was also much more common in patients with cancer and PSC. Polypoid lesions caused by carcinoma were larger than the mural irregularities that occur in PSC, being 1 cm or greater in diameter. Serial cholangiograms were available in 66 patients, and 4 of 15 patients with progressive strictures, as well as 4 of 5 patients with progressive ductal dilation had carcinoma. A retrograde cholangiographic pattern of multiple cystic dilations of the bile duct in a patient with PSC and chronic ulcerative colitis was proposed by Gluskin and Payne[110] as being strongly suggestive of cholangiocarcinoma occurring in association with PSC.

Some authors maintain that PSC can be a focal disorder and therefore resemble a carcinomatous stricture. However, only a few case reports support this concept, and the existence of focal PSC should not be regarded as established at this time. Golematis et al.[111] described a localized stricture at the bifurcation of the hepatic duct in a 23-year-old man that was thought to be due to PSC. Smadja et al.[112] described 2 patients with localized strictures in the region of the hilum of the liver that were initially misdiagnosed as cholangiocarcinoma. However, only benign stricturing was found on histologic study of the resected specimens, and further bile duct stricturing that was consistent with PSC developed in these patients. A similar clinical picture was reported by Panes et al.[113] of a 56-year-old man who underwent resection of a stricture and follow-up of 3 years, at which time liver biopsy findings were consistent with PSC. Cholangiocarcinoma may also be difficult to recognize microscopically if it has a marked sclerosing or fibrotic component.

Treatment

There is no proven treatment of PSC. Although there are anecdotal reports of response to corticosteroids, it has not been demonstrated conclusively that this therapy favorably influences the course of PSC. Colectomy has been suggested for patients with ulcerative colitis. In one report of 4 patients colectomy and prolonged biliary stenting plus daily saline irrigation and antibiotics improved their condition.[114] However, most authorities do not accept that colectomy alters the course of PSC in patients with ulcerative colitis. Other proposed treatments include aggressive surgical, percutaneous, or endoscopic dilation and stenting.

T-tube surgical drainage in sclerosing cholangitis is outmoded. Percutaneous transhepatic drainage is difficult; the sclerosed intrahepatic ducts are minute because of typically "rock-hard" periductal fibrosis and the common association of cirrhosis. Endoscopic drainage is technically difficult and rarely succeeds above the hepatic duct bifurcation. Percutaneous drainage into the duodenum can result in contamination of the intrahepatic biliary tree and gallbladder by virtue of duodenal reflux through the indwelling stent. Endoscopic drainage may have similar effects due to siphonage around the nasobiliary drain or stent. Balloon dilation would seem an attractive alternative, but the smallest 7-French dilating balloons are too large to pass pathophysiologically important areas of stenosis that measure less than 1 mm in diameter. In our experience, dilation with a stent or nasobiliary drain is almost always required before balloon dilation.

PANCREATIC DUCT STENOSIS

When pancreatic ductal obstruction is considered as a cause of pain in a patient with chronic pancreatitis, temporary decompression with an endoscopic or percutaneous drain defines ductal anatomy clearly, and symptom relief with successful decompression can be accepted as evidence of pathologic ductal obstruction (Fig. 31–4). Since chronic pancreatitis is not curable, therapeutic intervention of this type is palliative and must therefore be achieved with minimal risk and cost.

An endoscopically approachable pancreatic duct stenosis that appears to be the cause of symptoms is uncommon. With stenoses due to pancreatic cancer, the dangers in attempting pancreatic duct decompression appear to outweigh any potential benefit. Occasionally a single stenotic segment or even multiple stenoses may appear to be the cause of intolerable postprandial pain in patients with chronic pancreatitis. Some patients may respond to placement of a pancreatic duct stent (Fig. 31–4). Although pseudocysts that communicate with the main duct have been drained endoscopically, the number of cases reported is small and this technique should be considered investigational at present.[115] Endoscopic drainage of a communicating pseudocyst is rarely indicated, and because of significant hazards of pancreatitis and sepsis such a procedure should be attempted only when there is a clear therapeutic goal that cannot be achieved by other accepted methods.

Editor's note: References 116 to 120 are some recent reports of interest in relation to the subject matter in this chapter.

References

1. Bornman PC, Marks IN, Girdwood AH, et al. Is pancreatic duct obstruction or stricture a major cause of pain in calcific pancreatitis? Br J Surg 1980; 67:425–8.
2. Nagai H, Ohtsubo K. Pancreatic lithiasis in the aged. Its clinicopathology and pathogenesis. Gastroenterology 1984; 86:331–8.
3. Howard JM, Nedich A. Correlation of the histologic observations and operative findings in patients with chronic pancreatitis. Surg Gynecol Obstet 1971; 132:387–95.

 4. Warshaw AL, Popp JW Jr, Schapiro RH. Long-term patency, pancreatic function and pain relief after lateral pancreaticojejunostomy for chronic pancreatitis. Gastroenterology 1980; 79:289–93.

 5. Mahour GH, Wakim KG, Soule EH, Ferris DO. Structure of the common bile duct in man: Presence or absence of smooth muscle. Ann Surg 1967; 166:91–4.

 6. Niederau C, Sonnenberg NC, Mueller AJ. Comparison of the extrahepatic bile duct size measured by ultrasound and by different radiographic methods. Gastroenterology 1984; 87:615–21.

 7. Hamilton I, Ruddell WS, Mitchell CJ, et al. Endoscopic retrograde cholangiograms of the normal and post-cholecystectomy biliary tree. Br J Surg 1982; 69:343–5.

 8. Alonso-Lej F, Rever WB Jr, Pessagno DJ. Collective review: congenital choledochal cysts, with a report of 2, and an analysis of 94 cases. Int Abstr Surg 1959; 108:1–30.

 9. Arthur GW, Stewart JOR. Biliary cysts. Br J Surg 1964; 51:671–5.

10. Engle J, Salmon PA. Multiple choledochal cysts. Arch Surg 1964; 88:345–9.

11. Tsardakas E, Robnett AH. Congenital cystic dilatation of the common bile duct. Arch Surg 1956; 72:311–22.

12. Powell CS, Sawyers JL, Reynolds VH. Management of adult choledochal cysts. Ann Surg 1981; 191:666–74.

13. Saito S, Yura J, Yano H, et al. A proposal of a new classification of congenital biliary dilation. J Jpn Soc Pediatr Surg 1980; 16:319.

14. Todani T, Watanabe Y, Fujii T, Uemura S. Anomalous arrangement of the pancreaticobiliary ductal system in patients with a choledochal cyst. Am J Surg 1984; 147:672–6.

15. Deeg HJ, Rominger JM, Shah AN. Choledochal cyst and pancreatic carcinoma demonstrated simultaneously by endoscopic retrograde cholangiopancreatography. South Med J 1980; 73:1678–9.

16. Flanigan DP. Biliary cysts. Ann Surg 1975; 182:635–43.

17. Thatcher BS, Sivak MV Jr, Hermann RE, et al. ERCP in the evaluation and diagnosis of choledochal cyst. Report of five cases and a review of the literature. Gastrointest Endosc 1986; 32:27–31.

18. Todani T, Narusue M, Watanabe Y, et al. Management of congenital cyst with intrahepatic involvement. Ann Surg 1978; 187:272–80.

19. Glenn F, McSherry C. Congenital segmental cystic dilatation of the biliary ductal system. Ann Surg 1973; 177:705–13.

20. Babbitt DP. Congenital choledochal cysts: new etiological concept based on anomalous relationships of the common bile duct and pancreatic bulb. Ann Radiol 1969; 12:231–40.

21. Ono J, Sakoda K, Akita H. Surgical aspect of cystic dilatation of the bile duct—an anomalous junction of the pancreaticobiliary tract in adults. Ann Surg 1982; 195:203–8.

22. Miyano T, Suruga K, Shimomura H, et al. Choledochopancreatic elongated common channel disorders. J Pediatr Surg 1984; 19:165–70.

23. Muller EL, Miyamoto T, Pitt HA, et al. Anatomy of the choledochopancreatic duct junction in primary sclerosing cholangitis. Surgery 1985; 97:21–7.

24. Rattner DW, Schapiro RH, Warshaw AL. Abnormalities of the pancreatic and biliary ducts in adult patients with choledochal cysts. Arch Surg 1983; 118:1068–73.

25. Shiloni E, Lebensart P, Durst AL, et al. Type I choledochal cyst in adults. Isr J Med Sci 1983; 19:209–11.

26. Klein GM, Frost SS. Newer imaging modalities for the preoperative diagnosis of choledochal cyst. Am J Gastroenterol 1981; 76:148–52.

27. Paramsothy M, Somasundram K. Technetium 99m-diethyl-IDA hepatobiliary scintigraphy in the pre-operative diagnosis of choledochal cyst. Br J Radiol 1981; 54:1104–7.

28. Han BK, Babcock DS, Gelfand MH. Choledochal cyst with bile duct dilatation: sonography and ^{99m}Tc IDA cholescintigraphy. AJR 1981; 137:1075–9.

29. Huang MJ, Liaw YF. Intravenous cholescintigraphy using Tc-99m-labeled agents in the diagnosis of choledochal cyst. J Nucl Med 1982; 23:113–6.

30. Atkinson GO, Gay BB Jr. Choledochal cysts in children: radiologic features. South Med J 1982; 75:1215–21.

31. Araki T, Itai Y, Tasaka A. CT of choledochal cyst. AJR 1980; 135:729–34.

32. Efremidis SC, Lehr-Janus C, Yeh H-C, et al. Choledochal cyst: case report and review of the literature. Mt Sinai J Med 1980; 47:45–8.

33. Bloustein PA. Association of carcinoma with congenital cystic conditions of the liver and bile ducts. Am J Gastroenterol 1977; 67:40–6.

34. Flanigan DP. Biliary carcinoma associated with biliary cysts. Cancer 1977; 40:880–3.

35. Kimura K, Ohto M, Saisho H, et al. Association of gallbladder carcinoma and anomalous pancreaticobiliary ductal union. Gastroenterology 1985; 89:1258–65.

36. Gallagher PJ, Millis RR, Mitchinson MJ. Congenital dilatation of the intrahepatic bile ducts with cholangiocarcinoma. J Clin Pathol 1972; 25:804–8.

37. Thistlewait J, Horwitz A. Choledochal cyst followed by carcinoma of the hepatic duct. South Med J 1967; 60:872–4.

38. Attar S, Obeid S. Congenital cyst of the common bile duct—a review of the literature and a report of two cases. Ann Surg 1955; 142:289–95.

39. Lilly JR. The surgical treatment of choledochal cyst. Surg Gynecol Obstet 1979; 149:36–42.

40. Farkas IE, Patko A, Szebeni A, Tulassay Z. Diverticulum of the bile duct. Am J Gastroenterol 1980; 73:310–4.

41. Scholz FJ, Carrera GF, Larsen CR. The choledochocele: correlation of radiological, clinical and pathological findings. Radiology 1976; 118:25–8.

42. Jensen W. Intraduodenal cyst containing bile and stones "choledochocele" in an accessory bile duct. Report of a case with recurrent pancreatitis. Gastroenterology 1970; 58:397–401.

43. Greene FL, Brown JJ, Rubinstein P, et al. Choledochocele and recurrent pancreatitis. Diagnosis and surgical management. Am J Surg 1985; 149:306–9.

44. Hart MJ, White TT. Choledochocele associated with acute hemorrhagic pancreatitis. West J Med 1980; 133:340–4.

45. Goldberg PB, Long WB, Oleaga JA, et al. Choledochocele as a cause of recurrent pancreatitis. Gastroenterology 1980; 78:1041–5.

46. Marshall JB, Halpin TC. Choledochocele as the cause of recurrent obstructive jaundice in childhood: diagnosis by ERCP. Gastrointest Endosc 1982; 28:88–90.

47. Ozawa K, Yamada T, Matumoto Y, et al. Carcinoma arising in a choledochocele. Cancer 1980; 45:195–7.

48. Iriyama K, Mori T, Takenaka T, et al. Choledochocele: report of a case and review of the literatures. Jpn J Surg 1980; 10:149–55.

49. Burton FJ, Bamforth J. Intraluminal diverticulum of the duodenum and choledochocele. Gut 1972; 13:207–10.

50. Pollack M, Shirkhoda A, Charnsangavej CMD. Computed tomography of choledochocele. J Comput Assist Tomogr 1985; 9:360–2.

51. Brodey PA, Fisch AE, Fertig S, Roberts GS. Computed tomography of choledochocele. J Comput Assist Tomogr 1984; 8:162–4.

52. Siegel JH, Hardin GT, Chateau F. Endoscopic incision of choledochal cysts (choledochocele). Endoscopy 1981; 13:200–2.

53. Venu RP, Geenen JE, Hogan WJ, et al. Role of endoscopic retrograde cholangiopancreatography in the diagnosis and treatment of choledochocele. Gastroenterology 1984; 87:1144–9.

54. Zimmon DS, Falkenstein DB, Manno BV, et al. Choledochocele: radiologic diagnosis and endoscopic management. Gastrointest Radiol 1978; 3:348–51.

55. Ludwig J, Wiesner RH, LaRusso NF. Focal dilatation of intrahepatic bile ducts (Caroli's disease), cholangiocarcinoma, and sclerosis of extrahepatic bile ducts: a case report. J Clin Gastroenterol 1982; 4:53–7.

56. Menu Y, Lorphelin JM, Scherrer A, et al. Sonographic and computed tomographic evaluation of intrahepatic calculi. AJR 1985; 145:579–83.

57. Tulassay Z, Papp J, Szebeni A, et al. Caroli's disease: diagnosed by ERCP and ultrasonography. Endoscopy 1978; 10:211–4.

58. Kaiser JA, Mall JC, Salmen BJ, et al. Diagnosis of Caroli disease by computed tomography: report of two cases. Radiology 1979; 132:661–4.

59. Moody FG, Berenson MM, McCloskey D. Transampullary septectomy for post-cholecystectomy pain. Ann Surg 1977; 186:415–23.

60. Nichols DA, MacCarty RL, Gaffey TA. Cholangiographic evaluation of bile duct carcinoma. AJR 1983; 141:1291–4.

61. Roberts-Thomson IC, Hobbs JB. Cytodiagnosis of pancreatic and biliary cancer by endoscopic duct aspiration. Med J Aust 1979; 1:370–2.

62. Nguyen GK. Primary extranodal non-Hodgkin's lymphoma of the extrahepatic bile ducts. Report of a case. Cancer 1982; 50:2218–22.

63. Severini A, Bellomi M, Cozzi G, et al. Lymphomatous involvement of intrahepatic and extrahepatic biliary ducts. PTC and ERCP findings. Acta Radiol [Diagn] (Stockh) 1981; 22:159–63.

64. Gudjonsson B, Livstone EM, Spiro HM. Cancer of the pancreas: diagnostic accuracy and survival statistics. Cancer 1978; 42:2494–506.

65. Cooperman A. Periampullary CA—1983. Semin Liver Dis 1983; 3:181–92.

66. Neff RA, Fankuchen EK, Cooperman AM, et al. The radiological management of malignant biliary obstruction. Clin Radiol 1983; 34:143–6.

67. Osnes M. Endoscopic choledochoduodenostomy for common bile duct obstructions. Lancet 1979; 1:1059–60.

68. Braasch JW, Warren KW, Blevins PK. Progress in biliary stricture repair. Am J Surg 1975; 129:34–7.

69. Blumgart LH, Kelley CJ. Hepaticojejunostomy in benign and malignant high bile duct stricture: approaches to the left hepatic ducts. Br J Surg 1984; 71:257–61.

70. Mueller PR, Ferrucci JT Jr, Simeone JF, et al. Detection and drainage of bilomas: special considerations. AJR 1983; 140:715–20.

71. Molnar W, Stockum AE. Relief of obstructive jaundice through a percutaneous transhepatic catheter—A new therapeutic method. Am J Roentgenol Radium Ther Nucl Med 1974; 122:356–67.

72. Foutch PG, Sivak MV Jr. Therapeutic endoscopic balloon dilatation of the extrahepatic biliary ducts. Am J Gastroenterol 1985; 80:575–80.

73. Siegel JH, Guelrud M. Endoscopic cholangiopancreatoplasty: hydrostatic balloon dilation in the bile duct and pancreas. Gastrointest Endosc 1983; 29:99–103.

74. Wiesner RH, LaRusso NF. Clinicopathologic features of the syndrome of primary sclerosing cholangitis. Gastroenterology 1980; 79:200–6.

75. Schrumpf E, Fausa O, Kolmannskog F, et al. Sclerosing cholangitis in ulcerative colitis. A follow up study. Scand J Gastroenterol 1982; 17:33–9.

76. Tobias R, Wright JP, Kottler RE, et al. Primary sclerosing cholangitis associated with inflammatory bowel disease in Cape Town, 1975–1981. S Afr Med J 1983; 63:229–35.

77. Naveh Y, Mendelsohn H, Spira G, et al. Primary sclerosing cholangitis associated with immunodeficiency. Am J Dis Child 1983; 137:114–7.

78. Spivak W, Grand RJ, Eraklis A. A case of primary sclerosing cholangitis in childhood. Gastroenterology 1982; 82:129–32.

79. Werlin SL, Glicklich M, Jona J, Starshak RJ. Sclerosing cholangitis in childhood. J Pediatr 1980; 96:433–5.

80. Steckman M, Drossman DA, Lesesne HR. Hepatobiliary disease that precedes ulcerative colitis. J Clin Gastroenterol 1984; 6:425–8.

81. Chapman RWG, Burroughs AK, Bass NM, et al. Long-standing asymptomatic primary sclerosing cholangitis. Report of three cases. Dig Dis Sci 1981; 26:778–82.

82. Danzi JT, Makipour H, Farmer RG: Primary sclerosing cholangitis. A report of nine cases and clinical review. Am J Gastroenterol 1976; 65:109–16.

83. Sivak MV Jr, Farmer RG, Lalli AF. Sclerosing cholangitis: its increasing frequency of recognition and association with inflammatory bowel disease. J Clin Gastroenterol 1981; 3:261–6.

84. Brooke BN, Dykes PW, Walker FC. A study of liver disorders in ulcerative colitis. Postgrad Med J 1961; 37:245–51.

85. Bucuvalas JC, Bove KE, Kaufman RA, et al. Cholangitis associated with *Cryptococcus neoformans*. Gastroenterology 1985; 88:1055–9.

86. Waldram R, Kopelman H, Tsantoulas D, Williams R. Chronic pancreatitis, sclerosing cholangitis, and sicca complex in two siblings. Lancet 1975; 1:550–2.

87. Viteri AL, Hardin WJ, Dyck WP. Peyronie's disease and sclerosing cholangitis in a patient with ulcerative colitis. Dig Dis Sci 1979; 24:490–1.

88. Sjogren I, Wengle B, Krosgren M. Primary sclerosing cholangitis associated with fibrosis of the submandibular glands and the pancreas. Acta Med Scand 1979; 205:139–41.

89. Bodenheimer HC, LaRusso NF, Thayer WR, et al. Elevated circulating immune complexes in primary

sclerosing cholangitis: pathogenetic implications. (Abstr) Hepatology 1981; 1:497.

90. Thomas TI, Ochs HD, Wedgwood RJ. Liver disease and immunodeficiency syndromes. Lancet 1974; 1:311.

91. Thompson HH, Pitt HA, Lewin KJ, et al. Sclerosing cholangitis and histiocytosis X. Gut 1984; 25:526–30.

92. Schrumpf E, Fausa O, Forre O, et al. HLA antigens and immunoregulatory T cells in ulcerative colitis associated with hepatobiliary disease. Scand J Gastroenterol 1982; 17:187–91.

93. Chapman RW, Varghese Z, Gaul R, et al. Association of primary sclerosing cholangitis with HLA B8. Gut 1983; 24:38–41.

94. Alpert LI, Jindrak K. Idiopathic retroperitoneal fibrosis and sclerosing cholangitis associated with reticulum cell sarcoma. Gastroenterology 1972; 62:111–7.

95. Chapman RWG, Marbough BA, Rhodes JM, et al. Primary sclerosing cholangitis: a review of its clinical features, cholangiography, and hepatic histology. Gut 1980; 21:870–7.

96. Ludwig J, Barham SS, LaRusso NF, et al. Morphologic features of chronic hepatitis associated with primary sclerosing cholangitis and chronic ulcerative colitis. Hepatology 1981; 1:632–40.

97. Barbatis C, Grases P, Shepherd HA, et al. Histological features of sclerosing cholangitis in patients with chronic ulcerative colitis. J Clin Pathol 1985; 38:778–83.

98. Blackstone MA, Nemchausky B. Cholangiographic abnormalities in ulcerative colitis–associated pericholangitis which resemble sclerosing cholangitis. Dig Dis 1978; 23:579–85.

99. Galambos JT, Brooks WS Jr. Atypical biliary cirrhosis or sclerosing cholangitis. J Clin Gastroenterol 1980; 2:43–52.

100. Rohrmann CA Jr, Ansel HJ, Freeny PC, et al. Cholangiographic abnormalities in patients with inflammatory bowel disease. Radiology 1978; 127:635–41.

101. MacCarty RL, LaRusso NF, Wiesner RH, et al. Primary sclerosing cholangitis: findings on cholangiography and pancreatography. Radiology 1983; 149:39–44.

102. Epstein O, Chapman RWG, Lake-Bakaar G, et al. The pancreas in primary biliary cirrhosis and primary sclerosing cholangitis. Gastroenterology 1982; 83:1177–82.

103. Palmer KR, Cotton PB, Chapman M. Pancreatogram in cholestasis. Gut 1984; 25:424–7.

104. Summerfield JA, Elias E, Hungerford GD, et al. The biliary system in primary biliary cirrhosis. A study by endoscopic retrograde cholangiopancreatography. Gastroenterology 1976; 70:240–3.

105. Rohrmann CA Jr, Ansel HJ, Ayoola EA, et al. Endoscopic retrograde intrahepatic cholangiogram: radiographic findings in intrahepatic disease. AJR 1977; 128:45–52.

106. Falkenstein DB, Riccobono C, Sidhu G, et al. The endoscopic intrahepatic cholangiogram. Clinicopathologic correlation with postmortem cholangiograms. Invest Radiol 1975; 10:358–65.

107. MacCarty RL, LaRusso NF, May GR, Ludwig J. Cholangiocarcinoma complicating primary sclerosing cholangitis: cholangiographic appearances. Radiology 1985; 156:43–6.

108. Wee A, Ludwig J, Coffey RJ Jr, et al. Hepatobiliary carcinoma associated with primary sclerosing cholangitis and chronic ulcerative colitis. Hum Pathol 1985; 16:719–26.

109. Curzio M, Bernasconi G, Gullotta R, et al. Association of ulcerative colitis, sclerosing cholangitis and cholangiocarcinoma in a patient with IgA deficiency. Endoscopy 1985; 17:123–5.

110. Gluskin LE, Payne JA. Cystic dilatation as a radiographic sign of cholangiocarcinoma complicating sclerosing cholangitis. Am J Gastroenterol 1983; 78:661–4.

111. Golematis B, Giannopoulos A, Papchristou DN, Dreiling DA. Sclerosing cholangitis of the bifurcation of the common hepatic duct. Am J Gastroenterol 1981; 75:370–2.

112. Smadja C, Bowley NB, Benjamin IS, et al. Idiopathic localized bile duct strictures: relationship to primary sclerosing cholangitis. Am J Surg 1983; 146:404–8.

113. Panes J, Bordas JM, Bruguera M, et al. Localized sclerosing cholangitis. Endoscopy 1985; 17:121–2.

114. Wood RAB, Cuschieri A. Is sclerosing cholangitis complicating ulcerative colitis a reversible condition? Lancet 1980; 2:716–8.

115. Kozarek RA, Brayko CM, Harlan J, et al. Endoscopic drainage of pancreatic pseudocysts. Gastrointest Endosc 1985; 31:322–68.

116. Aabakken L, Karesen R, Serck-Hanssen A, Osnes M. Transpapillary biopsies and brush cytology from the common bile duct. Endoscopy 1986; 18:49–51.

117. Bruggen JT, McPhee MS, Bhatia PS, Richter JM. Primary adenocarcinoma of the bile ducts. Clinical characteristics and natural history. Dig Dis Sci 1986; 31:840–6.

118. Siegel JH, Snady H. The significance of endoscopically placed prostheses in the management of biliary obstruction due to carcinoma of the pancreas: results of nonoperative decompression in 277 patients. Am J Gastroenterol 1986; 81:634–41.

119. Huibregtse K, Katon RM, Tytgat GN. Endoscopic treatment of postoperative biliary strictures. Endoscopy 1986; 18:133–7.

120. Mir-Madjlessi SH, Farmer RG, Sivak MV Jr. Bile duct carcinoma in patients with ulcerative colitis. Relationship to sclerosing cholangitis. Report of six cases and review of the literature. Dig Dis Sci 1987; 32:145–54.

Chapter 32

THE INTRAHEPATIC BILE DUCTS AND GALLBLADDER

JARL Å. JAKOBSEN, M.D.
MAGNE OSNES, M.D.

Endoscopic retrograde cholangiography (ERC) has brought about major improvements in the diagnosis and therapy of diseases of the biliary tract. The most important advances are exactness in diagnosis of extrahepatic biliary diseases, especially those involving the common bile duct, and differentiation between benign and malignant conditions. There has also been remarkable progress in endoscopic therapeutic intervention in diseases involving the common bile duct. Despite this emphasis on the extrahepatic bile ducts, endoscopic cannulation has also enhanced the diagnosis of gallbladder disease and diseases affecting the intrahepatic ductal system.

A major restriction in the recognition of abnormalities in the gallbladder and intrahepatic ducts is that the endoscopic and radiologic techniques are difficult to master; accurate diagnosis requires considerable experience. This chapter focuses on the main technical principles, radiologic and endoscopic, of performance of examinations that permit exact diagnosis and successful treatment. The typical cholangiographic findings of diseases in the gallbladder, liver and intrahepatic ducts in which ERC plays or may play an important role will be described.

TECHNIQUE

Endoscopic Equipment

Basic endoscopic equipment required for ERC is listed in Table 32–1. A side-viewing duodenoscope with a large-diameter instru-mental channel (4.2 mm) is preferable. This allows use of a relatively large-diameter forceps for intraductal biopsies. Although any flexible biopsy forceps can be used for biopsy in either the common bile duct or the intrahepatic ducts, one with a soft tip is preferable. This will pass the papilla and reach the target in the ductal system with greater ease. Sheathed brushes may be used to obtain cytologic specimens in some pathologic conditions that involve the intrahepatic ducts.

Catheters with distal tips of varying shapes and diameters may be useful when cannulation of the papilla of Vater is difficult. Several different configurations are shown in Figure 32–1, some of which are available commercially; others are "home-made." Certain standard catheters if heated carefully can be

TABLE 32–1. **Endoscopic Equipment for ERC**

For Diagnosis
1. Side-viewing duodenoscope with large biopsy channel (4.2 mm)
2. Biopsy forceps with "soft" tip
3. Sheathed cytology brush
4. Balloon catheter for occlusion and selective filling of intrahepatic ducts
5. Guide wires for selective cannulation of intrahepatic ducts

For Treatment
1. Balloon catheter for removal of intrahepatic calculi
2. Baskets for removal of intrahepatic calculi
3. Grundzig-type balloon catheters for dilation of strictures

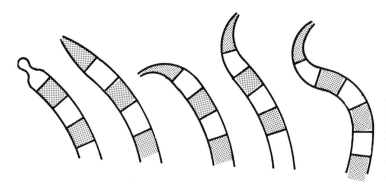

FIGURE 32–1. Catheters with variously shaped catheter tips, that may be useful when cannulation of the papilla of Vater is difficult. (Drawn by Per Engeseth. Reproduced with the permission of the Scandinavian Association for Digestive Endoscopy.)

shaped or drawn into different configurations; this depends, however, on the material of which the catheter is made.

For selective radiologic demonstration of an intrahepatic ductal segment, a balloon catheter may be of value. Contrast medium can be injected with gentle pressure and fluoroscopic monitoring when the balloon has been inflated to occlude the biliary system distal to the segment for selective study. In some instances a guide wire may also aid in cannulating the different intrahepatic ducts. Balloon and basket-type catheters may also be used for extraction of calculi from within the intrahepatic ducts. Grundiz-type balloon catheters can be used for dilation of strictures within the biliary system, in some cases with subsequent extraction of calculi lodged proximal to the stricture.

Peroral cholangioscopes are also being developed for use in conjunction with ERC for direct visualization of the ductal system. These instruments allow direct-vision biopsy of lesions within the ducts (see Chapter 10, Part 4).

Radiologic Equipment

The radiologic equipment needed for examination during ERC is listed in Table 32–2. The x-ray machine must be equipped with a movable table that allows x-ray exposures in different positions. A high resolution fluoroscopic unit is necessary for detection of small abnormalities. At any point in the examination it may be necessary to immediately document these fine variations of the normal anatomy. X-ray films may be made by using standard-size film and a conventional spot filming system, although a rapid camera system with smaller-size x-ray film provides a short exposure time and a fast method of documentation during filling of the duct system.

In addition to the standard compression apparatus of the x-ray machine, a compression device that operates on the principle of an inflatable rubber ball is useful.

The x-ray contrast agent should be a standard water-soluble iodine medium. The concentration of iodine should be low (200 mg/ml).

Gallbladder Examination During Endoscopy

Some important technical principles must be considered in order to obtain a satisfactory examination of the gallbladder with a high degree of diagnostic accuracy (Table 32–3). Following cannulation of the common bile duct, contrast material is injected under continuous fluoroscopic control. The main technical problem with demonstration of gallbladder disease is overfilling of the gallbladder with contrast agent. This often causes

TABLE 32–2. **Radiologic Equipment for Gallbladder and Intrahepatic Duct Examination During ERCP**

1. X-ray apparatus
   Tiltable, movable table
   Capability for horizontal beam x-rays
      (patient either upright or flat)

2. Standard fluoroscopy capability
   Additional monitor for endoscopist
   On/off foot pedal for endoscopist

3. Imaging system
   Spot-film system, standard film size (24 × 30 cm and 18 × 24 cm)
   Smaller-size film camera system (100 mm/70 mm)

4. Compression device
   Built into the x-ray apparatus
   Additional inflatable compression device

5. Standard contrast material (200 mg iodine/ml)

TABLE 32–3. **Radiologic Procedures for Gallbladder Examination During Endoscopy**

1. X-ray exposures when filling gallbladder
2. X-ray exposures with cystic duct filled
3. X-ray exposures in prone position with thin layer of contrast agent

dense opacification that consequently obscures the presence of small calculi.

The phenomenon of overopacification cannot be avoided by the use of contrast material with a low iodine concentration. The retrograde injection can be stopped when the cystic duct is filled or when the medium reaches the infundibulum of the gallbladder (Fig. 32–2), although sometimes excessive filling during the procedure cannot be avoided. Therefore, it may be necessary to interrupt the injection when a sufficient quantity of contrast medium has entered the gallbladder to obtain a series of x-rays before proceeding to complete opacification of the biliary system. Ordinarily the normal cystic duct and gallbladder will fill with contrast material automatically during the injection. However, lack of opacification does not necessarily indicate blockage of the cystic duct, and therefore cannulation of the cystic duct may be required to verify stenosis or occlusion (Fig. 32–3). During the endoscopic procedure it may also be necessary to change the patient's position from semi-prone (right shoulder raised) to prone to improve the radiologic view of the gallbladder.

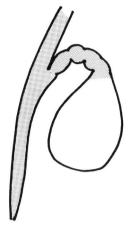

FIGURE 32–2. Contrast injection (shaded area) is stopped before it reaches the infundibulum of the gallbladder to avoid overfilling. (Drawn by Per Engeseth. Reproduced with the permission of the Scandinavian Association for Digestive Endoscopy.)

Gallbladder Examination After Endoscopy

The radiologic examination of the gallbladder after completion of the endoscopic phase of the procedure is summarized in Table 32–4. After removal of the endoscope, the patient is turned supine and a series of x-rays are made while gradually changing the subject's position from recumbent to half-upright or to standing (Fig. 32–4). During elevation toward the standing position, the gallbladder will fill with contrast agent, if not already opacified, unless an occlusion or ste-

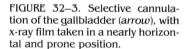

FIGURE 32–3. Selective cannulation of the gallbladder (*arrow*), with x-ray film taken in a nearly horizontal and prone position.

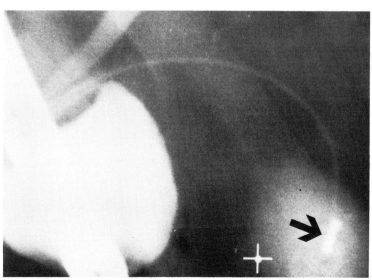

nosis of the cystic duct is present. Ideally, the first x-ray film should be taken when the gallbladder is coated with a thin layer of contrast. By elevating the patient toward the upright position it is not difficult to demonstrate movement of a filling defect(s). This confirms the diagnosis of calculi. Compression over the area of the gallbladder will move contrast material or air-filled loops of bowel from the x-ray field.

If after these procedures the status of the gallbladder is still unclear or the diagnosis uncertain, x-ray films should be obtained using a horizontal x-ray beam with the patient in a right lateral ducubitus position. The patient may be tilted upward and downward in this position (Fig. 32–5). Sometimes the best x-ray views are obtained when the patient executes a sustained expiration (Fig. 32–6). To demonstrate floating calculi it may be necessary to obtain delayed x-rays using the horizontal beam (Fig. 32–7).

After obtaining x-ray films utilizing the right lateral decubitus position, the patient may be turned to the supine position and further exposures made. As the contrast material shifts within the gallbladder, certain parts of the gallbladder will remain coated with a thin layer of contrast agent. This is ideal for x-ray study of the mucosal surface. By taking advantage of this phenomenon during the various changes in the patient's position, the entire mucosal surface of the gallbladder may be examined. With the use of the techniques described, it is unnecessary for the patient to ingest drugs or fatty meals in order to contract the gallbladder.

Examination of Intrahepatic Ducts During Endoscopy

The main technical points with reference to radiologic examination of the intrahepatic ducts during endoscopy are listed in Table 32–5. After injection of contrast medium by standard ERCP technique the intrahepatic ducts will be visualized in most cases. With the patient in the semi-prone position (right shoulder slightly raised), the left hepatic duct will fill with contrast material first. Sometimes significant filling of the intrahepatic ducts in the right lobe can be obtained with this technique. When this is not accomplished, the right ductal system may be filled by turning the patient to a prone or supine position during the endoscopic procedure. Although the right hepatic duct is generally oriented along the long axis of the body, it also has a somewhat posterior course. In the prone position this may mean that the course of the duct is upward and consequently the flow of contrast into the duct is opposed by gravity. Thus, in certain positions the left system may fill preferentially. Tilting the patient's head downward may also aid in filling the right hepatic system. Lack of filling of one of the intrahepatic systems based on these normal anatomic features can be misinterpreted as evidence of obstruction.

Generally the intrahepatic ducts fill more readily after cholecystectomy. When the gallbladder is present it often acts as a low-pressure reservoir. With standard injection technique with the catheter tip at the papilla, the gallbladder will fill in preference to the intrahepatic system; dense gallbladder opacification must then occur before the intrahepatic system begins to fill to any significant degree. Overdistention of the gallbladder may result in nausea and vomiting. When the intrahepatic ducts are the main object of the examination better filling may be achieved by deep cannulation to the bifurcation or selective cannulation of either of the intrahepatic ducts with the standard catheter (Fig. 32–8). If a higher injection pressure is required for satisfactory opacification, a balloon catheter may be used to occlude the distal biliary system during the injection (Fig. 32–9). A standard stone retrieval balloon catheter is suitable for this purpose. Depending on where the balloon is positioned, this catheter can also be used to prevent runoff of contrast material into the gallbladder. A guide wire can be useful if difficulty is encountered in correctly positioning either the standard catheter for selective opacification or the balloon catheter for occlusion and opacification. High-quality x-ray films should be obtained during the endoscopic procedure

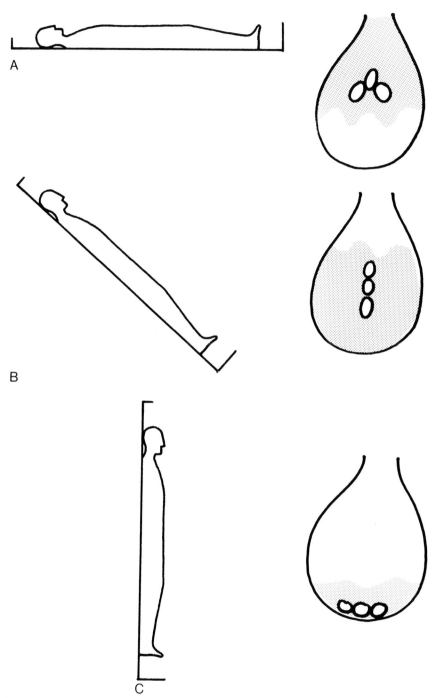

FIGURE 32–4. X-ray films of gallbladder are taken while gradually raising the patient from a horizontal (A) to a half-upright (B) to a standing (C) position in order to detect calculi and their motion. Also depicted is the movement of calculi in the gallbladder corresponding to the three patient positions. (Drawn by Per Engeseth. Reproduced with the permission of the Scandinavian Association for Digestive Endoscopy.)

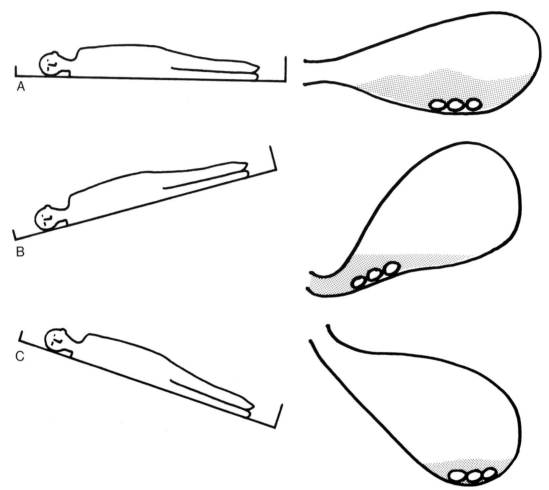

FIGURE 32–5. X-ray films of gallbladder are taken with the patient in right lateral decubitus position, either horizontal (A) or with head tilted downward (B) or upward (C). Also depicted is the movement of calculi in the gallbladder corresponding to the three patient positions. (Drawn by Per Engeseth. Reproduced with the permission of the Scandinavian Association for Digestive Endoscopy.)

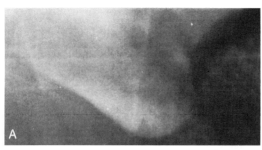

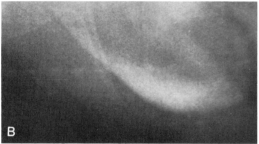

FIGURE 32–6. A, Contents of loop of bowel are shown overlying and obscuring the gallbladder. This can be avoided by having the patient exert maximum expiration while the x-ray film is being taken (B).

because of the relatively rapid emptying of the intrahepatic ducts when the injection is ended.

Examination of Intrahepatic Ducts After Endoscopy

Table 32–6 lists the main steps in the radiologic technique after the endoscopic phase of the procedure is completed. When the intrahepatic ducts are filled with contrast agent the endoscope is removed. The patient assumes a prone position and is then tilted head downward. Since contrast medium is heavier than bile, the effect of gravity will be advantageous in outlining various parts of the intrahepatic ductal system. With the pa-

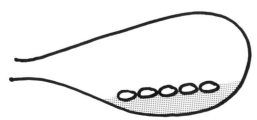

FIGURE 32–7. Diagram demonstrating position of floating calculi when x-ray film is taken on a delayed basis, using horizontal beam with the patient in right lateral decubitus position. (Drawn by Per Engeseth. Reproduced with the permission of the Scandinavian Association for Digestive Endoscopy.)

TABLE 32–5. Radiologic Procedures for Intrahepatic Duct Examination During Endoscopy

1. First spot film when contrast injection is nearly complete
2. Spot films when intrahepatic ducts are completely filled
3. Spot films after injection with occluding balloon catheter, after selective duct catheterization, or after positioning catheter in the mid-extrahepatic ductal system

tient in the prone, head-downward position the ventral and cranial parts of the bile ducts will be visualized (Fig. 32–10). When this maneuver does not produce complete filling of the upper aspect of the bile ducts, a pillow should be placed under the patient's abdomen. This position is also best for filling of the confluence of the right and left hepatic ducts (Figs. 32–10 and 32–11). The patient is then turned to the supine position, which results in opacification of the common bile duct and the dorsal parts of the intrahepatic ducts, particularly the right system (Figs. 32–10 and 32–12). X-ray films should also be taken under fluoroscopic guidance as the patient is raised toward an upright position. This ensures complete filling of the right posterior aspect of the intrahepatic ductal

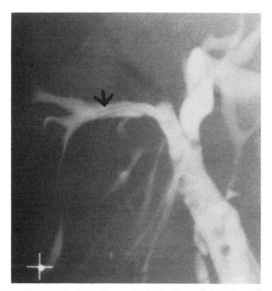

FIGURE 32–8. Selective catheterization of right hepatic duct (arrow indicates catheter) in patient with metastasis from papillary carcinoma. Air in biliary tree is due to endoscopic choledochoduodenostomy.

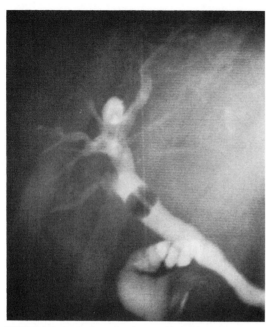

FIGURE 32–9. Catheterization and injection of contrast utilizing a balloon catheter to occlude the distal aspect of bile duct in a patient with cirrhosis.

system as well as the common bile duct (see Fig. 32–10).

Sometimes it is difficult to demonstrate the biliary ductal system proximal to an occlusion or stenosis. If the patient can be kept in a prone, head-downward position for a period of time, some contrast material may gradually flow into the proximal bile ducts. When this maneuver is successful, x-rays often reveal important information about the nature of the stenosis or obstruction (Figs. 32–10A and 32–13).

Some of the common sources of error in the radiologic examination of the gallbladder and intrahepatic ducts are listed in Table 32–7.

TABLE 32–6. Radiologic Procedures for Intrahepatic Duct Examination After Endoscopy*

1. First spot film with head tilted downward
2. Spot films after turning patient to supine position
3. Spot films with patient horizontal
4. Spot films while gradually tilting patient upright

*At each step, well-collimated exposures of regions of special interest must be taken. The entire duct system should be imaged in two projections to avoid false negative findings.

Other Diagnostic Procedures

There are many disorders of the bile ducts in which material for histologic examination is crucially important. Heretofore, such material was readily obtained at surgery. However, many nonsurgical methods of management have been introduced for a variety of pathologic conditions of the biliary tract. A number of techniques are available to obtain pathologic confirmation; our preference is transpapillary biopsy. The biopsy forceps is guided endoscopically through the papilla and then, under fluoroscopic control, to the lesion (Fig. 32–14). The main indication for this procedure is a lesion in the common bile duct (Fig. 32–15), but lesions in the intrahepatic ducts are also accessible. In some patients it may be necessary to perform an endoscopic papillotomy so that the forceps may be introduced more easily. In our experience with this technique, malignant disease of the bile ducts can be correctly diagnosed in 80% of cases with no false positive findings.

The use of a sheathed cytology brush may provide additional information. This accessory is especially helpful with stenotic lesions, the most common indication for its use. Following introduction through the papilla, the sheath is passed within or through the stenotic segment, and then the brush is advanced beyond the sheath and pushed and pulled several times through the pathologic segment before retracting it into the sheath. The results of brushing cytology of the bile ducts are, however, not entirely satisfactory.[1]

Intraductal cholangioscopy provides direct visualization of pathologic processes in the bile ducts. Peroral cholangioscopy is discussed in Part 4 of Chapter 10. Certain types of cholangioscopes have an accessory channel that makes it possible to obtain biopsies under visual control, and in a few instances to perform other therapeutic maneuvers. In our experience, the present instruments are heavy and difficult to use, although improvements in design can be expected.

DISEASES OF THE GALLBLADDER
Calculi

Cholecystolithiasis is usually diagnosed by methods other than ERC, most often ultrasonography and cholecystography. False negative findings may, however, be a problem with these examinations.[2] The use of intra-

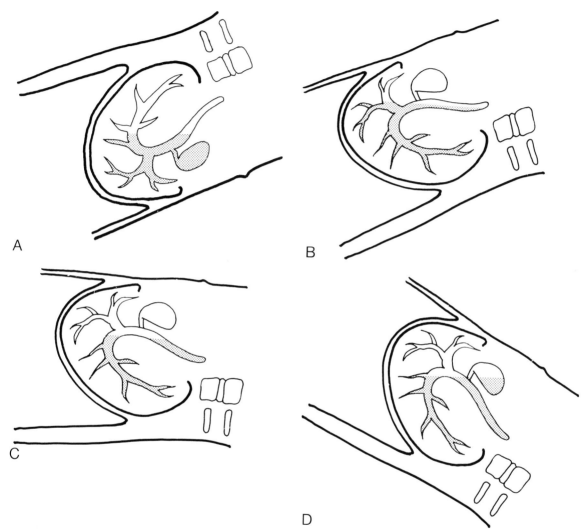

FIGURE 32–10. Diagrams of various essential positions for visualization of different parts of the intrahepatic ductal system. *A*, Patient prone, head downward; *B*, patient supine, head downward; *C*, patient supine and horizontal; *D*, patient supine, head upward. Note pooling of contrast (*shaded area*) within ducts, as a result of the influence of gravity. (Drawn by Per Engeseth. Reproduced with the permission of the Scandinavian Association for Digestive Endoscopy.)

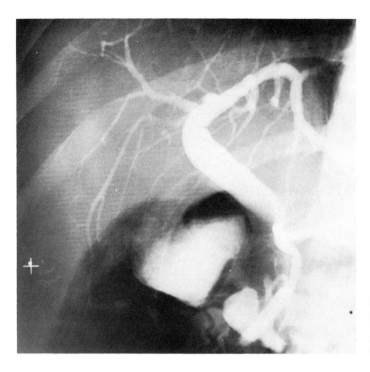

FIGURE 32–11. X-ray film of intrahepatic ducts made with patient in prone position with head tilted downward. Note good opacification of common bile duct and left hepatic ducts.

FIGURE 32–12. Intrahepatic cholangiogram with patient supine, head tilted downward. The right hepatic duct and right intrahepatic ducts (*arrowhead*) are well visualized (same examination as in Figure 32–11).

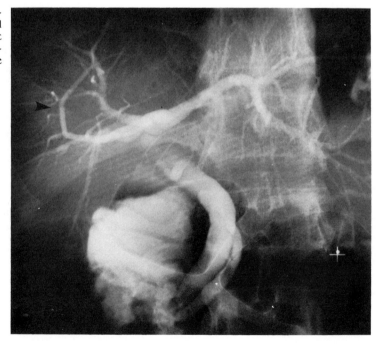

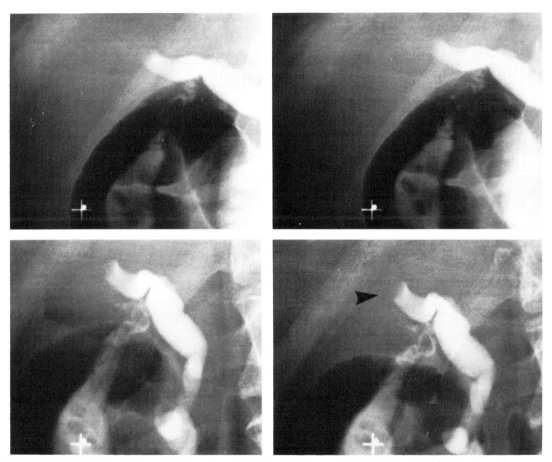

FIGURE 32–13. Malignant stenosis of common hepatic duct demonstrated while maintaining patient in prone, head-down position for a period of time. Sequence of x-ray films, which were taken over a course of several minutes, are arranged from left to right, top to bottom, with last film (*lower right*) demonstrating tumor (*arrowhead*). Calculi are also visible in gallbladder.

TABLE 32–7. **Technical Problems with Radiology of the Gallbladder and Intrahepatic Ducts**

Gallbladder
1. Overopacification with contrast medium
2. Contrast medium in the gut obscures view
3. Feces in right colon mimic small calculi
4. Contrast medium and bile fail to mix

Intrahepatic Cholangiogram
1. Insufficient filling of right hepatic ducts

venous cholangiography is steadily decreasing.

The ERC examination of the gallbladder is a very sensitive method for detection of stones, even when these are very small.[2, 3] This, however, requires adherence to the technical principles outlined in the previous section. The best opportunity for detection of small stones occurs with the early filling images of the gallbladder when there is only a thin layer of contrast material present (Fig. 32–16). Movement of small defects differentiate calculi from polyps (Fig. 32–17). Large stones are easily detectable, during both early and later filling of the gallbladder (Figs. 32–18 and 32–19). If calculi are adherent to the mucosa, their differentiation from polyps is impossible, and patients with this finding should undergo ultrasonographic examination since acoustic shadowing of the calculi may resolve this dilemma.

Calculi may occlude the cystic duct. This occlusion sometimes appears radiologically as a stenosis, or the flowing contrast material may halt abruptly in a concave contour. If the calculi are small, the contrast medium may completely outline the stones (Fig. 32–20). Occlusion of the cystic duct is clinically significant if this finding is verified by adequate filling of the duct (Fig. 32–21), either by injection under somewhat higher pressure or selective catheterization and injection of the cystic duct. Calculi within a cystic duct remnant after cholecystectomy are also detectable (Fig. 32–22). These may be difficult to differentiate from a suture granuloma.

The triad of cystic duct stone, cholecystitis, and benign stenotic occlusion of the common bile duct with icterus is termed the Mirizzi syndrome. The main ERC findings are smooth stenosis of the common hepatic duct, or a short, rounded indentation.[4] Depending on the degree of stenosis there may be dila-

tion of the intrahepatic ducts. In some instances it may be possible for contrast medium to enter the gallbladder, and thereby a stone and other abnormalities may be visualized. The main differential diagnosis is malignancy involving the gallbladder or common bile duct. The Mirizzi syndrome is also discussed in Chapter 32.

Chronic Cholecystitis

Cholelithiasis is the most common finding in chronic cholecystitis. Other abnormalities demonstrable by ERC are a shrunken gallbladder and an irregular, rigid wall (Fig. 32–23). Pseudopolyps that produce filling defects that do not move with changes in the patient's position may also be found. In some patients there is occlusion, either by inflammation or impacted stone in the cystic duct, that makes opacification of the gallbladder impossible (Fig. 32–24).

Tumors

Conventional radiologic examination in carcinoma of the gallbladder is difficult and neither sensitive nor specific.[5] A direct cholangiogram, as with ERC, will outline the entire biliary duct system if there is no occlusion. A tumor still localized to the gallbladder may be seen as a polyp or filling defect in a stiff, rigid, immobile gallbladder (Fig. 32–25). However, the tumor may infiltrate and occlude the cystic duct (Fig. 32–26). Often the common bile duct or the common hepatic duct or both may be involved, with infiltration or stenoses of either duct being the only finding. Infiltration of the liver is also frequent and may be detected with filling of the intrahepatic ducts (see Fig. 32–26).

The presence of calculi, either in the gallbladder or bile ducts, is a common finding with carcinoma of the gallbladder (see Fig. 32–26).

Transpapillary biopsies or material for cytologic examination should be obtained when possible. The diagnosis may also be established by guided transcutaneous biopsy or cytology, and further definition of the mass lesion may be obtained by computed tomography or ultrasonography. At ERC, direct inspection of the upper gastrointestinal tract may occasionally reveal involvement by the cancer, particularly in the duodenum.

A benign tumor of the gallbladder is an exceedingly rare finding during ERC. It is

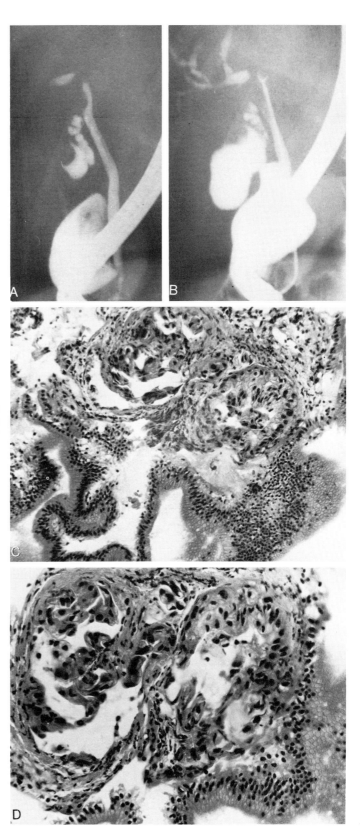

FIGURE 32–14. *A,* Radiograph of stenosis of bile duct. *B,* Transpapillary biopsy with forceps open at stenosis. *C,* Biopsy specimen (175×). *D,* Biopsy specimen (280×).

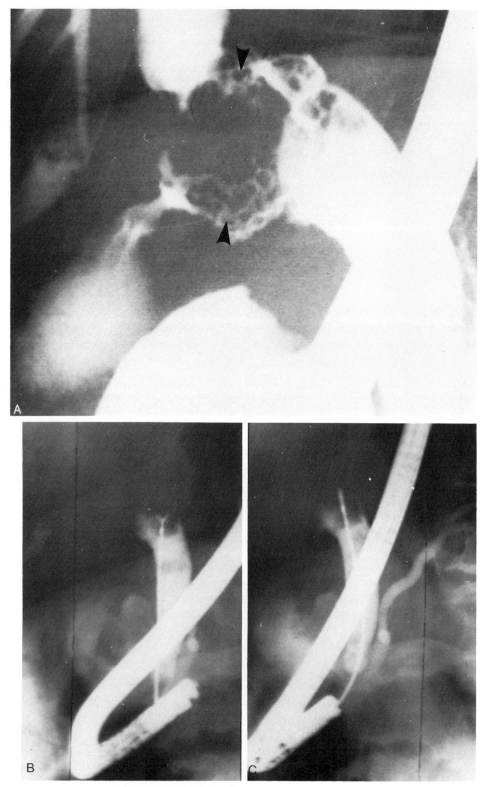

FIGURE 32–15. *A,* Adenoma (*arrowheads*) has irregular contour in common hepatic duct. *B,* Transpapillary biopsy with forceps open at lesion. *C,* Closure of forceps.

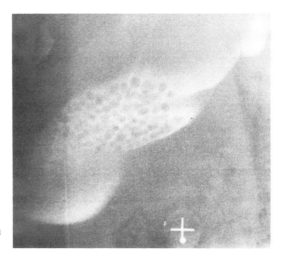

FIGURE 32–16. Cholelithiasis. Thin contrast material in gallbladder outlines multiple small filling defects.

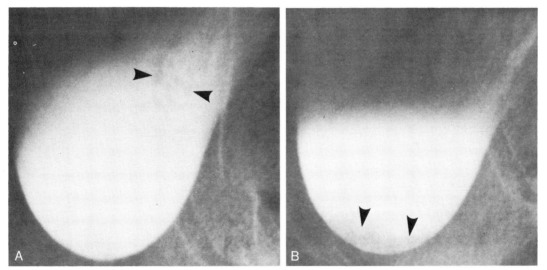

FIGURE 32–17. Small calculi in gallbladder. Position of calculi (*arrowheads*) within gallbladder changes as patient is raised from flat (*A*) to standing (*B*) position.

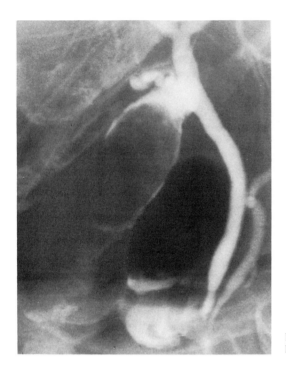

FIGURE 32–18. Cholelithiasis. Gallbladder contains a large stone.

FIGURE 32–19. Thin layer of contrast material demonstrates calculus in gallbladder (*arrow*). Cystic duct drains into an intrahepatic duct (*arrowhead*). Recognition of this anomaly is important to the operating surgeon.

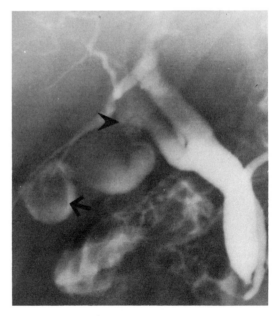

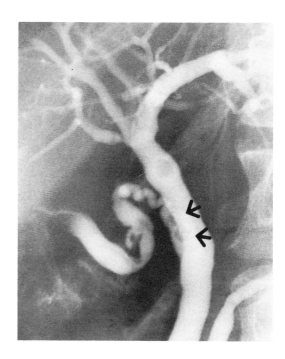

FIGURE 32–20. Calculi in cystic duct (*arrows*).

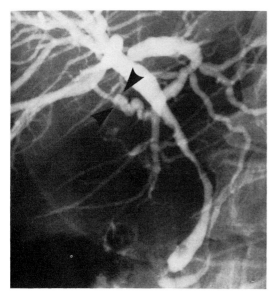

FIGURE 32–21. Occlusion of cystic duct (*between arrowheads*). Note relative stenosis of common duct due to inflammation of gallbladder.

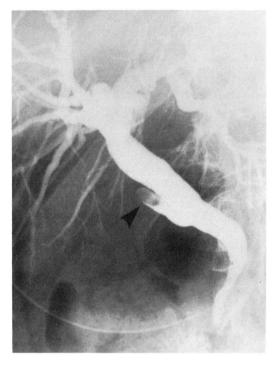

FIGURE 32–22. Calculus (*arrow*) in cystic duct remnant in patient who had undergone cholecystectomy. Calculus was removed after endoscopic papillotomy.

FIGURE 32–23. Chronic, acalculous cholecystitis. Gallbladder is shrunken and its wall is irregular (*arrowheads*).

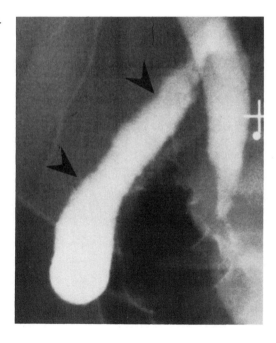

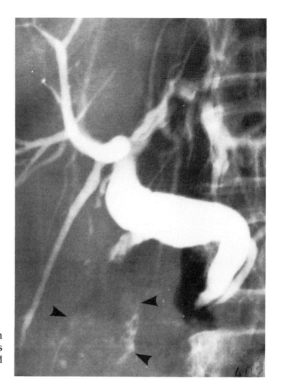

FIGURE 32–24. "Porcelain" gallbladder. Calcifications in wall are seen *en face* and in profile (*arrowheads*). There is occlusion of the cystic duct. Histologic study of resected specimen revealed chronic cholecystitis.

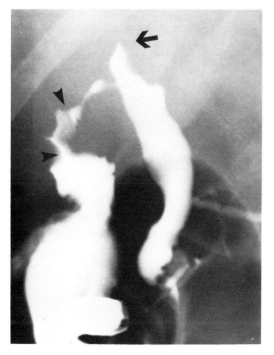

FIGURE 32–25. Carcinoma of gallbladder infiltrating gallbladder and cystic duct (*arrowheads*) as well as hilus (arrow).

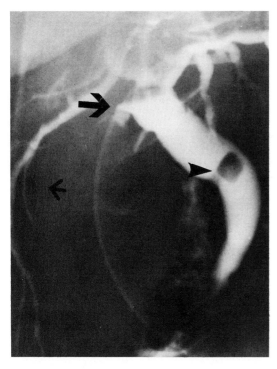

FIGURE 32–26. Carcinoma of gallbladder. Note occlusion of cystic duct by tumor (*large arrow*) and calculus (*arrowhead*) in common duct. Displacement of intrahepatic bile ducts is also present (*small arrow*).

probably impossible to differentiate such a lesion from a carcinoma by any method other than operation. There are no specific ERC findings for benign gallbladder tumors.

Cholesterolosis and Adenomyomatosis of the Gallbladder

The classification of cholesterolosis and adenomyomatosis is under discussion.[6] Mor-

phologically, the polypoid form of cholesterolosis and the annular (segmental) and localized form of adenomyomatosis are of interest here. The finding, which consists of one or more persistent filling defects, may be the same for both diseases (Fig. 32–27). Radiologic views of such lesions should be obtained *en face* as well as "profile." Compression must be utilized to determine whether the gallbladder wall is stiff or pliable. Both cholesterolosis and adenomyomatosis are

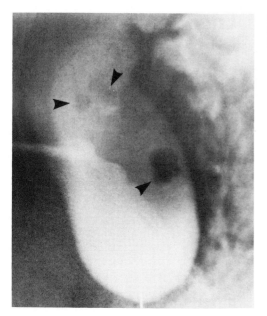

FIGURE 32–27. The defects shown (*arrowheads*), which did not move with changes in patient position, proved to be due to cholesterolosis of gallbladder.

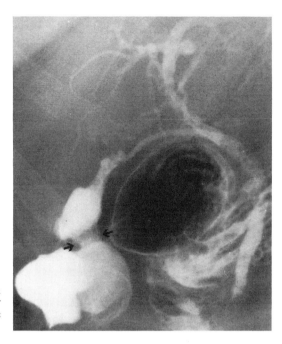

FIGURE 32–28. Cholecystocolonic fistula. Wide fistula (*between arrows*) present between shrunken gallbladder and hepatic flexure of colon. Numerous air bubbles are present in biliary ducts.

most often found in association with cholelithiasis.

Trauma

ERC may occasionally be indicated for the patient who has sustained acute trauma. The

gallbladder is injured in less than 2% of cases of major blunt injury to the abdomen.[7] However, delayed rupture has been reported.[8] This may occur directly into the peritoneal cavity and is diagnosed by leakage of contrast agent from the gallbladder during ERC. The rupture may also be into the liver, and this

FIGURE 32–29. Cholecystoduodenal fistula demonstrated by direct injection of contrast agent (*arrowheads*) through fistula into gallbladder.

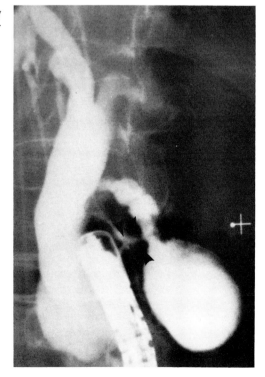

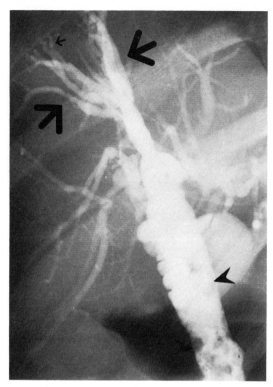

FIGURE 32–30. Numerous calculi are present in extra-hepatic bile ducts (*arrowheads*) of patient with chronic active hepatitis. Note approximation of ducts in right lobe (*large arrows*) as well as tortuosity (*small arrow*) and a short stenosis.

also may be recognized by ERC.[8] Perforation of the gallbladder may occur as a result of percutaneous liver biopsy.

Fistula

Usually a fistula between the gallbladder and neighboring organs forms as a result of infection or after operation. Occasionally it may occur in conjunction with a carcinoma in the region. The diagnosis is often confirmed by a barium meal or enema, but when the location or presence of fistula is in doubt it may be necessary to obtain contrast studies of the biliary system. After first achieving satisfactory opacification of the gallbladder (Fig. 32–28) or cystic duct, the course, direction, and termination of the escaping contrast medium may be studied. Endoscopy offers the possibility of direct cannulation and inspection of the fistula itself (Fig. 32–29) if it terminates in the duodenum or stomach. When carcinoma is suspected as the underlying cause, biopsy specimens from the intestinal terminus of the fistula may be positive.

DISEASES OF THE LIVER
Hepatitis

The major characteristic radiologic findings in the intrahepatic ducts in various diseases of the liver and bile ducts are summarized in Table 32–8. There are no significant radiologic changes in the intrahepatic biliary tree in acute hepatitis. In chronic active hepatitis, however, Rohrmann et al.[9] have described tortuosity of ducts in one patient and approximation of intrahepatic ducts in another. Changes in the intrahepatic ducts have also been reported by Hamilton and coworkers[10] in five patients, three of whom also had gallstones. The latter occurrence stresses the importance of direct cholangiography in patients with chronic liver disease and jaundice (Fig. 32–30).

Cirrhosis

Radiographic changes in the intrahepatic ducts are commonly found when ERC is performed in patients with cirrhosis.[11] A wide spectrum of ductal abnormalities are seen, the exact pattern being dependent on the degree and severity of cirrhosis rather than on specific causes (Fig. 32–31; also see Table 32–8). The most common finding is diminished branching, frequently termed "pruning" because of an appearance similar to that of a pruned tree.[9, 11] Multifocal stenoses of varying lengths and evidence of duct displacement are often present. The finer radicles may have a corkscrew shape, especially in micronodular cirrhosis. This same pattern of tortuous ducts with corkscrew-like changes is also found in primary biliary cirrhosis.[12] In this form of cirrhosis an external indentation or "notch" is found in the bile duct at the level of the porta hepatis more often than in other diseases.[10] This is thought to be due to enlargement of lymph glands in the liver hilum. However, neither this sign nor the other intrahepatic changes described are always present in cirrhosis, and a normal intrahepatic cholangiogram does not exclude cirrhosis. Gallstones are frequently found in primary biliary cirrhosis.[10, 12] The overall structure of the intrahepatic cholangiogram often suggests a decrease in the size of the liver in patients with cirrhosis (see Fig. 32–31B).

It is sometimes difficult to differentiate between the intrahepatic cholangiographic changes of cirrhosis and those of primary

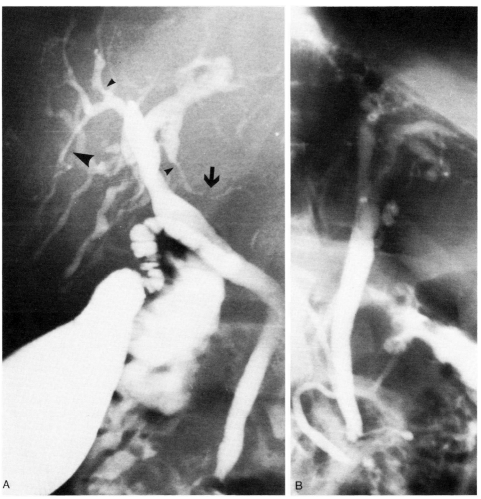

FIGURE 32–31. Contrast studies of patients with cirrhosis of liver. *A,* Intrahepatic bile ducts are tortuous, have multiple stenoses (*small arrowhead*), are somewhat displaced (*large arrow*), and exhibit stretching (*large arrowhead*). *B,* Outline of intrahepatic ducts indicates a liver of diminished size.

TABLE 32–8. Characteristic Intrahepatic Radiographic Findings in Liver and Biliary Diseases

Radiographic Finding*	Disease				
	Fatty Infiltration	Cirrhosis	PSC	Cholangitis	Tumors
Extrahepatic changes		(+)	+ +	+	
Displacement		+			+ +
Separation	+	+			+
Approximation		+			+
Stretching	+	+			
Pruning	+	+ +	+	(+)	
Obstruction		+			+ +
Focal stenosis		+ +	+ +	+	(+)
Focal dilation			+	+	+
Diffuse stenosis		+			+
Diffuse dilation				+	
Irregular wall		(+)	+		
Tortuosity		+			
Beading			+		

*Dilation with tumors usually occurs peripheral to stenosis caused by tumor. Numerous segments of focal stenosis and dilation in PSC produce the finding called "beading." In primary biliary cirrhosis lymph node compression of the bile duct in the portal region is often found.

PSC = primary sclerosing cholangitis; + = degree to which finding is encountered; (+) = variably present finding or one which is not a prominent feature.

sclerosing cholangitis confined to the intrahepatic ducts. Displacement of intrahepatic ducts, medium-length stenoses, and pruning are the more prominent features in cirrhosis. When signs of ductal displacement are prominent, however, the presence of multiple metastases must also be considered.

Fatty Infiltration

Cholangiographic findings have been reported in only a few patients with fatty infiltration of the liver. The intrahepatic ducts are straight and perhaps may appear stretched and separated.[13] A diffuse decrease in ductal caliber and diminished arborization (pruning) are also found.[9] Intrahepatic obstruction, which reportedly can be transient, also has been noted.[9] However, the use of proper radiologic and endoscopic opacification techniques must be stressed with respect to the appearance of obstructed ducts, since this finding may be false positive if filling is incomplete. Selective catheterization and the other techniques described in the preceding section will resolve this problem. In our experience the radiographic changes of fatty infiltration are usually discrete and focal and

not so fully developed as those that occur in cirrhosis.

Malignant Liver Tumors

There are no specific radiographic findings that differentiate between primary and metastatic liver tumors except for evidence of multiplicity. The most characteristic findings are displacement of the ducts, either alone or in combination with abrupt obstruction[9, 13] (Fig. 32–32). Stenosis is also found, especially when there is displacement of ducts. This most often appears as a gradually narrowing segment with smooth margins and is frequently associated with dilation of the more peripheral duct. These various findings taken together may give the impression of a mass lesion. In addition, separation or approximation of ducts may be observed, but irregularity of the walls of the intrahepatic ducts is usually not seen (Fig. 32–33).

Abscess

ERC is not usually a primary method of investigation when a liver abscess is suspected. However, if the abscess communi-

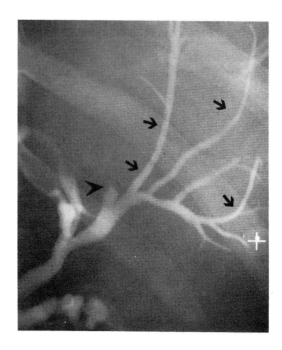

FIGURE 32–32. Multiple metastases at operation. There is occlusion of an intrahepatic bile duct (*arrowhead*) and displacement of other intrahepatic ducts (*arrows*).

cates with the biliary tree, it may fill with contrast medium during retrograde injection, in which case an irregular cavity will be demonstrated. The intrahepatic ducts leading to the necrotic area are often irregular (Fig. 32–34). When there is no communication with the biliary tree, the radiologic findings are those of a mass lesion. Depending on the causative agent, the abscess cavity may contain gas.

Trauma

A variety of other radiologic and clinical methods of investigation usually are more appropriate than ERC in diagnosis of trauma to the liver. However, a history of penetrating trauma may raise a question as to diagnosis and the exact nature of the injury. In stable patients ERC offers a unique opportunity for visualization of the biliary tree. Damage to

FIGURE 32–33. Displacement of bile duct by large liver cyst (*arrowheads*).

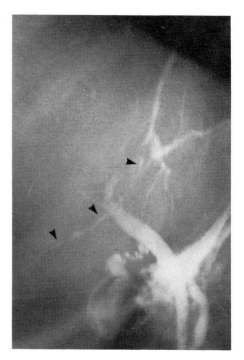

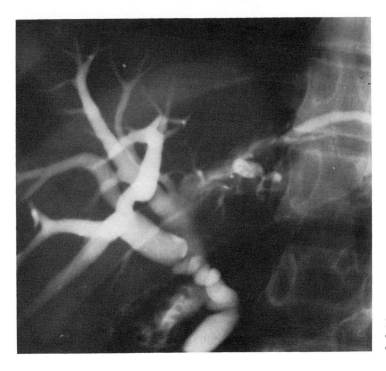

FIGURE 32–34. Abscess in left lobe of liver. Gross irregularities in bile ducts are notable.

FIGURE 32–35. Biliary-bronchial fistula as a result of gunshot trauma. Contrast material from bile ducts (*small arrowheads*) fills cavity (*large arrowheads*) and enters a bronchus (*arrows*).

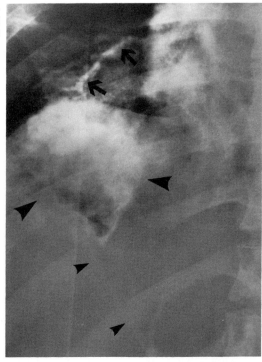

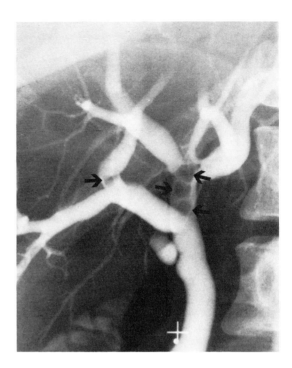

FIGURE 32–36. Calculi (*arrows*) in intrahepatic ducts.

DISEASES OF THE INTRAHEPATIC BILE DUCTS

Calculi

the extrahepatic ducts as well as intrahepatic fistulas can be defined (Fig. 32–35). In addition, the gallbladder and pancreas can be examined during the same procedure, and hematobilia may be recognized.[8]

Careful radiographic study of the intrahepatic ducts for calculi should be performed in patients with cholelithiasis, choledocholithiasis, cholangitis, stenoses and anomalies of the bile ducts, chronic hepatitis, and different forms of cirrhosis. Diagnosis is based upon the demonstration of a movable filling defect or defects (Figs. 32–36 and 32–37). An apparent filling defect in the column of contrast material in the region of the liver hilum can be caused by the right hepatic artery as it crosses the bile duct. This is sometimes termed a "pseudostone" and may be erroneously diagnosed as a tumor or stone.[14]

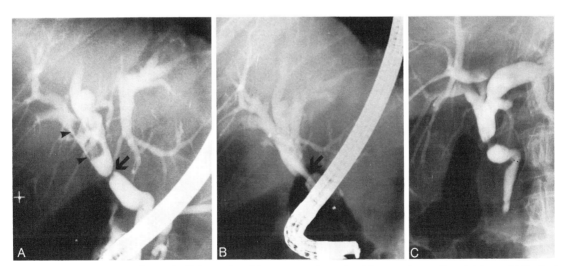

FIGURE 32–37. *A,* At least four calculi (*arrowheads*) are present proximal to a postoperative stricture of bile duct (*arrow*). *B,* Dilation of stricture by Grundzig-type hydrostatic balloon catheter (*arrow*). *C,* X-ray film taken after basket extraction of calculi.

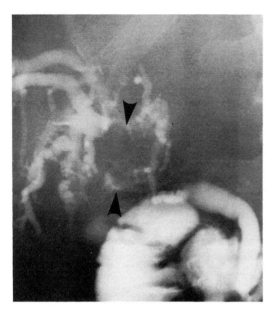

FIGURE 32–38. Large calculi (*arrowheads*) in region of hilus, with dilated intrahepatic ducts. Differentiation between stone and tumor in such cases is difficult.

Large stones in the region of the hilum may be difficult or impossible to differentiate from a tumor (Fig. 32–38); biopsy specimens can be of critical importance in such cases.

Primary Sclerosing Cholangitis

There has been a recent increase in interest and recognition of primary sclerosing cholangitis,[15] which is often associated with inflammatory bowel diseases, usually ulcerative colitis. Diffuse, multifocal, short stric-

tures with a patchy distribution throughout the liver, with involvement of both intrahepatic and extrahepatic ducts, are the most common radiographic findings.[16] Some degree of focal dilation is often found, producing the characteristic "beaded" appearance (Fig. 32–39). Slight irregularities in the wall of the intrahepatic ducts that produce a "shaggy" appearance may also be seen (Fig. 32–40). This is a relatively specific finding, although malignancy must be considered if the irregularities appear relatively coarse. Di-

FIGURE 32–39. Sclerosing cholangitis. There are changes in extrahepatic ducts (*arrow*) as well as intrahepatic ducts (*arrowhead*), with a "beaded" appearance in intrahepatic portion.

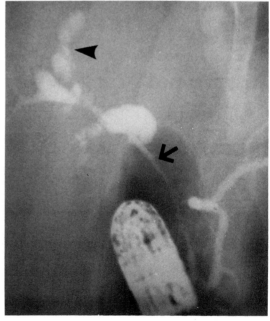

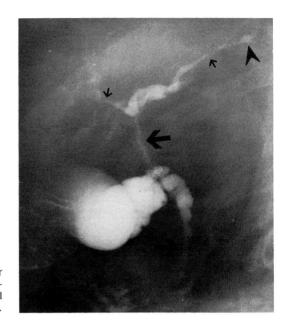

FIGURE 32–40. Sclerosing cholangitis. Multiple irregular areas of stenosis are present in intrahepatic (*small arrows*) and extrahepatic (*large arrows*) bile ducts. Focal dilation (*arrowhead*) of intrahepatic ducts is also notable.

lation peripheral to stenotic segments has a focal character, and diffuse dilation of the entire biliary tree is extremely uncommon. Some degree of pruning may occur.

Primary biliary cirrhosis may cause cholangiographic changes similar to those of primary sclerosing cholangitis, but in general stricturing is less pronounced and is more peripheral in location, and the extrahepatic ducts usually are not affected. In primary biliary cirrhosis there may also be ductal changes of concomitant cirrhosis.

Secondary Cholangitis

Secondary cholangitis may be associated with most diseases of the biliary tree or liver, such as cholelithiasis, cholangiocarcinoma, stricture, previous surgery in the region, and congenital abnormalities. The findings of the underlying disease usually dominate the radiologic picture. The primary disease process is usually located in the extrahepatic bile ducts and often causes dilation of these structures; consequently dilation of the intrahepatic biliary tree is the most common finding in association with secondary cholangitis.[9, 11] In some patients short stenoses and some degree of pruning may be seen (Fig. 32–41).

Bile Duct Carcinoma

About 4% to 8% of bile duct carcinomas arise in the intrahepatic ducts.[17, 18] The usual radiologic findings are those of a mass lesion. The size of the mass varies from a small discrete nodule to larger lesions several centimeters in diameter. Hence the appearance may be that of a small filling defect, although the most common findings are stricturing, displacement, and occlusion of the ducts (see Fig. 32–14). The stricture is often smooth and regular in contour (Fig. 32–42). A very unusual and uncommon diffuse infiltrating variant of bile duct carcinoma is difficult to distinguish from primary sclerosing cholangitis. Cholelithiasis is often found in association with ductal carcinoma.

Parasitic Diseases

One of the most common parasitic diseases encountered during ERC is the unilocular form of *Echinococcus granulosus*. The cholangiographic findings are those of a mass lesion; rupture into bile ducts also has been reported.[18]

Clonorchis sinensis infestation is common in Asia. ERC findings are not fully established or correlated with the clinical stages of this disease. However, cholangiography will demonstrate small or large filling defects as well as varying dilation of bile ducts[18] (Fig. 32–43).

The presenting symptoms of ascariasis may be jaundice or biliary colic. ERC may play a role in the evaluation of patients with these signs and symptoms. The radiographic pic-

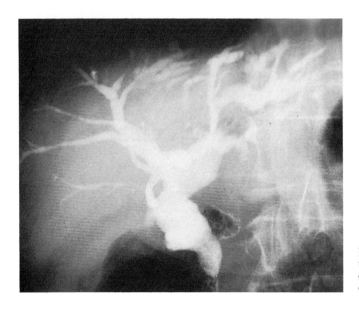

FIGURE 32–41. Secondary cholangitis due to gallstone disease. Stones were removed endoscopically. Note stenosis and some degree of pruning of intrahepatic ducts.

FIGURE 32–42. Infiltration by cholangiocarcinoma in hilus (*arrowhead*). Right lobe of liver had been resected.

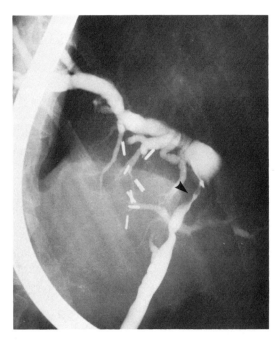

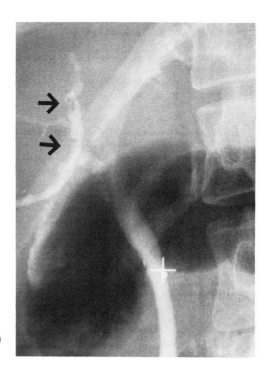

FIGURE 32–43. *Clonorchis sinensis.* Filling defects (*arrows*) were produced by worm in bile ducts.

ture is a characteristic filling defect caused by the adult worm (Fig. 32–44). Complications such as strictures, calculi, and abscesses may also be found. Sometimes the worm may be seen in the papillary orifice during the endoscopic procedure.

Caroli's Disease

Most authors now regard Caroli's disease as a variant of periportal fibrosis. This fibrosis results in dilation of the large subsegmental intrahepatic ducts and produces a character-

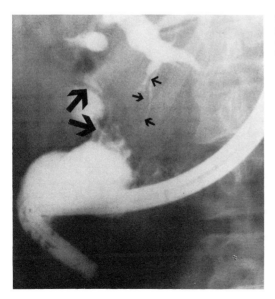

FIGURE 32–44. Intrahepatic ascariasis. Moving filling defects produced by worms are seen in both intrahepatic (*small arrows*) and extrahepatic (*large arrows*) bile ducts. Worms were later removed endoscopically.

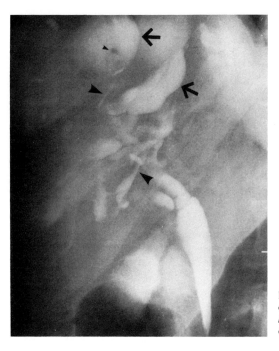

FIGURE 32–45. Caroli's disease. Subsegmental dilation of intrahepatic ducts (*arrows*) and stenoses (*large arrowheads*). A calculus (*small arrowhead*) is also visible within one dilated segment.

istic appearance sometimes likened to a "lollipop tree" (Fig. 32–45). Smooth-walled, long stenotic ductal segments may be present between dilated sections, and stone formation is common. Complications such as cholangitis and abscess formation may result in superimposition of other changes on the primary pattern and make interpretation of the cholangiogram difficult.

References

1. Harada H, Sasaki T, Yamamoto N, et al. Assessment of endoscopic aspiration cytology and endoscopic retrograde cholangio-pancreatography in patients with cancer of the hepato-biliary tract. Part II. Gastroenterol Jpn 1977; 12:59–64.
2. Osnes M, Gronseth K, Larsen S, et al. Comparison of endoscopic retrograde and intravenous cholangiography in diagnosis of biliary calculi. Lancet 1978; 2:230.
3. Venu RP, Geenen JE, Toouli J, et al. Endoscopic retrograde cholangiopancreatography. JAMA 1983; 249:758–61.
4. Kauffmann GW, Hoppe-Seyler P, Noldge G, Waninger J. Mirizzi syndrome. MMW 1982; 124:647–50.
5. Petterson H. Carcinoma of the gallbladder. Acta Radiol Diag 1974; 15:225–36.
6. Berk RN, van der Vegt JH, Lichtenstein JE. The hyperplastic cholecystoses: Cholesterolosis and adenomyomatosis. Radiology 1983; 146:593–601.
7. Mitre JR, Brodmerkel GJ Jr. Traumatic rupture of the gallbladder. Preoperative diagnosis by endoscopic retrograde cholangiopancreatogram (ERCP). Gastrointest Endosc 1979; 27:74–5.
8. Safrany L, van Husen N, Kautz G, et al. Endoscopic retrograde cholangiography (ERC) in surgical emergencies. Ann Surg 1978; 187:20–3.
9. Rohrmann CA Jr, Ansel HJ, Ayoola EA, et al. Endoscopic retrograde intrahepatic cholangiogram: Radiographic findings in intrahepatic disease. AJR 1977; 128:45–52.
10. Hamilton I, Lintott DJ, Rudell WSJ, Axon ATR. The endoscopic retrograde cholangiogram and pancreatogram in chronic liver disease. Clin Radiol 1983; 34:417–22.
11. Ayoola EA, Vennes JA, Silvis SE, et al. Endoscopic retrograde intrahepatic cholangiography in liver diseases. Gastrointest Endosc 1976; 22:156–9.
12. Summerfield JA, Elias E, Hungerford GD, et al. The biliary system in primary biliary cirrhosis. Gastroenterology 1976; 70:240–3.
13. Falkenstein DB, Riccobono C, Sidhu G, et al. The endoscopic intrahepatic cholangiogram. Invest Radiol 1975; 10:358–65.
14. Baer JW, Abiri M. Right hepatic artery as a cause of pseudocalculus in the biliary tree. Gastrointest Radiol 1982; 7:269–73.
15. Sivak MV Jr, Farmer RG, Lalli AF. Sclerosing cholangitis: its increasing frequency of recognition and association with inflammatory bowel disease. J Clin Gastroenterol 1981; 3:261–6.
16. MacCarty RL, LaRusso NF, Wiesner RH, Ludwig J. Primary sclerosing cholangitis: Findings on cholangiography and pancreatography. Radiology 1983; 149:39–44.
17. Berk RN, Ferrucci JT Jr, Leopold GRK. Radiology of the Gallbladder and Bile Ducts: Diagnosis and Intervention. Philadelphia: W. B. Saunders, 1983.
18. Hatfield PM, Wise RE. Parasitic diseases. In: Radiology of the Gallbladder and Bile Ducts. Baltimore: Williams & Wilkins, 1976.

Chapter 33

SPHINCTER OF ODDI

J. E. GEENEN, M.D.
W. J. HOGAN, M.D.
W. J. DODDS, M.D.

The sphincter of Oddi, located strategically at the choledochoduodenal junction, modulates the flow of bile and pancreatic secretion into the duodenum. Previously, because of its inaccessibility, the structure and function of the sphincter of Oddi in humans were of marginal interest to clinicians and clinical investigators. With the introduction of fiber-optic instruments and the development of advanced diagnostic and therapeutic capabilities, this once remote region of the gastrointestinal tract has been "rediscovered." This chapter is not a comprehensive presentation of the sphincter of Oddi's complex role as integrator of pancreaticobiliary flow dynamics; rather, it highlights anatomic, physiologic, and pathophysiologic features that are relevant to clinical problems encountered by the gastrointestinal endoscopist who performs endoscopic retrograde cholangiopancreatography (ERCP).

Much of the information included in this section is based upon the results of our clinical and laboratory studies of the sphincter of Oddi. Consequent to adopting this type of approach, a certain amount of bias pervades this discussion. Nevertheless, this offers the clinician a practical understanding of the function and dysfunction of the sphincter of Oddi.

STRUCTURE

Anatomy

Pancreaticobiliary Tract

The right and left hepatic ducts are the culmination of an extensive network of progressively larger tributaries originating within the liver that transport bile from the hepatocyte. These two main ducts fuse at the portal fissure to form the common hepatic duct. Four centimeters distal to the origin of the hepatic duct, the cystic duct branches off as a continuation of the gallbladder. From this juncture the common bile duct becomes the continuation of the hepatic duct. The common bile duct courses downward, encounters the posterior aspect of the pancreas, angles to the right, and enters the second portion of the duodenum. The anatomy of the biliary ducts and related structures is described in Chapter 27.

The intramural portion of the common bile duct ranges from 10 to 30 mm in length. The confluence of the distal common bile duct and the pancreatic duct usually occurs just before the ductal structures pierce the duodenal wall. The common bile duct and duct of Wirsung merge into a common channel (ampulla) in over 80% of patients. Two or more orifices in the same papilla or separate papillae for bile and pancreatic ducts occur rarely. The dimensions of the ampulla vary: length ranges from 2 to 17 mm, diameter from 2 to 7 mm.

Sphincter of Oddi

There is an interchange of fibers between the duodenal muscle layers and the intrinsic musculature of the distal bile duct as it traverses the wall of the duodenum; these "connecting" and "reinforcing" fibers are highly variable. Boyden's[1] meticulous dissection of the human sphincter of Oddi demonstrated the existence of an intrinsic choledochal muscle that is anatomically distinct from the surrounding duodenal musculature. There is now ample physiologic evidence to indicate that a zone of intrinsic electrical and contractile activity exists at the distal choledochus in man and most other mammals.

At anatomic dissection this intrinsic choledochal muscle is approximately 12 mm in length and is divided into two sphincteric zones: (1) a superior choledochal sphincter encircling the bile duct just proximal to the duodenum and (2) an inferior choledochal sphincter muscle surrounding the submucous portion of the duct.[2] The terminal end of the pancreatic duct is also surrounded by a muscle cuff that is continuous with that of the common bile duct (Fig. 33–1). Despite this anatomic arrangement, which suggests separate functioning sphincter zones, manometric studies of the human sphincter of Oddi have failed to identify discrete small sphincters, or "mini-sphincters," corresponding to those found by dissection. Rather, a contiguous zone of contractile activity and baseline pressure elevation is recorded over a ductal length of 6 to 8 mm, extending proximally from the aperture of the papilla of Vater. This segment is referred to as the "sphincter of Oddi zone."[3]

Embryology

The muscularis proprius of the distal choledochus first appears in the human fetus five weeks after the intestinal musculature. It arises de novo from the mesenchyme. In his definitive study of the embryology of the

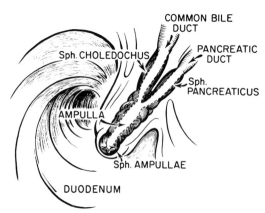

FIGURE 33–1. Schematic diagram depicting relative anatomic arrangement of intrinsic musculature of the sphincter of Oddi, in which the presence of "sphincter zones" is suggested. (Adapted from: Hess W. Manometry and radiography in the biliary system during surgery. In: Demling L, Classen M, eds. Endoscopic Sphincterotomy of the Papilla of Vater. Proceedings of the International Workshop of the World Congress of Gastroenterology, Munich, 1976. Stuttgart: Georg Thieme, 1978.)

sphincter of Oddi, Boyden remarked that the distal choledochus "is of a different order of musculature than the other (adjacent) structures."[1] It originates at the anatomic point where it subsequently penetrates the duodenal wall. The sphincter of Oddi segment, therefore, appears to be embryologically and anatomically distinct from the duodenal musculature.

Innervation

The extrahepatic bile ducts are innervated by sympathetic nerves originating from spinal segments 7 to 10 that reach the celiac ganglia via the splanchnic nerves.[4] The splanchnic nerves supply both motor and inhibitory fibers. Parasympathetic innervation is derived from the vagal nerves which supply both motor and sensory fibers. At the hiatus of the liver, parasympathetic fibers from both the right and left vagal nerves form the hepatic plexus, which subsequently supplies parasympathetic innervation to the extrahepatic bile ducts. The bulk of afferent nerve supply from the extrahepatic biliary system is believed to pass via the sympathetic afferents through both splanchnic nerves, and also through the right phrenic nerve in many cases.

The choledochoduodenal junction is innervated by both components of the autonomic nervous system via the gastroduodenal nerve, which ends in a plexus containing numerous ganglion cells within the sphincter of Oddi zone. Adrenergic nerves appear to be more sparse, but their fibers may directly innervate smooth muscle cells in the same pattern as described for the gut wall. The intrinsic cholinergic nerve apparatus of the sphincter of Oddi appears richly developed in comparison with that of the gut. The ganglion cells of the myenteric plexus and submucosal plexus appear to have a predominance of cholinergic nerves.

BLOOD SUPPLY

The major blood supply to the papillary region is derived from the retroduodenal artery, a branch of the inferior pancreaticoduodenal artery. Stolte[5] described variation of the arterial supply to the papillary region, using combined angiographic and histologic studies in 50 postmortem specimens (Fig. 33–2). A ventral and dorsal branch of the retroduodenal artery formed the arterial plexus

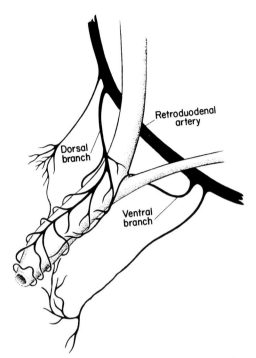

FIGURE 33–2. Diagram of blood supply to region of papilla of Vater. (Adapted from: Stolte M. Some aspects of the anatomy and pathology of the papilla of Vater. In: Classen M, Geenen J, Kawai K, eds. The Papilla Vateri and Its Diseases. Baden-Baden, Koln, New York: Witzstrock, 1979.)

of the papilla in over 50% of cases. The dorsal branch predominated in 25%; and the ventral branch was prevalent in 8%. In another 8% of cases, the arterial plexus was made up of small lateral vessels arising in the wall of the duodenum. In most specimens, the retroduodenal artery was located more than 35 mm from the papillary orifice; in 5%, the artery resided within the range of endoscopic papillotomy incision length. This latter variation therefore poses a threat of severe hemorrhage during endoscopic sphincterotomy. Doppler probes for determining the location of the retroduodenal artery are under development, and in the future these may be useful in assessing the potential for massive bleeding following endoscopic sphincterotomy.

STUDY TECHNIQUES

There have been investigators of biliary tract function for more than four centuries. In 1543 Vesalius noted a membrane at the orifice of the common duct which he postulated impeded bile flow and prevented regurgitation of duodenal contents. A possible sphincter mechanism at the distal choledochus was first described in 1879. Eight years later Rugero Oddi[6] performed such a thorough analysis of this tiny bundle of circular muscle fibers at the confluence of the choledochus and pancreatic ducts in animals that his name is given to this structure.

At the turn of this century attention was focused on research into the mechanisms of bile delivery into the duodenum. Many renowned physicians, including Krukenberg, Borghi, Aschoff, Meltzer, Judd, and Mann, studied gallbladder motor function and its interactions with the sphincter of Oddi and bile flow. This set the stage for considerable speculation about biliary tract function and the possibility that some symptoms and disease states were related to disordered function.

Experimental design, instrumentation, and methodology were relatively crude by present standards but improved during the decade from 1920 to 1930. During this period, humoral control mechanisms were suggested as primary modulating factors in biliary tract dynamics, particularly gallbladder evacuation of bile. For instance, it was found that specific food substances introduced into the duodenum prompted evacuation of bile and increased the contractile force of the gallbladder. Subsequently, Ivy and Oldberg[7] extracted a substance from hog mucosa that stimulated the evacuation of bile from the canine gallbladder. Ivy called this substance cholecystokinin (CCK); other investigators confirmed its status as a true hormone shortly thereafter.

In the next half-century important advances in experimental design and technology enabled more precise investigation and measurement of parameters of biliary tract dynamics in man. Intravenous cholangiography, cineradiography, operative and postoperative cholangiography, and various manometric recording techniques have been used to study pressure and flow dynamics of the extrahepatic biliary system. Some of these investigative techniques are described in the following section.

Cholangiographic Techniques

Bile flow kinetics have been studied by cholangiographic techniques that involve opacification of the bile ducts by intravenously administered contrast medium or by injection of contrast agent through a cannula at laparotomy or postoperatively. Radiomanometry consists of a sequence of bile duct radiographs obtained at low hydrostatic pressure sufficient to initiate common bile duct outflow (usually less than 15 cm of water) and at high hydrostatic pressure (approximately 40 to 50 cm of water).

Bile duct flow is measured by a drop counter during infusion of the common bile duct through a cannula. At a given pressure, flow is determined by the resistance at the sphincter of Oddi. It is assumed that the inflow rate of the infusate reflects the rate of outflow into the duodenum. Using a gravity fluid reservoir, the resting choledochal pressure and "passage pressure" (i.e., the pressure at which the sphincter yields) can be determined. Choledochal basal pressures of 5 to 10 cm of water and yield pressures of 12 to 15 cm of water have been measured. A contrast infusion pump has been added to the system and variable infusion rates have been used to study "sphincter activity." An infusion rate of 10 ml/min, associated with flow resistance in the tubing of 25 to 30 mm Hg, is commonly used. By substituting contrast material, continuous radiographic monitoring of the biliary tree can be performed during a period of dye injection. Average choledochal resting pressure of 6 ± 4 mm Hg has been measured in the human common bile duct. Cineradiographic imaging has shown phasic wave pressure activity, independent of respiration or heartbeat, in the sphincter of Oddi segment. Phasic pressure waves with an average amplitude of 6 mm Hg have been recorded. These were not accompanied by significant changes in intraduodenal pressure or contractile activity.[8]

A series of pressure/filling curves have been determined from these constant infusion studies of the biliary tract. The data obtained have been construed as reflecting sphincter of Oddi dynamics, that is, high common bile duct pressures are taken as indicating excessive sphincter of Oddi contraction, whereas low common duct pressures are thought to mean that little or no resistance to the flow of material into the duodenum is offered by the sphincter. Unfortunately, correlation by direct measurement of sphincter of Oddi motor activity and pressure has not accompanied this type of investigation.

ERCP Manometry

The measurement of pressures generated by the human sphincter of Oddi with a recording catheter is a logical evolution of diagnostic ERCP. Pressures from the distal choledochus were first measured by this method in 1974,[9] and in 1977 distinctive phasic wave contractions were described in the sphincter of Oddi zone using a minimally compliant catheter perfusion system.[10] There are several methods for ERCP manometry, including the use of small pressure transducers that are placed within the sphincter by endoscopic cannulation. Our technique utilizes an open catheter, constant perfusion system.

Pressure in the common bile duct, pancreatic duct, and sphincter of Oddi segment are recorded using a round, triple-lumen polyethylene catheter (O.D. 1.7 mm) with luminal diameters of 0.5 mm and a length of 200 cm, the entire catheter being extruded as a single tube (Medi-Tech, Inc., Watertown, Mass.). Each of the 3 recording lumens has a lateral recording orifice of 0.5 mm diameter. The distal orifice is located 5 mm from the end of the catheter. The 3 orifices are 2 mm apart and therefore span a length of 4 mm on the catheter. Six black rings, starting from the most proximal orifice, are etched on the catheter at 2 mm intervals to permit endoscopic determination of the depth of catheter insertion.

To obtain recordings from the biliary tree, the catheter is passed through the accessory channel in the fiberoptic endoscope. Continuous recording of intraduodenal pressure is obtained by a single-lumen catheter taped to the endoscope so that its recording side orifice is 4 mm proximal to the accessory channel opening (Fig. 33–3). During pressure recording, each catheter lumen is infused with bubble-free water at the rate of 0.25 ml/min by a minimally compliant hydraulic capillary infusion system driven by a constant reservoir pressure of 375 to 400 mm Hg.

The performance of the recording system at the reservoir pressure and infusion rate selected is tested as follows. The inherent postocclusion rise rate of the infused catheter system is determined by abruptly obstructing the recording orifice of each recording lumen. Under these conditions, the system will yield a postocclusion pressure rise rate of 400 mm Hg/sec or greater as measured during the initial 200 mm Hg pressure rise.

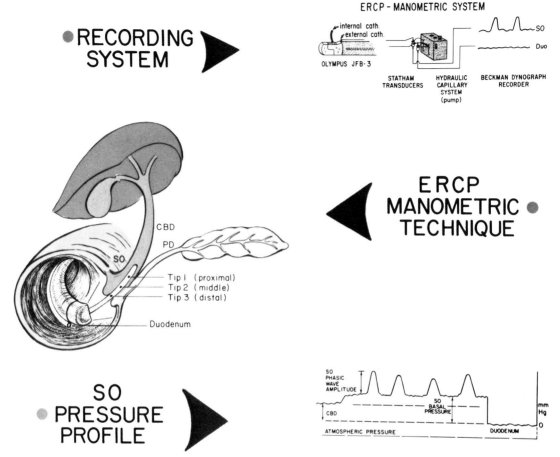

FIGURE 33–3. Overview of ERCP manometry. *Top,* Recording system showing internal/external catheters and noncompliant pump system. *Middle,* Manometric technique showing catheter oriented in common bile duct (CBD) with three recording tips within sphincter of Oddi (SO) zone. *Bottom,* SO pressure profile obtained during catheter pull-through from CBD to the duodenum. Appropriate reference points are indicated.

Preferably, patients who undergo ERCP manometry should receive either no sedation or only diazepam in small amounts (5 to 15 mg intravenously). Diazepam and water-soluble contrast media do not appear to alter the motor activity of the sphincter of Oddi.

After diagnostic ERCP, the manometric catheter is inserted through the endoscope into the papilla and directed toward either the common bile duct or the pancreatic duct. At the end of the manometric procedure, contrast material is instilled through the manometric catheter to verify its location. In each study the triple-lumen manometric catheter is passed into the appropriate duct and pressure is recorded. The catheter is withdrawn by 2 mm increments into the duodenum using the black marks on the catheter for orientation. At each station, pressure recordings are obtained for 2 to 3 minutes. When the catheter is positioned in the sphincter of

Oddi segment so that all 3 recording orifices record phasic contractions, a 3- to 5-minute recording is made with polygraph paper running at 1 cm/sec, this speed being best for demonstration of the onset of phasic wave contractions and their sequential relationship.

The specific value given to the baseline sphincter pressure depends on the zero reference. For example, a sphincter of Oddi basal pressure 8 mm Hg greater than that in the common bile duct might be 18 mm Hg above intraduodenal pressure and 28 mm Hg above atmospheric pressure.

PHYSIOLOGY OF THE SPHINCTER OF ODDI

The biliary tract is a low-pressure, low-flow system. Bile flow into the duodenum is determined mainly by the rate of bile production, contraction of the gallbladder, and motor activity of the sphincter of Oddi. Other factors such as cystic duct resistance, bile viscosity, duodenal contractions, and gravity are of lesser importance. There is ample evidence that sphincter of Oddi function is independent of duodenal contractile and electrical activity.[11] Furthermore, certain pharmacologic agents produce opposite effects in the sphincter and duodenum. For example, CCK in humans generally causes duodenal contraction and sphincter of Oddi relaxation.

The physiologic function of the sphincter of Oddi is threefold: (1) Regulation of bile flow into the duodenum; (2) diversion of hepatic bile into the gallbladder; and (3) prevention of reflux of duodenal contents into the biliary system. Traditionally, the sphincter of Oddi has been regarded solely as resisting bile flow. As a "resistor" it has active and passive components that gradually change during intervals of minutes to hours. These changes in tone, according to the established view, regulate bile flow during fasting and postprandial periods. However, the traditional explanation of sphincter of Oddi function ignores or is at odds with more recent information.

Sphincter of Oddi Contractile Activity

Since the 1950's, cineradiographic studies that provided rapid imaging of the sphincter of Oddi segment have demonstrated spontaneous, rhythmic contractions that were compared to intervals of "systolic contraction" separated by intervals of "diastolic relaxation" (Fig. 33–4). Direct pressure measurements from the human sphincter of Oddi were unavailable until the advent of ERCP. Subsequently, ERCP manometric pressure recording of sphincteric motor activity using a noncompliant infusion system has confirmed these radiographic observations and defined the pressure profile from within the sphincter of Oddi zone.

In patients judged to be normal, the sphincter of Oddi pressure profile obtained during pull-through across the sphincter has the following features (see Fig. 33–3). The sphincter of Oddi segment measures 4 to 6 mm in length. Within this zone there is a modest basal pressure that is measured between phasic contraction waves. In some subjects, sphincter of Oddi basal pressure may be isobaric with common bile duct pressure. We have never observed abrupt, transient

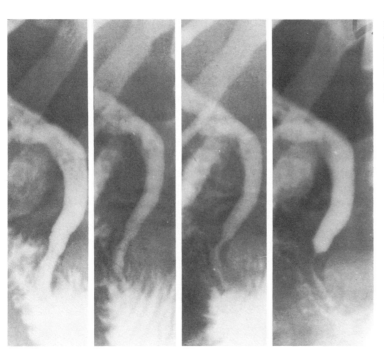

FIGURE 33–4. Radiographic sequence of sphincter of Oddi contractile activity (over 15 sec. interval) demonstrating opening (emptying) and closing (filling) of sphincter segment following retrograde contrast injection.

relaxations of sphincter of Oddi basal pressure comparable to transient relaxations that occur in the lower esophageal sphincter. The amplitude of the phasic contractions is calculated by subtracting the basal sphincteric pressure from the peak pressure. In one report, duodenal pressure recorded by this method averaged 6 mm Hg above atmospheric pressure, and common bile duct pressure averaged 8 mm Hg above duodenal pressure.[3] Basal sphincter pressure was 4 to 5 mm higher than common bile duct pressure and approximately 15 mm Hg higher than duodenal pressure.

Superimposed on the basal sphincter pressures were prominent phasic waves; the amplitude of these, averaged from the 3 recording tips, was 128 mm Hg above sphincter of Oddi basal pressure. Wave amplitudes did not differ statistically between multiple recording sites within the sphincter of Oddi segment (Fig. 33–5). There is no manometric evidence to support the existence of "minisphincters" within the pressure recording zone of the sphincter of Oddi. Frequency of the phasic contraction waves averaged 4 per minute, and the wave duration was about 6 seconds. Phasic contraction waves did not occur in the common bile duct.

The temporal relationship of the phasic contraction waves within the sphincter of Oddi zone has been analyzed.[12] In individuals with normal biliary and pancreatic ducts, 60% of sphincter of Oddi phasic contractions were oriented in an antegrade direction, i.e. toward the duodenum. About 14% of wave contractions were recorded in a retrograde direction and 26% occurred simultaneously. Comparison of phasic contraction sequence propagation between these individuals and patients with stones in the common bile duct is shown in Table 33–1. The antegrade orientation of most sphincter of Oddi phasic contractions suggests a propulsive role.

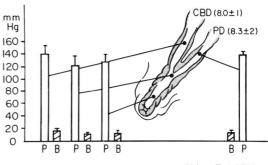

Values x̄ ± SEM

FIGURE 33–5. Sphincter of Oddi (SO) basal (B) and peak phasic (P) wave amplitudes obtained from multiple points within SO zone show no significant differences between recording sites whether catheter is directed into common bile duct (CBD) or pancreatic duct (PD). Pressures (mm Hg) are listed on vertical axis.

Sphincter of Oddi Electrical Activity

Myoelectrical recording from the human sphincter of Oddi has been obtained by positioning electrodes during laparotomy. Discrete electrical spike bursts were attributed to sphincter activity and clearly were not duodenal in origin (Fig. 33–6). Fluid flow through an indwelling T-tube was interrupted concurrently with sphincter of Oddi spike bursts.[11] Sphincter of Oddi electrical activity has been recorded recently in a few subjects by positioning catheter ring electrodes within the sphincter during ERCP.[13] However, information obtained from studies of the human sphincter of Oddi is limited by a number of clinical variables, so that comprehensive study of sphincter mechanisms requires an animal model.

Miniaturized bipolar electrodes implanted within the sphincter of Oddi segment of the opossum show omnipresent rhythmic spike bursts occurring at the rate of 1 to 8 per minute in the conscious fasted animal. Con-

TABLE 33–1. **Sphincter of Oddi: Phasic Contraction Sequence Propagation**

| Patient Group | Age (yrs)* | No. of Patients | Propagation (%)* | | |
			Antegrade	*Simultaneous*	*Retrograde*
Controls	42 ± 3	20	60 ± 4†	26 ± 3	14 ± 4‡
CBD stone	67 ± 4	15	18 ± 5†	29 ± 6	53 ± 9‡

*$\bar{x}$ ± SEM.
†$p < 0.001$.
‡$p < 0.005$.

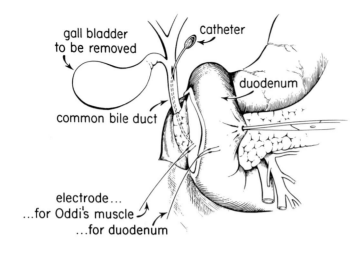

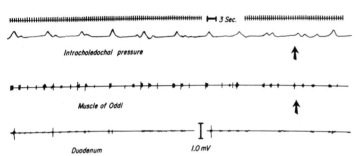

FIGURE 33–6. Myoelectrical recording from human sphincter of Oddi (SO). *Top,* Drawing showing electrodes positioned in SO (*Oddi's muscle*) and duodenum at time of laparotomy. *Below,* Phasic distal choledochal pressure recorded concurrent with discrete electrical spike bursts from SO zone. The latter clearly are not duodenal in origin. (From: Ono K, Watanabe N, Suzuki K. Bile flow mechanisms in man. Arch Surg 1968; 96:869–74. Reprinted with permission.)

current peristaltic contractions are recorded manometrically in the sphincter of Oddi zone as a propagating monophasic pressure wave. The spike bursts correspond to a peristaltic contraction that originates proximally in the sphincter and generally propagates to the sphincter-duodenal junction.[14]

Electrodes implanted within both the musculature of the opossum sphincter of Oddi and upper gastrointestinal tract provide a method for studying the relationship of biliary tract and gastrointestinal function in awake animals over the course of time. During Phase II of the duodenal migrating myoelectrical complex (MMC) activity, the rate of sphincter of Oddi spike bursts increases gradually and culminates in a 5-minute interval of maximal activity concurrent with the passage of the Phase III MMC activity through the duodenum. After feeding, the rate of sphincter of Oddi spike bursts increases during a 45-minute interval to reach a plateau of about 6 spike bursts per minute that lasts a minimum of 3 hours.[14] Thus, contractile activity in the opossum sphincter of Oddi is coordinated with patterns of gastrointestinal contractility occurring during the fasted and

fed states. Whether a similar coordination exists in the human remains undetermined.

Sphincter of Oddi Flow Studies

There is a consensus that fluid outflow from the common bile duct stops during each sphincter of Oddi phasic contraction. This observation has resulted in a controversy as to whether the phasic sphincter activity enhances or retards common bile duct emptying. The results of cineradiographic studies with simultaneous measurements of common bile duct pressure and flow are of interest in this regard. At resting common bile duct pressure (10–12 cm of water), sphincter of Oddi contractions occur at the rate of 3 to 5 per minute. When common bile duct flow occurs in the physiologic range (greater than 3.0 ml/min) the sphincter of Oddi contraction rate increases linearly with increases in flow rate, while the common bile duct pressure remains unchanged. At excessive common bile duct pressure of 40 to 50 cm of water, sphincter of Oddi contractions stop. The sphincter remains wide open and transsphincteric flow becomes entirely passive, being determined by sphincter diameter and fluid pressure.[15]

Sphincter of Oddi Control Mechanisms

The control mechanisms that regulate contractile activity of the sphincter of Oddi are incompletely defined. The prevalent concept is that the main controlling mechanism is hormonal, e.g. the reciprocal relationship between gallbladder contraction and sphincter of Oddi relaxation appears to be controlled by CCK released in response to a meal.[16] Neural mechanisms, however, may provide an important auxiliary function for controlling sphincter of Oddi contractile activity. Non-adrenergic inhibitory nerves, for example, are present in several mammalian animal species and may also be present in humans. Finally, vascular engorgement in the region of the sphincter can cause significant alteration in the spongelike network of mucosal folds lining this segment, thereby altering luminal resistance and influencing flow across the sphincter.[17]

Physiologic Role of the Sphincter of Oddi

The traditional concept of the physiologic role of the sphincter of Oddi in controlling delivery of bile into the duodenum is altered by current information. Our concept is as follows. The sphincter exhibits contraction waves as well as variable tone. Antegrade phasic contractions serve as a peristaltic pump and actively transport sphincter contents into the duodenum. The relative frequency of antegrade contractions may vary during the intestinal MMC cycle and after meals. The sphincter stroke volume relates to the degree of sphincter filling at the onset of a peristaltic sequence. The degree of sphincter filling is dependent upon sphincter basal pressure, rate of bile flow, common bile duct pressure, and the interval between sphincter of Oddi phasic contractions. Simultaneous or retrograde sphincter of Oddi phasic contractions may predominantly retard common bile duct emptying and subsequently promote gallbladder filling. The phasic contractions may prevent reflux of duodenal contents into the common bile duct and may play an important role in keeping the distal choledochus free of sludge and particulate matter.

The sphincter of Oddi basal pressure appears to provide a variable tonicity to the sphincteric mechanism that adds another element of complexity in understanding its function. Pharmacologic studies in the human show that sphincteric basal pressure and phasic contractions differ in their responses to intravenous doses of morphine.[18] Low doses increase the rate of phasic contractions, whereas higher doses increase basal pressure as well. These findings suggest a separation of function for these two components. In order for bile to flow into the duodenum, the basal pressure must be reduced to common bile duct pressure or the phasic contractions must transport bile against a resistance. The mechanisms regulating this feature of the sphincter of Oddi segment remain undefined.

SPHINCTER OF ODDI PHARMACOLOGY

Enteric Hormones

A number of enteric hormones have been administered to humans during direct manometric measurement of sphincter of Oddi motor activity. Cholecystokinin octapeptide (CCK-OP) promptly inhibits both tonic and phasic contractions in man (Fig. 33–7A) at an intravenous bolus dose of 20 to 40 µg/kg.[19] Studies in the cat indicate that CCK-OP releases a non-adrenergic neurotransmitter that inhibits sphincter motor activity. This inhibitory action masks a direct excitatory effect of CCK on the feline sphincter muscle that is observable after pharmacologic denervation of this segment.[20] This phenomenon is of particular interest because a possible counterpart in man is the paradoxical contraction of the sphincter of Oddi following CCK-OP administration. Such paradoxical responses have been observed in 8 patients with suspected sphincter of Oddi dyskinesia[21] (Fig. 33–7B). Continuous intravenous infusion of CCK-OP at a rate sufficient to reproduce physiologic blood levels has also been shown to inhibit human sphincter of Oddi motor activity.[22] Pentagastrin contracts the sphincter of Oddi in man following intravenous bolus administration, but this effect has not been analyzed carefully.

Secretin relaxes the human sphincter of Oddi, presumably by a direct effect on the muscle. Following intravenous bolus administration (GIH Secretin 1 µg/kg), there is a transient increase in phasic wave contractions

A. NORMAL RESPONSE

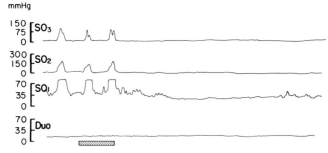

B. PARADOXICAL RESPONSE

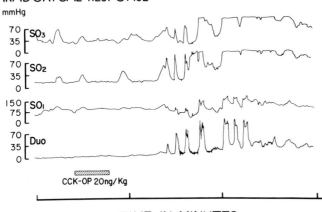

TIME IN MINUTES

FIGURE 33–7. Effect of CCK-OP on human sphincter of Oddi (SO) motor activity. *A,* Dramatic reduction in basal and phasic wave pressure recorded from three sites within SO segment (SO$_1$, SO$_2$, SO$_3$) immediately following intravenous bolus of CCK-OP (20 ng/kg). This is considered a normal response. *B,* Sustained contraction response recorded from three sites within SO segment (SO$_1$, SO$_2$, SO$_3$) following intravenous administration of CCK-OP. This is considered a paradoxical response and suggests possible SO denervation.

of the sphincter followed rapidly by inhibition of all motor activity for several minutes. Glucagon also inhibits sphincter of Oddi motor activity in man.

Drugs

In humans, intravenous administration of small doses of morphine increases the rate of phasic contractions of the sphincter of Oddi but has little effect on basal pressure. Larger doses of morphine cause "spasm" of the sphincter of Oddi segment. Naloxone abolishes the effect of morphine on the human sphincter of Oddi.[18] Meperidine, in clinical analgesia-producing doses, appears to cause an increase in sphincteric motor activity. Atropine decreases motor activity and also partially antagonizes the effect of morphine on the human sphincter of Oddi.[18] Amyl nitrite relaxes the sphincter of Oddi in all mammalian species. Administered as an inhalent (four "sniffs" from a ruptured pulvule), the inhibitory action of amyl nitrite has been used clinically to aid in distinguishing sphincter of Oddi spasm from stenosis (Fig. 33–8).

SPHINCTER OF ODDI DYSFUNCTION

The term sphincter of Oddi dysfunction is applied to a collection of symptoms and signs associated with either actual or presumed abnormalities of the sphincter of Oddi. In different parts of the world this syndrome is diagnosed in 1% to 40% of patients with postcholecystectomy pain.

Sphincter of Oddi dysfunction may be caused by structural narrowing of the sphincter segment as a result of direct trauma during passage of a common bile duct stone or injury at the time of an operative procedure, or it may be secondary to pancreatitis. Sphincter of Oddi dysfunction may also result from a functional motor abnormality with associated spasm that persistently produces intermittent bile or pancreatic duct obstruction.

Clinical Features

The clinical features of sphincter of Oddi dysfunction are as follows:

1. All patients experience recurring bouts of epigastric or right upper quadrant pain

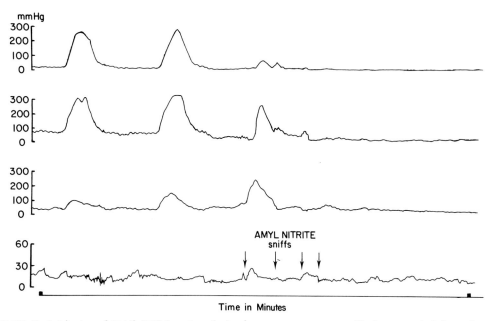

FIGURE 33–8. Sphincter of Oddi (SO) basal and phasic wave pressure amplitudes recorded from three sites within SO segment are suddenly and profoundly reduced following inhalation of amyl nitrite by patient.

that often radiates to the back and may be precipitated by meals.

2. Some patients may have intermittent or constant abnormalities in liver enzymes, particularly serum alkaline phosphatase, or they may have intermittent elevation of serum amylase levels.

3. The common bile duct may be dilated, as demonstrable by contrast material injection at ERCP, for example. A common bile duct diameter >12 mm or a pancreatic duct diameter >7 mm is considered abnormal.

4. Delayed emptying of contrast material from the biliary tree (>45 minutes) or pancreatic duct (>10 minutes) with the patient in the supine position may be present. If the emptying time is to be evaluated, the patient should not be given narcotics or anticholinergics, since these drugs influence sphincter of Oddi motor function.

Diagnosis

Unfortunately, there is no definitive standard by which the diagnosis of sphincter of Oddi dysfunction can be established with certitude. The current methods used to diagnose and treat patients with sphincter of Oddi dysfunction are unproven and most reports are based on results of uncontrolled studies or follow-up is incomplete. Nevertheless, it is logical to assume that this complex

sphincteric mechanism may be the object of motor dysfunction or structural narrowing.

In the past, several relatively crude methods were used to "confirm" the diagnosis of sphincter of Oddi dysfunction at operation. The decision for or against surgical sphincterotomy was based on these findings:

1. The resistance to flow of a column of fluid introduced through a T-tube into the distal common bile duct has been used as a measure of sphincter of Oddi resistance. A presumptive diagnosis of sphincter "stenosis" is suggested if measured resistance is in excess of 30 cm of water and stones are not present in the bile duct.

2. The inability of the surgeon to pass a size 3 Bakes (3 mm) dilator via the common bile duct through the sphincter of Oddi and into the duodenum or the inability to pass a 2 mm lacrimal duct probe into the pancreatic duct has been used as a definition of papillary "stenosis."

The inception of ERCP provided a nonsurgical method for diagnoses of sphincter of Oddi dysfunction. Subsequently, the development of endoscopic sphincterotomy offered a nonoperative treatment of this disorder. The methods for diagnosing sphincter of Oddi dysfunction at the time of ERCP study have included the following:

1. Assessment of the ease of cannulation of the papilla or, more precisely, the endos-

copist's estimate of "tightness" encountered during insertion of the catheter.

2. Anatomic definition by instillation of contrast agent into the pancreaticobiliary ducts and evaluation of ductal emptying rate.

3. Direct measurement of the pressure and pressure patterns of the sphincter of Oddi zone by ERCP manometric techniques.

In our experience, the endoscopist's ability to define a "tight" strictured sphincter or his difficulty in cannulating the ducts does not correlate with the presence or absence of recognizable sphincteric disease. Also, radiologic evaluation of a "strictured segment" and the opening and closing of the sphincteric segment has not yielded definitive information relative to sphincter of Oddi function or dysfunction.

Classification

With the use of a high-fidelity perfusion system, we have attempted to correlate sphincter of Oddi pressures obtained at ERCP manometry with the clinical syndrome of sphincter of Oddi dysfunction. It is not possible, however, to separate those patients with a strictly functional motility disorder of the sphincter (dyskinesia) from those with an anatomic stricture (papillary stenosis). Nonetheless, for the purpose of further study, patients have been subdivided categorically into three classes, and clinical criteria for sphincter of Oddi dysfunction has been redefined as follows:

Group I. Definitive sphincter of Oddi dysfunction.

Patients in this group must meet all the following criteria:

1. Pain that is typical for a biliary tract disorder.

2. Elevated serum alkaline phosphatase, bilirubin or both ($2\times$ normal values) on at least two occasions.

3. Dilated common bile duct with a diameter >12 mm on x-ray contrast study.

4. Delayed drainage of contrast material from the common bile duct (>45 minutes) after ERCP injection with the patient in supine position.

Group II. Presumptive sphincter of Oddi dysfunction.

Patients in this category must meet the following criteria:

1. Pain that is typical for a biliary tract disorder.

2. One or two of criteria numbers 2 through 4 listed above for group I.

Group III. Unexplained idiopathic recurrent pancreatitis.

Patients in this group must meet the following criteria:

1. Two or more documented episodes of clinical pancreatitis.

2. No structural abnormalities of the biliary tree or pancreas, with the possible exceptions of a dilated pancreatic duct or delayed drainage from this duct or both. All patients in this group have had a cholecystectomy, and those with biliary tract stones or a history of alcohol abuse are excluded.

Study Results

A total of 103 patients who fulfilled the criteria described in the previous section received the following evaluation. A detailed history was obtained including completion of a questionnaire for scoring the frequency and severity of symptoms. A battery of liver function tests and serum amylase levels were obtained. ERCP manometry of the sphincter of Oddi was performed, and, when possible, sphincter pressures were recorded following intravenous CCK-OP or amyl nitrate inhalation or both. After these studies were completed, either endoscopic or surgical sphincterotomy was performed. Following sphincterotomy the questionnaire was again completed for comparison with the first one.

Twenty-two patients met all 4 criteria for the diagnosis of sphincter of Oddi dysfunction (group I). ERCP manometry was obtained in 20 patients; 18 had elevated sphincter of Oddi basal pressure, as shown in Table 33–2. All patients underwent sphincterotomy, and 17 of the patients with elevated sphincter of Oddi basal pressure were relieved of pain and had normal liver function tests during a 6-month to 5-year follow-up. Two of these patients had recurrent pain and abnormal liver function tests. Re-stenosis of the papillary opening was found by ERCP, and both patients were successfully treated by repeated endoscopic sphincterotomy.

Of the 103 patients, 56 met the criteria for presumptive sphincter of Oddi dysfunction (group II). As shown in Table 33–2, 35 of these patients had elevated sphincter of Oddi basal pressures (>30 mm Hg above common bile duct pressure); 29 of the 35 had relief of pain following endoscopic sphincterotomy; 12 patients in group II had normal basal sphincter pressures, and only 3 of these experienced symptom improvement following endoscopic sphincterotomy.

TABLE 33–2. **Sphincter of Oddi (SO) Basal Pressure vs. Clinical Course with Sphincterotomy**

Patient Group*	No. of Patients	Clinical Course	
		Improved	*No Change*
I. Definitive dysfunction			
Elevated SO basal pressure	18	17	1
Normal SO basal pressure	2	1	1
II. Presumptive dysfunction			
Elevated SO basal pressure	35	29	6
Normal SO basal pressure	21	3	18
III. Idiopathic recurrent pancreatitis			
Elevated SO basal pressure	13	10	3
Normal SO basal pressure	12	4	8

*See text for explanation of patient groups I, II, and III.

In group III, 25 patients with a history of recurrent pancreatitis had a normal diagnostic ERCP examination. All underwent sphincter of Oddi manometry. Thirteen of these patients had elevated sphincter of Oddi basal pressures, and 10 of these were symptomatically improved following sphincterotomy (see Table 33–2). Eight of the 12 patients with normal pressures continued to have pain or recurrent attacks of pancreatitis following sphincterotomy.

In Table 33–3, elevated sphincter of Oddi basal pressures of patients from all three groups are compared with sphincter of Oddi basal pressures of 41 patients who served as a control population.

Complications of Endoscopic Sphincterotomy

The complication rate associated with endoscopic sphincterotomy for sphincter of Oddi dysfunction has been reported to be higher than that for treatment of common bile duct stones. A 9% complication rate and 2% mortality rate for patients with "papillary stenosis" following endoscopic sphincterotomy has been reported from Germany.[23] In our series, complications developed in 5 of 80 patients (6.3%) who underwent endoscopic sphincterotomy. There were no

deaths. This is similar to our complication rate with patients who have undergone endoscopic sphincterotomy for common bile duct stones.

Speculation on the Pathophysiology of Sphincter of Oddi Dyskinesia

The following list of abnormalities in sphincter of Oddi motor dysfunction, derived from our clinical observations, could represent examples of sphincter of Oddi dyskinesia.

Sphincter of Oddi Hypertonicity or Spasm. Elevation of basal and phasic wave contraction pressures has been recorded at ERCP manometry in patients with suspected sphincter of Oddi motor dysfunction (Fig. 33–9). This does not of itself indicate a smooth muscle abnormality, although a transient decrease in sphincter of Oddi pressure has been demonstrated in several of these patients after intravenous administration of glucagon or CCK-OP or following inhalation of amyl nitrate.

Sphincter of Oddi Denervation (Fig. 33–7B). A paradoxical elevation of sphincter of Oddi pressure in response to intravenous administration of CCK-OP has been demonstrated in a subset of patients with biliary disease–like pain. Eight patients with this

TABLE 33–3. **Basal Pressures in Sphincter of Oddi (SO) Dysfunction**

	Patient Group			
	Control	*Definitive SO Dysfunction*	*Presumptive SO Dysfunction*	*IRP*
No. of Patients	41	18	35	13
Basal Pressure (mm Hg)	15 ± 3	57 ± 12	42 ± 7	55 ± 11

IRP = Idiopathic recurrent pancreatitis.

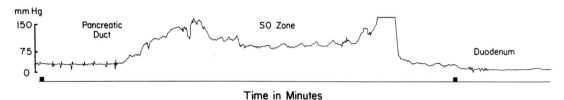

FIGURE 33–9. Example of sphincter of Oddi (SO) basal pressure hypertonicity recorded during catheter pull-through from pancreatic duct through SO zone and into duodenum.

type of pain demonstrated a paradoxical rise in sphincter of Oddi basal pressure following the intravenous bolus administration of CCK-OP during ERCP manometry. Whether this atypical response indicates a neuromuscular abnormality of the sphincter is not known. A similar paradoxical response to intravenous CCK has been shown in the denervated feline sphincter of Oddi[20] and lower esophageal sphincter (LES)[24] and in the LES in a majority of patients with achalasia.[25] This type of response suggests a defect in inhibitory innervation of the sphincter that "unmasks" a direct stimulatory effect of CCK on the smooth muscle of the sphincter of Oddi.

Sphincter of Oddi Phasic Wave Sequence Abnormality (Fig. 33–10). Normally the majority of phasic wave sequences in the sphincter of Oddi zone appear to propagate antegrade. The phasic wave sequence is altered in patients with common bile duct stones; there is a significant increase in the frequency of retrograde sphincter of Oddi phasic waves.[12] Conceivably alteration in the direction of phasic contraction wave propagation could impede bile flow and subsequently produce pain.

Sphincter of Oddi "Tachyoddia." The frequency of sphincter of Oddi phasic contractions appears to regulate the rate of common bile duct emptying in the opossum. Increasing this contraction rate appears to shorten the "diastolic" filling phase of the ampullary region. Theoretically, high-frequency sphincter of Oddi contraction waves could preclude emptying of the common bile duct in this model. Phasic contraction waves have been recorded at a frequency up to 12 per minute in the human during ERCP manometry (Fig. 33–11). Morphine causes a profound increase in the rate of phasic contraction waves. Theoretically, a prolonged, high rate of sphincter of Oddi contractions could disrupt the flow of bile into the duodenum and cause symptoms.

Clinical Relevance of Sphincter of Oddi Manometry

For the everyday evaluation of patients with symptoms and signs suggestive of sphincter of Oddi dysfunction, manometric pressure study may not be necessary prior to endoscopic sphincterotomy. For example, manometry may be unnecessary for patients

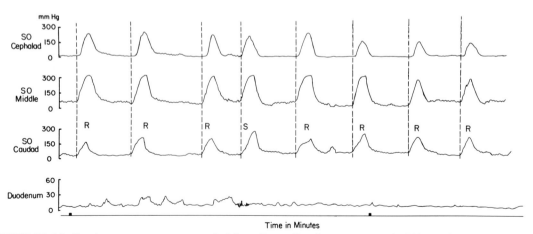

FIGURE 33–10. Phasic wave sequences recorded from three sites (4 mm segment) within sphincter of Oddi (SO) zone in patient with retained common bile duct stone. The majority of sequences shown here are retrograde in direction.

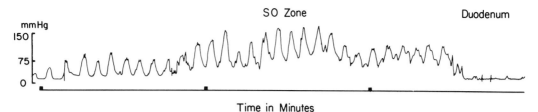

FIGURE 33–11. Rapid sphincter of Oddi (SO) phasic wave contractions of 12 per minute (tachyoddia) recorded during catheter pull-through from pancreatic duct into duodenum. The SO basal pressure is elevated in proximal segment of sphincter zone.

FIGURE 33–12. Sphincter of Oddi (SO) basal and phasic wave amplitudes recorded at three sites over 4 mm segment of SO prior to endoscopic sphincterotomy.

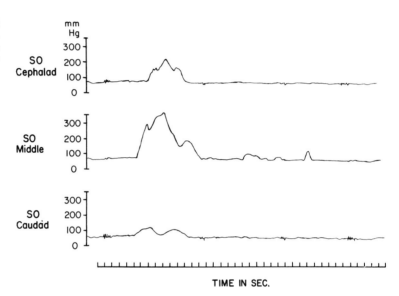

FIGURE 33–13. Following initial sphincterotomy incision (5.0 mm), sphincter of Oddi (SO) basal and phasic wave amplitudes, although reduced, are still significantly elevated.

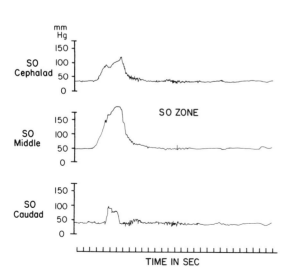

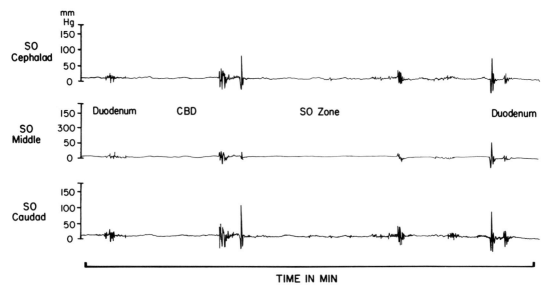

FIGURE 33–14. Extension of endoscopic sphincterotomy incision to 12 mm results in ablation of sphincter of Oddi (SO) basal and phasic pressures and eliminates duct-to-duodenal pressure gradient.

with all the criteria for inclusion in group I (see above). However, the effect of hormones or drugs on the sphincter of Oddi basal pressure may be useful in determining if sphincter dysfunction is the result of organic stricture or a primary motor disorder. Amyl nitrite and CCK lower the basal sphincteric pressure in patients with motor dysfunction or spasm of the sphincter segment but do not affect the elevated sphincter of Oddi basal pressure caused by an actual stricture.

Sphincter of Oddi manometry is also useful in evaluating the effectiveness of endoscopic sphincterotomy. If the common bile duct–to–duodenal pressure gradient does not approximate zero, or if phasic waves are not completely abolished, the sphincterotomy may not be adequate to alter sphincter dynamics and affect symptoms (Figs. 33–12, 33–13, and 33–14).

In group II and group III patients, manometric studies of the sphincter of Oddi segment may be an objective method for selecting those patients who may benefit from endoscopic or surgical sphincterotomy. At the present time, without manometric studies we find it difficult to determine which patients should undergo sphincterotomy. Although sphincter of Oddi manometry is useful in selecting patients who may benefit from sphincterotomy, it is conceivable that the sphincter dysfunction may be intermittent and may be missed during a manometric study. A reliable, provocative motor response

by the abnormal sphincter of Oddi to a pharmacologic agent or hormone would be extremely useful in identifying patients with suspected sphincter of Oddi motor dysfunction.

SUMMARY

The sphincter of Oddi is a superlatively adaptive structure that possesses ejecting as well as occluding mechanisms. Its primary physiologic role is regulation of flow pressure within the biliary and pancreatic system. Irrespective of the flow rate, pressure within the bile duct or pancreatic duct is maintained within a narrow range of low pressure that allows hepatic or pancreatic secretion to proceed against negligible hydrostatic pressure. Structural abnormalities of the sphincter of Oddi can occur as the result of passage of biliary calculi or injury at the time of operation. These abnormalities can be more easily identified and can be helped by appropriate relief of the obstruction.

The true incidence of primary sphincter of Oddi dysfunction in clinical practice is unknown; it is not a common disorder. Possible causes of primary sphincter of Oddi motor dysfunction include sphincter of Oddi spasm, denervation, and an abnormality of phasic contraction wave sequencing or rate. The majority of patients with suspected sphincter of Oddi dysfunction and elevated sphincter of Oddi basal pressure appear to be aided by sphincterotomy. A continuing scientific approach to this clinical problem is mandatory.

References

1. Boyden EA. The anatomy of the choledochoduo-denal junction in man. Surg Gynecol Obstet 1957; 104:641–52.
2. Boyden EA. The sphincter of Oddi in man and certain representative mammals. Surgery 1937; 1:25–37.
3. Geenen JE, Hogan WJ, Dodds WJ, et al. Intraluminal pressure recording from the human sphincter of Oddi. Gastroenterology 1980; 78:317–24.
4. Burnett W, Gairns FW, Bacsich P. Some observations on the innervation of the extrahepatic biliary system in man. Ann Surg 1964; 159:8–26.
5. Stolte M. Some aspects of the anatomy and pathology of the papilla of Vater. In: Classen M, Geenen J, Kawai K, eds. The Papilla Vateri and Its Diseases. Baden-Baden, Koln, New York: Witzstrock, 1979.
6. Oddi R. D'une disposition à sphincter speciale de l'ouverture du canal cholidoque. Arch Ital Biol 1887; 8:317–22.
7. Ivy AC, Oldberg E. A hormone mechanism for gallbladder contraction and evacuation. Am J Physiol 1928; 86:599–613.
8. Cushieri A, Hughes JH, Cohen M. Biliary pressure studies during cholecystectomy. Br J Surg 1972; 59:267–73.
9. Vondrasek P, Eberhardt G, Classen M. Endoscopic semiconductor manometry. Int J Med 1974; 3:188–92.
10. Geenen JE, Hogan WJ, Shaffer RD, et al. Endoscopic electrosurgical papillotomy and manometry in biliary tract disease. JAMA 1977; 237:2075–8.
11. Ono K, Watanabe N, Suzuki K, et al. Bile flow mechanisms in man. Arch Surg 1968; 96:869–74.
12. Toouli J, Geenen JE, Hogan WJ, et al. Sphincter of Oddi motor activity: A comparison between patients with common bile duct stones and controls. Gastroenterology 1982; 82:111–7.
13. Salducci J, Naudi B, Pin G, et al. Papilla electromyography: Endoluminal recording performed in man by perduodenoscopic cannulation. In: The Sphincter of Oddi. Proceedings of the Third Gastroenterological Symposium, Nice. New York: S. Karger, 1976.
14. Honda R, Toouli J, Dodds WJ, et al. Relationship of sphincter of Oddi spike bursts to gastrointestinal myoelectric activity in conscious opossums. J Clin Invest 1982; 69:770–8.
15. Hess W. Manometry and radiography in the biliary system during surgery. In: Demling L, Classen M, eds. Endoscopic Sphincterotomy of the Papilla of Vater. Proceedings of the International Workshop of the World Congress of Gastroenterology. Munich, 1976. Stuttgart: Georg Thieme, 1978.
16. Lin TM. Actions of gastrointestinal hormones and related peptides on the motor function of the biliary tract. Gastroenterology 1975; 69:1006–22.
17. Tansy MF, Salkin L, Innes DL, et al. The mucosal lining of the intramural common bile duct as a determinant of ductal opening pressure. Am J Dig Dis 1975; 20:613–25.
18. Venu R, Toouli J, Geenen JE, et al. Effect of morphine on motor activity of the human sphincter of Oddi. (Abstr) Gastroenterology 1983; 84:1342.
19. Toouli J, Hogan WJ, Geenen JE, et al. Action of cholecystokinin-octapeptide on sphincter of Oddi basal pressure and phasic wave activity in humans. Surgery 1982; 92:497–503.
20. Behar J, Biancani P. Effect of cholecystokinin and the octapeptide of cholecystokinin on the feline sphincter of Oddi and gallbladder. Mechanisms of action. J Clin Invest 1980; 66:1231–9.
21. Hogan WJ, Geenen JE, Dodds WJ, et al. Paradoxical motor response to cholecystokinin (CCK-OP) in patients with suspected sphincter of Oddi dysfunction. (Abstr) Gastroenterology 1982; 82:1085.
22. Jensen DM, Weiss S, Tapia JI, Beilin DB. Control of motility and pressures of the human sphincter of Oddi. Proceedings of the 4th Annual Meeting of the International Biliary Association. Paris, June 10–12, 1982.
23. Siefert E, Gail K, Weismueller J. Langzeitresultate nach endoskopischer Sphinkterotomie. Dtsch Med Wochenschr 1982; 107:610–4.
24. Behar J, Biancani P. Effect of cholecystokinin-octapeptide on the lower esophageal sphincter. Gastroenterology 1977; 73:57–61.
25. Dodds WJ, Dent J, Hogan WJ, et al. Paradoxical lower esophageal sphincter contraction induced by cholecystokinin-octapeptide in patients with achalasia. Gastroenterology 1981; 80:327–33.

Chapter 34

CHOLEDOCHOFIBEROSCOPY

KOJI GOCHO, M.D.
SHINOBU KAMEYA, M.D.
NOBORU IIJIMA, M.D.

OVERVIEW

Endoscopic examination of the bile ducts is performed for accurate diagnosis and extraction of foreign bodies such as calculi, indications that are essentially the same as in other endoscopic examinations of the gastrointestinal tract. Fiberoptic and rigid choledochoscopy can be used as an adjunct to surgery in the diagnosis and treatment of pathologic conditions of the bile ducts such as calculi. However, choledochoscopy has only limited application for removal of calculi during surgery, especially the removal of intrahepatic stones, for which the procedure is often difficult and lengthy. For this reason choledochofiberoscopy has been developed for use in the postoperative period.[1, 2]

There are several possible endoscopic approaches to the bile ducts. Peroral cholangioscopy by several methods is discussed in Chapter 10, part 4. A fiberoptic endoscope may be inserted into the bile ducts via a percutaneous transhepatic approach. There are also a number of avenues for endoscopic entry into the bile ducts in postoperative patients: via a T-tube tract, via a jejunostomy tract when fixed to the abdominal wall after choledochojejunostomy, and through the cystic duct after cholecystostomy or cystic duct drainage. This variety of avenues for access to the bile ducts has brought about modifications in the fiberscope and the development of special accessory instruments. As a result, diagnostic and therapeutic capabilities have become far greater than would have been possible using the rigid choledochoscope.[3–11]

APPROACHES TO THE BILE DUCTS

Choledochofiberoscopy may be classified according to the several possible approaches to the bile ducts. These are depicted diagrammatically in Figure 34–1.

Preoperative and Nonoperative Choledochoscopy

We consider this approach to be less invasive than surgery. Repeated examinations are possible, and the procedures are particularly useful in aged and high-risk patients who are not suitable candidates for surgery.[8, 11]

Percutaneous Transhepatic Cholangioscopy

Percutaneous transhepatic cholangiography (PTC) and external drainage (PTCD) under fluoroscopic guidance must be performed first.[12–14] Then, the intrahepatic tract is dilated using a fibrous tract dilator, and a 6- to 7-mm diameter tube is inserted into the intrahepatic bile duct and left in place. After approximately 3 weeks, a solid intrahepatic fibrous tract will form, and then a flexible fiberoptic choledochoscope can be inserted via this tract into the intrahepatic bile duct and distally to the common bile duct (Fig. 34–2).

Percutaneous transhepatic cholangioscopy can be performed in patients with dilated intrahepatic bile ducts and intrahepatic duct calculi or in patients in whom obstruction of the extrahepatic bile duct distal to retained calculi precludes extraction via endoscopic sphincterotomy. Biopsies may also be ob-

752

SURGERY	APPROACH ROUTE	SCHEME
Before Surgery (Preoperative Choledochoscopy)	Percutaneous Transhepatic Cholangioscopy	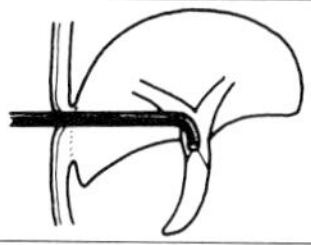
Without Surgery (Nonoperative Choledochoscopy)	Percutaneous Transhepatic Cholecystoscopy	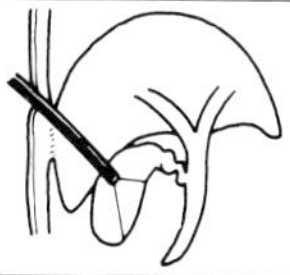
During Surgery (Operative Choledochoscopy)	Direct approach to the common bile duct	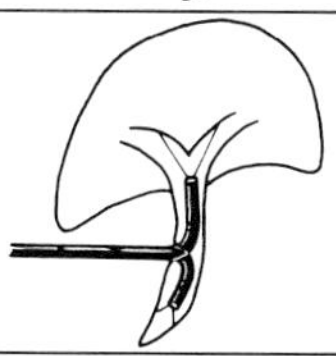
After Surgery (Postoperative Choledochoscopy)	T-tube Tract	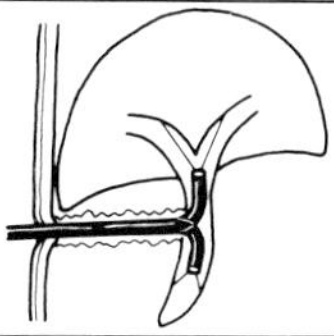
	Jejunostomy Tract	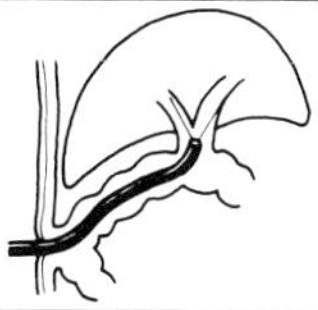
	Cystic Duct (after Cholecystostomy)	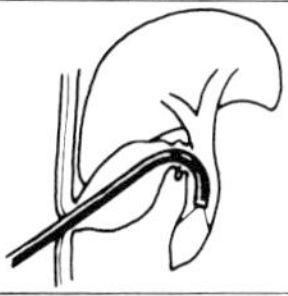
	Cystic Duct (after Cystic Duct Drainage)	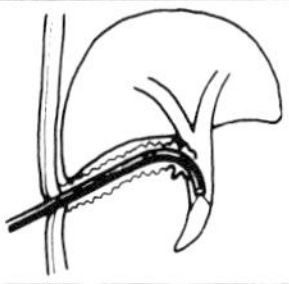

FIGURE 34–1. Diagrammatic illustration of endoscopic approaches to the biliary system before, during, and after surgery.

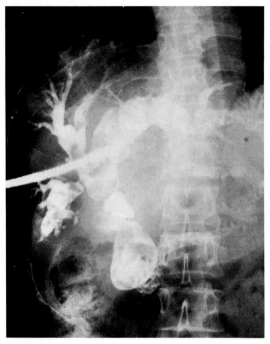

FIGURE 34–2. Percutaneous transhepatic cholangioscopy.

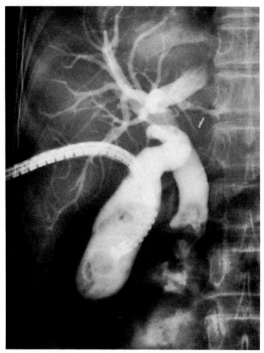

FIGURE 34–3. Percutaneous transhepatic cholecystoscopy.

tained of obstructing lesions such as bile duct carcinoma, and selective cholangiography can be performed.

Percutaneous Transhepatic Cholecystoscopy

Percutaneous transhepatic drainage of the gallbladder is first performed under ultrasonography. The fibrous tract is prepared in the same manner as for percutaneous transhepatic cholangioscopy. This secures the approach for routing the fiberoptic choledochoscope into the gallbladder[15–18] (Fig. 34–3). With this method of cholecystoscopy, biopsies of the gallbladder may be obtained under direct vision, and stones may be removed.

Operative Choledochoscopy

A choledochoscope can be inserted directly into the bile duct after opening the common duct during laparotomy. Operative choledochoscopy is usually performed as a method of exploration of the bile duct in patients with dilated ducts due to choledocholithiasis, in order to remove stones or to confirm the absence of residual stones. Both flexible fiberoptic and rigid choledochoscopes are available.[19–37]

One of the advantages of operative choledochoscopy is that any abnormalities discov-

ered endoscopically can be dealt with during the operation. However, the technique also adds to the length of the operative procedure. Another disadvantage is that operative choledochoscopy does not provide a method for clearing the intrahepatic ducts of stones.

Postoperative Choledochoscopy

In this method, an approach route to the bile duct is secured during the surgery, and endoscopic examination of the bile duct is performed at some point after operation.[1, 2, 38–45] One major advantage of postoperative choledochoscopy is that although the time of each examination may be limited, the procedure may be repeated many times using the fibrous tract.[36, 46, 47]

T-Tube Tract Choledochoscopy

A T-tube left in place in the common bile duct at laparotomy provides access to the biliary system. After a period of time, the tract of the T-tube becomes solid and fibrotic. Various authors differ as to how much time is necessary for formation of a solid tract. We introduce a flexible fiberoptic choledochoscope after about 3 weeks[48–50] (Fig. 34–4). This method makes possible the endoscopic exploration of the distal common bile duct as well as the intrahepatic ducts. It is the

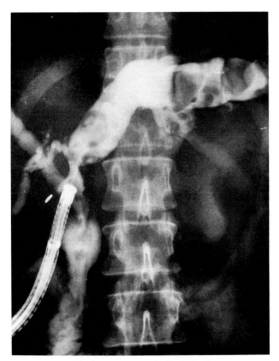

FIGURE 34–4. T-tube tract choledochoscopy.

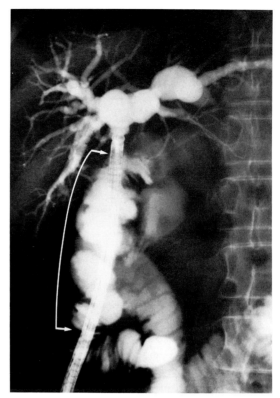

FIGURE 34–5. Jejunostomy tract choledochoscopy. Section of the fiberscope within the jejunal loop is indicated by arrows.

simplest and most commonly used of the different postoperative choledochoscopy procedures. The technical details are discussed below.

Jejunostomy Tract Choledochoscopy

This technique for postoperative choledochoscopy requires that a jejunostomy tract be constructed at the time of laparotomy; a choledochojejunostomy is performed and part of the jejunum is fixed to the parietal peritoneum.[51–54] A flexible fiberoptic choledochoscope is introduced into the bile duct through this jejunostomy tract after the operation (Fig. 34–5). Jejunostomy tract choledochoscopy is especially useful when residual intrahepatic stones are expected to be a problem after operation or recurrence of intrahepatic gallstones is anticipated.[55, 56] Endoscopic examination of the bile duct may be repeated long after the tract to the jejunostomy is closed because this may easily be reopened by making a small incision in the skin.[53]

Cystic Duct Choledochoscopy

After cystic duct drainage or cholecystostomy, the cystic duct can be dilated and a flexible fiberoptic choledochoscope introduced into the common bile duct through this tract[57, 58] (Figs. 34–6 and 34–7). The distal

common bile duct can be reached easily by means of this procedure, but the common hepatic duct is not accessible.

CHOLEDOCHOFIBERSCOPE AND ACCESSORIES

Fiberoptic Choledochoscope

The choledochofiberscope should have several attributes for satisfactory examination of the bile ducts. It should have a large forceps channel suitable for passage of a variety of accessories for biopsy or gallstone extraction[9, 59–62] (Fig. 34–8). Commercially available fiberoptic choledochoscopes have tip angulation systems that are similar to those of other types of fiberscopes. Because bile and floating debris in the biliary tract impair endoscopic observation, a channel for saline irrigation is also necessary.

Excessive irrigation of the bile ducts with saline during choledochoscopy increases the internal pressure within the ductal system and causes discomfort to patients. This may also result in diarrhea and vomiting after the examination. Therefore, instruments should

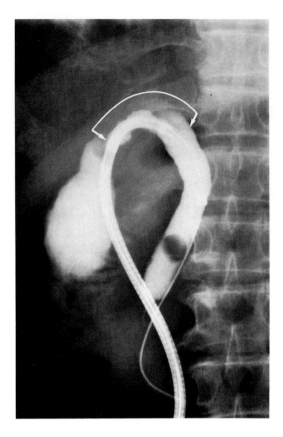

FIGURE 34–6. Cystic duct choledochoscopy after chole-cystostomy. Section of the fiberscope within the cystic duct is indicated by arrows.

FIGURE 34–7. Cystic duct choledochoscopy after cystic duct drainage.

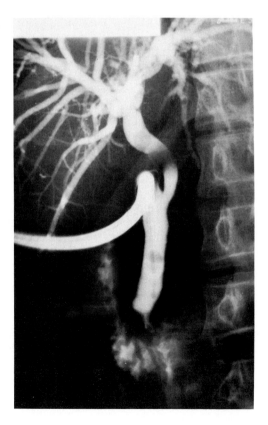

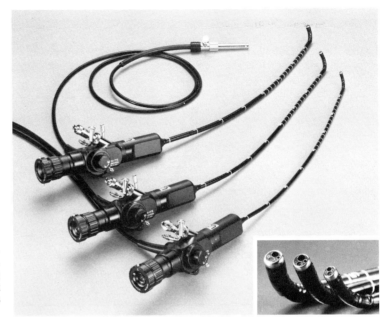

FIGURE 34–8. Fiber choledocho-scopes (Machida, Inc.) with inser-tion tubes of varying diameters and accessory channels of different diameters. All choledochoscopes shown are immersible.

have an aspiration mechanism by which excess saline can be removed from the system.

Accessories

A variety of accessory instruments are needed for maximum effectiveness during choledochoscopy. The essential items are a stone-holding basket forceps (Fig. 34–9; Plate 34–1) and biopsy forceps. Other optional accessories that increase therapeutic capability and aid in surmounting technical problems are a flushing tube (catheter for washing), alligator forceps, three-pronged grasping forceps, loop-type stone-crushing forceps, basket-type crushing forceps, biopsy forceps with stylet, electrosurgical cutting knife, and a guide wire (Fig. 34–10).

Two characteristics are indispensible for the stone-holding basket forceps. It should

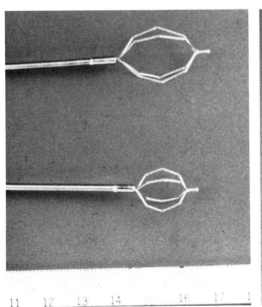
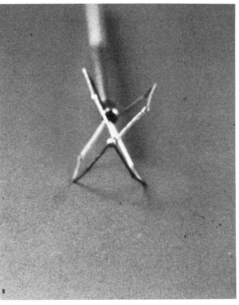

FIGURE 34–9. Basket forceps of a new design that makes it easier to hold stones.

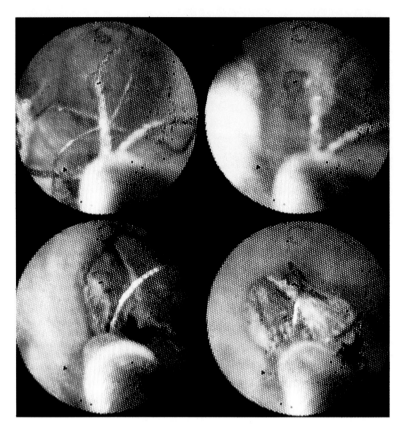

PLATE 34–1. Endoscopic views of process of grasping and removing stone with new type basket forceps.

permit easy capture of a stone, and it should not allow the stone to slip from within the basket during extraction. To meet these requirements, new mechanical basket forceps were developed that differ from existing forceps[46, 63, 64] (see Figs. 34–9 and 34–10). Basket forceps are available with baskets of various sizes, and the basket should be selected according to the size, characteristics, and position of the stone(s) to be extracted.

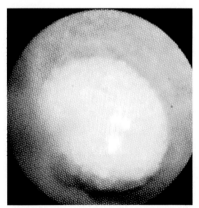

PLATE 34–2. Endoscopic view of retained stone demonstrated in Figure 34–2.

The epithelium of the biliary tract is harder and more resistant to endoscopic "pinch-type" biopsy than other mucosal surfaces of the gastrointestinal tract. Therefore a biopsy forceps with a needle bayonet or stylet within the forceps cups is useful for targeting and fixing the forceps in position to obtain a specimen (see Fig. 34–10).

It is common to encounter unusual circumstances and technical problems during any endoscopic procedure. Other accessories of various types are frequently useful during choledochoscopy. Some recommended items are shown in Figure 34–10.

When thick fluid, sludge, and floating debris are present in the bile ducts, a flushing tube can be used to wash out the material from the endoscopic field.[46, 63] Various types of crushing forceps should be available for grasping and crushing large, impacted, and/or hard calculi.[46, 63, 65] These include an alligator-type grasping forceps, a three-armed basket, and a loop-type snare. Nd:YAG laser energy has been used in conjunction with a choledochofiberscope to break stones in the bile ducts.[15, 66, 67] Shock waves produced by a high-voltage electrical discharge (electrohydraulic lithotripsy) have

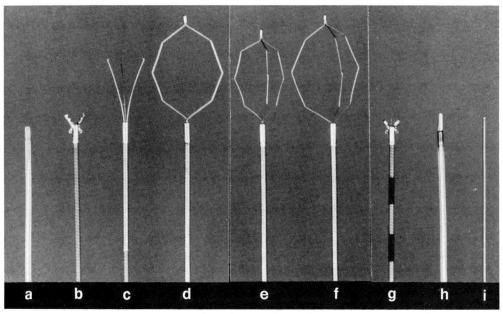

FIGURE 34–10. Optional accessories. *a*, Flushing tube; *b*, alligator forceps; *c*, three-armed forceps; *d*, loop-type stone crushing forceps; *e* and *f*, basket-type stone-crushing forceps; *g*, biopsy forceps with needle; *h*, cutting knife for use with high-frequency electrosurgical generator; *i*, guide wire.

also been used in conjunction with choledochoscopy to shatter stones.[68, 69] Strictures have been incised using an electrosurgical cutting knife.[46] Grüntzig-type balloons are useful for dilating strictures or tortuous branches of the bile ducts.[70] The fibrous tract through which the choledochoscope must pass to enter the biliary system may become narrowed, in which case either rigid or flexible dilators may be used to open the channel.[8, 17, 56]

TECHNIQUE OF POSTOPERATIVE CHOLEDOCHOFIBEROSCOPY VIA T-TUBE TRACT

A T-tube tract of sufficient diameter is required for passage of the choledochoscope into the bile duct. Generally this means that the portion of the T-tube that exits to the skin must have a diameter of 18 French. The tract produced by a tube of this diameter will allow a fiberscope with an insertion tube diameter of 6 mm to pass without difficulty after the tract has become fibrotic over the course of about 3 weeks.

It is preferable to perform flexible choledochoscopy under fluoroscopic control since it is useful to know the position of the instrument tip as well as the stone or stones within the bile duct. X-ray and endoscopic views are complementary and increase the reliability and thoroughness of the procedure, so that residual stones and other lesions are less

likely to be overlooked when both methods of observation are used.

Premedication and anesthesia are not necessary, as percutaneous choledochoscopy is seldom associated with discomfort. However, sedatives may be administered parenterally if necessary. Atropine is given intramuscularly before the examination.

The skin around the fibrous tract is sterilized in the same manner as for any operative procedure, and other than at the fibrous tract the patient is covered with a sterile drape.

Cholangiography is then performed by injecting a 30% solution of an iodinated contrast agent through the T-tube. The use of more concentrated solution such as the standard 60% concentration will result in dense opacification that may obscure small stones. Cholangiography provides a clear representation of the configuration of the bile ducts, residual stones, and any areas of narrowing or stricture formation. The contrast medium must be well mixed with the bile so that all areas of the biliary system are opacified, including the more peripheral intrahepatic ducts.

After satisfactory radiographs of the entire biliary system are obtained, the contrast material is washed out of the duct with saline, and then the T-tube is carefully withdrawn.

The fiberscope is inserted under direct vision, observing the inner wall of the fibrous tract as it is passed toward and into the bile duct (Fig. 34–11). During insertion, saline is injected through the irrigation channel of the fiberscope to maintain patency of the fibrous tract and bile duct and to provide a good visual field by eliminating bile and floating substances that obscure the view. One of the major merits of the choledochofiberscope is that it provides an excellent visual field. This allows the endoscopist to proceed using direct vision at all times. The fiberscope must be inserted carefully; the tip angulation mechanism should be used to maintain a satisfactory visual field. The endoscope should never be inserted blindly or forcefully. Abnormal endoscopic findings are documented by endoscopic photography.

Once floating stones are discovered and their sizes estimated, a basket forceps of comparable size is introduced through the accessory channel of the fiberscope. With the basket in the closed position, it is passed into the bile duct beyond the stone. Then the basket is opened and drawn back toward the stone. Generally, stones can be easily caught with the basket. It is then closed slowly until the stone is encountered, and then a firm, steady force is maintained. The basket must not be closed with too much force since this will crush the stone(s), and it will then be more difficult and time-consuming to remove the fragments. If the stone(s) cannot be captured, the basket size is often unsuitable and a larger basket should be used. Once the stone(s) is

(are) secure in the basket, the choledochoscope is removed slowly from the bile duct and through the T-tube tract.

If stones are too large to capture with a stone-holding basket forceps, they must be crushed using a stone-crushing forceps. If impacted, a stone may be crushed with an alligator forceps or three-armed forceps. Those that are too hard to crush with these mechanical devices may sometimes be shattered with a laser beam. After crushing a stone or stones, the flushing tube should be used to wash the duct. Otherwise fine particles and debris from the crushed stone(s) will obscure the visual field. Fragments of stones must be removed with a stone-holding forceps.

When there are many stones or stone fragments, crushing and extraction must be repeated as necessary until the bile duct has been completely cleared. This may be repeated usually for 1 to 2 hours. If the duct cannot be cleared during this time, the procedure should be repeated at another time. To facilitate subsequent procedures, the patency of the fibrotic T-tube tract must be maintained by reinsertion of the T-tube. This is relatively easy to accomplish. Damage to the bile duct wall by the tip of the tube occurs less often with a T-tube than with a straight tube.

After reinsertion of the T-tube, small stones and debris should be washed from the bile duct by introducing saline through the

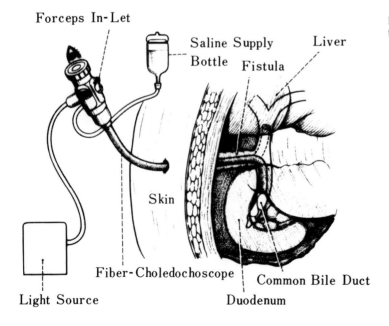

Forceps In-Let

Saline Supply Bottle

Liver

Fistula

Skin

Fiber-Choledochoscope

Common Bile Duct

Light Source

Duodenum

FIGURE 34–11. Schema of T-tube tract choledochoscopy.

reinserted T-tube. A final cholangiogram should be obtained to demonstrate either that no stones are present, or the number and position of any residual stones.

If the T-tube is left in place after the procedure to provide future access, it must be fixed securely to the skin to prevent dislodgement. If this should occur, the fibrous tract will close in a few days. It is possible to insert a thin tube through the tract within 24 hours of dislodgement. This can be followed by dilation, using a fibrous tract dilator so that eventually the T-tube may be reinserted.

Once there is confirmation that the bile duct is free of stones, the T-tube can be removed permanently. Bile leakage may be avoided by changing the T-tube to one with a smaller diameter before permanent removal. Thereafter the fibrous tract will close completely within a few days.

INDICATIONS FOR CHOLEDOCHOFIBEROSCOPY

Choledocholithiasis

When choledocholithiasis has been diagnosed preoperatively, the combined use of conventional surgical exploration and operative choledochoscopy reduces the frequency of postoperative retained bile duct stones.[71–74] However, small stones may stray into the intrahepatic ducts. Impacted stones may require a considerable amount of time for removal by operative choledochoscopy. If these problems excessively increase operation time or if there is a possibility of residual stones, then biliary drainage should be established. This also provides endoscopic access during the postoperative period. Biliary drainage should also be done when common duct stones are discovered by chance during surgery and a choledochoscope is not at hand. Stones can then be removed safely by postoperative choledochoscopy (Fig. 34–12; Plate 34–2).

There are a number of methods for treatment of choledocholithiasis via a T-tube or T-tube tract including dissolution therapy of various types and extraction under fluoroscopic control using a steerable catheter as introduced by Burhenne.[75] The latter method is frequently used in many countries and has a good success rate in experienced hands. However, this method also has some disadvantages. Radiation exposure can be considerable, especially if there are numerous stones and the procedure is prolonged

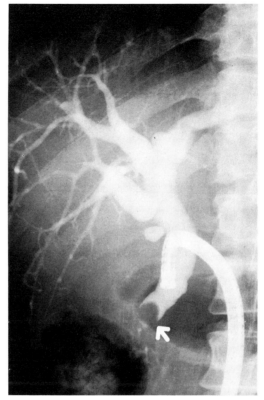

FIGURE 34–12. Cholangiogram demonstrating choledochofiberscope in relation to retained stone (*arrow*) in distal common bile duct.

or must be repeated. Calculi smaller than 5 mm may be difficult to define radiographically; they may be obscured as increasing amounts of contrast in the ducts produce denser opacification. It may also be difficult to remove impacted intrahepatic stones by the method of Burhenne, and it is sometimes necessary to allow a period of time for these to pass into the more distal intrahepatic or extrahepatic ducts. Some technical problems are common to both the endoscopic and fluoroscopically guided methods of stone extraction. For example, some stones may be too large to be withdrawn through the existing T-tube tract. The choice between endoscopic and fluoroscopically guided stone extraction depends on the clinical and anatomic circumstances and expertise in one or both procedures. Among different methods currently used to remove residual stones in the common bile duct, we consider endoscopic extraction under direct visual control to be the least traumatic to the ductal epithelium.[12, 75–79]

Birkett and Williams[44] performed choledochoscopy via a T-tube tract in 28 patients;

59 stones were extracted in 22 patients. In 6 patients, choledochoscopy resolved the nature of filling defects noted by T-tube cholangiography that proved to be due to findings other than calculi. The endoscopic findings in 3 of these patients were multiple papillary adenocarcinomas, malignant stricture, and a benign polyp. No abnormalities were found at endoscopy in a fourth patient, and in the last 2 patients the radiographic abnormalities were explained by the presence of normal mucosal folds.

Yamakawa et al.[38] performed 808 choledochoscopies via a T-tube tract in 292 patients; 104 patients had bile duct stones; the bile ducts were cleared of stones in 101 cases. The average number of sessions for removal of stones from the extrahepatic bile ducts was 1.5. If the stones were in the intrahepatic ducts, from 3 to 58 sessions were necessary, with a mean of 15.4. Failure of stone extraction was attributed to improper insertion of the T-tube, a long, narrow, and/or tortuous T-tube tract, giant stones, and stones lodged in the peripheral intrahepatic ducts.

Intrahepatic Stones

The problem of intrahepatic bile duct stones is encountered more frequently in some areas of the world, parts of the Orient, for example, than in others. Unilateral intra-

hepatic stones have been treated by left hepatic lobectomy.[80, 81] Bilateral intrahepatic stones can be even more troublesome because they frequently cannot be completely removed by conventional surgical stone extraction procedures.[82–84] These technical problems and more drastic methods of treatment are now obviated by operative and nonoperative stone extraction procedures. The use of a flexible fiberoptic choledochoscope makes it possible to completely remove intrahepatic stones in the majority of cases, and choledochoscopy is considered by numerous authors to be a satisfactory method for the treatment of intrahepatic stones.[2, 39, 46, 56, 85–87]

When intrahepatic stones are discovered preoperatively, cholangiography may not reveal the entire biliary system because the intrahepatic ducts are often packed with stones and sludge. The degree and extent of stone impaction may not be demonstrated, since the contrast medium does not penetrate beyond the impacted stones and debris. In such cases, preoperative choledochofiberoscopy can be performed to eliminate some stones, debris, and turbid bile (Fig. 34–13; Plate 34–3). Then, endoscopic selective cholangiography can be performed to outline the entire intrahepatic bile duct system; the operative approach can then be planned based on accurate radiographic assessment.[55, 86]

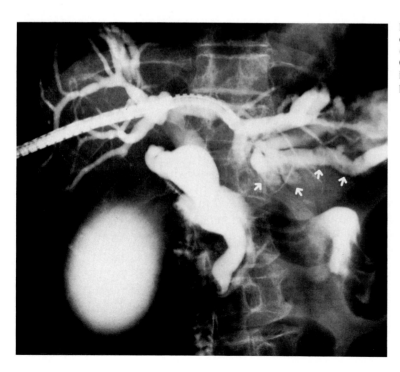

FIGURE 34–13. Cholangiogram demonstrating retained stones (*arrows*) in left hepatic bile duct. Choledochofiberscope has been inserted into biliary system via a percutaneous approach.

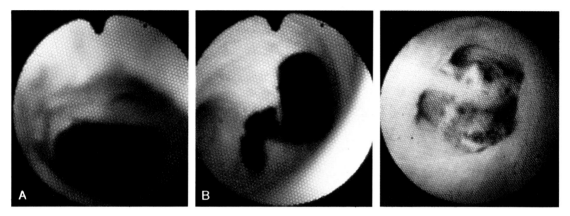

PLATE 34—3. PLATE 34—4.

PLATE 34—3. Endoscopic views A, B of stones demonstrated by cholangiography in Figure 34-3.
PLATE 34—4. Endoscopic view of impact stone demonsestrated by cholangiography in Figure 34-15.

Hwang et al.[39] treated intrahepatic stones in 30 patients with a 7-mm diameter fiberoptic choledochoscope via T-tube tracts. Complete extraction of all stones present was achieved in 25 cases (83%). The average number of sessions required was 4.3 with a range of 1 to 15. Chen et al.[88] performed endoscopic extraction of calculi via T-tube tracts in 66 patients. In 48 of these, the stones were located in the intrahepatic ducts, and the authors successfully extracted these in 38 patients.

Murata et al.[55] successfully extracted intrahepatic stones via T-tube tracts in 6 of 9 patients. In 3 other patients, these authors extracted intrahepatic calculi with the aid of percutaneous transhepatic cholangioscopy. The average number of procedures for these 3 patients was 5.3. Murata et al.[55] noted that the percutaneous approach had advantages in some circumstances, and considered it indicated when surgery was precluded by dense adhesions as a result of multiple prior operations, and when other methods of extraction, via a T-tube tract, for example, had failed. The latter circumstance may be due to impaction of stones beyond a stricture. The procedure may also be considered when technical problems such as a prior partial gastrectomy with a Billroth II anastomosis or

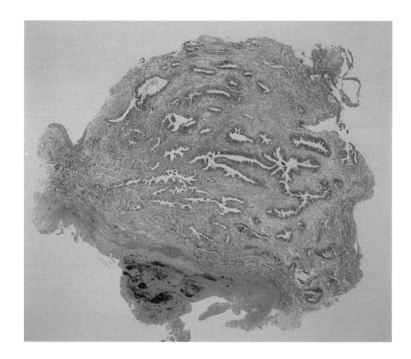

PLATE 34—5. Microscopic view of biopsy specimen pertaining to Figure 34-17.

Roux-Y anastomosis renders endoscopic sphincterotomy and extraction of stones difficult or impossible.[89]

Orii et al.[67] have used the Nd:YAG laser to fragment stones in the bile ducts. In a report of 11 cases, there were 8 patients with intrahepatic stones. Both the percutaneous cholangioscopic approach and choledochoscopy via T-tube tracts were utilized in this series. These authors noted that the Nd:YAG laser was especially useful for removal of stones impacted in the intrahepatic ducts that could not be removed by the usual methods of choledochofiberoscopy. In their technique, the laser wave guide is placed near the stone and a 5-second pulse of laser energy is delivered at a power of 40 watts. This may be repeated several times for one stone. Orii et al.[67] have also pointed out that YAG laser energy is suitable for fragmenting bilirubinate stones, but that cholesterol stones resist fracturing.

When intrahepatic stones are discovered intra-operatively, removal of as many as possible should be attempted at surgery. However, if the stones are numerous and impacted into many of the peripheral intrahepatic radicles, removal of all stones may necessitate excessive operating time. If complete removal is precluded because of the length of surgery, or if there is uncertainty that the biliary system has been cleared of stones, then an access route to the biliary system should be established so that postoperative choledochofiberoscopy can be performed.

T-tube choledochofiberoscopy can be performed when intrahepatic stones have been discovered postoperatively by T-tube cholangiography (Figs. 34–14, 34–15, and 34–16; Plate 34–4). As stones are removed, the status of the intrahepatic ducts and any remaining stones can be defined by repeated T-tube cholangiography.[2, 39, 42, 46, 90]

If postoperative recurrence of intrahepatic stones is expected, a provision can be made at surgery for jejunostomy tract choledochoscopy by performing a choledochojejunostomy and then fixing a portion of the jejunum near the biliary enteric anastomosis to the parietal peritoneum. This provides an access route to the intrahepatic ducts via the jejunostomy tract that can be used in the event of a recurrence of intrahepatic stones long after closure of the choledochojejunostomy.[91]

Cholangiocarcinoma

The cause of obstructive jaundice by percutaneous transhepatic cholangiography may sometimes remain in doubt. Impacted stones

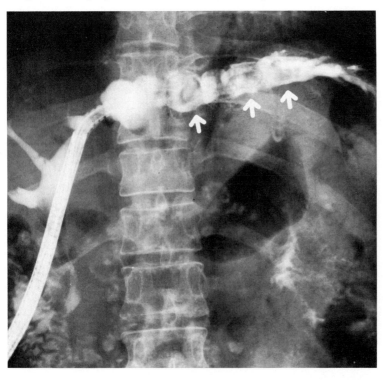

FIGURE 34–14. Choledochoscopic approach to retained stones (*arrows*) in left hepatic duct.

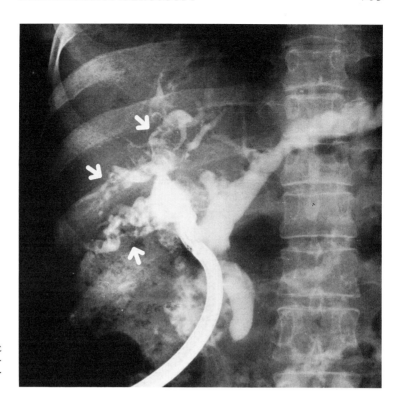

FIGURE 34–15. Choledochoscopic approach via T-tube tract to retained stones (*arrows*) in right hepatic bile ducts.

with complete obstruction may occasionally resemble cholangiocarcinoma. In such cases, the diagnosis may be facilitated by percutaneous transhepatic cholangioscopy. After a period of percutaneous drainage, a flexible choledochoscope can be introduced through the intrahepatic fibrous tract.[92, 93] If the obstruction is not due to gallstones, biopsy under direct vision from the area of obstruction will establish the diagnosis of cholangiocarcinoma[94–98] (Fig. 34–17; Plate 34–5). Operative and postoperative choledochoscopy have also been reported as useful in the diagnosis of cholangiocarcinoma.[99] However, preoperative definitive diagnosis and a determination of the extent of malignant infiltration are preferable, so that the proper management can be decided before surgery, or in some cases without resorting to operation.[98]

Other Findings by Choledochofiberoscopy

In addition to calculi and cholangiocarcinoma, parasites, benign tumors, xanthoma, compression ulcers, and granulomas discovered by choledochofiberoscopy have been reported.[100–103]

CONTRAINDICATIONS AND COMPLICATIONS

There are no absolute contraindications except for a bile duct that has too small a diameter to introduce a choledochofiberscope.

Relatively few complications have been reported.[24, 38, 44, 104–106]

In the series of Birkett and Williams,[44] of 28 patients treated by T-tube choledochoscopy, transient fever developed in 5 patients, and pancreatitis developed in 2. Of the 218 procedures performed by Chen et al.[88] there were subsequently 8 episodes of abdominal pain, 6 of fever and chills, and 2 of bleeding from the fistula tract. A duodenocutaneous fistula developed in 1 patient. Yamakawa et al.[38] performed 808 endoscopic procedures via T-tube tracts in 292 patients. Limited extravasation of contrast occurred in 5 patients, 3 of whom had retained stones. Free extravasation of contrast from the T-tube tract occurred in 4 patients, with formation of a subhepatic collection of bile in 2, a subphrenic bile collection in 1, and free intra-abdominal extravasation in 1 patient. Fistula formation between the T-tube tract and duodenum occurred in 1 patient. In the report of 30 cases by Hwang et al.,[39] fever and chills

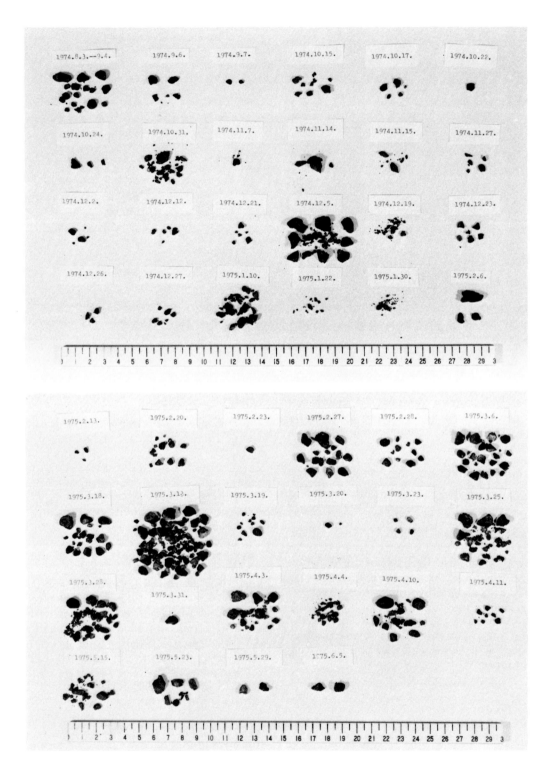

FIGURE 34–16. *Top,* Stones removed from left hepatic bile duct shown in Figure 34–14. *Bottom,* Stones removed from right hepatic bile duct shown in Figure 34–15.

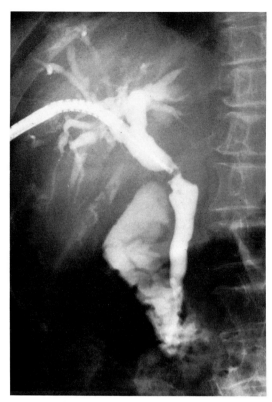

FIGURE 34–17. Cholangiogram demonstrating endo-scopic biopsy of cholangiocarcinoma of the common hepatic duct.

developed in 6 patients, and a pyogenic liver abscess occurred in 1. Moss et al.[43] performed T-tube choledochoscopy in 17 patients (19 procedures) and encountered 1 episode of post-procedure bacteremia and 1 episode of bacteremia after dilation of the T-tube tract.

References

1. Gocho K, Ikezawa H, Hiratsuka H. Endoscopic approaches in intrahepatic calculi: report 1, significance of preoperative and postoperative choledochoscopy. Abstracts of the 8th Congress of the Japanese Society of Gastroenterological Surgery, Amori, Japan, 1975; 24.
2. Gocho K, Hiratsuka H, Yamakawa T. Endoscopic management of intrahepatic calculi using the choledochofiberscope. Proceedings of the 2nd Asian Pacific Congress of Endoscopy, Singapore, 1976; 214–8.
3. Shore JM, Lippman HN. A flexible choledochoscope. Lancet 1965; 1:1200–1.
4. Shore JM, Berci G. Operative management of calculi in the hepatic ducts. Am J Surg 1970; 119:625–30.
5. Takada T, Hanyu F, Kobayashi S, et al. Percutaneous transhepatic cholangiodrainage and cholangioscopy for the cases of severe obstructive jaundice caused by pancreatic tumor. Proceedings of the 18th World Congress of the International College of Surgeons. Amsterdam: Excerpta Medica, 1972; 478.
6. Takada T, Suzuki S, Nakamura K, et al. Percutaneous transhepatic cholangioscopy as a new approach to the diagnosis of the biliary diseases. Gastroenterol Endosc (Jpn) 1974; 16:106–11.
7. Gocho K, Hiratsuka H, Hasegawa M, et al. Percutaneous intrahepatic fistula dilation for nonoperative choledochoscopy in intrahepatic stones. Jpn J Gastroenterol 1974; 71:526.
8. Gocho K, Hiratsuka H. Percutaneous intrahepatic fistula dilation—case report of intrahepatic stones. Diagnosis and treatment of obstructive jaundice cases. Tokyo: Igakutosho Shuppan, 1976; 85–90.
9. Yamakawa T, Mieno K, Gocho K, Shikata J. Improved choledochoscopes. Gastroenterol Endosc (Jpn) 1975; 17:459–67.
10. Yamakawa T, Mieno K, Shikata J. Improved choledochofiberscopes and non-surgical removal of retained biliary calculi under direct visual control. (Abstr) Gastroenterology 1975; 68:1051–2.
11. Nimura Y, Hayakawa N, Toyoda S, et al. Percutaneous transhepatic cholangioscopy (PTCS). Stomach and Intestine (Jpn) 1981; 16:681–9.
12. Tsuchiya Y. A new safer method of percutaneous transhepatic cholangiography. Jpn J Gastroenterol 1966; 66:438–55.
13. Takada T, Hanyu F, Kobayashi S, Uchida Y. Percutaneous transhepatic cholangial drainage: Direct approach under fluoroscopic control. J Surg Oncol 1976; 8:83–97.
14. Nakayama T, Ikeda A, Okuda K. Percutaneous transhepatic drainage of the biliary tract: Technique and results in 104 cases. Gastroenterology 1978; 74:554–9.
15. Ichikawa K, Hayashi S, Ema Y, et al. Percutaneous transhepatic cholangioscopic laser lithotomy (PTCS-LL) and percutaneous transhepatic cholecystoscopy (PTCCS). Gastroenterol Endosc (Jpn) 1982; 24:2022.
16. Ichikawa K, Nakazawa S, Naito Y, et al. Percutaneous transhepatic cholecystoscopy (PTCCS)—the second report. Gastroenterol Endosc (Jpn) 1983; 25:798.
17. Miyoshi T, Yamakawa T, Itoh S, et al. Percutaneous transhepatic cholangioscopy for malignant biliary tract diseases—PTCS or PTCCS. Gastroenterol Endosc (Jpn) 1983; 25:537–41.
18. Inui K, Nakae Y, Nakamura J, et al. Percutaneous transhepatic cholecystoscopy (PTCCS). Gastroenterol Endosc (Jpn) 1983; 25:636–41.
19. Nora PF, Berci G, Dorazio RA, et al. Operative choledochoscopy: results of a prospective study in several institutions. Am J Surg 1977; 133:105–10.
20. Broadie TA, Lowe DK, Glover JL, et al. Intraoperative choledochoscopy: an efficacious adjunct to common duct exploration in calculous biliary tract disease. Am Surgeon 1981; 47:121–4.
21. Feliciano DV, Mattox KL, Jordan GL Jr. The value of choledochoscopy in exploration of the common bile duct. Ann Surg 1980; 191:649–54.
22. Cooperman A, Gelbfish G, Zimmon DS. Choledochoscopy. Surg Clin North Am 1982; 62:853–9.
23. Finnis D, Rowntree T. Choledochoscopy in exploration of the common bile duct. Br J Surg 1977; 64:661–4.
24. Kappas A, Alexander-Williams J, Keighley MRB, Watts GT. Operative choledochoscopy. Br J Surg 1979; 66:177–9.

25. Ashby BS. Fiberoptic choledochoscopy in common bile duct surgery. Ann R Coll Surg (Engl) 1978; 60:399–403.

26. Motson RW, Wood AJ, DeJode LR. Operative choledochoscopy: experience with a rigid choledochoscope. Br J Surg 1980; 67:406–9.

27. Leslie D. Endoscopy of the bile duct: an evaluation. Aust NZ J Surg 1974; 44:340–2.

28. Botticher R, Knoch M. Diagnostischr und therapeutischr Stellenwert der intraoperativen Choledochusrevisionen. Langenbecks Arch Chir 1980; 351:17–22.

29. Michot F, Champault G, Patel JCL. La choledocoscopie en chirurgie biliaire. Med Chir Dig (Fr) 1979; 8:333–5.

30. Olivero S, Ibba F, Foco A, Viglione GC. Intraoperative choledochoscopy. Minerva Chir (Suppl) (It) 1978; 23–4:1773–86.

31. Yap PC, Atacador M, Yap AG, Yap RG. Choledochoscopy as a complementary procedure to operative cholangiography in biliary surgery. Am J Surg 1980; 140:648–52.

33. Wang YH. The use of operative choledochoscope. J Formosan Med Assoc 1982; 81:1140–3.

34. Lin SC. Clinical application of fiber choledochoscope: report of 15 cases. (Author's translation) Chung Hua Wai Ko Tsa Chih 1980; 18:446–7.

35. Shikata J, Yamakawa T, Watanabe, et al. Clinical evaluation of choledochofiberscope. Jpn J Gastroenterol 1976; 73:1222–31. (English Abstr)

36. Okabe N, Kawai K, Kondo O, et al. Operative and postoperative choledochofiberoscopy. Am J Surg 1979; 137:816–20.

37. Arai T. Practice of operative choledochoscopy. J Clin Surg (Jpn) 1978; 33:857–62.

38. Yamakawa T, Komaki F, Shikata J. The importance of postoperative choledochoscopy for management of retained biliary tract stones. Jpn J Surg 1980; 10:302–9.

39. Hwang MH, Yang JC, Lee SA. Choledochofiberoscopy in the postoperative management of intrahepatic stones. Am J Surg 1980; 139:860–4.

40. Chen MF, Chou FF, Wang CS. Removal of retained biliary stone by choledochofiberscope. J Formosan Med Assoc 1979; 78:761–6.

41. Ho LC. Postoperative choledochofiberoscopy: an experience of 39 patients. Southeast Asian J Surg 1980; 3:65–71.

42. Ker CG, Sheen PC. Postoperative choledochofiberscopic removal of retained intrahepatic stones. Taiwan I Hseuh Hui Tsa Chi 1981; 80:158–69.

43. Moss JP, Whelan JG Jr, Dedman TC III, Voyles RG. Postoperative choledochoscopy through the T-tube tract. Surg Gynecol Obstet 1980; 151:807–9.

44. Birkett DH, Williams LF Jr. Postoperative fiberoptic choledochoscopy. Ann Surg 1981; 194:630–4.

45. Siegel JH, Mayer LF. Percutaneous choledochoscopy and cholecytoscopy: diagnostic and therapeutic uses. Endoscopy 1981; 13:124–7.

46. Gocho K, Hiratsuka H. Postoperative choledochofiberscopic removal of intrahepatic stones. Jpn J Surg 1977; 7:18–27.

47. Gocho K, Ikezawa H, Hasegawa M, et al. Postoperative choledochoscopic follow-up of a common bile duct cancer. Prog Dig Endosc (Jpn) 1977; 10:244–6.

48. Yamakawa T, Komaki F, Shikata J. Experience with routine choledochoscopy via the T-tube sinus tract. World J Surg 1978; 2:379–85.

49. Moss JP, Whelan JG Jr, Powell RW, et al. Postop-

erative choledochoscopy via the T-tube tract. JAMA 1976; 236:2781–2.

50. Birkett DH, Williams LF. Choledochoscopic removal of retained stones via a T-tube tract. Am J Surg 1980; 139:531–4.

51. Miyazaki I, Nagakawa T, Kurachi M, et al. Choledochojejunostomy (end-to-side anastomosis) for postoperative choledochofiberoscope. Reports on Hepatic Duct Disorder, Japanese Research Group, 1979; 30–3.

52. Hwang MH, Kuo RJ. Modified Roux-en-Y choledochojejunostomy with postoperative choledochofiberoscopy in the treatment of intrahepatic stones. J Formosan Med Assoc 1980; 79:631–6.

53. Sheen PC, Ker CG. Intrahepatic stones (II: Clinical study). J Formosan Med Assoc 1981; 80:1217–26.

54. Ho LC. Surgical treatment of intrahepatic stones: clinical significance of additional procedure. J Chun Shan Med Dent Coll 1981; 3:95–9.

55. Murata N, Beppu T, Bandai Y, et al. Treatment of intrahepatic lithiasis using the choledochofiberscope. Endoscopy 1981; 13:240–2.

56. Nimura Y, Hayakawa N, Toyoda S, et al. Endoscopic treatment for intrahepatic stone. Surgical Therapy (Jpn) 1982; 46:577–86.

57. Amberg JR, Chun G. Transcystic duct treatment of common bile duct stones. Gastrointest Radiol 1981; 6:361–2.

58. Mason RR, Shorvon PJ, Cotton PB. Percutaneous descending biliary sphincterotomy with a choledochoscope passed through the cystic duct after cholecystostomy. Br J Radiol 1982; 55:595–7.

59. Iseli A, Marshall VC. Choledochoscopy: a comparison of a rigid and a flexible fiberoptic instrument. Med J Aust 1978; 1:131–2.

60. Siegel JH, Sherman HI, Davis RC Jr, Webb WA. Modification of a bronchoscope for percutaneous choledochoscopy. Gastrointest Endosc 1981; 27:179–81.

61. Oishi N, Yamakawa T, Miyoshi T, et al. Experience with postoperative choledochoscopy using Olympus CHF type 4B. Gastroenterol Endosc (Jpn) 1982; 24:1910–6.

62. Gocho K, Ikezawa H, Kameya S, et al. Experience using Machida fiberoptic choledochoscope FCH-6T. Gastroenterol Endosc (Jpn) 1981; 23:1862.

63. Gocho K, Hasegawa M, Masuda H, et al. Endoscopic approaches in intrahepatic calculi: (2nd report) in special reference to developments of forceps of choledochoscopy. Prog Dig Endosc (Jpn) 1975; 7:170–3.

64. Gocho K, Iizuka K, Ishimoto K, et al. Development and improvement of basket forceps for choledochofiberscopy. Prog Dig Endosc (Jpn) 1979; 14:65–8.

65. Komaki F, Yamakawa T, Shikata J. Newly devised forceps for non-surgical removal of intrahepatic stones. Prog Dig Endosc (Jpn) 1976; 9:65–8.

66. Orii K, Nakahara A, Takase Y, et al. Choledocholithotomy by Yag laser with a choledochofiberscope: case reports of two patients. Surgery 1981; 90:120–2.

67. Orii K, Ozaki A, Takase Y, Iwasaki Y. Lithotomy of intrahepatic and choledochal stones with YAG laser. Surg Gynecol Obstet 1983; 156:485–8.

68. Manegold BC, Mennicken C, Jung M. Endoscopic electrohydraulic disintegration of common bile duct concrements. (Abstr) Scand J Gastroenterol (Suppl 78) 1982; 17:144.

69. Nakajima M, Fujimoto S, Imaoka W, et al. Endo-

scopic electrohydraulic lithotripsy (EEL) of biliary tract stones. Gastroenterol Endosc (Jpn) 1982; 24:1391–9.

70. Grüntzig A, Kumpe DA. Technique of percutaneous transluminal angioplasty with the Grüntzig balloon catheter. AJR 1979; 132:547–52.

71. Samama G, Dupuis F, Descamps L. Cent lithiases du choledoque sans lithiase residuelle. Interet de la choledocoscopie. Med Chir Dig (Fr) 1981; 10: 575–6.

72. Rattner DW, Warshaw AL. Impact of choledochoscopy on the management of choledocholithiasis: experience with 499 common duct explorations at the Massachusetts General Hospital. Ann Surg 1981; 194:76–9.

73. Bauer JJ, Salky BA, Gelernt IM, Kreel I. Experience with the flexible fiberoptic choledochoscope. Ann Surg 1981; 194:161–6.

74. Berci G, Shore JM, Morgenstern L, Hamlin JA. Choledochoscopy and operative fluorocholangiography in the prevention of retained bile duct stones. World J Surg 1978; 2:411–27.

75. Burhenne HJ. Percutaneous extraction of retained biliary tract stones: 661 patients. AJR 1980; 134:888–98.

76. Mazzariello RM. A fourteen-year experience with nonoperative instrument extraction of retained bile duct stones. World J Surg 1978; 2:447–55.

77. Pepe RG, Havrilla TR, Meaney TF. Percutaneous retrieval of retained common bile duct stones. Cleve Clin Q 1977; 44:35–40.

78. Ellman BA, Berman HL. Treatment of a common duct stone via transhepatic approach. Gastrointest Radiol 1981; 6:357–9.

79. Choi TK, Lee NW, Wong J, Ong GB. Extraperitoneal sphincteroplasty for residual stones. Ann Surg 1982; 196:26–9.

80. Huang CC. Partial resection of the liver in treatment of intrahepatic stones. Chinese Med J 1959; 79:40–5.

81. Longmire WP, Tompkins RK. Manual of Liver Surgery. New York: Springer-Verlag, 1981; 190–8.

82. Maki T, Sato T, Matsushiro T. A reappraisal of surgical treatment for intrahepatic gallstones. Ann Surg 1972; 175:155–65.

83. Warshaw AI, Bartlet MK. Technic for finding and removing stones from intrahepatic bile ducts. Am J Surg 1974; 127:353–4.

84. Takada T, Uchida Y, Fukushima Y, et al. Classification and treatment of intrahepatic calculi. Jap J Gastroenterol Surg 1978; 11:769–74.

85. Yamakawa T, Mieno K, Kasai T, et al. Two cases of hepatic calculi detected by selective cholangiography under direct visual guidance by improved choledochofiberscope. Prog Dig Endosc (Jpn) 1975; 6:196–9.

86. Nimura Y, Maeda S, Kamiya J, et al. Endoscopic treatments of intrahepatic stones. Operation (Jpn) 1982; 36:161–8.

87. Chen MF, Chou FF, Wang CS, et al. Surgical treatment of intrahepatic gallstone—An experience of 194 operations. (Abstr 1547) Scand J Gastroenterol (Suppl) 1982; 17:389.

88. Chen M-F, Chou FF, Wang CS, Jang YI. Experience with and complications of postoperative choledochofiberoscopy for retained biliary stones. Acta Chir Scand 1982; 148:503–9.

89. Shimada H, Nakagawara G, Abe T, et al. Extraction of retained gallstones using a fiber-choledochoscope through a PTC-drainage fistula. Jpn J Surg 1983; 13:415–9.

90. Yamakawa T, Komaki F, Kitano Y, et al. Intrahepatic stones and postoperative choledochoscopy. Gastroenterol Jpn 1980; 15:577–83.

91. Hwang MH. Clinical experience of choledochoscopy in residual and recurrent intrahepatic stones. The Postgraduate Course: Choledochoscope and Gallstone. The 4th Biennial General Scientific Meeting of Association of Surgeons of Southeast Asia. Kaohsiung, Republic of China, April 1, 1983.

92. Nimura Y, Kamiya J, Hasegawa H, et al. Percutaneous transhepatic cholangioscopy (PTCS) for diagnosis of obstructive jaundice. (Abstr 493) Scand J Gastroenterol (Suppl) 1982; 17:124.

93. Yasui K, Mukoyama T, Toyota S, et al. Percutaneous transhepatic cholangioscopy and bile duct biopsy. Abstracts of 28th Congress of Societe International de Chirurgie. San Francisco: 1979; 73.

94. Hattori T, Yasui K, Hayakawa N, et al. Percutaneous transhepatic biopsy of the bile duct and percutaneous transhepatic cholangioscopy. Abstracts of 4th World Congress of Digestive Endoscopy. Madrid, 1987; 178.

95. Nimura Y. Cholangioscopic diagnosis of cholangiocarcinoma. Diag Imag Abd (Jpn) 1982; 2:73–8.

96. Nimura Y. Importance of preoperative biopsy in bile duct carcinoma cases. Path Clin Med (Jpn) 1983; 1:206–7.

97. Yoshida T, Fukuda S, Iwasaki T, et al. The utility of percutaneous transhepatic cholangio-scope (PTCS) and percutaneous transhepatic cholangio-biopsy (PTCB). Gastroenterol Endosc (Jpn) 1983; 25:392–9.

98. Inui K, Nakae R, Sato T, Nimura Y. A case of common bile duct carcinoma, superficial spreading type, whose invasive extent was diagnosed by cholangioscope before operation. Gastroenterol Endosc (Jpn) 1981; 23:1176–80.

99. Tompkins RK, Johnson J, Storm FK, Longmire WP Jr. Operative endoscopy in the management of biliary tract neoplasms. Am J Surg 1976; 132:174–82.

100. Ker CG, Sheen PC, Kuo MC, Chen ER. Choledochoscopic findings in clonorchiasis. J Surg Assoc, Republic of China 1982; 15:173–80.

101. Ker CG, Huang TJ, Sheen PC, Chen CY. Postoperative choledochofiberoscopy in icteric type hepatoma. Proceedings of the Third Asian-Pacific Congress of Digestive Endoscopy, Taipei, Republic of China 1980; 755–9.

102. Gocho K, Toyoda T, Ishimoto K, et al. A few problems on postoperative choledochoscopy. Prog Dig Endosc (Jpn) 1977; 11:57–9.

103. Shoda Y, Kogure Y, Horikawa T, et al. Benign tumor of the common bile duct detected by intraoperative choledochoscopy—case report. J Clin Surg (Jpn) 1980; 35:1335–9.

104. Chen MF, Chou FF, Wang CS, Jang YY. Experience with and complications of postoperative choledochofiberoscopy for retained biliary stones. Acta Chir Scand 1982; 148:503–9.

105. Weller RM. The choledochoscope—two hazards. (Correspondence) Anaesthesia 1982; 37:606.

106. Griffin WT. Choledochoscopy. Am J Surg 1976; 132:697–8.

Chapter 35

CONGENITAL ANOMALIES OF THE PANCREAS

HARRISON W. PARKER, M.D.

Congenital anomalies of the pancreas are rarely of clinical importance. Prior to the advent of endoscopic retrograde cholangio-pancreatography (ERCP), pancreatic anomalies were found infrequently by the surgeon or as a curiosity at autopsy. With the ability to cannulate the pancreatic duct and obtain pancreatograms preoperatively, some congenital anomalies have been recognized more frequently. Pancreas divisum, annular pancreas, ectopic pancreas, and ductal anomalies have generated the most interest, but other types of anomalies have also been described.

The embryology of the pancreas in relation to developmental anomalies, the classification of these anomalies, a description of pertinent radiographic and endoscopic features, and the clinical relevance of pancreatic anomalies will be discussed in this chapter.

EMBRYOLOGY

The anatomy and embryology of the pancreas are discussed in detail in Chapter 27. Because knowledge of pancreatic embryology is essential to the understanding of the origin of congenital pancreatic anomalies, the main points of this development will be reviewed.

The pancreas is an endocrine/exocrine organ that develops as part of the hepato-pancreatico-duodenal complex. Most information regarding its organogenesis comes from experimental studies in animals.[1] During the fourth week of intrauterine life, the hepatic bud develops from the ventral aspect of the foregut. By the fifth week the ventral anlage of the pancreas arises from the liver bud. The dorsal pancreatic anlage originates directly from the foregut. The ventral portion is initially bilobed, but the left lobe disappears by the fifth week of development.

Fusion of the ventral and dorsal anlagen occurs in the sixth to seventh week. This takes place after the ventral bud has rotated with the common duct behind the duodenum to fuse with the dorsal bud. The ventral anlage contributes the caudal portion of the head and uncinate process to the adult pancreas. The dorsal aspect produces the cephalad portion of the head as well as the body and tail of the pancreas.

With complete fusion of the gland, drainage occurs along the main pancreatic duct, the duct of Wirsung, through the major papilla Vater. The duct of Santorini is a remnant of the dorsal ductal system that opens to the minor papilla, which is 2 to 3 cm proximal to the major papilla. In 7% of the population, however, there is no communication between the duct of Santorini and the duodenum.

CLASSIFICATION OF PANCREATIC ANOMALIES

During organogenesis, a number of embryologic "mistakes" can occur (Table 35–1). Pancreatic anomalies can be classified as failures of migration or fusion, and as anomalies of ductal duplication either as variations in number of ducts or unusual variations of form. A fourth miscellaneous group of anomalies reflects complex developmental problems. Most of these have little significance to the endoscopist but are discussed for completeness. Anomalies of migration, fusion, or duplication are more likely to be encountered during endoscopic examination.

770

TABLE 35–1. **Classification of Pancreatic Anomalies**

1. Migration anomalies
    Annular pancreas
    Ectopic pancreas

2. Fusion anomalies
    Pancreas divisum

3. Ductal duplication anomalies
    Number variations
    Form variations

4. Miscellaneous
    Agenesis
    Hypoplasia
    Cystosis
    Pancreatic "bladder"
    True accessory pancreas

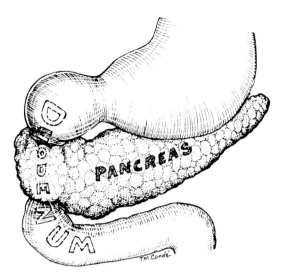

FIGURE 35–1. Annular pancreas.

Annular Pancreas

Annular pancreas, first described by Ecker in 1862,[2] is an unusual occurrence. Fifty per cent of patients with annular pancreas will develop symptoms before the age of one year.[3] This condition is frequently associated with other congenital defects, including malrotation of the intestine, duodenal and esophageal atresia, intestinal webs, Down's syndrome, Meckel's diverticulum, and certain types of congenital heart disease.[4, 5] There is a strong correlation between the presence of annular pancreas and duodenal ulcer disease and also pancreatitis.[6] According to published series, male children are more commonly affected.

At least three theories have been proposed to explain the development of annular pancreas. First, the most popular theory is persistence and fixation of the ventral lobe of the pancreas which grows around the left side of the duodenum to fuse with the dorsal pancreas.[7] Second, atypical growth of the pancreatic ductal system may account for this anomaly. Third, an embryologic defect of the foregut may lead to the development of an annular pancreas.

In a symptomatic patient an annular pancreas constricts the duodenum by encircling the gut tube (Fig. 35–1). Histologically, pancreatic tissue involves the muscular layers of the duodenal wall. Eighty-five per cent of cases are found in the second portion of the duodenum, the majority being positioned proximal to the major papilla (suprapapillary) and totally surrounding the duodenum. Occasionally the anomaly is located in the first or third part of the duodenum.

In children vomiting is the usual presenting symptom. In adults colicky, postprandial epigastric pain, with or without vomiting, has been frequently reported.[8] Jaundice is uncommon, but chronic pancreatitis is a recognized complication. On physical examination, particularly of children, abdominal distention and visible peristalsis may be detected. Annular pancreas can also remain asymptomatic throughout life.

In the newborn or infant, plain x-ray films of the abdomen often show dilation of the duodenum and stomach, producing the "double-bubble" sign.[9] This finding, as well as the duodenal "cut-off" sign, suggests a high degree of mechanical obstruction. The differential diagnosis includes duodenal atresia, webs, and stenosis.

Barium contrast radiography usually reveals a concentric constriction of the second part of the duodenum. The proximal duodenum and stomach may be symmetrically dilated, with effacement of the mucosa.[10] Radiographically the length of the constricted duodenal segment varies from 0.8 cm to 5 cm. Reverse peristalsis proximal to the annulus is often detectable fluoroscopically.

Annular pancreas may not be detected endoscopically. Sometimes a smooth, concentric compression effect with various degrees of stenosis may be recognized. An intraluminal web or an ulcer may be associated with the anomaly. The valvulae conniventes are generally not thickened in appearance and the mucosa looks normal.

Pancreatography, either by ERCP or at operation, will visualize the ductal system of an annular pancreas (Fig. 35–2). The annulus of pancreatic tissue has a single main duct

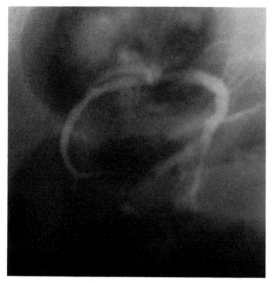

FIGURE 35–2. Retrograde pancreatography demonstrates an annular pancreatic duct. The dorsal portion of the duct is not visualized.

originating in the portion that overlies the left anterior surface of the duodenum. The duct crosses the duodenum posteriorly from right to left and opens into the pancreatic duct near the papilla.[11] Variations of this pattern have been reported by Heymann and Whelan,[12] including direct communication of the annular duct with both the major and minor papilla.

The time-honored management of symptomatic annular pancreas is surgical bypass. Division of the annulus has been fraught with a high incidence of complications (55%), including pancreatitis and pancreatic fistula.[13] Simple bypass procedures such as duodenojejunostomy, duodenoduodenostomy, and gastroenterostomy with vagotomy have an acceptable morbidity rate (10%) and will alleviate the proximal bowel obstruction.

Pancreatic Rest

Ectopic (aberrant or heterotropic) pancreatic tissue is occasionally noted on upper gastrointestinal x-rays and at esophagogastroduodenoscopy. Aberrant pancreatic tissue, often referred to as a pancreatic rest, can be found anywhere along the foregut and proximal midgut and usually causes no symptoms.[14] This entity is defined as the presence of pancreatic tissue which lacks anatomic and vascular continuity with the main body of the pancreas.[15] The frequency of ectopic pancreas in autopsy series ranges from 0.6% to 14%. It is encountered once in

every 500 operations on the upper abdomen.[16]

Three theories have been developed to explain the origin of aberrant pancreas. According to Barbosa et al.,[16] Horgan suggested that small portions of the dorsal and ventral anlagen become attached to the gut wall prior to fusion and coalescence. As the main bodies of pancreatic tissue pull away to complete growth and development, "islands" of pancreatic tissue are left attached to the gut wall. According to these same authors, Warthin proposed, in a second theory, that lateral buds of rudimentary pancreatic ducts penetrate the bowel wall and are eventually severed from the main pancreatic body. It has also been suggested that multipotential cells, capable of specialized differentiation, exist in the primitive gut tube and can form pancreatic rests.

Heterotropic pancreatic tissue has been found throughout the gastrointestinal tract, including within a Meckel's diverticulum. The most common locations are the stomach and duodenum. In the stomach, the pancreatic rest has a predilection for the prepyloric region, often the greater curvature aspect; 75% are found in the submucosa, 15% in the muscular layers, and 10% in the subserosa.[17] Histologically, aberrant pancreas can contain the full complement of lobular structures including acini, islets, and ducts, although any combination of structures may exist.

A pancreatic rest is usually asymptomatic; the incidence is highest in the fifth and sixth decades. A number of nonspecific gastrointestinal symptoms have been attributed to heterotropic pancreatic tissue, including epigastric pain, distention, eructation, nausea, and vomiting (Table 35–2). In most cases it is difficult to prove that a patient's symptoms are secondary to a small mass of tissue which

TABLE 35–2. **Clinical Features of Pancreatic Rest**

1. Usually asymptomatic
2. Incidental discovery common
3. Incidence highest in fifth and sixth decades
4. Obstructive jaundice rare
5. Duodenal obstruction
   Stenosis
   Mass effect
6. Bleeding
7. Intussusception
8. Epigastric pain
9. Malignant degeneration

may or may not be functional. However, malignant degeneration, cyst formation, pancreatitis, islet cell tumors, bleeding, obstructive jaundice, intussusception, and obstruction are infrequently reported as complications of pancreatic rest.[18]

Pancreatic rests appear as round, smooth submucosal filling defects with a central umbilication on barium contrast studies of the upper gastrointestinal tract (Fig. 35–3). In several series, 80% of lesions were located on the greater curvature in the prepyloric region of the stomach. The differential diagnosis includes leiomyoma which closely mimics aberrant pancreas.

Endoscopically, a pancreatic rest appears as a round, sometimes yellow, firm, intramural lesion from 2 mm to 4 cm in diameter with a central mucosal depression that may be ulcerated (Plate 35–1). The relationship of aberrant pancreas to diverticular formation in humans is not clear despite animal studies supporting this association.

Operative treatment is reserved for complicated problems such as recurrent bleeding, obstruction, or malignant degeneration. Less than half the patients operated on for nonspecific symptoms will show clinical improvement.

Pancreas Divisum

Pancreas divisum is an anomaly caused by failure of fusion of the ventral and dorsal

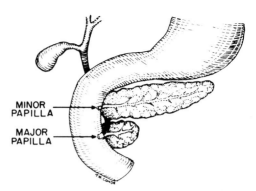

FIGURE 35–4. Completed rotation of ventral pancreas. Non-fusion of ventral and dorsal ducts (pancreas divisum).

anlagen. As a result, the major portion of the pancreas drains through the duct of Santorini and the minor papilla; usually, the duct of Wirsung drains only a small ventral pancreas (Fig. 35–4). In 2% to 3% of cases, the ventral system is rudimentary or absent, and no ductal system can be demonstrated by pancreatography. This may account for some cases of failed pancreatograms during ERCP. Rarely, a narrow-diameter communication exists between the ducts of Wirsung and Santorini (Fig. 35–5).

Pancreas divisum is diagnosed by ERCP or operative pancreatography. Ultrasound and abdominal computed tomography (CT) can be normal or interpreted as showing nonspecific enlargement of the head of the pancreas. The pancreatogram in pancreas divisum demonstrates the immediate appearance of fine branching of the duct of Wirsung following injection of the major papilla (Fig. 35–6).

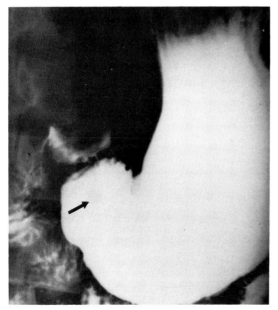

FIGURE 35–3. Barium study of the upper gastrointestinal tract shows a round filling defect (arrow) representing a pancreatic rest in the antrum of the stomach.

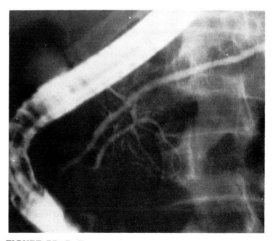

FIGURE 35–5. Pancreatogram showing short, narrow-diameter connecting duct between dorsal and ventral pancreatic ducts. (Courtesy of M. V. Sivak, Jr., M.D.)

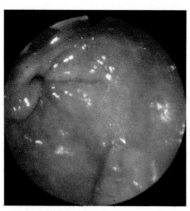

PLATE 35–1. Endoscopic appearance of an antral pancreatic rest, with characteristic central mucosal depression. Note proximity to pylorus. (Courtesy M.V. Sivak, Jr., M.D.)

The radiographically opacified duct is much shorter than expected, and its diameter may also be relatively small. Parenchymal blushing, the result of filling of the ductal system completely to the acini, often occurs because the anatomic variant is not recognized immediately. The patient may experience pain as a result, and acute pancreatitis of the ventral portion of the gland is a possibility. The major differential diagnosis of pancreas divisum is cancer of the pancreas as well as any other process that results in obstruction of the pancreatic duct, including chronic pancreatitis and pseudocyst. In malignancy of the pancreas, the ductogram shows encasement of the main duct or abrupt termination of the flow of contrast medium, with elimination of the normal side-branching pattern. In contrast, the pattern in pancreas divisum is that of a delicately branching structure that gradually and smoothly approaches a terminal point.

Pancreas divisum is the most common anomaly of the pancreas and the most frequent anomaly of the pancreaticobiliary system with the exception of periampullary diverticulum.[19] In autopsy series, it is present in 5% to 10% of the population.[20] Retrospective endoscopic series have a 1.3% to 5% incidence (Table 35–3).

Ideally, the minor papilla should be cannulated to visualize the dorsal portion of the pancreatic ductal system when ERCP is being performed because of suspected pancreatic disease (Fig. 35–7). Radiographic demonstration of the ventral system alone does not eliminate the presence of pancreatic disorders since virtually any pathologic process can involve the larger dorsal portion to the exclusion of the smaller ventral component. Cannulation of the minor papilla is technically difficult due to its small orifice and superior location on the duodenal wall. The average success rate is only about 40% (Table 35–4). The use of tapered or blunt needle-tipped catheters[21] facilitates cannulation and has produced a success rate of 85% in one small series.[22] Catheters with fine metal tips should be used with care, since a significant degree of trauma may be caused with the tip including submucosal injection of contrast medium (Fig. 35–8).

The clinical significance of pancreas divisum remains uncertain. The major question is whether pancreas divisum predisposes to idiopathic pancreatitis because of a relative degree of obstruction at the minor papilla. Cotton[23] found a 16% incidence of pancreas divisum in patients with pancreatitis versus a 3.6% incidence (virtually the same as the incidence in the general population) in patients with biliary tract disease. The incidence of pancreas divisum was even higher (26%) in patients with idiopathic pancreatitis. In a number of reports it has been suggested that acute pancreatitis occurs more often in individuals with pancreas divisum than in their normal counterparts (Table 35–5). The largest series reported (over 4,000 patients), however, showed no increased incidence of pancreas divisum in patients with pancreatitis over those with normal anatomy.[24]

It is tempting to conclude that non-fusion of the pancreatic ductal system predisposes to recurrent episodes of acute pancreatitis, that perhaps in some cases ends in permanent pancreatic damage, and that some type of drainage procedure of the dorsal pancreas would be of therapeutic benefit. Endoscopic sphincterotomy, surgical sphincteroplasty, and pancreatojejunostomy have been performed with mixed results. At least two authors and associates[25, 26] have reported success with transduodenal operative sphincteroplasty and one endoscopist obtained satisfactory results in 50% patients undergoing endoscopic sphincterotomy of the minor papilla.[27]

The clinical implications of pancreas divisum remain uncertain at the present time. Further study is clearly required to substantiate the claim that the anomaly has clinical significance in terms of the pathogenesis of acute pancreatitis in patients who have this

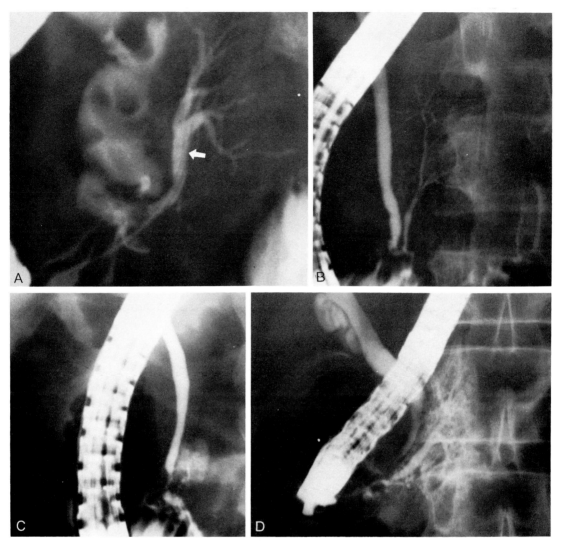

FIGURE 35–6. Ventral pancreas. A, Cannulation of the major papilla shows a ventral pancreas (*arrow*). Adjacent to the attenuated duct of Wirsung is a dilated, calculus-filled common bile duct. B, Short, narrow-diameter, smoothly tapering duct with delicate side-branching pattern. C, A small rudimentary ventral pancreas with extremely short duct. Blush is produced by filling the entire structure with contrast medium to the acini. D, Overopacification of the ventral pancreas prior to recognizing its presence. (B and D, courtesy of M. V. Sivak, Jr., M.D.)

TABLE 35–3. **Incidence of Pancreas Divisum in Endoscopic Series**

Author(s)	Year	No. of Patients	Patients with PD*	% with PD
Delhaye et al.[24]	1982	4186	209	5.0
Richter et al.[25]	1981	519	26	5.0
Cotton[23]	1980	810	47	5.8
Tulassay and Papp[35]	1980	2410	33	1.3
Mitchell et al.[36]	1979	499	21	4.7
Gregg et al.[26]	1977	1100	33	3.0
Ravitch[18]	1973	314	21	6–7

*Pancreas divisum.

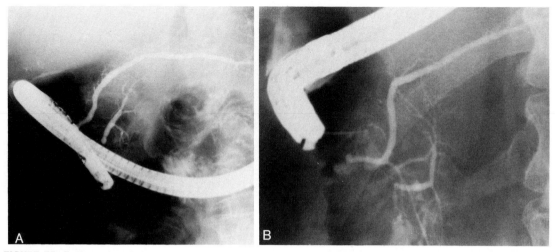

FIGURE 35–7. Ventral and dorsal pancreas. *A*, Retrograde pancreatography demonstrates the ventral pancreas and the dorsal duct after cannulation of both major and minor papillae. *B*, Cannulation of minor papilla followed rapidly by cannulation and injection of major papilla demonstrates duality of ductal system.

TABLE 35–4. **Cannulation of the Minor Papilla**

Author(s)	Attempted	Successful	% Successful
Delhaye et al.[24]	45	35	77
Mitchell et al.[36]	21	1	4
Richter et al.[25]	26	3	11
Cotton[23]	35	18	51
Gregg et al.[26]	15	4	26
Belber and Kazuko[28]	6	0	
Total	148	61	41

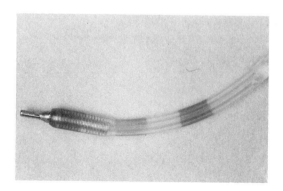

FIGURE 35–8. Blunt, fine-tipped metal cannula (Wilson-Cook, Inc.) of Cremer type. (Courtesy of M. V. Sivak, Jr., M.D.)

TABLE 35–5. **Incidence of Pancreatitis**

	Pancreas Divisum		Normal Fusion	
Author(s)	*Patients with Pancreatitis (%)*	*Patients with IP (%)**	*Patients with Pancreatitis (%)*	*Patients with IP (%)**
Delhaye et al.[24]	15	—	13	—
Ravitch[18]	38	75	—	—
Richter et al.[25]	58	33	21	36
Cotton[23]	62	66	27	28
Tulassay and Papp[35]	42	—	8	—
Mitchell et al.[36]	19	—	27	—
Gregg et al.[26]	45	—	—	—

*Percentage of patients with pancreatitis considered to have idiopathic pancreatitis (IP).

finding. These uncertainties make it difficult to interpret response to therapeutic intervention, and controlled studies of patients with idiopathic pancreatitis are necessary.

Ductal Duplication Anomalies

ERCP studies, together with several autopsy investigations, have demonstrated a number of pancreatic duct variations of the fused gland[28] (Fig. 35–9). Since variations of ductal anatomy are common and usually mi-

nor, it is difficult to define the "normal pancreatic duct system." Certain duplication anomalies may produce considerable deviation from the "normal" configuration, but they are primarily a radiographic curiosity and generally of little clinical importance.

The primitive pancreas is composed of a plexus of small ducts, one of which normally becomes dominant and assumes the role of the main duct. If there is failure to form a main duct, the plexus pattern persists as

FIGURE 35–9. Normal and aberrant pancreatic duct development.

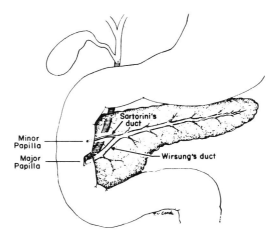

NORMAL PANCREATIC DUCTS

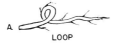

A. LOOP

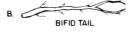

B. BIFID TAIL

C. SPIRAL

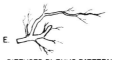

D. MAIN DUCT DUPLICATION IN THE BODY

E. DIFFUSED PLEXUS PATTERN COMMUNICATING THROUGH BOTH ANLAGEN

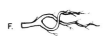

F. RING-LIKE DUPLICATION OF MAIN DUCT IN THE BODY

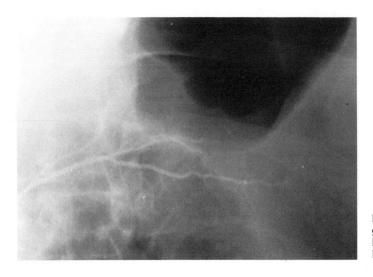

FIGURE 35–10. Retrograde pancreato-gram demonstrating bifid ductal system in tail. (Courtesy of M. V. Sivak, Jr., M.D.)

multiple channels, particularly in the head of the pancreas (Fig. 35–9E). Symmetric duplication of ducts causes ring- or fork-shaped segments[29] (Fig. 35–9F). The most common symmetric anomaly is a bifid duct in the tail of the pancreas (Figs. 35–9B and 35–10). Duplication of channels can lead to the formation of spiral (Fig. 35–9C) or loop (Fig. 35–9A) configurations.[30]

Duplication variations (Fig. 35–9D) of all types have been associated with a greater than normal amount of pancreatic tissue that sometimes produces a "pseudo-mass effect" that can be detected by CT. ERCP is necessary to define the ductal anatomy.

Miscellaneous Anomalies

Several complex anomalies of the pancreas are recognized.

Total agenesis of the pancreas is usually associated with multiple congenital anomalies including acardia and anencephaly.[31] Complete agenesis has also been reported as an isolated finding. Partial agenesis can include either the exocrine or endocrine portion of the gland. Agenesis of either the dorsal or ventral anlage has been described.[32] Hypoplasia of the exocrine pancreas is characterized histologically by a diminished ductal system, normal acinar elements, and islet cells surrounded by lipomatous tissue. The poorly developed ductal system results in pancreatic insufficiency. Interestingly, the pancreas may maintain normal size and shape with hypoplasia.[33]

Congenital cystosis of the pancreas is frequently associated with polycystic kidney and liver disease, as well as situs inversus, and various central nervous system malformations. Histologically, the pancreas appears normal except for multiple small cysts. Pancreatic exocrine insufficiency is the usual clinical expression of cystosis.

The pancreatic "bladder" anomaly is extremely rare in man. A bud arises from the left lobe of the ventral pancreas and grows into the lesser omentum, parallel to the hepatic duct.[34] This growth becomes an isolated cystic structure in the right upper quadrant of the abdomen. Pancreatic bladder may be mistaken for duplication of the gallbladder or cystic duct.

True accessory pancreas must not be confused with aberrant or heterotropic pancreas. The true accessory pancreas is a lobular unit connected to the papilla Vater by its own duct system.

SUMMARY

With the exception of annular pancreas, the clinical significance of various pancreatic anomalies requires further study. Despite advances in ultrasound and CT imaging of the pancreas, ERCP is required for delineation of ductal anatomy. With pancreas divisum, a complete demonstration of the pancreatic ductal system requires cannulation of the minor papilla. Knowledge of ductal variations may spare an individual from unnecessary exploratory surgery.

Editor's note: Pancreas divisum is a controversial topic and the object of considerable investigative effort. Whether it is an anomaly or a congenital pathologic condition remains problematic. References 37 to 44 are recent articles of interest.

References

1. Richardson KE, Spooner BS. Mammalian pancreas development: Regeneration and differentiation in vitro. Dev Biol 1977; 58:402–20.
2. Ecker A. Bildungsfehler des Pancreas und des Herzens. Z rat Med 1862; 14:354–6.
3. Ravitch MM. The pancreas in infants and children. Surg Clin North Am 1975; 55:377–85.
4. Warkany J, Passarge E, Smith LB. Congenital malformations in autosomal trisomy syndromes. Am J Dis Child 1971; 112:502–17.
5. Jackson JM. Annular pancreas and duodenal obstruction in the neonate: A review. Arch Surg 1963; 87:379–83.
6. Drey NW. Symptomatic annular pancreas in the adult. Ann Intern Med 1957; 46:750–72.
7. Howard NJ. Annular pancreas. Surg Gynecol Obstet 1930; 50:533–40.
8. Lloyd-Jones WL, Mountain JC, Warren KW. Annular pancreas in the adult. Ann Surg 1972; 176:163–70.
9. Dodd GD, Nafis WA. Annular pancreas in the adult. Am J Roentgenol 1956; 75:333–42.
10. Mast WH, Tello LD, Turek RO. Annular pancreas; errors in diagnosis and treatment of eight cases. Am J Surg 1957; 94:80–9.
11. Clifford KM: Annular pancreas diagnosed by endoscopic retrograde choledochopancreatography (ERCP). Br J Radiol 1980; 53:593–5.
12. Heymann RL, Whelan TJ Jr. Annular pancreas: Demonstration of the annular duct on cholangiography. Ann Surg 1967; 165:470–2.
13. Thomford NR, Knight PR, Pace WG, Madura JA. Annular pancreas in the adult: Selection of operation. Ann Surg 1972; 176:159–62.
14. McLean JM. Embryology of the pancreas. In: Howat HT, Sarles H, eds. The Exocrine Pancreas. Philadelphia: W. B. Saunders, 1979.
15. Dolan RV, ReMine WH, Docherty MB. The fate of heterotropic pancreatic tissue. A study of 212 cases. Arch Surg 1974; 109:762–5.
16. Barbosa JJdeC, Dockerty MB, Waugh JM. Pancreatic heterotrophy: Review of the literature and report of 41 authenticated surgical cases of which 25 were clinically significant. Surg Gynecol Obstet 1946; 82:527–42.
17. Palmer ED. Benign intramural tumors of the stomach: Review with special reference to gross pathology. Medicine 1951; 30:81–181.
18. Ravitch MM. Anomalies of the pancreas. In: Cary LC, ed. The Pancreas. St. Louis: C. V. Mosby, 1973.
19. Phillip J, Koch H, Classen M. Variation anomalies of the papilla of Vater, the pancreas, and the biliary system. Endoscopy 1974; 6:70–7.
20. Dawson W, Langman J. An anatomical-radiological study on pancreatic duct pattern in man. Anat Rec 1961; 39:59–68.
21. Elmore MF, Lehman GA, Meadows JR. Endoscopic retrograde cannulation of the accessory papilla. Gastrointest Endosc 1977; 23:170.
22. O'Connor KW, Lehman GA. Accessory papilla (AP) cannulation at endoscopic retrograde pancreatography aided by intravenous (IV) secretin and needle-tipped cannula. (Abstr) Gastrointest Endosc 1983; 29:172.
23. Cotton PB. Congenital anomaly of pancreas divisum as cause of obstructive pain and pancreatitis. Gut 1980; 21:105–14.
24. Delhaye M, Cremer M, Dunham F. Pancreas divisum in pancreatitis. Abstract presented to ASGE. Digestive Disease Week, May 1982, Chicago, Ill.
25. Richter JM, Schapiro RH, Mulley AG, Warshaw AL. Association of pancreas divisum in pancreatitis and its treatment by sphincteroplasty of the accessory ampulla. Gastroenterology 1981; 81:1104–10.
26. Gregg JA, Monaco AP, McDermott WV. Pancreas divisum: Results of surgical intervention. Am J Surg 1983; 145:488–92.
27. Liquory C. Unpublished data, presented at the World Congress of Gastroenterology. Stockholm, Sweden, 1982.
28. Belber JP, Kazuko B. Fusion anomalies of the pancreatic ductal system: Differentiation from pathological states. Radiology 1977; 122:637–42.
29. Bernard C: Memoire sur le pancrease. Paris: J. B. Bailliere, 1856.
30. Yatto RP, Siegel JH. Variant pancreatography. Am J Gastroenterol 1983; 78:115–8.
31. Warkany J. Congenital Malformations. Chicago: Year Book Medical Publishers, 1971.
32. Seifert G. Die Pathologie des Kindlichen Pankreas. Leipzig: Georg Thieme, 1956.
33. Bodien M. Fibrocystic Disease of the Pancreas. New York: Grune and Stratton, 1953.
34. Keefe A. Human Embryology and Morphology. London: Edward Arnold, 1948.
35. Tulassay Z, Papp J. New clinical aspects of pancreas divisum. Gastrointest Endosc 1980; 26:143–6.
36. Mitchell CJ, Lintott DJ, Ruddell WS, et al. Clinical relevance of an unfused pancreatic duct system. Gut 1979; 20:1066–71.
37. Cotton PB. Pancreas divisum—curiosity or culprit? Gastroenterology 1985; 89:1431–5.
38. Soehendra N, Kempeneers I, Nam VC, Grimm H. Endoscopic dilatation and papillotomy of the accessory papilla and internal drainage in pancreas divisum. Endoscopy 1986; 18:129–32.
39. Delhaye M, Engelholm L, Cremer M. Pancreas divisum: congenital anatomic variant or anomaly? Contribution of endoscopic retrograde dorsal pancreatography. Gastroenterology 1985; 89:951–8.
40. O'Connor KW, Lehman GA. An improved technique for accessory papilla cannulation in pancreas divisum. Gastrointest Endosc 1985; 31:13–7.
41. Russell RC, Wong NW, Cotton PB. Accessory sphincterotomy (endoscopic and surgical) in patients with pancreas divisum. Br J Surg 1984; 71:954–7.
42. Blair AJ III, Russell CG, Cotton PB. Resection for pancreatitis in patients with pancreas divisum. Ann Surg 1984; 200:590–4.
43. Jacocks MA, ReMine SG, Carmichael DH. Difficulties in the diagnosis and treatment of pancreas divisum. Arch Surg 1984; 119:1088–91.
44. Warshaw AL, Richter JM, Schapiro RH. The cause and treatment of pancreatitis associated with pancreas divisum. Ann Surg 1983; 198:443–52.

Chapter 36

ERCP IN ACUTE AND CHRONIC PANCREATITIS

WOLFGANG RÖSCH, M.D.

Cannulation of the papilla of Vater with injection of a radiographic contrast medium was initially intended for the study of patients with suspected pancreatic disorders. It has come about that as many or perhaps more patients undergo endoscopic retrograde cholangiopancreatography (ERCP) for disorders of the biliary system. However, endoscopic ductography remains an indispensable diagnostic method in patients with pancreatitis when surgical intervention is indicated. Other imaging methods such as ultrasonography and computed tomography are valuable adjuncts in screening for chronic pancreatitis or differential diagnosis between inflammatory and neoplastic changes within the pancreas, but for precise definition of pancreatic ductal anatomy opacification of the main pancreatic duct is mandatory.

In 1963 the Marseille conference[1] proposed a clinical classification of pancreatitis that grouped patients into four categories: (1) acute pancreatitis, (2) relapsing acute pancreatitis, (3) chronic relapsing pancreatitis, and (4) chronic pancreatitis. Although the primary objectives of the symposium were a consideration of the pathologic anatomy and etiology of chronic pancreatitis, without reference to correlations of function and anatomy, the classification has been widely adopted for clinical purposes. The classification is useful from the conceptual point of view; acute and relapsing acute pancreatitis were regarded as non-progressive disorders provided their primary cause could be eliminated. Chronic and chronic relapsing pancreatitis implied residual pancreatic damage (either anatomic or functional); chronic pancreatitis was regarded as the result of chronic relapsing pancreatitis. Only occasionally was chronic disease thought to follow the acute

form. In clinical practice it can be difficult to separate patients with pancreatic inflammatory disease into these precise categories. The classification of pancreatitis adopted by the Marseille conference requires revision. In particular our experience suggests that diffuse and focal pancreatic changes should be considered as separate entities. A useful classification that reflects our experience with retrograde pancreatography is outlined in Table 36–1. At an international workshop at King's College in Cambridge another classification was suggested, the main features of which are summarized in Table 36–2.[2]

ERCP IN ACUTE PANCREATITIS

ERCP During the Acute Episode

For many years acute pancreatitis, at least early after onset, was considered a contraindication to ERCP. Some endoscopists per-

TABLE 36–1. **Classification of Pancreatitis**

Diffuse pancreatitis (with or without impaired secretory function)
    Acute pancreatitis
        Single episode
        Recurrent (acute recurrent pancreatitis)
    Chronic pancreatitis
        Recurrent chronic pancreatitis
        Primary chronic pancreatitis

Focal (segmentary) Pancreatitis (with or without impaired secretory function)
    Segmentary pancreatitis (tail, body, head, uncinate process)
    Pancreatitis in pancreas divisum (ventral or dorsal pancreas)

Special forms of pancreatitis
    Groove pancreatitis

TABLE 36–2. **Classification of Pancreatograms in Chronic Pancreatitis***

Terminology	MPD	Abnormal MPDB	Additional Features
Normal	Normal	None	None
Equivocal	Normal	< 3	None
Mild chronic pancreatitis	Normal	3 or more	None
Moderate chronic pancreatitis	Abnormal	> 3	None
Marked chronic pancreatitis	Abnormal	> 3	One or more: large cavity, obstruction, filling defects, severe dilation, or irregularity

MPD = Main pancreatic duct; MPDB = main pancreatic duct branches.

*If pathologic changes are limited to one third or less of gland, they are classified as "local" and designated as being in the head, body, or tail; if more than one third of gland is involved, changes are classified as "diffuse."

form ERCP after a few weeks even if serum amylase or lipase levels have not returned to normal. Fatal pancreatic necrosis, even in apparently normal glands, is thought to occur in 0.1% of retrograde pancreatography procedures.[3] Safrany et al.[4] have presented convincing data that inadvertent instillation of contrast medium into the pancreatic duct does not have an untoward effect in patients undergoing endoscopic sphincterotomy for gallstone-induced pancreatitis. Although reservations concerning ERCP during acute pancreatitis are based on an assumed hazard, there are only limited data to support the view that deliberate retrograde injection of the pancreas during acute pancreatitis is innocuous. Presently, the only indication for ERCP in acute pancreatitis is relief of gallstone-induced pancreatitis by endoscopic sphincterotomy in certain clinical situations. Other than this, virtually no gain in patient management is achieved by retrograde pancreatography during the acute phase of pancreatitis.

ERCP During the Recovery Phase of Acute Pancreatitis

Pancreatic function does not return to normal at the time when the clinical symptoms of acute pancreatitis have subsided. Tympner et al.[5] demonstrated a dissociation between clinical and biochemical recovery; subnormal pancreatic secretion of bicarbonate, amylase, lipase or trypsin may persist for many months, even though normal ductal anatomy is demonstrated by retrograde pancreatography. Hamilton and associates[6] performed elective ERCP in 31 patients who had sustained an attack of acute pancreatitis. No cause was evident by either cholecystography

or intravenous cholangiography, and ERCP was carried out only after the serum amylase levels had been normal for at least 6 weeks. Four of the patients studied were found to have previously unrecognized gallstones, 2 patients with known cholelithiasis were found to have common duct calculi that were treated by endoscopic sphincterotomy, and evidence of chronic pancreatitis was found in 8 patients. If ERCP is performed within a few days of an attack, opacification of the pancreatic parenchyma may occasionally take place (Fig. 36–1). This degree of opacification may possibly be indicative of tissue necrosis that may finally result after several months in pseudocyst formation. It is advisable to follow by ultrasonography patients who exhibit this phenomenon.

ERCP in Acute Recurrent Pancreatitis

Some patients sustain repeated attacks of acute pancreatitis. The clinical classification of these patients is problematic in that they may have relapsing acute pancreatitis without structural changes in the pancreas, or they may have chronic relapsing pancreatitis, which implies permanent pathologic changes within the pancreas. ERCP is indicated in patients who have documented recurrences of acute pancreatitis, in order to define any anatomic lesion or lesions that could be responsible for the repeated episodes. Cotton and Beales[7] studied 31 such patients; 12 definite lesions amenable to surgical therapy, such as stricturing or obstruction of the main pancreatic duct and pseudocysts, were found among 25 patients in whom pancreatography was successful. Similar results were reported by Zimmon and coworkers[8] and Cooperman et al.[9] in idiopathic acute recurrent pancrea-

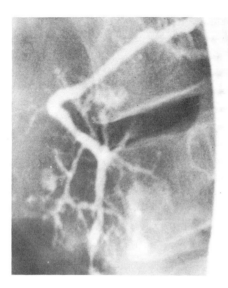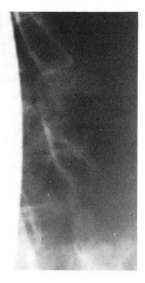

FIGURE 36–1. "Spontaneous" parenchymography in acute pancreatitis.

titis in which ERCP established the existence and precise nature of potentially correctable abnormalities. Because of the possibility of finding potentially correctable anatomic lesions, ERCP should be considered in any patient who has had two or more attacks of acute pancreatitis.

Serial endoscopic pancreatograms over the course of time may show marked changes of chronic pancreatitis within a few years after a demonstration of normal ductal anatomy in patients with recurrent episodes of pancreatitis, including patients who do not misuse alcohol[10] (Fig. 36–2). The latter point is in contrast to the work of Nagata et al.[11] These authors performed serial pancreatograms in patients with known or suspected chronic pancreatitis. Progressive changes were demonstrated in the pancreatic ducts of patients with pancreatitis related to misuse of alcohol. Abstinence from alcohol or a reduction in intake had no apparent effect on this evolution in the radiographic findings. However, patients whose pancreatitis was regarded as idiopathic or related to causes other than alcohol demonstrated no radiographic progression to more severe chronic pancreatitis. Although most patients in this study had abdominal pain, its clinical pattern was not described. Presumably many had unremitting pain rather than discrete episodes.

ERCP in Hemorrhagic Necrotizing Pancreatitis

Many authors regard hemorrhagic necrotizing pancreatitis as a contraindication to ERCP. Generally patients with this disease are extremely ill, their prognosis is poor, and surgical debridement is considered as a desperate measure. Even if the question of exacerbation of the disease by ERCP is disregarded, the procedure can be extremely difficult, special problems will arise with respect to support of the patient during the procedure, and any information gained by ERCP will be of minimal value for the immediate management and survival of the patient. However, Gebhardt et al.[12] argued in favor of ERCP in hemorrhagic necrotizing pancreatitis once a decision is made to operate. By means of postmortem pancreatography, these investigators found that in many fatal cases where operative debridement had been performed, pancreatic fistulas had been overlooked. These were thought to contribute to the demise of these patients. ERCP was performed in 8 patients in whom conservative management had failed, despite various technical problems such as endotracheal intubation and performance of ERCP with patients in a supine position. The following conclusions were drawn in regard to guiding surgical treatment: If a normal pancreatic duct system is demonstrated without evidence of a fistula, only peripancreatic debridement is necessary. If there is leakage of contrast medium via a fistula from the pancreatic duct, then a partial resection including removal of the fistulous area is indicated. If the ductal system is normal but there is complete parenchymal staining, then a partial resection should be performed. In some cases, a perforation into the duodenum from a necrotic cavity in the head of the pancreas

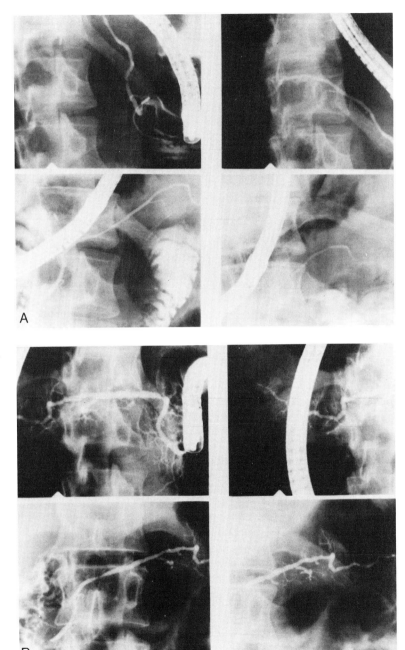

FIGURE 36–2. A, Normal pancreatogram following acute attack of pancreatitis. B, Minimal change pancreatitis with impaired secretory function 1 year after pancreatogram in A.

was demonstrated. Surgery was deferred because recovery was anticipated in view of the established drainage. None of the patients subjected to preoperative ERCP in the series of Gebhardt et al. died; in contrast, the mortality was at least 35% in most series of patients. ERCP cannot at present be recommended in this clinical situation until further studies confirm the safety and efficacy of this approach.

ERCP IN CHRONIC PANCREATITIS

Diagnostic ERCP

Diffuse Chronic Pancreatitis

The staging of the pancreatographic changes in chronic pancreatitis as suggested by Kasugai et al.[13] has proved to be of value. According to this system, three categories of chronic pancreatitis may be recognized by endoscopic pancreatography. These are minimal, moderate, and advanced (also referred to as grades I, II and III, respectively). In minimal chronic pancreatitis the radiographic findings are limited to the main pancreatic duct branches and subbranches and consist of irregular distribution, dilation, stenosis, and obstruction. Dilation to cystic proportions and calculi are not present. In moderate pancreatitis all of these changes are present but to a more advanced degree, and in addition there may be cystic dilation of the main pancreatic duct branches. However, the main difference between this and minimal pancreatitis is that alterations are also found in the main pancreatic duct. These consist of tortuosity, dilation, and stenosis of a mild degree. In advanced pancreatitis all of the findings cited thus far are present in a more severe degree, and in addition there may be obstruction and/or dilation of the main pancreatic duct to cystic proportions. Also, the main duct and its branches will contain calculi, there is coarse opacification of the acini, and the size of the pancreas appears diminished. This classification is depicted schematically in Figure 36–3.

The Kasugai radiographic classification of chronic pancreatitis correlates well with the degree of pancreatic dysfunction as determined by pancreatic stimulation testing,[14] the anatomic extent of disease, and clinical symptomatology. The presence of calcification of the pancreas and stenosis of the common bile duct increases with each of the successive stages in the classification (Table 36–3).

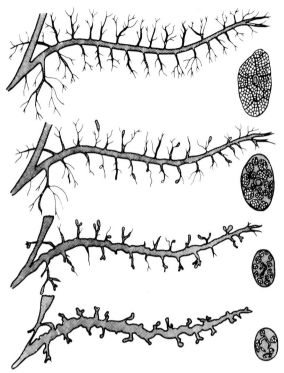

FIGURE 36–3. Schematic representation of pancreatographic changes in Kasugai classification of chronic pancreatitis. The diagrams illustrate (*top to bottom*) normal pancreatography and findings in minimal, moderate, and advanced pancreatitis. The corresponding appearance of the pancreatic acinus (*right*) is depicted schematically for each stage.

It is debatable whether the ductogram or the secretin-pancreozymin stimulation test of pancreatic function is more sensitive in the early detection of chronic inflammatory changes in the pancreas.[15–18] Braganza et al.[19] studied the relation between pancreatic duct morphology as demonstrated by retrograde pancreatography and the results of the secretin-pancreozymin test in 45 patients with chronic pancreatitis. Pancreatograms were graded according to the Kasugai classification, except that changes of advanced pan-

TABLE 36–3. **Relation of Common Bile Duct Stenosis and Pancreatic Calcification to Radiographic Grade of Chronic Pancreatitis (Kasugai Classification) in 265 Patients**

Chronic Pancreatitis	CBD Stenosis	Calcification
Grade I (minimal	0	0
Grade II (moderate)	42%	6%
Grade III (advanced)	66%	34%

creatitis were also divided into subcategories of main duct dilation, segmentation ("chain of lakes"), and obstruction. These authors found a negative correlation between radiographic classification of chronic pancreatitis and the secretory volume as well as the amounts of bicarbonate and enzyme secreted. Because of broad overlap between the various subgroups, the appearance of the pancreatogram could not be predicted on the basis of the pancreatic stimulation test, nor the results of the stimulation test by the appearance of the pancreatogram. In contrast to the study by Di Magno et al.[20] Braganza et al.[19] found no correlation between the length of patent main pancreatic duct and pancreatic secretion in patients with advanced pancreatitis and obstruction of the main duct.

Braganza et al.[19] suggested that a combination of factors probably explain these results. Chronic pancreatitis is by nature a "patchy" process that may affect acinar and ductular portions of the gland to varying degrees in a given patient. Abnormalities of the main pancreatic duct branches and smaller ducts are commonly found in association with a relatively normal main duct. The pathologic state of the pancreas varies over the course of time; function might be temporarily altered by a subclinical attack of acute pancreatitis. Finally, relatively uninvolved areas of the pancreas may hypertrophy in response to damage elsewhere in the gland.

Secretory function was markedly reduced in some patients with normal or nearly normal ducts and was preserved in occasional patients with incomplete duct obstruction. Both the secretin-pancreozymin test and pancreatography failed to identify 5 patients (11%) with chronic pancreatitis at operation. Reduction of bicarbonate identified 3 of 8 patients with chronic pancreatitis and normal ductograms. In one of the 45 patients studied, pancreatography correctly diagnosed chronic pancreatitis, although the results of function testing were normal.

In our experience, an occasional patient may have severe exocrine insufficiency and a normal ductogram, that is, lacking at least radiographic evidence of severe structural damage to the pancreas; chronic calcifying pancreatitis may sometimes be associated with normal secretory function.[21]

In some patients with chronic pancreatitis, ERCP may fail to opacify the pancreatic duct. This may be the result of faulty technique but can also be due to stenosis or obstruction of the main pancreatic duct near the papilla of Vater. If the bile duct is visualized, the presence of a long, distally tapering, smooth stricture is characteristic of the bile duct narrowing that occurs in association with chronic pancreatitis and suggests the presence of chronic pancreatitis[22–24] (Fig. 36–4).

The interpretation of the radiographic findings when there is a minimal degree of chronic pancreatitis may be difficult. Correct opacification of the main pancreatic duct branches requires careful attention to ERCP technique. Even when this is optimal, minor differences in the appearance of the main pancreatic duct branches may occur as a result of slight differences in injection pressure or timing of the x-ray exposure. In some cases, certain changes that suggest chronic pancreatitis can be attributed to the age of the patient (see Chapter 28). These factors account for the variation in interpretation when the ERCP diagnosis of minimal pacreatitis is being considered (Fig. 36–5). According to Caletti et al.,[25] who examined 1179 pancreatograms of patients with chronic pancreatitis, difficulty in distinguishing a normal pancreatogram from one displaying minimal pancreatitis occurs in 6.8% of ERCP procedures. As duration of the disease increased, the ability to recognize it by pancreatography also increased, although the presence of extensive calcification and calculi made it more difficult to obtain a satisfactory pancreatogram.

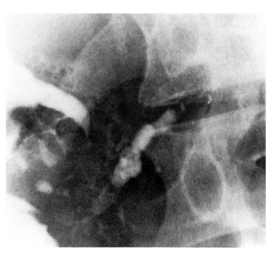

FIGURE 36–4. Chronic calcifying pancreatitis with narrowing of common bile duct.

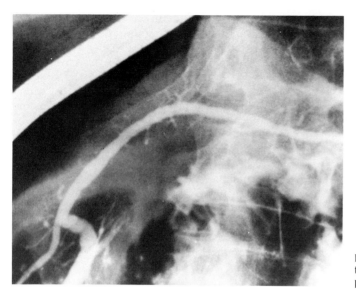

FIGURE 36–5. Minimal change pancreatitis (grade I) with cystic dilation of main pancreatic duct branches.

When chronic pancreatitis is well developed, the retrograde pancreatogram is usually pathognomonic (Fig. 36–6). However, the differential diagnosis between pancreatic carcinoma and severe chronic pancreatitis can be problematic.

Caletti and associates[25] encountered difficulty in distinguishing cancer and chronic pancreatitis in 11.3% of pancreatograms. Both diseases can cause similar radiographic abnormalities; this is especially a problem when stricturing or obstruction appears to be an isolated finding. Of a group of 500 pancreatograms, Rohrmann and coworkers[26] studied 50 which showed incomplete opacification of the main pancreatic duct that suggested obstruction. The status of the pancreas was known in each case either by surgery or autopsy, or in some cases a repeat study was normal and clinical follow-up extended at least one year. Chronic pancreatitis was the actual cause of the obstruction in 8 cases; other causes included carcinoma in 15 cases, pseudocyst in 15, acute pancreatitis in 3, and pancreatic abscess in 2 instances. Seven patients proved to have normal pancreases. The apparent obstruction in these 7 patients could be partly accounted for by faulty technique, although physiologic or anatomic factors such as compression by lymph nodes, vascular structures, or the vertebral column were suggested as playing a role. Others have

FIGURE 36–6. Moderate chronic pancreatitis (grade II) with irregularities of main pancreatic duct.

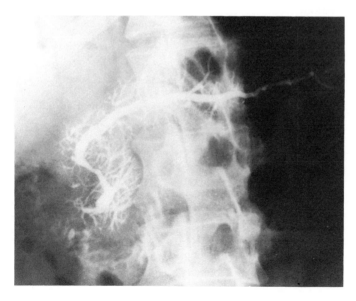

pointed out this occasional difficulty with differential diagnosis between benign and malignant pancreatic lesions.[27]

A difficult differential diagnosis between chronic pancreatitis and carcinoma can often be resolved by correlating the history and physical examination, the results of other imaging procedures including guided aspiration cytology, and the appearance of the pancreatogram; however, surgical exploration is still indicated in cases where the differential diagnosis remains problematic despite a comprehensive investigation. In some cases, the appearance of the pancreatogram itself may be sufficient indication for exploration even if the etiology of the radiographic findings cannot be determined. Obstruction of the bile duct, for example, might occur with either chronic pancreatitis or carcinoma, and in itself is an indication for operation (Fig. 36–7).

Focal Pancreatitis

At least 10% of pancreatograms, if carefully examined, will have evidence of focal or focally accentuated chronic pancreatitis; resected specimens as well will exhibit localized chronic inflammation. The pancreatographic findings of focal chronic pancreatitis are those described in the Kasugai classification except that they are localized to one area of the pancreas, the radiographic appearance being normal elsewhere. Usually more than just minor alterations in the main pancreatic duct branches (minimal pancreatitis) will be found, and circumscribed pseudocyst formation as well as intracanalicular calcifica-

tions are characteristic. Pancreatic stimulation tests, however, will usually show normal secretory function.

Focal pancreatitis may be confined to the head of the pancreas, although in our experience with 77 patients with focal pancreatitis, the abnormality was limited to the tail of the gland in two thirds[28] (Fig. 36–8 and Plate 36–1). In an occasional patient the segmentary abnormality may be limited to the uncinate process (Fig. 36–9 and Plate 36–2); the anatomic features in this area present a special technical problem when surgery is undertaken because of intractable pain. A special form of focal pancreatitis may occur in association with pancreas divisum, in which only the ventral or the dorsal ductal system displays ductal changes of chronic pancreatitis[28] (Fig. 36–10); occasionally both anlagen show chronic inflammatory changes.[29]

Pancreas divisum is discussed in Chapter 35. It is still debatable whether this fusion anomaly of the pancreas is especially prone to acute pancreatitis and/or chronic relapsing pancreatitis.[30–33] Although it is difficult to explain the localization of chronic inflammatory changes to either the dorsal or ventral anlagen, in some cases of pancreas divisum, no increase in the incidence of pancreatitis was found in a combined series of Cremer and ourselves (unpublished data) comprising 350 cases of pancreas divisum. It is still speculative whether or not abdominal pain can be caused by impaired flow of pancreatic juice through the small accessory papilla. Nevertheless, there does appear to be an occasional patient in whom improved drain-

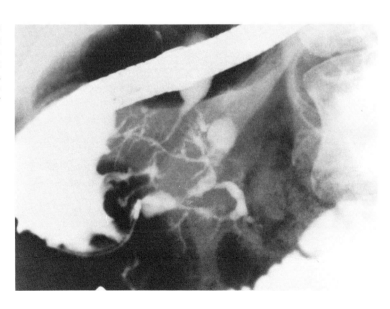

FIGURE 36–7. Advanced or severe chronic pancreatitis with common bile duct obstruction and obstruction of main pancreatic duct with cystic alterations in head region. A preoperative diagnosis of malignancy on the basis of this study was not confirmed at operation.

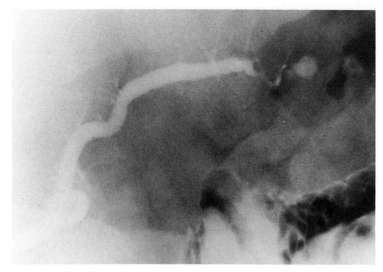

FIGURE 36–8. Segmental pancreatitis in tail region.

FIGURE 36–9. Chronic calcifying pancreatitis of uncinate process in a patient with normal pancreatic secretory function.

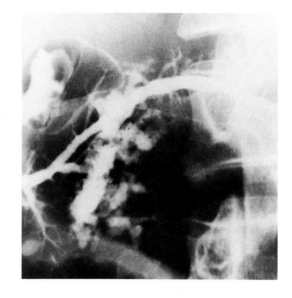

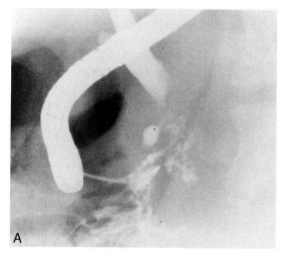

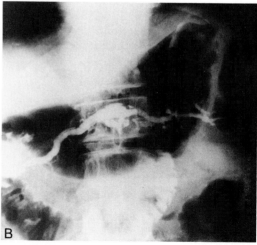

FIGURE 36–10. *A,* Focal chronic pancreatitis of ventral pancreas with narrowing of common bile duct. *B,* Chronic pancreatitis of dorsal pancreas.

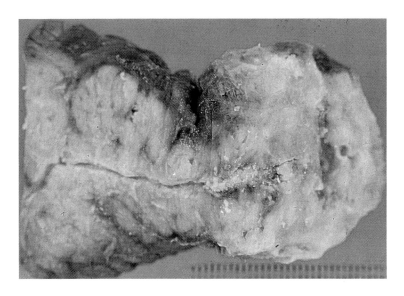

PLATE 36–1. Segmental pancreatitis in tail region. Surgical specimen with sharp demarcation between healthy and inflamed tissue.

PLATE 36–2. Pancreatitis of uncinate process. Surgical specimen after Whipple procedure was performed because of intractable pain.

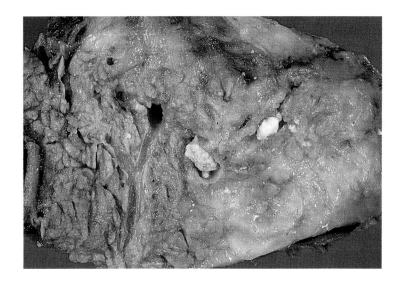

PLATE 36–3. Operative view of congenitally small pancreas (5 cm diameter) with chronic pancreatitis.

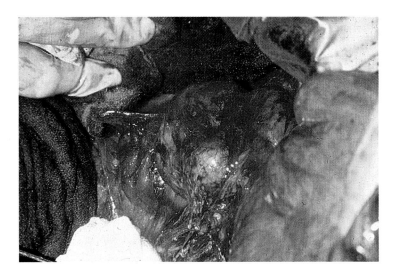

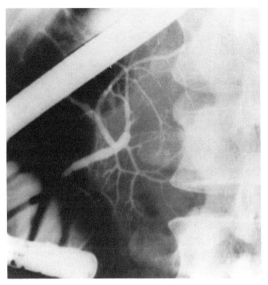

FIGURE 36–11. Congenitally small pancreas.

age at the minor papilla by endoscopic sphincterotomy may relieve pain. This procedure has not been thoroughly evaluated and requires the highest degree of expertise in endoscopic sphincterotomy.

Other anomalies, such as a congenitally small pancreas (Fig. 36–11 and Plate 36–3), may also be susceptible to chronic inflammatory changes, but they are so rare that no reliable data are available.

Groove Pancreatitis

Groove pancreatitis is a special and unusual form of focal pancreatitis affecting the head of the pancreas. The inflammatory fibrotic changes are localized to the groove between the head of the organ and the duodenum. The main clinical symptoms relate to duodenal stenosis and compression of the common bile duct. Symptoms may also be those of chronic pancreatitis, and ultrasonography and computed tomography will often suggest the presence of a tumor in the head of the pancreas. The pancreatic duct is normal radiographically, although it is displaced by the fibrotic process (Fig. 36–12). Extensive surgical resection has been performed for this disorder.[34] Histologically, pronounced fibrosis and cicatrization of the parenchyma are found in resected specimens. Groove pancreatitis probably arises as a sequela of a localized acute necrotizing pancreatitis limited to the head of the pancreas.

ERCP and Other Imaging Procedures

It is difficult to compare ERCP in the diagnosis of chronic pancreatitis with other imaging modalities such as ultrasonography and computed tomography with respect to sensitivity and specificity.[35–38] The type of information derived by each study is different; the technical problems encountered by each procedure also differ but nevertheless can influence results; the technologies of ultrasound and computed tomography are constantly evolving, a factor that makes earlier investigations irrelevant; and the experience and ability of the examiner, especially for

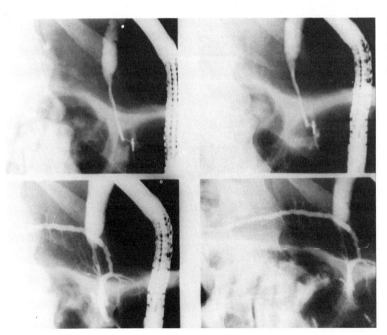

FIGURE 36–12. Groove pancreatitis with duodenal stenosis, common bile duct obstruction, and displacement of normal pancreatic duct.

ERCP and ultrasonography, are critical but unquantifiable variables.

Cotton et al.[35] reported experience with ultrasonography and ERCP in patients with known or suspected pancreatic disease. Ultrasonography failed for technical reasons in 6% of patients, and ERCP did not provide an adequate image of the pancreatic duct in 5%. There were 34 patients with chronic pancreatitis in this report. Ultrasonography was falsely normal in 3 patients, pancreatography in 5. Both studies were falsely normal in only 1 patient. There were 5 patients with a pseudocyst, all of which were detected by ultrasonography, whereas ERCP demonstrated filling of the cyst in 1 patient and pancreatic duct obstruction in the other 4 patients. The authors concluded that the combination of both studies constituted a comprehensive approach to diagnosis.

Swobodnik and associates[38] reported experience with ultrasonography, computed tomography, and ERCP in 81 patients with suspected pancreatic disease. Final diagnosis was established by surgery or autopsy in about one fourth of patients and the remainder by clinical follow-up. Technically unsatisfactory results were obtained in 2.5% of sonograms, 1.2% of CT scans, and 3.7% of retrograde pancreatographies. With regard to chronic pancreatitis, the sensitivities of ultrasonography, computed tomography, and ERCP were 52%, 74%, and 93%, respectively; the specificities were 100%, 98%, and 100%, respectively.

ERCP is the best diagnostic method in patients with suspected chronic pancreatitis when the morphology of the pancreatic ductal system is of interest. This is particularly important when there is a possibility of coexistent or associated biliary tract disease, and when pancreatic surgery is contemplated. The main diagnostic problems, as noted, arise in relation to recognition of minimal degrees of chronic pancreatitis, and in the differential diagnosis of chronic pancreatitis and pancreatic cancer.

ERCP may contribute to the diagnosis of mucoviscidosis or hereditary chronic pancreatitis. The number of reported cases, however, is relatively small.[39, 40]

Endoscopic Therapy in Chronic Pancreatitis
Endoscopic Sphincterotomy

In contrast to its use in the management of biliary tract disorders, endoscopic sphinc-

terotomy in the treatment of chronic pancreatitis is an experimental procedure. There are occasional reports of successful management of circumscribed ductal stenosis or the extraction of a pancreatic calculus situated close to the papillary orifice, but a prospective study on the efficacy of this type of maneuver is urgently required. Anecdotal reports indicate that in some patients normal secretory function may return after correction of prepapillary obstacles to flow; the experience with surgical sphincteroplasty in chronic pancreatitis is in general disappointing. Although endoscopic sphincterotomy of the pancreatic duct can be performed safely, there is seldom an indication for the procedure.

Pancreatic Duct Occlusion

Ligation of the main pancreatic duct near the papilla of Vater is known to produce pancreatic atrophy. In 1977 Little et al.[41] produced atrophy of the gland by instillation of an alkyl-alpha-cyanoacrylate glue into the main pancreatic duct. Gebhardt and Stolte[42] carried out pancreatic duct injection studies in dogs with an alcoholic prolamine solution. They found this solution suitable because it was radiopaque, moderately viscous and easy to inject, and biologically inactive. We have carried out duct occlusion studies using this solution in patients with chronic pancreatitis and intractable pain. The initial results were encouraging.[43] However, the long-term outcome has been disappointing, with less than 50% of patients being relieved of their pain. A recent survey reported that 73 patients had been treated by injection of an occlusive material into the main pancreatic duct in an effort to enhance "burning-out" of the inflammatory process.[21]

The main technical difficulty with endoscopic occlusion of the main pancreatic duct remains the rapid hardening of the occlusive substance. This makes it extremely difficult to fill the entire ductal system, including the branches of the main pancreatic duct and their tributaries. For this reason, this investigational procedure must at present be limited to patients who have had a partial left pancreatectomy. Pseudocysts, intraductular calculi, and narrowing of the common bile duct constitute contraindications to the procedure, since duct occlusion will not improve these conditions and further obstruction may worsen the problem of poor drainage.

ERCP IN DIAGNOSIS OF
UNEXPLAINED ABDOMINAL PAIN

Abdominal pain is a common clinical problem. In some cases, such as postcholecystectomy pain, the pain may be related to the prior surgery. The possibility of recurrent choledocholithiasis and papillary stenosis, for example, provides relatively definite indications for ERCP. However, there remains a large group of patients with pain in whom multiple imaging procedures and x-ray contrast studies as well as upper gastrointestinal endoscopy are negative or nonrevealing. In such cases the problem is to distinguish an organic etiology from symptoms that have a purely functional or psychological basis. ERCP is frequently considered at this point. It is difficult to weigh the complication rate, albeit low, and the cost of ERCP against the potential benefit. This problem requires considerable clinical acumen in virtually every case.

There are only a few reports of the diagnostic yield of ERCP in the investigation of unexplained abdominal pain.[44] Ruddell et al.[45] performed ERCP in 140 patients with undiagnosed severe abdominal pain. This represented 14% of their total number of patients undergoing ERCP over a period of 3 years. The minimal criterion for admission to this study was severe pain of 3 months' duration. All patients had undergone numerous investigative procedures. ERCP was diagnostic in 34 patients (24%). The duration of time that patients had complained of pain had no relation to the ERCP findings, either positive or negative. Eight patients had peptic ulcers and previously unrecognized gallstones were discovered in 5. Pancreatography was abnormal in 25 patients (18%), one pancreatogram revealing a pancreatic cancer. Twenty-five patients, or 18% of the total number studied, gave a history of past or ongoing misuse of alcohol. The incidence of pancreatographic abnormalities in this subgroup was 60%, the majority being classified as minimal pancreatitis. The highest diagnostic yield for ERCP in patients with pain of obscure origin occurred in those with a history of excessive alcohol ingestion.

SUMMARY

ERCP is usually not indicated in acute pancreatitis. Recurrent attacks raise the possibility of an anatomic lesion as an etiologic factor, in which case ERCP can be of value.

Although ERCP has been proposed for the preoperative evaluation of the pancreas in hemorrhagic necrotizing pancreatitis, this indication requires further evaluation. ERCP is the procedure of choice for defining ductal anatomy when surgical therapy is planned for chronic pancreatitis. Although the relative value of ERCP, pancreatic stimulation testing, and other studies such as ultrasonography in the diagnosis of early-stage chronic pancreatitis is not known, it is clear that false positive and negative studies may occur with any of these procedures. Therefore, ERCP can be of additional value even when only a minimal degree of pancreatitis is present. The long-term results of endoscopic occlusion of the main pancreatic duct for intractable pain related to chronic pancreatitis have been disappointing. Endoscopic sphincterotomy has a very limited role in the management of chronic pancreatitis. In an occasional patient, endoscopic sphincterotomy of the minor papilla may be of value in pancreas divisum, although this procedure is difficult and has not been thoroughly evaluated in relation to this anomaly. ERCP is occasionally indicated in patients with undiagnosed chronic abdominal pain when other diagnostic methods including ultrasonography and computed tomography fail to reveal an etiology. The yield for ERCP in patients in this latter category is highest when the history suggests misuse of alcohol.

References

1. Perrier CV. Symposium on the etiology and pathological anatomy of chronic pancreatitis: Marseilles, 1963. Am J Dig Dis 1964; 9:371–6.
2. Axon ATR, Classin M, Cotton PB, et al. Pancreatography in chronic pancreatitis: international definitions. Gut 1984; 25:107–12.
3. Ebner F, Hofler H, Kratochvil P, et al. Pankreasnekrose nach endoskopisch retrograder Pankreatikographie. Dtsch med Wochenschr 1982; 107:453–5.
4. Safrany L, Neuhaus B, Krause S, et al. Endoskopische Papillotomie bei akuter biliarer Pankreatitis. Dtsch med Wochenschr 1980; 105:115–9.
5. Tympner F, Domschke W, Rösch W, et al. Verlauf der hydrokinetischen und ekbolen Pankreasfunktion nach akuter Pankreatitis. Z Gastroenterologie 1976; 14:684–7.
6. Hamilton I, Bradley P, Lintott DJ, et al. Endoscopic retrograde cholangiopancreatography in the investigation and management of patients after acute pancreatitis. Br J Surg 1982; 69:504–6.
7. Cotton PB, Beales JSM. Endoscopic pancreatography in management of relapsing acute pancreatitis. Br Med J 1974; 1:608–11.
8. Zimmon DS, Falkenstein DB, Abrams RM, et al. Endoscopic retrograde cholangiopancreatography

(ERCP) in the diagnosis of pancreatic inflammatory disease. Radiology 1974; 113:287–92.

9. Cooperman M, Ferrara JJ, Carey LC, et al. Idiopathic acute pancreatitis: The value of endoscopic retrograde cholangiopancreatography. Surgery 1981; 90:666–70.

10. Rösch W, Schaffner O, Tympner F, Koch H. Endoskopisch radiologische Verlaufsbeobachtungen bei Pankreatitis. In Lindner H, ed. Fortschritte der gastroenterologischen Endoskopie. Baden-Baden: Witzstrock, 1975.

11. Nagata A, Homma T, Tamai K, et al. A study of chronic pancreatitis by serial endoscopic pancreatography. Gastroenterology 1981; 81:884–91.

12. Gebhardt CH, Riemann JF, Lux G. The importance of ERCP for the surgical tactic in haemorrhagic necrotizing pancreatitis (preliminary report). Endoscopy 1983; 15:55–8.

13. Kasugai T, Kuno N, Kizu M, et al. Endoscopic pancreatocholangiography. II. The pathological endoscopic pancreatocholangiogram. Gastroenterology 1972; 63:227–34.

14. Tympner F, Rösch W, Lutz H, Koch H. Diagnostische Methoden bei chronischer Pankreatitis. Stellenwert von endoskopisch retrograder Pankreatikographie, volumenverlustkorrigiertem Sekretin. Dtsch med Wochenschr 1978; 103:805.

15. Nakano S, Horiguchi Y, Takeda T, et al. Comparative diagnostic value of endoscopic pancreatography and pancreatic function tests. Scand J Gastroenterol 1974; 9:383–9.

16. Sawabu N, Makino H, Nakajima S, et al. Diagnostic value of endoscopic pancreatography in comparison with pancreatic function tests. Jpn J Gastroenterol 1976; 73:248–56.

17. Rolny P, Lukes PJ, Gamklou R, et al. A comparative evaluation of endoscopic retrograde pancreatography and secretin CCK test in the diagnosis of pancreatic disease. Scand J Gastroenterol 1978; 13:777–81.

18. Ashton MG, Axon AT, Lintott DJ. Lundh test and ERCP in pancreatic disease. Gut 1978; 19:910–5.

19. Braganza JM, Hunt LP, Warwick F. Relationship between pancreatic exocrine function and ductal morphology in chronic pancreatitis. Gastroenterology 1982; 82:1341–7.

20. Di Magno EP, Malagelada J-R, Go VLW. The relationship between pancreatic ductal obstruction and pancreatic secretion in man. Mayo Clin Proc 1979; 54:157–62.

21. Rösch W. The value of endoscopic occlusion of the pancreatic duct. Endoscopy 1983; 15 (suppl 1):175–7.

22. Siegel JH, Sable RA, Ho R, et al. Abnormalities of the bile duct associated with chronic pancreatitis. Am J Gastroenterol 1979; 72:259–66.

23. Gregg JA, Carr-Locke DL, Gallagher MM. Importance of common bile duct stricture associated with chronic pancreatitis. Diagnosis by ERCP. Am J Surg 1981; 141:199–203.

24. Wisloff F, Jakobsen J, Osnes M. Stenosis of the common bile duct in chronic pancreatitis. Br J Surg 1982; 69:52–4.

25. Caletti G, Brocchi E, Agostini D, et al. Sensitivity of endoscopic retrograde pancreatography in chronic pancreatitis. Br J Surg 1982; 69:507–9.

26. Rohrmann CA Jr, Silvis SE, Vennes JA. The significance of pancreatic ductal obstruction in differential diagnosis of the abnormal endoscopic retrograde pancreatogram. Radiology 1976; 121:311–4.

27. Tulassay Z, Papp J, Kollin E, et al. Das pathologische endoskopische Pankreatogramm: Wertigkeit der rontgenmorphologischen Veranderungen. Rontgen-blatter 1981; 34:205–11.

28. Rösch W. Die segmentare Pankreatitis. Leber Magen Darm 1983; 13:49–54.

29. Rösch W, Koch H, Schaffner O, Demling L. The clinical significance of the pancreas divisum. Gastrointest Endosc 1976; 22:206–7.

30. Cotton PB, Kizu M. Malfusion of dorsal and ventral pancreas; a cause of pancreatitis? (Abstr) Gut 1977; 18:A400.

31. Mitchell CJ, Lintott DJ, Ruddell WSJ, et al. Clinical relevance of an unfused pancreatic duct system. Gut 1979; 20:1066–71.

32. Richter JM, Schapiro RH, Mulley AG, Warshaw AL. Association of pancreas divisum and pancreatitis, and its treatment by sphincteroplasty of the accessory ampulla. Gastroenterology 1981; 81:1104–10.

33. Sahel J, Cros R-C, Bourry J, Sarles H. Clinicopathological conditions associated with pancreas divisum. Digestion 1982; 23:1–8.

34. Stolte M, Weiss W, Volkholz H, Rösch W. A special form of segmental pancreatitis: "groove pancreatitis." Hepatogastroenterology 1982; 29:198–208.

35. Cotton PB, Lees WR, Vallon AG, et al. Gray-scale ultrasonography and endoscopic pancreatography in pancreatic diagnosis. Radiology 1980; 134:453–9.

36. Foley WD, Stewart ET, Lawson TL, et al. Computed tomography, ultrasonography and endoscopic retrograde cholangiopancreatography in the diagnosis of pancreatic disease. Gastrointest Radiol 1980; 5:29–35.

37. Gmelin E, Weiss HD, Fuchs HD, Reiser M. Vergleich der diagnostischen Treffsicherheit von Ultraschall, Computertomographie und ERCP bei der chronischen Pankreatitis und beim Pankreas karzinom. ROEFO 1981; 134:136–41.

38. Swobodnik W, Meyer W, Brecht-Kraus D, et al. Ultrasound, computed tomography and endoscopic retrograde cholangiopancreatography in the morphological diagnosis of pancreatic disease. Klin Wochenschr 1983; 61:291–6.

39. Rohrmann CA, Surawicz CM, Hutchinson D, et al. The diagnosis of hereditary pancreatitis by pancreatography. Gastrointest Endosc 1981; 27:168–73.

40. Perrault J, Gross JB, King JE. Endoscopic retrograde cholangiopancreatography in familial pancreatitis. Gastroenterology 1976; 71:138–44.

41. Little JM, Lauer C, Hogg J. Pancreatic duct obstruction with an acrylate glue: a new method for producing pancreatic exocrine atrophy. Surgery 1977; 81:243–9.

42. Gebhardt CH, Stolte M. Pankreasgang Okklusion durch Injektion einer schnellhartenden Aminosaurenlosung. Langenbecks Arch klin Chir 1978; 346:149–66.

43. Rösch W, Phillip J, Gebhardt CH. Endoscopic duct obstruction in chronic pancreatitis. Endoscopy 1979; 11:43–6.

44. Bull J, Keeling PW, Thompson RP. Endoscopic retrograde cholangiopancreatography for unexplained upper abdominal pain. Br Med J 1980; 1:764.

45. Ruddell WSJ, Lintott DJ, Axon ATR: The diagnostic yield of ERCP in the investigation of unexplained abdominal pain. Br J Surg 1983; 70:74–5.

Chapter 37

THE INTRADUCTAL SECRETIN TEST (IDST)—AN ADJUNCT TO THE DIAGNOSIS OF PANCREATIC DISEASE AND PANCREATIC PHYSIOLOGY

JAMES A. GREGG, M.D.

Various pancreatic function tests have been employed for many years to determine the presence of pancreatic inflammatory disease, pancreatic cancer, and the degree of pancreatic functional impairment. All have certain limitations.

The most widely used test has been the secretin test introduced by Chiray et al[1] or its later modifications by Lagerlof[2] and others.[3-12] Secretin has been administered intravenously either as a bolus or by constant infusion, with or without cholecystokinin (CCK), the latter being given as a bolus or by constant infusion prior to, concurrent with, or following secretin. These tests are time consuming and require intubation and proper fluoroscopic placement of a multilumen tube. The loss of unknown quantities of duodenal juice, and the admixture of duodenal juice with gastric juice and particularly bile if CCK is administered, make interpretation problematic, especially with respect to volume flow and also bicarbonate concentration in view of its low concentration in bile.

With the more physiologic Lundh test meal it is impossible to determine secretory volume and bicarbonate concentration, and frequently only one pancreatic enzyme is measured in duodenal juice.[13] Bile admixture is also a problem, and the Lundh test does not stress the pancreas to its secretory limits as can be achieved with the secretin or augmented secretin-CCK test. The results may also be abnormal in some patients with primary malabsorptive disorders of the small intestine because of impaired release of secretin and/or CCK from intestinal mucosa.

Tubeless, noninvasive studies, such as the pancreolauryl and NBT-PABA tests, require ingestion of a synthetic compound that can be hydrolyzed by pancreatic enzymes to produce a low molecular weight substance that is easily absorbed from the small intestine and then secreted in the urine in a measurable form.[14] Other noninvasive tests require the absorption of foodstuffs, such as the two-stage triolean and the rice-flour breath tests. Stool tests measuring nitrogen or fat or both or chymotrypsin are unpleasant and, like the breath tests, time consuming and insensitive except in advanced pancreatic insufficiency; all may be abnormal in malabsorptive disorders of the small intestine. Lankisch et al.[14, 15] have reviewed the methodology, accuracy, and associated problems of these various tests.

Endoscopic retrograde cholangiopancreatography (ERCP) not only provides a method for defining pancreatic and bile duct morphology but also permits pancreatic function testing by direct access to intraductal secretions. The intraductal secretin test (IDST) obviates most of the problems associated with the various pancreatic function tests. The pure pancreatic juice (PPJ) obtained is uncontaminated by bile or gastric juice. This permits the determination of true concentrations of bicarbonate and enzymes as they are secreted by the pancreas in response to a wide variety of exogenous and endogenous stimuli. PPJ can be obtained after administration of secretin,[16–53] secretin plus CCK,[29, 53–62] and secretin plus caerulein.[61, 62] Basal flow rates,[34, 63] peak secretory flow rates (PSFR),[25, 26, 32–37, 39, 48, 54, 57, 61, 62] electrolyte content,[28, 29, 32, 34, 35, 39, 48, 61] enzymes,[23, 24, 26, 33, 35, 38–40, 44, 47–57, 59–62] tumor markers and nonspecific markers of pancreatic disease,[18, 19, 22, 38, 39, 41, 43, 49–53, 58, 59, 63] pancreatic fluid cytology,[16, 17, 20, 21] PPJ viscosity,[45, 46] bacterial content,[30] and the secretion of antibiotics[64, 65] have been studied using the IDST.

A standard IDST with secretin or secretin/CCK can easily be performed at the time of ERCP or in conjunction with upper gastrointestinal endoscopy in a fraction of the time required for a duodenal secretin test (DST). Secretin testing can be used to assess the magnitude of secretory impairment in patients with known pancreatic disease and also to establish the presence of pancreatic disease when the results of other studies have been negative in patients who are nevertheless thought to have a disorder of the pancreas.

METHODOLOGY OF THE INTRADUCTAL SECRETIN TEST (IDST)

The preparation of the patient for the IDST is the same as for gastroscopy or ERCP and can be done in conjunction with either examination, except that no antispasmodics, ganglionic blocking agents,[66, 67] or glucagon[26] can be used, since these compounds significantly reduce secretory flow rates and enzyme concentration in the PPJ. Diazepam does not appear to affect these parameters.[67] If the IDST is performed prior to ERCP, the subsequent injection of contrast agent will result in immediate efflux of the contrast material from the duct, making it difficult to obtain a complete pancreatogram and impossible to determine pancreatic duct drainage time. These problems are avoided when the IDST is done after the ERCP phase of the procedure.

After proper orientation of the duodenoscope to the papilla, a standard secretin IDST is done by administering secretin, 1 U/kg body weight, as a bolus without skin testing. A measurable increase in pancreatic secretion begins within 30 to 60 seconds, and PSFR is reached within several minutes and continues essentially at this same rate for at least 10 minutes, after which time it gradually decreases.

The pancreatic juice secreted during the first few minutes should not be used for diagnostic purposes since it contains mainly preformed enzymes that are "washed out" from the duct. This fluid has high concentrations of protein and enzymes and low amounts of bicarbonate.[28, 48, 54] From 5 to 10 minutes after secretin administration, PSFR is stable,[35, 48, 54] but protein secretion may vary.[54] To avoid minute-to-minute variations in protein concentration, it is best to obtain a 5-minute collection of PPJ 5 to 10 minutes after secretin injection. This can be done by gentle aspiration with a 10 ml syringe attached to the ERCP cannula, the tip of which has been positioned 5 to 20 mm into the pancreatic duct, or by siphonage. The cannula tip must be positioned properly within the duct so that free flow of PPJ occurs by either method, both for the safety of the patient and for obtaining the most accurate PSFR.

Aspiration is preferable, particularly in hypersecretory states; in this situation siphonage may greatly underestimate actual flow rates. In patients with very low PSFR, siphonage is generally preferred. It decreases the possibility that excessive suction with the syringe will result in aspiration of pancreatic duct epithelium into the cannula tip. In rare instances this causes pancreatitis.

Since secretin is absorbed by plastic surfaces[68] it should be prepared just prior to use and administered with a glass syringe through the shortest possible length of intravenous plastic tubing. Pancreatic secretion can also be studied by constant infusion of secretin at doses of 0.5 or 1 U/kg body weight per hour. Since constant infusion requires intravenous tubing between syringe and patient, the secretin should be dissolved in dilute human serum albumin for stabilization[35] to ensure that the intended dose is actually received by the patient.

To study PPJ high in protein and enzyme concentration, CCK (1 U/kg) can be administered as a bolus concurrent with, or 10 to 20 minutes after, administration of the secretin bolus. CCK can also be administered as a constant infusion at the same dosage. Bolus administration of CCK results in a rapid increase in the secretion of protein and enzymes.[32, 35, 54, 57, 61, 62] This increase is transient, lasting several minutes, and is followed by a gradual decline to pre-CCK levels within 15 to 20 minutes. Its effect on the small bowel may result in intestinal cramps, nausea, and occasionally vomiting, factors that should be considered if CCK is to be used. It has not been established that the information obtained with combined secretin/CCK stimulation provides greater diagnostic capability than that with secretin stimulation alone.

Caerulein appears to have properties similar to CCK.[61, 62] In addition to side effects similar to those of CCK as mentioned, its additional cost and the time required for use in conjunction with secretin must be considered.

The PPJ obtained during an IDST should be analyzed for PSFR, and concentrations of chloride, bicarbonate, amylase, lipase, gamma-glutamyltransferase (GGT), and total protein. In certain situations, culture of the pancreatic juice, and cytologic study may be useful. Determinations of trypsinogen, chymotrypsinogen, and other enzymes may provide additional information if the methodology for these studies is available.

An IDST cannot be done in all patients, although a success rate of at least 90% is possible with experience. Stenosis of the major pancreatic sphincter may preclude cannulation of the pancreatic duct in a few patients. In patients with pancreas divisum, it is usually possible to cannulate satisfactorily only the ventral duct, and great care must be exercised in aspirating PPJ because of the small duct caliber and low PSFR. After sphincteroplasty of the minor papilla, however, PPJ can usually be aspirated from the dorsal ductal system during the IDST.

SECRETORY FLOW DURING THE IDST

Volume of PPJ

Although the IDST provides uncontaminated PPJ for study, it may not provide exact secretory flow rates. Loss of PPJ through the minor ampulla is probably negligible or nonexistent, since this structure is minute and not patent in the majority of patients. Loss of PPJ from around the ERCP cannula cannot be measured but is probably small in most cases. Osnes,[69] using a double lumen ERCP cannula, demonstrated that the recovery of an intraductally infused marker, Cobalt-57–labeled vitamin B_{12}, administered as a constant infusion through one lumen of

the cannula within the pancreatic duct, ranged from 78% to 96% (mean, 84%), even at high flow rates of PPJ when PPJ was aspirated through the other cannula channel after secretin administration. Denyer et al.[28] compared the volume recovery rates of pancreatic and duodenal juice during an IDST and DST in the same subjects on different occasions. Using a marker, they found that the mean volume of duodenal juice recovered during the DST to be 69%, with a range of 12.5% to 100%. The corrected mean duodenal juice volumes exceeded PPJ volumes by a ratio of 2.3 to 1 in normal individuals. These lower recovery rates of PPJ were presumably due to incomplete recovery of PPJ during the IDST as well as to volume enhancement of duodenal juice by admixture with intestinal secretions and bile during the DST. The use of siphonage rather than aspiration of PPJ with a syringe during the IDST may also have contributed to low PPJ recovery rates. The duodenal juice recovery rates in this study are similar to those reported for the DST by Tympner et al.[10] in paired studies. Escourrou et al.[61] reported no significant difference between the volumes of duodenal juice and PPJ during a secretin test, the mean volume of PPJ being 104 ml/ 30 min collection.

Basal Secretory Flow Rates of PPJ

Basal secretory flow rates (BSFR) have been reported. Domschke et al.[32, 34] found BSFR of approximately 4 µl/kg or 0.03 ml/min for a 70 kg subject. In our experience with 10 normal subjects the BSFR were similar, ranging from 0.02 to 0.07 ml/min when PPJ was collected for 20-minute periods beginning 5 minutes after cannulation. Likewise, the BSFR found by Osnes et al.[63] had a range of 0.06 to 0.07 ml/min beginning at 5 minutes after cannulation of the pancreatic duct. The first 5-minute specimen demonstrated higher flow rates of 0.17 to 0.47 ml/min. These authors believed that this was due to release of secretin from duodenal mucosa during cannulation, since a slight rise in plasma immunoreactive secretin was noted immediately after cannulation.

Effect of Graded Doses of Secretin on PPJ

Very small doses of secretin administered intravenously, either as a bolus or by constant infusion, elicit a significant flow of PPJ (Fig. 37–1). Domschke et al.[34] demonstrated that as little as 8 ng (0.031 U)/kg/hr increased secretory flow rates and that maximal flow was reached at 0.5 U/kg/hr. Denyer and Cotton[35] obtained PPJ secretory flow rates of 1.6 ml/min with a bolus dose of only 0.014 U/kg, and 2.3 ml/min with a dose of 0.057 U/kg; PSFR occurred with a dose of 1 U/kg. The secretin used in this study was stabilized in dilute albumin for optimum accuracy. In studies such as these, increasing doses of secretin every 10 minutes may have some cumulative effect on flow rates. An intravenous infusion of albumin-stabilized secretin at 0.06 U/kg/hr (16 ng) produces plasma secretin levels similar to those of the postprandial state in man and thus produces physiologic rather than pharmacologic secretory response.

Normal Pancreatic Secretory Flow Rates

The reported PSFR after bolus administration of secretin as shown in Table 37–1 range from 2.5 to 6.5 ml/min,[25, 32, 34, 35, 37, 39, 48, 54, 61] although the majority are in the range of 3.0 to 5.5 ml/min. Gregg and Sharma[25, 37] initially determined PSFR to be 4.13 ml/min (±0.88) and more recently, 4.19 (±0.73) ml/min for the IDST. The results of Cotton and Heap[27] and Denyer and Cotton[35] are similar, as are those of Domschke et al.[34] The PSFR reported by Rinderknecht et al.[54] are significantly lower using the same dose of secretin. The PSFR of Robberecht et al.[62] are even lower, but these authors administered an anticholinergic agent prior to secretin. The administration of CCK with secretin results in a slight but significant increase in PSFR

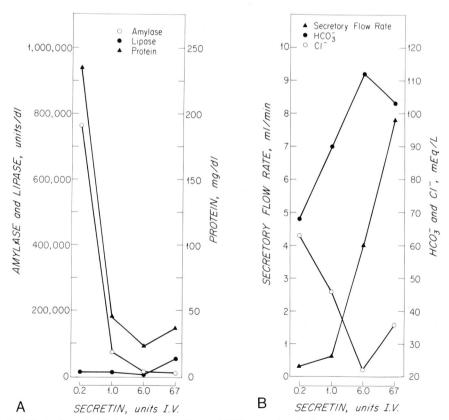

FIGURE 37–1. Effect of graded infusion of secretin on PPJ flow rate and electrolyte and enzyme concentrations. A, Secretion of amylase, lipase, and total protein in PPJ in a patient with chronic pancreatitis. The amylase concentration is low and secretion of amylase and lipase is nonparallel. B, Pancreatic hypersecretion and low bicarbonate ion concentration in the same patient as in A. Note the reciprocal secretion pattern of bicarbonate and chloride ions.

TABLE 37–1. **PPJ Flow Rates After Secretin or Secretin/CCK Stimulation in Normal Humans.**

Author(s)	No. Subjects	Flow Rate (ml/min)	Secretin (units)	CCK (units)
Gregg and Sharma[25, 37]	18	4.13 ± 0.88 (2.8–5.5)	90	
Denyer and Cotton[35]	19	3.92	70	1/kg
Cotton and Heap[27]	16	2.6–6.5	1/kg	
Rinderknecht et al.[54]	15	3.15 ± 0.24 (2.0–5.6)	1/kg	
	15	3.40 ± 0.29	1/kg	
Escourrou et al.[61]	7	4.15	0.5/kg	1/kg
Gregg[48]	27	4.19 ± 0.73 (3.0–6.5)	1/kg	
Domschke et al.[34]	7	50 μl/min/kg	0.5/kg	

above that obtained by secretin alone.[54, 61] The PSFR obtained by the DST are generally in agreement with those obtained by the IDST. Using 10-minute collection periods, PSFR reported with the DST are as follows: Wormsley,[8] 51 ml (±2); Burton et al.,[4] 57 ml; and Hartley et al.,[7] 35 ml (±6). With a 20-minute collection period, PSFR reported by Dreiling and Janowitz[3] was 66 ml, and by Petersen,[9] 110 ml (±23).

Secretory Flow Rates in Pancreatic Disease

Pancreatic PSFR in patients with chronic pancreatitis have been shown by Dreiling and Bordalo[70] to have a bimodal distribution; this has also been demonstrated by the author.[36, 37, 39] Patients with chronic pancreatitis in its early stages may have normal pancreatic secretion or hypersecretion,[39, 70] whereas those with advanced chronic disease usually have a marked decrease in PSFR; an occasional patient may have no demonstrable pancreatic secretion by the IDST. Some patients with advanced chronic pancreatitis have particulate matter in the pancreatic juice that is precipitated proteinaceous material. In some patients with acute or chronic pancreatitis PSFR after secretin administration may not be reached for as long as 10 minutes. An IDST during an acute episode of pancreatitis may show very low PSFR; the same study a week later may demonstrate almost total functional recovery with nearly normal PSFR.

Low flow rates are commonly encountered in patients with cancer of the head of the pancreas[11, 17, 19] and body[59]; normal flow rates commonly occur in patients with cancer of the tail of the pancreas during either the

IDST[11, 19] or the DST.[71] The author has not encountered a PSFR greater than 3.3 ml/min in patients with pancreatic cancer, including those with cancer of the tail of the pancreas.

OTHER COMPONENTS OF PPJ

Electrolytes

The concentrations of sodium and potassium ions in PPJ determined by the IDST are similar to those found in duodenal juice by means of the DST. The duodenal juice values of 145–160 and 138–143 mEq/l for sodium reported by Wormsley[8] and by Dreiling and Janowitz[3] respectively compare closely with PPJ sodium ion concentrations of 150.63 mEq/l (± 1.90) found by this author (unpublished data); the potassium ion concentration of 3.5 (±4.5) reported by Wormsley[8] is also similar to the value of 3.95 mEq/l (±0.31) for PPJ found by this author (unpublished data). The concentrations of potassium and sodium ions are unaffected by flow rate or pancreatic disease. In our laboratory, chloride ion concentration in PPJ after secretin administration (1 U/kg) was 25.78 mEq/l (±7.64); the bicarbonate plus chloride ion concentration in PPJ was 155.41 mEq/l (±9.12) at all flow rates and in all clinical conditions. This correlates closely with the value of 155–157 mEq/l for chloride plus bicarbonate in duodenal juice during the DST reported by Dreiling and Janowitz.[3]

After secretin stimulation, bicarbonate concentrations in PPJ exceed those of duodenal juice (Table 37–2). Denyer et al.,[28] using a DST and IDST in the same subjects, found a mean increase in bicarbonate ion concentration in PPJ over that in duodenal juice of 34 mEq/l. Escourrou et at.,[61] using constant secretin infusion (0.5 U/kg/hr), reported a

TABLE 37–2. **Normal PPJ Bicarbonate Concentration.**

Author(s)	No. Subjects	Bicarbonate (mEq/l)	Secretin (units/kg)
Denyer and Cotton[35]	9	124 (median) (108–126)	1
Escourrou et al.[61]	7	124.5 ± 11.32	0.5
Domschke et al.[34]	7	135 ± 9	0.5
Gregg[48]	27	129.63 ± 6.23 (119–146)	1

difference of 48 mEq/l. Domschke et al.,[34] using a constant infusion of secretin, and the author,[25, 48] using both constant infusion and bolus doses of secretin, have reported similarly higher values for bicarbonate concentration in PPJ compared with duodenal juice.

As the dose of secretin is increased during the IDST, bicarbonate concentrations rise to a maximum and then begin to fall, even as the actual bicarbonate output per minute increases in association with increasing flow rates.[34, 35] Similar findings were reported by Wormsley[8] using the DST. Domschke et al.[32] demonstrated that infusions of secretin in doses as small as 0.06 U/kg/hr can produce a bicarbonate concentration of 117 mEq/l with PSFR of 1.41 ml/min; the concentration increases as the secretin dosage is increased (Table 37–2). These small infused dosages, as is the case with the small doses of secretin used by Denyer and Cotton,[35] produce plasma immunoreactive secretin levels that are similar to those found in humans after a meal, and thus more accurately duplicate the physiologic response to secretin. Domschke et al.[34] reported maximal bicarbonate secretion of 338 uEq/kg/hr (± 79) at a secretin dose of 0.5 U/kg/hr. The bicarbonate concentration correlated closely with levels of cyclic AMP in PPJ.

Bicarbonate concentrations below the normal range (see Table 37–2) are indicative of pancreatic disease. Bicarbonate concentrations in PPJ[20] or duodenal juice[71, 72] of patients with pancreatic cancer may be normal or low and are not diagnostic.

Pancreatic Proteins

PPJ collected during the first few minutes after administration of secretin has a very high concentration of protein, presumably due in part to washout of enzymes from within the duct. Denyer and Cotton[35] observed that a small bolus of secretin repeated at 10-minute intervals gave distinct, albeit progressively smaller, transient elevations in protein and enzyme values. This suggests that these secondary rises are not solely due to a "washout phenomenon." It has also been demonstrated that the initial fractions of PPJ contain active proteolytic enzymes,[23, 54] presumably due to the introduction of minute amounts of enterokinase-containing duodenal mucosa into the pancreatic duct, probably by the tip of the cannula.

Robberecht et al.[62] noted a total protein of 50 to 100 mg/dl in PPJ after secretin administration, although in this study an anticholinergic agent had been administered just prior to the procedure. Protein concentrations in PPJ of approximately 50 mg/dl,[54] 38.13 mg/dl, (± 10.13), and 200 mg/dl[32] in response to secretin administration have been reported.

The addition of CCK to the secretin infusion or secretin bolus produces an abrupt increase in PPJ enzymes and protein output. A mean 12.2-fold (range, 3- to 24-fold) increase in protein output,[54] and a five- to tenfold increase[61] have been noted. This markedly increased protein secretion lasts only several minutes, gradually returning to pre-CCK levels within 15 to 20 minutes. In normal individuals, there is a parallel increase in some but not all enzymes.[42, 54, 61]

PPJ from patients with acute or subsiding pancreatitis contains active proteolytic enzymes throughout long collection periods,[23, 24, 55] well beyond the levels expected in healthy individuals. Geokas and Rinderknecht[50] reported similar findings in studies of PPJ obtained by catheter drainage after surgery.

The concentrations of amylase and lipase in PPJ during PSFR after secretin stimulation were 46,017 Somogyi units/dl (± 25,380 units) and 32,976 Roe-Byler-Well units/dl (± 19,852 units), respectively, in a recent study.[48] Rinderknecht et al.[54] found amylase levels of approximately 120,000 IU/dl in PPJ which, with application of the appropriate conversion factor, translates to a mean amylase in PPJ, after secretin, of 64,900 Somogyi units/dl, a value similar to the author's.

Trypsin inhibitor was studied by Renner et al.,[57] who noted that the ratio of trypsinogen to trypsin inhibitor in PPJ of chronic alcoholics without pancreatitis was much higher than in normal persons, thus suggesting that low trypsin inhibitor levels may favor intraductal activation of trypsinogen and other enzymes. Elias et al.[24] reported an absence of trypsin inhibitor in PPJ of two patients with nonalcoholic pancreatitis. Lysosomal enzymes were demonstrated in PPJ of normal humans and chronic alcoholics in one study,[56] but there was no statistical difference in these various enzymes between the two groups except for increased secretion of B-D glucuronidase in alcoholics.

Recently, Scheele et al.[40] identified 15 different pancreatic exocrine proteins with enzymatic activity using gel electrophoresis. One of these, a third form of trypsinogen, was also demonstrated in PPJ and in pancreatic tissue by Rinderknecht et al.[60] This active protease, mesotrypsin, is of particular interest because it is almost totally resistant to biologic trypsin inactivators and can activate trypsinogen even in the presence of excess trypsin inhibitor. By its action on trypsinogen it also induces activation of other enzymes. Its potential role, if any, in the pathogenesis of pancreatitis remains to be determined.

Pancreatic polypeptide has been demonstrated in PPJ by Carr-Locke and Track.[47] There was no statistical difference between the concentration of this protein in PPJ of normal individuals and of patients with chronic pancreatitis or cancer.

PANCREATIC HYPERSECRETION

Pancreatic hypersecretion has been reported to occur during a DST in some patients with cirrhosis[73,74] and/or pancreatitis,[70,75] and also more recently in chronic alcoholics without known cirrhosis or pancreatitis.[76] Gregg and Sharma,[36] using the IDST, confirmed that at least a part of the large duodenal aspirate encountered in these clinical disorders is due to pancreatic hypersecretion. It has also been demonstrated using the DST in some patients with Zollinger-Ellison syndrome.[77] The author has studied pancreatic secretion in two patients with Zollinger-Ellison syndrome using the IDST and PPJ. The

PSFR as well as bicarbonate and enzyme concentrations were within normal ranges.

In the author's experience with PPJ,[36] hypersecretion was encountered in 6 of 12 patients with cirrhosis, all alcoholics. Three of the six with hypersecretion also had pancreatitis. Secretory rates ranged from 7.8 to 26 ml/min after administration of secretin. Two of three patients with hypersecretion and no clinical, pancreatographic, or ultrasonographic evidence of pancreatitis, were found at autopsy several years later to have had chronic pancreatitis, the probable cause of the hypersecretion. Hypersecretion may be sustained and prolonged for many years; one of the author's patients had PSFR as high as 27.5 ml/min over a 30-minute period after bolus administration of secretin; another patient had secretin-stimulated PSFR of 11.5 to 30.0 ml/min on four examinations during a 5-year period. Pancreatic hypersecretion may also occur in the presence of pancreatic duct obstruction; another of our patients had a PSFR of 10.0 ml/min, even though the pancreatic duct was totally obstructed at the junction of the head and body of the gland. None of the 15 patients with pancreatic hypersecretion that we have studied has had either steatorrhea or pancreatic calcification, although several did have chronic pancreatitis and dilated pancreatic ducts.

Renner et al.[78] also reported pancreatic hypersecretion of PPJ in cirrhotic patients, none of whom had evident pancreatitis. It would seem that some of these patients must have had occult pancreatitis since all were chronic alcoholics. The hypersecretory rates of 5.19 ml/min (± 0.33) were much lower than those the author has observed, but the normal flow rates of 3.12 ml/min reported by Renner and colleagues were also lower than those found by the author.

Studies of pancreatic hypersecretory states in humans by the DST, particularly by combined secretin/CCK stimulation, must be interpreted with caution. Although secretin is a weak stimulant of bile and biliary bicarbonate secretion in humans,[79, 80] hypersecretion of bile may occur in response to secretin in some cirrhotic patients. The author encountered bile flow rates of 5.0 to 12.5 ml/min during the first 10 minutes after secretin administration when bile was aspirated directly from the common ducts of three patients with cirrhosis who had undergone cholecystectomy. This volume of dilute bile when added to pancreatic secretion as a component of the duodenal juice obtained during the DST could easily lead to an incorrect conclusion of pancreatic hypersecretion. The biliary component of duodenal juice adds an unknown but potentially significant error to any DST performed in a cirrhotic patient.

The occurrence of hypersecretion of bile or pancreatic juice after physiologic doses of secretin has not been demonstrated. The dosages administered during secretin stimulation testing produce plasma levels of immunoreactive secretin well in excess of those that occur after meals.

In the presence of pancreatic hypersecretion, the concentrations of pancreatic enzymes obtained by a DST may be proportionately low, although the bicarbonate concentration usually remains normal.[75, 76] The author's experience with PPJ obtained by IDST is similar. Renner et al.[57] demonstrated a significantly higher output of trypsin in PPJ after CCK was added to a secretin infusion in patients with alcoholic cirrhosis. The increased bicarbonate levels in duodenal aspirates of cirrhotic subjects, especially those with hemochromatosis, may be due to an increase in bile bicarbonate secretion in association with bile hypersecretion, in addition to an element of pancreatic hypersecretion.[75]

Hypersecretion of pancreatic juice appears to be unrelated to portosystemic shunting, since pancreatic secretion is unaffected by a splenorenal shunt.[81] It is also not related to delayed clearance of secretin from the plasma, since secretin clearance is normal in cirrhotic subjects.[82] It is possible that the pancreatic hypersecretion observed in cirrhotic patients, especially those with known pancreatitis, is due to some element of pancreatic ductular reduplication as has been documented in some patients with pancreatitis.[70]

Ductal reduplication has been documented in the liver[70] and may be responsible for the increased bile flow in response to secretin observed in patients with cirrhosis. Combined hypersecretion of bile and pancreatic juice could account for the large duodenal aspirates encountered during the DST in patients with hemochromatosis as suggested by Dreiling et al.,[75] since this disease affects both organs. The observation that patients with nonalcoholic cirrhosis and no evidence of chronic pancreatitis have duodenal aspirates during a DST only slightly above that in normal subjects[75] is also consistent with this hypothesis.

PPJ AND THE DIAGNOSIS OF PANCREATIC CANCER

Diagnosis of pancreatic cancer using PPJ has not been notably successful. Early studies by the author and colleagues[17] and Kozu[16] focused on PPJ cytology in normal individuals and in patients with pancreatitis and pancreatic cancer. Although PPJ collected during the IDST contains a large number of pancreatic duct columnar cells and occasionally sheets of these cells, the author and coworkers obtained positive cytologic findings in only 5 of 49 patients with pancreatic cancer; accordingly, PPJ cytology was abandoned in 1977 because of its low yield. Kawanishi et al.[20] demonstrated positive cytologic findings in four of eight patients using "relatively uncontaminated" PPJ. In a study by Hatfield et al.,[21] 14 of 26 patients with pancreatic cancer had positive PPJ cytologic results. In some patients the cytologic material for study was actually duodenal juice, since PPJ could not be obtained. In several patients there was transmural extension of the cancer into the duodenum.

Percutaneous aspiration biopsy of the pancreas under CT or ultrasonographic guidance results in a positive diagnosis of malignant cells in 75% to 80% of patients with pancreatic cancer.[83, 84] The false-positive rate of diagnosis is negligible. These factors, plus the general availability and ease of percutaneous aspiration biopsy, favor this approach to the cytologic diagnosis of pancreatic cancer provided there is no transmural tumor extension that would lend itself to endoscopic biopsy or brushing for cytologic material.

Other methods for diagnosis of pancreatic carcinoma by analysis of noncellular components of PPJ have been proposed. Early attempts utilized carcinoembryonic antigen (CEA) levels in PPJ.[18, 19, 22] CEA-like activity was first demonstrated in PPJ by Sharma et al.[18] in 1974. Although the PPJ levels of CEA are usually elevated in patients with pancreatic cancer, they are also increased in patients with chronic pancreatitis, and the degree of overlap is such that CEA determinations are not diagnostic.

Schneider et al.[41] isolated a glycoprotein from PPJ of 73% of patients with chronic pancreatitis and 93% of patients with pancreatic cancer. The protein is found in normal individuals and is distinct from CEA. Like CEA, it is a nonspecific marker for pancreatic disease.

Schmiegel et al.[43] demonstrated the presence of an oncofetal antigen in pancreatic juice that differs from the one that was initially described in serum. The antigen, which is also distinct from CEA, was demonstrated in PPJ of 59 of 74 patients with pancreatic cancer and in 16% to 26% of those with other pancreatic disorders. Although this determination appears to be more specific than CEA for pancreatic cancer, the overlap with values found in other pancreatic disorders remains substantial.

Scheele[44] studied PPJ from normal individuals and from patients with pancreatic cancer using an isoelectric focusing technique to separate proteins. Patients with cancer had abnormal pancreatic protein profiles, but patients with chronic pancreatitis were not studied for comparison.

Rinderknecht et al.[59] studied PPJ secretory profiles for 11 pancreatic enzymes and proteins in nine patients with pancreatic cancer after secretin/CCK stimulation. Because of low PSFR, minute-to-minute collections for study were successful in less than 25% of the patients. The activity of lysosomal enzymes remained within or above the normal range, whereas total protein secretion and the secretion of trypsin inhibitor and digestive enzymes were either at the lowest end of the normal range or below normal. The ratio of lysosomal enzyme activity to digestive enzyme activity was greater than normal for ten different enzyme ratios. In a similar study of 25 patients with chronic pancreatitis, these enzyme ratios were similar to those associated with cancer in only three patients.

PPJ secretory flow rates in patients with pancreatic cancer are usually low[19, 37, 59] except in those with cancer involving the tail of the pancreas,[37] in which case they may be in the low range of normal; these findings agree with those obtained by the DST.[71, 72]

Other nonspecific markers of pancreatic disease in PPJ include alkaline phosphatase,[38, 39, 52] gamma-glutamyltransferase (GGT),[38, 39, 53] and glutamic oxaloacetic transaminase (GOT).[39] Elevated concentrations of these enzymes have been found with pancreatic cancer and with chronic pancreatitis. In one study there was considerable overlap between the elevated levels in malignant and benign disease.[38] In the author's experience,[39] unlike that of Carr-Locke and Davies,[38] many subjects with and without chronic pancreatitis have no detectable alkaline phosphatase in PPJ. This may be accounted for by differences in methodology. Dyck et al.[52] demonstrated that the alkaline phosphatase in PPJ is distinct from that of hepatic or bony origin. The levels of GGT and GOT in PPJ bear no relationship to serum GGT or GOT levels.[38, 39]

Lactoferrin in PPJ has been given considerable attention since the initial demonstration of this nondigestive iron-containing protein in duodenal juice by Colomb et al.[85] in 1973. Multigner et al.[58] demonstrated increased secretion of lactoferrin in the PPJ of almost all patients with chronic pancreatitis whether or not there was pancreatic calcification or pancreatic insufficiency. Hayakawa et al.[49] noted a gradual increase in PPJ lactoferrin content as chronic pancreatitis increased in severity. Elevated secretion of lactoferrin was also found to be associated with elevated amounts of albumin in PPJ.[58] However, only three patients with pancreatic cancer were studied and no attempt was made at differential diagnosis. The study of lactoferrin in PPJ by Fedail et al.[51] demonstrated similar findings and also showed that the concentration of lactoferrin in PPJ of patients with pancreatic cancer was in the range encountered in normal individuals. Tympner[45] reported elevated levels of lactoferrin in PPJ of patients with chronic pancreatitis, but levels in pancreatic cancer for comparison were not determined. In summary, the place of PPJ lactoferrin in the diagnosis of pancreatic disease is not yet established.

VISCOSITY OF PPJ

Tympner and Rösch[46] reported that the viscosity of secretin-stimulated PPJ of normal controls is similar to that of water, but that there was a marked increase in PPJ viscosity in patients with pancreatitis. This increased viscosity was still present after the PPJ had been centrifuged to remove all visible precipitated protein particles. These results were confirmed by Tympner[45] in a much larger number of subjects. The protein concentration in centrifuged PPJ of patients with chronic pancreatitis did not differ from that of normal controls, although the amount of dissolved and precipitated protein material taken together was much higher in patients with chronic pancreatitis. These studies confirmed similar findings in the duodenal juice of patients with chronic pancreatitis as described by Leonhardt and Reinhardt.[86] These studies suggest that factors other than dissolved protein in PPJ are responsible for the increased viscosity.

In patients with chronic pancreatitis, the endoscopist may note mucus plugs in the ampulla of patients with chronic pancreatitis, or thick mucus-like material in the syringe during an IDST. Occasionally it may be impossible to aspirate this thick mucoid material farther than the tip of the ERCP cannula. These observations suggest that mucus may be responsible for the increased viscosity. The studies of Wakabayashi and Takeda[87] support this hypothesis. They reported higher amounts of hexosamine, a mucosubstance, in the duodenal aspirate after CCK-secretin stimulation in patients with chronic pancreatitis than in normal subjects. The highest levels occurred in patients with non-calcifying pancreatitis with only mild to moderate disturbances in pancreatic function. The smallest elevations were found in patients with chronic calcific pancreatitis and severe exocrine dysfunction. Further study of PPJ-mucus may prove rewarding.

COMPARISON OF THE IDST AND ERCP IN DIAGNOSIS OF CHRONIC PANCREATITIS

There are several studies that compare ERCP to the Lundh test,[88, 89] secretin stimulation,[90] and secretin/CCK stimulation[91] in the diagnosis of pancreatitis. The selection of patients varies from series to series. In most investigations, only patients with severe chronic pancreatitis were studied by ERCP and a pancreatic secretion test, and in all patients a DST was performed rather than an IDST. There were also differences in the parameters measured as well as the number of parameters used in the various studies. In general, 80% to 100% of patients with severe chronic pancreatitis and ERP abnormalities will have an abnormal Lundh, secretin, or secretin/CCK test.[88, 91] In several studies,[88] 35% of patients with chronic pancreatitis and a normal ERP had one or more abnormal parameters of pancreatic secretion. In one small study,[90] 57% of patients with chronic pancreatitis had abnormal secretion.

The author,[39] using ERCP and the IDST, studied 87 patients with a history strongly suggestive of pancreatitis in whom serum amylase and lipase levels, plain radiographs of the abdomen, and abdominal ultrasonography were normal. Thirty patients had abnormal secretory volumes by IDST. Seven

had pancreatic hypersecretion with PSFR of 7 to 30 ml/min; the remaining 23 patients had PSFR of less than 2.5 ml/min. Low concentrations of bicarbonate ion were present in 37, low amylase levels in 25 of 82 patients tested, low lipase in 34 of 78 patients, and high GGT in 9 of 36 patients so tested. Forty patients had one or more secretory abnormalities indicative of chronic pancreatitis. Pancreatography demonstrated pancreatic duct abnormalities in 25 of 87. The IDST confirmed the diagnosis of chronic pancreatitis in 24 patients with normal pancreatograms. Based on these results, it appears that the IDST is more sensitive than pancreatography in the diagnosis of chronic pancreatitis.

Although there are no studies that compare retrograde pancreatography, ultrasonography and CT of the pancreas with the IDST, in the author's experience, some patients have only an abnormal IDST even in the presence of severe chronic pancreatitis. Ultrasound, CT, retrograde pancreatography, and the IDST should be used as complementary studies. These investigative techniques provide different information about the pancreas, and in a given patient with chronic pancreatitis only one may be abnormal. The IDST is easy to perform and can be used almost routinely after ERCP if the pancreatogram is normal in a patient with suspected chronic pancreatitis.

ENDOGENOUS STIMULATION TESTS OF PANCREATIC FUNCTION

Osnes et al.[31] stimulated pancreatic secretion by introducing dilute hydrochloric acid into the descending duodenum of a patient for 5 minutes through a separate cannula attached to the duodenoscope after the pancreatic duct had been cannulated with another cannula. There was a rapid rise in PPJ bicarbonate ion concentration to approximately 135 mEq/l and in volume flow to almost 5 ml/min.

Osnes[92] also stimulated PPJ production endogenously by introduction of human bile into the duodenum using the same technique as with hydrochloric acid. When bile with a high bile acid concentration was placed into the duodenum, there was an increase in PPJ volume and bicarbonate ion concentration in the three subjects studied.

Gregg and Chey[93] stimulated pancreatic secretion by placing 20 gm of cottonseed oil

(Neocholex, Fleet's Co.) at the inferior angle of the duodenum by means of the duodenoscope. PPJ was aspirated 10 to 20 minutes later as during a standard IDST. This time period corresponded to maximal release of CCK from the small intestinal mucosa. In this stimulation test, PSFR ranged from 0.6 to 1.0 ml/min in five normal subjects. Bicarbonate concentrations in PPJ stimulated by this method were 76 to 110 mEq/l in the five normal individuals and from 40 to 76 mEq/l in six patients with chronic pancreatitis. With this method of pancreatic stimulation, there was a 3- to 30-fold increase in PPJ amylase concentrations and a 4- to 16-fold increase in PPJ lipase concentrations over the values obtained during an IDST in the same subjects. The increases in the two enzymes are not always parallel, especially in patients with chronic pancreatitis.

Other methods for stimulating endogenous release of CCK include intraduodenal infusion of an essential amino acid[94] and infusion of an elemental diet,[95] both of which result in pancreatic secretion. With this approach it is not possible to measure pancreatic secretory rates, and bicarbonate ions in bile make interpretation of bicarbonate concentrations difficult during a DST. It is possible, however, that endogenous methods of pancreatic stimulation such as these might be used in conjunction with an IDST.

ANTIBIOTICS IN PPJ

Infection of the pancreatic duct with gram-negative organisms has been demonstrated in patients with chronic pancreatitis[30]; these organisms can be eradicated by systemically administered cephalothin. This study also suggested that beta-lactam antibiotics were secreted in PPJ. Subsequent work has confirmed the secretion of cephalothin in PPJ after secretin stimulation. Antibiotic concentrations up to 1.8 μg/ml in PPJ are found in normal persons and in patients with pancreatitis.[65] Cephalothin secretion occurs only during the first 15 minutes after termination of the antibiotic infusion. In the same study, cefoxitin was not detected in PPJ, but the assay was insensitive below 4 μg/ml.

Roberts and Williams[64] studied the secretion of ampicillin in PPJ after intramuscular administration and found a concentration of less than 1.0 μg/ml in one subject and no detectable antibiotic level in the other six subjects in this report.

Although appropriate antibiotic therapy will probably eradicate pancreatic duct infection at least temporarily, there is no definitive information on antibiotic levels in the pancreatic parenchyma, and no evidence that antibiotic therapy alters the course of chronic pancreatic disease.

FUTURE OF THE IDST

The administration through the duodenoscope of endogenous substances (e.g., hydrochloric acid, elemental diet, lipid meal) that stimulate pancreatic secretion duplicates most closely the physiologic function of the pancreas. However, this approach has limitations. The stimulant may not stress the pancreas enough to reveal minor degrees of secretory impairment. There is a risk of introducing the stimulating substance into the pancreatic duct. Since intraductal introduction of even a minute amount of hydrochloric acid would be hazardous, this is a major deterrent to the use of this stimulant of pancreatic secretion. The safety of other substances such as Neocholex or an elemental diet is unknown. Use of a large stimulant volume, as is the case with the elemental diet, or use of an opaque emulsion (Neocholex, for example) may interfere with visualization and cannulation of the pancreatic duct. Retrograde flow of a small but unknown amount of the stimulant into the stomach may also alter the outcome of the test.

The use of exogenous stimulants such as intravenous CCK or secretin or a combination of these ensures that a precise amount of hormone is administered, although this approach is not as physiologic as those that utilize endogenous stimulants. Precise secretin dosage is problematic if administered as a constant infusion, since plastic surfaces absorb this hormone. Ideally it should be dissolved in dilute serum albumin to obviate this problem. The exogenous methods of stimulation also make it possible to stimulate the pancreas to varying degrees including maximal secretory capacity, although this only occurs with pharmacologic amounts of the hormones. Despite the limitations of both exogenous and endogenous methods, each has advantages for particular purposes.

The IDST has many distinct advantages over the DST but also some risk that does not occur with the DST. Any manipulation of the pancreatic sphincter or cannulation of the pancreatic duct, with or without injection of contrast material, can produce pancreatitis, and the IDST is no exception. In the author's experience, acute pancreatitis developed in four of 402 patients who underwent IDST. In two of the four patients this occurred when the IDST was done in conjunction with ERCP. In the other two it occurred after IDST alone, and in one of these patients acute pancreatitis occurred after a seemingly nontraumatic Neocholex IDST. All four patients had underlying chronic pancreatitis and two of the four had very low PSFR. Possible explanations for this complication include the presence of active proteolytic enzymes in the pancreatic duct, duct mucosa damage from the ERCP cannula, transport of an exogenous stimulant into the pancreatic duct, or any combination of these.

As with any diagnostic study, the information to be gained along with its applicability to patient management must be weighed against the risks of the procedure. Although many of the applications of the IDST are currently investigational, this test provides certain refinements in endoscopic diagnosis, particularly with respect to recognition of mild and early chronic pancreatitis when the pancreatic ducts appear to be normal radiographically. The IDST provides a unique method for studying pancreatic physiology that circumvents many of the limitations of the DST. The study of pancreatic function by means of this direct access to PPJ is limited only by considerations of safety for each method, laboratory capabilities for various biochemical determinations, and the imagination of endoscopists.

References

1. Chiray M, Jeandel A, Salmon A. L'exploration clinique du pancréas et l'injection intraveineuse de secretine purifée. Presse Med 1930; 38:977–82.
2. Lagerlof HO. Pancreatic function and pancreatic disease studies by means of secretin. Acta Med Scandinav (Suppl) 1942; 128:1–289.
3. Dreiling DA, Janowitz HD. The measurement of pancreatic secretory function. In: deReuck AVS, Cameron MP, eds. Ciba Foundation Symposium on the Exocrine Pancreas: Normal and abnormal functions. Boston: Little, Brown, and Co., 1962; 225–58.
4. Burton P, Evans DG, Harper AA, et al. A test of pancreatic function in man based on the analysis of duodenal contents after administration of secretin pancreozymin. Gut 1960; 1:111–24.
5. Sun DCH. Normal values for pancreozymin-secretin test. Gastroenterology 1963; 44:602–6.
6. Banwell JG, Northam BE, Cooke WT. Secretory responses of the human pancreas to continuous intravenous infusion of secretin. Gut 1967; 8:50–7.
7. Hartley RC, Gambill EE, Summerskill WH. Pancreatic volume and bicarbonate output with augmented doses of secretin. Gastroenterology 1965; 48:312–7.
8. Wormsley KG. Response to secretin in man. Gastroenterology 1968; 54:197–209.
9. Petersen H. The duodenal aspirate following secretin stimulation. A variance study in man. Scand J Gastroenterol 1969; 4:407–12.
10. Tympner F, Domschke S, Domschke W, et al. Reproducibility of the response to secretin and secretin plus pancreozymin in man. Scand J Gastroenterol 1974; 9:377–81.
11. Dreiling DA, Messer J. The secretin story: a saga in clinical medicine and gastrointestinal physiology. Am J Gastroenterol 1978; 70:455–79.
12. Rolny P. Diagnosis of pancreatic disease with special reference to the secretin-CCK test. Scand J Gastroenterol (Suppl 60) 1980; 15:1–33.
13. Oliver J. Progress report: The Lundh test. Gut 1973; 14:582–91.
14. Lankisch PG, Schreiber A, Otto J. Pancreolauryl test. Evaluation of a tubeless pancreatic function test in comparison with other indirect and direct tests for exocrine pancreatic function. Dig Dis Sci 1983; 28:490–3.
15. Lankisch PG. Progress report: Exocrine pancreatic function tests. Gut 1982; 23:777–98.
16. Kozu T. Duodenoscopic collection of intraductal pure pancreatic juice and its application to the cytodiagnosis. In: Endoscopy of the small intestine with retrograde pancreatocholangiography. International workshop at Erlangen. Stuttgart: Thieme, 1972.
17. Gregg JA, Mann BF, Middleton M. The cytology of secretin stimulated pure pancreatic juice in normals, patients with pancreatitis and pancreatic cancer obtained during endoscopic cannulation of the pancreatic duct. Presented at the annual meeting of the American Cytology Society, New Orleans, LA, November 2, 1972.
18. Sharma MM, Gregg JA, McCabe RP, et al. Carcinoembryonic antigen (CEA)-like activity in pancreatic juice of patients with pancreatic carcinoma and pancreatitis. (Abstr) Gastroenterology 1974; 66:A-122/776.
19. Sharma MM, Gregg JA, Lowenstein MS, et al. Carcinoembryonic antigen (CEA) activity in pancreatic juice of patients with pancreatic carcinoma and pancreatitis. Cancer 1976; 38:2457–61.
20. Kawanishi H, Sell JE, Pollard HM. Combined endoscopic pancreatic fluid collection and retrograde pancreatography in the diagnosis of pancreatic cancer and chronic pancreatitis. Gastrointest Endosc 1975; 22:82–5.
21. Hatfield AR, Smithies A, Wilkins R, et al. Assessment of endoscopic retrograde cholangiopancreatography (ERCP) and pure pancreatic juice cytology in patients with pancreatic disease. Gut 1976; 17:14–21.
22. Carr-Locke DL. Pancreatic juice analysis, carcinoembryonic antigen (CEA) and endoscopic retrograde cholangiopancreatography (ERCP) in the diagnosis of pancreatic disease. (Abstr) Gut 1977; 18: A980–1.
23. Gregg JA, Sipos T, Sharma MM, et al. Enzymatic analysis of pure pancreatic juice (PPJ) obtained during the endoscopic cannulation of the main pancreatic duct (ECMPD). (Abstr) Gastroenterology 1975; 68:A-47/904.

24. Elias E, Southcott J, Marten A, et al. The trypsin inhibitory activity of pure pancreatic juice. (Abstr) Gut 1976; 17:A385.

25. Gregg JA, Sharma MM. The effect of secretin on pancreatic juice flow rates during endoscopic cannulation of the main pancreatic duct. (Abstr) Gastroenterology 1975; 68:A-48/905.

26. Fontana G, Costa DL, Tessari R, et al. Effect of glucagon on pure human exocrine pancreatic secretion. Am J Gastroenterol 1975; 63:490–4.

27. Cotton PB, Heap TR. The analysis of pancreatic juice. Br J Hosp Med 1975; 14:658–66.

28. Denyer ME, Cotton PB, Kyne M, et al. Paired pancreatic function studies using pure pancreatic juice and duodenal juice. (Abstr) Gut 1977; 18:A980.

29. Gregg JA. Pancreas divisum: its association with pancreatitis. Am J Surg 1977; 134:539–43.

30. Gregg JA. Detection of bacterial infection of the pancreatic ducts in patients with pancreatitis and pancreatic cancer during endoscopic cannulation of the main pancreatic duct. Gastroenterology 1977; 73:1005–7.

31. Osnes M, Hanssen LE, Myren J. An endoscopic method for the study of the exocrine pancreatic secretion in man. Endoscopy 1976; 8:124–6.

32. Domschke S, Domschke W, Rösch W, et al. Inhibition by somatostatin of secretin-stimulated pancreatic secretion in man: a study with pure pancreatic juice. Scand J Gastroenterol 1977; 12:59–63.

33. Cremer M, Robberecht P, Toussaint J, et al. La secretion pancreatique pure chez l'homme. Endosc Dig 1976; 1:117–27.

34. Domschke S, Domschke W, Rösch W, et al. Bicarbonate and cyclic AMP content of pure human pancreatic juice in response to graded doses of synthetic secretin. Gastroenterology 1976; 70:533–6.

35. Denyer ME, Cotton PB. Pure pancreatic juice studies in normal subjects and patients with chronic pancreatitis. Gut 1979; 20:89–97.

36. Gregg JA, Sharma MM. Pancreatic hypersecretion in liver disease. Am J Dig Dis 1978; 23:9–11.

37. Gregg JA, Sharma MM. Endoscopic measurement of pancreatic juice, secretory flow rates, and pancreatic secretory pressures after secretin administration in human controls and in patients with acute relapsing pancreatitis, chronic pancreatitis, and pancreatic cancer. Am J Surg 1978; 136:569–74.

38. Carr-Locke DL, Davies TJ. Pancreatic juice gamma-glutamyltransferase, alanine transaminase, and alkaline phosphatase in pancreatic disease. Dig Dis Sci 1980; 25:374–8.

39. Gregg JA. Intraductal secretin test of pancreatic function in suspected pancreatitis. (Abstr) Gastroenterology 1981; 80:1163.

40. Scheele G, Bartelt D, Bieger W. Characterization of human exocrine pancreatic proteins by two-dimensional isoelectric focusing/sodium dodecyl sulfate gel electrophoresis. Gastroenterology 1981; 80:461–73.

41. Schneider MU, Rösch W, Domschke S, Domschke W. Pancreatic juice protein associated with chronic pancreatitis and adenocarcinoma of the pancreas. Scand J Gastroenterol 1984; 19:139–44.

42. Dagorn JC, Sahel J, Sarles H. Nonparallel secretion of enzymes in human duodenal juice and pure pancreatic juice collected by endoscopic retrograde catheterization of the papilla. Gastroenterology 1977; 73:42–5.

43. Schmiegel WH, Becker WM, Arndt R, et al. Pancreatic oncofetal antigen in pancreatic juices. Partial chemical characterization and diagnostic application of a pancreatic cancer-associated antigen. Scand J Gastroenterol 1981; 16:1033–9.

44. Scheele GA. Human pancreatic cancer: analysis of proteins contained in pancreatic juice by two-dimensional isoelectric focusing/sodium dodecyl sulfate gel electrophoresis. Cancer 1981; 47(6 suppl):1513–5.

45. Tympner F. Selectively aspirated pure pancreatic secretion. Viscosity, trypsin activity, protein concentration and lactoferrin content of pancreatic juice in chronic pancreatitis. Hepatogastroenterology 1981; 28:169–72.

46. Tympner F, Rösch W. Viskosität des reinen Pankreassekretes bei chronischer Pankreatitis. Klin Wochenschr 1978; 56:421–2.

47. Carr-Locke DL, Track NS. Human pancreatic polypeptide in pancreatic juice. Lancet 1979; 1:151–2.

48. Gregg JA. The intraductal secretin test; an adjunct to ERCP. Gastrointest Endosc 1982; 28:199–203.

49. Hayakawa T, Harada H, Noda A, et al. Lactoferrin in pure pancreatic juice in chronic pancreatitis. Am J Gastroenterol 1983; 78:222–4.

50. Geokas MC, Rinderknecht H. Free proteolytic enzymes in pancreatic juice of patients with acute pancreatitis. Am J Dig Dis 1974; 19:591–8.

51. Fedail SS, Salmon PR, Harvey RF, et al. Radioimmunoassay of lactoferrin in pancreatic juice as a test for pancreatic diseases. Lancet 1978; 1:181–3.

52. Dyck WP, Spiekerman AM, Ratliff CR. Pancreatic secretory isoenzyme of alkaline phosphatase (40312). Proc Soc Exp Biol Med 1978; 159:192–4.

53. Renner IG, Juttner HU. A new nonspecific marker of early pancreatic disease. (Abstr) Gastroenterology 1976; 70:A-71/929.

54. Rinderknecht H, Renner IG, Douglas AP, et al. Profiles of pure pancreatic secretions obtained by direct pancreatic duct cannulation in normal healthy human subjects. Gastroenterology 1978; 75:1083–9.

55. Renner IG, Rinderknecht H, Douglas AP. Profiles of pure pancreatic secretions in patients with acute pancreatitis: the possible role of proteolytic enzymes in pathogenesis. Gastroenterology 1978; 75:1090–8.

56. Rinderknecht H, Renner IG, Koyama HH. Lysosomal enzymes in pure pancreatic juice from normal healthy volunteers and chronic alcoholics. Dig Dis Sci 1979; 24:180–6.

57. Renner IG, Rinderknecht H, Valenzuela JE, et al. Studies of pure pancreatic secretions in chronic alcoholic subjects without pancreatic insufficiency. Scand J Gastroenterol 1980; 15:241–4.

58. Multigner L, Figarella C, Sahel J, et al. Lactoferrin and albumin in human pancreatic juice. A valuable test for diagnosis of pancreatic diseases. Dig Dis Sci 1980; 25:173–8.

59. Rinderknecht H, Renner IG, Stace NH. Abnormalities in pancreatic secretory profiles of patients with cancer of the pancreas. Dig Dis Sci 1983; 28:103–10.

60. Rinderknecht H, Renner IG, Abramson SB, et al. Mesotrypsin: a new inhibitor-resistant protease from a zymogen in human pancreatic tissue and fluid. Gastroenterology 1984; 86:681–92.

61. Escourrou J, Frexinos J, Ribet A. Biochemical studies of pancreatic juice collected by duodenal aspiration and endoscopic cannulation of the main pancreatic duct. Am J Dig Dis 1978; 23:173–7.

62. Robberecht P, Cremer M, Vandermeers A, et al.

Pancreatic secretion of total protein and of three hydrolases collected in healthy subjects via duodenoscopic cannulation. Effects of secretin, pancreozymin, and caerulcin. Gastroenterology 1975; 69:374–9.

63. Osnes M, Hanssen LE, Larsen S. The unstimulated pancreatic secretion obtained by endoscopic cannulation and the plasma secretin levels in man. Scand J Gastroenterol 1979; 14:503–12.

64. Roberts EA, Williams RJ. Ampicillin concentrations in pancreatic fluid bile obtained at endoscopic retrograde cholangiopancreatography (ERCP). Scand J Gastroenterol 1979; 14:669–72.

65. Gregg JA, Maher L, DeGirolami PC, et al. Secretion of B-lactam antibiotics in pure human pancreatic juice. Am J Surg 1985; 150:333–5.

66. Dreiling DA, Janowitz HD. Inhibitory effect of new anticholinergics on the basal and secretin-stimulated secretion in patients with and without pancreatic disease. Therapeutic and theoretic implications. Am J Dig Dis 1960; 5:639–54.

67. Saunders JHB, Masoero G, Wormsley KG. Effect of diazepam and hyoscine butylbromide on response to secretin and cholecystokinin-pancreozymin in man. Gut 1976; 17:351–3.

68. Miyata M, Rayford PL, Thompson JC. Loss of secretin from plastic infusion systems. (Letter to the editor) N Engl J Med 1979; 300:95.

69. Osnes M. Studies on recovery and variation of pancreatic juice obtained by endoscopic cannulation of the main pancreatic duct in man. Scand J Gastroenterol 1981; 16:39–44.

70. Dreiling DA, Bordalo O. Secretory patterns in minimal pancreatic pathologies. Am J Gastroenterol 1973; 60:60–9.

71. Dreiling DA. Secretion analysis: secretin testing in pancreatic cancer. J Surg Oncol 1975; 7:101–5.

72. Dimagno EP, Malagelada JR, Moertel CG, et al. Prospective evaluation of immunoreactive carcinoembryonic antigen, enzyme, and bicarbonate in patients suspected of having pancreatic cancer. Gastroenterology 1977; 73:457–61.

73. Van Goidsenhoven GE, Henke WJ, Vacca JB, et al. Pancreatic function in cirrhosis of the liver. Am J Dig Dis 1963; 8:160–73.

74. Gross JB, Comfort MW, Wollaeger EE, et al. External pancreatic function in primary parenchymatous hepatic disease as measured by analysis of duodenal contents before and after stimulation with secretin. Gastroenterology 1950; 16:151–61.

75. Dreiling DA, Greenstein AJ, Bordalo O. The hypersecretory states of the pancreas: implications in the pathophysiology of pancreatic inflammation and the pathogenesis of peptic ulcer diathesis. Am J Gastroenterol 1982; 77:817–20.

76. Neves MM, Borges DR, Vilela MP. Exocrine pancreatic hypersecretion in Brazilian alcoholics. Am J Gastroenterol 1983; 78:513–6.

77. Dyck WP. Pancreatic hypersecretion in the Zollinger-Ellison syndrome. Gastroenterology 1971; 60: 90–5.

78. Renner IG, Rinderknecht H, Wisner JR. Pancreatic secretion after secretin and cholecystokinin stimu-lation in chronic alcoholics with and without cirrhosis. Dig Dis Sci 1983; 1089–93.

79. Jorpes JF, Mutt V, Jonson G, et al. The effect of secretin on bile flow. Gastroenterology 1963; 45:786–8.

80. Grossman MI, Janowitz HD, Ralston H, et al. The effect of secretin on bile formation in man. Gastroenterology 1949; 12:133–8.

81. Lee SP, Lai KS. Exocrine pancreatic function in hepatic cirrhosis. Am J Gastroenterol 1976; 65: 244–8.

82. Justus PG, Wheeldon SH, Kolts ME. Secretin half-life in cirrhotics with high secretory volumes to a secretin test. Proc Soc Exp Biol Med 1979; 162: 351–3.

83. Hancke S, Holm HH, Koch F. Ultrasonically guided percutaneous fine needle biopsy of the pancreas. Surg Gynecol Obstet 1975; 140:361–4.

84. Clouse ME, Gregg JA, McDonald DG, et al. Percutaneous fine needle aspiration biopsy of pancreatic carcinoma. Gastrointest Radiol 1977; 2:67–9.

85. Colomb E, Estevenson JP, Clemente F, et al. Comparison between the pancreatic juice of normals and subjects with chronic calcific pancreatitis. Biol Gastroenterol 1973; 6:83–4.

86. Leonhardt H, Reinhardt I. Viscosity of duodenal juice examined in patients with excretory pancreas insufficiency by the pancreocymin secretin test compared to a control group and patients with cholelithiasis. Acta Hepatogastroenterol 1978; 25:45–8.

87. Wakabayashi A, Takeda Y. The behavior of mucopolysaccharide in the pancreatic juice in chronic pancreatitis. Am J Dig Dis 1976; 21:607–12.

88. Seligson U, Cho JW, Ihre T, et al. Evaluation of the diagnosis pancreatitis. Scand J Gastroenterol 1982; 17:905–11.

89. Elsborg L, Bruusgaard A, Strandgaard L, et al. Endoscopic retrograde pancreatography and the exocrine pancreatic function in chronic alcoholism. Scand J Gastroenterol 1981; 16:941–4.

90. Braganza JM, Hunt LP, Warwick F. Relationship between pancreatic exocrine function and ductal morphology in chronic pancreatitis. Gastroenterology 1982; 82:1341–7.

91. Dobrilla G, Fratton A, Valenti M, Vantini I, et al. Endoscopic retrograde pancreatography and secretin-pancreozymin test in diagnosis of chronic pancreatitis: a comparative evaluation. Endoscopy 1976; 8:118–23.

92. Osnes M. Does human bile stimulate the exocrine pancreas? Scand J Gastroenterol 1981; 16:45–7.

93. Gregg JA, Chey WY. The effects of intraduodenal lipid on the secretion of pure pancreatic juice. Correlation with plasma immunoreactive cholecystokinin. (submitted for publication)

94. Owyang C, Vinik AI, Kothary P, et al. Cholecystokinin is not the major intestinal stimulus of pancreatic enzyme secretion. (Abstr) Gastroenterology 1983; 84:1268.

95. Watanabe S, Shiratori K, Tackeuchi T, et al. Release of cholecystokinin (CCK) and exocrine pancreatic secretion in response to an elementary diet in humans. (Abstr) Gastroenterology 1983; 84:1346.

Chapter 38

PANCREATIC TRAUMA, ASCITES, FISTULA, AND PSEUDOCYST

STEPHEN E. SILVIS, M.D.

A common theme in this chapter is the extravasation of pancreatic juice into extrapancreatic areas. Pancreatic fluid outside the acinar tissue, ductules, or major pancreatic ducts produces acute inflammation. This can occur as a result of direct pancreatic injury, blunt trauma to the abdomen, or acute pancreatitis from any cause. With abdominal trauma, fracture of the pancreas and disruption of the main pancreatic duct may occur and result in either leakage of pancreatic juice into the retroperitoneal space with formation of a large fluid collection, or into the peritoneal cavity to produce pancreatic ascites. The form that this fluid takes will depend on the extent of ductal injury and the tissue with which the fluid comes in contact.

PANCREATIC TRAUMA

The pancreas is a fragile organ that contains concentrated, highly destructive enzymes. Despite this, serious pancreatic trauma is relatively uncommon. In man the organ is entirely retroperitoneal. The head of the pancreas nestles in the duodenal loop and is posterior to the spine. In patients of normal weight it is cushioned by retroperitoneal fat. Although the tail of the pancreas varies markedly in its anatomic position, it almost invariably lies superior to the left kidney and posterior to the stomach within the retroperitoneal space (Figs. 38–1 and 38–2). Lateral views of retrograde pancreatograms demonstrate that the pancreatic duct curves anteriorly over the spine in the region of the body of the pancreas so that the head and tail sections are posterior to the vertebral bodies. In the anterior-posterior x-ray projection, these relationships are not apparent, although the position of the body and tail to the right and left of the spine will be demonstrated. Exceptions to this normal anatomic position occur with pancreatic anomalies such as annular pancreas, in which the pancreas may encircle the duodenum (Fig. 38–3). In this location, the pancreas is more vulnerable to trauma.

There are two major forms of pancreatic trauma. Direct injury, such as occurs with bullet or stab wounds or during surgery, may produce a contusion of the gland or disruption of a duct, with enzymes leaking into the peripancreatic tissue. External compression, however, is the more common cause of trauma to the pancreas. The region of the body of the pancreas that lies over the vertebrae is most subject to blunt or external compressive trauma. Steering wheel compression of the abdomen during an auto accident or a blow to the abdomen in a fight are common causes of this type of injury. In one report, 21% of pancreatic cysts resulted from traffic accidents.[1] A number of cases have been reported in which the patients appeared to have sustained relatively minor abdominal trauma that resulted in major pancreatic injury.[1, 2] Compression injury to the pancreas may occur without damage to any other abdominal organs or vital structures.

The onset and severity of symptoms following external compression injury to the pancreas are extremely variable. The result may be catastrophic with disruption of the main pancreatic duct and outpouring of pancreatic enzymes into the abdomen. This degree of

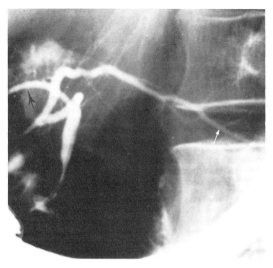

FIGURE 38–1. Normal pancreatogram made in lateral position. Filling of main pancreatic duct branches is adequate. Position of tail of pancreas posterior to vertebral bodies is demonstrated (*small arrow*); Santorini branch is prominent (*large arrow*).

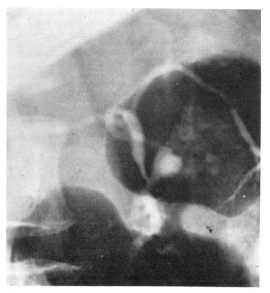

FIGURE 38–3. Pancreatogram demonstrates annular pancreas. Gland encircles duodenum and is more vulnerable to blunt trauma. Although patients with this anomaly may have symptoms of duodenal obstruction, this particular pancreatogram was an incidental finding in a patient with biliary tract disease.

trauma plus associated injury to other organs usually requires laparotomy. After severe trauma, as can occur in auto accidents, for example, pancreatic trauma is frequently associated with other intra-abdominal injuries such as splenic rupture and lacerations of the liver or kidney. In such cases, injury to the

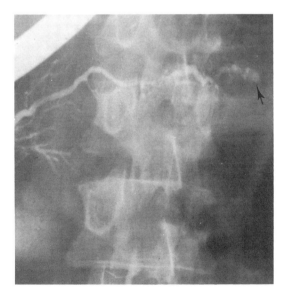

FIGURE 38–2. Posterior/anterior x-ray of pancreatic duct. Bowing of pancreas over spine is not apparent. There are changes of a chronic pancreatitis plus small pseudocyst (*arrow*) in tail of pancreas. Patient sustained blunt abdominal trauma with injury to main pancreatic duct where it crosses the spine.

pancreas is frequently less an immediate threat to life than the trauma to other organs. Surgical management of pancreatic trauma depends on the location and extent of injury. At a minimum, it is necessary to insure adequate drainage from the area of the pancreas. Resection of the portion of the pancreas distal to a point of disruption of the main duct may be indicated.[3] When extensive damage to several organs is found at laparotomy, pancreatic injury may also be overlooked or underestimated.

At the opposite end of the clinical spectrum of pancreatic injury is mild, self-limiting pancreatitis with upper abdominal pain and elevated amylase levels, all of which may subside within a few days. Generally, this clinical picture occurs in patients with isolated pancreatic injury, although it may also appear postoperatively after surgical repair of other extensive injuries. A patient may have relatively mild upper abdominal pain that either decreases or subsides completely within a few days after the injury, only to be followed days or even weeks later by the appearance of a tender abdominal mass that has resulted from the accumulation of extravasated pancreatic secretion and digestion of peripancreatic tissue. The evolution of this type of mass is variable. It may be absorbed spontaneously with time, or it may acquire a thick-walled capsule which, with liquefaction of its contents, will become a pancreatic pseudocyst.

The initial treatment of pancreatic injury with the more protracted clinical picture is usually conservative, although this must include a search for trauma to other organs and surgical management of these associated injuries when necessary. Total parenteral nutrition has been reported to be beneficial[4, 5]; however, results of a study in animals suggest that large intravenous fluid volumes produce similar results.[6]

The indications for endoscopic retrograde cholangiopancreatography (ERCP) in pancreatic trauma are limited, but ERCP is reported to be of value in certain patients.[7] Usually these patients have a more protracted course than those who have more severe pancreatic injury. Some may have had surgical exploration and even pseudocyst drainage. They may have recurrent or persistent abdominal pain, persistent high fluid volumes with high concentrations of amylase by surgical drainage catheters, or pancreatic ascites with or without evidence of a pseudocyst. These findings may indicate more extensive pancreatic injury than was estimated at operation or on initial medical evaluation. In such circumstances, ERCP can establish either disruption or continuity of the main pancreatic duct (Fig. 38–4).

If a pancreatic mass develops, its size and characteristics should be documented by ultrasonography or computed tomography (CT). There are certain limitations and complications inherent to ERCP when used in the investigation of pancreatic pseudocysts (vide infra). Therapy for a pseudocyst may be surgical; a number of reports demonstrate that time is required for the wall of a pseudocyst to become fibrotic and therefore satisfactory for suturing to the bowel.[8–11] If the patient is stable and the size of the mass is not increasing, it is advisable to wait 4 to 6 weeks before undertaking internal cyst drainage surgically.

PANCREATIC ASCITES

Pancreatic ascites should be suspected in patients with marked ascites of unknown etiology. These patients often have a history of pancreatic disease or abdominal trauma, although in some patients, symptomatic ascites develops with no history of other pancreatic disease. Pancreatic ascites can easily be overlooked in the alcoholic patient who, not infrequently, already has ascites as a result of alcoholic liver disease. Its presence is readily confirmed by paracentesis with measurement of amylase content in the ascitic fluid; the amylase level is usually extremely high.

In essence, pancreatic ascites represents a fistula from the pancreas to the peritoneal

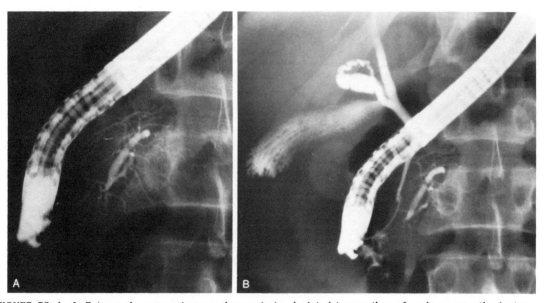

FIGURE 38–4. A, Retrograde pancreatogram demonstrates isolated transection of main pancreatic duct as a result of compression injury by steering wheel. B, Integrity of adjacent bile duct and biliary system is confirmed by retrograde cholangiography. (Courtesy of M. V. Sivak, Jr., M.D.)

cavity. The main concerns are therefore disruption of a major pancreatic duct or leakage of pancreatic fluid via a pancreatic pseudocyst. Approximately one third of patients with pancreatic ascites respond to conservative therapy.

The value of ERCP has been well documented in management of pancreatic ascites.[12–22] ERCP should be performed only when surgical intervention is contemplated, since there is no advantage to precise definition of the point of leakage from the pancreatic duct until this time. Furthermore, the ascitic fluid may become infected by injection of contrast material into the pancreatic duct or a pseudocyst.

Surgery for pancreatic ascites consists of drainage or excision of the pseudocyst or closure of the pancreatic fistula with a Roux-Y jejunal limb over the point of the pancreatic duct disruption. Smith et al.[20] described eight cases and reviewed previous reports of 62 patients. They recommended internal drainage via a Roux-Y jejunostomy as the surgical treatment of choice. External drainage may be indicated as a temporary initial procedure in some poor-risk patients. If the site of leakage of pancreatic juice is not precisely known preoperatively, it will also not be identified at surgery in approximately 30% of patients undergoing operation.[23, 24] Therefore, accurate preoperative identification of the site of duct disruption by ERCP provides a marked advantage to the operating surgeon.

Sankaran et al.[13] reported ERCP findings in six patients with pancreatic ascites. Single or multiple pseudocysts that filled with contrast were demonstrated in five patients and presumed to be the cause of the ascites. Leakage of contrast agent into the ascitic fluid was observed in only one of these patients, probably because of rapid dilution of the contrast by the large volumes of ascitic fluid. One patient had stenosis of the pancreatic duct; she responded to the distal pancreatic resection. The other patients were managed successfully by pseudocyst drainage. Davis and Graham,[14] and Rawlings et al.[15] reported a total of four cases; two patients had ductal narrowing and one had an intraductal calculus at the site of extravasation of contrast material into pseudocysts. Although pancreatic ascites is an uncommon condition, prompt diagnosis will lead to effective therapy.

PANCREATIC FISTULA

Fistulas between the pancreas and other intra-abdominal organs are described; the latter include the duodenum, spleen, and various vascular structures. Fistulas into the pleural spaces, the mediastinum, and the subphrenic cavity may occur (Figs. 38–5, 38–6, and 38–7). Percutaneous pancreatic fistulas also occur, either spontaneously or as a postoperative complication of external pancreatic drainage. It is frequently difficult to determine whether a fistula tract represents primary fistulization or is a result of rupture of a previously formed pancreatic pseudocyst. The diagnosis of pancreatic fistula is suggested by a fluid collection with a high amylase content in any actual or potential body space. Although such collections may be suspected clinically and are usually recognized by imaging techniques such as CT or ultrasonography, ERCP is frequently indicated to demonstrate the source and extent of the fistula.[25–38] Precise definition of the fistula and any associated pancreatic pathology can be invaluable at the time of surgery.

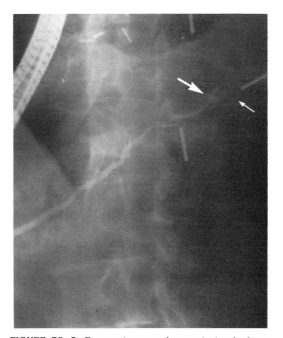

FIGURE 38–5. Pancreatogram demonstrates leakage of contrast from main pancreatic duct in tail of pancreas into cavity (*large arrow*) and then into cutaneous drainage tube (*small arrow*). There is contrast material within acinar tissue in head and body. This occurred inadvertently because attention was directed fluoroscopically to region of tail. After ERCP, patient underwent resection of fistula tract and tail of pancreas.

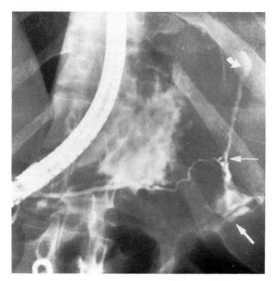

FIGURE 38–6. Pancreatogram demonstrates pancreatic fistula (*narrow arrow*) that developed as a result of severe episode of acute pancreatitis. Leakage of contrast material occurs toward surgical drain (*wide arrow*) at lower right of photograph and also to left subphrenic collection (*curved arrow*). (Courtesy of M. V. Sivak, Jr., M.D.)

Fistulization may be much more extensive and complicated than suspected, and complete assessment, especially in anticipation of surgery, may require a combination of imaging techniques.

A marked decrease in the incidence of pancreatic cutaneous fistulas is due to greater utilization of internal drainage of pancreatic pseudocysts. External drainage may be unnecessary with the advent of percutaneous needle drainage of acute pseudocysts.

The initial therapy for pancreatic fistula is conservative and supportive, since spontaneous closure may occur during a period of observation. For example, an unusual spontaneous closure of a pancreatico-pleural fistula has been documented.[4, 11] Greenwald et al.[38] reported successful treatment with radiation therapy (500 rads) to the pancreas in high surgical risk patients. Radiation is known to reduce transiently pancreatic secretion in animals and man[39–41]; this is the proposed mechanism for its influence on pancreatic fistulas and pancreatic ascites. Fistulas between a pseudocyst and the stomach or duodenum may be self-draining and may require no further therapy.[42, 43] Fistula tracts into other locations generally necessitate resection of the tract with drainage of the pseudocyst or pancreatic fistula tract with a jejunostomy.[25, 42, 43] If spontaneous closure does not occur after a few weeks of observation and conservative therapy, then surgical resection of the fistula (with or without pancreatic resection and drainage into the intestinal lumen) is indicated.

PSEUDOCYST OF THE PANCREAS

Pseudocyst is one of the complications of idiopathic acute pancreatitis or acute pancreatitis from any cause (e.g., trauma, gallstones, alcohol). It is formed by pancreatic juice that enters the retroperitoneal space as a result of necrosis or rupture of one or more of the pancreatic ducts. Ongoing pancreatic secretion extends and enlarges this space until resistance of the thickening cyst wall

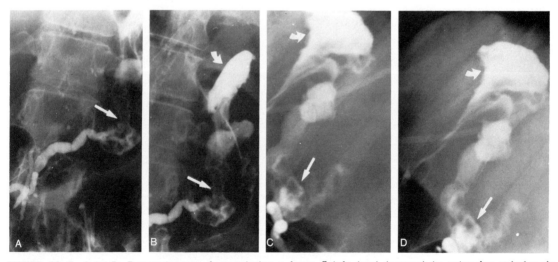

FIGURE 38–7. A to D, Pancreatogram demonstrates a large fistula tract (*arrows*) to extensive subphrenic collection (*curved arrow*). C and D are lateral views. (Courtesy of M. V. Sivak, Jr., M.D.)

and the surrounding tissue balances the resistance to pancreatic secretion by the sphincter of Oddi. Therefore, a stabilized pseudocyst occupies a part of the peripancreatic space. It may be full of old blood, necrotic tissue, or pancreatic juice. It is frequently in communication with the major pancreatic ducts.[44-47] The exact frequency of pseudocyst formation following pancreatitis is not established, but is probably about 1% to 2%. The frequency of pseudocyst formation appears to be increasing, but this may be artifactual because the sophistication of relevant diagnostic tests is also improving.[48-52]

A palpable abdominal mass in a patient who has had pancreatitis should engender a suspicion of pancreatic pseudocyst. This finding, however, is highly nonspecific. For example, Czaja et al.[53] showed that abdominal masses developed in 19 of 78 patients with acute alcohol-induced pancreatitis. The mass persisted longer than 3 weeks in 11 of these patients, but surgical drainage for a pancreatic pseudocyst was required in only 3 cases.

The presence of a mass in the region of the pancreas on either plain x-rays of the abdomen or an upper gastrointestinal barium study has the same lack of specificity as a palpable mass. These studies demonstrate only large pseudocysts that compress the abdominal viscera and they do not differentiate between solid and cystic masses.[49]

Prolonged elevation of the serum or urine amylase may direct attention to the possibility of a pseudocyst. Ebbesen and Schonebeck[54] demonstrated that 33 of 79 patients with prolonged elevated amylase levels had pancreatic pseudocysts. Usually the serum amylase returns to normal within 3 to 5 days after an attack of acute pancreatitis, although elevated levels may occasionally persist for 6 to 7 days.[55-58] In a series of 295 cases of acute pancreatitis reported by Wenckert,[58] 30 patients had persistent elevated amylase levels on the fourth day, but only 2 on the sixth day. These authors defined prolonged elevation of the amylase as persisting for longer than 1 week. Although this is a reasonable indication for the development of pseudocyst, more than 50% of the patients with this finding do not develop pancreatic pseudocysts. In contrast, Vajcner and Nicoloff[59] found that 5 of 25 patients with confirmed chronic pancreatic pseudocysts did not at any time show elevation of the urine amylase levels. In addition, they demonstrated that it is common for the amylase values to fluctuate

to a marked degree. In one of their patients, 12 urinary amylases were measured during the preoperative period, of which 8 were normal and 1 was 1400 units per hour. Prolonged elevated amylase levels, therefore, are suggestive of pseudocysts, although this abnormality is highly nonspecific. Lipase, isoamylase, and amylase clearance measurements yield similar information but are probably somewhat more specific tests for a pancreatic abnormality.[60]

Although the ability to diagnose pancreatic pseudocysts has improved, there are remaining difficulties for a number of reasons. During an attack of pancreatitis, the total size of the pancreas frequently increases by virtue of swelling and edema. It is difficult to differentiate between the large phlegmon of pancreatitis and a developing pseudocyst, except by observing the patient for a period of time to determine whether the mass develops into a cystic space or is absorbed gradually. For example, CT in a patient who had acute pancreatitis may show massive phlegmon. CT scans over a period of time may demonstrate stabilization of the size of the mass and, finally, cyst formation within the mass (Fig. 38–8).

Over the past decade and a half, the diagnostic capabilities of abdominal ultrasonography, CT, and ERCP have increased with regard to pancreatic pseudocyst and edematous pancreatitis.[8-10, 48-52] Each of these procedures has advantages and disadvantages. In most institutions, ultrasonography is probably the procedure of first choice (Fig. 38–9).

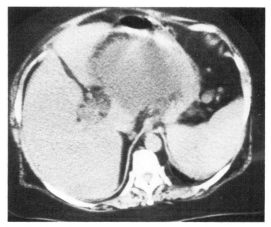

FIGURE 38–8. Computed tomography demonstrates large pseudocyst posterior to stomach at level of spleen and liver. Thick cyst wall is clearly seen. It is mature enough to hold sutures and allow successful internal drainage.

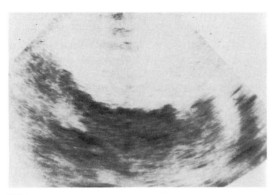

FIGURE 38–9. Ultrasonographic demonstration of large pseudocyst. Cyst wall can be visualized under ideal conditions, although most often wall is not so clearly defined as shown here. A small number of internal echoes is a fairly common finding.

Under optimal conditions it will clearly show the cyst space and wall. Its major disadvantage is that images are frequently unsatisfactory because of interposed air-containing loops of bowel. Patients with acute and subacute pancreatic disease frequently have some degree of ileus. Furthermore, interpretation of the findings as well as many technical aspects of the performance of the procedure are highly subjective. Nevertheless, ultrasonography has several advantages: it is noninvasive and relatively inexpensive; also using ultrasonography, the pancreas can be imaged in multiple planes.

CT is not compromised by gas in the bowel. The results of CT are usually more satisfactory in somewhat obese patients, since fat

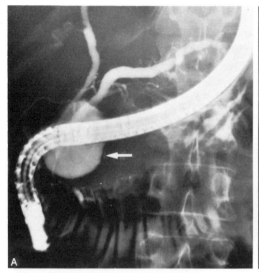

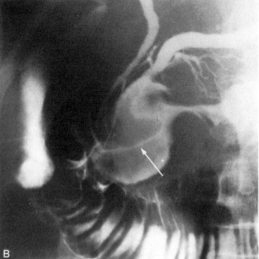

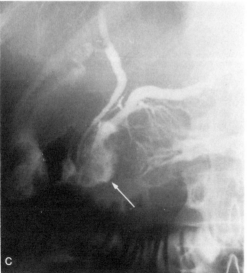

FIGURE 38–10. A, Retrograde pancreatogram demonstrates pseudocyst in head of pancreas (arrow). B, After removal of endoscope, remaining contrast material demonstrates bile duct deviation due to presence of pseudocyst as well as the relation of pseudocyst to air-filled duodenal bulb (arrow). C, Opacification of pseudocyst is less dense (arrow), indicating communication with and drainage into main duct. Note distortion of main pancreatic duct branches in head of pancreas. (Courtesy of M. V. Sivak, Jr., M.D.)

between tissue planes results in better separation of organ structures. Its disadvantages are the high cost of the equipment, significant radiation exposure, and the inability to scan the pancreas in planes other than transverse.

The role of ERCP in the diagnosis and therapy of pancreatic pseudocyst is still debated. Retrograde pancreatography has significantly advanced our knowledge of the course and evolution of pseudocysts. In the 1950's Doubilet[61] recognized that pseudocysts frequently communicate with one of the pancreatic ducts, often the main pancreatic duct. This has been confirmed by ERCP in many studies.[42-50] From 50% to 75% of pseudocysts will fill with contrast material during retrograde pancreatography (Fig. 38–10). ERCP studies have clearly shown that some pseudocysts are gradually absorbed and disappear spontaneously. For diagnosis the injection of contrast agent must be adequate for visualization. At the same time, there is a distinct possibility that opacification will convert the pseudocyst into a pancreatic abscess, the latter having a significantly worse prognosis. Two principles guide the performance of ERCP in patients with pseudocysts: the injected volume of contrast should be no more than the minimum necessary for demonstration of the presence of the pseudocyst, and drainage must be prompt.

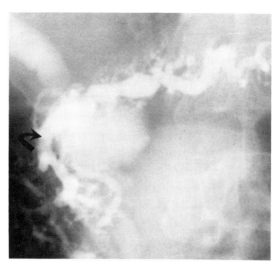

FIGURE 38–12. ERCP demonstrates large cystic mass in head of pancreas. This causes compression and dilation of bile duct. Marked changes of chronic pancreatitis are present in pancreatic duct including dilation and tortuosity of main duct. Dilation and terminal beading of main pancreatic duct side branches are shown. Diameter of main duct appears to increase as it crosses over pseudocyst (*arrow*), probably indicating compression of duct by the pseudocyst. Symptoms resolved after cyst-duodenostomy.

In our experience with surgically confirmed pseudocysts, retrograde pancreatography resulted in filling of a cystic space in 68% (unpublished data). The failure rate was 8%. However, the main pancreatic duct may also be compressed by the developing cyst wall, in which case it is usually impossible to inject contrast material past the point of obstruction and into the cystic space (Fig. 38–11). A pseudocyst may compress either the common bile duct or main pancreatic duct or both (Figs. 38–12 and 38–13). When the pancreatographic findings are those of main pancreatic duct obstruction or displacement of ductal or other normal structures and the cyst cavity is not filled, the radiographic differential diagnosis includes most of the common disorders of the pancreas such as carcinoma, a true cyst, or chronic pancreatitis. Usually the clinical history and findings by other imaging techniques will resolve this problem.

Rarely, a pancreatic carcinoma may cavitate and this may be demonstrated by ERCP. As a differential point, the size of this type of cavity is seldom large. Reference to other findings on the pancreatogram, such as the presence of a normal ductal structure up to a point of cavitation or evidence of chronic pancreatitis in the opacified portions of the ductal system, may aid in differential diag-

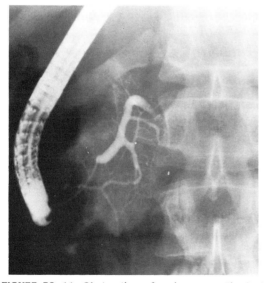

FIGURE 38–11. Obstruction of main pancreatic duct by pseudocyst. Attempted injection of contrast beyond point of obstruction has resulted in filling of pancreatic ductal system to level of the acini (acinarization). This finding on the radiograph cannot be differentiated from other causes of pancreatic duct obstruction. (Courtesy of M. V. Sivak, Jr., M.D.)

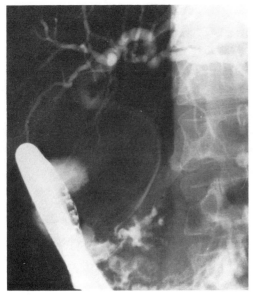

FIGURE 38–13. Retrograde cholangiography demonstrates compression and deviation of common duct and an obstructed main pancreatic duct that is also dilated and irregular. At operation a large pseudocyst was present in the head of pancreas, in addition to chronic pancreatitis. (Courtesy of M. V. Sivak, Jr., M.D.)

nosis (Fig. 38–14). However, differentiation of a small pseudocyst from a cavitating carcinoma cannot be made with certainty by pancreatographic findings alone. Again, reference to the results of other imaging procedures and the patient's history will resolve this problem.

Since the presence of a pancreatic pseudocyst can almost always be recognized by CT and ultrasonography, ERCP is usually not essential for diagnosis. Its main value is precise localization of the cyst and demonstration of its relation to other structures. If the pseudocyst appears to be resolving, this degree of precision may not be necessary. However, if surgical therapy must be considered, retrograde pancreatography and, cholangiography can add significant information that can be essential in planning the operation (Figs. 38–15, 38–16, and 38–17; see also Fig. 38–2).

An example is shown in Figure 38–2 in which precise definition and localization by ERCP of a small pseudocyst in the tail proved to be essential. The patient had been in an auto accident about 4 years earlier and had continued to have intermittent abdominal pain with no positive findings. At operation, the surgeon was unable to locate the pseudocyst until the area had been dissected and splenic vessels ligated. The operation consisted of splenectomy and resection of the distal pancreatic pseudocyst with Roux-Y jejunal drainage. The patient has remained asymptomatic since surgery.

It is difficult to measure the impact on

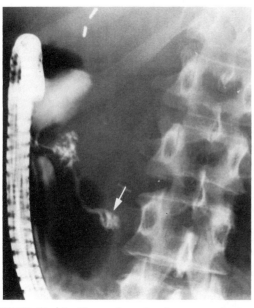

FIGURE 38–14. Obstruction of main pancreatic duct due to carcinoma. The tumor has cavitated and a small cystic space (arrow) is demonstrated at point of obstruction. (Courtesy of M. V. Sivak, Jr., M.D.)

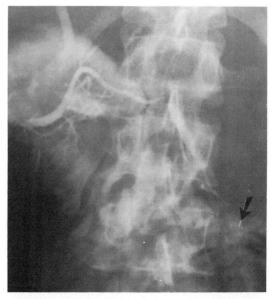

FIGURE 38–15. ERCP demonstrates normal bile duct and short segment of normal pancreatic duct up to spine. A large cyst fills via one branch in head of pancreas. Fistula tract (arrow) leads downward to second pseudocyst in left flank. Knowledge of presence of two cysts was important to surgical procedure.

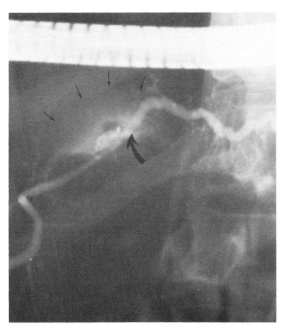

FIGURE 38–16. Huge, faintly opacified pseudocyst (*small arrows*). Tract leading upwards into mediastinal area is also demonstrated. There is pancreatic duct dilation beyond point of compression (*curved arrow*) of duct by pseudocyst. Leakage of contrast material into pseudocyst probably occurs at this point. Treatment was by cystgastrostomy and was without further complications.

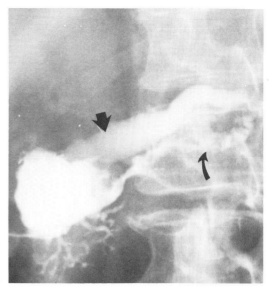

FIGURE 38–17. Large cystic cavity demonstrated in head of pancreas. Pancreatic duct (*short arrow*) is markedly dilated. Long fistula tract (*long curved arrow*) follows lower edge of pancreas but does not enter another structure. Cyst-duodenostomy resulted in resolution of patient's symptoms.

surgical therapy of this radiographic information. We have the same opinion as Sankaran et al.[13]: it is primarily a subjective impression of surgeons that knowledge of the precise location and anatomic connections of the cystic space is of benefit.

ERCP must be a preoperative procedure if a pancreatic pseudocyst is suspected or known to be present. The frequency of sepsis following ERCP and filling of the cystic cavity is approximately 10% to 20%, unless drainage is performed within 24 hours.[62, 63] Because of possible conversion of a pseudocyst into a pancreatic abscess by injection of contrast, ERCP must not be performed for suspected pancreatic pseudocyst until surgical therapy has actually been scheduled and drainage of the opacified cyst is assured within a specified time. When done as a preoperative procedure the morbidity is low.

ERCP may occasionally be useful in evaluating patients who have had surgery for a pancreatic pseudocyst. This indication usually applies to patients with persistent pain after surgery. Any question concerning the adequacy of surgical drainage of the pancreatic duct can usually be resolved by ERCP (Fig. 38–18).

COURSE AND THERAPY OF PANCREATIC PSEUDOCYST

The clinical course of pancreatic pseudocyst is highly unpredictable. As the attack of

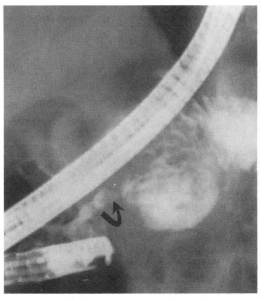

FIGURE 38–18. Pancreatogram shows short dilated duct with flow of contrast into attached jejunal limb. Although there is slight narrowing of pancreatic duct (*arrow*) at anastomosis with jejunum, no obstruction to flow of contrast is apparent. Further surgery was not considered.

acute pancreatitis begins to subside, there is usually an initial and relatively short period during which the diagnosis is uncertain. A pancreatic mass may be present during this interval, but whether this is a pancreatic phlegmon or a pseudocyst remains in question. During the acute period, satisfactory fluid and nutritional status must be maintained. The diagnosis is usually then confirmed by ultrasonography or CT. It is desirable to wait 4 to 6 weeks for maturation of the cyst wall before undertaking internal surgical drainage, provided the patient remains stable, the pseudocyst is not enlarging, or acute abdominal pain does not develop. Percutaneous needle aspiration of the acute pseudocyst has been performed under ultrasound or CT guidance in a small number of patients.[64-66] In some instances a cyst has been aspirated repeatedly. There is a single report[67] of endoscopic transgastric aspiration of a pseudocyst with apparently satisfactory results. At present, these measures should be considered as temporary to allow time for maturation of the cyst. However, if fluid does not re-accumulate in the cyst, drainage is not indicated.

The options for surgical therapy of pancreatic pseudocyst include cyst-gastrostomy, cyst duodenostomy, cyst-jejunostomy, resection of the pancreatic pseudocyst, or external drainage. These have been extensively reviewed.[68-71] External drainage is reserved for the patient with an immature pseudocyst in which the cyst wall will not hold sutures. It is to be avoided if possible, since results, including lower morbidity and mortality, are much better with internal drainage. There is disagreement as to whether jejunostomy or direct drainage into an adjacent organ is preferable. Unless the pseudocyst is directly adherent to the duodenum or stomach, drainage into these organs should not be attempted. For cyst-jejunostomy most surgeons prefer a devitalized jejunal limb (Roux-Y) for internal drainage. Operative and postoperative mortality varies according to the procedure, being as high as 25% with external drainage, and as low as 3% to 4% with drainage into the gastrointestinal tract. Probably the differences in mortality are not inherent to the procedures themselves but reflect the selection of one procedure over another according to the condition of the patient. An external drainage procedure, for example, is most likely to be performed on an urgent basis in a seriously ill patient.

The most serious complications of pancreatic pseudocyst are infection and hemorrhage. Infection of the cyst may occur either spontaneously or through instrumentation. Fistulization into various other organs may occur. Mortality from hemorrhage secondary to pancreatic pseudocyst is high, probably in the range of 60% to 80%.[72-74] Abdominal angiography appears to be of value preoperatively in a patient with hemorrhage from the pseudocyst.[75]

Early diagnosis and careful follow-up and observation should reduce the complications from pancreatic pseudocyst. There are several accurate imaging methods including CT, ultrasonography, and ERCP. These can eliminate the majority of diagnostic errors, so that surgical exploration of patients with immature pseudocysts or pancreatic phlegmons should be largely unnecessary.

Editor's note: References 76 and 77 are recent publications of interest in relation to points covered in this chapter.

References

1. Hollender LF, Marrie D, Alexiu D, et al. Pseudocyst of the pancreas. J Coll Surg Edinb 1975; 20:42–8.
2. Karatzas GM. Pancreatic pseudocysts. Br J Surg 1976; 63:55–9.
3. Bohlman TW, Katon RM, Lee TG, et al. Use of endoscopic retrograde cholangiopancreatography in the diagnosis of pancreatic fistula. Gastroenterology 1976; 70:582–4.
4. Dudrick SJ, Wilmore DW, Steiger E, et al. Spontaneous closure of traumatic pancreatoduodenal fistulas with total intravenous nutrition. J Trauma 1970; 10:542–53.
5. Hamilton RF, Davis WC, Stephenson DV, et al. Effects of parenteral hyperalimentation on upper gastrointestinal tract secretions. Arch Surg 1971; 102:348–52.
6. Adwers JR, Davis WC. Adjuvant treatment of blunt pancreatic trauma. Surg Gynecol Obstet 1974; 139:514–8.
7. Taxier M, Sivak MV Jr, Cooperman AM, Sullivan BH JR. Endoscopic retrograde pancreatography in the evaluation of trauma to the pancreas. Surg Gynecol Obstet 1980; 150:65–8.
8. Bradley EL III, Gonzalez AC, Clements JL Jr. Acute pancreatic pseudocysts: incidence and complications. Ann Surg 1976; 184:734–7.
9. Thomford NR, Jesseph JE. Pseudocyst of the pancreas: a review of 50 cases. Am J Surg 1969; 118:86–94.
10. Warren KW, Athamassiades S, Frederick P, et al. Surgical treatment of pancreatic cysts: review of 183 cases. Ann Surg 1966; 163:886–91.
11. Cerilli J, Farris TD. Pancreatic pseudocysts: delayed versus immediate treatment. Surgery 1967; 61:541–3.
12. Satake K, Cho K, Sowa M, et al. Demonstration of a pancreatic fistula by endoscopic pancreatography

in a patient with chronic pleural effusion. Am J Surg 1979; 136:390–2.

13. Sankaran S, Sugawa C, Walt AJ. Value of endoscopic retrograde pancreatography in pancreatic ascites. Surg Gynecol Obstet 1979; 148:185–92.

14. Davis RE, Graham DY. Pancreatic ascites: the role of endoscopic pancreatography. Am J Dig Dis 1975; 20:977–80.

15. Rawlings W, Bynum TE, Pasternak G. Pancreatic ascites: diagnosis of leakage site by endoscopic pancreatography. Surgery 1977; 81:363–5.

16. Ward PA, Raju S, Suzuki H. Preoperative demonstration of pancreatic fistula by endoscopic pancreatography in a patient with pancreatic ascites. Ann Surg 1977; 185:232–4.

17. Levine JB, Warshaw AL, Falchuk KR, et al. The value of endoscopic retrograde pancreatography in the management of pancreatic ascites. Surgery 1977; 81:360–2.

18. Bretholz A, Lammli J, Corrodi P, Knoblauch M. Ruptured pancreatic pseudocysts: diagnosis by endoscopy. Report of 3 cases. Endoscopy 1978; 10: 19–23.

19. Anderson MC. Management of pancreatic pseudocysts. Am J Surg 1972; 123:209–21.

20. Smith RB 3rd, Warren WD, Rivard AA Jr, et al. Pancreatic ascites. Diagnosis and management with particular reference to surgical technics. Ann Surg 1973; 177:538–46.

21. Russell DM, Roberts-Thomson IC, Macrae FA, et al. Recurrence of pancreatic ascites due to a second leak demonstrated radiologically. Br J Surg 1981; 68:381–2.

22. Bozymski EM, Orlando RC, Holt JW III. Traumatic disruption of the pancreatic duct demonstrated by endoscopic retrograde pancreatography. J Trauma 1981; 21:244–5.

23. Eldrup J, Burcharth F, Stadil F. Pancreatic ascites. Intraoperative localization of the pancreatic fistula. Acta Chir Scand 1980; 146:301–2.

24. Sugawa C, Walt AJ, Sankaran S. Pancreatic pseudocysts communicating with the stomach: demonstration by endoscopic retrograde pancreatography. Arch Surg 1977; 112:1050–3.

25. Ellenbogen KA, Cameron JL, Cocco AE, et al. Fistulous communication of a pseudocyst with the common bile duct: demonstration by endoscopic retrograde cholangiopancreatography. Johns Hopkins Med J 1981; 149:110–1.

26. Hoff G, Heldaas J. Pancreatic pseudocyst and pancreaticoduodenal fistula diagnosed by endoscopic fistulography. Endoscopy 1981; 13:221–2.

27. Heiss FW, Shea JA, Cady B, Scholz FJ. Pancreatic pseudocyst with mediastinal extension and pleural effusion. Demonstration of pathologic anatomy by endoscopic pancreatography. Dig Dis Sci 1979; 24:649–51.

28. Carr-Locke DL, Salim KA, Lucas PA. Hemorrhagic pancreatic pleural effusion in chronic relapsing pancreatitis. ERCP demonstration of internal pancreatic fistula. Gastrointest Endosc 1979; 25:160–2.

29. Sottomayor M, Nam Chang R, Dawson M. Use of ERCP in the diagnosis of internal pancreatic fistula. GUT 1978; 19:244–6.

30. Darras T, Gulbis A, Khazzaka E, et al. Endoscopic retrograde pancreatography in the diagnosis of pancreatic pleural fistula. J Belge Radiol 1977; 60: 423–6.

31. Paloyan D, Simonowitz D, Blackstone M. Pancreatic fistula. Management guided by endoscopic retro-grade cholangiopancreatography. Arch Surg 1977; 112:1139–40.

32. Greiner L, Prohm P. Pancreatico-pleural fistula with chronic pleural effusion—endoscopic-retrograde visualization and therapy by ultrasonically-guided drainage. Endoscopy 1983; 15:73–4.

33. Yamamoto S, Takeshige K, Aradawa T, et al. Case report of a pancreatic pseudocyst ruptured into the splenic vein causing extrahepatic portal hypertension. Jpn J Surg 1982; 12:387–90.

34. Aagaard J, Matzen P, Thorsgaard Pederson N. The role of endoscopic pancreatography in pancreatic ascites. Acta Chir Scand 1982; 148:93–5.

35. Tumen JJ, Wade Sutton W, Dewey Dunn G. Bilateral pancreatic pleural effusions: a case report and literature review. Am J Gastroenterol 1983; 78: 84–6.

36. Angeras U, Munthe SH, Swedenborg J, Jarhult J. Pancreatico-pleural fistulae. Presentation of a case and review of the literature. Ann Chir Gynaecol 1982; 71:178–83.

37. Panitch N, Piken E, Hanelin L, Grinker J. The value of endoscopic pancreatography in the diagnosis of pancreatic pleural effusion: direct demonstration of pancreaticopleural fistula. Am J Gastroenterol 1982; 77:574–5.

38. Greenwald RA, Deluca RF, Raskin JB. Pancreaticpleural fistula: demonstration by endoscopic retrograde cholangiopancreatography (ERCP) and successful treatment with radiation therapy. Dig Dis Sci 1979; 24:240–4.

39. Rauch FR, Stenstrom KW. Effects of x-ray radiation on pancreatic function in dogs. Gastroenterology 1952; 20:595–603.

40. Orndoff BH, Farrell JI, Ivy AC. Studies on the effect of roentgen rays on glandular activity. V. The effect of roentgen rays on external pancreatic secretion. Am J Roentgenol 1926; 16:349–54.

41. Wachtfeidl V, Vitez M. X-ray therapy for acute pancreatitis. Am J Surg 1968; 116:853–67.

42. Hatfield AR, Hately W. Resolution of a pancreatic pseudocyst by spontaneous drainage into the stomach. Br J Radiol 1980; 53:595–7.

43. Takayama T, Kato K, Katada N, et al. Radiological demonstration of spontaneous rupture of a pancreatic pseudocyst into the portal system. Am J Gastroenterol 1982; 77:55–8.

44. Silvis SE, Vennes JA, Rohrmann CA. Endoscopic pancreatography in the evaluation of patients with suspected pancreatic pseudocysts. Am J Gastroenterol 1974; 61:452–9.

45. Sugawa C, Walt AJ. Endoscopic retrograde pancreatography in the surgery of pancreatic pseudocysts. Surgery 1979; 86:639–47.

46. Tim LO, Thompson PM, Segal J, Lawson HK. Endoscopic retrograde cholangiopancreatography in the management of traumatic pancreatic pseudocysts. A report of 2 cases. S Afr Med J 1979; 55:767–70.

47. Seifert E. X-ray findings of pancreatic cysts diagnosed by endoscopic pancreatocholangiography. Endoscopy 1974; 6:77.

48. Andersen BN, Hancke S, Nielsen SA, et al. The diagnosis of pancreatic cyst by endoscopic retrograde pancreatography and ultrasonic scanning. Ann Surg 1977; 185:286–9.

49. Feinberg SB, Schreiber DR, Goodale R. Comparison of ultrasound pancreatic scanning and endoscopic retrograde cholangiopancreatogram: a retrospective study. J Clin Ultrasound 1977; 5:96–100.

50. Gonzalez AC, Bradley EL, Clements JL Jr. Pseudo-cyst formation in acute pancreatitis: ultrasonographic evaluation of 99 cases. Am J Roentgenol 1976; 127:315–7.

51. Duncan JG, Imrie CW, Blumgart LH. Proceedings: Ultrasound in the management of acute pancreatitis. Br J Radiol 1976; 49:731.

52. Kressel HY, Margulis AR, Gooding GW, et al. CT scanning and ultrasound in the evaluation of pancreatic pseudocysts: a preliminary comparison. Radiology 1978; 126:153–7.

53. Czaja A, Fisher M, Marin GA. Spontaneous resolution of pancreatic masses (pseudocysts?) appearing after acute alcoholic pancreatitis. (Abstr) Gastroenterology 1973; 64:714.

54. Ebbesen KE, Schonebeck J. Prolonged amylase elevation. Acta Chir Scand 1967; 133:61–5.

55. Jordan GL, Howard JM. Pancreatic pseudocysts. Am J Gastroenterol 1966; 45:444–53.

56. Veith FJ, Filler RM, Berard CW. Significance of prolonged elevation of the serum amylase. Ann Surg 1963; 158:20–6.

57. Malinowski T. Clinical value of serum amylase determination. JAMA 1952; 149:1380–5.

58. Wenckert A. Longstanding increase of urine-amylase in acute pancreatitis with the development of a pseudocyst. Studies in Surgery, 1963; 163.

59. Vajcner A, Nicoloff DM. Pseudocysts of the pancreas: value of urine and serum amylase levels. Surgery 1969; 66:842–5.

60. Johnson SG, Ellis CJ, Levitt MD. Mechanism of increased renal clearance of amylase/creatinine in acute pancreatitis. N Engl J Med 1976; 295:1214–7.

61. Doubilet H. Pancreatic pseudocysts: present concept as to etiology and treatment. Surgery 1957; 41:522–3.

62. Bilbao MK, Dotter CT, Lee TG. Complications of endoscopic retrograde cholangiopancreatography (ERCP). Gastroenterology 1976; 70:314–20.

63. Silvis SE, Nebel O, Rogers G, et al. Endoscopic complications. Results of the 1974 American Society for Gastrointestinal Endoscopy Survey. JAMA 1976; 235:928–30.

64. Hancke S, Pedersen JF. Percutaneous puncture of pancreatic cysts guided by ultrasound. Surg Gynecol Obstet 1976; 142:551–2.

65. MacErlean DP, Bryan PJ, Murphy JJ. Pancreatic pseudocyst: management by ultrasonically guided aspiration. Gastrointest Radiol 1980; 5:255–7.

66. Weinrauch LA, Aoki T, Arky R, D'Elia JA. Insulin resistance with pancreatic pseudocyst relieved by percutaneous drainage. Arch Intern Med 1983; 143:1244–5.

67. Rogers BHG, Cicurel NJ, Seed RW. Transgastric needle aspiration of pancreatic pseudocyst through an endoscope. Gastrointest Endosc 1975; 21:133–4.

68. Sandy JT, Taylor RH, Christensen RM, et al. Pancreatic pseudocyst: changing concepts in management. Am J Surg 1981; 141:574–6.

69. Bodurtha AJ, Dajee H, You CK. Analysis of 29 cases of pancreatic pseudocyst treated surgically. Can J Surg 1980; 23:432–4.

70. Martin EW Jr, Catalano P, Cooperman M, et al. Surgical decision-making in the treatment of pancreatic pseudocysts: internal versus external drainage. Am J Surg 1979; 138:821–4.

71. Bradley EL III, Clements JL Jr, Gonzalez AC. The natural history of pancreatic pseudocysts: a unified concept of management. Am J Surg 1979; 137:135–41.

72. Wu TK, Zaman SN, Gullick HD. Spontaneous hemorrhage due to pseudocysts of the pancreas. Am J Surg 1977; 134:408–10.

73. Cogbill CL. Hemorrhage in pancreatic pseudocysts: a review of literature and report of two cases. Ann Surg 1968; 167:112–5.

74. Stanley JC, Frey CF, Miller TA, et al. Major arterial hemorrhage: a complication of pancreatic pseudocysts and chronic pancreatitis. Arch Surg 1976; 111:435–40.

75. Kadell BM, Riley JM. Major arterial involvement by pancreatic pseudocysts. Am J Roentgenol 1967; 3:632–6.

76. O'Connor M, Kolars J, Ansel H, et al. Preoperative endoscopic retrograde cholangiopancreatography in the surgical management of pancreatic pseudocysts. Am J Surg 1986; 151:18–24.

77. Iglehart JD, Mansback C, Postlethwait R, et al. Pancreaticobronchial fistula. Case report and review of the literature. Gastroenterology 1986; 90:759–63.

Chapter 39

ENDOSCOPIC DIAGNOSIS OF CANCER OF THE PANCREAS

KEIICHI KAWAI, M.D.
KENJIRO YASUDA, M.D.
MASATSUGU NAKAJIMA, M.D.

The pancreas is one of the most difficult intra-abdominal organs to evaluate. By the time symptoms indicate the presence of carcinoma of the pancreas the disease is well advanced in the majority of cases; usually the tumor is unresectable and the prognosis for the patient is poor.

Tumor markers in the serum such as elastase 1, pancreatic oncofetal antigen (POA), carcinoembryonic antigen (CEA), and carbohydrate antigen (CA 19–9) have been proposed as screening tests for the detection of pancreatic malignancy; those evaluated thus far are insensitive and nonspecific. Morphologic examinations including body imaging techniques are, therefore, still essential for the diagnosis of cancer of the pancreas. Recent advances in linear scanning ultrasonography, computed tomography (CT), and selective celiac angiography have increased the accuracy of diagnosis of pancreatic disorders. Endoscopic retrograde cholangiopancreatography (ERCP), now used worldwide,[1–4] is considered one of the most reliable diagnostic procedures for biliary and pancreatic diseases, especially cancer of the pancreas.[5–10] Moreover, advanced endoscopic instruments coupled with retrograde cannulation of the papilla of Vater have brought about direct visualization of the biliary and pancreatic ductal systems.

In this chapter, the retrograde pancreatographic diagnosis of pancreatic cancer will be considered, including some remaining problems. New endoscopic techniques for diagnosis of pancreatic cancer will also be presented.

DIAGNOSIS OF PANCREATIC CARCINOMA

ERCP is usually performed for precise or differential diagnosis of biliary and pancreatic diseases, for which purposes it has a number of advantages. It combines endoscopic and radiologic examinations and thus provides direct information about the stomach and duodenum as well as the biliary and pancreatic ductal systems. Evidence of pancreatic carcinoma can often be detected, as secondary alterations in the stomach, duodenum, and bile duct produced by the tumor. Direct biopsy of the papilla of Vater and aspiration of bile and pancreatic juice for cytologic study are possible[11–13] (see Chapter 37). Biopsies under direct vision may be obtained of periampullary tumors that invade the duodenal wall (see Chapter 23 for a discussion of primary and secondary duodenal tumors). However, the diagnosis of cancer of the pancreas by ERCP depends mainly on the interpretation of pancreatograms. Therefore, a knowledge of normal pancreatography as well as the ductal changes produced by various diseases is important for correct interpretation.[4, 14] The normal pancreatogram is discussed in Chapter 28.

ENDOSCOPIC RETROGRADE CHOLANGIOPANCREATOGRAPHY (ERCP)

ERCP Results

During the past 13 years, we attempted ERCP in 252 patients with cancer of the

821

TABLE 39–1. **Ductal Opacification by ERCP in
Cancer of the Pancreas**

Cancer Site	No. of Patients	Successful			Unsuccessful		
		BD & PD	PD	BD	Papillary Invasion	Duodenal Stenosis	Technical Error
Head	137	73	31	14	9	8	2
Body or tail	97	70	25	1	0	0	1
Whole	18	11	6	1	0	0	0
Total	252	154	62	16	9	8	3

BD = bile duct; PD = pancreatic duct.

pancreas, the majority confirmed by laparotomy or autopsy; 54.2% had cancer of the head of the pancreas, 38.5% of the body or tail, and 7.1% had cancer of the entire pancreas (Table 39–1). ERCP was successful in 232 patients (92%); this provided cholangiopancreatography in 154 patients, pancreatography alone in 62 patients, and cholangiography alone in 16 patients, the pancreatic duct being, therefore, visualized in 216 patients (85.7%) (Table 39–1). A pancreatogram was not obtained in 36 patients (14.3%); the malignant tumors in the latter group were located mainly in the head of the pancreas, where involvement of the duodenal wall and/or papilla of Vater prevented adequate pancreatography.

The results of ERCP in terms of correct diagnosis are shown in Table 39–2. Carcinoma was diagnosed in 239 of 252 patients (94.8%); in 207 patients this was by interpretation of the pancreatograms alone, and in 32 patients by cholangiographic and/or duodenoscopic findings with or without biopsy and/or cytology. A misdiagnosis was made in 8 patients (3.2%) in whom there were no marked abnormalities of the ductal systems (false-negatives). In the remaining 5 patients (2.0%), no diagnosis was made because of technical or anatomic difficulties encountered during ERCP.

Silvis et al.[6] reported 84 cases of pancreatic or bile duct carcinoma in 1976. ERCP was successful in 73 cases, and the tumor was correctly diagnosed in 67 (92%). The procedure was successful in 40 of 43 patients with pancreatic cancer and the diagnosis was correct in 37 patients based on the presence of stenosis (16 patients) or obstruction (14 patients) of the pancreatic duct. In 7 patients the diagnosis of pancreatic cancer was based on abnormalities noted in the common bile duct; in 5 of these the pancreatic duct was normal. The authors noted that in some or all of these 5 cases the tumor may have originated in the bile duct itself or perhaps in the accessory pancreatic duct.

Moss et al.[15] compared ERCP and CT in the diagnosis of pancreatic cancer in a prospective, blind clinical evaluation of 61 patients. ERCP had an accuracy of 62% with a 30% failure rate and gave a false-negative diagnosis in 8%. If ERCP failures were excluded, accuracy was 88%. CT provided a correct diagnosis in 76%, a false-negative diagnosis in 13%, and a false-positive diagnosis in 5%. The CT diagnosis was indeterminate in 6%. The CT and ERCP diagnoses agreed in 67%, in which case diagnostic accuracy was 93%, i.e., greater than either study alone.

DiMagno et al.[8] prospectively evaluated 70 patients with suspected pancreatic cancer, 68 of whom underwent laparotomy. The final diagnosis was carcinoma in 30 patients, pancreatitis in 7, other neoplasm in 9, and nonneoplastic disease or no disease in 24 patients. These investigators found that ultrasonography and pancreatic function testing using cholecystokinin-stimulated enzyme output were the best tests for detection of pancreatic disease. They recommended ultrasonography as a first procedure in suspected pancreatic disease, and if the result was negative that pancreatic function testing be performed. A positive result by either test was considered an indication for ERCP. This sequence of procedures correctly identified pancreatic cancer in 88% of cases.

Freeny and Ball[9] found the sensitivity and specificity of ERCP in pancreatic cancer to be 94% and 97%, respectively; the predictive value of a positive ERCP study was 83%, and the predictive value of a negative examination was 99%. However, the sensitivity and specificity of CT were 95% and 92%, respectively, with the predictive value of a positive

TABLE 39–2. **Results of ERCP in Cancer of
the Pancreas**

Cancer Site	No. of Patients	Diagnosis			
		Positive	Suspected Positive	Missed	Un-diagnosed
Head	137	91	38 (31)*	6	(2)
Body or tail	97	88	4	2	(3)
Whole	18	15	3 (1)		
Total	252	194	45 (32)	8	(5)

*( ) = No visualization of the pancreatic duct.

result being 76% and the predictive value of a negative CT being 99%. These authors concluded that CT should be the initial procedure of choice in the diagnosis of pancreatic cancer and that ERCP should be reserved for the evaluation of patients with equivocal or technically unsatisfactory CT studies or normal CT results when symptoms nevertheless suggest pancreatic carcinoma.

Frick et al.[16] studied ERCP in patients with suspected pancreatic cancer and indeterminate CT results. ERCP explained the CT finding of equivocal pancreatic enlargement in 10 of 12 cases by making the diagnoses of carcinoma in 5, chronic pancreatitis in 2, and ductal variation in 3; the pancreatogram was normal in 2 patients with pancreases beyond the normal size limits for CT. Four patients with a pancreatic mass by CT and known malignancy originating elsewhere underwent ERCP. In all 4 cases the ERCP was normal, and the abnormal CT results were explained at laparotomy by peripancreatic lymphadenopathy due to lymphoma in 2 patients and metastatic testicular carcinoma in 2 patients. In 10 patients CT showed evidence of chronic pancreatitis and a noncalcified mass. ERCP correctly diagnosed carcinoma in one of these patients and confirmed the presence of chronic pancreatitis in the other 9 patients, although in 1 of the latter patients a carcinoma was overlooked by ERCP.

Radiographic Findings

Pancreatic ductal changes in cancer of the pancreas are of two kinds.[4] Either there are significant changes in the main pancreatic duct or an abnormality occurs only in the branch ducts or the acinar field of the pan-

FIGURE 39–1. Obstruction of main pancreatic duct (type I) in cancer of pancreas. A, Abrupt obstruction with irregular appearance (arrow); B, obstruction with tapering (arrow); C, obstruction with cystic dilation (arrow).

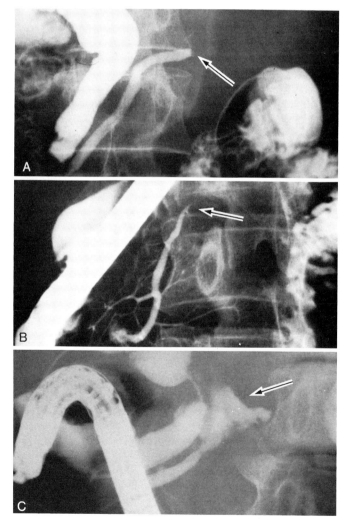

creas. From this standpoint, pancreatograms in cancer of the pancreas can be classified into the following types: (I) obstructive, (II) stenotic, (III) diffuse narrowing, (IV) abnormal branching, and (V) cyst formation.[17, 18] In the first of these, there is complete obstruction of the main pancreatic duct, and characteristically the terminal end of the obstructed portion is irregular, tapered, or shows cystic dilation (Fig. 39–1). The stenotic type, in which there is a localized stricture of the main duct, is often accompanied by dilation of the duct upstream from the stenosis (Fig. 39–2), this being correctly termed prestenotic dilation (see Chapter 28 for a discussion of the terms proximal and distal as applied to the main pancreatic duct). Pancreatograms of the diffuse narrowing type reveal generalized or segmental narrowing of the main pancreatic duct, which also has an irregular contour in the region of the tumor (Fig. 39–3). The abnormal branching type, in which there is no marked change in the main duct, demonstrates only abnormally shaped main duct branches; findings such as filling defects, obstruction, stenosis, or cystic dilation are included (Fig. 39–4). Cyst formation, in which there is cystic dilation of the main duct or one or more of its branches,

is characteristic of cystadenocarcinoma (Fig. 39–5). Silvis et al.,[6] however, reported that contrast medium filled an extraductal cavity in 5 of 43 cases of pancreatic cancer. This led to an incorrect diagnosis of pseudocyst in 1 case, the only one in which the malignancy-associated cavity was greater than 2 cm in diameter. Other classifications of the pancreatographic findings in carcinoma are similar to ours.[2, 4, 5, 19, 20]

In our 216 patients with pancreatic cancer who had successful pancreatography, the most common alterations of the pancreatic ductal system were obstruction (type I) and stenosis (type II) of the main pancreatic duct (Table 39–3). These findings are essentially the same as those of other investigators.[18–22] The number of examples of pancreatographic types III, IV, and V was small. There was no relation between any of the pancreatographic findings and resectability of the tumor.

Pancreatic diseases may produce secondary changes in the bile duct because of the anatomic relation of these two structures (see Chapters 27 and 28). Cholangiographic abnormalities include displacement, effacement, stenosis, and obstruction. Freeny et al.[21] termed the cholangiographic findings of

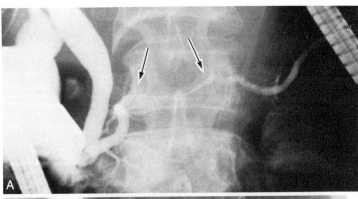
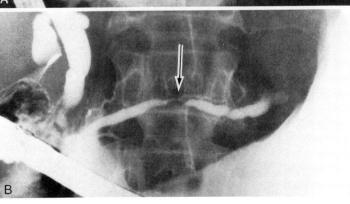

FIGURE 39–2. Stenosis of main pancreatic duct (type II) in cancer of pancreas. *A*, Long stenosis (*arrows*) of duct in body; *B*, short stenotic segment (*arrow*) in body, due to small carcinoma.

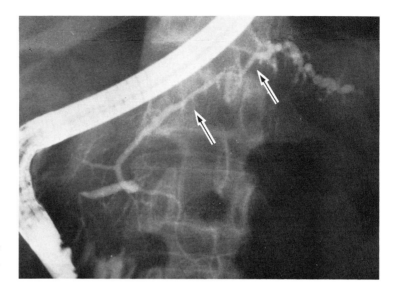

FIGURE 39–3. Diffuse narrowing of main pancreatic duct (*arrows*) in cancer of pancreas (type III).

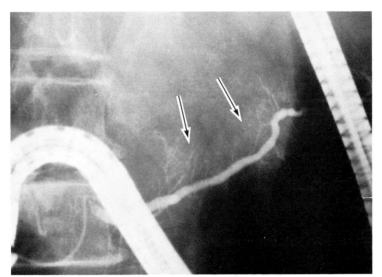

FIGURE 39–4. Abnormal main pancreatic duct branches (*arrows*) in cancer of pancreas (type IV).

FIGURE 39–5. Cyst formation (*arrow*) in pancreas, due to cancer (type V).

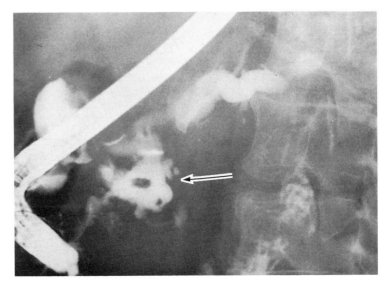

TABLE 39–3. **Pancreatographic Classification of Cancer of the Pancreas**

			Site of Cancer		
	Type	No. of Patients	Head	Body or Tail	Whole
I.	Obstruction of the MPD	126	51	68	7
II.	Stenosis of the MPD	63	45	16	2
III.	Diffuse narrowing of the MPD	16	3	17	6
IV.	Abnormal branching	9	4	3	2
V.	Cyst formation	2	1	1	
Total		216	104	95	17

MPD = Main pancreatic duct.

secondary biliary involvement in pancreatic carcinoma the "double-duct" sign. In a blind review of 40 pancreatograms these authors correctly diagnosed 11 cases of pancreatic cancer. They found that diagnostic accuracy increased in pancreatic cancer when the bile duct also showed evidence of encasement with an irregular margin. They also found secondary biliary involvement in other pancreatic diseases, but disorders other than cancer tended to produce smooth and symmetrical stenoses of the bile duct. Plumley et al.[23] encountered the double-duct sign in 52 of 1180 pancreatograms. This was caused by pancreatic cancer in 30 and by benign pancreatic disease in 22 patients. Although they regarded this radiographic sign as not disease specific, they found that certain characteristics favored a malignant or benign process. Ductal obstruction, especially of the common bile duct, close proximity radiographically of the abnormalities in both ducts, a short stenotic segment of the common duct, and an abrupt and irregular transition from normal to an obstructed or stenotic bile duct favored the diagnosis of carcinoma. All cases of complete obstruction of the common bile duct were due to carcinoma (Fig. 39–6). Long, smooth stenotic bile duct segments were more characteristic of benign pancreatic disease such as chronic pancreatitis.

There have been a few reports in which the main pancreatic duct appeared to be normal in the presence of proved pancreatic cancer.[3, 5, 6] Special care is required for the diagnosis of cancer in the uncinate portion of the pancreas, because this location is relatively blind in terms of pancreatographic visualization.

Metastatic malignancy may occasionally involve the pancreas and the main pancreatic

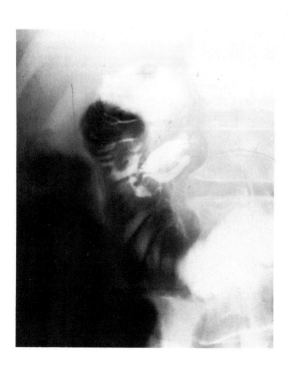

FIGURE 39–6. Retrograde cholangiopancreatogram demonstrates complete obstruction of both common bile and pancreatic ducts ("double-duct" sign) in cancer of head of pancreas. (Courtesy of M. V. Sivak, Jr., M.D.)

duct. The main pancreatographic findings, stenosis and obstruction of the main duct, are indistinguishable from those of pancreatic carcinoma[24] (Fig. 39–7).

Differential Diagnosis

As noted, pancreatic carcinoma may have several pancreatographic appearances. Similar radiographic patterns occasionally occur in other benign diseases including chronic pancreatitis.[2–4, 6, 18] Pancreatograms in elderly patients without any pancreatic disease may mimic abnormal findings.[3, 25] Ductal changes in older individuals can include widening of the main duct and ectatic and/or cystic changes in the main duct branches, changes that simulate the findings of chronic pancreatitis or the type IV pattern of carcinoma.[25] Apparent radiographic defects in the pancreatic ducts can be caused by compression by arteries, lymph nodes, or bony structures. Anatomic anomalies of the pancreas and pancreatic ducts can also cause problems in diagnosis.[26] Atypical papillary hyperplasia of the pancreatic ductal epithelium causing obstruction of the main pancreatic duct has led to an incorrect diagnosis of pancreatic carcinoma.[27] Pancreatic ductal distortion simulating pancreatic carcinoma has been reported after gastric surgery.[28]

Precise study of the appearance of the pancreatogram at the point of obstruction or stenosis is of assistance in differentiating benign from malignant causes.[22] The main points of differentation are illustrated schematically in Figure 39–8. Carcinoma causes the outline or shape of the column of contrast material at the point of main duct obstruction to be flat or blunt, serrated, pointed or cone shaped, or irregular; branches of the main duct are poorly outlined or not visible at all near the occluded end of the main duct (Fig. 39–9A). By contrast, the pancreatographic appearance of ductal obstruction due to chronic pancreatitis has a relatively smooth contour with a shape that can be described as hemispheric, either concave or convex, (in some cases produced by a pancreatic duct calculus) or spindle, flat, or rod-like (Fig. 39–9B). Main pancreatic duct branches in the region of the obstruction often fill with contrast material and so are visualized by pancreatography, although they are usually irregular, dilated, and/or ectatic.

In malignant stenosis of the main pancreatic duct the narrowed segment is usually localized and the contour of the duct within this region is irregular; main pancreatic duct branches are not opacified near the stenosis (Fig. 39–10A). The contour of the main duct changes abruptly at the point of stenosis. Between the papilla and the stenotic segment the main duct and its branches are usually

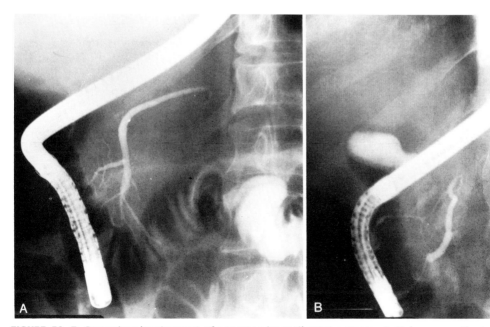

FIGURE 39–7. Secondary involvement of pancreas by malignant process. A, Main pancreatic duct obstruction due to lymphadenopathy in lymphoma; B, main pancreatic duct obstruction due to metastatic breast carcinoma. (Courtesy of M. V. Sivak, Jr., M.D.)

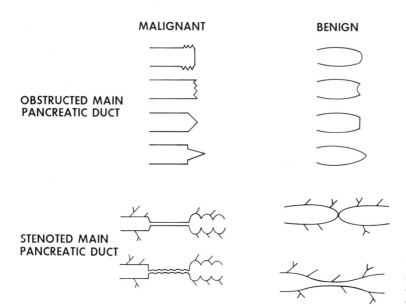

MALIGNANT   BENIGN

OBSTRUCTED MAIN
PANCREATIC DUCT

STENOTED MAIN
PANCREATIC DUCT

FIGURE 39–8. Basic pancreatographic patterns used to differentiate malignant and benign disorders.

FIGURE 39–9. Pancreatographic
patterns of obstruction in cancer
and chronic pancreatitis. *A*, Irregular, saw-like obstruction (*arrow*)
of duct in body, due to cancer; *B*,
smooth, blunt obstruction (*arrow*)
of duct in body, due to chronic
pancreatitis.

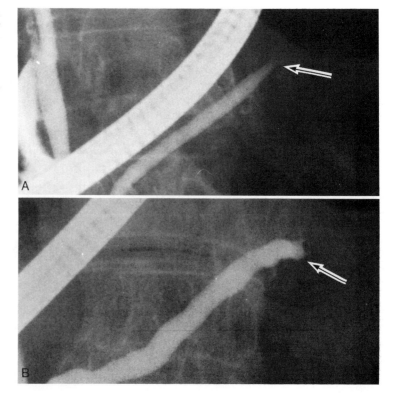

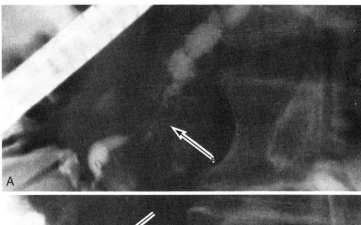

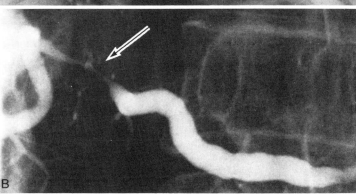

FIGURE 39–10. Pancreatographic patterns of stenosis in cancer and chronic pancreatitis. A, Irregular stenosis (arrow) of main duct in head of pancreas, due to cancer. Note lack of branch ducts in stenotic section. B, Smoothly tapered stenosis of main duct (arrow), due to chronic pancreatitis. Note presence of main duct branches in the region of stenosis.

normal. Main pancreatic duct stenosis produced by chronic pancreatitis is either extremely short and localized or relatively long. The transition from the normal-diameter portion of the duct to the stenotic segment is relatively smooth and gradual, and branches are demonstrated in the region of the stenosis (Fig. 39–10B). The pancreatogram of the main duct and branches between the stenosis and the papilla of Vater often reveals additional changes of chronic pancreatitis, including dilation and tortuosity.

Pancreatic cancer may also cause diffuse narrowing of the main duct (type III) and abnormalities in the pattern of main pancreatic duct branching (type IV), findings that are relatively uncommon. These patterns not only are difficult to recognize but also present problems with differential diagnosis. Provided that the minute branches within the parenchyma of the pancreas are shown, the following findings suggest carcinoma: displacement and obstruction of branches, and sparse or absent branching in the region of the tumor. When contrast medium has been injected to the level of the pancreatic acinus, a radiographic outline of the entire pancreas known as a parenchymogram may obtained. In rare instances a filling defect in the par-

enchymogram may be seen in pancreatic cancer.

Diagnostic Problems

More than 80% of pancreatic cancers are ductal carcinomas originating in the epithelial cells of the pancreatic ducts. The growth of the acinar cell carcinomas of pancreatic parenchymal origin also affects the pancreatic ducts. Since the great majority of pancreatic malignancies produce changes in the ductal system, ERCP is one of the most sensitive and reliable methods for demonstrating findings due to cancer. When ERCP has been evaluated in prospective trials, diagnostic accuracy has been found to be high.[7, 8] However, with the widespread use of ERCP, several problems and some limitations have become apparent.[4, 17–19]

Differential Diagnosis

The first of these problems is concerned with pancreatographic interpretation. There are cases in which it is difficult to differentiate pancreatic cancer from other pancreatic disorders; both false-negative and false-positive diagnoses of malignancy may occur.[7] For example, there were 8 false-negative diag-

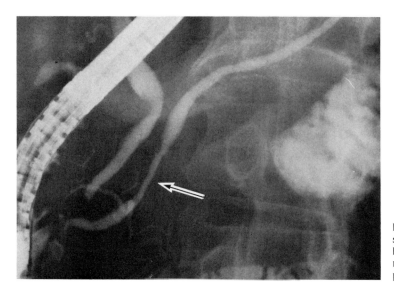

FIGURE 39–11. Slight irregular stricture (*arrow*) of main duct in head of pancreas, due to carcinoma. Pancreatogram was interpreted as normal (false-negative).

noses of pancreatic cancer in our series of 252 cases (Fig. 39–11). In addition, 16 cases of chronic pancreatitis including 10 confirmed by laparotomy were misdiagnosed (false-positive cases) as pancreatic carcinoma (Fig. 39–12). Furthermore, it is possible that some pancreatic cancers, particularly early cancer, may have been overlooked among the cases diagnosed as chronic pancreatitis or regarded as normal. In general, an effort to discover early pancreatic cancer by ERCP may result in an increased number of false-positive cases, whereas an attempt to diagnose only unequivocal cases or cases of advanced cancer may result in an increased number of false-negative cases.[4]

In some cases, biopsy and/or cytologic di-

agnosis can enhance the accuracy of ERCP.[11–13] Furthermore, the approach to diagnosis must be comprehensive and must consider the history and physical findings as well as the results of other investigations.

In an effort to resolve problems in differential diagnosis, ductal changes can also be studied carefully for findings that are characteristic of different pancreatic diseases.

Rohrmann et al.[22] found main pancreatic duct obstruction by pancreatography in 50 of 500 ERCP studies, of which 15 proved to be neoplastic. In two thirds of the cases of malignancy the obstruction had a tapered, eccentric or irregular radiographic configuration. Other authors have found this type of observation to be useful in the diagnosis

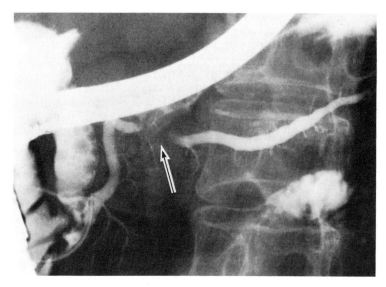

FIGURE 39–12. Localized stenosis of main pancreatic duct (*arrow*), due to chronic pancreatitis but misdiagnosed as cancer of the head of pancreas (false-positive).

of pancreatic cancer.[21, 29] However, Ralls et al.[30] found the characteristic pancreatographic changes of chronic pancreatitis and carcinoma to be less useful in differentiating benign from malignant disorders. In this blind study of pancreatic ductograms from 49 patients with ductal narrowing, there were 8 with carcinoma and 41 with chronic pancreatitis. Eccentric, nodular, narrowed segments occurred in both groups, and the authors concluded that morphologic ductal changes alone were unreliable with regard to differential diagnosis. Their most reliable criterion for chronic pancreatitis was multiple stenoses in the pancreatic duct, and they considered the diagnosis of pancreatic cancer unreliable if evidence of chronic pancreatitis was also present.

Frick et al.[29] studied the accuracy of ERCP in the differentiation between benign and malignant pancreatic disease. ERCP x-rays from 71 patients were reviewed in random order and without reference to other clinical, laboratory, or radiologic data. Final diagnosis was confirmed by laparotomy or 2-year clinical follow-up. Pancreatic carcinoma was diagnosed in 33 cases. Accuracy in the detection of pancreatic cancer was 88%; in the detection of chronic pancreatitis, 85%. The findings by ERCP correctly differentiated benign from malignant disease in 90% of the patients. Carcinoma had developed in a gland already affected by chronic pancreatitis in 3 patients and was misdiagnosed as only chronic pancreatitis in all of these patients.

Gilmore et al.[31] evaluated 400 ERCP x-rays to determine the accuracy of ERCP in the diagnosis of pancreatic cancer. ERCP findings were positive in 62% of the 32 patients with proved pancreatic carcinoma. There were 4 false-negative and 4 false-positive diagnoses. Of the false-positive results, 2 occurred in patients with chronic pancreatitis, 1 was due to main pancreatic obstruction produced by an abdominal aortic aneurysm, and 1 was due to a congenitally short pancreas. The procedure was not diagnostic in 12 patients (38%). In 8 of these the pancreatic duct was not opacified. In 4 of these 8 patients abnormalities of the duodenal mucosa or papilla suggested carcinoma, but biopsies were negative. In the other 4 patients cannulation was successful but there was no opacification of the ductal system. The remaining 4 of the 12 nondiagnostic studies consisted of the group with a false-negative diagnosis, although retrospectively there was evidence of carcinoma on the pancreatogram

of 1 of these 4. Endoscopy, pancreatography, and cholangiography were unequivocally normal in only 1 of the 32 patients. In this patient a 5 × 5 cm inoperable tumor mass was found in the body of the pancreas.

Early Diagnosis

A second problem with ERCP diagnosis of carcinoma of the pancreas is that in the majority of cases the diagnosed cancer is far advanced and surgically unresectable.[3, 4] In our series, resection was possible in only 25 of 252 cases (9.9%); in 20 of these patients the cancer was in the head, and in 5 its origin was the body or tail. The prognosis for patients undergoing resection, however, remains poor in most cases. Although serendipitous detection of pancreatic cancer in a relatively unadvanced stage has been reported,[32] early detection by ERCP has been essentially unsuccessful. As a screening test, ERCP is impractical, and the complication rate, albeit low, is prohibitive. At present, there is no effective screening method that detects early or small pancreatic cancers or leads to their detection by ERCP (Figs. 39–13 and 39–14).

Extent of Pancreatic Cancer

The third problem with respect to ERCP in pancreatic cancer is difficulty in evaluating the extent of invasion or resectability of the cancer. This is beyond the capability of ERCP at the present stage of development. In 1975 Clouse et al.[33] suggested the combined use of angiography and CT as an effective way to define the size, extension, and resectability of the cancer. Another approach is to consider that most pancreatic carcinomas are unresectable or that on the whole, surgical resection leads at best to a small improvement in survival of patients with pancreatic cancer. This has led to less invasive methods of management such as CT or ultrasonographically guided fine-needle aspiration cytology for tissue diagnosis, coupled with endoscopic endoprosthesis placement for biliary obstruction and sophisticated methods of pain management. This end-stage approach to the disorder reflects the want of a method of early diagnosis.

Another approach is the aggressive use of available diagnostic methods in an effort to define resectable lesions. Mackie et al.[34] studied the value of ultrasonography, CT, scintiscanning, ERCP, secretin-stimulated duodenal aspiration cytology, and angiography

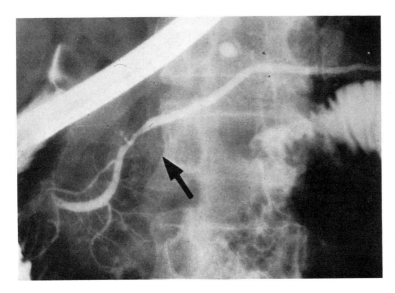

FIGURE 39–13. Mild irregularity of the main pancreatic duct with abnormal branches (*arrow*) in head of pancreas, due to small cancer of pancreas.

in 186 patients with symptoms suggestive of pancreatic carcinoma. The final diagnosis was pancreatic cancer in 73 patients (39%), other malignancy in 31 (17%), and other benign disorders in 82 patients (44%). In 28 patients the pancreatic carcinoma was resectable. In these patients the mean diameter of the tumor was 3.35 cm (range 1.4 to 6.5 cm); the majority had obstructive jaundice. The frequency of resectable tumors identified by the various studies was as follows: ultrasonography 96%, ERCP 87%, cytology 75%, angiography 75%, and scintiscan 47%. Ultrasonography was also found to be more sensitive and CT considerably less sensitive in the diagnosis of resectable as opposed to unresectable lesions. The technical failure rates for ultrasonography, CT, and ERCP were 8%, 10% and 15%, respectively.

Nix et al.[35] reported the results of a 10-year study of 123 patients with carcinoma of the head of the pancreas who underwent ERCP. Many patients had "early," nonspecific complaints such as the sudden onset of diabetes mellitus (33.3%), weight loss (80.5%), tiredness and malaise (42.3%), change in bowel habits (41.5%), and upper abdominal discomfort (22.0%). Jaundice (88.6%) and pain typical of pancreatic cancer (70.7%) were considered late symptoms. The diagnostic accuracy of ERCP was 92.7% and was considerably higher than that of CT (58.5%) or ultrasonography (54.4%). The patients were divided into three groups according to tumor diameter; group 1, diameter 2.5 to 4 cm (44 patients); group 2, diameter 4.5 to 6 cm (45 patients); and group 3, diameter 7 to 15 cm (34 patients). Resection for cure was possible in 22% of the patients, and in these the 4-year survival was 44%. Four-year survival for the entire group of patients was 7.9%. Over the decade-long study period there was a tendency toward diagnosis of smaller tumors that had a higher chance of resectability. The authors suggested that aggressive use of ERCP in patients with nonspecific, "early" symptoms might improve the results of treatment of pancreatic cancer.

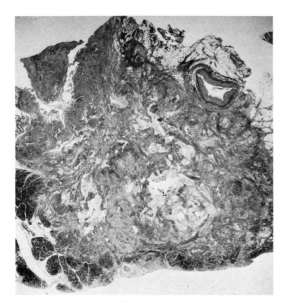

FIGURE 39–14. Photomicrograph of cross section of resected pancreas showing small cancer (18 × 15 × 13 mm) from same patient as Figure 39–13.

Endoscopic Retrograde Parenchymography of the Pancreas (ERPP)

Visualization of the pancreas by present ERCP technology is usually limited to the main pancreatic duct and secondary or tertiary branch ducts. Opacification of the ductal system to a greater degree has been thought to be associated with an increased incidence of post-ERCP acute pancreatitis.[3, 4] This means that detection of a tumor requires that the lesion arise in the main duct or in a branch duct near the main duct, such that the main duct becomes obstructed or stenotic. However, a small tumor located away from the main duct would be difficult to recognize even if some abnormality of a branch duct or ducts could be localized.

To overcome these limitations of standard pancreatography in the detection of small cancers and the differential diagnosis of cancer of the pancreas, it would be advantageous to opacify the parenchyma of the entire pancreas provided this would not cause pancreatitis. A small tumor would then appear radiographically as a filling defect in the pancreatic field. Parenchymography of the pancreas (ERPP) was first performed safely by Yoshimoto et al.[36] We have also evaluated the practical applications and usefulness of this method of pancreatic imaging.[37]

Technique

The technique of ERPP is similar to that of ERCP. However, a nonionic surfactant is mixed with the contrast medium to increase permeability. The medium used is a 20 ml solution of sodium iothalamate or sodium diatrizoate mixed with 100 to 500 mg of Menoquinon 4 (Eisai Co.), which contains a surfactant, HCO-60. After pancreatic ductograms have been obtained by standard injection technique, this contrast medium is also injected by hand into the pancreatic duct via the ERCP cannula. Total opacification of the acini occurs in 10 to 50 seconds, at which point the parenchymogram x-ray may be obtained. The modified contrast medium usually disappears rapidly upon withdrawal of the catheter, even in cases where a dense radiographic shadow of the pancreas is produced.

Minute pancreatic detail can be demonstrated by pancreatic parenchymography (Fig. 39–15). In our experience of more than 500 cases, a parenchymogram was obtained using the technique described above in 73.3% of cases. A similar x-ray picture could only be produced with the standard technique in 26.5% of cases, a statistically significant difference. The success of parenchymography and the extent of visualization of the pancreatic parenchyma depend on injection pressure, the amount of contrast medium–surfactant solution injected, and also on the degree of abnormality of the pancreatic ducts. With severe abnormalities visualization has been poor; when changes in the pancreatic ducts are less severe, better opacification of the parenchyma of the entire pancreas can be obtained.[37] In our series of ERPP procedures, serum amylase levels were elevated afterwards more often (60% of cases)

FIGURE 39–15. Normal parenchymograph of pancreas produced by ERPP.

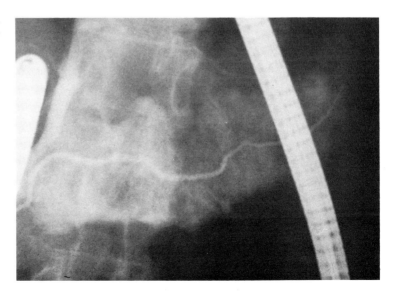

than after standard pancreatography, but these high levels did not persist. There has been no evidence of acute pancreatitis as a complication of ERPP using a surfactant-containing contrast medium.

Visualization of the Pancreas

No minute or early cancer of the pancreas has yet been detected by ERPP alone; however, advanced cancers were clearly demonstrated in 70% of the cases with the use of the surfactant method (Table 39–4). The characteristic parenchymographic finding with pancreatic carcinoma is a filling defect in the pancreatic field (Fig. 39–16). In contrast, an irregular pancreatic contour or minimal visualization of the parenchyma are the usual findings in chronic pancreatitis. Thus, ERPP has been of assistance in the pancreatographic differentiation of carcinoma and chronic pancreatitis when malignancy is either suspected or in doubt. In a few cases, minute filling defects in the pancreatic field have been recognized in patients with localized chronic pancreatitis with fibrosis. This suggests that minute cancers of the pancreas might be detectable using this technique.

Retrograde Pancreatography with Computed Tomography (CT)

Several authors have performed CT of the pancreas shortly after retrograde injection of contrast medium into the pancreatic duct.[38, 39] This technique is based on the finding that small amounts of contrast medium remain in the peripheral pancreatic acini and ducts after opacification, and that the presence of this material enhances pancreatic CT scans. This technique has been proposed as useful in differential diagnosis—the differentiation of chronic pancreatitis from pancreatic cancer, for example—and for the demonstration of the extent of pancreatic carcinoma.[38, 39] However, no extensive clinical trials have been reported.

TABLE 39–4. **Results of Endoscopic Retrograde Parenchymography (ERPP) in Cancer of the Pancreas**

Contrast Medium	No. of Patients	Visualization		
		Good	*Poor*	*Not Obtained*
With surfactant	25	16 (64%)	4 (16%)	5 (20%)
Without surfactant	25	6 (24%)	9 (36%)	10 (40%)

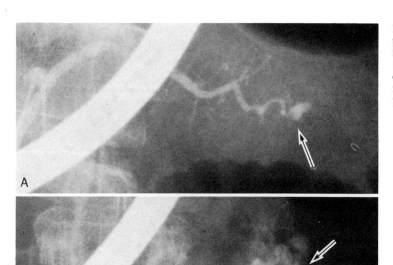

FIGURE 39–16. Cancer of tail of pancreas. *A,* Standard ERCP showing irregularity and cystic dilation (*arrow*) of main duct in tail; *B,* ERPP of same region demonstrates irregular filling defects (*arrows*) in pancreatic field in tail.

NEW ENDOSCOPIC METHODS FOR DIAGNOSIS OF PANCREATIC CANCER

Peroral Cholangiopancreatoscopy (PCPS)

Peroral cholangiopancreatoscopy (PCPS) is the result of recent improvements in the design of small-caliber fiberoptic instruments. The technical and practical aspects of PCPS are discussed in Chapter 10, part 4. PCPS can provide reasonably good visualization of both the bile and pancreatic ductal systems, although there are still certain mechanical and technical limitations. PCPS may be useful in the interpretation of doubtful or suspiciously abnormal ductograms provided by ERCP, PTC, or other radiographic studies. In our experience, tumors of the pancreas can be readily inspected using this new endoscopic technique. Findings include irregular stenosis, obstruction, or polypoid lesions of the main pancreatic duct.

Endoscopic Ultrasonography (EUS)

In recent years, abdominal ultrasonography (US) has been widely used as a diagnostic tool. Because of its noninvasiveness, US has special value in the visualization of tumors of the liver, bile duct, and pancreas. However, ultrasonographic detection of small cancers of the pancreas remains difficult because of technical restrictions presented by intraabdominal gas, subcutaneous fatty tissue, bone, and the anatomically deeper position of the pancreas.

Intraluminal ultrasonography is presently under development as a method to circumvent some of these problems. Since the initial reports of EUS by Hisanaga et al.[40] and DiMagno et al.,[41] the instruments and techniques for EUS have evolved rapidly.[42, 43] We have found EUS to be valuable clinically, especially in the diagnosis of cancer of the pancreas.[44, 45] EUS is discussed in Chapter 10, part 1.

Instruments and Techniques

The echoendoscope we use is a forward oblique-viewing instrument that contains a sector scan transducer at the tip (Olympus Co). EUS is performed after the introduction of the echoendoscope into the stomach and

FIGURE 39–17. Demonstration of pancreas by endoscopic ultrasonography (EUS). *A*, Transduodenal approach (GB = gallbladder, CBD = common bile duct, PV = portal vein, P = pancreas); *B*, Transgastric approach (p. duct = main pancreatic duct, SV = splenic vein, L.K. = left kidney).

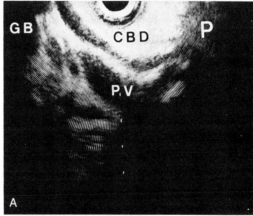

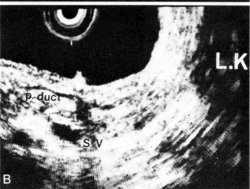

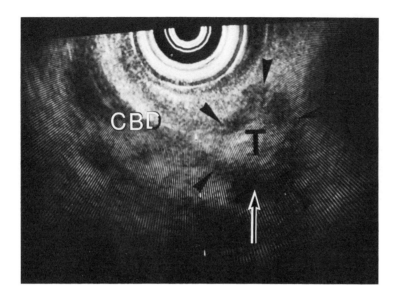

FIGURE 39–18. Small cancer in head of pancreas (*arrow, arrowheads*) that was only detected by EUS (T = tumor, CBD = common bile duct).

duodenum, using standard local pharyngeal anesthesia and intravenous premedication. Two EUS scanning methods are available: In the balloon-tip method a water-filled balloon is placed on the tip of the instrument over the transducer in order to provide good contact with the gastroduodenal wall. We have used this method mainly for imaging the bile duct and entire pancreas through the gastroduodenal wall. In the water-filled stomach method, 300 to 800 ml of deaerated water are placed in the stomach. We find this technique to be useful for visualization of the body and tail of the pancreas.

Demonstration of the Pancreas

Images of the gallbladder, bile duct, portal vein, splenic vein, pancreas, pancreatic duct, and kidneys can be obtained by EUS (Fig. 39–17). Tumors of the pancreas are usually shown as hypoechogenic lesions. In our series of 15 patients with cancer of the pancreas examined by EUS, all tumors were clearly demonstrated. In three of these cases the cancer was less than 30 mm in size, and none of these were detected by conventional US. EUS revealed a small, hypoechogenic mass (18 × 14 mm) within the head of the pan-

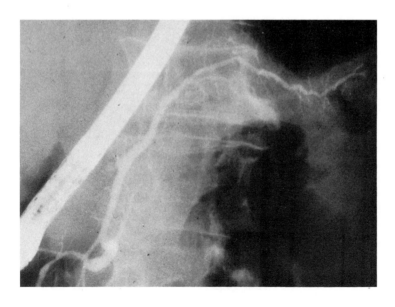

FIGURE 39–19. Retrograde pancreatogram from same patient as in Figure 39–18, showing no abnormality.

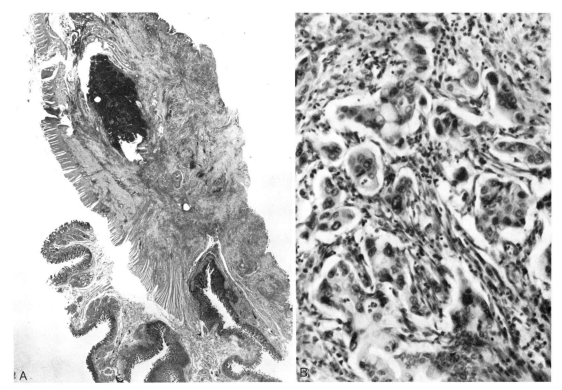

FIGURE 39–20. Photomicrographs of resected specimen from same patient as in Figures 39–18 and 39–19. A small (20 × 20 × 15 mm) carcinoma is present.

creas in one of these patients, who had a small pancreatic cancer and slight jaundice (Fig. 39–18). ERCP in this patient did not define any abnormality in the pancreatic ducts (Fig. 39–19), nor was there any evidence of the tumor by US, CT, and angiography. The resected specimen was an 18 × 13 × 15 mm histologically well-differentiated adenocarcinoma of the pancreas (Fig. 39–20).

EUS appears to be a safe and effective procedure that can provide excellent visualization of the pancreas as well as other organs. However, the technique has not undergone extensive clinical trials and should be considered investigational at the present time. Although it has certain advantages over conventional ultrasonography, EUS also has technical limitations that currently restrict its use. It is expected that newer-generation instruments will overcome some of the present restrictions. It is possible that the more frequent use of a technique such as EUS may lead to detection of small cancers of the pancreas that might be overlooked by present standard procedures such as conventional ultrasonography.

References

1. Zimmon DS, Breslaw J, Kessler RE. Endoscopy with endoscopic cholangiopancreatography. The combination as a primary diagnostic procedure. JAMA 1975; 233:447–9.
2. Kasugai T. Recent advances in the endoscopic retrograde cholangiopancreatography. Digestion 1975; 13:76–99.
3. Cotton PB. Progress report, ERCP. Gut 1977; 18:316–41.
4. Takemoto T, Kasugai T, eds. Endoscopic Retrograde Cholangiopancreatography. Tokyo, New York: Igakushoin, 1979.
5. Zonca M, Schuman BM, Wong KH. The diagnosis of cancer of the biliary tract and pancreas by endoscopic retrograde cannulation. Gastrointest Endosc 1975; 21:129–32.
6. Silvis SE, Rohrmann CA, Vennes JA. Diagnostic accuracy of endoscopic retrograde cholangiopancreatography in hepatic, biliary, and pancreatic malignancy. Ann Intern Med 1976; 84:438–40.
7. Wood RAB, Moossa AR, Blackstone MO, et al. Comparative value of four methods of investigating the pancreas. Surgery 1976; 80:518–22.
8. DiMagno EP, Malagelada JR, Taylor WF, Go WLW. A prospective comparison of current diagnostic tests for pancreatic cancer. N Engl J Med 1977; 297:737–42.
9. Freeny PC, Ball TJ. Endoscopic retrograde cholangiopancreatography (ERCP) and percutaneous transhepatic cholangiography (PTC) in the evaluation of suspected pancreatic carcinoma: diagnostic

limitations and contemporary roles. Cancer 1981; 47:1666–78.

10. Mackie CR, Cooper MJ, Lewis MH, Moossa AR. Non-operative differentiation between pancreatic cancer and chronic pancreatitis. Ann Surg 1979; 189:480–7.

11. Endo Y, Morii T, Tamura H, et al. Cytodiagnosis of pancreatic malignant tumors by aspiration under direct vision using a duodenal fiberscope. Gastroenterology 1974; 67:944–51.

12. Kawanishi H, Sell JE, Pollard HM. Combined endoscopic pancreatic fluid collection and retrograde pancreatography in the diagnosis of pancreatic cancer and chronic pancreatitis. Gastrointest Endosc 1975; 22:82–5.

13. Tsuchiya R, Henmi T, Kondo N, et al. Endoscopic aspiration biopsy of the pancreas. Gastroenterology 1977; 73:1050–2.

14. Robbins AH, Messian RA, Widrich WC, et al. Endoscopic pancreatography. An analysis of the radiologic findings in pancreatitis. Radiology 1974; 113: 293–6.

15. Moss AA, Federle M, Shapiro HA, et al. The combined use of computed tomography and endoscopic retrograde cholangiopancreatography in the assessment of suspected pancreatic neoplasm: a blind clinical evaluation. Radiology 1980; 134:159–63.

16. Frick MP, Feinberg SB, Goodale RL. The value of endoscopic retrograde cholangiopancreatography in patients with suspected carcinoma of the pancreas and indeterminate computed tomographic results. Surg Gynecol Obstet 1982; 155:177–82.

17. Fukumoto K, Nakajima N, Murakami K, et al. Diagnosis of pancreatic cancer by endoscopic pancreatocholangiography. Am J Gastroenterol 1974; 62:210–3.

18. Nakajima M, Yamagichi Y, Akasaka Y. Endoscopic retrograde cholangiopancreatography (ERCP) in the diagnosis of pancreatic cancer. In: Kawai K, ed. Early Diagnosis of Pancreatic Cancer. Tokyo, New York: Igakushoin, 1979; 140–5.

19. Stadelmann O, Safrany L, Loffler A, et al. Endoscopic retrograde cholangiopancreatography in the diagnosis of pancreatic cancer. Endoscopy 1974; 6:84–93.

20. Norton RA, Ogoshi K, Hara Y, et al. Pancreatographic abnormalities due to pancreatic cancer. Gastrointest Endosc 1973; 20:13–4.

21. Freeny PC, Bilbao MK, Katon RM. "Blind" evaluation of endoscopic retrograde cholangiopancreatography (ERCP) in the diagnosis of pancreatic carcinoma; The "double duct" and other signs. Radiology 1976; 119:271–4.

22. Rohrmann CA Jr, Silvis SE, Vennes JA. The significance of pancreatic ductal obstruction in differential diagnosis of the abnormal endoscopic retrograde pancreatogram. Radiology 1976; 121:311–4.

23. Plumley TF, Rohrmann CA, Freeny PC, et al. Double duct sign: reassessed significance in ERCP. AJR 1982; 138:31–5.

24. Swensen T, Osnes M, Serck-Hanssen A. Endoscopic retrograde cholangio-pancreatography in primary and secondary tumours of the pancreas. Br J Radiol 1980; 53:760–4.

25. Kreel L, Sandin B. Changes in pancreatic morphology associated with aging. Gut 1973; 14:962–70.

26. Rösch W, Koch H, Schaffner O, et al. The clinical significance of the pancreatic divisum. Gastrointest Endosc 1976; 22:206–7.

27. Ferrari BT, O'Holloran RL, Longmire WP Jr, Lewin KJ. Atypical papillary hyperplasia of the pancreatic duct mimicking obstructing pancreatic carcinoma. N Engl J Med 1979; 301:531–2.

28. Meakins JL, Stein LA. Postgastrectomy distortion of the pancreatic ducts simulating carcinoma. AJR 1976; 127:675–7.

29. Frick MP, O'Leary JF, Walker HC Jr, Goodale RL. Accuracy of endoscopic retrograde cholangiopancreatography (ERCP) in differentiating benign and malignant pancreatic disease. Gastrointest Radiol 1982; 7:241–4.

30. Ralls PW, Halls J, Renner I, Juttner H. Endoscopic retrograde cholangiopancreatography (ERCP) in pancreatic disease. A reassessment of the specificity of ductal abnormalities in differentiating benign from malignant disease. Radiology 1980; 134:347–52.

31. Gilmore IT, Pemberton J, Thompson RPH. Retrograde cholangiopancreatography in the diagnosis of carcinoma of the pancreas. Gastrointest Endosc 1982; 28:77–8.

32. Parke R, Sivak M, Cohen M, Talbert W Jr. Pancreatitis with coexistent pancreatic duct stone and carcinoma. Arch Intern Med 1977; 137:924–6.

33. Clouse ME, Gregg JA, Sedgwick CE. Angiography vs. pancreatography in the diagnosis of carcinoma of the pancreas. Radiology 1975; 114:605–10.

34. Mackie CR, Dhorajiwala J, Blackstone MO, et al. Value of new diagnostic aids in relation to the disease process in pancreatic cancer. Lancet 1979; 2:385–8.

35. Nix GAJJ, Schmitz PIM, Wilson JHP, et al. Carcinoma of the head of the pancreas. Therapeutic implications of endoscopic retrograde cholangiopancreatography findings. Gastroenterology 1984; 87:37–43.

36. Yoshimoto S, Doi S, Arao M, et al. A new method for the radiological opacification of the pancreas. Endoscopy 1978; 24:141–5.

37. Akasaka Y, Nakajima M, Yamaguchi K, et al. Diagnosis of pancreatic cancer by endoscopic retrograde parenchymography of the pancreas (ERPP). In: Kawai K, ed. Early Diagnosis of Pancreatic Cancer. Tokyo, New York: Igakushoin, 1980:155–63.

38. Frick MP, O'Leary JF, Salomonowitz E, et al. Pancreas imaging by computed tomography after endoscopic retrograde pancreatography. Radiology 1984; 150:191–4.

39. Jaffe MH, Glazer GM, Amendola MA, et al. Endoscopic retrograde computed tomography of the pancreas. J Comput Assist Tomogr 1984; 8:63–6.

40. Hisanaga K, Hisanaga A, Nagata K, et al. High speed rotating scanner for transgastric sonography. AJR 1980; 135:627–9.

41. DiMagno EP, Buxton JL, Regan RT, et al. Ultrasonic endoscope. Lancet 1980; 22:629–31.

42. Strohm WD, Phillip J, Haganmüller F, et al. Ultrasonic tomography by means of ultrasonic fiberendoscope. Endoscopy 1980; 12:241–4.

43. Lux G, Heyder N, Lutz H, et al. Endoscopic ultrasonography—technique, orientation and diagnostic possibilities. Endoscopy 1982; 14:220–5.

44. Yasuda K, Tanaka Y, Fujimoto S, et al. Use of endoscopic ultrasonography in small pancreatic cancer. Scand J Gastroenterol 1984; 19(suppl 102):9–17

45. Tanaka Y, Yasuda K, Aibe T, et al. Anatomical and pathological aspects in ultrasonic endoscopy for GI tract. Scand J Gastroenterol 1984; 19(suppl 94): 43–50.

Section IV

COLONOSCOPY

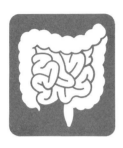

Chapter 40

TECHNIQUE OF COLONOSCOPY

YOSHIHIRO SAKAI, M.D., D.M.Sc.

Fiberoptic examination of the colon was introduced in routine endoscopic practice approximately 15 years ago. During this period, the colonoscope has been transformed by improvements in design and construction. The technique of colonoscopy has also changed with technologic improvement in the instrument. Fifteen years ago endoscopic examination of the colon was considered a special and difficult examination. Now it is more appropriate to use the term "lower panendoscopy" rather than colonoscopy since it is customary to insert the instrument tip beyond the ileocecal valve into the terminal ileum as far as 20 to 30 cm. The greater ability and knowledge of colonoscopists coupled with superior instrument design has led to the use of colonoscopy in lieu of x-ray constrast study of the colon in many clinical situations.

The endoscopist must know the indications and contraindications for lower panendoscopy; a thorough knowledge of the complications, the countermeasures for dealing with potential complications, and the clinical management of untoward results are also prerequisites. These are discussed in Chapter 41. The technique of lower panendoscopy is described in this chapter.

ANATOMY OF THE COLON AND RECTUM

The intestines are tubular organs that are placed in the abdominal cavity in a systematic way. The small intestine, transverse colon, and sigmoid colon are mobile by virtue of attachment to the mesentery. These segments shift position freely, being limited only by their length and the length of the mesenteric attachment. Their positions and configurations are uncertain and variable and are determined by extrinsic factors such as the influence of surrounding organs, adjacent segments of intestine or masses, the presence of adhesions or invasion by various pathologic processes, and the contents of the intestinal segment itself. Frequently the parts of the colon with a mesenteric attachment will be located close to the abdominal wall. The ascending and descending colon have no mesentery and are attached to the retroperitoneal wall; this attachment results in a relatively fixed configuration for these segments. The rectum differs from the aforementioned segments in that it passes through the pelvic connective tissue from the anus to the peritoneal reflection. Only a short segment of the proximal rectum is within the abdominal cavity.

Beginning at the anus and following the course of the colon in a retrograde fashion, the rectum turns posteriorly at the lower end of the coccyx to lie anterior to the sacrum and follows the gently curved course of this bony structure. After passing through the peritoneal reflection, the rectum joins the sigmoid colon to form a bend that projects anteriorly and toward the left and the sigmoid colon proper. The configuration and length of the sigmoid are extremely variable. In joining the descending colon, it often forms a bend that projects inferiorly and leftward. The descending colon has a relatively straight course ending at the splenic flexure where there is always an acute angulation as the colon changes direction abruptly to the right and anteriorly. In contrast to the course at the splenic flexure, the direction of the colon is posterior and then inferior at the hepatic flexure. The configuration of the mobile transverse colon segment between these two fixed flexures is variable. The course of the ascending colon and cecum is almost a straight line. The ileocecal valve marks the junction of the latter two segments, is usually located in the medial-posterior wall of the colon, and is usually oriented in an inferior direction. The cecum may vary in length and can occasionally be mobile. At each junction point of the several segments of the colon the nature of the colonic attachment changes from fixed to mobile or from mobile to fixed (Fig. 40–1).

Endoscopically, a regular arrangement of folds demarcates the haustra, or sacculations, of the colon (Fig. 40–2). The characteristic segmentation of the colon is produced by the longitudinal muscle of the bowel. This is less complete in comparison with the longitudinal muscle of the small intestine. Rather, there are three longitudinal muscle bands, each about 1.2 cm in diameter, that are parallel to the long axis of the colon. These teniae coli are superficial to the circular muscle and mucosa and are readily observed on the surface of the colon beneath the serosa. The teniae coli are slightly shorter than the colon proper, and therefore account for the sacculated, or haustrated, shape of the colon. They are usually not apparent endoscopically, although one or more can occasionally

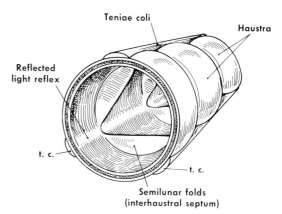

FIGURE 40–2. Gross anatomic structure of colon.

be seen in mobile segments of the colon when the lumen is maximally distended and there is tension on the wall, such as occurs when a colonic loop is formed during colonoscopy. When visible, the teniae coli always run parallel to the lumen and so indicate its course when this is not apparent at a flexure or acute angulation; generally the teniae coli, if observed, are perpendicular to the more familiar circular segmenting folds. They have their origin at the base of the appendix (the appendix has a complete coat of longitudinal muscle) and may be seen endoscopically as converging at the appendiceal orifice.

Crescentic folds, termed semilunar folds, also contribute to the pattern of regular segmentation of the colon that characterizes its endoscopic appearance (see Fig. 40–2). These folds, or septa, are sometimes incorrectly termed haustral folds. In the mobile segments of the colon each fold is circumferential; they are usually semilunar in shape in the fixed colonic segments. Endoscopically, the folds in the transverse colon form a triangular pattern due to tension in the longitudinal muscle fibers of the teniae coli. This appearance is characteristic of the transverse colon, although it is sometimes observed in other segments. Usually, three transverse plicae (valves of Houston) are found in the rectum; the proximal and distal plicae are on the right side of the rectum, with the middle one to the left.

The average caliber of the colon is 7.5 cm; the segment with the greatest diameter is usually the cecum, followed by the ascending colon and rectum. The wall of the colon is composed of four layers: mucosa, submucosa, muscle layer, and serosa (Fig. 40–3). There is a muscularis mucosae between mucosa and submucosa. The mucosal surface is

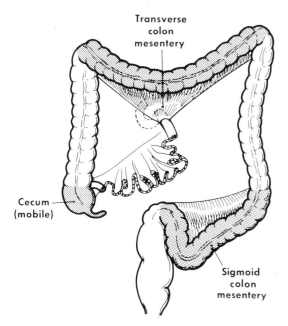

FIGURE 40–1. Position of colon within abdomen. Note that attachments of various sections alternate between fixed and mobile.

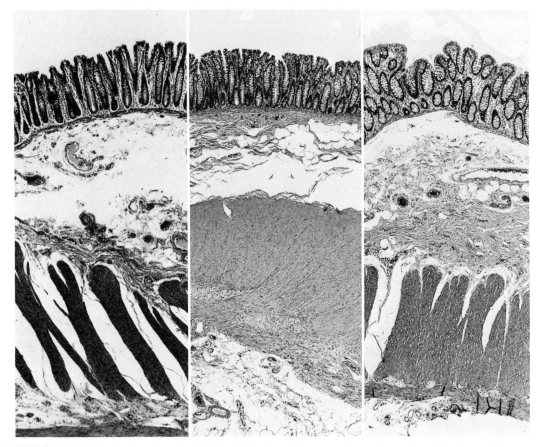

FIGURE 40–3. Histologic structure of colonic wall. *Left to right*, ascending colon, sigmoid colon, and rectum.

smooth and devoid of villi. Scattered solitary lymph follicles may be found, especially in the rectum and near the ileocecal valve, but these are less numerous than in the terminal ileum. The serosal coat is complete in the mobile portions of the colon except at the point of attachment to the mesentery; the serosa is incomplete over the ascending and descending colonic segments where they meet the posterior abdominal wall, and over the rectum.

INSTRUMENTS FOR COLONOSCOPY

More than 20 fiberoptic colonoscopes are available commercially. These have different purposes and capabilities.

Instruments for routine examinations are available in four insertion tube lengths; these are approximately 180 cm, 140 cm, 100 cm and 70 cm. Selection of an instrument depends on the segment of colon to be examined. The short instrument is used for endoscopy of the rectum and sigmoid colon in most cases; the longest is used for total colon-

oscopy and lower panendoscopy. When the patient has a short sigmoid colon, a medium length instrument (140 cm) is usually satisfactory for examination of the whole colon. Many endoscopists prefer this length of instrument for most routine examinations of the colon and terminal ileum. However, routine use of an intermediate length instrument requires meticulous technique with a constant effort to maintain the colon in as straight a configuration as possible.

Sometimes it is not possible to reach into the right side of the colon with an intermediate length instrument because the sigmoid colon is long and redundant or the transverse colon is especially long and ptotic in position, or both. For this type of technical problem some colonoscopists use a stiffening tube.

The stiffening tube must be placed over the insertion tube of the colonoscope before beginning the procedure. It is drawn backward to a position just ahead of the control section. Nevertheless, placement of the stiffening tube on the shaft of the endoscope reduces the usable length of the insertion tube. Therefore, the longer instrument (180 cm) is preferable if the stiffening tube is to be used.

Some colonoscopists also prefer the longer length instrument for lower panendoscopy, especially when the colon is long and redundant. The technique of colonoscopy does not differ in relation to differences in the length of available instruments; the technique for insertion is precisely the same whether the instrument is short or long.

Most currently available colonoscopes are about 13 mm in diameter. There are certain limitations with respect to the manufacture of colonoscopes; it is difficult to diminish caliber and still maintain satisfactory tip angulation, image quality, and an accessory channel of at least 2.8 mm diameter. The interrelations of the various components in an insertion tube are discussed in Chapter 2. Development of a narrow diameter instrument entails a penalty with respect to some other function—for example, a decrease in illumination or accessory channel diameter.

Some narrow diameter instruments have less torque or rotatory stability relative to standard diameter instruments. Rotatory (torque) stability refers to the ability of the insertion tube to transmit rotational motion from proximal to distal. When rotatory stability is poor, a twist at the mid-point of the insertion tube or a point nearer the control section results in a less than equal motion at the distal tip of the instrument; that is, some of the rotatory motion has been absorbed by the flexible shaft.

A small diameter insertion tube does not necessarily provide an advantage during insertion of the instrument. It does not, for example, provide greater capability for control of loop formation during the procedure. The use of the 11 mm diameter pediatric colonoscope in adult patients does not reduce discomfort. Patient discomfort is related to the difficulty of the examination and the skill of the operator. Some colonoscopists, however, find that it is possible to insert the pediatric colonoscope for a greater distance into the terminal ileum than is possible with a standard diameter instrument in adult patients; therefore they consider this type of instrument essential for lower panendoscopy.

Almost all modern colonoscopes have a 4-way tip angulation system. The maximal up/down deflection of the instrument tip is usually 180 degrees. However, if lateral bending of the tip is added after maximum upward (or downward) deflection, the bending angle of the fiberscope reaches 230 degrees (Fig. 40–4). This is more than adequate for most acute angulations that will be encountered, although in practice it is sometimes impossible to sufficiently angulate the instrument tip. When the insertion tube is formed into a loop of any kind, the wires that control deflection of the tip are stretched, and there is an increase in the frictional force that the wires encounter. As a result of these inherent properties of the endoscope, the maximum bending angle that may be achieved when the insertion tube is looped is diminished. This may be reduced

FIGURE 40–4. Distal aspect of insertion tube after maximal deflection using up/down and right/left deflection simultaneously. Narrow diameter (''pediatric'') instrument (*top*) and standard instrument with biopsy forceps (*bottom*) are shown.

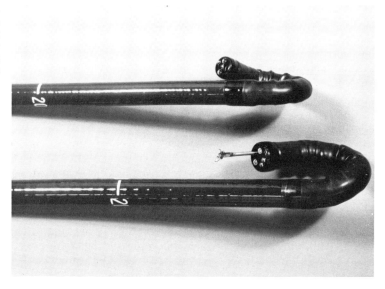

to as little as 150 degrees when looping is extreme.

The flexibility of the insertion tube varies over its length. Usually the distal portion is made more flexible than the middle and proximal sections. Ideally, the flexibility would gradually decrease, proceeding from distal tip to control section. However, it is technically difficult to make an instrument with a gradual change in flexibility. Therefore, presently available instruments have only two or three different degrees of flexibility built into the insertion tube. Furthermore, the point on the shaft where the more flexible distal section meets the more rigid middle section differs from model to model. This transitional point is usually placed 35 cm or 40 cm from the distal tip in an intermediate length instrument.

The flexibility characteristics of insertion tubes differ, depending on the manufacturer, and may not even be the same for different models produced by the same manufacturer. Flexibility refers to the inherent ability of the insertion tube to resist (or permit) bending. (This does not refer to the distal bending section of the shaft where tip deflection takes place.)

The flexibility of an instrument is an extremely important characteristic. In general, a high degree of insertion tube flexibility results in a decrease in torque (rotatory) stability. Instruments with greater flexibility tend to allow loop formation more readily. An instrument with high flexibility can also be pushed forward in the colon in spite of the loop, since the insertion tube will conform to the shape of the loop. Advancement of the instrument when there is a loop in the colon (and hence the instrument) is referred to as "pushing through the loop." A less flexible or stiffer instrument tends to resist loop formation.

The flexibility of any instrument can be altered somewhat during the examination by rotating or torquing the insertion tube. Part of the inner construction of an insertion tube consists of a metal tube made up of helical, interdigitating steel bands as well as a layer of steel mesh (see Chapter 2). This is the actual supporting framework of the insertion tube that gives it its shape and protects the inner vital parts. It is also the component that determines the flexibility and torque stability qualities of the instrument. When the instrument is rotated the metal compo-

nents tend to lock, so that this maneuver imparts a greater degree of rigidity to the shaft. This also produces some wear and tear, so that with usage over the course of time, an insertion tube tends to acquire a greater degree of flexibility.

Expert colonoscopists often have a preference for certain characteristics in an insertion tube. Generally, these preferences are related to their insertion technique. Those colonoscopists who attempt to straighten and pleat the colon over the insertion tube in an accordion-like fashion will usually prefer a shorter, "stiffer" insertion tube.

Improvements in the objective lens system of colonoscopes have made the endoscopic examination much easier. The angle of view was 60 degrees in the earliest models and was later increased to 100 degrees. Current instruments provide an angle of view of about 120 degrees. This ultra-wide lens system results in some distortion of the image at the periphery and slight exaggeration of distance in long tubular sections of the colon. Fortunately, these aberrations do not interfere with the examination, and the disadvantages are outweighed by some advantages.

With the wide-angle field small abnormalities at the periphery of the endoscopic field can be seen without difficulty. It is also easier to determine the course of the colon by observation of mucosal characteristics. Therefore, less maneuvering and tip deflection are required to orient the tip of the instrument in the proper direction, and insertion can be more precise and quick. Various endoscopic manipulations such as polypectomy can be accomplished more easily, and this improved optical system probably increases the reliability and safety of the procedure. Although a further increase in the angle of view is possible, the present systems are adequate.

In other respects, colonoscopes are similar to other standard endoscopes. Generally, there are two co-axial, independently locking control knobs for deflection of the tip, and push-button type valves for air and carbon dioxide insufflation, washing, and suction. All instruments have an accessory channel for insertion of various devices. The diameter of the accessory channel, and hence the size and type of accessory it will accommodate, varies from one instrument model and manufacturer to another. Most standard instruments have a channel diameter between 3 and 4 mm. The larger channel diameters are useful for quick aspiration of intestinal contents.

For examination of pediatric-age patients, the small diameter pediatric colonoscope is preferable (Fig. 40–4), although colonoscopic technique is the same as that for adults after the colonoscope is passed beyond the anus. Pediatriac colonoscopy is discussed in Chapter 48.

In addition to preparation of the fiberscope itself, it is advisable to prepare all the related accessories and equipment that will be needed for the procedure prior to beginning. The biopsy forceps, polypectomy snare (with extra wires), and electrosurgical generator should be ready for use at all times. Other necessities are the "hot-biopsy" forceps, specimen containers, polyp retrieval devices, and coagulating electrode. A loaded camera and extra film should also be at hand to make photographic records.

I prefer glycerin for lubrication of the anus. If Vaseline or olive oil is used for this purpose, the outer rubber coat over the distal bending section of the fiberscope tube will swell and gradually expand. This may lead to cracks in its surface that will allow water to enter and damage the instrument.

A stiffening tube (splinting device, overtube, sliding tube) is sometimes useful, especially when the patient is thought to have a long and redundant sigmoid colon (Fig. 40–5). A stiffening tube is a hollow tube about 40 cm long. It tapers slightly at its distal end so that its inner diameter approximates that of the insertion tube with a few millimeters to spare. The main purpose of this device is to maintain the sigmoid colon in a straightened configuration. This will make examination of the more proximal segments of the colon easier. The endoscope may also be withdrawn through the stiffening tube and removed from the colon, leaving the stiffening tube in place. This facilitates examination when it is necessary to reinsert the instrument several times as, for example, to remove numerous polyps.

The stiffening tube cannot be inserted prior to insertion of the colonoscope because for safe insertion it is necessary that the sigmoid be in a straight alignment with the descending colon and rectum. This configuration can only be maintained with the colonoscope inserted to the splenic flexure. If a loop has developed in the sigmoid colon during insertion, the loop must be removed and the sigmoid colon straightened before attempting to insert the stiffening tube. The stiffening tube must be placed on the colonoscope prior to insertion; it is not possible to do so after insertion.

Although it is essential that the sigmoid colon be straight during advancement of the stiffening tube along the outside of the insertion tube of the colonoscope, it is advisable that fluoroscopy be used to monitor placement of the stiffening tube. Some expert colonoscopists may occasionally use the stiffening tube without the aid of fluoroscopy, but this requires considerable expertise and experience. If the sigmoid colon cannot be straightened, the stiffening tube should not be used.

An internal stiffening wire-like device has been used to circumvent some of the disad-

FIGURE 40–5. Devices for "stiffening" the insertion tube: stiffening wire (*top*) and stiffening tube (*bottom*).

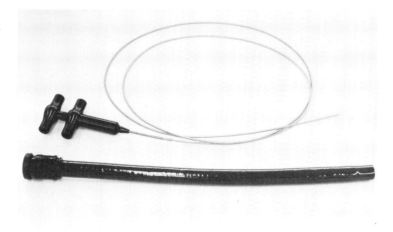

vantages of the stiffening tube (see Fig. 40–5). This device is inserted through the accessory channel of the endoscope. When the wire is tightened it imparts a greater degree of stiffness to the insertion tube. This type of stiffening device does not reduce the working length of the endoscope, but the degree of stiffening imparted to the endoscope is not great. It is also not possible to use the accessory channel for other purposes when the stiffening wire is in place. Some endoscopists have found that this instrument can damage the glass fiber bundle. For these reasons, the internal stiffening wire is not used widely.

The use of fluoroscopy during colonoscopy is not necessary in the majority of examinations. It is recommended, however, that colonoscopy be performed with the aid of fluoroscopy until the examiner gains adequate experience. Fluoroscopy demonstrates the configuration of the instrument within the colon, including any loops that have formed. This gives the student a more immediate picture and understanding of the consequences of various maneuvers and motions. With greater experience, the colonoscopist learns to anticipate and recognize the configurations that the colon takes in response to the maneuvers that are part of the insertion technique. When fluoroscopy is in use the endoscope should never be advanced by reference to the x-ray image alone; the x-ray image provides a view in only one plane, making it hazardous to push the instrument forward while simply referring to the fluoroscopic image.

Fluoroscopy shortens the learning period, but it must be used judiciously to minimize x-ray exposure to the patient, colonoscopist, and assisting personnel. Over the course of time x-rays also damage the fiberoptic bundles of the endoscope, and excessive use of fluoroscopy will shorten the useful life of the instrument.

Expert colonoscopists will sometimes resort to fluoroscopy during colonoscopy in especially difficult cases in which the colon is long and redundant, in order to minimize patient discomfort and shorten the time required for the examination. When a lesion has been identified within the colon, it can be located precisely by fluoroscopic reference to the position of the tip of the colonoscope within the colon.

Meticulous care must be taken to avoid contamination of the examining table and room. When an infectious disease is suspected—for example, amebic colitis, dysentery, or tuberculosis—a mask, gown, and gloves should be worn by all personnel. The use of disposable drapes and pads under the patient's hip and thigh is advisable in such situations. As the instrument is moved in and out of the patient's anus during insertion, and during the concluding withdrawal and examination of the colon, an assistant can clean the insertion tube with swabs soaked in alcohol.

PREPARATION AND PREMEDICATION

Preparation

For satisfactory lower panendoscopy, the intestinal contents must be removed completely. Large amounts of stool compromise endoscopic observation and make insertion of the fiberscope difficult. When observation is limited, the risk and the possibility of overlooking important pathologic findings are increased. Once stool adheres to the objective lens a great deal of effort and time may be required to remove it. Generally this necessitates additional maneuvering and extra use of the air-water insufflation and perhaps supplemental washing of larger quantities of water directly through the accessory channel. Liquid stool can be aspirated through the accessory channel, but also increases examination time. Large quantities of mucus are sometimes encountered; although this does not hinder insertion, it may make observation more difficult.

When problems with the preparation of the colon are encountered, the bowel tends to become overinflated as the colonoscopist struggles to clear the endoscopic field. Overinflation of the more proximal segments of the colon increases patient discomfort and produces a greater degree of angulation at the bends and flexures that increases the technical difficulty of the procedure.

Unfortunately, there is no completely reliable preparation method. Castor oil and other laxatives have been used, but poor results may occur with almost any method. One of the essential elements for good bowel preparation is the cooperation of the patient. If patients are to prepare themselves, they must be aware of the necessity of good bowel preparation, must understand what is expected of them, and must have specific, preferably written instructions.

If the colon is not especially redundant, the use of repeated saline cleansing enemas alone will adequately prepare the greater part of the colon. However, this is time-consuming and laborious and requires a patient nursing staff who are able to coach the patient through this troublesome process.

I have had good results with a modification of a bowel preparation method introduced by Brown[1] for x-ray examination of the colon. Enemas are not required with this method (Table 40–1), which has become popular in Japan. Magnesium citrate is required in this method (see Table 40–1); since it is a little bitter and induces some degree of nausea in most patients, in the modified method, one half the original dose is administered along with 10 ml of 0.75% sodium picosulfate.

Brown's method is most useful for removing the contents of the left side of the colon but is less reliable for complete cleansing of the right side. Thick fluid or sticky mucus may sometimes remain in the ascending colon and cecum. Small lesions in these segments may be overlooked if the examination is cursory. When diminutive lesions are suspected, it is sometimes necessary to change the patient's position to move fluid away from the area to be examined or to spray the surface with lukewarm water by means of a catheter introduced through the accessory channel.

A relatively standard preparatory procedure consists of a clear liquid diet for 24 to 48 hours prior to the examination, a laxative during the late afternoon of the day before the procedure, and the use of enemas beginning about 2 hours before colonoscopy. Citrate of magnesia (10 ounces) is the commonly used laxative.

If the patient is to self-administer the enemas, a pre-prepared type in a disposable administration container is most satisfactory. Self-administered enemas are often less effective than those supervised by the nursing staff. The results may be improved by having the patient give himself a second enema. Some patients may be anxious concerning the enema and fearful that it will cause some injury to the anus or rectum. This reservation must be identified by the endoscopist or assistant staff beforehand if poor preparation of the colon is to be avoided. In such cases it is best that the enemas be given by an experienced member of the endoscopy staff. Some colonoscopists prefer that this is done in all cases, since the results are generally better. Warm tap water or saline enemas given until the return is clear are suitable for this purpose. About 500 ml are required in the average patient.

Colonic lavage has also become a commonly used method of preparation. A large volume of appropriate fluid is ingested or instilled via a nasogastric tube at a fast rate until clear watery diarrhea results. One of the main advantages of this method is that the colon can be fully prepared in 4 to 6 hours.

The first attempts at lavage preparation of the bowel utilized saline or electrolyte solutions balanced to reflect the concentration of electrolytes in the serum. Although effective for cleansing the colon, these solutions, including the balanced electrolyte solution, produced a net gain in weight and absorption of significant quantities of sodium and chlo-

TABLE 40–1. **Preparation of the Colon by Modified Brown's Method***

12 Noon	Lunch—1 cup of bouillon soup with crackers; 1 white-meat chicken sandwich (no butter, lettuce, mayonnaise, or other additive); ½ glass of clear apple or grape juice; 1 serving of plain gelatin dessert (no cream, fruit, or other additive); 1 glass of skimmed or non-fat dry milk.
1 PM	1 Full glass or more of water.
3 PM	1 Full glass or more of water.
5 PM	Supper—1 cup of bouillon soup; 1 glass of clear apple or grape juice; 1 serving of plain gelatin dessert (no cream, fruit, or other additive).
7 PM	1 Full glass or more of water.
8 PM	250 ml bottle of magnesium citrate (cold).
10 PM	3 Bisacodyl tablets with full glass or more of water.
Midnight	1 Full glass or more of water.
7 AM	1 Bisacodyl rectal suppository.

*Adapted from Brown GR. A new approach to colon preparation for barium enema. Univ Mich Med Bull 1961; 27:225–230.

ride.[2, 3] Fluid and electrolyte retention makes these solutions hazardous for certain patients, such as those with renal failure or congestive heart failure.

To circumvent the problem of fluid and electrolyte absorption, other lavage solutions have been developed that contain sodium sulfate and other osmotically active agents such as mannitol or polyethylene glycol (PEG).[4] The substitution of a sulfate salt for the chloride salt of sodium markedly reduces the active absorption of sodium that normally takes place in the intestine. However, the use of this divalent compound results in a hypotonic solution that if used alone would result in water absorption. In order to make the solution isosmotic with the plasma, a nonabsorbable solute is required. Mannitol is converted to hydrogen by bacterial action in the colon, and this creates an explosion hazard if electrosurgery devices are being employed, unless an inert gas such as carbon dioxide is used for insufflation.[5] The substitution of PEG for mannitol avoids this problem, and it is used in most of the commercially available colonic lavage solutions. Although it is likely that some electrolyte shifts between the plasma and the gut occur with these whole-gut lavage solutions, the net absorption or loss of fluid and electrolytes is minimal.

Colonic lavage preparation has some disadvantages. Many patients have an aversion to the nasogastric tube method of instillation. The patient may simply ingest the lavage solution, but this must be done at the rate of at least one liter per hour. It has a salty taste that can be disguised by chilling or by addition of lemon flavoring. However, patients often feel chilly and uncomfortable from drinking a large quantity of cold liquid. Rapid ingestion of large volumes of fluid also produces nausea and sometimes vomiting. To reduce these side effects, many authors recommend administration of metaclopramide by mouth or intramuscularly 30 to 45 minutes before the patient begins to ingest the solution.[6-8] Ernstoff et al.[9] found this to be unnecessary with most patients. Many authors indicate that the lavage preparation is well tolerated and preferred by the majority of patients.

It is difficult to determine whether one method of preparation is superior to the others. Ernstoff et al.[9] compared colonic lavage with the established method comprising three days of clear liquid diet; 240 ml of magnesium citrate and 10 mg of bisacodyl by mouth on the second and third nights; and, on the morning of the procedure, enemas until return of clear fluid. In this blind clinical trial, the lavage solution provided a significantly better colon preparation. These investigators also found that examination time was shorter with the lavage method.

The method of preparation should in practice be tailored to the personality and condition of the patient. For those who are habitually constipated, it may be necessary to extend the period of clear liquid intake and to use additional doses of laxatives. If the patient has diarrhea—for example, associated with inflammatory bowel disease—it is often necessary to eliminate laxatives from the preparation and rely on liquid diet and gentle cleansing enemas. Motivated, impatient individuals may prefer the lavage preparation; others may prefer the longer method with clear liquid diet, laxatives, and enemas. If any degree of obstruction is suspected, tap water enemas alone may be suitable. In clinical situations in which expeditious endoscopic examination would be useful, such as recent or persistent colonic hemorrhage, the lavage preparation is ideal.

Premedication

Most patients experience some discomfort, usually abdominal cramps, during colonoscopy. This results from stretching of the bowel and its mesentery and is impossible to avoid completely. To minimize pain and discomfort, it is customary to administer a narcotic agent intravenously, such as meperidine (50 to 100 mg), prior to beginning the procedure. Diazepam is often given intravenously either alone on in conjunction with meperidine. There have been attempts to utilize inhalation of nitrous oxide for sedation and analgesia during colonoscopy, but this is complicated and the results are often unsatisfactory. Rectal administration of sedative agents (e.g., diazepam, 20 mg) has also been introduced recently. Diazepam given by this route is absorbed relatively quickly and reaches a peak serum level after about 15 minutes. Rectal administration usually provides adequate sedation and avoids some of the side effects inherent to the intravenous approach, such as thrombophlebitis.

With the use of small amounts of sedative drugs, the procedure can be performed with minimal discomfort if the insertion technique is skillful and the instrument is introduced slowly and carefully. The dosages of sedative and analgesic agents should be kept to a minimum. Deep sedation and analgesia may blunt responsiveness so completely that the patient does not complain when unacceptable and inept techniques are being used to insert the instrument. The experienced colonoscopist judges the level of discomfort and makes appropriate changes in technique in the lightly sedated patient with mild to moderate analgesia for pain. In the obtunded patient the use of excessive force may not be appreciated and a complication becomes more probable. The amounts of sedative and analgesic drugs administered should be tailored to the patient's size, condition, anxiety level, and ability to tolerate discomfort. Inexperienced examiners tend to titrate the medication according to their lack of skill. This often leads to repeated dosages during prolonged procedures. It is far better to equate patient safety and comfort with the skill of the operator rather than with the dosage of medication.

Anticholinergic drugs are not effective for decreasing pain and discomfort. In addition, the hypotonicity they induce in the bowel enhances loop formation of the colon. In fact, difficulty with insertion of the endoscope may be compounded by hypotonicity of the colon. However, anticholinergic agents are occasionally useful when contractile activity disturbs observation of fine mucosal detail or renders polypectomy difficult. If this type of drug is to be used, it should be administered only after reaching the cecum or terminal ileum.

TECHNIQUES OF LOWER PANENDOSCOPY

General Methods

An endoscope can be manipulated in a limited number of ways. These are forward and backward movement of the insertion tube, rotatory or twisting motion, tip deflection, air insufflation and suction, application of external pressure on the insertion tube, and changes in the relative position of the instrument by changing the position of the patient. The number of options is sufficient, however, to permit a substantial number of combinations. The skilled colonoscopist accomplishes the procedure with the smallest number of choices. These manipulations can be performed by one person alone or two working together.

In the two-person technique, one individual operates the tip deflection controls and the other advances and withdraws the instrument. Good technique requires simultaneous and coordinated use of the different ways in which the instrument can be manipulated. This is difficult to achieve with the two-person technique and can only be done when both individuals understand the technique of colonoscopy. The worst method is to allow an assistant with little or no understanding of the nuances of the procedure to advance and withdraw the instrument. This discards all the information that can be gained from the behavior of the insertion tube; more importantly the chief operator has no awareness of how hard the assistant is pushing.

In the one-person technique, the left hand operates the up/down deflection control (never the lateral deflection); the right hand advances and withdraws the instrument. The lateral deflection control may be used, but this is done by shifting the right hand back and forth between the insertion tube and the control knob. During the early stages of the insertion procedure, the shaft may be held by an assistant when the operator wishes to use lateral deflection to prevent the instrument from falling out of the rectum. But the assistant never advances or withdraws the instrument.

Although it would seem that the one-person technique sacrifices some of the ability to turn the instrument tip to the left or right, it is nevertheless possible to move the tip in a 360-degree arc just as if the two control knobs were being used. This is accomplished by a combination of rotation and upward (or downward) tip deflection. For example, if the operator wishes to turn right, this can be accomplished by rotating the insertion tube 90 degrees to the right (clockwise) while turning the tip upward (Fig. 40–6). Furthermore, advancement or withdrawal can be added to this maneuver as desired.

Since the closer the right hand is to the tip, the greater the control of the end of the instrument, it is best to grasp the insertion tube with the right hand about 20 cm from the anus. Thus positioned, the right hand can also move the insertion tube forward as needed.

The one-person technique works best if the height of the examining table is about level to the colonoscopist's hip. The length of the insertion tube external to the patient should not be allowed to lie on the table and

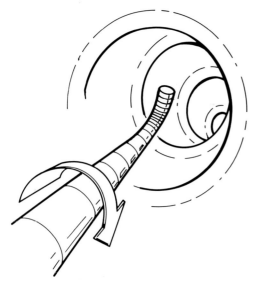

FIGURE 40–6. Tip deflection and rotation to direct endoscope tip toward lumen.

form a loop. In order to be able to rotate the insertion tube both left and right, it is necessary that the control section, the insertion tube, and the patient's anus be more or less within the same plane. When the insertion tube is allowed to lie on the examination table it is in effect being rotated to either the left or right. This may or may not be desirable at a given point in the insertion procedure. Some colonoscopists avoid this by bringing the patient close to the edge of the table and allowing the insertion tube to drape over the edge.[10] To prevent the instrument from falling out by virtue of the weight of the insertion tube, the operator holds it against the side of the table with his right hip when he wishes to use the lateral deflection knob with the right hand. However, colonoscopists of normal height can usually keep the insertion tube within the desired plane by keeping it close to their right side as they stand at the table.

Insertion into the Rectum

The examination is usually begun with the patient in a left lateral position on the examination table. Some colonoscopists prefer to keep the patient in this position throughout the procedure, while others find it advantageous to periodically change the patient's position, especially to the supine. The anus should be inspected (see Chapter 47) and a digital examination of the rectum and anus

performed. During the digital examination, particular attention should be given to the anterior wall of the distal rectum, as this area is not seen well during lower panendoscopy.

The tip of the fiberscope may then be inserted through the anus and into the rectum after lubrication of the distal half of the insertion tube. It may be necessary to apply lubricant to the insertion tube and anus periodically throughout the procedure. The lubricant tends to dry and to be rubbed away as the insertion tube moves in and out at the anus. If there is insufficient lubrication, the amount of resistance to advancement and withdrawal will increase. If the operator does not recognize that this has happened, he may incorrectly assume that advancement of colonoscope is meeting with increasing resistance within the colon.

The anal canal is about 2 to 3 cm long. From a vantage point at the anus, the canal is directed anteriorly toward the umbilicus. The rectum follows a posterior course toward the curve of the sacrum. As a result, the junction of the rectal ampulla and the anus forms an angle of about 90 degrees.

Standing at the patient's back, the examiner should grasp the distal end of the insertion tube with the right hand, with the index finger extended so that its tip is about 2 cm from the end of the insertion tube. The instrument tip is then placed at a 90-degree angle on the anal ring; the patient is asked to bear down as if about to have a bowel movement, and the instrument is advanced into the rectum while simultaneously changing the angle of insertion so that the insertion tube points toward the umbilicus at the conclusion of the maneuver. The right index finger need not enter the anus. This "turning into" the anus reduces the chance that lubricant will cover the distal tip of the instrument and produces a more gradual opening of the anal sphincteric muscles, in contrast with insertion of the instrument directly along the axis of the anal canal. When the patient "bears down," this pushes the pelvic floor muscles outward and reduces the patient's normal tendency to contract the pelvic and gluteal muscles in response to insertion of an instrument into the rectum.

The instrument should not be advanced more than 2 or 3 cm into the canal, since the tip encounters the anterior wall of the rectum beyond this distance. Generally, it is easy to know when the tip has passed the anal canal, because there is a sudden decrease in resistance to the inserting force. Advancement of the instrument from this point is performed under direct vision. Since the course of the lumen turns posteriorly proximal to the anal canal, it is usually necessary to rotate the insertion tube left and deflect the tip upward. This orients the instrument in the center of the rectal lumen. If this does not occur and there is a "red-out" of the image, the instrument tip is usually against the anterior wall of the rectum and should be withdrawn 1 to 2 cm, and the leftward maneuver should be repeated.

Air insufflation into the rectum should be kept to a minimum. This makes advancement of the instrument a little more difficult because the Houston valves and normal anatomic curvature give the collapsed rectum a degree of tortuosity that is not apparent when the rectum is distended. However, rapid distention of the rectum not only results in patient discomfort, but more importantly any excess insufflation makes the proximal flexures and bends in the colon more acute and difficult to negotiate with the instrument tip.

Even in the well-prepared patient a small amount of fluid and/or stool will be found in the rectum. It is usually unnecessary to hastily suction out the rectal contents since the rectum can be examined completely during withdrawal. Insertion should proceed without being too particular about rectal contents unless the mucosa appears friable or abnormal.

The fiberscope should be introduced through the rectum using upward angulations of the tip and left and right torquing or rotatory motions of the insertion tube (see Fig. 40–6). Whenever the tip passes a bend, the fiberscope would be withdrawn slowly. Since the bending section of the insertion tube is usually angulated after passing the bend, withdrawal will reduce the redundancy of the insertion tube and straighten the axis of the lumen.

The proximal margin of the rectum is located about 15 cm from the anus. It is impossible to know by observation alone whether or not the tip of the fiberscope has left the pelvis and entered the colon within the abdominal cavity. The rectosigmoid junction is usually located 15 to 20 cm from the anus, where there is usually a bend. Depending on the degree of angulation of this rectosigmoid bend, the walking stick phenomenon may develop (Fig. 40–7).

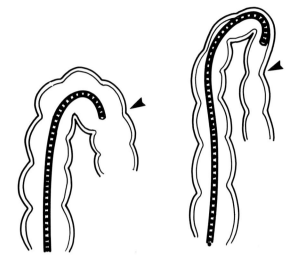

FIGURE 40–7. Walking stick phenomenon. The end of the instrument moves backward despite deeper insertion.

The term "walking stick" describes the configuration of the inserted section of the instrument. Viewed fluoroscopically, the outline of the insertion tube suggests a cane or walking stick. This phenomenon always comes about as the instrument is advanced in one of the mobile sections of the colon with the tip deflected. This occurs when negotiating a corner or bend, such as the rectosigmoid junction, where it is necessary to angulate the bending section of the instrument to view the lumen ahead. If tip deflection must be maintained to view the lumen during advancement, then the walking stick phenomenon will inevitably take place.

There are several ways in which the operator appreciates that this is happening. The patient usually experiences discomfort from stretching of the bowel and its mesentery. An experienced colonoscopist anticipates the walking stick phenomenon because of the fact that it is necessary to maintain tip deflection to view the lumen. With this configuration, a great deal or all of the forward force exerted on the insertion tube will be transmitted against the wall of the colon. This results in increasing resistance to forward motion, and the instrument tip may not advance unless a significant increment of forward force is added. Endoscopically, the lumen ahead may appear to recede as the mobile section of colon is stretched into a larger loop; even though the instrument is being advanced externally, the tip appears to be moving backward. This phenomenon is sometimes referred to as "paradoxical motion." All of these clues indicate loop formation of the colon.

Insertion into the Sigmoid Colon

The rectosigmoid junction previously presented a greater technical problem than it does now because of the limited field of observation of earlier colonoscopes. This made it difficult to determine the center and course of the lumen at this bend. The current wide-angle lens systems make it easier to recognize the correct direction. Tip deflection of earlier colonoscopes was more limited than that possible with newer models, and this also made the rectosigmoid junction a more formidable problem.

When the angle of view is less than 100 degrees and tip deflection is limited, the instrument is advanced by repeatedly confirming that it is directed toward the proximal colon. Since it is difficult to obtain a tubular view of the colon with an instrument with this limited capability, it was necessary to withdraw the instrument after every few centimeters of forward motion to confirm that the tip was aligned in the correct direction. As the instrument was advanced gently, the usual endoscopic view was only that of mucosa slipping past the endoscopic field. This is termed "slide-by." Endoscopic observation often showed only a red-out, indicating that the tip was in contact with the mucosa.

Advancement of the instrument had to be halted when the mucosa was no longer sliding or began to appear white ("white-out") as compression decreased blood perfusion to the mucosa. Both of these observations indicate excessive pressure against the colonic wall. The fiberscope must be withdrawn at this point. If insertion is continued in a careless or rough manner, a free perforation may occur. Most examiners who have produced free perforations relate that at the time of the accident they did not feel any unusual resistance to advancement of the instrument and that the only observed changes were a red-out or white-out of the mucosa.

Fortunately, the design of newer instruments reduces some of these technical problems, and the slide-by technique should not be used. But even with better instruments, the inexperienced operator may encounter difficulties at the rectosigmoid junction similar to those found with early instrument

models, and he must be aware of the signs of impending perforation.

The rectosigmoid junction is in a sense the key to the colon. If it can be negotiated successfully, skillfully and quickly, the remainder of the examination will often be proportionately less difficult. Even with the best of colonoscopes, this junction can be a formidable obstacle. The problem is sometimes compounded by adhesions due to previous surgery or radiation, or by carcinomatous invasion of the pelvis. Patience and meticulous attention to technique are worthwhile at this point in the examination. Air insufflation should be minimized when negotiation of the rectosigmoid is time-consuming, since excessive inflation will compound any difficulty with later stages of the procedure.

With angulation and tip rotation at the rectosigmoid, a view will be obtained of the sigmoid colon. Beginning from the walking stick configuration at the retosigmoid junction, it is usually possible to advance the instrument into the mid- and proximal sigmoid. The patient will experience discomfort or pain as advancement begins to stretch the sigmoid and its mesentery into a loop configuration. Frequently a long tunnel view will be obtained in the mid-sigmoid as the loop is being formed (Plate 40–1). When advancement is persistent and uninterrupted by attempts to straighten and control the loop, the loop may become large enough to accommodate 50 to 60 cm of the length of the insertion tube entirely within the sigmoid colon.

There are several common types of loop that may develop (Fig. 40–8). Descriptive terms have been attached to these, based on their shape as if viewed fluoroscopically in an anteroposterior direction. Thus, the alpha loop resembles the Greek letter α and the N loop resembles the letter N. Every loop has two components: an upward (cephalad) directed convex curvature that is oriented in an anteroposterior direction; and a downward (caudad) directed convex curved line that is oriented in an anterior–left posterior plane. As a result, each of the common sigmoid loops have exactly the same configuration when viewed laterally (Fig. 40–9). In addition to the more common loop configurations, various complex shapes, such as the double alpha and double reverse alpha loops, may be formed on rare occasions (Fig. 40–10). It is not possible to know the shape that

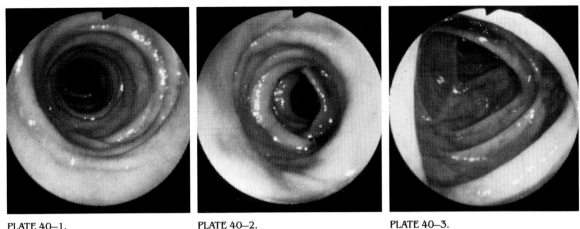

PLATE 40–1.   PLATE 40–2.   PLATE 40–3.

PLATE 40–1. Long tunnel endoscopic view of the sigmoid colon.
PLATE 40–2. Endoscopic view of the descending colon.
PLATE 40–3. Endoscopic view of the transverse colon. Note the triangular pattern of semilunar folds.

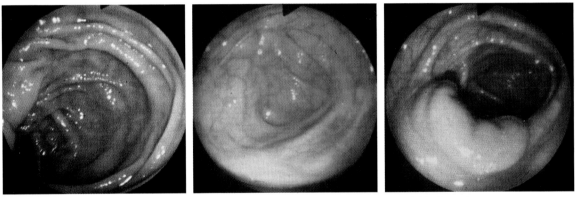

PLATE 40–4.   PLATE 40–5.   PLATE 40–6.

PLATE 40–4. Endoscopic view of the ascending colon.
PLATE 40–5. Endoscopic view of orifice of the appendix.
PLATE 40–6. Endoscopic view of the ileocecal valve (papillary form).

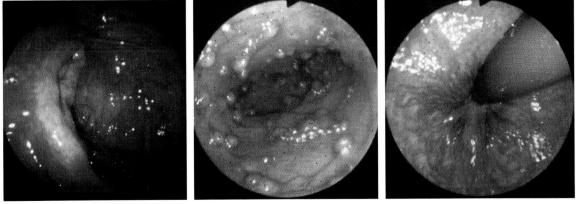

PLATE 40–7.   PLATE 40–8.   PLATE 40–9.

PLATE 40–7. Endoscopic view of the ileocecal valve (labial form).
PLATE 40–8. Endoscopic view of lymph follicle hyperplasia in the terminal ileum.
PLATE 40–9. Endoscopic view of rectal ampulla.

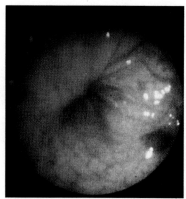

PLATE 40–10. Endoscopic view of colon at twisted part of the volvulus. The instrument tip must be gently inserted through this constricted segment.

the sigmoid loop has taken without fluoroscopy.

With experience, it is possible to advance the instrument from the rectosigmoid junction to the descending colon without formation of a large sigmoid loop. This requires repeated backward and forward motions of the fiberscope in order to telescope the sigmoid colon onto the insertion tube. Each time the tip of the instrument reaches a bend or turn in the lumen the tip is deflected at the bend and the instrument is withdrawn. In addition, it is usually advantageous to rotate the insertion tube as it is withdrawn (see Fig. 40–6). Rightward or clockwise rotation usually works best.

Since the rotation, tip deflection, and withdrawal motions are most effective when performed in a smooth and coordinated manner, the right hand must grasp the insertion tube. Then, tip deflection with the left thumb must of necessity be either upward or downward.

The instrument should be withdrawn up to the point that it appears that further withdrawal will result in the instrument slipping backward. Generally, the resisting force or tension on the colon and mesentery increases rapidly at this point and the patient may experience discomfort. Withdrawal (with rotation/tip deflection) should stop just short of this point. This may occur after only a few centimeters of insertion tube has been withdrawn, or if a large loop has formed as much as 20 to 30 cm or more will be withdrawn before the sigmoid is straightened.

During withdrawal/rotation the endoscopic view of the lumen should remain relatively stationary. Upon completion of each withdrawal/rotation, the instrument tip is repositioned to look for and advance to the next turn. A certain degree of torquing or rotation of the instrument during advancement, especially to the right (clockwise), may also be useful in preventing excessive loop formation (Fig. 40–11).

Less than one-to-one motion, increasing resistance to forward motion, or worsening patient discomfort during advancement usually indicates that a loop is reforming, and withdrawal/rotation should be repeated at the first opportunity. Usually the maneuvers of tip angulation/withdrawal/rotation and advancement/clockwise rotation are repeated numerous times as small segments of the sigmoid are straightened and shortened during the approach to the descending colon (Fig. 40–12).

This method of insertion through the sigmoid is the most ideal. Patient discomfort is minimized, excessive air insufflation of the proximal colon is avoided, and certain other technical problems such as entry into the descending colon are avoided or minimized.

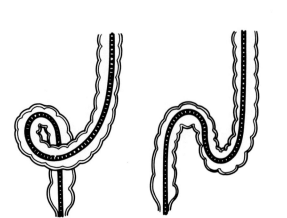
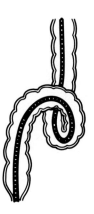

FIGURE 40–8. Common configurations of fiberscope in sigmoid colon: Alpha loop (*left*), N-loop (*middle*), reverse alpha loop (*right*).

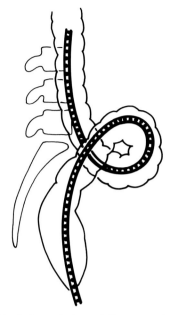

FIGURE 40–9. Lateral view of fiberscope in sigmoid. Each of the common loops has this appearance on lateral view.

With experience, it is generally possible to utilize this method, provided that the sigmoid colon is not too redundant.

Insertion into the Descending Colon

There is no endoscopic landmark that indicates the junction of the sigmoid and descending colon. Depending on the presence and type of sigmoid loop, the junction may have a relatively sharp angulation. Endoscopically, the descending colon may have a somewhat lesser diameter than the sigmoid, the interhaustral septa are occasionally more semilunar in shape than their circular counterparts in the sigmoid, and a long tunnel

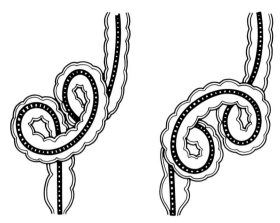

FIGURE 40–10. Complex sigmoid loop: Double alpha loop (*left*) and double reverse alpha loop (*right*).

view of the lumen may be obtained upon entry (Plate 40–2). Because of the descending colon's dependent location with lateral and supine patient positions, some increase in intestinal contents will often be encountered upon entry into the descending colon.

Because of the marked deflection capability of the distal tip of newer colonoscopes, it is usually not difficult to direct the instrument into the descending colon, even if the angle at the sigmoid–descending colon junction is relatively acute owing to formation of a sigmoid loop. If the sigmoid colon is straight, insertion to the proximal descending colon usually proceeds smoothly; advancement to the mid- and proximal descending colon may be more problematic depending on the type of sigmoid loop.

If a sigmoid loop is present, it may be necessary to remove it in order to advance further into the descending colon. Depending on the type of loop, advancement without first straightening the sigmoid colon may

FIGURE 40–11. Repeated clockwise rotation/withdrawal maneuver tends to keep sigmoid straight. This illustration demonstrates maneuver in which a small reverse alpha loop is tending to form.

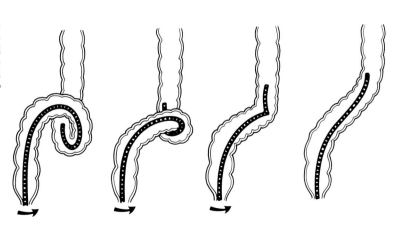

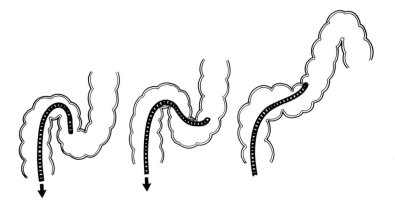

FIGURE 40–12. "Jiggling" (repeated withdrawal of short segments with clockwise rotation and tip angulation) and straightening keep sigmoid relatively straight during insertion.

encounter a marked degree of resistance, increased patient discomfort, and little or no advancement of the tip of the instrument. This usually means that most of the forward force exerted with the insertion tube is being directed against the apex of the loop itself, which in consequence becomes even larger. These events are commonly encountered with the N-shaped loop. By contrast, formation of an alpha loop preserves a minimally angulated transition from sigmoid to descending colon. As a result, smooth and gentle advancement of the instrument tip to the splenic flexure is possible with a minimum of patient discomfort, although the alpha loop itself may widen.

Formation of an N sigmoid loop may cause the angle formed at the junction of the mobile sigmoid and fixed descending colon to become acute to the point that it is not possible to direct the instrument tip around this bend and into the descending colon. It may be necessary to convert the loop to another configuration. This can be done by withdrawing the insertion tube to the mid-sigmoid. With tip deflection and left rotation (counterclockwise) during advancement, the loop can often be converted to an alpha loop that meets the descending colon at a less acute angle.

Removal of the Sigmoid Loop

It is always necessary at some point in the procedure to straighten the sigmoid by removing any loop that has formed if the instrument is to be inserted to the proximal colon. As noted above, excessive looping reduces the range of deflection of the bending section and almost always increases patient discomfort during advancement. When marked resistance is encountered in attempting to advance proximally into the descend-

ing colon as a result of loop formation, rough and forceful persistence with forward motion may endanger the patient. Excessive force on the sigmoid loop can eventually result in ischemia and a tear along the antimesenteric border of the sigmoid. It is necessary, therefore, that the colonoscopist be capable of straightening the sigmoid loop.

Clockwise rotation and withdrawal are usually sufficient to remove an alpha loop (Fig. 40–13); formation of this loop often occurs when upward angulation and counterclockwise rotation has been used in passing the instrument through the sigmoid. Removal of the reverse alpha loop may require either counterclockwise (left) or clockwise (right) rotation plus withdrawal (Fig. 40–14); the reverse alpha loop tends to form if downward tip deflection and left rotation have been employed in negotiating the sigmoid.

Since the precise configuration of the sigmoid loop cannot be known without fluoroscopy, straightening the sigmoid is a trial-and-error process. If the tip of the instrument is in the descending colon, withdrawal and rotation are almost always required. Because formation of the alpha loop is common, clockwise (right) rotation should be attempted first. During the straightening maneuver, the tip of the instrument must be kept in the center of the lumen of the descending colon. As the maneuver proceeds, the tip may become directed into the wall; this should be corrected with the deflection controls. When withdrawal/rotation is effective, the instrument tip will remain at the same level in the colon or it may actually move forward. Successful reduction of the loop in this manner produces a characteristic "feel" from the instrument as the sigmoid comes into a linear configuration. If the straightening maneuver is ineffective, increasing resistance to withdrawal will usually

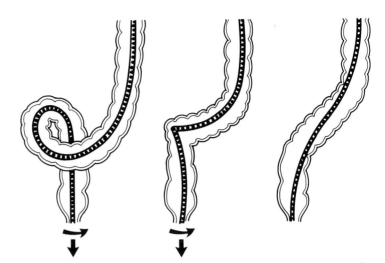

FIGURE 40–13. Removal of alpha loop by withdrawal and clockwise rotation.

be encountered, the patient may experience discomfort, and the tip will often slip backward into the sigmoid colon. When an attempt at reduction of the loop is ineffective, a lesser or greater degree of rotation should be used, or rotation in the opposite direction may be attempted.

Depending on the shape of the loop there may be a lesser or greater margin for error with the straightening maneuver. With an alpha loop, for example, it is usually possible to insert the instrument tip as far as the splenic flexure without producing undue patient discomfort, since the tip will pass the sigmoid–descending colon junction without significant difficulty. As the instrument is withdrawn, several corrections can be made in the degree and direction of rotation before the instrument slips below the sigmoid–descending colon junction. By contrast, it may only be possible to get the distal few centimeters of the bending section of the insertion tube into the descending colon if there is a large N loop. As the instrument is withdrawn, there is less opportunity to make corrections in rotation and tip deflection because the tip may abruptly return to the sigmoid colon. This is more likely to happen if the angulation of the tip at the sigmoid–descending colon junction is not very acute, that is, if the junction has not been "hooked" with the bending section of the insertion tube.

If the sigmoid is in an N-loop configuration, withdrawal without rotation is usually

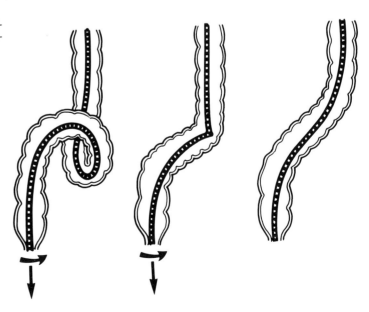

FIGURE 40–14. Removal of reverse alpha loop, in this case by clockwise rotation with withdrawal.

adequate to straighten the sigmoid. The presence of the N loop can be recognized only by trial and error. If, in fact, the sigmoid loop is in some configuration other than the N shape, withdrawal without rotation will usually result in backward motion of the instrument tip, which will be evident endoscopically. Withdrawal of about 20 cm of the insertion tube without rotation should be tried (Fig. 40–15). If by endoscopic observation this action appears to be effective—that is, if the level of the tip in the colon is maintained or even moved forward slightly—then the withdrawal maneuver should be continued until it seems that the instrument is straight. With a large N loop, 40 cm or more may be withdrawn before the insertion tube is straight.

If and when the instrument is straight within the sigmoid, withdrawal will also move the tip backward. Also, advancement of the insertion tube results in prompt and proportionally equal advancement of the tip within the colon (one-to-one motion). Rotatory motions and use of the deflection controls will also be transmitted and reproduced at the instrument tip with predictable and equal fidelity. By both tactile sensation and visual observation of the action of the tip, the experienced colonoscopist will "feel" that the instrument is in a straightened position. When this is achieved, and the tip of the instrument is in the descending colon, the insertion tube has usually been withdrawn to a point at which only 30 or 40 cm remain within the colon.

External pressure on the abdominal wall is sometimes helpful in negotiating the sigmoid colon. Generally, this requires that the patient be relatively thin and able to relax the muscles of the abdominal wall. Gentle but firm caudally and posteriorly directed pressure must be maintained by an assistant as the instrument is advanced. It is often possible for an experienced assistant to palpate the colonoscope within the sigmoid loop if the patient is thin. If so, the counterpressure on the sigmoid loop will be better localized and the maneuver will more likely be successful.

Insertion into the Transverse Colon

Sometimes passage of the instrument tip into the transverse colon is relatively easy. However, several problems may arise. A straightened sigmoid colon is prerequisite for entry and passage of the transverse colon. When this has been accomplished, the length of the insertion tube within the colon will be only about 50 or 60 cm even in the largest patients. When the tip reaches the splenic flexure, transillumination of the abdominal wall in the left upper quadrant will occur in all but the most obese patients.

As an attempt is made to advance the tip into the transverse colon, the paradoxical motion phenomenon is frequently noted; that is, the lumen appears to be receding or the instrument tip seems to be moving backward. This is the same walking stick phenomenon noted at the rectosigmoid junction, except that the splenic flexure is relatively more fixed in position, and upward (cephalad) movement of the flexure is limited by the diaphragm (Fig. 40–16). Most of the external forward force exerted on the insertion tube is actually directed through the deflected bending section toward the outer wall of the flexure. If the instrument remains straight in the sigmoid, the flexure will be pushed in a cephalad direction.

At this point one of two things may occur. If the sigmoid remains straight, the instrument may eventually move forward into the distal transverse colon. This may be accompanied by discomfort localized to the left upper quadrant.

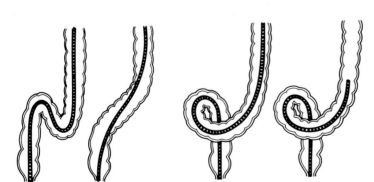

FIGURE 40–15. Trial withdrawal to differentiate N-loop from other types. Withdrawal without rotation reduces N-loop (*left*). Withdrawal without rotation with alpha loop (*right*) causes the instrument tip to slip back.

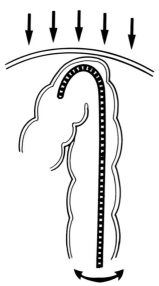

FIGURE 40–16. Procedure for passing splenic flexure. Deep inspiration, clockwise rotation, and changing patient to right lateral or supine position are useful at this acute bend.

Several things can be done to facilitate advancement. Because the transverse colon is anterior in position and the descending colon is posterior, some degree of rotation of the insertion tube is usually helpful. Clockwise or right rotation is usually more effective; this also assists in keeping the sigmoid colon straight. Changing the patient's position from left lateral to supine may also be helpful. In effect, this means that the insertion tube is being rotated to the right, although actually the patient is being rotated to the colonoscopist's left.

With lesser degrees of tip deflection at the splenic flexure, more force can be exerted in the forward direction. This reduces the laterally directed force being transmitted through the bending section and decreases the walking stick phenomenon. It is necessary that these three components (advancement, rotation, and opening of the angle of deflection) are carried out in a coordinated and to some degree simultaneous manner. The positions of the transverse colon and splenic flexure change with respiration, and this can sometimes be used to advantage. A deep, sustained inspiration by the patient may diminish the acuteness of the splenic flexure angle and facilitate passage of the instrument (see Fig. 40–16). This maneuver, however, is usually more effective at the hepatic flexure.

If the flexure is not passed, the instrument should be withdrawn gently and gradually until it is certain that the sigmoid colon is as straight as possible. Then another attempt can be made with greater or lesser rotation. Occasionally, leftward rotation or no rotation at all will be effective. After these steps are repeated several times, the proper degree of rotation and tip deflection may be found by trial and error, in which case the instrument tip will advance readily to the mid-transverse colon.

Some colonoscopists make use of the prone or right lateral position when an unusual degree of difficulty is encountered when advancing into the transverse colon. However, there are problems with these positions. For example, with the right lateral position the colonoscopist faces the patient and must either reach over the patient's legs to manipulate the insertion tube or move himself and the light source to the opposite side of the table. This is thus an awkward solution at best and not very effective in practice.

The second problem that may occur when attempting to advance beyond the splenic flexure is re-formation of the sigmoid loop. This can be anticipated if the sigmoid has already been found to be redundant and is more difficult to straighten and maintain in a straightened position than usual. The first evidence of this is that the insertion tube advances a considerable distance (30 or 40 cm), but endoscopically the instrument tip has not moved. If the tip is hooked across the flexure it will usually not slip backward as the sigmoid loop forms. Almost always this loop will be an N loop. This also causes the patient some discomfort, which is the second clue that the sigmoid loop has re-formed. The insertion tube must be withdrawn and another attempt made. Rotation of the insertion tube is helpful in this situation, especially clockwise or right rotation, as this aids in keeping the sigmoid straight. Counterpressure in the left lower quadrant may also be useful.

Occasionally, all attempts to pass the splenic flexure may be frustrated because of repeated formation of the sigmoid N loop. In such a case the stiffening tube must be used to hold the sigmoid colon straight as the instrument tip is advanced past the flexure. As noted previously, there are clearly defined requirements for use of the stiffening tube. It is of paramount importance that the sigmoid colon is in a straight configuration between the rectum and the descending colon during insertion. With the instrument tip at the splenic flexure, this usually means that the insertion tube has been withdrawn to the 40 or 50 cm mark. Lubrication, internally and externally, of the stiffening tube is essential. Insertion with a left and right twisting motion generally facilitates placement (Fig. 40–17).

If the fiberscope has not been straightened, advancement of the stiffening tube along the insertion tube will meet resistance at the point of loop formation before it is fully inserted (Fig. 40–18). Usually this means that the end of the stiffening tube will be against the wall of the bowel rather than positioned within the lumen. In this position it is more likely that mucosa will become trapped between the insertion tube and inner wall of the stiffening tube as the colonoscope is moved forward and backward. Therefore, partial insertion of the stiffening tube into the sigmoid loop is unsafe and the device should be withdrawn if it cannot be positioned properly.

If full insertion of the stiffening tube brings its end up to the tip of the fiberscope (this may occur in a small patient), motion of the bending section of the instrument will be compromised. Therefore, insertion of the overtube should be halted when it reaches the mid-descending colon. In a small patient, 5 to 10 cm may therefore remain external to the anus.

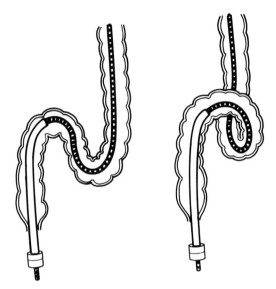

FIGURE 40–18. Problems with insertion of stiffening tube due to insufficient straightening of sigmoid loop.

Advancement to the Hepatic Flexure

After the bending section of the instrument has passed the splenic flexure, there is usually little difficulty in advancing to the mid-transverse colon. The tip of the fiberscope actually follows a caudally directed course from posterior to anterior toward the midpoint of the transverse colon, and then in an upward and anterior to posterior direction in approaching the hepatic flexure.

Generally, transillumination will be more or less continuous as the instrument traverses the transverse colon, since this segment is relatively close to the anterior abdominal wall. The lumen of the transverse colon has a characteristic triangular shape (Plate 40–3). Transmitted aortic pulsations are a consistent endoscopic finding in the distal transverse colon.

Depending on the length of the transverse colon, a U-shaped loop may be formed as the instrument is advanced. The apex of this loop forms at the midpoint of the transverse colon and is directed toward the pelvis. This is in effect a manifestation of the walking stick phenomenon, although the direction of the loop is opposite to that which occurs at the rectosigmoid junction. Formation of this transverse loop will be evident endoscopically as an abrupt angulation in the course of the lumen at the midpoint of the transverse colon. In some cases the transverse loop will not form and the instrument can be steadily advanced to the hepatic flexure without much difficulty or additional maneuvering.

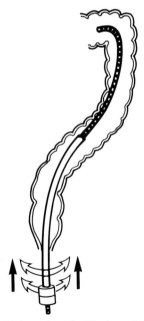

FIGURE 40–17. Insertion of stiffening tube. Alternating twists to left and right make insertion easier. The sigmoid must be straight before this procedure is begun.

If the transverse loop does form, it is best that this section be straightened before attempting to negotiate the hepatic flexure. After deflecting the tip at the acute bend in the mid-transverse colon, the instrument is withdrawn to the point that it seems that further withdrawal will cause the tip to slip backward. Often, a small degree of right (sometimes left) rotation facilitates straightening.

Since the splenic flexure is fixed to the retroperitoneal space, a fulcrum-like effect may occur in which the tip makes a closer approach to the hepatic flexure as the instrument is being withdrawn. At this point it is useful to suction as much air from the colon as possible. This will cause the walls of the colon to collapse in a more or less symmetric fashion, since any given segment of inflated colon is analogous to an inflated sphere. If the internal air pressure is decreased, the walls must necessarily collapse uniformly. Use of the suction while withdrawing the transverse loop will therefore draw the hepatic flexure closer to the tip of the instrument.

The combination of withdrawal (with a slight degree of rotation), the effect of suction, and the fulcrum-like effect produced by the fixed splenic flexure is often enough to position the tip right at the hepatic flexure (Fig. 40–19). This sequence of events occurs so commonly that this maneuver is relatively standard in a procedure that for the most part has little in the way of standard maneuvers.

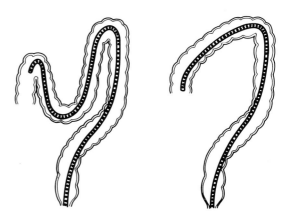

FIGURE 40–20. Deep U-shaped transverse loop (*left*) formed by "pushing-through" loop to hepatic flexure. After hooking hepatic flexure, colonoscope is withdrawn to straighten the loop.

If, as a result of the transverse straightening maneuver, the tip of the instrument reaches the hepatic flexure, quick and precise deflection of the tip will be required if the flexure is to be hooked with the bending section.

In some cases it may be necessary to repeat the mid-transverse withdrawal/suction/rotation maneuver several times to get close enough to the flexure to turn the tip into the ascending colon. However, if the transverse colon is especially ptotic, this maneuver may not work. Manual counterpressure on the abdominal wall may also straighten the loop; maintenance of this pressure may aid advancement past this point by preventing reformation of the loop. When these maneuvers fail, it is usually possible to advance the instrument tip to the flexure in spite of transverse loop formation, provided the sigmoid colon remains straight. This may cause the patient some discomfort, and it is not the best method for reaching the hepatic flexure. Formation of a deeper and wider loop in effect makes the angle at the hepatic flexure more acute and more difficult to negotiate (Fig. 40–20).

Insertion into the Ascending Colon and Cecum

The outer wall of the hepatic flexure is frequently denoted by a bluish mucosal tint. This is usually ascribed to its proximity to the liver and gallbladder, although a similar color, albeit somewhat less definite, can be seen in other areas of the colon. One or more of the teniae coli may be seen in the approach

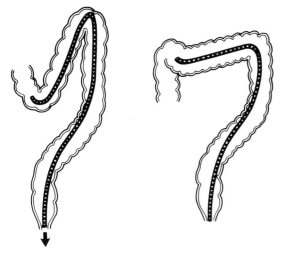

FIGURE 40–19. Withdrawal and lifting of transverse colon loop.

to the flexure if the transverse colon has been stretched by loop formation.

It is usually necessary to make use of the deflection controls to turn the tip of the instrument into the ascending colon. As a general rule, the greater the depth of insertion of the shaft of the instrument, the less responsive the tip will be to rotation or torquing, especially if there is loop formation.

Turning the tip in the anticipated direction of the ascending colon will result in either a tubular view of the lumen (Plate 40–4) or a red-out if the tip is against the wall. Gentle withdrawal may result in alignment of the tip in the axis of the ascending colon if a U-shaped loop is still present in the transverse colon. A small degree of right or left rotation may also be helpful. Sometimes withdrawal at this point will result in advancement of the instrument as the transverse colon straightens. If, however, the transverse is already straight, the tip may slip backward into the distal transverse colon.

Once the tip is aligned with the ascending colon, the instrument can be advanced cautiously until it can be determined how the instrument will behave if the motion is continued. The addition of torque to the forward motion may also facilitate advancement into the ascending colon. If, however, the transverse U-shaped loop is still present, or if it re-forms during the attempt to advance the tip into the ascending colon, the tip will either not advance or may even slip backward as stretching of the transverse loop causes the colon to lengthen. Upward-directed manual compression in the right upper quadrant may occasionally be helpful in this situation.

A much more complex loop may occasionally form in the transverse colon, especially if this section is unusually long. This may have a gamma configuration (i.e., having the outline of the Greek letter γ) (Fig. 40–21). Removal of this type of loop is usually difficult. Rotation and withdrawal under fluoroscopic control should be tried, but the success rate for reduction of this type of loop is not high because the loop is often large and rotatory, and torquing motions are poorly transmitted to the loop. Sometimes the gamma loop can be advantageous in that it straightens the hepatic flexure, but it is difficult to deliberately produce a transverse gamma loop. It is sometimes possible to continue to advance and "push through" the gamma loop to reach the ascending colon.

It is useful to remove as much air from the

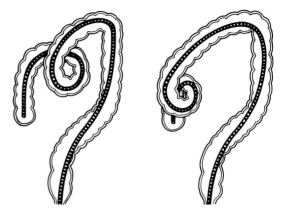

FIGURE 40–21. Complex gamma loops in transverse colon.

colon as possible in negotiating the hepatic flexure. Since this segment of the insertion technique is near the last of the maneuvers to be performed, it is likely that the colon has become overinflated. Suction will shorten the colon and cause the cecum to move upward toward the instrument tip as the colon collapses (Fig. 40–22). This is analogous to the effect described for the approach to the hepatic flexure.

Since the hepatic flexure is confined to a greater degree than the splenic flexure by virtue of its proximity to the liver, deep inspiration can be effective in pushing the instrument downward toward the cecum

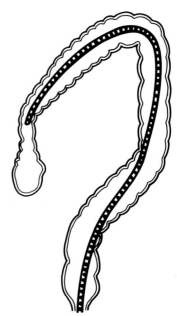

FIGURE 40–22. Suction of air from ascending colon shortens distance to cecum.

once the instrument tip has turned the hepatic flexure. It may also be useful to change the patient's position if entry into the ascending colon is difficult. Just as at the splenic flexure, the greater the degree of deflection of the bending section, the greater the proportion of the force of advancement that is transmitted laterally against the wall of the colon. Therefore, the instrument will advance past the flexure with less difficulty if the degree of tip angulation is kept to a minimum. With sharp angulation at the flexure, most of the forward force may be directed toward the right flank so that endoscopically it appears as if the lumen is receding as the colon is stretched toward the point of contact of the lateral wall with the bending section of the colonoscope.

Negotiation of the hepatic flexure is usually the most difficult colonoscopic problem, except for that of the sigmoid. Once the bending section has passed the flexure, however, it is relatively easy to advance to the cecum, provided there are no loops proximally in the colon. If the ascending colon is especially long, a loop may form, usually in the transverse colon, as the instrument is advanced. It may be necessary to withdraw and advance repeatedly, gaining a net few centimeters with each forward motion, until the cecum is reached. Generally, the addition of some degree of torque, either left or right, will also help in this maneuver.

If there is to be any difficulty with the preparation of the colon it will occur upon entry into the ascending colon, since complete cleansing of the right colon is the most difficult part of the preparation procedure. Repeated washing of the lens, suction of intestinal contents, and washing of the mucosa by means of catheters inserted through the accessory channel can easily lead to overinflation. The presence of stool limits maneuverability and makes it difficult to recognize the correct direction of the lumen; also, clogging of the suction channel eliminates the use of suction as a means of maneuvering the cecum closer to the instrument tip as described previously.

Since the ascending colon is fixed to the retroperitoneal wall and is posterior in position, transillumination is often lost after the tip passes the hepatic flexure. However, when the tip reaches the somewhat more mobile cecum, transillumination again occurs in the right lower quadrant (Fig. 40–23). If the preparation is adequate, the orifice of the

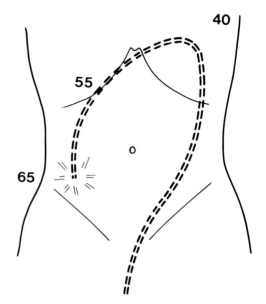

FIGURE 40–23. Transillumination occurs in right lower quadrant just above inguinal ligament when instrument tip is in cecum. When instrument is perfectly straight it has shape of number 7.

appendix can be seen as a round opening or a slit behind a fold (Plate 40–5). The teniae coli converge at the tip of the cecum, and this may also be evident.

Once the colonoscope has been inserted fully to the cecum, its overall configuration within the abdomen should have the shape of the number 7 (see Fig. 40–23). If all segments are straight, 60 to 70 cm of the insertion tube will be within the colon.

Insertion into the Terminal Ileum

If the colonoscope is withdrawn about 5 cm from the tip of the cecum, the ileocecal valve is usually observable. When the valve protrudes into the lumen in a papillary form (Plate 40–6), or when intestinal contents issue from the valve, endoscopic confirmation of its location is not difficult. On occasion, however, the valve may be located on the distal side of a relatively large semilunar fold, in which case it is more difficult to view the entire valve or its opening. A close-up view of the orifice will reveal either a narrow opening or a closed opening represented only by a small depression in the center of the ileocecal ring (Plate 40–7).

Fine, precise tip control is required for entry into the ileum. The position and appearance of the valve is less obvious and the opening is more likely to be closed when the cecum is maximally distended with air. Therefore, it is helpful to partially collapse the cecum, using suction. Once the instrument tip is positioned at the ileocecal orifice, however, an increase in air pressure may be necessary to open the valve.

If the ileum is not entered, the fiberscope should be introduced to the tip of the cecum and withdrawn gently while maintaining an approximate 90-degree tip angulation in the anticipated direction of the ileocecal valve (Fig. 40–24). This maneuver is designed to catch the proximal edge of the valve with the receding tip of the fiberscope. If the maneuver is performed properly, the ileocecal mucosa will suddenly appear as the backward motion and tension on the instrument catches and opens the valve. Slight adjustments in tip deflection may be necessary for better alignment, but generally it is possible to advance the instrument into the terminal ileum. If, however, the insertion tube has been withdrawn 10 cm and the endoscopic view is still that of a red-out of the colonic mucosa, then most likely the direction of tip angulation was wrong and the maneuver should be repeated.

If a narrow-diameter fiberscope is being used, it is possible to make a U-turn at the tip of the cecum, in which case entry into the ileum can often be performed under direct vision as the instrument is withdrawn, since the ileocecal valve is viewed more readily from this position (Fig. 40–25).

It is customary to examine to a distance of about 10 cm from the ileocecal junction, although as much as 40 cm of the ileum may be examined with skill and experience. To some degree this is dependent on keeping the more proximal portion of the instrument straight (see Fig. 40–23).

The appearance of the ileal mucosa differs from that of the colon. Hemispheric elevations 2 to 4 mm in diameter may be seen

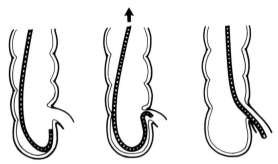

FIGURE 40–25. Insertion into terminal ileum by U-turn method, using pediatric colonoscope.

normally (Plate 40–8). These are lymphoid follicles. They tend to decrease in number and prominence with increasing age. The characteristic circular folds of the small intestine are less prominent in the terminal ileum than in the distal duodenum during upper panendoscopy.

Observation

Endoscopic examination of the colon is conducted principally as the instrument is withdrawn. If spastic contractions disturb the orderly endoscopic examination, administration of an anticholinergic agent may sometimes be necessary to avoid a false negative diagnosis. The bowel is a tubular organ but is tortuous and winding and has characteristic semilunar folds. Those areas that are illuminated by the fiberscope can be seen without difficulty, but areas behind folds and acute angles such as at the flexures may be difficult to examine completely.

To examine the mucosa behind a fold it is necessary to hook the instrument tip proximal to the fold and then gradually withdraw the insertion tube so that the fold is pulled distally and flattened against the wall to some degree (Fig. 40–26). With an especially large

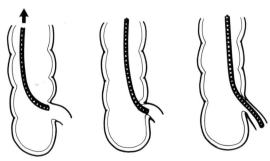

FIGURE 40–24. Insertion into terminal ileum by hooking and withdrawal.

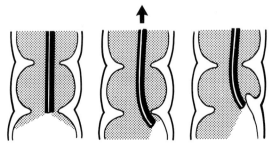

FIGURE 40–26. Method of tip angulation and withdrawal to flatten semilunar fold and view behind fold.

fold, it may be necessary to repeat this maneuver several times to be certain that a lesion has not remained hidden. Instruments with wide-angle lens systems facilitate this procedure.

The junctional points between mobile and fixed segments of the colon occur as flexures or acute angulations in the shape of the colon. Because of this angulation, certain areas of mucosa, such as the inner aspect of each flexure, may be difficult to observe. These blind areas occur at the rectosigmoid, in the proximal inner aspect of the splenic flexure, and at the hepatic flexure. If there is a mid-transverse loop, the inner aspect of this angulation may also be a blind area.

Observation of the mucosa at these turns during simple withdrawal may not be sufficient, especially if the tip of the endoscope slips rapidly backward from the flexure. Sharp angulation of the tip with advancement of the insertion tube will often change the view of the inner aspect of flexure as the instrument is pushed against the outer curvature of the flexure. This maneuver takes advantage of the walking stick phenomenon.

The hepatic flexure may be especially difficult to examine completely. Frequently the instrument tip must be deflected quickly into the ascending colon and hooked. Gentle withdrawal and concomitant straightening of the transverse colon may cause the tip to jump forward into the ascending colon (Fig. 40–27A). As a result of these rapid maneuvers the hepatic flexure may be observed only poorly during insertion. As the tip of the

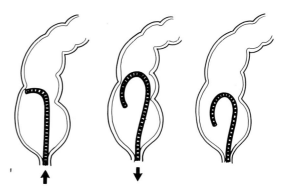

FIGURE 40–28. U-turn maneuver in rectum to view rectal ampulla.

fiberscope passes the hepatic flexure during withdrawal, there is a tendency for the instrument to slip rapidly backward when the bending section is straightened to orient the tip with the axis of the transverse colon. Once the hepatic flexure is unhooked, the transverse colon will return to its natural position. The length of the fiberscope in the straightened transverse colon is much shorter than the normal length of the transverse colon (Fig. 40–27B), and thus the tip often falls backward toward the mid-transverse colon. Therefore, it is often necessary to reinsert the tip past the flexure and make observations during both insertion and withdrawal.

The distal end of rectum is also difficult to observe clearly because of poor distensibility. This problem can be circumvented with the U-turn technique. As the colonoscopy procedure is nearing its conclusion and when the tip of the instrument has been withdrawn to the level of the middle valve of Houston, the tip of the instrument is maximally deflected using both the up/down and left/right deflection controls, and then the insertion tube is advanced to approximately the 20 cm mark on the insertion tube. This will turn the tip completely so that the rectal ampulla can be viewed as the insertion tube is slowly withdrawn (Fig. 40–28 and Plate 40–9). Rotation of the insertion tube with the instrument tip in this configuration permits a complete examination of the circumference of the dentate line and the lower end of the rectum. The bending section should be straightened before drawing the insertion tube through the anus.

Fiberscopic Treatment in the Bowel

There are numerous opportunities for therapeutic procedures during colonoscopy,

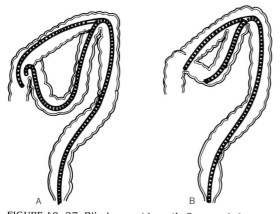

FIGURE 40–27. Blind area at hepatic flexure. A, Instrument tip jumps past flexure as transverse colon U-loop is straightened during insertion. B, Instrument tip slips backward from hepatic flexure as bending section is straightened and transverse colon assumes its normal position.

polypectomy being a prime example. Many of these procedures are discussed in other chapters.

Sigmoid volvulus can be treated by colonoscopic manipulation. Generally this can be differentiated clinically and by x-ray study from other acute conditions that require emergency surgery. Plain x-rays of the abdomen will reveal a large, reverse U-shaped intestinal gas shadow, sometimes accompanied by a fluid level (Fig. 40–29). If there are clinical signs of peritonitis, colonoscopy is contraindicated.

A small-volume tap water or saline enema may be used with care to prepare the distal colon. Usually the procedure must be done with little or no sedation. The colonoscope is introduced into the rectum and sigmoid colon in the usual fashion, except that air insufflation must be limited to the smallest amount necessary to determine the course of the lumen, and air should be frequently removed from the colon. Visualization of the

point of torsion will usually reveal an edematous and nontransparent mucosa in which the normal vascular pattern is not discernible (Plate 40–10). The tip of the fiberscope should be introduced very carefully into the narrow segment in short steps with frequent but minimal degrees of tip deflection. A wide-angle endoscope usually makes it easier to determine the course of the lumen.

After the tip of the fiberscope is passed through the constricted segment, it enters the proximal distended segment, where a large amount of gas and fluid will often be found. This should be evacuated immediately. An endoscope with a large accessory channel is most suitable for this purpose. This decompression will itself frequently reduce the volvulus to some degree so that subsequent maneuvers will be less difficult.

The mucosa should be observed for ischemic damage. If, after entry and evacuation of the distended segment, the mucosa is observed to be friable and there is tissue

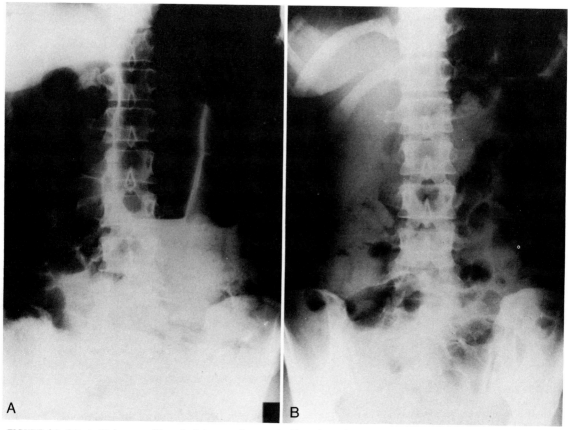

FIGURE 40–29. A, Plain x-ray film of abdomen demonstrating sigmoid volvulus. B, Plain x-ray film of abdomen soon after colonoscopic reduction of volvulus.

slough, the mucosa is undoubtedly ischemic and further colonoscopic manipulation will be hazardous. If this can be ruled out, the fiberscope can be inserted into the descending colon and then the sigmoid may be straightened. Fluoroscopy is useful since this shortens the period of maneuvering to straighten the sigmoid; the configuration of the loop and its response to maneuvers with the colonoscope will be readily apparent, and it will not be necessary to perform a series of trial-and-error maneuvers.

Some patients have repeated episodes of sigmoid volvulus. Although colonoscopic reduction of the volvulus is relatively easy, such patients should be referred for surgery, provided their general condition will permit this.

Editor's note: Colonoscopy as a therapeutic measure in acute colonic pseudoobstruction, referred to as Ogilvie's syndrome, is not covered extensively in this volume. References 11 to 17 pertain to colonoscopic decompression in this disorder.

References

1. Brown GR. A new approach to colon preparation for barium enema. Univ Mich Med Bull 1961; 27:225–30.
2. Levy AC, Benson JW, Hewlett EL, et al. Saline lavage: a rapid, effective and acceptable method for cleaning the gastrointestinal tract. Gastroenterology 1976; 70:157–61.
3. Crapp AR, Powis SJA, Tillotson P, et al. Preparation of the bowel by whole-gut irrigation. Lancet 1975; 2:1239–40.
4. Davis GR, Santa Ana CA, Morawski SG, et al. Development of a lavage solution associated with minimal water and electrolyte absorption or secretion. Gastroenterology 1980; 78:991–5.
5. Bigard M-A, Gaucher P, Lassalle C. Fatal colonic explosion during colonoscopic polypectomy. Gastroenterology 1979; 77:1307–10.
6. Goldman J, Reichelderfer M. Evaluation of rapid colonoscopy preparation using a new gut lavage solution. Gastrointest Endosc 1982; 28:9–11.
7. Rhodes JB, Engstrom J, Stone KF. Metaclopramide reduces the distress associated with colonic cleansing by an oral electrolyte overload. Gastrointest Endosc 1978; 24:162–3.
8. Minervini S, Alexander-Williams J, Donovan IA, et al. Comparison of three methods of whole bowel irrigation. Am J Surg 1980; 140:400–2.
9. Ernstoff JJ, Howard DA, Marshall JB, et al. A randomized blinded clinical trial of a rapid colonic lavage solution (Golytely) compared with standard preparation for colonoscopy and barium enema. Gastroenterology 1983; 84:1512–6.
10. Waye JD. Colonoscopy intubation techniques without fluoroscopy. In: Hunt RH, Waye JD, eds. Colonoscopy. Techniques, Clinical Practice and Colour Atlas. London: Chapman and Hall, 1981; 147–78.
11. Nanni C, Garbini A, Luchetti P, et al. Ogilvie's syndrome (acute colonic pseudo-obstruction): Review of the literature (October 1948 to March 1980) and report of four additional cases. Dis Colon Rectum 1982; 25:157–66.
12. Bode WE, Beart RW Jr, Spencer RJ, et al. Colonoscopic decompression for acute pseudoobstruction of the colon (Ogilvie's syndrome). Report of 22 cases and review of the literature. Am J Surg 1984; 147:243–5.
13. Kukora JS, Dent TL. Colonoscopic decompression of massive nonobstructive cecal dilation. Arch Surg 1977; 112:512–7.
14. Bernton E, Myers R, Reyna T. Pseudoobstruction of the colon: case report including a new endoscopic treatment. Gastrointest Endosc 1982; 28:90–2.
15. Nivatvongs S, Vermeulen FD, Fang DT. Colonoscopic decompression of acute pseudoobstruction of the colon. Ann Surg 1982; 196:598–600.
16. Robbins RD, Schoen R, Sohn N, Weinstein MA. Colonic decompression of massive cecal dilatation (Ogilvie's syndrome) secondary to cesarian section. Am J Gastroenterol 1982; 77:231–2.
17. Nakhgevany KB. Colonoscopic decompression of the colon in patients with Ogilvie's syndrome. Am J Surg 1984; 148:317–20.

Chapter 41

INDICATIONS, CONTRAINDICATIONS, AND COMPLICATIONS OF COLONOSCOPY

GEORGE B. RANKIN, M.D.

For the past decade, colonoscopy has played an increasingly important role in the diagnosis and treatment of patients with diseases of the colon and rectum. The indications, contraindications, and complications of colonoscopy are outlined and discussed in this chapter.

The various indications for colonoscopy can be considered in two major categories: (1) diagnostic or clinical indications and (2) therapeutic or operative indications. These are listed in Table 41–1.

DIAGNOSTIC (CLINICAL) INDICATIONS

Unexplained Gastrointestinal Signs and Symptoms (with Normal Barium Enema)

A complete history and physical examination will provide enough information in some patients to make a tentative diagnosis. Colonoscopy is usually considered only when conventional studies such as proctosigmoidoscopy and barium enema as well as stool examinations fail to confirm a diagnosis. Unexplained diarrhea and abdominal pain with or without weight loss are the major indications for colonoscopy in as many as 20% of patients.[1]

Unexplained Rectal Bleeding

All patients with unexplained rectal bleeding should undergo colonoscopy unless it is contraindicated.[2] The causes of rectal bleeding are numerous and the major ones are listed in Table 41–2. Rectal bleeding is most often chronic but may also be acute and massive and at times life-threatening. In this situation, colonoscopy has been shown to be an important diagnostic study because of the

TABLE 41–1. **Indications for Colonoscopy**

Diagnostic (Clinical) Indications
Unexplained gastrointestinal symptoms and signs
  (with normal barium enema)
Unexplained rectal bleeding
Nondiagnostic radiographic examination
Polyp and cancer follow-up
Inflammatory bowel disease
Stricture or colonic narrowing
  (with and without inflammatory bowel disease)
Diverticular disease
Infectious colitides
Radiation colitis
Ischemic colitis
Endometriosis
Pneumatosis cystoides intestinalis
Evaluation of ureterosigmoidostomy
Decompression of pseudo-obstruction
Evaluation of experimental colitis

Therapeutic (Operative and Intraoperative) Indications
Polypectomy
Foreign body removal
Identification of bleeding sites (small intestine)
Hemostasis
Tumor palliation
Colonic decompression

TABLE 41–2. Causes of Rectal Bleeding

Hemorrhoids	Inflammatory bowel disease
Anal fissure	Crohn's disease
Polyp	Ulcerative colitis
Carcinoma	Infectious colitides
Diverticular disease	Radiation colitis
Solitary ulcers	Ischemic colitis
Vascular abnormality	Endometriosis
Angiodysplasia	Causes above ileocecal
Arteriovenous	valve
malformation	Meckel's diverticulum
Angioma	Upper gastrointestinal
Varices	bleeding

recognized limitations of rigid sigmoidoscopy and the barium enema.[3] A number of investigators have demonstrated that in some groups of ambulatory patients with chronic bleeding, colonoscopy will be diagnostic when a previous barium enema has been reported as entirely normal. Results of several reported series are listed in Table 41–3.[4–9]

A more challenging group of patients are those whose presenting symptom is acute bleeding. In some of the initial reports[9, 10] colonoscopy was considered to be unsuitable in acute bleeding; however, more recent studies have shown that colonoscopy is extremely valuable.[11–13] The limitation of colonoscopy in acute bleeding relates to the frequent inability to visualize clearly the colonic mucosa when the lumen is filled with blood. Newer instruments with large suction channels and effective methods of rapid preparation such as colonic lavage have significantly reduced this problem.

Colonoscopy in lower gastrointestinal bleeding is discussed in Chapter 6.

Nondiagnostic Radiographic Examination

Colonoscopy is performed commonly in patients in whom the barium enema examination is interpreted as being abnormal or possibly abnormal, but not diagnostic.[13–15] The most common types of real or spurious radiologic abnormalities that lead to endoscopy are colonic filling defects, nonspecific mucosal irregularities, segmental narrowing, and colon polyps.

Polyps and Cancer Follow-up

One of every five patients with neoplastic disease of the large bowel when first examined has more than one tumor, either an adenoma or an adenocarcinoma.[16] It has also been shown that in approximately 6% of those patients with a single tumor, one or more additional colonic neoplasms will subsequently develop. Neoplastic lesions are multiple in at least 25% of patients.

In most large series of patients with cancer of the colon or rectum, about 5% will have more than one cancer as either a synchronous or a metachronous lesion.[17, 18] Since patients with prior adenomas or carcinomas of the colon and rectum are at high risk for additional or new lesions, they should be kept under surveillance and have regularly scheduled follow-up colonoscopy examinations. Special attention should be given to those patients who have had a colon resection with an anastomosis. Colon cancers recur in the anastomotic line in 1% to 2% of postoperative colon cancer patients. Recognizable changes at the anastomosis may be present 3 to 6 months postoperatively. Follow-up colonoscopy with biopsy and brush cytology has been recommended.[19]

The question of how often to screen patients who have had previous adenomas or colorectal cancers cannot be answered with certainty at this time. Various protocols and schedules are used at present in which the interval between examinations ranges from 12 to 48 months. The problem of colorectal

TABLE 41–3. Colonoscopy in Patients with Chronic Gastrointestinal Bleeding and Negative Barium Enema

Author	No. Patients	Cancer	Polyps	IBD*	Other	Total
Waye[4] (1976)	93	15	14	10	17	56 (60%)
Tedesco et al.[5] (1978)	258	29	39	19	15	102 (39.5%)
Brand et al.[6] (1980)	306	25	43	11	13	92 (30%)
Swarbrick et al.[7] (1978)	239	23	39	24	9	95 (39.7%)
Knutson and Max[8] (1980)	168	5	—	—	—	46 (27%)
Gilbert et al.[9] (1984)	2797	311	926	265	1538	—

*IBD = Inflammatory bowel disease.

neoplasia in relation to colonoscopy is considered extensively in Chapter 45.

Inflammatory Bowel Disease (IBD)

Colonoscopy can be an extremely useful procedure in the diagnosis and management of patients with inflammatory bowel disease (IBD); however, the majority of patients with IBD do not require colonoscopy. There is rarely a clear indication for colonoscopy in acute severe colitis,[20] and it is contraindicated in the presence of fulminant colitis, toxic megacolon, and suspected perforation or peritonitis.[21] The specific indications for colonoscopy in patients with inflammatory bowel disease are listed in Table 41–4.[22–27] Additional aspects of colonoscopy in IBD are discussed in Chapters 42 and 43.

Strictures or Colonic Narrowing

The demonstration of a colonic stricture or narrowing must be considered a pathologic condition that requires further evaluation. Colonoscopy permits direct examination of strictured areas and a histologic diagnosis can be made in most cases.[28–31] The common causes of colonic stricture and narrowing are listed in Table 41–5. If the stricture has caused partial obstruction, colonoscopy can be performed after minimal preparation with enemas and usually provides a diagnosis. Colonoscopy is not required for all colonic strictures; the value of each proposed study should be considered in relation to the clinical setting. The history and physical findings together with the appearance of the barium contrast x-ray films may make endoscopy unnecessary. In general, colonoscopy is indicated when malignancy is possible but uncertain, if surgery is considered but not inevitable, or if clinical management might be altered by the results of the procedure. Con-

TABLE 41–4. Specific Indications for Colonoscopy in Patients with Inflammatory Bowel Disease

1. Differential diagnosis
2. Determine extent and severity of disease
3. Resolution of radiographic abnormalities (e.g., filling defects and narrowed or strictured areas)
4. Preoperative and postoperative evaluation in Crohn's disease
5. Examination of stomas
6. Screening for premalignant and malignant changes

TABLE 41–5. Common Causes of Colonic Stricture

1. Carcinoma (primary or recurrent)
2. Spasm
3. Ischemia
4. Trauma
5. Radiation
6. Diverticulitis
7. Adhesions
8. Inflammatory bowel disease
9. Infectious bowel disease
10. Extracolonic pathology
    Endometriosis
    Pneumatosis coli

traindications in these settings are few and similar to those applicable to any colonoscopic procedure.

Diverticular Disease

Diverticula and the various manifestations of diverticular disease can usually be well documented radiographically, and in most clinical situations colonoscopy is not indicated.[30] It has been shown that x-ray examination of the colon often fails to document the total number of diverticula and also characteristically tends to minimize the intensity of the inflammatory changes.[32] The major limitation of the barium contrast x-ray of the colon, however, is the inability to distinguish between changes due to diverticulitis and those due to carcinoma.

Colonoscopy should not be performed in patients when acute diverticulitis is suspected, but it is indicated primarily when the radiographic appearance of the colon raises doubt as to the possible presence of underlying malignancy or an inflammatory condition which fails to respond to medical treatment. The relatively small number of reports on the use of colonoscopy in diverticular disease are summarized in Table 41–6.[33–37] This shows that in diverticular disease there is a minority of patients in whom unsuspected carcinomas are found. Of equal importance is the ability to exclude endoscopically the presence of carcinoma with a high degree of confidence.

Even though colonoscopy may be extremely difficult in some patients with diverticular disease, it is performed primarily because of the inherent inaccuracy of even good-quality air contrast studies of the colon in the diagnosis of polyps and carcinoma.[30, 38]

TABLE 41–6. **Colonoscopy in Diverticular Disease**

Author(s)	No. Patients	Unexpected Cancer Found	Failed Examination
Dean and Newell[33] (1973)	36	4 (11%)	17 (47%)
Forde[34] (1977)	40	2 (5%)	
Glerum et al.[35] (1977)	30	2 (7%)	3 (10%)
Max and Knutson[36] (1978)	26	2 (8%)	7 (27%)
Hunt[37] (1979)	44	6 (13%)	6 (13%)

The true incidence of bleeding from diverticular disease is not known. It is generally agreed that occasionally patients bleed massively from ulceration of a diverticulum. Colonoscopic diagnosis in these patients may be helpful in localizing the source of bleeding.

Infectious Colitis

Since most infectious colitides tend to be self-limited, rarely do patients with these diseases require colonoscopy. In acute infections of the colon due to *Salmonella*, *Shigella*, and *Campylobacter*, the colonoscopic findings may be difficult to differentiate from those of ulcerative colitis or Crohn's disease.

In antibiotic associated colitis due to *Clostridia difficile*, colonoscopy may be helpful in identifying the classic plaques or membranes. These often do not involve the colon in a uniform distribution, and may be confined to the right colon instead of the rectosigmoid colon.[39, 40]

Tuberculosis can involve any portion of the large bowel or ileum and produce changes indistinguishable from those of Crohn's disease.[41–44]

Amebiasis typically produces an intense inflammatory reaction in the colon that may resemble Crohn's disease. Positive biopsy specimens can be obtained from any area of the mucosa.[45]

Schistosomiasis, although rarely encountered in temperate climates, may alert the colonoscopist to the possibility of this diagnosis by the presence of inflammatory polyps, especially in a patient from an endemic area. Calcified polyps that have the appearance of white nodules are a unique feature of this condition.[46]

Yersinia enterocolitica has the appearance of small diffuse ulcerations throughout the colon and may be mistaken for Crohn's colitis.[47]

The subject of inflammatory and infectious colitides is considered extensively in Chapter 42.

Radiation-Induced Colitis

Radiation-induced colitis is a common complication of modern megavoltage radiotherapy. Damage may occur to either the large or small intestine, and with colonic involvement rectal bleeding is usually the presenting symptom. A history of radiation therapy should increase one's suspicion as to the diagnosis, but often the severe changes induced by radiation may not become symptomatic until many years after therapy.[48] Radiation-induced colitis is considered in Chapter 44.

Ischemic Colitis

Ischemic colitis is a well-recognized entity, usually in elderly patients, in most of whom the presenting symptoms are hematochezia, abdominal pain, and diarrhea. Until recently, the diagnosis of ischemic colitis was based on the clinical presentation and the barium enema and proctosigmoidoscopy examinations. There is limited experience with the endoscopic evaluation of patients with ischemic colitis.[49, 50] From available studies, it can be concluded that colonoscopy is an alternative and a reasonably safe modality for diagnosis of ischemic colitis that has proved to be more accurate than conventional x-ray or proctosigmoidoscopy examinations.[51, 52] The risks of excessive air insufflation and the potential for instrument-induced perforation of the necrotic bowel have been considered contraindications to colonoscopy.[23] The subject of ischemic colitis is developed in Chapter 44.

Endometriosis

Colonic involvement occurs in about 30% to 35% of female patients with endometriosis, and its differentiation from neoplasm may be difficult.[53, 54] Colonoscopy is an important adjunctive tool in the diagnosis and management of colorectal endometriosis. The colonoscopic findings of a reduction of the lumen of the bowel and extrinsic compression in the presence of an intact mucosa are strongly suggestive of this diagnosis.[55] Endometriosis is discussed in Chapter 46.

Pneumatosis Cystoides Intestinalis

A variety of disorders have been associated with pneumatosis cystoides intestinalis, albeit usually without a clear cause-and-effect relation. It has been suggested that many of the disorders of the gastrointestinal tract with which pneumatosis cystoides intestinalis has been associated have the common element of partial intestinal obstruction. The marked alteration of the mucosa that occurs with this disorder often raises the question of another underlying disease, such as inflammatory bowel disease or malignancy. Colonoscopy therefore can be considered as a potentially useful adjunct in the evaluation of these patients.[56] Further discussion is found in Chapter 46.

Miscellaneous

Other clinical indications for colonoscopy include the evaluation and surveillance of ureterosigmoidostomies, decompression of pseudo-obstruction of the colon,[57, 58] emergency reduction of sigmoid volvulus,[59] and evaluation of experimental forms of colitis in animal models.[60]

THERAPEUTIC (OPERATIVE) INDICATIONS

Therapeutic colonoscopy, which includes both operative and intra-operative uses in this discussion, is reported to be of value in almost every situation in which it has been employed.[61, 62] The indications for therapeutic colonoscopy are listed in Table 41–7.

Intra-operative colonoscopy refers to fiberoptic colonoscopy per anus during intra-abdominal surgical procedures without a colotomy. Intra-operative colonoscopy can be

TABLE 41–7. **Indications for Therapeutic Colonoscopy**

Polypectomy
Foreign body removal
Identification of bleeding sites (small intestine)
Hemostasis
Tumor palliation
Colonic decompression

used to avoid a colotomy or resection and to determine whether or not a planned resection should be extended or limited; it can also suggest unplanned but necessary surgical resection.[63]

Polypectomy

Polypectomy is the most important procedure in this group of indications and accounts for more than 95% of all therapeutic colonoscopies. This is discussed in Chapter 45.

Foreign Body Removal

In contrast to the removal of foreign bodies from the upper gastrointestinal tract, the use of colonoscopy for removal of foreign bodies from the colon and rectum is less common.[61] However, many different objects have been extracted from the colon and rectum with the use of various accessories (see Chapter 14).

Identification of Bleeding Sites (Small Intestine)

Colonoscopy has considerable potential value in the examination of patients with unexplained recurrent gastrointestinal bleeding and permits complete examination of the small bowel during a laparotomy without the need for a colotomy or an enterotomy.

Hemostasis

The need for colonoscopic hemostasis is rare. A variety of methods have been successful including electrocoagulation and photocoagulation. The sources of bleeding that may require endoscopic hemostasis include polypectomy sites, solitary ulcers, solitary angiomas, and various angiodysplastic lesions. Circumscribed bleeding from radiation injury may also require endoscopic hemostasis.

Tumor Resection (Palliative)

There is limited experience with the application of colonoscopy to tumor resection of the colon and rectum. At present this is considered investigative and essentially palliative. Methods such as laser photodestruction for relief of obstruction and for reduction of bleeding from tumors are being studied.

Colonic Decompression

Colonoscopy has been reported as being effective for the reduction of sigmoid volvulus and intussusceptions of the colon (see Chapter 40). The published experience consists largely of case reports; there are no large prospective series.

CONTRAINDICATIONS TO COLONOSCOPY

Although there are few absolute contraindications for colonoscopy, there are a number of relative contraindications, as listed in Table 41–8.

Colonoscopy should not be attempted by unskilled and poorly trained individuals who lack thorough knowledge of the equipment and proper techniques.[62] In all instances, the endoscopist must assess the age and general condition of the patient being considered for colonoscopy. He must select the appropriate method of bowel preparation, with modifications as necessary, and be familiar with the uses and hazards of medications that will be administered.

COMPLICATIONS AND HAZARDS OF COLONOSCOPY

Just as the diagnostic and therapeutic potential of colonoscopy has progressed over the years, the awareness of the potential complications and hazards associated with the procedure has also increased. Table 41–9 is a complete listing of the recognized complications and hazards.

It has been stated repeatedly that colonoscopy requires a combination of sound clinical judgment; development of manipulative

TABLE 41–8. **Contraindications to Colonoscopy**

1. Acute inflammation of colon (fulminant), including ulcerative colitis, Crohn's colitis, ischemic colitis, diverticulitis and radiation colitis
2. Peritonitis
3. Pregnancy (2nd and 3rd trimester)
4. Uncooperative patient
5. Bleeding disorder
6. Acute cardiorespiratory disease
7. Recent myocardial infarction
8. Pulmonary embolus
9. Shock
10. Large aortic or ileac aneurysm
11. Recent pelvic or colonic surgery

TABLE 41–9. **Complications of Colonoscopy**

Diagnostic Colonoscopy	Therapeutic Colonoscopy
Related to preparation	Perforation
Related to medication	Hemorrhage
Bacteremia	Serosal burns
Hemorrhage	Incomplete polypectomy
Perforation	Explosion
Diastatic serosal tears	Accidental removal of ureterosigmoidostomy stoma
Post-colonoscopy distention	
Vasovagal reflex	Accidental removal of intussuscepted appendix
Splenic avulsion	
Cardiac and ECG abnormalities	Electrical perforation of ileum
Volvulus	
Colonic obstruction	
Adynamic ileus	
Pneumocystoides intestinalis	
Incarceration of instrument in hernia	
Impaction of instrument in hernia	
Aortic aneurysm dissection	
Cardiopulmonary problems	

skills; a working knowledge of the anatomy, especially that of the colon; extreme patience; and safe and functional equipment. Despite these prerequisites, complications are inevitable in colonoscopy because the slightest misjudgment, momentary loss of control, malfunction of equipment, anatomic variation, or pathologic alteration can lead to untoward results.[63]

The major complications of colonoscopy are hemorrhage, perforation, and death. The incidence rates of these complications in several large series are listed in Table 41–10.[64–67] Other large reported series show comparable figures.[68–72]

An interesting correlation between the complication rate and the experience of the endoscopist has been documented in several series.[64, 66, 68] As might be expected, the highest complication rate occurs with inexperienced examiners during their first 50 to 100 colonoscopies.[66]

Complications of Diagnostic Colonoscopy

Bowel Preparation

The potential hazards of the preparation process include fluid and electrolyte imbalance. Although fluid overload may occur, dehydration and hypovolemia are more com-

TABLE 41–10. **Incidence Rates of Complications of Colonoscopy Reported in ASGE and ASCRS Surveys and a Series in the Federal Republic of Germany (FRG)***

	ASGE[64] (1975)		ASCRS[65] (1976)		FRG[66]		ASGE[67] (1984)	
	No. Patients	(%)	No. Patients	(%)	No. Patients	(%)	No. Patients	(%)
Perforation								
Diagnostic	25,298	(0.22)	12,746	(0.26)	35,892	(0.14)	4,713	(0.17)
Polypectomy	6,214	(0.29)	9,238	(0.42)	7,365	(0.34)	1,901	(0.11)
Hemorrhage								
Diagnostic	25,298	(0.05)	12,746	(0.07)	35,892	(0.008)	4,713	(0.01)
Polypectomy	6,214	(0.77)	9,228	(1.0)	7,365	(2.24)	1,901	(2.16)
Deaths								
Diagnostic	25,298	(0.008)	12,746	(0.03)	35,892	(0.02)	4,713	(0)
Polypectomy	6,214	(0)	9,238	(0.01)	7,365	(0.1)	1,901	(0.05)

*ASGE = American Society for Gastrointestinal Endoscopy; ASCRS = American Society of Colon and Rectal Surgeons.

mon. Mannitol is an excellent agent for bowel preparation,[73] but because bacterial action produces hydrogen, there is a potential for explosion within the colon. Mannitol should never be used when electrosurgery is contemplated unless carbon dioxide is used for bowel insufflation.[74] More suitable alternative solutions are available.[75, 76]

Premedication

The most commonly used premedication regimen consists of the use of diazepam in conjunction with a narcotic analgesic such as meperidine (pethidine). The most frequent serious side effect of diazepam is respiratory depression; rapid intravenous administration can lead to respiratory arrest.[77] Individual sensitivity to diazepam varies widely and seems to increase with the age of the patient. Thrombophlebitis at the site of the intravenous injection of diazepam is a known complication, and the reported incidence ranges from 3.5% to 10%.[64, 68, 69, 78, 79]

Adverse reactions to narcotic analgesics such as meperidine are not uncommon and may include respiratory depression, hypotension, bradycardia, nausea, vomiting, and sweating. Respiratory depression can be quickly reversed by intravenous administration of naloxone (Narcan).

Bacteremia and Antibiotic Prophylaxis

During colonoscopic procedures, a transient bacteremia may occur,[64] but bacterial endocarditis has not been reported. The bacteremia associated with colonoscopy has been studied by many authors, and yet no specific precautions have been recommended.[80–85]

Some authors believe that even though the risk of bacteremia is negligible in healthy and low-risk patients, it is probably beneficial, based on current information, to prescribe antibiotics to high-risk patients until better prospective, double-blind controlled studies are available.[68, 86–88] The high-risk category would, in particular, include patients with prosthetic heart valves and other prosthetic devices.

Colonoscopy is not mentioned directly in the publications of the American Heart Association concerning the prevention of bacterial endocarditis in patients with cardiac disease, but prophylaxis is recommended by the American Heart Association for patients who are undergoing proctosigmoidoscopy, and it is generally agreed that similar recommendations seem appropriate for colonoscopy.[89] Prophylaxis has been recommended for patients with known valvular heart disease or prostheses,[68] for immunosuppressed patients, and for cirrhotic patients with ascites.

If antibiotics are used, ampicillin and an aminoglycoside or vancomycin (alone or with an aminoglycoside) should be used in the dosages suggested by the American Heart Association.[90]

Hemorrhage

Hemorrhage is a rare complication of diagnostic colonoscopy, occurring in 0.008% to 0.17% of procedures in large series (see Table 41–10). Bleeding in such instances usually is intra-abdominal and is the result of excessive force during manipulation.[73] The source may be a seromuscular tear,[91-93] rupture of the liver or spleen,[94, 95] or tearing of the mesentery.[96] It is important to ascertain prior to colonoscopy whether a patient has a history of a bleeding diathesis or is receiving anticoagulant therapy.

Perforation

Perforation is the most common complication of diagnostic colonoscopy, with a reported incidence of 0.14% to 0.26% in large surveys (see Table 41–10). Perforations are most often the result of mechanical pressure resulting from the direct force of the colonoscope tip or shaft. The majority of perforations occur during mechanical manipulations of the sigmoid loop including slide-by, the alpha maneuver, and straightening of the loop.[96] The most common sites of these perforations, which are usually mural perforations, are the rectosigmoid and the junction of the sigmoid and descending colon. Extraperitoneal perforations also occur and are caused by pneumatic pressure or a combination of mechanical and pneumatic pressure. These most commonly occur in the rectum or the posterior wall of the descending colon.

Correlative anatomic-radiologic studies have established the characteristic distribution of extraperitoneal gas according to the site of perforation.[97] The gas may dissect its way into many areas, including the upper renal poles, adrenal glands, the medial border of the liver and spleen, the medial crus of the diaphragm, and the immediate subphrenic tissue. Extension of gas into the flank fat stripes, anterior abdominal wall, scrotum, mediastinum, and chest may occur.

Perforations are more likely to occur in patients with adhesions, severe diverticular disease, areas of severe transmural inflammation, or a strictured segment of the colon. Free perforation is four times more common than closed perforation.[64]

Diastatic Serosal Tears

There is considerable evidence that diastatic serosal tears occur during colonoscopy.[91-93] The frequency of this complication is not known, since the diagnosis is confirmed only when patients subsequently undergo a laparotomy. In the laboratory model, increasing the segmental intraluminal pressure results in sequential seromuscular stripping, mucosal herniation, and ultimate mucosal rupture.

A combination of factors is responsible for serosal and seromuscular tears of the colon during colonoscopy. Among the contributing factors are the volume of air, rate of insufflation, location of the insufflated air, and localized mechanical stretching and bowing of the antimesenteric wall of the sigmoid colon during insertion of the colonoscope.

Post-Colonoscopy Distention Syndrome

Post-colonoscopy distention syndrome has been reported by many authors. This complication is characterized by an uncomfortably distended abdomen occurring toward the end of colonoscopy. The symptoms can mimic perforation but x-ray films show only distended loops of both large and small intestine. In some cases post-colonoscopy distention is thought to be related to patency of the ileocecal valve. Overdistention of the bowel can be prevented by the cautious use of air insufflation. Most instances of post-colonoscopy distention syndrome resolve rapidly without specific treatment; however, cases of adynamic ileus have been reported that required nasogastric suction and intravenous fluids.[65, 98]

Vasovagal Reflex

The vasovagal reflex is characterized by bradycardia, hypotension, and cold, clammy skin; it is thought to be caused by stretching the mesentery to the point that pain results. It is less likely to occur in the patients who receive narcotic analgesics as premedication. The incidence of this complication in one large series was 0.72%.[67]

Cardiac and Electrocardiographic Abnormalities

Transient electrocardiographic abnormalities have been described in various endoscopic procedures. In one study the incidence was 40% in patients undergoing colonoscopy.[99] The majority of abnormalities noted were new or exaggerated electrocardiographic abnormalities, such as frequent premature atrial and ventricular beats, sinus tachycardia, and ST-T segment depression. A large number of these patients had recognized heart disease. The arrhythmias that occurred in patients with known heart disease were more frequent and serious.[99]

Myocardial infarction has been documented during or shortly after colonoscopy.[65]

The possibility that patients who have cardiac pacemakers may experience dangerous electrical interference with their pulse generators during colonoscopic electrosurgery has been suggested.[100] Recent improvement in pacemaker design minimizes this risk. Nonetheless, the use of electrosurgery in this setting should be approached with caution.[101] Knowledge of the type of pacemaker may be helpful in assessing the risk; unipolar units appear to be more susceptible to electrical interference than bipolar units.[102] Some manufacturers recommend special safeguards such as magnetic conversion to a fixed rate (see Chapter 7 for a discussion of electrosurgery and pacemakers).

Volvulus

Although colonoscopy has been used to reduce sigmoid volvulus, this condition may also be a complication of the procedure.[63] Sigmoid volvulus as a result of the alpha maneuver has been reported;[65] a transverse colon volvulus apparently occurred when insufflated air was trapped by the angulation of the hepatic and splenic flexures; cecal volvulus has occurred after colonoscopy.[103] Surgery is usually needed for decompression.[65]

Miscellaneous Complications

Other complications of colonoscopy include incarceration of a previously reducible long-standing incisional hernia after colonoscopy,[104] and impaction of the colonoscope in a hernial sac.[105] Dissection of a large aortic aneurysm has been reported. Partial colonic obstruction has been converted to complete obstruction, apparently by overinsufflation of air. Colonic obstruction in a patient with extensive diverticulosis also has been noted. Pneumatic ileal perforation necessitating urgent resection of the bowel has been described in a patient with multiple distal adhesions of the small intestine and a competent ileocecal valve.[106] Pneumatosis cystoides coli is a rare complication of colonoscopy.[107, 108]

Complications of Therapeutic Colonoscopy

Hemorrhage

The major complication of colonoscopic polypectomy is hemorrhage. The reported incidence in large surveys (see Table 41–10) ranges from 0.77% to 2.24%. Most bleeding occurs immediately after transection of the pedicle,[63, 64, 66] and most delayed hemorrhages are manifested within the first 24 hours, although delays up to 21 days have been reported.[64, 109]

As a rule, bleeding after polypectomy results from inadequate coagulation of the vessels that supply the polyp. The most common technical error is mechanical transection of the pedicle of the polyp before adequate electrocoagulation has occurred. Special caution is advised in approaching larger pedunculated polyps.[110]

Analysis of collected data shows an increased incidence of postpolypectomy hemorrhage among inexperienced colonoscopists.[64]

The management of postpolypectomy hemorrhage is primarily expectant. In most instances bleeding will stop spontaneously. If it persists and the area is still visible endoscopically, attempts to re-snare the pedicle remnant and repeat the electrocoagulation are said to be successful in some instances.[111] This should be done cautiously because overcoagulation can result in perforation.[71] A collection of blood at the bleeding site may interfere with attempts at electrocoagulation, and the instillation of a vasoconstrictive solution such as epinephrine (1:10,000) via an endoscopic catheter may stop or slow the bleeding.[63] Other methods such as selective intra-arterial vasoconstrictive infusions for the control of postpolypectomy bleeding have been successful in some instances.[112] Most postpolypectomy hemorrhages do not require transfusions or surgical intervention. Death in these circumstances is extremely rare.

Perforation

Perforation associated with colonoscopic polypectomy is also a major complication, which has a frequency from 0.11% to 0.42% (see Table 41–10). The risk of perforation increases during removal of sessile polyps.[65] The various factors that contribute to perforation are cutting through bowel wall, which has been inadvertently pulled into the snare loop; application of too much power, ending in eventual necrosis of a transmural burn; and mechanical or pneumatic pressures on bowel wall already weakened by electrocoagulation.[63]

Perforation may also occur from the forceful passage of the instrument in the absence of an adequate view of the lumen or as a result of rotating or straightening maneuvers during the procedure.

Perforation can occur without the patient experiencing acute abdominal pain, especially in the case of a small retroperitoneal perforation. Endoscopic visualization of an open defect in the bowel wall, visible fatty tissue such as the omentum, or actual abdominal organs indicates a perforation.

Most commonly, the symptoms of perforation are the onset of persistent abdominal pain that may be accompanied by generalized tenderness (a sign of peritoneal irritation apparently due to bacterial contamination in the abdominal cavity), and abdominal distention. Documentation of free air under the diaphragm by x-ray studies is confirmatory evidence.

When a colon perforation occurs, the adequacy of the bowel preparation, the underlying pathologic process prompting colonoscopy, the size of the perforation, and other medical factors that collectively influence the anesthetic and operative risks must be weighed in deciding on the course of management.

In most instances of frank perforation, the degree of immediate contamination of the abdomen is minimal, as fecal liquids and solids in the colon are markedly reduced by mechanical cleansing prior to endoscopy. However, when a major perforation of the bowel wall is apparent, prompt surgical intervention is advisable to control the spread of intraperitoneal or extraperitoneal contamination. When performed within several hours, operative treatment can be definitive and should include local debridement and primary closure of the colonic rent. If operative therapy is delayed, abscess formation or extensive peritonitis may result, and a procedure to divert the fecal stream with limited resection may then be necessary.[113] In all operative cases antibiotic coverage is indicated.

There is evidence that some small colonic leaks may heal spontaneously without untoward sequelae, thereby obviating the need for surgical closure.[114–117] This approach merits consideration, especially in well-prepared patients with benign colonic disease and when medical factors weigh strongly against surgery.[117] This course of action requires that the patient's status be observed closely. On occasion, rapid decompression of the abdomen by needle or trocar for a post-colonoscopy pneumoperitoneum is required to relieve compromised cardiorespiratory function.[116]

Transmural Burn

A presumptive diagnosis of a transmural burn is made when a patient who has undergone polypectomy develops abdominal pain, leukocytosis, and fever without evidence of a perforation.[64] The presumptive diagnosis is strengthened if the patient experienced pain at the time of polypectomy or electrocoagulation.[49] Conservative therapy is indicated.

Incomplete Polypectomy

Incomplete polypectomy, especially with large polyps, is a distressing and time-consuming complication.[63] The cause is usually an incarcerated snare wire. This may occur with braided-wire snares when the current density is too low or the ratio of coagulation to cutting power is too high. The situation may require the removal of the snare handle, withdrawal of the colonoscope while leaving the snare wire attached to the polyp, reinsertion of the colonoscope, insertion of a second snare, and a repeat attempt at polypectomy.[118] Alternative piecemeal polypectomy has been recommended as the initial technique for large lesions, or surgery may be considered.[49]

Explosion of Colonic Gases

Two cases of intracolonic explosion during endoscopic electrosurgery have been reported.[119, 120] In both cases, a mannitol solution was used for bowel preparation. Only one patient recovered after surgery. As a result of such cases, there is little doubt that the use of mannitol or other carbohydrate solutions (sorbital, lactose) is contraindicated in the routine bowel preparation if there is any possibility of electrosurgery.

Death

Death as a complication of therapeutic or diagnostic colonoscopy is extremely rare. The incidence in large series ranges from 0 to 0.3%.[64–68] The causes of death include overmedication, peritonitis, and operative complications.

Miscellaneous Complications

As with any endoscopic procedure, therapeutic misadventures may occasionally occur. Some of those reported include accidental removal of a ureterosigmoidostomy stoma,[121] endoscopic removal of an intussuscepted appendix mimicking a polyp,[122] and perforation of the ileum related to the use of electrosurgery.[123]

Prevention of Complications

Only a qualified colonoscopist should use electrosurgery during colonoscopy. Skill in diagnostic colonoscopy should be a prerequisite in undertaking colonoscopic electrosurgery.[72] A colonoscopist must have a thorough understanding of the principles of electrosurgery, and be familiar with the type of electrosurgical equipment used, which must also be kept in good repair.[63]

It is imperative that pertinent information in each patient's medical history be obtained prior to colonoscopy, with particular emphasis on the history of bleeding tendencies, allergies, and cardiopulmonary disease.

References

1. Dybdahl JH, Myren J, Serck-Hanssen A. Routine colonoscopy, a retrospective evaluation. J Oslo City Hosp 1978; 28:65–72.
2. Williams CB, Teague RH. Progress report colonoscopy. Gut 1973; 14:990–1003.
3. Forde KA. Colonoscopy in the diagnosis and management of colonic bleeding. Bull NY Acad Med 1983; 59:301–5.
4. Waye JD. Colonoscopy in rectal bleeding. S Afr J Surg 1976; 14:143–9.
5. Tedesco FJ, Waye JD, Raskin JB, et al. Colonoscopic evaluation of rectal bleeding. A study of 304 patients. Ann Intern Med 1978; 89:907–9.
6. Brand EJ, Sullivan BH Jr, Sivak MV Jr, et al. Colonoscopy in the diagnosis of unexplained rectal bleeding. Ann Surg 1980; 192:111–3.
7. Swarbrick ET, Fevre DI, Hunt RH, et al. Colonoscopy for unexplained rectal bleeding. Br Med J 1978; 2:1685–7.
8. Knutson CO, Max HH. Value of colonoscopy in patients with rectal blood loss unexplained by rigid proctosigmoidoscopy and barium contrast enema examinations. Am J Surg 1980; 139:84–7.
9. Gilbert DA, Shaneyfelt SL, Silverstein FE, et al. The National ASGE Colonoscopy Survey—Analysis of colonoscopic practices and yield. Gastrointest Endosc 1984; 30:143.
10. Sivak MV Jr, Sullivan BH Jr, Rankin GB. Colonoscopy. A report of 644 cases and review of the literature. Am J Surg 1974; 128:351–7.
11. Hedberg SE. Endoscopy in gastrointestinal bleeding. A systematic approach to diagnosis. Surg Clin North Am 1974; 54:549–59.
12. Rossini HG, Ferrari A. Emergency colonoscopy. Acta Endosc Radiochim 1976; 6:165.
13. Jensen DM, Machicado GA, Tapia JI. Emergent colonoscopy in patients with severe hematochezia. (Abstr) Gastrointest Endosc 1983; 29:177.
14. Knutson CO, Max MH. Diagnostic and therapeutic colonoscopy: a critical review of 662 examinations. Arch Surg 1979; 114:430–5.
15. Schmitt MG Jr, Wu WC, Geenen JE, et al. Diagnostic colonoscopy. An assessment of the clinical indications. Gastroenterology 1975; 69:765–9.
16. Muto T, Bussey HJR, Morson BC. The evolution of cancer of the colon and rectum. Cancer 1975; 36:2251–70.
17. Heald RJ, Bussey HJR. Clinical experiences at St. Mark's Hospital with multiple synchronous cancers of the colon and rectum. Dis Colon Rectum 1975; 18:6–10.
18. Winawer SJ. Colon cancer. In: Hunt RH, Waye JD, eds. Colonoscopy: Techniques, Clinical Practice, and Colour Atlas. London: Chapman and Hall, 1981; 327–42.
19. Overholt BF. Colonoscopy and colon cancer: Current clinical practice. CA 1982; 32:180–6.
20. Hogan WJ, Hensley GT, Geenen JE. Endoscopic evaluation of inflammatory bowel disease. Symposium on inflammatory bowel disease. Med Clin North Am 1980; 64:1083–1102.
21. Waye JD. The role of colonoscopy in the differential diagnosis of inflammatory bowel disease. Gastrointest Endosc 1977; 23:150–4.
22. Teague RH, Waye JD. Inflammatory bowel disease. In: Hunt RH, Waye JD, eds. Colonoscopy: Techniques, Clinical Practice, and Colour Atlas. London: Chapman and Hall, 1981; 343–62.
23. Williams CB, Waye JD. Colonoscopy in inflammatory bowel disease. Clin Gastroenterol 1978; 7:701–17.
24. Lennard-Jones JE, Morson BC, Ritchie JK, et al. Cancer in colitis: assessment of the individual risk by clinical and histological criteria. Gastroenterology 1977; 73:1280–9.
25. Yardley JH, Bayless TM, Diamond MP. Cancer in ulcerative colitis. Gastroenterology 1979; 76:221–5.
26. Nugent FW, Haggitt RC, Colcher H, et al. Malignant potential of chronic ulcerative colitis: preliminary report. Gastroenterology 1979; 76:1–5.
27. Fuson JA, Farmer RG, Hawk WA, et al. Endoscopic surveillance for cancer in chronic ulcerative colitis. Am J Gastroenterol 1980; 73:120–6.
28. Rozen P, Ratan J, Gilat T. Colonoscopy in the differential diagnosis of colonic strictures. Dis Colon Rectum 1975; 18:425–9.
29. Aste H, Pugliese V, Munizzi F, et al. Left-sided stenosing lesions in colonoscopy. Gastrointest Endosc 1983; 29:18–20.
30. Williams CB. Diverticular disease and strictures. In: Hunt RH, Waye JD, eds. Colonoscopy: Techniques, Clinical Practice, and Colour Atlas. London: Chapman and Hall, 1981; 363–81.
31. Forde KA, Lebwohl O, Seaman WB. Colonoscopy as an adjunctive technique in evaluating acquired colonic narrowing. Surgery 1980; 87:243–7.
32. Marks G, Moses ML. The clinical application of flexible fiberoptic colonoscopy. Surg Clin North Am 1973; 53:735–56.
33. Dean ACB, Newell JP. Colonoscopy in the differential diagnosis of carcinoma from diverticulitis of the sigmoid colon. Br J Surg 1973; 60:633–5.
34. Forde KA. Colonoscopy in complicated diverticular disease. Gastrointest Endosc 1977; 23:192–3.
35. Glerum J, Agenant D, Tytgat GN. Value of colonoscopy in the detection of sigmoid malignancy in patients with diverticular disease. Endoscopy 1977; 9:228–30.
36. Max MH, Knutson CO. Colonoscopy in patients with inflammatory colonic strictures. Surgery 1978; 84:551–6.

37. Hunt RH. The role of colonoscopy in complicated diverticular disease. Acta Chir Belg 1979; 78:349–53.

38. Teague RH, Manning AP, Thornton JR, et al. Colonoscopy for investigation of unexplained rectal bleeding. Lancet 1978; 1:1350–1.

39. Seppala K, Hjelt L, Sipponen P. Colonoscopy in the diagnosis of antibiotic-associated colitis. A prospective study. Scand J Gastroenterol 1981; 16:465–8.

40. Anderson DL, Cammerer RC, Boyce HW Jr: Pseudomembranous enterocolitis: clinical spectrum and endoscopic findings. (Abstr) Gastroenterology 1974; 66:803.

41. Hiatt GA. Miliary tuberculosis with ileocecal involvement diagnosed by colonoscopy. JAMA 1978; 240:561–2.

42. Aoki G, Nagasako K, Nakae Y, et al. The fibrecolonoscopic diagnosis of intestinal tuberculosis. Endoscopy 1975; 7:113.

43. Bretholz A, Strasser H, Knoblauch M. Endoscopic diagnosis of ileocecal tuberculosis. Gastrointest Endosc 1978; 24:250–1.

44. Franklin GO, Mohapatra M, Perrillo RP. Colonic tuberculosis diagnosed by colonoscopic biopsy. Gastroenterology 1979; 76:362–4.

45. Crowson TD, Hines C Jr. Amebiasis diagnosed by colonoscopy. Gastrointest Endosc 1978; 24:254–5.

46. Nebel OT, El-Masry NA, Castell DO, et al. Schistosomal colonic polyposis: Endoscopic and histologic characteristics. Gastrointest Endosc 1974; 20:99–101.

47. Vantrappen G, Ponette E, Geboes K, et al. Yersinia enteritis and enterocolitis: gastroenterological aspects. Gastroenterology 1977; 72:220–7.

48. Reichelderfer M, Morrissey JF. Colonoscopy in radiation colitis. Gastrointest Endosc 1980; 26:41–3.

49. Sugarbaker PH, Vineyard GC, Lewicki AM, et al. Colonoscopy in the management of diseases of the colon and rectum. Surg Gynecol Obstet 1974; 139:341–9.

50. Teague RH, Salmon PR, Read AE. Fibreoptic examination of the colon: a review of 255 cases. Gut 1973; 14:139–42.

51. Scowcroft CW, Sanowski RA, Kozarek RA. Colonoscopy in ischemic colitis. Gastrointest Endosc 1981; 27:156–61.

52. McNeil C, Green G, Bannayan G, et al. Ischemic colitis diagnosed by colonoscopy. Gastrointest Endosc 1974; 20:124–6.

53. Kratzer GL, Salvati EP. Collective review of endometriosis of the colon. Am J Surg 1955; 90:866–9.

54. Mihas AA, Mihas TA. Colorectal endometriosis: the importance of preoperative diagnosis by colonoscopy. (Abstr) Gastrointest Endosc 1983; 29:178.

55. Farinon AM, Vadora E. Endometriosis of the colon and rectum: an indication for preoperative coloscopy. Endoscopy 1980; 12:136–9.

56. Forde KA, Whitlock RT, Seaman WB. Pneumatosis and cystoides intestinalis. Report of a case with colonoscopic findings of inflammatory bowel disease. Am J Gastroenterol 1977; 68:188–90.

57. Strodel WE, Nostrant TT, Eckhauser FE, et al. Therapeutic and diagnostic colonoscopy in nonobstructive colonic dilatation. Ann Surg 1983; 197:416–21.

58. Feinstat T, Gilbert V, Burns M, et al. The role of colonoscopic decompression in patients with acute pseudo-obstruction of the colon (Ogilvie's syndrome). (Abstr) Gastrointest Endosc 1982; 28:147.

59. Joergensen K, Kronborg O. The colonoscope in volvulus of the transverse colon. Dis Colon Rectum 1980; 23:357–8.

60. Mann NS, Demers LM. Experimental colitis studied by colonoscopy in the rat: effect of indomethacin. Gastrointest Endosc 1983; 29:77–82.

61. Fruhmorgen P. Therapeutic colonoscopy. In: Hunt RH, Waye JD, eds. Colonoscopy: Techniques, Clinical Practice, and Colour Atlas. London: Chapman and Hall 1981; 199–235.

62. Panish JF. Limitations and complications of colonoscopy. Gastrointest Endosc 1980; 26:205–6.

63. Rogers BHG. Complications and hazards of colonoscopy. In: Hunt RH, Waye JD, eds. Colonoscopy: Techniques, Clinical Practice, and Colour Atlas. London: Chapman and Hall 1981; 237–64.

64. Rogers BHG, Silvis SE, Nebel OT, et al. Complications of flexible fiberoptic colonoscopy and polypectomy. An analysis of the 1974 ASGE survey. Gastrointest Endosc 1975; 22:73–7.

65. Smith LF. Symposium. Fiberoptic colonoscopy: complications of colonoscopy and polypectomy. Dis Colon Rectum 1976; 19:407–12.

66. Fruhmorgen P, Demling L. Complications of diagnostic and therapeutic colonoscopy in the Federal Republic of Germany. Results of an inquiry. Endoscopy 1979; 11:146–50.

67. Gilbert DA, Hallstrom AP, Shaneyfelt SL, et al. The National ASGE Colonoscopy Survey Complications of Colonoscopy. (Abstr) Gastrointest Endosc 1984; 156.

68. Macrae FA, Tan KG, Williams CB. Towards safer colonoscopy: a report on the complications of 5000 diagnostic or therapeutic colonoscopies. Gut 1983; 24:376–83.

69. Berci G, Panish JF, Schapiro M, et al. Complications of colonoscopy and polypectomy. Report of the Southern California Society for Gastrointestinal Endoscopy. Gastroenterology 1974; 67:584–5.

70. Davis RE, Graham DY. Endoscopic complications. The Texas experience. Gastrointest Endosc 1979; 25:146–9.

71. Geenen JE, Schmitt MG Jr, Wu WC, et al. Major complications of colonoscopy: Bleeding and perforation. Am J Dig Dis 1975; 20:231–5.

72. Wolff WI, Shinya H. A new approach to colonic polyps. Ann Surg 1973; 178:367–78.

73. Hunt RH. Towards safer colonoscopy. Gut 1983; 24:371–5.

74. LaBrooy SJ, Avgerinos A, Fendick CL, et al. Potentially explosive colonic concentrations of hydrogen after bowel preparation with mannitol. Lancet 1981; 1:634–6.

75. Davis GR, Santa Ana CA, Morawski SG, et al. Development of a lavage solution associated with minimal water and electrolyte absorption or secretion. Gastroenterology 1980; 78:991–5.

76. Goldman J, Reichelder M. Evaluation of rapid colonoscopy preparation using a new gut lavage solution. Gastrointest Endosc 1982; 28:9–11.

77. Hall SC, Ovassapian A. Apnea after intravenous diazepam therapy. JAMA 1977; 238:1052.

78. Langdon DE. Thrombophlebitis following diazepam. JAMA 1973; 225:1389.

79. Langdon DE, Harlan JR, Bailey RL. Thrombophlebitis with diazepam used intravenously. JAMA 1973; 223:184–5.

80. Rafoth RJ, Sorenson RM, Bond JH Jr. Bacteremia following colonoscopy. Gastrointest Endosc 1975; 22:32–3.

81. Norfleet RG, Mulholland DD, Mitchell PD, et al. Does bacteremia follow colonoscopy? Gastroenterology 1976; 70:20–1.

82. Norfleet RC, Mitchell PD, Mulholland DD, et al. Does bacteremia follow colonoscopy? II. Results with blood cultures obtained 5, 10, and 15 minutes after colonoscopy. Gastrointest Endosc 1976; 23:31–2.

83. Dickman MD, Farrell R, Higgs RH, et al. Colonoscopy associated bacteremia. Surg Gynecol Obstet 1976; 142:173–6.

84. Hartong WA, Barnes WG, Calkins WG. The absence of bacteremia during colonoscopy. Am J Gastroenterol 1977; 67:240–4.

85. Coughlin GP, Butler RN, Alp MH, et al. Colonoscopy and bacteremia. Gut 1977; 678–9.

86. Pelican G. Hentges D, Butt J, et al. Bacteremia during colonoscopy. Gastrointest Endosc 1976; 23:33–5.

87. Kumar S, Abcarian H, Prasad ML, Lakshmanin S. Bacteremia associated with lower gastrointestinal endoscopy, fact or fiction? I. Colonoscopy. Dis Colon Rectum 1982; 25:131–4.

88. Liebermann TR. Bacteremia and fiberoptic endoscopy. Gastrointest Endosc 1976; 23:36–7.

89. American Heart Association Committee Report: Prevention of bacterial endocarditis. Circulation 1977; 56:139A–43A.

90. Meyer GW. Prophylaxis of infective endocarditis during colonoscopy: report of a survey. Gastrointest Endosc 1981; 27:58–9.

91. Livstone EM, Cohen GM, Troncale FJ, et al. Diastatic serosal lacerations: an unrecognized complication of colonoscopy. Gastroenterology 1974; 67:1245–7.

92. Rogers BHG. (Letter) Serosal lacerations during coloscopy. Gastroenterology 1975; 69:276–7.

93. Livstone EM, Kerstein MD. Serosal tears following colonoscopy. Arch Surg 1976; 111:88.

94. Telmos AJ, Mittal VK. (Letter) Splenic rupture following colonoscopy. JAMA 1977; 237:2718.

95. Ellis WR, Harrison JM, Williams RS. Rupure of spleen at colonoscopy. Br Med J 1979; 1:307–8.

96. Geenen JE, Schmitt MG Jr, Hogan WJ. Complications of colonoscopy. (Abstr) Gastroenterology 1974; 66:812.

97. Meyers MA. Radiologic features of the spread and localization of extraperitoneal gas and their relationship to its source. An anatomical approach. Radiology 1974; 111:17–26.

98. Ramakrishnan T. Adynamic ileus complicating colonoscopy. South Med J 1979; 72:92–3.

99. Alam M, Schuman BM, Duvernoy WFC, et al. Continuous electrocardiographic monitoring during colonoscopy. Gastrointest Endosc 1976; 22:203–5.

100. Marino AWM. Complications of colonoscopy. Dis Colon Rectum 1978; 21:15–9.

101. O'Donoghue JK. Inhibition of a demand pacemaker by electrosurgery. Chest 1973; 64:664–6.

102. Fein RL. Transurethral electrocautery procedures in patients with cardiac pacemakers. JAMA 1967; 202:101–3.

103. Anderson JR, Spence RAJ, Wilson BG, et al. Gangrenous caecal volvulus after colonoscopy. Br Med J 1983; 286:439–440.

104. Rees BI, Williams LA. Incarceration of hernia after colonoscopy. (Letter) Lancet 1977; 1:371.

105. Waye JD. Colonoscopy: A clinical view. Mt. Sinai J Med 1975; 42:1–34.

106. Razzak IA, Millan J, Schuster MM. Pneumatic ileal perforation: an unusual complication of colonoscopy. Gastroenterology 1976; 70:268–71.

107. Heer M, Altorfer J, Pirovino M, et al. Pneumatosis cystoides coli: A rare complication of colonoscopy. Endoscopy 1983:15:119–20.

108. Wertkin MG, Wetchler BB, Waye JD, et al. Pneumatosis coli associated with sigmoid volvulus and colonoscopy. Am J Gastroenterol 1976; 65:209–14.

109. Norfleet RG. Colonoscopy experience in 100 examinations. Wis Med J 1974; 73:S66–8.

110. Dagradi AE, Riff DS, Norum TM, et al. A complication of colonoscopic (cecal) polypectomy. Am J Gastroenterol 1976; 65:449–53.

111. Spencer RJ, Coates HL, Anderson MJ Jr. Colonoscopic polypectomies. Mayo Clin Proc 1974; 49:40–3.

112. Carlyle DR, Goldstein HM. Angiographic management of bleeding following transcolonoscopic polypectomy. Am J Dig Dis 1975; 20:1196–1201.

113. Schwesinger WH, Levine BA, Ramos R. Complications in colonoscopy. Surg Gynecol Obstet 1979; 148:270–81.

114. Smith LE, Nivatvongs S. Complications in colonoscopy. Dis Colon Rectum 1975; 18:214–20.

115. Gordon MJ. Retroperitoneal emphysema from colonoscopy of the distal limb of a Hartmann colostomy. Gastrointest Endosc 1975; 22:101–2.

116. Jacobsohn WZ, Levy A. Colonoscopic perforation: its emergency treatment. Endoscopy 1976; 8:15–7.

117. Taylor R, Weakley FL, Sullivan BH Jr. Non-operative management of colonoscopic perforation with pneumoperitoneum. Gastrointest Endosc 1978; 24:124–5.

118. Stearns MW Jr, moderator. Symposium. Evaluation of colonoscopic examination. Dis Colon Rectum 1975; 18:365–85.

119. Bigard MA, Gaucher P, Lassalle C. Fatal colonic explosion during colonoscopic polypectomy. Gastroenterology 1979; 77:1307–10.

120. Raillat A, Desaintjulien J, Abgrall J. Colonic explosion during endoscopic electrosurgery after bowel preparation with mannitol (translation from the French). Gastrointest Clin Biol (Abstr). 1982; 6:68.

121. Williams CB, Gillespie PE. Accidental removal of ureteral stoma at colonoscopy. Gastrointest Endosc 1979; 25:109–10.

122. Fazio RA, Wickremesinghe PC, Arsura EL, et al. Endoscopic removal of an intussuscepted appendix mimicking a polyp—an endoscopic hazard. Am J Gastroenterol 1982; 77:556–8.

123. Erdman LH, Boggs HW Jr, Slagle GW. Electrical ileal perforation: an unusual complication of colonoscopy. Dis Colon Rectum 1979; 22:501–2.

Chapter 42

THE DIFFERENTIAL DIAGNOSIS OF INFLAMMATORY AND INFECTIOUS COLITIS

JEROME D. WAYE, M.D.

Diarrhea is a common symptom for which patients frequently seek medical attention. Information from several sources is necessary to determine its cause. Most important is the detailed history of pertinent events leading to the onset of illness, including travel, diet, antibiotic use, and sexual preferences.

Difficulty may arise in differentiating an infectious colitis from idiopathic inflammatory bowel disease because of the many features common to both types of disease. With chronic idiopathic inflammatory bowel disease, the patient's history usually includes previous episodes of gastrointestinal illness, often with chronic malaise that persists for months or years, and with diarrhea a prominent and probably intermittent feature. By contrast, the history of acute infectious colitis may include fever and debility, but characteristically lacks the element of chronicity. Although diarrhea is the hallmark of infectious colitis, rectal bleeding is relatively common. If not voluminous, this should not prompt any extraordinary investigative methods beyond those indicated in the usual evaluation for a suspected infectious etiology.

Unfortunately, the visual appearance of the mucosal lining of the rectum and colon in infectious and inflammatory colitis may be indistinguishable, as is also true for many histologic features in tissue specimens obtained at endoscopy. Because of this similitude among many conditions that affect the large bowel, the astute endoscopist must always consider numerous diagnostic possibilities even when "typical" evidence of nonspecific inflammatory bowel disease is encountered. Such findings do not necessarily exclude an infectious etiology.[1]

When a patient presents with acute colitis, the differential diagnosis must include viral and bacterial etiologies in addition to the heralding siege of chronic inflammatory bowel disease. Characteristically, the illness caused by bacterial toxins and most bacterial infections is a short-term diarrheal syndrome with a rapid onset. The various viral etiologies for diarrhea usually produce a similar self-limited illness that rarely lasts more than a few days. With prolonged symptoms, especially diarrhea, the probability of an infectious process is lessened, and the probability of idiopathic inflammatory disease becomes greater. However, the differential diagnosis is more complex than this because some infections may cause long-standing diarrheal illnesses[2]; these include Campylobacter infections, tuberculosis, schistosomiasis, and amebiasis. Although most patients with the acute onset of diarrhea respond to symptomatic therapy, those who do not respond or become debilitated require an intense search for a treatable infecting agent.

A treatable infectious cause of any diarrheal illness must always be considered, even if the diagnosis of idiopathic inflammatory bowel disease is well established for a considerable period; there is always a possibility that an acute exacerbation of a chronic illness may be provoked by superimposed infection.[3]

"Inflammatory bowel disease" is usually a clinical diagnosis, but one must be wary of this diagnosis until infectious etiologies have been eliminated. For example, in one institution in the southern United States, approximately 38% of all patients with a diarrheal illness of 6 weeks' duration, considered clinically as having inflammatory bowel disease, were found to have colitis with infectious etiologies when extensive laboratory studies were performed.[4]

When a bacterial etiology for colitis is suspected, colonoscopy is usually not the investigative procedure of choice and can never be the only procedure employed for diagnosis. However, endoscopic evaluation of the rectum and sigmoid colon is frequently undertaken to evaluate the status of the mucosa in patients with the acute onset of diarrhea. Since sigmoidoscopy may now be performed with either the rigid or flexible instrument, the physician who introduces any instrument for visualization of the large bowel mucosa must be able to determine which of various infectious and inflammatory bowel diseases may be present. Guidelines that aid in this differential diagnosis and the specific idiopathic inflammatory and infectious diseases that must be considered will be presented in this chapter.

NORMAL APPEARANCE OF THE COLORECTAL MUCOSA

Endoscopically, the normal colorectal mucosa has a transparent, glistening surface that is uniformly salmon-pink in color throughout the colon with the exception of an occasional blue tint in some areas, particularly the region of the hepatic flexure. The surface normally reflects the light of the endoscope.

A progressively branching vascular network is present throughout the colon and should be immediately obvious on observation.[5] The vessels that compose this visible vasculature rest on the surface of the submucosa just beneath the superficial mucosal layer. Arborization of the superficial vascular pattern is characteristic of the surface topography and is present in the normal mucous membrane. Vascularity is more prominent in the rectum than in any other area; there, large blood vessels are present whose caliber increases in diameter distally.

One characteristic that never varies in healthy subjects is the smoothness of the surface. No nodules or irregular projections should be seen with the exception of the small nodules that may be found in an occasional adolescent or young adult patient with lymphoid hyperplasia (see Chapter 48 for a discussion of lymphoid hyperplasia). Throughout the entire colon, the interhaustral septa are ordinarily "paper-crease" sharp in their semicircular or triangular configuration.

No bleeding will be seen in the normal large intestine, nor is there pus or mucus on the bowel wall. Only rarely does the preparation process for the examination cause alterations in the surface mucosa. These changes may consist of mild erythema or slight edema, recognized as loss of the normal bright, glistening appearance of the mucosal surface. Bleeding in response to gentle contact with the instrument tip or another device (contact bleeding, "friability") never develops as a result of preparation with cathartics and enemas.

Response of the Colorectal Mucosa to Injury

The intestinal lining can respond in only a limited number of ways to any process that disrupts its integrity. Any inflammatory condition that affects the colon may alter the smoothness of the surface lining, may change its color, or may affect the delicate branching vascular pattern, any or all of which may be observed endoscopically. In addition there may be bleeding or ulceration of the mucosa as well as pus or purulent exudate on the surface, or any combination of these.

The initial response of the mucosa is often an increase in the local blood supply that is seen endoscopically as erythema. Edema frequently accompanies mucosal inflammation and may be appreciated endoscopically as loss of the usually visible mucosal vascular architecture. Edema also alters the contour of the mucosa. Normally smooth and flat, it takes on a granular surface that colonoscopically resembles wet sandpaper. This is often given the descriptive term "granularity." Granularity is also evident by observing the mucosal reflection of the endoscopic light. The individual mounds of edematous tissue are punctuated by the colon crypts so that the reflection of light, i.e., the light reflex, is broken up as multiple small reflections.

Because of vascular engorgement or the presence of minute ulcerations, or both, the mucosa may bleed either spontaneously or in response to gentle contact with the tip of the endoscope or other instrument. This response to contact is often termed "contact bleeding" or "friability." Ulcers may have a variety of shapes and sizes ranging from large and grossly evident to minute and unobservable; spontaneous and contact bleeding episodes are consequences of minute and microscopic ulcerations.

The formation of pseudopolyps is a nonspecific reaction that occurs in many inflammatory diseases of the colon. Their presence signifies that the process has gone through at least one healing phase. Although technically polyps, they are not neoplastic in character: thus the qualified term *pseudopolyp*. They represent overgrowth of normal remaining mucosa during the healing phase of an inflammatory disease. Although they may be small and hemispheric in shape (Plate 42–1), pseudopolyps are characteristically somewhat elongated. They usually have a maximum dimension of less than 1 cm but can be quite large. Clusters of pseudopolyps or extremely large ones may be confused with other lesions such as tumors or adenomas when demonstrated by barium contrast radiography (Plate 42–2).

Mucosal bridges may also occur (Plate 42–3). They share a common pathogenesis with pseudopolyps, being created when two adjacent ulcerations meet by burrowing beneath a piece of inflamed mucosa instead of destroying it; as healing occurs there is re-epithelialization of the ulcer bed as well as of the undersurface of the mucosal strip, thereby producing a mucosal tube connected at both ends.

Depending on the type and stage of disease, any or all of the above features may be present or absent. Furthermore, certain diseases, Crohn's colitis for example, may have nonmucosal components. Unfortunately, the observable changes in the colonic mucosa are rarely specific for any particular etiologic factor or disease, so that differential diagnosis can be difficult or impossible on an endoscopic basis alone. Furthermore, the microscopic features of tissue specimens may also be remarkably similar, making biopsy of limited assistance in differentiating between various entities.

CROHN'S DISEASE AND ULCERATIVE COLITIS

Differential Diagnosis

The most complete descriptions of endoscopic patterns of colonic inflammation are those of the major idiopathic inflammatory bowel diseases: ulcerative colitis and Crohn's disease (granulomatous, transmural colitis).[6] Despite the many known differences in clinical, radiologic, and sigmoidoscopic findings between ulcerative and granulomatous colitis, differentiation may be difficult. Because endoscopy allows visualization of the total colon and can provide tissue for histologic study, it is frequently undertaken to assist with the correct diagnosis in inflammatory bowel disease. In some instances even the most sophisticated methods of investigation may not provide a definitive answer as to the type of colitis. However, ulcerative and granulomatous colitis affect the colon differently, and usually the gross appearances of the two are sufficiently distinct to enable the endoscopist to distinguish between them.

Ulcerative colitis primarily affects the mucosal layer, whereas Crohn's disease involves the submucosa as well as the mucosa.

Because mucosal involvement is not prominent early in the course of Crohn's disease, there is a tendency for the surface vascular pattern to remain intact. One of the earliest lesions of Crohn's disease is a small aphthous-type ulcer. This ulcer is usually not more than 3 to 4 mm in diameter and is characteristically surrounded by a narrow red border of erythematous mucosa (Plate 42–4). It has been demonstrated by scanning electron microscopy that the aphthous ulcers of granulomatous colitis originate in the submucosal lymphatic follicles and penetrate the mucosa with an inflammatory eruption through the superficial layer.[7] This results in a tiny ulcer on an otherwise completely normal mucosal surface.

The earliest manifestation of colonic involvement by ulcerative colitis is an increase in mucosal blood flow that appears endoscopically as diffuse erythema. Concomitant edema causes inability to visualize the vascular architecture along with granularity and disruption of the normal light reflex (vide supra) (Plates 42–5 and 42–6). The engorged mucosa is friable, i.e. bleeds readily with minor trauma (Plates 42–7 and 42–8). As the inflammation progresses, minute surface ulcerations occur. In combination with mucosal hyperemia these ulcers cause the spontaneous bleeding so characteristic of this disease. Large ulcerations are not uncommon in ulcerative colitis but always occur in a bed of surrounding inflammation; they represent coalescence of the myriad smaller surface erosions.

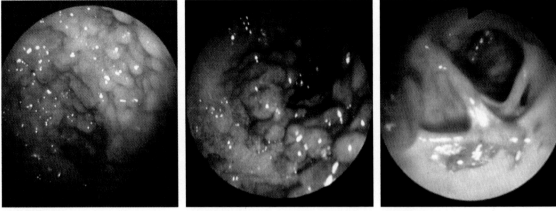

PLATE 42–1.　　　　　　　　PLATE 42–2.　　　　　　　　PLATE 42–3.

PLATE 42–1. Dense carpet of pseudopolyps in a patient with longstanding chronic ulcerative colitis. (Courtesy of M.V. Sivak, Jr., M.D.)

PLATE 42–2. Dense cluster of pseudopolyps that simulated the appearance of tumors in barium enema studies in a patient with chronic ulcerative colitis. (Courtesy of M.V. Sivak, Jr., M.D.)

PLATE 42–3. Mucosal bridging in a patient with chronic ulcerative colitis. (Courtesy of M.V. Sivak, Jr., M.D.)

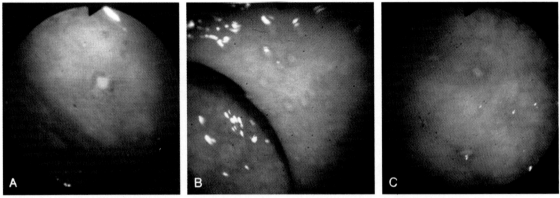

PLATE 42–4. A, Solitary aphthous ulcer of Crohn's disease. B, Multiple small aphthous ulcers on interhaustral septum of the sigmoid colon in a patient with Crohn's colitis. C, Small aphthous ulcers of early Crohn's colitis. Each ulcer has a surrounding "halo" characteristic of erythema. Normal vessels can still be seen in the surrounding mucosa. (Courtesy of M.V. Sivak, Jr., M.D.)

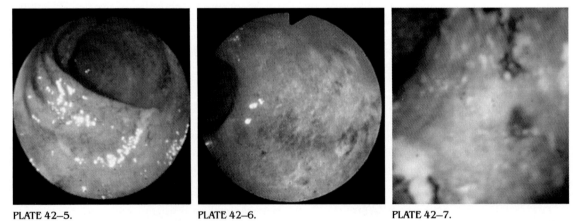

PLATE 42–5.　　　　　　　　PLATE 42–6.　　　　　　　　PLATE 42–7.

PLATE 42–5. Acute ulcerative colitis. There is erythema and loss of vascular pattern. Note the granular appearance of interhaustral septum and the "break-up" of light reflection. (Courtesy of M.V. Sivak, Jr., M.D.)

PLATE 42–6. Acute ulcerative colitis. There is loss of vascular pattern, erythema, and exudate over the mucosal surface. The linear bleeding pattern was caused by contact with the tip of the endoscope (contact bleeding, friability). (Courtesy of M.V. Sivak, Jr., M.D.)

PLATE 42–7. Moderately severe ulcerative colitis. There is loss of vascular pattern, exudate over the mucosal surface, and small areas of spontaneous bleeding. (Courtesy of M.V. Sivak, Jr., M.D.)

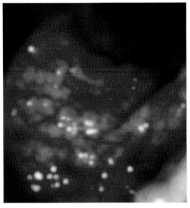
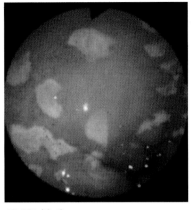

PLATE 42–8. Severe acute ulcerative colitis. No vascular pattern is discernible. There is a severe degree of spontaneous bleeding. (Courtesy of M.V. Sivak, Jr., M.D.)
PLATE 42–9. Somewhat larger ulcers of Crohn's colitis. (Courtesy of M.V. Sivak, Jr., M.D.)

PLATE 42–8.   PLATE 42–9.

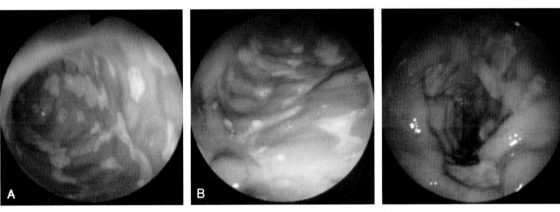

PLATE 42–10.   PLATE 42–11.

PLATE 42–10. A, Linear ulcers of Crohn's colitis. B, Mucosa surrounding the ulcers is nodular (cobblestoning). (Courtesy of M.V. Sivak, Jr., M.D.)
PLATE 42–11. Deep ulcers in Crohn's colitis. Note also the marked cobblestoning of the surrounding mucosa. (Courtesy of M.V. Sivak, Jr., M.D.)

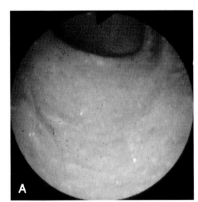
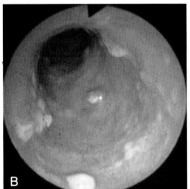
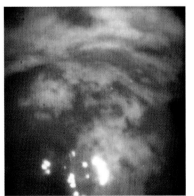

PLATE 42–12.   PLATE 42–13.

PLATE 42–12. A, Chronic ulcerative colitis. B, The inflammatory process has subsided, leaving a tubular colon with blunting of interhaustral septa, a pale featureless mucosa with loss of vascular pattern, and pseudopolyps. (Courtesy of M.V. Sivak, Jr., M.D.)
PLATE 42–13. Shigella colitis. Patchy areas of erythema, spontaneous bleeding, and loss of the normal vascular pattern are evident. (Courtesy of Dr. Francis Tedesco.)

Large surface ulcers are more common in Crohn's disease but their pathogenesis differs completely from that of ulcerative colitis. The small aphthous inflammatory erosions in granulomatous colitis tend to enlarge concentrically and encroach upon the normal surrounding mucosal surface as they increase in diameter (Plate 42–9). Unless the disease has spread to a broad area of the colonic surface, large ulcers in Crohn's disease will be typically surrounded by normal appearing mucosa. Progression of Crohn's colitis usually results in larger ulcers. These are often elongated, with their long axis oriented parallel to the luminal axis (Plate 42–10). Such longitudinal ulcers may extend several centimeters to produce deep fissures. Rarely, Crohn's ulcers may have a deep "punched out" appearance; these bleed easily, may perforate, and are associated with a poor prognosis.

Cobblestoning is a manifestation of submucosal involvement in Crohn's disease; the term has different meanings for pathologists and endoscopists. From the gross pathology viewpoint, cobblestoning refers to a segment of colon ravaged by severe ulcerative inflammation; criss-crossing furrowed ulcerations demarcate an area of inflamed mucosa that represents the cobblestoning in this descriptive lexicon. Endoscopists use the term cobblestoning to refer to uniform nodules caused by submucosal edema. Although ulcers might be present in an area that exhibits cobblestoning, they do not themselves define the cobblestoned mucosa (Plate 42–11). In endoscopic cobblestoning, the nodules are characteristically low in height with a broad base and bear little relation to ulcers. This nodular mucosa of Crohn's disease is easily recognized and is unlikely to be mistaken for the small nubby mucosal surface irregularities indicative of dysplasia in ulcerative colitis. Cobblestoning must be distinguished from multiple pseudopolyps projecting into the lumen in inflammatory bowel disease. The length of pseudopolyps is characteristically greater than the width of their base, and the immediately adjacent mucosa is usually flat, whereas the low nodules of cobblestoning are distinctly contiguous.

Several endoscopic features can be used to differentiate between ulcerative colitis and Crohn's disease with a high degree of certainty.[8] The most important are the following:

1. Ulcers never occur in ulcerative colitis in an area of otherwise normal mucosa. Ulcers may occur in diffusely abnormal mucosa in both forms of colitis, but if the surrounding mucosa is normal, the diagnosis is never ulcerative colitis.

2. Aphthous ulcers are pathognomonic of Crohn's colitis.

3. Cobblestoning is pathognomonic of Crohn's colitis.

4. Granularity and friability are common early in ulcerative colitis, but may be late findings in granulomatous colitis.

In most instances, these distinctive features will correctly differentiate between ulcerative and Crohn's colitis, although the late stages of both may so closely resemble one another that correct differentiation may be impossible. Although there are exceptions to most of the distinguishing criteria, two may be accepted as absolutes:[9] (1) in ulcerative colitis, ulcerations are never seen in an area of normal appearing mucosa with intact vascularity; and (2) true cobblestoning occurs only in Crohn's disease.

Many mucosal abnormalities are common to both diseases and therefore are not helpful in differentiating between them. Pseudopolyps occur in both forms of colitis and their presence does not favor the diagnosis of one particular type of inflammatory bowel disease. Mucosal bridges are seen in both types of idiopathic colonic inflammatory bowel disease; these may rarely prevent passage of the colonoscope. Other similarities between the two in their healing phases include loss or blunting of the shape of the interhaustral septa, and the presence of fibrotic strictures and linear mucosal surface scars (Plate 42–12).

The actual severity of ulcerative colitis tends to correlate with the endoscopic visual estimation of the mucosal reaction. In ulcerative colitis, gross ulcerations are a manifestation of severe disease and do not occur in mildly inflamed portions of the colon.

Colonoscopic Biopsy

Despite the colonoscopic capability for providing an unlimited number of biopsy specimens in any specified area of the colon, histopathology often provides little assistance in differentiating between ulcerative colitis and granulomatous colitis. One reason is that granulomas in colonoscopic biopsy specimens are seen infrequently, usually less than 10%, in patients with Crohn's colitis.[10, 11] Some authors, however, report a surprisingly high frequency of granulomas in biopsy material.[12] This discrepancy may be due to the type of patients referred for colonoscopy, since biopsies from aphthous ulcerations in the early stage of Crohn's colitis tend to have the highest yield of granulomas. Granulomas are most likely to be found if biopsies are taken from the center of small ulcers; as the ulcers enlarge they tend to engulf and destroy the original epithelioid cluster of cells.

Whenever colonoscopy is utilized in the differential diagnosis of inflammatory bowel diseases, several biopsies should be obtained for histopathologic identification. Each specimen or group of specimens should be labeled as to location in the colon. Although a biopsy may not provide a specific diagnosis, several biopsies from different areas may define a pattern of inflammation. This mapping of the inflammatory process provides additional information that may be of assistance in unraveling the diagnostic problems. For example, a pattern of biopsies showing increasing inflammation progressing distally toward the rectum is consistent with ulcerative colitis, whereas a patchy distribution of inflammatory changes throughout the colon or even variations of the distribution in inflammatory cells within one of the tiny tissue specimens is more characteristic of Crohn's disease.[13] Although biopsy material is of limited value in differentiating between ulcerative colitis and Crohn's colitis, it can be more helpful in the recognition of other types of colitis such as certain infectious varieties (vide infra). Biopsy has greater significance, therefore, in distinguishing idiopathic inflammatory colitis from infectious colitis.

The microscopic pathologic findings must be interpreted with the knowledge that colonoscopic biopsy samples represent only the smallest fraction of the total surface area of the colon. These tiny tissue specimens require closer scrutiny than when a surgical specimen is studied pathologically. Many of the microscopic features are meaningful only when considered as a part of the overall evaluation; a number of nonspecific histologic features may actually assist in the differential diagnosis because of known patterns of inflammation associated with various types of specific and nonspecific inflammatory bowel disease. For example, two known characteristics of inflammatory bowel disease, microabscesses and the amount of goblet cell mucus, may differ quantitatively in mucosal biopsies of ulcerative colitis and granuloma-

tous colitis. Microabscess formation is twice as common in ulcerative colitis as in Crohn's disease; a marked increase in goblet cell mucus in severely inflamed mucosa is suggestive of Crohn's disease. In some cases of longstanding granulomatous disease, amyloid may be found; this is not present in biopsy specimens from patients with ulcerative colitis.

Colonoscopic assessment of the extent of colon involvement by inflammatory bowel disease is accurate and usually not difficult. However, this may be of limited benefit to the patient, since therapeutic decisions, with certain exceptions, are based on clinical criteria without regard to the extent of involvement; the type or dosage of drug therapy as well as the decision for surgery should not be based on the amount of bowel involved by the inflammatory process.

One exception is the patient with proctosigmoiditis who is not responding to standard topical therapy. Colonoscopy in this circumstance may show the proximal extent of colon involvement to be greater than appreciated by double contrast radiography; colonoscopic biopsy may also demonstrate an even greater degree of involvement than can be appreciated from endoscopic observation of the mucosa alone.[14] In this circumstance, management and the choice of therapeutic methods may be altered by the endoscopic findings.

Another exception is the endoscopic assessment of Crohn's colitis prior to operation. Colonoscopy may be used to ascertain which areas of large bowel are actually affected by the granulomatous process. The results of this endoscopic assessment may lead to modifications in planning the surgical approach. Colonoscopy can be used to confirm the anastomotic recurrence of Crohn's disease, but the decision for surgical or medical therapy remains a clinical one.

Although it is well known that the risk of carcinoma in patients with chronic ulcerative colitis is greater when the entire colon is involved, the parameter for determination of pancolitis has always been the barium enema x-ray study. The diagnosis of total colon involvement can also be made by colonoscopy. Often the findings by colonoscopy indicate a significantly greater extent of disease than can be determined from a corresponding barium enema study. Furthermore, colonoscopic biopsies may indicate a greater extent of involvement than can be appreciated by visual endoscopic assessment. With respect to cancer risk, there is no current information concerning the significance of total colitis diagnosed by either colonoscopic observation or colonoscopic biopsy when the severity of the disease process has not been sufficient to produce radiographic changes in the entire colon.[15] The problem of cancer in association with ulcerative colitis is discussed in Chapter 43.

INFECTIOUS COLITIS

All the endoscopic and histologic abnormalities previously described as characteristic of the two major types of idiopathic inflammatory bowel disease may also be seen in patients with infectious colitis. Some infections of the colon are primarily mucosal inflammatory processes and thereby produce an endoscopic picture similar to that of ulcerative colitis, whereas others affect deeper portions of the colon wall and appear identical to Crohn's disease. In many circumstances the endoscopic view is nondiagnostic and the etiology of the colitis must be determined by integrating data from multiple sources, primary elements being the patient's history coupled with the results of stool cultures and biopsy specimens.

The results of stool cultures may be unavailable at the time of endoscopic examination, and an infectious etiology must always be considered when a patient presents with diarrhea. Fortunately, most of the infective diarrheal illnesses are self-limiting, and for this reason total colonoscopy is rarely performed in these patients. It is usual, however, to examine the rectum and sigmoid colon with a sigmoidoscope during the acute phase of diarrheal illness. Any physician who looks at the colon mucosa with either a rigid or flexible sigmoidoscope or colonoscope must be familiar with the endoscopic characteristics of all types of proctitis and colitis.

General Endoscopic Characteristics of Infectious Colitis

Endoscopy often reveals a yellowish, tenacious exudate that may partially or completely cover the mucosal surface in diarrheal illnesses due to infectious causes. Free pus, detectable by its thick consistency and off-white color, may be seen in the lumen; the presence of pus is unusual with any of the idiopathic inflammatory bowel diseases.

Visible ulceration, common in Crohn's disease and less frequently seen in ulcerative colitis, is not usually found in association with most of the infectious colitides. Many infections cause the mucosal surface to be intensely red, almost magenta-colored, in contrast to the deeper red of idiopathic inflammatory bowel disease. Since mucosal edema is responsible for the granularity so characteristic of inflammatory bowel disease, it is not surprising that granularity may also be present in infectious disease of the colon. One of the most characteristic findings in the endoscopic appearance of infectious colitis is its distinct pattern of patchy involvement within the same colon segment.[4] In a single visual field, many small areas may be obviously inflamed while the intervening mucosa appears entirely normal.

Confusion in the differentiation between specific and nonspecific inflammatory bowel diseases has occurred because various authors ascribe different endoscopic descriptions to the same infectious agent. Some observers have found one agent to produce a picture resembling Crohn's disease, whereas others state that the same organism produces the endoscopic appearance of ulcerative colitis. This can be accounted for by variations in mucosal response to the same infection. Differences in response are undoubtedly related to several factors, including the actual degree of aggressiveness of a particular organism in individual patients, the duration of the infection, the stage of the disease, and the host's response to inflammation.

The endoscopic appearance of many of the types of infectious colitis will be discussed. Their visual presentation will be characterized whenever possible as resembling either ulcerative colitis or granulomatous colitis.

Types of Infectious Colitides
Shigellosis

Shigellosis, commonly known as bacillary dysentery, may resemble ulcerative colitis.[1] The infection primarily affects the large intestine and is caused by the gram-negative bacterium *Shigella dysenteria*. The onset of the disease is sudden and characterized by fever, crampy abdominal pain, tenesmus, and mucoid diarrhea that frequently contains gross blood. The endoscopic features range from erythema and mild granularity to multiple

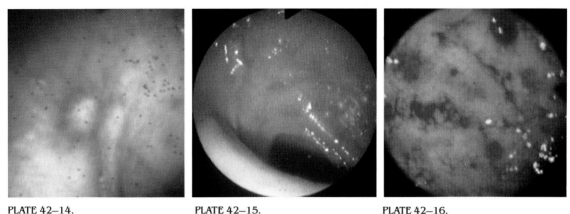

PLATE 42–14.   PLATE 42–15.   PLATE 42–16.

PLATE 42–14. *Shigella* colitis. A discrete punched-out ulcer with intense surrounding erythema is present. Mucosa adjacent to the ulcer is normal (Courtesy of Dr. Jose Romeu.)

PLATE 42–15. *Shigella* colitis. The patient presented with acute diarrheal illness. Multiple discrete aphthous ulcers, each surrounded by intense zone of erythema, can be seen. (Courtesy of Dr. Myron Goldberg.)

PLATE 42–16. *Salmonella* colitis. There is diffuse erythema, spontaneous bleeding, and loss of vascular pattern with formation of telangiectasis. (Courtesy of Dr. Francis Tedesco.)

ulcers with considerable exudate (Plates 42–13, 42–14, and 42–15). The pattern of mucosal involvement is characteristically patchy, but may otherwise closely resemble the endoscopic findings in ulcerative colitis. Crypt abscesses may be found on biopsy in addition to the changes of acute inflammation. In this infection the erythema of the bowel wall is particularly intense and often magenta-hued, a clue to the astute endoscopist that an infectious etiology may be present rather than the usual inflammatory bowel disease.

Salmonellosis

Salmonellosis, a bacterial infection that may resemble Crohn's disease, primarily involves the small intestine but often affects the colon.[16] Ulceration is unusual; however, ulcers have been reported as occurring proximal to the sigmoid colon. Although the disease may spare the rectum, there is often segmental involvement throughout the colon. Early endoscopic findings include edema, erythema, and granularity; progression of

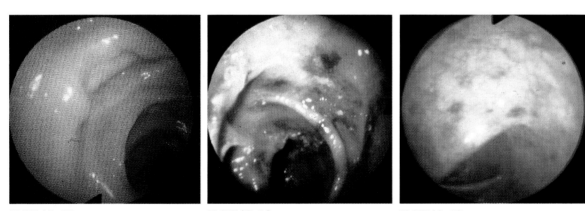

PLATE 42–17.   PLATE 42–18.   PLATE 42–19.

PLATE 42–17. *Salmonella* colitis, which presented as a segmental colitis with a discrete, punched-out ulcer in the zone of edema. Little or no erythema is present. (Courtesy of Dr. Peter Rubin.)

PLATE 42–18. *Campylobacter* enteritis. Areas of ulceration, patchy erythema, and edema alternate with normal segments of colon. (Courtesy of Dr. Francis Tedesco.)

PLATE 42–19. *Campylobacter* colitis. Diffuse erythema and well-defined hemorrhagic areas are present. Spontaneous bleeding is absent. (Courtesy of Dr. Stuart Finkel.)

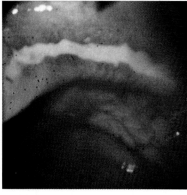 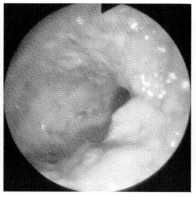 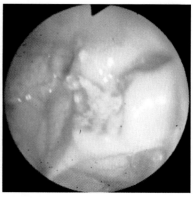

PLATE 42–20. PLATE 42–21. PLATE 42–22.

PLATE 42–20. Tuberculosis. Linear ulceration can be seen running circumferentially along interhaustral septum, with tiny satellite ulcerations. This must be distinguished from longitudinal ulcerations in inflammatory bowel disease. (Courtesy of Dr. Francis Tedesco.)

PLATE 42–21. Tuberculosis. Note the irregular flat ulcerations at the 12 o'clock position. Diffuse submucosal elevations in the lower half of the field are due to tuberculosis. (Courtesy of Dr. Jose Romeu.)

PLATE 42–22. Atypical *Mycobacterium* infection. Culture of biopsy material showed that the irregular stallate ulceration with surrounding zone of erythema was due to atypical mycobacteria. (Courtesy of Dr. Jack Walfish.)

the disease may result in mucosal friability with petechial hemorrhages (Plate 42–16). Deep ulcerations and concomitant strictures have been reported but are distinctly rare (Plate 42–17).

Yersinia enterocolitica *Colitis*

Yersinia enterocolitica colitis may resemble either ulcerative colitis or Crohn's disease.[17] This infection can produce diffuse granularity, erythema, and friability throughout the entire colon in about one half of affected patients and may therefore resemble ulcerative colitis. However, some patients may have a patchy or right-sided distribution that includes involvement of the terminal ileum. Aphthous ulcers may occur adjacent to areas of normal mucosa, a finding considered diagnostic of Crohn's disease. Normal rectal mucosa is often encountered with the rigid proctosigmoidoscope, since 40% of affected patients have endoscopic manifestations of

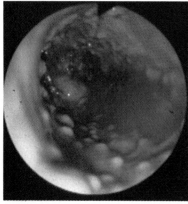 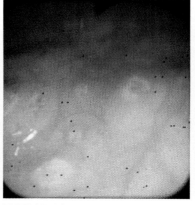 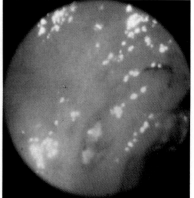

PLATE 42–23. PLATE 42–24. PLATE 42–25.

PLATE 42–23. Tuberculosis. Multiple discrete submucosal nodules project into the lumen. The reddish mound in the distance is the ileocecal valve. Biopsies of nodules demonstrated tubercle bacilli on acid-fast staining. (Courtesy of Dr. Jose Romeu.)

PLATE 42–24. Amebiasis. Discrete punched-out ulcerations appear to be superficial.

PLATE 42–25. Amebiasis. Several punched-out ulcers appear to be superficial. Some are surrounded by a narrow border of erythema. Mucosal edema is evident. (Courtesy of Dr. Francis Tedesco.)

the disease only proximal to the rectosigmoid area.[3] Symptoms of *Yersinia enterocolitica* may persist for months, and several weeks may be required for cultures to demonstrate growth of the organism. If the disease is suspected, specific growth media should be inoculated to enhance the probability of a positive culture for this bacterium. This may not be a routine laboratory procedure in some institutions.

Campylobacter fetus *Subspecies Infection*

This agent was formerly known as *Vibrio fetus*. Infection by *Campylobacter fetus* subspecies at endoscopy resembles either ulcerative colitis or Crohn's disease. It has been recognized as capable of producing an acute form of colitis that is indistinguishable from acute ulcerative colitis.[18, 19] The findings consist of erythema and friability, along with granularity, spontaneous bleeding, and a diffuse exudate over the mucosal surface (Plates 42–18 and 42–19). In addition to these usual endoscopic findings of inflammation there may also be an inflammatory mass lesion within the lumen. The rectum is usually involved; the right colon is rarely affected.

Some patients do not have the "typical," ulcerative colitis–like endoscopic findings. Rather, the endoscopic picture may simulate Crohn's disease in that involvement is segmental and patchy and consists of erythema, friability, edema, and occasionally small ulcers. In most patients the disease is of short duration, but organisms may persist as long as 7 weeks after the onset of symptoms.[20]

Tuberculosis

Mycobacterium tuberculosis can infect any part of the large bowel or terminal ileum, although the right side of the colon and especially the ileocecal area are most commonly affected. The rectum and sigmoid are frequently spared so that flexible or rigid proctosigmoidoscopy findings are usually normal. The endoscopic findings are so similar to those of Crohn's disease that the two disorders may be indistinguishable by endoscopic observation alone.

Colonoscopy may demonstrate diffuse linear ulcerations and stricture formation. The ulcers usually have a surrounding border of erythema and edema and are frequently located in an area of otherwise normal-appearing mucosa, findings that are also typical for the ulcerations of Crohn's disease (Plates 42–20, 42–21, and 42–22). In this chronic infec-

tion, mass lesions or tuberculomas can also be present and fistulization may occur between loops of bowel. Cobblestoning due to submucosal involvement with thickening of the bowel walls has been reported, and inflammatory pseudopolyps may also be seen throughout the colon (Plate 42–23).

The colonoscopic differentiation between Crohn's disease and tuberculosis can be difficult for even the experienced endoscopist since the endoscopic findings are so similar. There are, however, some findings that assist correct visual diagnosis. In both diseases there are segments of normal colon interposed between diseased segments. These so-called "skip areas" tend to be shorter in the colon infected with *M. tuberculosis* than in Crohn's colitis. In tuberculous colitis, the ulcers may have a rolled edge and lack the sharp definition usually associated with the ulcers of Crohn's disease. Tubercle bacilli can be found in colonoscopic biopsy specimens in cases of tuberculous colitis if an acid-fast stain is employed.[21] However, this is not entirely reliable. Because the organisms may be difficult to demonstrate, their absence in tissue specimens does not eliminate the possibility of tuberculous colitis. It is essential to the diagnosis of *M. tuberculosis* colitis that this possibility be considered clinically in conjunction with a high index of suspicion on the part of the endoscopist and histopathologist.

Antibiotic-Associated Colitis (Pseudomembranous Colitis)

Antibiotic-associated colitis is a specific type of colitis caused by *Clostridia difficile*.[22, 23] Although it may resemble ulcerative colitis, its appearance in the colon is relatively distinct and it can usually be recognized endoscopically. The rectum is usually involved, but the distribution is not always uniform and the disease may be confined to the right colon or to the sigmoid.[24]

The main endoscopic characteristic is a yellow membrane that covers much of the mucosal surface. This usually consists of multiple, elevated, creamy yellowish plaques, 2 to 5 mm in diameter, that dot the surface of a moderately inflamed mucosa. These are usually distinct but may become confluent and are firmly adherent to the underlying mucosa. The mucosa between plaques is not ulcerated; its inflammatory changes range from granular and friable to hemorrhagic, features that are similar to those of ulcerative colitis. Because the characteristic exudates may be diffuse, the area of involvement is not sharply demarcated. Bleeding may follow biopsy of the plaques.

Biopsy specimens reveal a pseudomembrane overlying an inflamed mucosa. The pseudomembrane is made up of polymorphonuclear leukocytes, fibrin, chronic inflammatory cells, and epithelial debris. While necrosis of the mucosal surface is frequent, true ulcers are not present. A microscopic section downward through the center of a plaque and into the underlying mucosa may reveal the typical "volcano" lesion. This profile view shows the membrane to be adherent to the mucosa at a central point and to have an expanding, overhanging, and nonadherent edge. With some imagination this suggests the outline of an erupting volcano. Since colonoscopic biopsy specimens are small and often distorted, the volcano shape of the lesion may not be evident. The essential pseudomembrane over an inflamed mucosa is always present in a properly placed biopsy, so that histopathologic confirmation should not be difficult.

It appears that this form of colitis can be associated with the administration of virtually any antibiotic with the exception of vancomycin and perhaps parenterally administered aminoglycosides. However, cases of pseudomembranous colitis are reported in which there has been no associated prior use of antibiotics. Even in these instances, however, the endoscopic findings are typical for the disease, and the histopathologic appearance of the pseudomembrane is characteristic.

Amebic Colitis

This protozoan infection primarily affects the large bowel. Any portion of the colon can be involved, although involvement is usually segmental. The most common location is the right colon and cecum followed by the left colon and rectum. Amebiasis of the colon may resemble either Crohn's disease or ulcerative colitis.[25] Symptoms vary from none to an acute fulminating course, with explosive bloody diarrhea, abdominal cramps, tenesmus, and fever. The majority of patients are asymptomatic or have relatively mild complaints.

Endoscopy during the acute phase of the infection may demonstrate diffuse granularity and friability that resembles ulcerative colitis. With chronic amebiasis, 80% to 90% of patients will have cecal involvement. The most characteristic appearance of chronic amebiasis is that of discrete ulcers with undermined edges in a bed of normal mucosa (Plates 42–24 through 42–27). The ulcers may be covered with a yellowish-white exudate. The amebic ulcer often has a red rim[26]; this characteristic may be of assistance in the endoscopic differentiation between amebiasis and Crohn's disease. Biopsy specimens should be taken from the ulcer margin, since this area provides the best yield for demonstration of trophozoites.

In some cases of chronic amebiasis, a fibrous reaction may occur that involves layers of the bowel wall deep to the mucosa. The fibrous component is dense and there may be associated granulomatous changes. The pathogenesis of this type of reaction is unknown. It produces a segmental narrowing of the colon, called an ameboma, that can closely resemble colonic carcinoma.

Because amebiasis is curable it should always be considered in any case of acute diarrheal illness when x-ray films and endoscopic findings resemble those of Crohn's disease. Patients with amebic infection must be treated for this condition, even though the appearance may be absolutely "characteristic" of Crohn's colitis. The administration of corticosteroids to a patient with amebic infection of the colon because of the mistaken diagnosis of Crohn's colitis or acute ulcerative colitis can have catastrophic consequences.

Schistosomiasis

Schistosomiasis, a parasitic infection of the colon, may resemble ulcerative colitis and is encountered only rarely in temperate climates. The presence of large, inflammatory polypoid lesions marked by a whitish surface exudate should alert the colonoscopist to the possibility of this infestation.[27] These polyps, which may involve the entire colon, are produced by the hyperplastic inflammatory response to degenerating ova. Mucosal changes most commonly affect the proximal colon; the rectum and sigmoid may be completely normal. When the rectum is affected, the manifestations are similar to those of ulcerative colitis, including erythema, friability, and granularity of the mucosa with shallow ulcerations. The histologic finding of encysted schistosomes in a resected polyp or biopsy specimen is a unique feature of this disease.[27]

Histoplasmosis

Histoplasmosis rarely affects the colon but may produce a type of colitis that resembles

Crohn's disease.[28] The ileum and cecum are the most common sites of involvement; the rectum is frequently spared.

The endoscopic findings consist of ulcers and pseudopolyps along with erythema and friability. If the rectum is involved, discrete, granular, plaque-like lesions may be seen in small patches. Biopsy specimens of the plaques usually demonstrate the organism. The patchy nature of the inflammation and the predominantly right-sided distribution of this mycotic infection cause it to be mistaken for granulomatous colitis.

Cytomegalovirus Infection

The cytomegalovirus is an opportunistic infectious agent that is seen in immunosuppressed patients, especially those with malignant disease who are receiving cytotoxic drugs or corticosteroids. Recently, infection by this organism has also been identified in homosexual males with the acquired immunodeficiency syndrome (AIDS). Patients may be asymptomatic or may complain of abdominal pain and intermittent diarrhea that contains occult blood or is grossly bloody. Perforation of the colon has been described in association with cytomegalovirus infection.[29]

The endoscopic appearance of the rectum and sigmoid may resemble ulcerative colitis with granularity or mucosal friability (Plate 42–28). The hallmark of the disease, however, is the occurrence of discrete punched-out shallow ulcerations. These may be present in the cecum in otherwise normal mucosa and thus resemble the ulcers of Crohn's disease (Plates 42–29, 42–30, and 42–31). In contrast to granulomatous colitis, however, the cytomegalovirus ulcers are usually solitary and vary in size from 2 to 6 mm. Biopsy specimens taken from the edges of the ulcerations will reveal the cytomegalic inclusion cells on routine hematoxylin and eosin staining.

Balantidium coli Infection

Infection of the colon by *Balantidium coli* is an unusual occurrence that resembles amebiasis in all its characteristics.[30] The endoscopic findings may therefore resemble ulcerative colitis and Crohn's disease as well. The diagnosis is thus especially difficult by endoscopic characteristics alone. However, trophozoites may be found in tissue specimens, especially scrapings from rectal ulcers, and these may be distinguished from amebiasis by their histologic characteristics.

"Gay Bowel Syndrome"

A number of colon infections are related to rectal intercourse and are frequently associated with homosexual activity in men.[31] A variety of infectious agents are responsible for the manifestations of the so-called gay bowel syndrome. The endoscopic appearance produced by each agent is relatively nonspecific. Therefore, whenever "nonspecific proctitis" is diagnosed in any patient, a history of sexual activity and practices should be obtained since anal intercourse transmits rectal infections that will be overlooked unless specifically sought.

Homosexual men are particularly susceptible to unusual diseases affecting the large bowel and to some illnesses that have not been proved infectious in etiology. Some of the diseases described thus far in this chapter may occur as a part of the gay bowel syndrome; for example, amebiasis and shigellosis are frequent infections in homosexual men and cytomegalovirus is a fairly common opportunistic invader in the immunologically deficient person.

The diseases that are specifically venereal and therefore directly transmitted by sexual contact will be discussed.

Gonorrhea

Infection with *Neisseria gonorrhoeae* is the most common cause of acute proctitis in the male homosexual population.[32] Patients will have a moderate degree of tenesmus and a copious rectal mucous discharge. The endoscopic findings are those of a "nonspecific proctitis," although the appearance is characterized by the presence of a considerable quantity of creamy mucous exudate. Only rarely are ulcerations present in this acute illness. Frequently, the organism may be present in the asymptomatic male with no visible abnormalities on sigmoidoscopic examination.

Anorectal Herpes Simplex Infection

Herpes simplex virus is also a frequent cause of acute proctitis.[33] The presenting symptoms are usually severe anorectal pain accompanied by constipation, tenesmus, and rectal discharge of blood and pus. There may be an accompanying paresthesia of the buttocks and thighs. Many patients with this infection will have perianal vesicles or ulcerations.

The endoscopic findings are again those of a "nonspecific proctitis." Sigmoidoscopy will reveal a friable mucosa with ulceration and

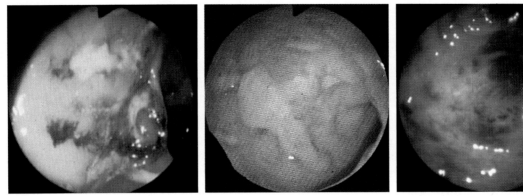

PLATE 42—26.   PLATE 42—27.   PLATE 42—28.

PLATE 42—26. Amebiasis. There are multiple irregular punched-out ulcers with spontaneous bleeding. Note the absence of significant erythema around the ulcers. (Courtesy of Dr. Jose Romeu.)

PLATE 42—27. Amebiasis. A large ulceration is present in a patient with granulomatous colitis who had secondary infection with amebiasis. Biopsies revealed amebae, but the underlying disease did not respond to anti-amebic therapy.

PLATE 42—28. Cytomegalovirus infection. Patchy erythema and spontaneous bleeding proved on biopsy to be secondary to cytomegalovirus in a man with acquired immune deficiency syndrome (AIDS).

erosions. Intranuclear inclusions may be present in rectal biopsy specimens.

Syphilis

The proctosigmoidoscopic findings may also be those of "nonspecific proctitis." The rectal mucosa may be granular and friable. Anal ulcers or fissures or discrete rectal ulcers (syphilitic chancre) may be present. The latter are usually associated with rectal discomfort, tenesmus, and mucoid discharge that may progress to bloody diarrhea. The base of the ulcers may become fibrotic as the chronic phase develops. Smooth, lobulated masses may also be found in the rectum.

Syphilis has long had the reputation as a "great imitator." Anorectal syphilitic disease may easily be confused with anal fissure, perianal Crohn's disease, cryptitis, and solitary rectal ulcer unless the endoscopist maintains a constant awareness of this disease and entertains suspicion when a lesion compatible with the diagnosis is encountered. Specific

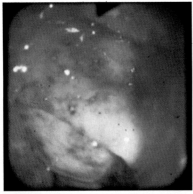 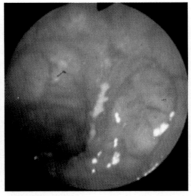 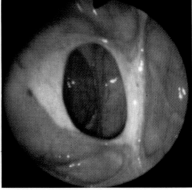

PLATE 42—29.   PLATE 42—30.   PLATE 42—31.

PLATE 42—29. Cytomegalovirus infection. Small, discrete aphthous-appearing ulcerations can be seen in the right colon of a patient with acquired immune deficiency syndrome (AIDS). Biopsies revealed the presence of cytomegalovirus.

PLATE 42—30. Cytomegalovirus infection. A series of circumferentially arranged irregular ulcers was demonstrated to contain cytomegalovirus by colonoscopic biopsies. Patient underwent colonoscopy because of diarrhea that developed while on long-term corticosteroid therapy.

PLATE 42—31. Cytomegalovirus infection. An ulcer circumferentially involves interhaustral septum in the right colon. The more proximal interhaustral septum noted in the distance has a similar but smaller ulcer on its edge.

immunofluorescent staining of biopsy specimens from rectal lesions will reveal the presence of *Treponema pallidum*.[34]

Lymphogranuloma Venereum (LGV)

Infection by *Chlamydia trachomatis*, a microorganism that is probably closely related to bacteria, is transmitted mainly through sexual contact. The disease can take several forms.[35] LGV, the most common venereal form, consists of a primary vesicular genital lesion that ulcerates and then heals without scarring. This is followed by a second stage that is characterized by inguinal and femoral lymphadenopathy and systemic symptoms including fever, chills, and typically headache. In about one fourth of patients, however, the rectum is the primary site of infection. Rectal infections may be due to non-LGV immunotypes of *Chlamydia* that may produce a milder course or may even be asymptomatic in comparison to the more severe proctitis due to infection with LGV immunotypes. In homosexual men, infection is not usually accompanied by enlargement of inguinal lymph nodes.

Infection of the rectum usually produces an acute illness that lasts less than 4 weeks and is associated with anorectal pain, discharge, rectal bleeding, and tenesmus. There is often a change in stool frequency.

Endoscopic examination in symptomatic patients usually reveals purulent exudate, friability, and discrete ulcers. The findings are most common in the rectum, but may extend to the sigmoid colon or even to the descending colon. If the disease is not treated, strictures may occur; these are usually located close to the anal margin. Fistulas and perirectal abscesses may also develop, so that the disease simulates Crohn's disease of the rectum (Plate 42–32). The distinction between the granulomatous colitis of Crohn's disease and *Chlamydia* infection is compounded by remarkable similarities in the microscopic findings. Biopsies in patients with LGV infections reveal a granulomatous proctitis with crypt abscesses and granulomas containing giant cells.

Serologic testing is generally not useful for diagnosis unless seroconversion or an increase in titer is demonstrated. Since the endoscopic and biopsy findings mimic Crohn's disease, diagnosis rests mainly on isolation of *Chlamydia* from the rectum.

Kaposi's Sarcoma

Kaposi's sarcoma may be an infectious disease of the entire gastrointestinal tract in patients with AIDS, although it is usually considered to be a spontaneously occurring malignant tumor.[36]

Colonic involvement is recognized endoscopically by the presence of a typical dark, magenta-colored nodule that is only slightly elevated and occurs in the midst of otherwise normal appearing mucosa (Plates 42–33 and 42–34). When grasped with the biopsy forceps the mucosa is not "bound down" and can easily be moved over the deeper layers of submucosa. Biopsies are positive in only 50% of patients because of the submucosal characteristic of the lesion. The disease may have a patchy distribution with infrequently occurring nodules involving the distal large bowel.

Cryptosporidiosis

Cryptosporidial involvement of the colon is caused by an unusual parasite, *Cryptosporidium*, which has previously been reported in the intestinal tracts of various vertebrates including reptiles, birds, and mammals. It is associated with a subacute or chronic diarrheal illness in patients with AIDS.[37] Colonoscopy may be completely normal (Plate 42–35), but cultures and biopsies of the mucosa are frequently positive for the presence of tiny dot-like organisms on the mucosal border of the cells. Weight loss is a prominent clinical feature despite the absence of gross morphologic changes consistent with a diarrheal illness.

OTHER INFLAMMATORY CONDITIONS OF THE COLON

The pathophysiologic response of the colon to injury is limited. Therefore the overall appearance of the reaction to any specific offending agent may be grossly and microscopically identical to that caused by a variety of other etiologic agents.

In preceding sections the endoscopic appearance of the colonic mucosa in many different types of specific infections was described in relation to the known responses found in idiopathic inflammatory bowel disease. There are other inflammatory conditions that affect the large bowel, and the reactions to most of them will be similar to those noted previously.

The importance of the patient's history of the illness cannot be overemphasized, since early in the course of an inflammatory process the mucosal response may produce a pattern that resembles ulcerative colitis. The

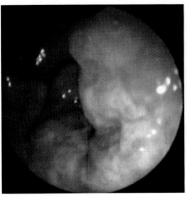 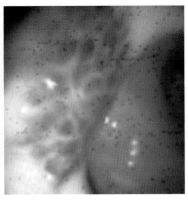

PLATE 42–32. Lymphogranuloma venereum. Rectal pseudotumor has many features of carcinoma, including nodularity, ulceration, fixation, and friability. Biopsies proved the diagnosis of lymphogranuloma venereum. (Courtesy of Dr. Jose Romeu.)

PLATE 42–33. Kaposi sarcoma. Mottled, reddish submucosal polypoid projection typical of intracolonic Kaposi sarcoma is seen in the sigmoid colon of a patient with acquired immune deficiency syndrome (AIDS).

PLATE 42–32.   PLATE 42–33.

progression of that disease to a later stage can cause damage to the colon's deeper layers that results in an appearance similar to Crohn's colitis.

Diverticular Disease

Diverticular disease of the colon has a wide pathophysiologic spectrum with only a few responses that relate to this chapter. The known muscular hypertrophy of this disorder is usually not associated with any true "inflammatory" reaction, but sequelae of the hypercontractile state may closely resemble inflammatory bowel disease.[38]

Although uncomplicated diverticulosis, even with severe luminal narrowing, is not associated with a visible mucosal inflammatory response, certain mucosal abnormalities may be present. Patchy, mottled red areas may be noted on the tips of several adjacent hypertrophied folds in the sigmoid colon in patients with diverticulosis. These small areas

almost never bleed spontaneously and are usually not friable. The redness is characteristically uniform and confluent on the edge of folds and becomes discontinuous over a distance of a few millimeters proceeding toward the haustral pouches. When viewed closely, the red areas consist of myriad tiny red dots, each of which resembles petechiae.

The pathogenesis of these red areas is unclear, but it is thought that contractile pressure generated by muscular activity in the narrowed sigmoid colon may actually cause capillary ruptures or diapedesis of red cells across intact capillary walls. Biopsy specimens of the reddened mucosa do not demonstrate any inflammation; however, hemosiderin, a product of corpuscular hemoglobin, is frequently found in the extravascular tissues. When a broad segment of mucosa is involved, friability may develop, and rarely spontaneous bleeding may occur. If either of these is present, the endoscopic appearance may suggest an isolated segment

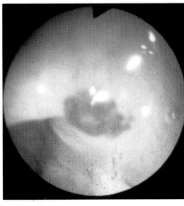 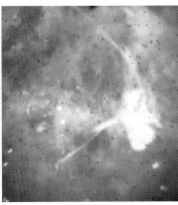

PLATE 42–34. Kaposi sarcoma. Discrete, mottled nodular submucosal projection characteristic of colonic involvement with Kaposi sarcoma is present in a patient with acquired immune deficiency syndrome (AIDS).

PLATE 42–35. Cryptosporidiosis. Patchy erythema was the only endoscopic abnormality in the transverse colon of a homosexual man with a 3-month history of diarrhea. Typical histopathological finding of cryptosporidia was present in endoscopic biopsy specimens.

PLATE 42–34.   PLATE 42–35.

of inflammatory bowel disease, but biopsy samples are characteristic for their hemorrhagic infiltration and lack of inflammatory cell response.

A more extensive discussion of diverticular disease of the colon is presented in Chapter 46.

Ischemic Colitis

Ischemic colitis has a varied endoscopic appearance according to the severity of the ischemic process. It has similarities to both ulcerative colitis and Crohn's disease.[39–41] With mild ischemia there may be only slight granularity and loss of vascular pattern; in severe cases the blue-black coloration of incipient gangrene may be seen. The mucosa may be hemorrhagic, friable, and ulcerated and sharply demarcated from normal mucosa at each end of the involved segment. A pseudomembrane may overlie the ischemic area and when removed reveals a reddened, friable mucosa with contact bleeding. The healing phase of ischemia may be manifested by patchy ulceration in otherwise normal-appearing mucosa, in which case the history of a short clinical disease with accompanying rectal bleeding may be the only clue that the underlying disease is not Crohn's colitis. The ulcers of ischemic colitis may resemble aphthous ulcerations or may be linear and irregular. The development of a stricture may accompany the healing process and can cause marked luminal constriction.

A syndrome of induced bowel ischemia has been described in women taking oral contraceptives, estrogens, or progesterone.[42] The clinical course resembles ischemic bowel disease. Endoscopic findings include normal mucosa in the rectum and discrete ulcers in otherwise normal-appearing mucosa proximal to the rectum, or there may be confluent friability and edema in the involved segment.

Ischemic colitis is discussed in detail in Chapter 44.

Solitary Ulcers

Solitary ulcers are most often found in the rectum during the investigation of rectal bleeding.[43] They are usually superficial, irregularly shaped with an intensely red margin, and may be several centimeters in diameter. Characteristically there is no surrounding inflammation, and they are usually located on the lip of the rectosigmoid fold; they are rarely found in the dilated rectal ampulla. Isolated ulcers may be present throughout the remainder of the bowel, most commonly in the cecum. Ischemia may be the cause in elderly patients with fecal stasis and rectal prolapse; in younger patients self-induced trauma may be the cause. Solitary colon and rectal ulcers are discussed in Chapter 46.

Radiation Colitis

The colonic mucosa is more sensitive to injury from inadvertent x-ray exposure than the deeper components of the colonic wall. A colitic response of short duration frequently follows radiotherapy of the pelvic organs, and may include diarrhea and tenesmus with the passage of mucous and occasionally blood. Endoscopy is rarely requested for this well-recognized and self-limiting phenomenon; endoscopic features include granularity, erythema, loss of vascular pattern, and multiple small bleeding sites.

The acute reaction to radiation exposure usually heals spontaneously, but even in the absence of immediate damage there may be long-lasting tissue destruction that may remain unrecognized for a considerable time. Rectal bleeding becomes evident within 6 months or as long as 20 years after treatment. The endoscopic appearance consists of mucosal friability, spontaneous bleeding, granularity and multiple telangiectasias, findings that are also typical of "nonspecific proctitis" and ulcerative colitis.

Radiation-induced colitis is considered in detail in Chapter 44.

COMPLICATIONS OF INSTRUMENTATION

There are three aspects to consider with regard to complications that may occur in association with colonoscopy in infectious and inflammatory colitis; complications related to the procedure itself, transmission of infections via the colonoscope, and infection of the endoscopy staff via contaminated materials and equipment.

The broad aspect of complications from instrumentation is beyond the scope of this discussion (see Chapter 41). The inflamed large bowel is probably less able than the normal colon to adapt to the stress of stretching and distention imposed by the passage of the colonoscope. Every effort must be made to maintain the insertion tube in as straight a configuration as possible with a minimum of loop formation (see Chapter 40); air insufflation should be kept to a minimum.

Although the number of reports of transmission of infection from patient to patient via a fiberoptic endoscope are few,[44] it is prudent to disinfect equipment after each use in cases of infectious or inflammatory colitis. In addition to meticulous mechanical cleansing, the instrument and accessories should be soaked in the disinfectant solution recommended by the endoscope manufacturer.[45] After examination of a patient with known or suspected AIDS, the current recommendation is that the colonoscope and all ancillary equipment be gas-sterilized. Gas sterilization is not currently recommended following endoscopy for any other condition.

General standards of cleanliness are required whenever endoscopy is performed in a patient with potentially infectious colitis, but the technique of "reverse isolation" with gowns, gloves, and masks is not recommended except for cases of AIDS. When cultures are necessary, colonic secretions can be collected in a bronchoscopic-type suction trap and sent to the microbiology laboratory in that sealed container without the need to inoculate specimens in the endoscopy suite.

Editor's note: References 46 to 52 are some recent publications of interest in relation to the topics presented in this chapter.

References

1. Tedesco FJ, Moore S. Infectious diseases mimicking inflammatory bowel disease. Am Surg 1982; 48:243–9.
2. Tedesco F. Differential diagnosis of ulcerative colitis and Crohn's ileocolitis and other specific inflammatory disease of the bowel. Med Clin North Am 1980; 64:1173–83.
3. Rutgeerts P, Geboes K, Ponette E, et al. Acute infective colitis caused by endemic pathogens in Western Europe: Endoscopic features. Endoscopy 1982; 14:212–9.
4. Tedesco FJ, Hardin RD, Harper RN, et al. Infectious colitis endoscopically simulating inflammatory bowel disease: a prospective evaluation. Gastrointest Endosc 1983; 29:195–7.
5. Waye JD. Colonoscopy intubation technique without fluoroscopy. In: Hunt RH, Waye JD, eds. Colonoscopy. Techniques, Clinical Practice and Colour Atlas. London: Chapman & Hall, 1981; 174–6.
6. Waye JD, Hunt RH. Colonoscopic diagnosis of inflammatory bowel disease. Surg Clin North Am 1982; 62:905–13.
7. Rickert RR, Carter HW. The gross, light microscopic and scanning electron microscopic appearance of the early lesions in Crohn's disease. Scann Electron Microsc 1977; 2:179–86.
8. Waye JD. The role of colonoscopy in the differential diagnosis of inflammatory bowel disease. Gastrointest Endosc 1977; 23:150–4.
9. Teague RH, Waye JD. Inflammatory bowel disease. In: Hunt RH, Waye JD, eds. Colonoscopy. Techniques, Clinical Practice and Colour Atlas. London: Chapman & Hall, 1981; 343–62.
10. McGovern VJ, Goulston SJM. Crohn's disease of the colon. Gut 1968; 9:164–76.
11. Geboes K. The value of endoscopic biopsies in the diagnosis of Crohn's disease. Tijdschr Gastroenterol 1978; 21:87–97.
12. Lux G, Fruhmorgen P, Phillip J, et al. Diagnosis of inflammatory disease of the colon—comparative endoscopic and roentgenological examinations. Endoscopy 1978; 10:279–84.
13. Rotterdam H, Sommers SC. Biopsy diagnosis of the digestive tract. New York: Raven Press, 1981.
14. Das KM, Farid T, Berkowitz JM. Value of colonoscopy in the investigation of inflammatory bowel disease. (Abstr) Gastroenterology 1974; 66:681.
15. Williams CB, Waye JD. Colonoscopy in inflammatory bowel disease. Clin Gastroenterol 1978; 7:701–17.
16. Saffouri B, Bartolomeco RS, Fuchs B. Colonic involvement in salmonellosis. Dig Dis Sci 1979; 24:203–8.
17. Vantrappen G, Ponette E, Geboes K, et al. *Yersinia* enteritis and enterocolitis: gastroenterological aspects. Gastroenterology 1977; 72:220–7.
18. Blaser MJ, Parsons RB, Wang WL. Acute colitis caused by *Campylobacter fetus* ss. *jejuni*. Gastroenterology 1980; 78:448–53.
19. Loss RW Jr, Mangla JC, Pereira M. *Campylobacter* colitis presenting as inflammatory bowel disease with segmental colonic ulcerations. Gastroenterology 1980; 79:138–40.
20. Karmoli M, Fleming PC. *Campylobacter enteritis*. Can Med Assoc J 1979; 120:1525–32.
21. Franklin GO, Mohapatra M, Perillo RP. Colonic tuberculosis diagnosed by colonoscopic biopsy. Gastroenterology 1979; 76:362–4.
22. Bartlett JG, Chang TW, Gurwith M, et al. Antibiotic-associated pseudomembranous colitis due to toxin-producing clostridia. N Engl J Med 1978; 298: 531–4.
23. Peikin SR, Galdibini J, Bartlett JG. Role of *Clostridium difficile* in a case of nonantibiotic-associated pseudomembranous colitis. Gastroenterology 1980; 79:948–51.
24. Tedesco FJ. Antibiotic associated pseudomembranous colitis with negative proctosigmoidoscopy examination. Gastroenterology 1979; 77:295–7.
25. Tucker PC, Webster PD, Zachary M, et al. Amebic colitis mistaken for inflammatory bowel disease. Arch Intern Med 1975; 135:681–5.
26. Blumencranz H, Kasen L, Romeu J, et al. Role of endoscopy in suspected amebiasis. Am J Gastroenterol 1983; 78:15–8.
27. Nebel OT, El-Masry NA, Castell DO, et al. Schistosomal colonic polyposis: endoscopic and histologic characteristics. Gastrointest Endosc 1974; 20:99–101.
28. Haws CC, Long RF, Caplan GE. *Histoplasma capsulatum* as a cause of ileocolitis. AJR 1977; 128:692–4.
29. Goodman ZD, Boitnott JK, Yardley JH. Perforation

of the colon associated with cytomegalovirus infection. Dig Dis Sci 1979; 24:376–80.

30. Knight R. Giardiasis, isosporiasis and balantidiasis. Clin Gastroenterol 1978; 7:31–47.

31. Quinn TC, Correy L, Chaffee RG, et al. The etiology of anorectal infections in homosexual men. Am J Med 1981; 71:395–406.

32. Lebedeff DA, Hochman EB. Rectal gonorrhea in men: diagnosis and treatment. Ann Intern Med 1980; 92:463–6.

33. Goldmeier D. Proctitis and Herpes simplex virus in homosexual men. Br J Vener Dis 1980; 56:111–4.

34. Quinn TC, Lukehart SA, Goodell SE, et al. Rectal mass caused by *Treponema pallidum:* confirmation by immunofluorescent staining. Gastroenterology 1982; 82:135–9.

35. Quinn TC, Goodell SE, Mkrtichian E, et al. *Chlamydia trachomatis* proctitis. N Engl J Med 1981; 305:195–200.

36. Levy JA, Zeigler JL. Acquired immunodeficiency syndrome is an opportunistic infection and Kaposi's sarcoma results from secondary immune stimulation. Lancet 1983; 2:78–81.

37. Petras RE, Carey WD, Alanis A. Cryptosporidial enteritis in a homosexual male with an acquired immunodeficiency syndrome. Cleve Clin Q 1983; 50:41–5.

38. Williams CB. Diverticular disease and stricture. In: Hunt RH, Waye JD, eds. Colonoscopy. Techniques, Clinical Practice, and Colour Atlas. London: Chapman & Hall, 1981; 363–81.

39. Hunt RH, Buchanan JD. Transient ischaemic colitis—colonoscopy and biopsy in diagnosis. J R Nav Med Serv 1979; 65:15–9.

40. Scowcroft CW, Sanowski RA, Kozarek RA. Colonoscopy in ischemic colitis. Gastrointest Endosc 1981; 27:156–9.

41. McNeill C, Green G, Bannayan G, et al. Ischemic colitis diagnosed by early colonoscopy. Gastrointest Endosc 1974; 20:124–6.

42. Tedesco FJ, Volpicelli NA, Moore FS. Estrogen- and progesterone-associated colitis: a disorder with clinical and endoscopic features mimicking Crohn's colitis. Gastrointest Endosc 1982; 28:247–9.

43. Rutter KRP, Riddell RK. The solitary ulcer syndrome of the rectum. Clin Gastroenterol 1975; 4:505–30.

44. Dean AG. Transmission of *Salmonella typhi* by fiberoptic endoscopy. Lancet 1977; 2:134.

45. Geenen JE, Pfeifer M, Simonsen L. Cleaning and disinfection of endoscopic equipment. Gastrointest Endosc 1978; 24:185–6.

46. Pera A, Bellando P, Caldera D, et al. Colonoscopy in inflammatory bowel disease. Diagnostic accuracy and proposal of an endoscopic score. Gastroenterology 1987; 92;181–5.

47. Gomes P, du Boulay C, Smith CL, Holdstock G. Relationship between disease activity indices and colonoscopic findings in patients with colonic inflammatory bowel disease. Gut 1986; 28:92–5.

48. Bo Linn GW, Vendrell DD, Lee E, Fordtran JS. An evaluation of the significance of microscopic colitis in patients with chronic diarrhea. J Clin Invest 1985; 75:1559–69.

49. Meiselman MS, Cello JP, Margaretten W. Cytomegalovirus colitis. Report of the clinical, endoscopic, and pathologic findings in two patients with the acquired immune deficiency syndrome. Gastroenterology 1985; 88:171–5.

50. Luterman L, Alsumait AR, Daly DS, Goresky CA. Colonoscopic features of cecal amebomas. Gastrointest Endosc 1985; 31:204–6.

51. Bhargava DK, Tandon HD, Chawla TC, et al. Diagnosis of ileocecal and colonic tuberculosis by colonoscopy. Gastrointest Endosc 1985; 31:68–70.

52. Radhakrishnan S, Al Nakib B, Shaikh H, Menon NK. The value of colonoscopy in schistosomal, tuberculous, and amebic colitis. Two-year experience. Dis Colon Rectum 1986; 29:891–5.

Chapter 43

SPECIAL PROBLEMS IN CHRONIC ULCERATIVE COLITIS

FRANCIS J. TEDESCO, M.D.

Specific and frequently unique clinical problems may arise in the natural course of patients with a chronic illness. Some special problems inherent in the management of patients with chronic ulcerative colitis will be discussed in this chapter. Included are the evaluation of strictures, surveillance for cancer by means of sigmoidoscopy and colonoscopy, an attempt at defining the significance of dysplasia as well as management of this finding, and the role of colonoscopy in determining the extent of involvement of the colon in ulcerative disease of the colonic mucosa.

STRICTURES

The development of one or more colonic strictures is a common problem in patients with long-standing ulcerative colitis.[1, 2] Most strictures in patients with inflammatory bowel disease are benign. They occur with about equal frequency in ulcerative colitis and granulomatous colitis and may be the result of fibrosis, muscular hypertrophy, spasm, or carcinoma. Strictures can be associated with the active phase of inflammatory bowel disease; these are secondary to mucosal and submucosal inflammation and edema in contrast to those of the more chronic phase that result from muscular spasm, fibrosis or both. Any stricture occurring in a patient with ulcerative colitis raises the question of carcinoma and therefore requires further evaluation.

A stricture may be identified by barium contrast radiography. Colonoscopy is the best method available for investigation of these radiographic abnormalities, as it provides multiple biopsies and specimens for cytologic examination in addition to direct inspection of the stricture. Most strictures demonstrated by barium contrast radiography can be approached with a standard diameter colonoscope, including those that appear to markedly narrow the lumen. In many cases this type of endoscope can be passed through and beyond such strictures because air insufflation during colonoscopy distends the narrowed lumen, especially when the stricture is due to spasm or muscular hypertrophy. However, on certain occasions a smaller diameter "pediatric" fiberscope is required if the endoscope is to be passed through a tight stricture to adequately inspect the entire inner aspect of the stricture and the bowel beyond. Sometimes radiographically demonstrated strictures may be difficult or impossible to identify at endoscopy because air insufflation expands the narrowed area and because the spherical aberration associated with modern "wide angle" optics makes it difficult to appreciate small changes in the diameter of the colon.

As a general rule, fibrotic strictures appear thin, short, and web-like, whereas strictures secondary to active inflammation, muscular thickening, or spasm are smooth and tapered. Mucosal ulcerations, friability, and erythema are frequently noted (Plates 43–1 and 43–2). Endoscopic features suggestive of malignancy are firmness and fixation of the involved colonic segment ("rigidity"), a shelf-like proximal edge, and an inability to negotiate the colonoscope through the narrowed segment (Plates 43–3 and 43–4).

900

Endoscopic evaluation of a stricture is equal in importance to histologic and cytologic assessment. At times the endoscopist may suspect malignancy although biopsy and cytologic specimens are negative or inconclusive. This suspicion is sometimes reinforced by the histologic finding of dysplastic changes in biopsies from either the strictured area or the epithelium proximal or distal to the stricture. Malignant strictures have also been incorrectly diagnosed as benign by endoscopic examination. Since maneuverability may be limited, a carcinoma located just proximal or distal to an apparently smooth stricture can be easily overlooked at endoscopy. This emphasizes the desirability of cytologic study as an adjunct to both endoscopic observation and biopsy. The ability of the barium x-ray examination to demonstrate all aspects of a stricture must also be emphasized, especially in cases where the entire area of narrowing and the adjacent mucosa are not well seen at colonoscopy. Although most carcinomas associated with ulcerative colitis appear to originate from the mucosal surface, there is one report of carcinoma spreading submucosally that yielded biopsy specimens negative for malignancy.[3]

Although endoscopic appearance, biopsy, and cytology are the best available means for evaluation of strictures in ulcerative colitis, it is reasonable that surgery be performed in preference to repeated colonoscopic examinations if any malignancy is suspected based on radiographic, colonoscopic, histologic, or cytologic assessment; if the stricture cannot be examined thoroughly; or if biopsy and cytologic specimens are inadequate.

The endoscopic examination of strictures in patients with ulcerative colitis should be performed with caution, since the colonic wall in such patients is usually thinned and the mucosa may be markedly friable. As a result of these factors, the colon may not permit the same degree of longitudinal stretching that can be tolerated by the normal large bowel. Only minimal pressure should be exerted when attempting to pass the endoscope through these strictures lest excessive bowel trauma and perforation occur.

CANCER SURVEILLANCE AND DYSPLASIA

The occurrence of carcinoma in the colon of patients with long-standing ulcerative colitis is well documented. However, the magnitude of this problem has only recently been recognized.[4, 5] It is postulated that cancer of the colon will develop in 40% to 50% of patients who have total involvement of the colon and have had the disease for 25 years or more. Although there is virtually universal agreement that chronic ulcerative colitis leads to an increased incidence of colorectal carcinoma, the precise incidence remains the subject of considerable debate. For example, Katzka et al.[6] utilized both the classic life-table and a generalized life-table approach to estimate the risk of colorectal cancer. This provocative paper reported that this risk was even less than previously reported for hospitalized patients. In an accompanying editorial by Yardley et al.[7] some of the more serious deficiencies of this retrospective study were pointed out, especially with respect to patient selection, follow-up procedures, and methods used for detection of neoplastic disease. Yardley et al. pleaded for prospective studies that are lacking and are necessary if we are to increase our understanding of the variables that affect the incidence of cancer in ulcerative colitis. If one is fully aware of the lack of prospective data, some reasonable statements about cancer and dysplasia in ulcerative colitis are possible.

Carcinoma associated with chronic ulcerative colitis tends to occur at an earlier age relative to that for colorectal carcinoma in the general population. Its distribution is uniform throughout the colon, and carcinoma is at times multifocal. These facts, coupled with the markedly limited ability to diagnose early malignancy by radiologic means, have led to a search for "premalignant" changes that would permit therapeutic intervention before metastases occur. Twenty years have passed since Morson and Pang[8] reported the presence of a precancerous lesion in the colonic and rectal mucosa of patients with chronic ulcerative colitis. Since this publication, intense interest has focused on epithelial dysplasia as the marker for increased cancer risk and the necessity for colectomy in ulcerative colitis. To have a better understanding of this complex area of investigation, it is important that the following terms be defined: atypia, dysplasia, and carcinoma in situ.

Atypia signifies any epithelial change in which there is deviation from the normal. In fact, most atypical epithelial alterations are reactive, that is, secondary to inflammation, and not neoplastic. It is imperative that pathologists separate reactive from neoplastic atypia.

Dysplasia signifies neoplastic epithelium that is confined within the basement membrane and therefore has no potential to metastasize. Dysplasia is divided into low-grade and high-grade categories based on the degree of atypia or deviation from normal. Dysplastic epithelium has the potential for malignant transformation (i.e., to become invasive and to metastasize); this potential is presumed to be greater for high-grade dysplasia.

Carcinoma in situ designates neoplastic epithelium in which the cells show marked atypia resembling that of carcinoma, but these cells are confined to the mucosa superficial to the basement membrane.

The evidence supporting the concept of dysplasia as a premalignant lesion in ulcerative colitis comes for the most part from two methods of investigation. First, retrospective analysis of resected colons harboring carcinomas from patients with ulcerative colitis has demonstrated the presence of dysplasia either adjacent to or remote from the carcinoma.[9–12] Second, prospective studies in which colectomy was performed because of the biopsy finding of dysplasia have demonstrated that 30% to 70% of patients with dysplasia will have a clinically unsuspected pre-existing carcinoma in the resected specimen.[11, 13–16]

It appears that dysplasia comprises a sequence of events from increasing degrees of atypia to frankly invasive carcinoma. Although definitive data to support this hypothesis are still being gathered, circumstantial evidence does suggest that carcinomas are more often associated with the more advanced degrees of dysplasia. It must be noted, however, that carcinoma may arise from epithelium with less than the highest degree of dysplasia. Therefore, it appears possible that invasive malignancy may develop without necessarily progressing through increasing degrees of atypia.

Another significant concern is that recognition and grading of dysplasia is to a considerable extent subjective, and even experienced pathologists will sometimes disagree as to both the presence and severity of dysplasia. A non-unanimous consensus concerning diagnostic criteria for recognizing and grading dysplasia has been developed.[16] Table 43–1 reviews this biopsy classification and its implications for management.[16, 17]

TABLE 43–1. Biopsy Classification and Suggested Approach to Clinical Management

Biopsy Classification	Recommended Management
Negative	
Normal	
Inactive Disease	Continue regular follow-up
Active Disease	
Indefinite (with respect to dysplasia)	
Probably inflammatory	
Probably Dysplasia	Short interval follow-up (3 to 6 months)
Low-grade Dysplasia	Short interval follow-up or Consider colectomy (especially with gross lesion)
High-grade Dysplasia	After confirmation, advise colectomy

Modified from: Haggitt RC. American Society for Gastrointestinal Endoscopy. Postgraduate Endoscopy Course II, December 1982.

Cancer surveillance in patients with chronic ulcerative colitis has focused on the use of dysplasia as an indication of malignancy. Although the original studies of the relation between cancer and dysplasia were based on sigmoidoscopic biopsies in the intact colon or on colectomy specimens received at operation, the finding that only 66% of patients with carcinoma complicating ulcerative colitis had dysplasia in the rectum at the time of colectomy has led to the utilization of colonoscopy as the accepted method of surveillance.[11, 18]

Cancer surveillance in patients with ulcerative colitis is quite different from the use of colonoscopy to evaluate a barium enema x-ray abnormality. Patients are preselected for surveillance colonoscopy on the basis of clinical factors that include a previously and clearly established diagnosis of ulcerative colitis, a certain duration of disease, and in most cases universal involvement of the colon. The clinical course with respect to severity of disease and exacerbations and the degree and duration of inflammatory activity are not relevant.

Interpretation of the available retrospective data suggests that the occurrence of dysplasia within the colon does not follow a uniform distribution. As noted, only two thirds of patients with ulcerative colitis and cancer had dysplastic epithelium in the rec-

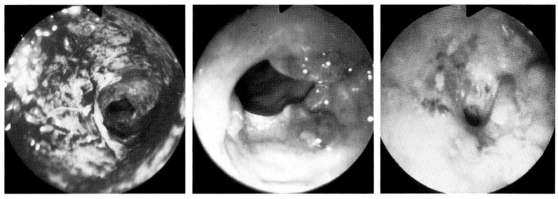

PLATE 43–1.   PLATE 43–2.   PLATE 43–3.

PLATE 43–1. Colonoscopic appearance of inflammatory stricture. Note the mucosal ulcerations and friability proximal to the stricture.

PLATE 43–2. Inflammatory stricture with adjacent pseudopolyps.

PLATE 43–3. Colonoscopic appearance of fibrotic stricture. Note the shelf-like edge on the right. This is a "suspicious" stricture.

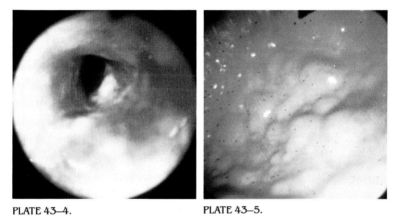

PLATE 43–4.   PLATE 43–5.

PLATE 43–4. Malignant stricture. Cancer was detected at surgery. Preoperative biopsy specimens revealed dysplasia.

PLATE 43–5. Bumpy mucosa in a patient with ulcerative colitis. Biopsy confirmed dysplasia.

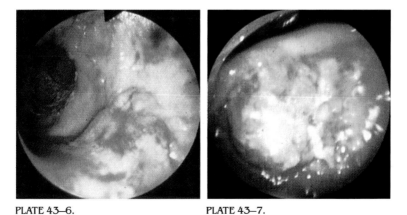

PLATE 43–6.   PLATE 43–7.

PLATE 43–6. Dysplasia associated lesion or mass (DALM). Note the mass-like elevation against background changes of chronic ulcerative colitis.

PLATE 43–7. Mass below ileocecal valve in a patient with chronic ulcerative colitis. Dysplasia (DALM) was demonstrated by biopsy.

tum at the time of colectomy. In addition, study of specimens in which there is no cancer shows that dysplasia will be present in 13%. In general, dysplasia has been found in 80% to 88% of all colectomy specimens containing carcinoma.[18] More recent prospective data have likewise demonstrated that in one third of patients with moderate to severe dysplasia on biopsy, a colon cancer will be discovered when colectomy is performed.[18] Although with the majority of cancers there is associated dysplasia elsewhere in the colon, biopsy specimens that do not reveal dysplastic changes are no assurance that cancer does not exist—for example, in unexamined areas or proximal to strictures.

Some physicians recommend colectomy for patients with pancolitis after 10 years, although at present most physicians do not advise "prophylactic" colectomy solely on the basis of duration of disease. However, it is this group of unoperated patients for whom surveillance is mandatory. The surveillance program is usually started after ulcerative colitis has affected the colon for 10 years, although cancer of the colon has been documented when the disease has been present for only 8 years, and it has been suggested that surveillance should probably begin at the seventh to eighth year of disease.[10, 15, 19] There is evidence that patients with left-sided colitis also are at increased risk, but it appears that the precancerous phase of this disease is longer; therefore in these cases long-term surveillance probably can be initiated in the 15th year of illness.[20]

A major reason for advocating evaluation of the total colon rather than reliance on repeated proctosigmoidoscopies with biopsies is that the right colon, where approximately 25% of all carcinomas occur in chronic ulcerative colitis, can be evaluated. Furthermore, one third of patients in whom the rectum is spared of dysplastic changes will have dysplasia in the colon.[20] In addition, precancerous dysplasia may be more readily differentiated histologically from the reactive epithelial changes of active colitis when biopsies are obtained sequentially from the cecum to the rectum because the inflammatory process is usually less marked in the proximal colon than in the rectum and sigmoid colon.

Colonoscopy permits a careful visual evaluation of minute lesions and bumpy mucosal irregularities demonstrated by barium contrast radiography (Plate 43–5). Biopsies may

also be obtained from such small lesions. Larger lesions may also be noted, especially at colonoscopy (Plates 43–6 and 43–7). The results of one study suggest that dysplasia found in association with any grossly visible lesion, especially a polypoid mass, indicates a high likelihood that cancer may already be present. This finding is sometimes given the abbreviation DALM, meaning dysplasia associated lesion or mass.[21] This suggests that dysplasia associated with a lesion or mass is in itself a strong indication for colectomy. This, however, is controversial. Since adenomas are common in individuals over 40 years of age, their coincidental occurrence in older patients with ulcerative colitis is to be expected. Some clinicians believe that an adenoma in a patient with chronic ulcerative colitis can be managed like any other adenoma provided it is recognized that the lesion may not be coincidental but rather indicative of a high risk for invasive cancer. That is, the adenoma may be representative of a generalized tendency for neoplastic transformation of the colonic mucosa.[17]

With the above as background to the rationale for using colonoscopy as the principal surveillance method, there are certain practical clinical questions that must be answered: How should the patient with chronic ulcerative colitis be prepared for colonoscopy? How often should he or she undergo colonoscopy? What are the sites for biopsy as well as the correct number of specimens?

Although there are no definitive answers with respect to the best schedule of procedures or the types of examination that should be performed, many recent reports recommend yearly total colonoscopy; others suggest that colonoscopy be performed every 2 years, with fiberoptic sigmoidoscopy and biopsies in the intervening years.[10, 11, 13, 15, 18] We recommend yearly colonoscopy and biopsy. If dysplasia is found, colonoscopy is repeated within 3 to 6 months for confirmation of this finding. If low-grade dysplasia is found, the interval between colonoscopic examinations is shortened. Colectomy should be considered if short-interval surveillance cannot be carried out. If high-grade dysplasia is found and confirmed at a second endoscopy, colectomy is recommended.

Because of the importance of visualization of minor aberrations of the mucosal contour, the colon must be well prepared for surveillance endoscopy. Although bowel preparation must be individualized for each patient, there are several general methods. In asymptomatic patients a 24- to 48-hour clear-liquid diet, 10 oz. of citrate of magnesia orally the evening before the procedure, and tap water enemas until the return is clear are satisfactory. Oral colon electrolyte lavage preparations have also been used successfully, and this method provides excellent preparation for detailed visualization of the colon.

The actual number of colonoscopic biopsies required for adequate sampling of the colorectal mucosa for dysplasia has not been determined. Based on some data derived from resected specimens from patients with ulcerative colitis and carcinoma, many endoscopists elect to obtain biopsies in eight standardized locations: (1) cecum, (2) ascending colon, (3) hepatic flexure/proximal transverse colon, (4) mid-transverse colon, (5) distal transverse colon/splenic flexure area, (6) descending colon, (7) sigmoid colon, and (8) rectum. In addition, biopsies are obtained of any other areas thought to be suspicious based on endoscopic assessment. Special attention should be given to mucosal areas that are heaped-up or thickened, that are slightly raised either as plaque-like or nodular configurations, or that have a villous-appearing texture.

EXTENT OF MUCOSAL INFLAMMATION

Determination of the proximal limit of disease in the colon is usually not required during the initial evaluation of most patients with ulcerative colitis, since this information is rarely of critical importance in the initial or early clinical management. Although endoscopic assessment of the rectum and distal sigmoid is mandatory, total colonoscopy is rarely indicated. However, colonoscopy may occasionally be of major importance in differentiating ulcerative and granulomatous colitis from other more specific types of colitis.[22] In general this type of differential diagnosis is not difficult with the aid of the patient's history and the results of sigmoidoscopy, rectal biopsy, and barium enema x-ray examination. Many infectious agents can mimic ulcerative colitis, and the use of appropriate culturing techniques as well as endoscopy is frequently necessary to establish a definitive diagnosis.[23]

Colonoscopy has a greater role in determining extent of disease in patients with suspected ulcerative proctosigmoiditis who do not respond to topical measures such as cortisone enemas. In this clinical setting, it must be considered that the inflammatory process may extend more proximally than the rectosigmoid regardless of normal barium x-ray findings for the left colon. Colonoscopy with multiple biopsies may provide useful clinical information that may alter the therapeutic approach to the patient's disease. It may also change the patient's prognosis if more extensive disease is demonstrated.

Editor's note: Information on colonoscopic surveillance for dysplasia in chronic ulcerative colitis continues to accumulate. References 24, 25, and 26 are recently published articles concerning this topics. Reference 27 is also of interest in relation to colonoscopy and the problem of cancer in chronic ulcerative colitis.

References

1. Hunt RH, Teaque RH, Swarbrick ET, et al. Colonoscopy in management of colonic strictures. Br Med J 1975; 3:360–1.
2. Waye JD. Colitis, cancer, and colonoscopy. Med Clin North Am 1978; 62:211–24.
3. Crowson TD, Ferrante WF, Gathright JB. Colonoscopy: Inefficacy for early carcinoma detection in patients with ulcerative colitis. JAMA 1976; 236:2651–2.
4. Devroede GJ, Dockerty MB, Sauer WG, et al. Cancer of the colon in patients with ulcerative colitis since childhood. Can J Surg 1972; 15:369–74.
5. Devroede G, Taylor WF. On calculating cancer risk and survival of ulcerative colitis patients with the life table method. Gastroenterology 1976; 71:505–9.
6. Katzka I, Brody RS, Morris E, et al. Assessment of colorectal cancer risk in patients with ulcerative colitis: experience from a private practice. Gastroenterology 1983; 85:22–9.
7. Yardley JH, Ransohoff DF, Riddell RH, et al. Cancer in inflammatory bowel diseases: How serious is the problem and what should be done about it? Gastroenterology 1983; 85:197–9.
8. Morson BC, Pang LS. Rectal biopsy as an aid to cancer control in ulcerative colitis. Gut 1967; 8:423–34.
9. Riddell RH. The precarcinomatous phase of ulcerative colitis. Curr Top Pathol 1976; 63:179–219.
10. Nugent FW, Haggitt RC, Colcher H, et al. Malignant potential of chronic ulcerative colitis. Gastroenterology 1979; 76:1–5.
11. Dobbins WO III. Current status of the precancer lesion in ulcerative colitis. Gastroenterology 1977; 73:1431–3.
12. Yardley JH, Keren DF. Precancer lesions in ulcerative colitis. A retrospective study of rectal biopsy and colectomy specimens. Cancer 1974; 34:835–44.
13. Fuson JA, Farmer RG, Hawk WA, et al. Endoscopic surveillance for cancer in chronic ulcerative colitis. Am J Gastroenterol 1980; 73:120–6.

14. Myrvold HE, Kock NG, Ahren CH. Rectal biopsy and precancer in ulcerative colitis. Gut 1974; 15:301–4.

15. Lennard-Jones JE, Morson BC, Ritchie JK, et al. Cancer in colitis: assessment of the individual risk by clinical and histological criteria. Gastroenterology 1977; 73:1280–9.

16. Riddell RH, Goldman H, Ransohoff DT, et al. Dysplasia in inflammatory bowel disease: standardized classification with provisional clinical implications. Hum Pathol 1983; 14:931–68.

17. Haggitt RC. Dysplasia in inflammatory bowel disease. American Society for Gastrointestinal Endoscopy. Postgraduate Endoscopy Course II, December 1982.

18. Waye JD. Role of colonoscopy in surveillance for cancer in patients with ulcerative colitis. In: Winawer SJ, Schottenfeld D, Sherlock P, eds. Colorectal cancer: prevention, epidemiology and screening. Prog Cancer Res Ther 1980; 13:387–92.

19. Yardley JH, Bayless TM, Diamond MP. Cancer in ulcerative colitis. Gastroenterology 1979; 76:221–5.

20. Greenstein AJ, Sachar DB, Prucillo A, et al. Cancer in universal colitis and left-sided colitis: clinical and pathologic features. Mt Sinai J Med 1979; 46:25–32.

21. Blackstone MO, Riddell RH, Rogers BHG, et al. Dysplasia-associated lesion or mass (DALM) detected by colonoscopy in long-standing ulcerative colitis: an indication for colectomy. Gastroenterology 1981; 80:366–74.

22. Tedesco FJ. Differential diagnosis of ulcerative colitis and Crohn's ileocolitis and other specific inflammatory diseases of the bowel. Med Clin North Am 1980; 64:1173–83.

23. Tedesco FJ, Hardin RD, Harper RN, et al. Infectious colitis endoscopically simulating inflammatory bowel disease. A prospective evaluation. Gastrointest Endosc 1983; 29:195–7.

24. Brostrom O, Lofberg R, Ost A, Reichard H. Cancer surveillance of patients with longstanding ulcerative colitis: a clinical, endoscopical, and histological study. Gut 1986; 27:1408–13.

25. Rosenstock E, Farmer RG, Petras R, et al. Surveillance for colonic carcinoma in ulcerative colitis. Gastroenterology 1985; 89:1342–6.

26. Ransohoff DF, Riddell RH, Levin B. Ulcerative colitis and colonic cancer. Problems in assessing the diagnostic usefulness of mucosal dysplasia. Dis Colon Rectum 1985; 28:383–8.

27. Mir-Madjlessi SH, Farmer RG, Easley KA, Beck GJ. Colorectal and extracolonic malignancy in ulcerative colitis. Cancer 1986; 58:1569–74.

Chapter 44

DISORDERS OF THE LARGE BOWEL HAVING A VASCULAR COMPONENT

B. H. GERALD ROGERS, M.D.

VASCULAR ABNORMALITIES OF THE MUCOSA AND SUBMUCOSA

Acquired Vascular Abnormalities of the Cecal Region

With the advent of angiography and colonoscopy, vascular abnormalities of the cecum have attracted considerable interest. These lesions have been given various names, including angiodysplasia, hemangioma, arteriovenous malformation, vascular ectasia, vascular malformation, vascular dysplasia, angioma, telangiectasia, and others. The appropriate name will probably remain controversial until its etiology is demonstrated. The lesion is easily recognized in the proper clinical setting because it is apparently part of a syndrome—that is, acquired mucosal vascular abnormalities of the gastrointestinal tract occurring in the elderly and associated with cardiac, vascular, or pulmonary disease. Colonoscopy has diagnostic and therapeutic roles in dealing with this lesion. The bright-red, flat, vascular abnormality is most easily seen endoscopically in vivo. Once found, endoscopic therapy is relatively easy. The success of endoscopic therapy often has added importance since many patients are elderly, and most have one or more associated medical conditions that increase operative morbidity and mortality.

Colonoscopic Diagnosis

The clinical setting should alert the colonoscopist to the possibility of a vascular abnormality in the cecal region. The diagnosis should be suspected in any patient older than 55 years whose gastrointestinal blood loss has been undiagnosed by other means. Almost all patients will have some obvious disease that is known to be associated with cecal vascular abnormalities such as atherosclerotic heart disease, valvular heart disease, atherosclerotic vascular disease, chronic obstructive pulmonary disease, hypertension, or diabetes mellitus. Many will have more than one of these conditions. Most patients will have gross rectal bleeding that is usually bright red when bleeding is rapid, and maroon when slower. Very slow bleeding from the right colon can result in melena. The lesions are equally divided between men and women.

Physical examination may show pallor as well as findings consistent with any of the associated diseases mentioned. Roentgenographic contrast studies of the entire gastrointestinal tract will be normal or demonstrate abnormalities unrelated to the patient's blood loss. If a vascular abnormality has been shown by angiography prior to colonoscopy, the colonoscopist may expect to encounter the largest lesion in a corresponding area. Even if the angiographic results are negative, total colonoscopy should be performed. Colonoscopy is the most reliable method for exclusion of a vascular abnormality in the cecal area; other disorders such as carcinoma, polyps, and inflammatory bowel disease that may have been overlooked radiographically may also be detected. If colonoscopic findings are negative, the lesion may be in the upper intestinal tract or small bowel, and a further search is warranted.

The largest and most highly developed vascular abnormality is usually located on the antimesenteric aspect of the cecum opposite the ileocecal valve; careful endoscopic inspection is required in this region. The vascular abnormality may be solitary, but more often several smaller lesions are found near the largest. The abnormalities may be scattered throughout the entire large bowel, but are seen less frequently and are less developed proceeding distally from the cecum. If the clinical circumstances are strongly suggestive of a vascular lesion but colonoscopy is negative, then the distal terminal ileum should be inspected because vascular lesions have been found in this region.[1]

Endoscopic recognition of a vascular abnormality is not difficult in the living patient because it is perfused by oxygenated blood that gives it a bright-red color (Plate 44–1). The center of the well-developed lesion is composed of a mass of vascular tissue so dense that individual vessels cannot be discerned. At the margin, individual vessels may be seen that gradually disappear into the mucosa. These vessels radiate from the center and, therefore, frequently give the lesion a stellate appearance. The shape can be irregular, especially when two large lesions are close together with vessels coursing between them. Vascular abnormalities vary in size from pinpoint to more than 2 cm in diameter. The lesion responsible for bleeding usually has a solidly red center and is 3 mm or more in diameter. Most are not bleeding actively when viewed endoscopically. The surface of the lesion is glistening when intact, but a white fleck near the center is occasionally seen and indicates that the surface is eroded (Plate 44–2). The presence of an erosion means that the lesion has probably bled recently. Most lesions will be flat and flush with the surrounding mucosa. Extremely well developed vascular abnormalities will be slightly raised 1 or 2 mm above the surrounding mucosal surface; these are more likely to be eroded. Elevation is difficult to appreciate unless the lesion is viewed tangentially.

Small mucosal vascular abnormalities of the large bowel bleed easily with minor trauma. This marked friability can result in brisk, bright-red bleeding in response to gentle contact. The lesions are easily differentiated from the bluish submucosal varix that yields a soft indentation (cushion sign) when probed. There should also be no difficulty with recognition of the much larger congenital vascular abnormalities of the colon.[2, 3] These usually occur in a much younger age group, and grossly deform the lumen. This deformity produces a characteristic appearance on x-ray studies. Endoscopic therapy is not recommended for congenital lesions.

Histologic Confirmation

Spontaneous ecchymoses, endoscope-induced submucosal hemorrhages, flat adenomas, and small foci of inflammation are indistinguishable endoscopically from vascular abnormalities. Since similar vascular lesions can occur in the small bowel and stomach, histologic confirmation in the colon has important implications, especially if blood loss continues after all colonic lesions have been destroyed or surgically removed. Although biopsies have been obtained from these lesions with ordinary forceps,[4] use of the insulated monopolar electrocoagulating forceps is recommended because this accessory allows simultaneous electrocoagulation and biopsy ("hot-biopsy").[5] When current is applied to this forceps, heat is generated in the surrounding mucosa by virtue of its electrical resistance. Because there is little or no resistance within the forceps, the enclosed tissue escapes coagulation.

If properly obtained, a biopsy will show large, abnormal, dilated, vascular channels in the mucosa coursing between colonic glands (Plate 44–3). The diameter of an intramucosal vessel can be compared with that of an adjacent colonic gland, and if the vessel diameter is the greater, then the vessel is definitely dilated. The vascular channels are typically lined by a thin wall of endothelial cells. Thick-walled vessels are seen less frequently and are thought to be due to arteriovenous shunting. Atheromatous emboli are found infrequently and are recognized by the cholesterol clefts seen in the mucosa and submucosa. Biopsies of small, acquired vascular abnormalities usually do not show inflammation or epithelial cell changes.

Electrocoagulation and Other Endoscopic Treatment Methods

Satisfactory visualization of a vascular abnormality is a prerequisite for proper electrocoagulation (Plate 44–4). Adequate preparation facilitates visualization and also tends to eliminate hydrogen and methane from the colon. Sparking during colonoscopic electrosurgery can ignite these explosive gases with disastrous consequences.[6] I insufflate carbon dioxide throughout colonoscopy, so that if

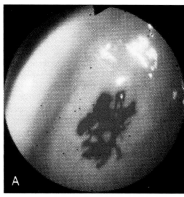 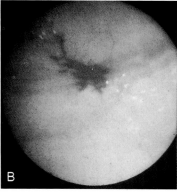 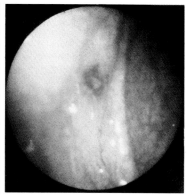

PLATE 44–1.   PLATE 44–2.

PLATE 44–1. *A*, Vascular abnormality is located in the proximal right colon. (Courtesy of Dr. J. Petrini). *B*, Bright red, flat, irregular, 6 x 8 mm vascular abnormality is located on the lateral wall of the cecum in an 82-year-old patient with anemia, stools positive for occult blood, and long-standing hypertension. Diagnosis and successful therapy were achieved simultaneously, utilizing electrocoagulating biopsy forceps.

PLATE 44–2. Vascular abnormality was found in a 65-year-old woman who had recently passed dark red blood per rectum and had a long history of atherosclerotic heart disease. The lesion was about 5 mm in diameter, located just below and somewhat lateral to the ileocecal valve. The white fleck in the center is an erosion that suggested recent bleeding. Diagnosis and successful therapy were achieved simultaneously, utilizing electrocoagulating biopsy forceps.

the preparation is not perfect, electrocoagulation can be performed without fear of an explosion. If air has been insufflated during colonoscopy, it can be exchanged with carbon dioxide just prior to electrocoagulation.

There are many types of electrosurgical generators and endoscopes that may be used safely to electrocoagulate vascular abnormalities, provided that all equipment is in working order. The amount of power needed to treat these lesions is low, usually 25 watts or less. The power output of virtually all commercially available electrosurgical generators used for endoscopic electrosurgery is adequate for this purpose. When the electrocoagulating biopsy forceps is used, it should be extended far enough into the endoscopic viewfield so that the insulated portion can be seen. This prevents a short circuit of current through the endoscope.

The largest vascular abnormality should be dealt with first. It is the most likely source of

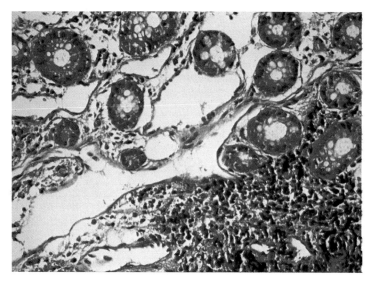

PLATE 44–3. Photomicrograph is of tissue obtained with electrocoagulating biopsy forceps from the lesion seen in Plate 44–2. Note that the colonic mucosa is laced with large, abnormal, thin-walled vascular channels.

the patient's bleeding and any reduction in its vascular tissue should decrease the chance of further bleeding. Frequently the first electrocoagulation biopsy, if taken from the center of the lesion, is the only one that is diagnostic. After biopsy, bleeding from the margin may obscure the field, so that the main lesion can no longer be located with certainty. If the electrocoagulation session is terminated prematurely, treating the largest lesion first results in the greatest benefit. If bleeding does become a problem before the treatment is completed, the entire procedure can be repeated 1 or 2 days later.

When confronted with an unusually large lesion, a circumferential electrocoagulation pattern working inward from the periphery of the lesion without biopsy is reasonable. With this circumferential approach the center of the lesion is treated last. The size of the lesion can be estimated by comparing it to the width of the open forceps.

When the electrocoagulation-biopsy technique is used, a small portion of the lesion is grasped with the forceps and pulled into the lumen to produce a tent of mucosa with the lesion at the apex (Plate 44–5). If too small an amount of tissue is grasped, it will be torn away and initiate bleeding. Too large a bite results in ineffective electrocoagulation and increases the possibility of post-treatment hemorrhage and perforation. The ideal amount of tissue to grasp is that which half fills the mouth of the forceps.

After the lesion has been grasped and elevated, approximately 10 watts of current are applied for 2 seconds or less. This amount of power usually corresponds to the lowest setting on endoscopic electrosurgical units. If conditions are ideal the vascular tissue held by the forceps at the apex of the "tent" turns white (Plate 44–6). When tissue whitening is observed the biopsy is obtained by quickly pulling the forceps into the endoscope.

If the conditions are not ideal, or if the patient is large or obese, more current will be required. Power should be increased to 15 watts and then to 25 watts if necessary. Current should not be applied for more than 2 seconds. The longer the application and the higher the power setting the greater the chance of a transmural burn or perforation. The cecum, it will be recalled, has the thinnest wall in comparison with other segments of the large bowel. The endoscopic field should be kept as clean as possible because monopolar electrosurgical therapy is less effective when the site is flooded with blood, feces, or residual enema fluid. After the biopsy specimen has been taken, residual vascular tissue is grasped, elevated, and coagulated in the same fashion. If the first biopsy is thought to be adequate for diagnosis, additional biopsies are not necessary.

Many endoscopists are cautious when considering treatment of small vascular abnormalities of the gastrointestinal tract because of potential hemorrhage. I have previously described the use of the electrocoagulation-biopsy technique for vascular abnormalities,[7, 8] and have applied it in more than 60 cases, without perforation or significant bleeding. Others have also reported success with this technique.[9, 10]

Although I prefer the electrocoagulating biopsy forceps, the dome-tip electrode can be used. The advantage of the dome-tip is that it can be effectively applied tangentially to mucosal lesions. One disadvantage is the tendency after application of current for coagulated tissue to break away with the electrode as it is withdrawn from the mucosal surface. This can be circumvented somewhat by keeping the electrode clean and by applying a "non-stick" cooking oil such as Pam (Boyle-Midway Inc., New York, NY) or some other oily substance to the electrode between electrocoagulations.

A second disadvantage of the dome-tip electrode is the tendency for the bowel wall to thin-out where this probe is applied. This makes a transmural burn and perforation more likely. In contrast, the electrocoagulation-biopsy forceps technique pulls the mucosal lesion away from the muscularis propria and decreases the chance of a transmural burn. When using the dome-tip electrode, applications of current should be given as the probe is applied with light pressure to the wall. Consequently, there will be less tissue destruction. More than one course of therapy may be necessary to eradicate the lesions, using a dome-tip device.

Another disadvantage of the dome-tip electrode is the lack of tissue for microscopic examination.

A variety of relatively new electrosurgical devices have been introduced for endoscopic electrosurgery. For example, the sticking of a coagulum to the electrode after electrocoagulation appears to be less of a problem with the hydroelectrocoagulator.[11] Treatment of small vascular abnormalities using bipolar or

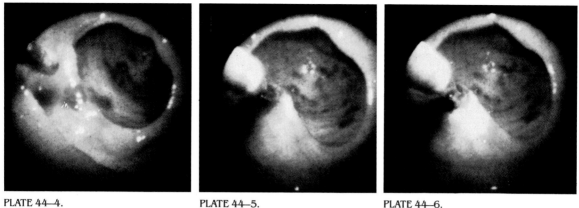

PLATE 44–4.   PLATE 44–5.   PLATE 44–6.

PLATE 44–4. Vascular abnormality found opposite ileocecal valve in a 70-year-old man with aortic stenosis and intermittent rectal bleeding. Electrocoagulating biopsy forceps has been passed through accessory channel of colonoscope and protrudes toward lesion.

PLATE 44–5. Lesion has been grasped with electrocoagulating biopsy forceps and elevated from bowel wall to produce "tent" of mucosa. Insulation of forceps is clearly in view.

PLATE 44–6. Apex of "tent" of mucosa including vascular abnormality turned white after electrocoagulation with 10 watts for 2 seconds. This was the only treatment necessary for this patient's single lesion. The mucosa remains pink and undamaged at the base of "tent".

multipolar probes or a thermal probe is also accepted. The Bicap (American Cystoscope Makers, Stamford, CT) appears to stick to coagulated tissue to a lesser degree. Another advantage is that the tissue damage is superficial and this makes the occurrence of a transmural burn and perforation unlikely. A disadvantage of the Bicap is that tissue is not obtained for microscopic confirmation. The Heat Probe (Olympus Corp.) has also been introduced recently. The problem of sticking to coagulated tissue is also reduced with this device, but there are few reports of its use at present. Endoscopic electrosurgery methods for control of gastrointestinal bleeding are also discussed in Chapter 8.

Theoretically, laser photocoagulation is ideally suited for treatment of small vascular abnormalities of the gastrointestinal tract. The most important advantage of laser therapy is the ability to treat a lesion without touching it. This usually results in bloodless destruction of the lesion, which is particularly helpful when there are multiple lesions as in

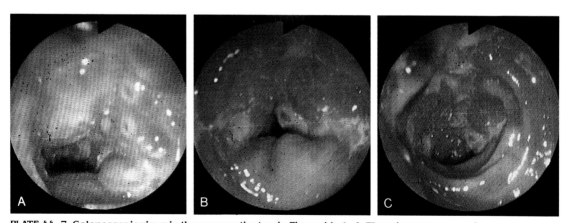

PLATE 44–7. Colonoscopic views in the same patient as in Figure 44–1. A, There is severe narrowing of lumen in the proximal descending colon due to submucosal hemorrhage. B, Narrowing is due to submucosal hemorrhage in the mid descending colon. C, Areas of submucosal hemorrhage appear as discrete "blebs" in the distal descending colon. There is early ulcer formation; therefore the findings might be classified as between an "acute" and "subacute" stage. The patient recovered with supportive measures alone. (Courtesy M.V. Sivak, Jr., M.D.)

hereditary hemorrhagic telangiectasia. Laser therapy has some disadvantages also. For example, no specimen is obtained for histologic confirmation. This can be overcome by obtaining a biopsy prior to treatment, but this adds an additional step and bleeding may obscure the location of the lesion. Other obvious disadvantages of laser include its expense, large size, and lack of portability; the need for special plumbing; and the possibility of ophthalmologic injury to the endoscopist.

The argon laser appears to be the most appropriate and safest laser for treating vascular abnormalities. Argon laser light is absorbed almost completely by hemoglobin and has a depth of penetration of only 1 mm. Treatment should be with low power and a short exposure time. When laser energy is applied, the lesion will blanch and shrink. When exposure time is excessively long, bleeding may result. Large lesions are best treated in several sessions, as the energy required to destroy them at one session may be enough to severely damage the external muscle layer and risk perforation. An interval of 1 to 2 weeks between treatments allows partial healing and reduces this risk. Assessing the extent of the area to treat during each session is difficult, but the final endoscopic appearance should be replacement of the entire vascular abnormality by scar and normal mucosa.[12] Satisfactory results with laser therapy have been reported by at least three groups.[12-14]

The Nd:YAG (neodymium:yttrium aluminum garnet) laser has also been used to treat vascular abnormalities of the gastrointestinal tract.[12] However, this laser is much more powerful than the argon laser. Its depth of penetration is 4 mm, enough to cause transmural coagulation in a distended cecum, which could easily result in perforation.

Surgery

Rational surgical therapy is dependent upon a preoperative demonstration of the vascular abnormality by angiography or colonoscopy. Right colectomy for lower gastrointestinal bleeding of undetermined cause is no longer recommended.[15] Unfortunately, what appears to be a vascular abnormality on angiography may be something quite different or even unrelated to the bleeding.[16, 17] Colonoscopy should be performed prior to exploration in any patient in whom bleeding

from a vascular lesion is suspected, since this may show unexpected lesions such as a carcinoma or inflammatory bowel disease and thereby alter the therapeutic approach. The major disadvantage of surgery is its associated morbidity and mortality in elderly patients with cardiac, vascular, and/or pulmonary diseases. The reported surgical mortality is as high as 7%.[18] At exploration the lesion will rarely be identified, and its demonstration in the excised specimen is extremely difficult unless laborious injection techniques are used. Bleeding recurs after surgery in at least 10% of patients.[16, 19] New or overlooked lesions in another part of the gastrointestinal tract should be suspected in this circumstance, and repeated upper and lower endoscopy and angiography should be helpful in localizing the bleeding site.

Hereditary Hemorrhagic Telangiectasia (Rendu-Osler-Weber Disease)

Patients with hereditary hemorrhagic telangiectasia (HHT) are easily recognized because of the several features of the disease, including recurrent epistaxis beginning early in life, a positive family history, and the presence of small telangiectases on the mucous membranes of the nose and mouth. Those with gastrointestinal bleeding often have numerous small lesions in the upper gastrointestinal tract. In addition, some patients have typical vascular abnormalities in the cecal region.[8, 20] The endoscopic and microscopic appearance of the small vascular abnormality that occurs in the right colon of elderly patients is indistinguishable from that of the telangiectasia of HHT.[21] Endoscopic treatment of all gastrointestinal telangiectases within the range of upper gastrointestinal endoscopy and colonoscopy is recommended. The technique is precisely the same as outlined above.

Kaposi's Sarcoma

Kaposi's sarcoma is a systemic neoplastic disease of pluripotential vascular endothelial cells. Violaceous skin lesions usually appear first and dominate the clinical picture. In the past it has been found in the United States in men in the fifth through seventh decades and had a 10% incidence of visceral involvement. However, there is a recent increase in reports of Kaposi's sarcoma in homosexual men with the acquired immune deficiency syndrome (AIDS). This group has been found by endoscopy to have a 48% incidence of visceral involvement.[22] When the disease is limited to the skin, the prognosis is good with life expectancy between 10 and 25 years, but when visceral involvement is proved, the prognosis is poor with life expectancy of only 1 to 2 years.[23]

The manifestation of Kaposi's sarcoma in the large bowel is primarily left-sided; most lesions are within the reach of the flexible sigmoidoscope.[22] They are usually multiple and vary between 5 and 10 mm in size. The tumors in an early stage are smooth, sessile, and bright red. They are primarily submucosal, so that biopsies will show only normal mucosa. More advanced lesions have a reticulated white surface and the largest lesions have central umbilications. Gastrointestinal involvement can be present without skin involvement.[24] Kaposi's sarcoma of the large bowel can mimic ulcerative colitis.[25] Kaposi's sarcoma is also discussed in Chapters 42 and 46.

Turner's Syndrome

About 10% of patients with Turner's syndrome (gonadal dysgenesis) have intestinal vascular abnormalities that can cause significant gastrointestinal bleeding.[26] The small vascular abnormalities in these patients appear to be amenable to endoscopic coagulation, whereas the large "bag of worms" malformation is treated surgically.[27, 28]

Blue Rubber-Bleb Nevus Syndrome

Bean[29] separated the blue rubber-bleb nevus syndrome from other cutaneous vascular lesions and gave the syndrome its name. These vascular lesions can involve all parts of the gastrointestinal tract and may result in significant bleeding. Treatment has been primarily surgical. Preoperative colonoscopy has been helpful in locating lesions in the large bowel that were later excised.[30]

Hemangiopericytoma

Hemangiopericytoma is a rare tumor arising from pericytes. These are primitive mesenchymal cells closely associated with capillary endothelial cells. This neoplastic lesion can involve the large bowel.[31] Bleeding after endoscopic biopsy should not be significant because the tumor contains only tiny vascular spaces. Microscopic examination of the biopsy will show sheets of spindle-shaped cells separated by endothelium-lined vascular spaces. Since malignancy occurs in a high percentage of cases the tumor should be removed surgically.

ISCHEMIC COLITIS

Ischemic colitis is divided into three categories: (1) gangrene due to transmural infarction, (2) ischemic stricture that results from near transmural infarction and bacterial invasion, and (3) transient ischemic colitis resulting from a localized ischemic insult that is completely reversible.[32, 33]

Clinical Presentation

The patient with symptoms of transient ischemic colitis is usually over age 50. Most elderly patients will have associated disease including cardiovascular disease, respiratory failure, diabetes mellitus, and chronic renal failure.[34, 35] In the elderly there seems to be an equal distribution between men and women. In younger women patients there may be a history of oral contraceptive use.[36–38] In many young patients there is no associated disease.[39, 40] Although rare, inferior mesenteric vein thrombosis can result in transient ischemic colitis.[41] It can occur long after abdominoperineal resection, after resection of abdominal aortic aneurysms, and after renal transplantation.[42–44] Transient ischemic colitis has been reported after intravenous vasopressin therapy and during sickle cell crisis.[45, 46] Ischemic colitis has also been reported with carcinoma of the colon, ergot ingestion, amyloidosis, vasculitis, polyarteritis nodosa, systemic lupus erythematosus, and rheumatoid arthritis.[47–54]

Transient ischemic colitis usually has an abrupt onset. Typically the first symptom is periumbilical pain. Ischemic bowel seems to react with hyperperistalsis that results in emptying of the colon. The patient then continues to make frequent trips to the toilet but passes only small amounts of blood and mucus. On physical examination the abdomen is usually nontender. If tenderness and rebound are present they indicate transmural ischemia that could progress to infarction. Bowel sounds are active shortly after the onset of pain and decrease as the disease progresses. Despite rectal bleeding the hemoglobin and hematocrit are usually slightly elevated; this probably reflects hemoconcentration. Leukocytosis is usually present, and fever is mild or absent.

Early Management

Transient ischemic colitis must be differentiated from acute diverticulitis, bacterial colitis, parasitic infestation, and inflammatory bowel disease (see also Chapter 42). In ischemic colitis the feces will contain leukocytes and occult blood, but cultures for pathogenic organisms and examinations for ova and parasites will be negative. Intravenous fluid infusion should be started promptly and antibiotics administered as soon as a stool specimen is obtained for culture. Endoscopic examination of the entire colon with biopsy is helpful in differentiating ischemic colitis from Crohn's disease, ulcerative colitis, and diverticulitis. Barium contrast radiography of the colon can suggest transient ischemic colitis in the proper clinical setting, but in mild cases the study will be normal or indicate spasm in the affected area. Mesenteric angiography has not been helpful in most cases, apparently because it is not sensitive enough to show small vessels where the ischemia originates. At the outset there is no way to predict whether the disease will be transient or whether it will progress to infarction with perforation. If clinical signs of peritoneal irritation and inflammation improve with bed rest, intravenous fluids, and antibiotics, then further conservative therapy is indicated. If there is increasing evidence of peritoneal irritation and bowel sounds diminish, then angiography and surgery should be considered.

Colonoscopy

Colonoscopy in patients with transient ischemic colitis is not difficult. Preparation is easy because the initial hyperperistalsis has already emptied the colon; tap water enemas alone are satisfactory. The rectum is almost always spared because of its profuse blood supply. The involved segment is clearly demarcated from adjacent normal mucosa, and when the colonoscope reaches this point the advisability of farther advancement of the instrument must be decided. A considerable degree of spasm is often present, and this usually means that the bowel wall is still viable. Intravenous glucagon is sometimes helpful in relaxing this associated spasm. Friability of the mucosa indicates that there is superficial necrosis and that advancement through the area should not be hazardous. Patient discomfort should be monitored carefully. If attempted advancement of the colonoscope through the affected area results in significant pain, it is wise to obtain representative biopsies and make a careful retreat. If black or green bowel is encountered, then transmural infarction is likely. Under these circumstances the colonoscope should be withdrawn and surgical consultation obtained.

Ischemic colitis has been divided into three endoscopic stages: acute, subacute, and chronic.[35]

Acute changes occur in the first 24 hours and include patchy areas of hyperemia alternating with areas of blanching. The hyperemic areas tend to ooze blood after contact with the colonoscope, whereas bleeding is minimal on biopsy of blanched areas. During the next 48 hours erythema becomes more generalized and involves larger areas of mucosa, and superficial 2 to 4 mm ulcerations often appear. Submucosal bleeding is manifested by petechiae or less commonly by bluish submucosal hemorrhage that correlates with the "thumb-printing" seen on barium enema x-rays (Fig. 44–1). Biopsies taken in the acute stage most often show nonspecific changes, but in some there are changes that support the diagnosis of ischemic bowel disease, including congestion of the microcirculation, mucosal edema, thrombosed submucosal capillaries, disruption of the surface epithelium, ghost crypts, and the early changes of focal areas of coagulative necrosis.

In the subacute stage the ulcerative process involves more of the mucosal surface (Plate 44–7). The ulcerated areas tend to elongate into well-defined longitudinal or serpentine ulcers, 1 to 2 cm wide and 3 to 4 cm long, that are reminiscent of Crohn's disease. Some patients may have a more diffuse exudative process. After 7 days there is usually no further progression of the ulcerative changes. Radiographic correlates during the subacute stage include ulcerations, nonspecific mucosal irregularity, and loss of haustrations. Histologic findings during the subacute stage show an exudative process of variable degree superimposed on underlying necrosis. Crypt abscesses, cryptitis, and destruction of normal glandular architecture are also seen.

In the chronic stage the disease may progress to stricture formation. Healing may occur as early as 2 weeks or as late as 3 months. With healing, normal mucosa may reappear or there may be residual fine granularity. The submucosal vascular pattern may be altered. Radiographic correlates include stricture, stenosis, and loss of haustrations of the involved segment. Biopsy specimens show mucosal atrophy, focal loss of mucosal thickness, and replacement of the normal submucosa by granulation tissue.

Late Management

After the diagnosis of ischemic colitis has been confirmed, conservative management is indicated as long as the patient's condition is stable or improving. Antibiotics are thought to play a role in the prevention of late stricture formation and should be continued until the mucosa has healed. Therefore follow-up colonoscopy is indicated at about 4 weeks after onset. Most patients who have had one episode of transient ischemic colitis do not

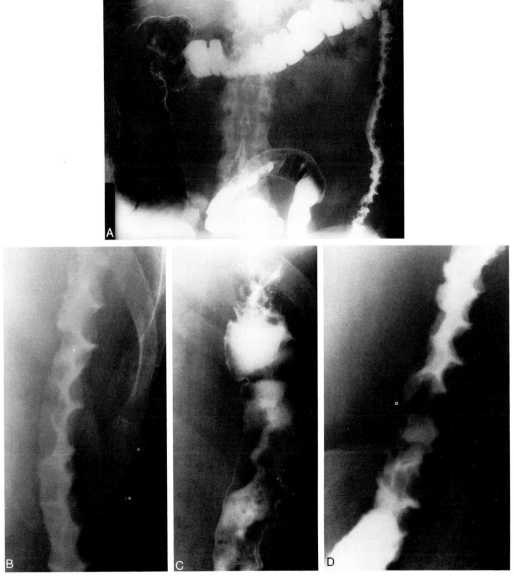

FIGURE 44–1. *A*, Barium enema x-ray shows "thumb printing" in a 70-year-old diabetic man with a brief history of hematochezia; *B*, proximal descending colon; *C*, mid descending colon; *D*, distal descending colon and proximal sigmoid. (Courtesty of M. V. Sivak, Jr., M.D.)

have subsequent episodes, but if the disease does recur, angiography is indicated. In those patients whose condition deteriorates and in whom signs of peritoneal inflammation worsen, colonoscopy has been used to monitor progressive ischemia to the point of infarction; these endoscopic findings have been used in planning surgery.[55]

RADIATION PROCTOCOLITIS

Radiation injury to the large bowel is almost always the result of therapy for a malignancy in an adjacent organ. Ionizing radiation results in acute (early) and chronic (delayed) forms of injury. These two reactions are distinctly different. The acute reaction is due primarily to injury of the crypt cells of the colonic glands and is transient. The chronic reaction is induced by a progressive endarteritis obliterans that can result in long-term morbidity and eventual death.

Acute (Early) Radiation Proctocolitis

Symptoms of acute radiation proctocolitis usually begin in the middle of the second week of therapy and include diarrhea, mucoid discharge, tenesmus, abdominal distention, and lower abdominal cramps. Proctosigmoidoscopy will usually show homogeneous involvement of the mucosa with duskiness and loss of vascularity. Friability and ulcers are usually not seen in the early stage.

Biopsy specimens frequently show crypt abscesses composed almost entirely of eosinophils along with focal tissue eosinophilia.[56] Surface-cells become less columnar and more cuboidal in shape. Nuclei lose their basal polarity and tend to become larger. Mitoses in the crypt epithelium diminish but do not disappear. Mucus production is reduced and polymorphonuclear neutrophils are scarce.

Acute radiation-induced proctocolitis is self-limited. Symptoms usually respond to a low-roughage diet, psyllium hydrophilic mucilloid, antidiarrheal agents, and perianal soaks (Sitz baths).

Chronic (Delayed) Radiation Proctocolitis

The latent period between treatment and the appearance of the delayed radiation reaction is usually 6 to 24 months but may be greater than 30 years. The incidence after radiation treatment ranges from 2% to 24%.[57, 58] The majority of patients have radiation proctocolitis due to treatment of a gynecologic malignancy. A small percentage of patients will have been treated for lymphoma or other malignancies such as carcinoma of the prostate, testis, bladder, kidney, or adrenal gland. In addition to radiation proctocolitis, other delayed reactions include ulceration, perforation, stricture, fistula, and rarely neoplasm.

Delayed radiation proctocolitis is caused by primary injury to the blood vessels that results in endarteritis, thrombosis, and subsequent infarction.[59] Localized ischemia produces ulceration of the mucosa, leaving single or multiple irregular, superficial erosions that may progress to deep, punched-out, discrete ulcers characterized by a ragged, grayish base and sharp margins. The surrounding mucosa becomes thickened and indurated with numerous telangiectases. An ulcer may perforate into the peritoneal cavity resulting in generalized peritonitis, or it may extend with fistula formation to the vagina or bladder. As ulcers heal, strictures may form that lead to obstruction. If most of the pelvic organs are involved, they become matted together and produce a "frozen pelvis" that severely restricts fiberoptic endoscopy.

Rectal bleeding may be the only symptom of chronic radiation proctocolitis. However, tenesmus and frequent stools are usually associated with bleeding. Crampy abdominal pain usually indicates disease proximal to the rectum.[60]

Endoscopic examination will reveal a narrowed lumen, loss of rectal valves, and very friable mucosa. Biopsy may show edema, fibrosis, atrophy, increased chronic inflammatory cells and telangiectases. The base of the crypts may be separated from the muscularis mucosa below by inflammatory cells and irregular collections of pale-staining macrophages.[61] The findings of thrombosis or vasculitis with the typical intimal foam cells in endoscopic biopsies strongly support the diagnosis of radiation proctocolitis, but these are rare findings because of the superficial nature of most endoscopic biopsies.

A rectal ulcer can produce persistent anorectal pain. If present, the ulcer is almost always located on the anterior wall about 8 cm from the anal sphincter in the vicinity of the posterior vaginal fornix.[62] The ulcer is flat with well-demarcated margins from which superficial endoscopic biopsies should be taken with a standard 2 mm flexible for-

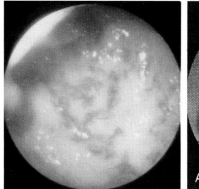
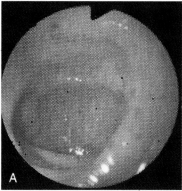
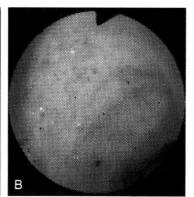

PLATE 44—8.   PLATE 44—9.

PLATE 44—8. Endoscopic view of chronic (delayed) radiation-induced proctocolitis shows patches of white mucosa due to scarring and fibrosis from ischemia.

PLATE 44—9. Chronic (delayed) radiation-induced proctocolitis. A, Pale mucosa in which normal submucosal vascular structures are replaced by petechial-size hemorrhages and abnormal vessels; B, areas of small spontaneous mucoasl hemorrahages. (Courtesy of M.V. Sivak, Jr., M.D.)

ceps. Biopsy should not be performed with a large rigid forceps because rectovaginal fistula may become manifest immediately afterward.[63] Ordinarily the ulcer will heal with conservative measures.

A stricture is sometimes associated with an ulcer and it may limit the extent of endoscopic examination. An attempt should be made to pass the endoscope through the stricture to obtain biopsy specimens at the upper margin, the middle portion, and lower margin. Collection of specimens for cytologic examination is also useful. If the stricture cannot be negotiated, then biopsy specimens should be taken from the lower margin and cytologic specimens taken from the narrowed area by brushing.

Colonoscopy

Colonoscopy in patients with radiation proctocolitis is frequently limited by patho-logic alterations.[64] If the patient has had a hysterectomy the sigmoid colon may adhere to the operative site and be injured during subsequent radiation therapy.[62] This results in a narrowed and sharply angulated mid-portion of the sigmoid that is difficult, if not impossible, to negotiate. Even if the colonoscope is passed through the diseased area, care should be exercised in moving the narrowed area during sigmoid straightening. When the endoscopist encounters such difficulties his enthusiasm for farther advancement of the instrument should be tempered by the realization that radiation-injured bowel is brittle, easy to perforate, and probably tethered to other organs by adhesions. Perforation in such patients carries a high mortality rate because surgery is difficult in an area that has been exposed to ionizing radiation.

All strictures encountered should be suspect, because carcinoma of the large bowel is

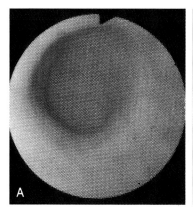
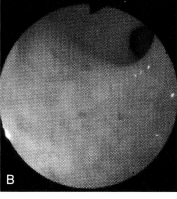

PLATE 44—10. Chronic (delayed) radiation-induced proctocolitis. A, Pale featureless mucosa with loss of interhaustral septae. B, abnormal telangiectatic vascular pattern with several small spontaneous mucoasl hemorrahages.

a known long-term complication of radiation therapy.[65, 66] A biopsy should be obtained of the stricture, and the stricture brushed to obtain a specimen for cytologic study.

If the patient has rectal bleeding, mucosa that is bleeding spontaneously or is markedly friable may be encountered. When the blood is washed away, patches of erythema will be seen against a background of pale white mucosa (Plate 44–8). The red patches usually represent ecchymoses, distorted mucosal vessels or telangiectases. The pale white areas are caused by scarring and fibrosis due to ischemia. When taking biopsies the mucosa itself will be found to be pliable, but the underlying bowel wall will be firm, rigid, and fairly fixed. The lumen is usually narrowed. Telangiectases are sometimes visible (Plates 44–9' and 44–10). Biopsies from the pale areas usually show drop-out of crypts. Hyalinization of the submucosa with numerous bizarre fibroblasts and abnormal collagen have also been found.[67]

Differential Diagnosis

A history of radiation therapy is essential to the diagnosis of radiation proctocolitis. If the typical colonoscopic findings mentioned above are present in the field of radiation and if malignancy has been excluded, the diagnosis is firmly established. Chronic ischemic colitis and chronic radiation proctocolitis have similar endoscopic appearances because their underlying pathophysiologic mechanisms are the same.

Most often the patient with radiation proctocolitis is referred for colonoscopy to exclude malignancy. Recurrent malignancy in the area of radiation therapy is difficult to recognize. A nodular mucosa suggests malignancy, but the diagnosis is confirmed only by a positive biopsy or cytology specimen. The differential diagnosis includes other diseases that present with hematochezia including polyps, diverticular disease, inflammatory bowel disease, and vascular abnormalities of the cecal area. Radiation injury to the large bowel is frequently associated with injury to the small bowel and this may explain some of the patient's symptoms. The urinary bladder, the ureters, and bone can also be injured by radiation therapy.

Endoscopic differentiation of Crohn's disease from radiation proctocolitis is usually not difficult. In Crohn's disease there are aphthoid ulcers with relatively normal intervening mucosa. In radiation proctocolitis the intervening mucosa is friable and may be pale as a result of ischemia or atrophy. In Crohn's disease there are linear ulcers and cobblestoning, but friability is minimal. It may be impossible to differentiate between radiation-related and Crohn's strictures, except that other aspects of the endoscopic findings may suggest a correct diagnosis.

Endoscopically, the changes of moderately severe ulcerative colitis and delayed chronic radiation proctocolitis are similar. In ulcerative colitis the mucosal exudate contains pus and mucus in addition to blood, whereas the exudate in radiation proctocolitis is almost entirely blood. Biopsies will show pyogenic crypt abscesses and mucus depletion, microscopic findings that are unusual in delayed radiation proctocolitis.

The endoscopic appearance in an excluded loop of colon can be similar to that of radiation colitis; both have loss of interhaustral septa, narrowing of the lumen and friable mucosa. Spontaneous bleeding in exclusion colitis is unusual but it is found frequently in radiation proctocolitis. The endoscopic findings of localized atrophy with pale mucosa and biopsy findings of crypt drop-out suggestive of radiation proctocolitis will not be present in exclusion colitis.

Treatment

Medical therapy for chronic radiation proctocolitis is directed at symptoms only. A low-roughage diet in conjunction with psyllium hydrophilic mucilloid may decrease rectal bleeding. Sulfasalazine and steroid enemas have been prescribed, but in most cases they appear to be of no benefit. A diverting colostomy may not stop rectal bleeding, but it may allow a fistula to heal. Direct surgical intervention should be discouraged because numerous adhesions make dissection extremely difficult and ischemic changes interfere with postoperative healing. Surgical excision is usually justified when dealing with biopsy-proved malignancy or when malignancy is strongly suspected on the basis of radiographic findings.

Editor's note: References 68, 69, and 70 are some recently published articles of interest in relation to topics covered in this chapter.

References

1. Whitehouse GH. Solitary angiodysplastic lesions in the ileocecal region diagnosed by angiography. Gut 1973; 14:977–82.

2. Blackstone MO, Rogers BHG, Baker AL. A cutaneous and pelvic lymphangioma with varices, lymphangiomas and capillary hemangiomas of the rectosigmoid colon. Gastrointest Endosc 1976; 23:39–41.
3. Lieberman DA, Krippaehne WW, Melnyk CS. Colonic varices due to intestinal hemangiomas. Dig Dis Sci 1983; 28:852–8.
4. Bartelheimer W, Remmele W, Ottenjann R. Coloscopic recognition of hemangiomas in the colon ascendens. Case report of so-called cryptogenic gastrointestinal bleeding. Endoscopy 1972; 4:109–14.
5. Williams CB: Diathermy-biopsy: a technique for endoscopic management of small polyps. Endoscopy 1973; 5:215.
6. Bigard M, Gaucher P, Lassalle C. Fatal colonic explosion during colonoscopic polypectomy. Gastroenterology 1979; 77:1307–10.
7. Rogers BHG, Adler F. Hemangiomas of the cecum: colonoscopic diagnosis and therapy. Gastroenterology 1976; 71:1079–82.
8. Rogers BHG. Endoscopic diagnosis and therapy of mucosal vascular abnormalities of the gastrointestinal tract occurring in elderly patients and associated with cardiac, vascular and pulmonary disease. Gastrointest Endosc 1980; 26:134–8.
9. Nuesch HJ, Kobler E, Buhler H, et al. Angiodysplasien des Kolons—Diagnose und Therapie. Schweiz med Wochenschr 1979; 109:607–8.
10. Howard OM, Buchanan JD, Hunt RH. Angiodysplasia of the colon: experience of 26 cases. Lancet 1982; 2:16–9.
11. Matek W, Fruhmorgen P, Kaduk B, et al. Modified electrocoagulation and its possibilities in the control of gastrointestinal bleeding. Endoscopy 1979; 11:253–8.
12. Brown SG. Endoscopic argon and Nd:YAG therapy of angiomata. (Postgraduate course). Endoscopic Laser Therapy, Cook County Hospital, Chicago, Oct. 20, 1982.
13. Waitman AM, Grant DZ, Chateau F. Argon laser photocoagulation treatment of patients with acute and chronic bleeding secondary to telangiectasia. (Abstr) Gastrointest Endosc 1982; 28:153.
14. Jensen DM, Machicado GA, Tapia JI. Endoscopic treatment of haemangiomata with argon laser in patients with gastrointestinal bleeding. Proceedings of Laser Tokyo '81, p 20.
15. Gianfrancisco JA, Abcarian H. Pitfalls in the treatment of massive lower gastrointestinal bleeding with "blind" subtotal colectomy. Dis Colon Rectum 1982; 25:441–5.
16. Baum S, Athanasoulis CA, Waltman AC, et al. Angiodysplasia of the right colon: A cause of gastrointestinal bleeding. AJR 1977; 129:789–94.
17. Tarin D, Allison DJ, Modlin IM, et al. Diagnosis and management of obscure gastrointestinal bleeding. Br Med J 1978; 2:751–4.
18. Boley SJ, Sammartano R, Brandt LJ, et al. Vascular ectasias of the colon. Surg Gynecol Obstet 1979; 149:353–9.
19. Richardson JD, Max MH, Flint LM, Jr, et al. Bleeding vascular malformations of the intestine. Surgery 1978; 84:430–6.
20. Halpern M, Turner AF, Citron BP. Hereditary hemorrhagic telangiectasia, an angiographic study of abdominal visceral angiodysplasias associated with gastrointestinal hemorrhage. Radiology 1968; 90:1143–9.
21. Wolff WI, Grossman MB, Shinya H. Angiodysplasia

of the colon: diagnosis and treatment. Gastroenterology 1977; 72:329–33.
22. Derezin M, Lewin KJ, Groopman J, et al. Gastrointestinal involvement with Kaposi's sarcoma in epidemic acquired immune deficiency syndrome (AIDS). (Abstr) Gastrointest Endosc 1983; 29:178–9.
23. Port JH, Traube J, Winans CS. The visceral manifestations of Kaposi's sarcoma. Gastrointest Endosc 1982; 28:179–81.
24. Hanno R, Owen LG, Callen JP. Kaposi's sarcoma with extensive silent internal involvement. Int J Dermatol 1979; 18:718–21.
25. Roth JA, Schell S, Panzarino S, et al. Visceral Kaposi's sarcoma presenting as colitis. Am J Surg Pathol 1978; 2:209–14.
26. Rosen KM, Sirota DK, Marinoff SC. Gastrointestinal bleeding in Turner's syndrome. Ann Intern Med 1967; 67:145–50.
27. Rutlin E, Wisloff F, Myren J, et al. Intestinal telangiectasia in Turner's syndrome. Endoscopy 1981; 13:86–7.
28. Schultz LS, Assimacopoulous CA, Lillehei RC. Turner's syndrome with associated gastrointestinal hemorrhage: A case report. Surgery 1970: 68:485–8.
29. Bean WB. Blue rubber bleb nevi of the skin and gastrointestinal tract. In: Bean WB, ed. Vascular Spiders and Related Lesions of the Skin. Springfield: Charles C Thomas, 1958:178–85.
30. Wong SH, Lau WY. Blue rubber-bleb nevus syndrome. Dis Colon Rectum 1982; 25:371–4.
31. Genter B, Mir R, Strauss R, et al. Hemangiopericytoma of the colon: Report of a case and review of literature. Dis Colon Rectum 1982; 25:149–56.
32. Boley SJ, Schwartz S, Lash J, et al. Reversible vascular occlusion of the colon. Surg Gynecol Obstet 1963; 116:53–60.
33. Marston A, Pheils MT, Thomas ML, et al. Ischaemic colitis. Gut 1966; 7:1–15.
34. Abel ME, Russell TR. Ischemic colitis: Comparison of surgical and nonoperative management. Dis Colon Rectum 1983; 26:113–5.
35. Scowcroft CW, Sanowski RA, Kozarek RA. Colonoscopy in ischemic colitis. Gastrointest Endosc 1981; 27:156–61.
36. Heron HC, Khubchandani IT, Trimpi HD, et al. Evanescent colitis. Dis Colon Rectum 1981; 24:555–61.
37. Barcewicz PA, Welch JP. Ischemic colitis in young adult patients. Dis Colon Rectum 1980; 23:109–14.
38. Ghahremani GG, Meyers MA, Farman J, et al. Ischemic disease of the small bowel and colon associated with oral contraceptives. Gastrointest Radiol 1977; 2:221–8.
39. Lewis MI. Reversible ischemic colitis. Dis Colon Rectum 1973; 16:121–6.
40. Clark AW, Lloyd-Mostyn RH, Sadler MRC: "Ischaemic" colitis in young adults. Br Med J 1972; 4:70–2.
41. Archibald RB, Burnstein AV, Knackstedt VE, et al. Ischemic colitis in a young adult due to inferior mesenteric vein thrombosis. Endoscopy 1980; 12:140–3.
42. Wittenberg J, Athanasoulis CA, Williams LF, Jr, et al. Ischemic colitis: Radiology and pathophysiology. Am J Roentgenol 1975; 123:287–300.
43. Launer DP, Miscall BG, Beil AR, Jr. Colorectal infarction following resection of abdominal aortic aneurysms. Dis Colon Rectum 1978; 21:613–7.

44. Arvantitakis C, Malek G, Uehling D, et al. Colonic complications after renal transplantation. Gastroenterology 1973; 64:533–8.

45. Lambert M, de Peyer R, Muller AF. Reversible ischemic colitis after intravenous vasopressin therapy. JAMA 1982; 247:666–7.

46. Gage TP, Gagnier JM. Ischemic colitis complicating sickle cell crises. Gastroenterology 1983; 84:171–4.

47. Whitehouse GH, Watt J. Ischemic colitis associated with carcinoma of the colon. Gastrointest Radiol 1977; 2:31–5.

48. Stillman AE, Weinberg M, Mast WC, et al. Ischemic bowel disease attributable to ergot. Gastroenterology 1977; 72:1336–7.

49. Perarnau JM, Raabe JJ, Courrier A, et al. A rare etiology of ischemic colitis-amyloid colitis. Endoscopy 1982; 14:107–9.

50. Korn JE, Weaver GA. Vasculitis of the colon diagnosed by colonoscopy. Gastrointest Endosc 1979; 25:156–8.

51. Matsuura H, Murai M, Hashimoto T, et al. C2 deficiency vasculitis: Complication of enterocolitis, cutaneous ulcers, and neuropsychiatric disorder. Am J Gastroenterol 1983; 78:1–5.

52. Wood MK, Read DR, Kraft AR, et al. A rare cause of ischemic colitis: Polyarteritis nodosa. Dis Colon Rectum 1979; 22:428–33.

53. Kistin MG, Kaplan MM, Harrington JT. Diffuse ischemic colitis associated with systemic lupus erythematosus—response to subtotal colectomy. Gastroenterology 1978; 75:1147–51.

54. Burt RW, Berenson MM, Samuelson CO, et al. Rheumatoid vasculitis of the colon presenting as pancolitis. Dig Dis Sci 1983; 28:183–8.

55. Hagihara PF, Parker JC, Griffen WO, Jr. Spontaneous ischemic colitis. Dis Colon Rectum 1977; 20:236–51.

56. Gelfand MD, Tepper M, Katz LA, et al. Acute irradiation proctitis in man: development of eosinophilic crypt abscesses. Gastroenterology 1968; 54:401–11.

57. Requarth W, Roberts S. Intestinal injuries following irradiation of pelvic viscera for malignancy. Arch Surg 1956; 73:682–8.

58. Aune EF, White BV. Gastrointestinal complications of irradiation for carcinoma of uterine cervix. JAMA 1951; 147:831–4.

59. Bacon HE. Radiation proctitis; a preliminary report of 39 cases. Radiology 1937; 29:574–7.

60. De Cosse JJ, Rhodes RS, Wentz WB, et al. The natural history and management of radiation induced injury of the gastrointestinal tract. Ann Surg 1969; 170:369–84.

61. Novak JM, Collins JT, Donowitz M, et al. Effects of radiation on the human gastrointestinal tract. J Clin Gastroenterol 1979; 1:9–39.

62. Stockbine MF, Hancock JE, Fletcher GH. Complications in 831 patients with squamous cell carcinoma of the intact uterine cervix treated with 3,000 rads or more whole pelvis irradiation. Am J Roentgenol 1970; 108:293–304.

63. Palmer JA, Bush RS. Radiation injuries to the bowel associated with the treatment of carcinoma of the cervix. Surgery 1976; 80:458–64.

64. Reichelderfer M, Morrissey JF. Colonoscopy in radiation colitis. Gastrointest Endosc 1980; 26:41–3.

65. Cunningham MP, Wilhoite R. Radiation-induced carcinoma of the transverse colon: Report of a case. Dis Colon Rectum 1973; 16:145–8.

66. Qizilbash AH. Radiation-induced carcinoma of the rectum: a late complication of pelvic irradiation. Arch Pathol 1974; 98:118–21.

67. May J, Loewenthal J. Irradiation injury to the colon. Gut 1965; 6:444–7.

68. Brandt LJ, Katz HJ, Wolf EL, et al. Simulation of colonic carcinoma by ischemia. Gastroenterology 1985; 88:1137–42.

69. Levine DS, Surawicz CM, Spencer GD, et al. Inflammatory polyposis two years after ischemic colon injury. Dig Dis Sci 1986; 31:1159–67.

70. Stamm B, Heer M, Buhler H, Ammann R. Mucosal biopsy of vascular ectasia (angiodysplasia) of the large bowel detected during routine colonoscopic examination. Histopathology 1985; 9:639–46.

Chapter 45

COLON POLYPS AND CARCINOMA

CHRISTOPHER B. WILLIAMS, B.M., F.R.C.P.
ASHLEY B. PRICE, B.M., F.R.C.PATH.

Any localized elevation above the intestinal mucosa is by definition a polyp. Polyps range from tiny, translucent, almost invisible mucosal bumps through stalked lesions with a diameter of 3 to 5 cm to sessile growths of 10 to 20 cm. They may be single, occur together in small numbers, or carpet the colon by the hundreds or thousands in the polyposis syndromes. It is often impossible to be certain about the histology of a polyp from its gross morphology, although a few lesions such as postinflammatory polyps or lipomas have characteristic appearances. Microscopy is necessary if histologic type is to be established. This usually requires an excision biopsy by electrosurgical snare polypectomy, except in the case of very small or extremely large lesions. Larger "polypoid" tumors on a broad base may ulcerate centrally or may spread circumferentially to form an annular or stricturing lesion; even these appearances are not necessarily diagnostic of malignancy.

Since an uncharacterized or nonspecific polyp, tumor, or stricture is the presenting clinical problem, general principles of diagnosis and therapy will be considered first; specific appearance and management of particular histologic types or conditions will then be discussed.

METHODS OF DIAGNOSIS OF POLYPS AND TUMORS

Clinical Presentation

Colonic polyps are commonly asymptomatic, although those over 1 cm in diameter may bleed intermittently.[1] On examination many patients with colorectal bleeding will by chance have another cause such as hemorrhoids in addition to polyps. It is unusual for polyps to cause pain or altered bowel habit, symptoms that are more often attributable to a coexistent functional bowel disorder when polyps are found in conjunction with these complaints. Larger sessile polyps and cancers can cause secondary alteration of bowel habit, flatulence, and excessive mucus production, which are symptoms that can mimic functional bowel disorder. Watery diarrhea with hypokalemia is a rare clinical presentation of villous adenomas of the rectosigmoid, most of which present without electrolyte disturbance. Anemia can occur in polyposis syndromes, but with one or two polyps it is more suggestive of a missed carcinoma or another unrelated cause elsewhere in the gastrointestinal tract.

That polyps are generally a chance finding is further borne out by the remarkably high incidence of adenomas in postmortem studies; these demonstrate that between 30% and 50% of subjects over age 55 have adenomas of some size, 10% being 1 cm or greater in diameter.[2, 3] This high incidence of "silent" neoplastic polyps, along with the hope of reducing colorectal cancer mortality in Western countries by removing them, has led to the current interest in screening examinations, follow-up programs and diagnostic methodology.[4]

Digital Examination and Rigid Proctosigmoidoscopy

Palpation of the distal third of the rectum must be performed in every patient because abnormalities in this area are easily overlooked during endoscopy. A skilled examiner obtains considerable information about the mobility of a tumor or sessile polyp including the presence or absence of perirectal lymph nodes. For visualization, and for biopsy or ablation of small lesions, the rigid proctosigmoidoscope is probably superseded by the superior view obtained with flexible instruments. For large lesions however, larger biopsy specimens can more easily be obtained using conventional forceps through the rigid instrument. With the operating proctosigmoidoscope or special anorectal retractors, the colorectal surgeon can resect even a 20 cm diameter villous adenoma in the rectum after infiltration of the submucosa with epinephrine (20 to 30 ml in 1:100,000 solution),[4] a procedure that is impossible with a fiberendoscope.

Fiberoptic Sigmoidoscopy

Fiberoptic sigmoidoscopy with the 60 cm length instrument reaches the proximal sigmoid or descending colon in a 5- to 7-minute examination. This procedure is a major gain in the preliminary assessment of patients at risk for polyps or tumors.[5] Pathologic findings are two to three times that of rigid instruments because of the greater length of colon examined[6-10] and because these instruments provide a close-up view of the mucosa that easily demonstrates 1 to 2 mm lesions for biopsy, lesions that would be invisible with the use of rigid instruments or x-ray (see dye-spray technique). The 35 cm length fiberoptic sigmoidoscope has protagonists who argue for its safety and easy mastery by non-endoscopist physicians.[7, 11, 12] Electrocoagulation, snare polypectomy, and snare loop biopsy techniques are safe during fibersigmoidoscopy only if carbon dioxide insufflation or rigorous air-exchange techniques are used to exclude the possibility of explosive gas concentrations after the limited bowel preparation commonly used for this procedure.[13] Fiberoptic sigmoidoscopy is discussed in Chapter 49.

Barium Enema

The first-line colonic screening technique of the past has been the barium enema,[14] all too frequently using the "single-contrast" method that Gilbertsen et al.[15] have pithily described as "an excellent technique for diagnosis of inoperable colon carcinoma." The air-contrast or double-contrast barium enema gives superior results when bowel preparation is meticulous; when enough x-ray films are taken in different positions, and the x-rays are studied immediately by the radiologist so that additional views will be obtained of dubious findings; and when the entire examination is reviewed subsequently by a second radiologist.[16, 17] Most overlooked abnormalities are visible on x-ray films in retrospect. Interpretation is subjective and often a matter of opinion. An inexperienced radiologist is apt to report "ring shadows" due to air bubbles or feces as polyps and more serious pathology as fecal material. Bowel deformity and ring shadows caused by muscular hypertrophy in diverticular disease, overlapping loops of redundant colon, and retained feces in the cecal pole are the most frequent causes of missed lesions on double-contrast enema studies.[18] The majority occur in the sigmoid colon and can be detected by fiberoptic sigmoidoscopy.[8, 19]

High-quality double-contrast barium enema performed by an expert radiologist is an accurate technique that is acceptable for demonstration of the proximal colon if colonoscopy is unavailable or technically difficult in a particular patient.[6] Barium enema examinations can safely be performed after colonoscopic biopsy,[20] after carefully performed biopsy with electrocoagulation ("hot-biopsy"), and probably after electrosurgical snare removal of small stalked polyps. If carbon dioxide insufflation is used during fiberoptic sigmoidoscopy or colonoscopy, a barium enema can be satisfactorily performed 30 minutes later, since this gas is rapidly reabsorbed.[21] Such a combination of endoscopy and radiology provides maximum accuracy and may be justified in the surveillance of some patients at high risk for polyps or cancer.[6, 22]

Colonoscopy

Colonoscopy demands greater dexterity than barium enema, and intravenous sedation is often required so that patients can tolerate the procedure.[23] It is, however, the more accurate technique, and interpretation of endoscopic findings is relatively easier. It also has the inestimable advantage of allowing immediate biopsy as well as destruction or removal of certain lesions.

The colonoscopist can miss large lesions in the vicinity of acute bends in the voluminous proximal colon or when the colon is fixed in position or difficult to examine. Direct comparison of colonoscopy and double-contrast barium enema using both procedures in patients with polyps has suggested 91% specificity for endoscopy and 72% for barium enema in detection of lesions 7 mm or more in diameter.[6] In all probability the endoscopist misses at least 20% to 30% of 2 to 5 mm polyps, particularly when attention is focused on removal of large lesions; therefore a second endoscopy is usually advised one year after polypectomy, but thereafter follow-up colonoscopy is scheduled at longer intervals.[24]

Whereas colonoscopy limited to the left colon (limited colonoscopy) or fiberoptic sigmoidoscopy is quick and easy (except sometimes in diverticular disease or after pelvic surgery), total colonoscopy is very difficult in 20% to 30% of patients, usually those with an uncontrollably mobile colon. With heavier sedation and occasional recourse to technical dodges such as the overtube or use of fluoroscopy, it should be possible to reach the cecum in more than 95% of patients when there is a known or strongly suspected lesion. It is doubtful that extreme efforts, usually traumatic for the patient, are justified for

screening or follow-up after polypectomy in asymptomatic patients. Colonoscopy is always preferable to double-contrast enema for cancer screening in patients with long-standing chronic extensive ulcerative colitis, since mucosal dysplasia often occurs in flat mucosa and this abnormality is undetectable radiographically.[25]

Intramucosal carcinoma, extracolonic cancer, or metastatic carcinoma infiltrating submucosally appears benign endoscopically because the mucosal surface over such lesions may be normal. Similarly, some malignant strictures are difficult to assess at colonoscopy. Even if the colonoscope passes through the stricture its maneuverability may be restricted to the point that adequate biopsies cannot be obtained.[26] Endoscopic diagnosis is inadvisable if the instrument will not pass through the stricture; the distal aspect of a malignant stricture may appear normal because the tumor has infiltrated the submucosa. Small-diameter pediatric endoscopes can be invaluable for assessment of tight strictures (Fig. 45–1). Biopsies carefully directed onto the most irregular area should show dysplastic tissue even if there is no

FIGURE 45–1. *A*, Barium enema radiograph of sigmoid colon stricture that raises suspicion of malignancy. *B*, The stricture is passable only with pediatric colonoscope. Endoscopy demonstrated findings to be those of uncomplicated diverticular disease.

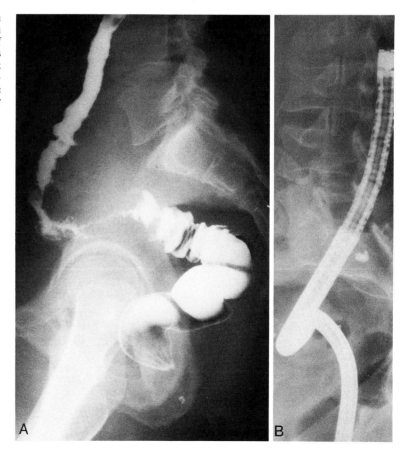

actual tumor invasion at the biopsy site. Washings from the stricture and cell specimens obtained by endoscopic brushing also assist in diagnosis.

Scanning Techniques

Scanning techniques such as computed tomography (CT) have no relevance in assesssing intracolonic lesions such as polyps but are important in estimating the local spread of carcinoma and the possibility of distant metastases.[27]

ENDOSCOPIC MANAGEMENT OF POLYPS

Snare Polypectomy

The principles for the safe use of electrosurgery are discussed in Chapter 7. Most colorectal polyps are easy to remove, since they are either on a relatively narrow stalk of normal tissue or the underlying mucosa and submucosa can be pulled apart with the snare loop to make a narrow pseudopedicle. In either case the configuration of the stalk makes electrocoagulation and excision beneath the limit of pathologic tissue technically easy. Excepting removal of sessile polyps, the main problem during snare polypectomy is to prevent bleeding. The arteries or arterioles of a polyp stalk form a plexus drawn up from the submucosa, and the vessels, being thickwalled, are the last part of the stalk to be affected by the heat of electrocoagulation (Plate 45–1). Probably the main factor in achieving hemostasis is the physical compression of these vessels produced by the tissue swelling that occurs as the stalk is heated. Heat also causes muscle tissue to contract, and this tends to constrict the arterioles until the clotting cascade and the platelet-aggregating effect associated with tissue damage combine to cause thrombosis. Sufficient heating of the polyp stalk before severance is thus the fundamental point of endoscopic polypectomy.

The mechanics of snare polypectomy require some practice and dexterity. The opened snare loop must be maneuvered over the head of the polyp by movements of the colonoscope controls, slid down onto the narrowest part of the stalk (usually near the top), and gently closed (Plate 45–2). At this point it is helpful to move the polyp back and forth with the snare to obtain a better view and to prove that a portion of the adjacent normal mucosa or bowel wall has not been entrapped in the snare. Further pressure is used to tighten the snare and "neck" the tissue to ensure local current concentration and thus localized heating.[23] Coagulating current alone is used by most endoscopists, since the particular characteristics of cutting current do not favor controlled heating of a sufficient depth of stalk tissue. Any electrosurgical unit can be used, but those designed for endoscopic purposes are safer. A low power setting is preferred (equivalent to 15 to 25 watts); 15 to 30 seconds of current application may be needed before visible whitening and swelling of the stalk indicate that the polyp can be severed safely. The stalk is usually severed by steadily increasing tension on the snare loop and sometimes by slightly turning up the power output of the electrosurgical generator. Polyp stalks of larger diameter require a longer duration of current flow for sufficient heating, and may also require a slightly higher power setting. Impatience, overly aggressive tightening of the snare, and excessively high power settings may result in cutting of the core too quickly, which risks immediate or delayed hemorrhage.[28]

Large or Broad-Based Polyps

Stalks to about 1.5 cm in diameter can be safely electrocoagulated and severed. Polypectomy in this manner gives the pathologist a single specimen that is easier to assess than a collection of smaller pieces. However, larger or sessile polyps may have bases in which the volume of tissue is too great to permit adequate heating without resorting to a power setting and duration of electrocoagulation that seriously increase the risk of perforation. Piecemeal removal of the polyp head in three to six portions is comparatively easy and safe, although it may be necessary that colonoscopy be repeated at 2- to 3-week intervals to be certain that all tissue has been removed[29] (Plate 45–3). Large polyps judged to be difficult to remove endoscopically have been snared and intussuscepted from the midsigmoid colon to the anus for local surgical management.[30] It is difficult to specify a size limit for endoscopic polypectomy, since much depends on the clinical situation and the experience of the endoscopist. It is usually best to attempt at least partial removal of a large polyp, regardless of size, since the procedure may prove to be unexpectedly

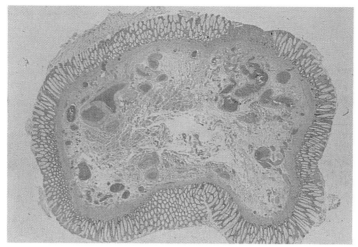

PLATE 45–1. Transverse section of polyp stalk showing central electrocoagulation necrosis but inadequate coagulation of peripheral vessels.

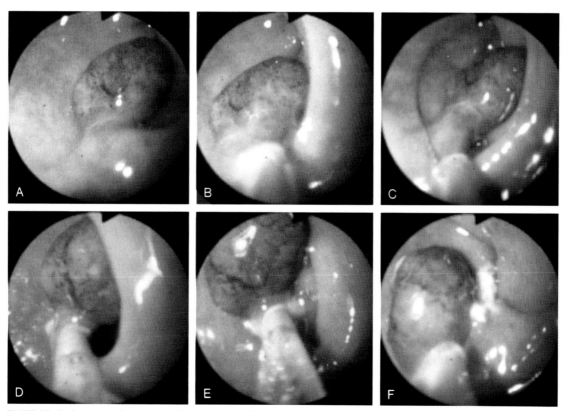

PLATE 45–2. Sequence in snaring, electrocoagulation, and severance of a stalked polyp. *A,* Stalked polyp; *B,* snare sheath protruding into visual field; *C,* snare wire placed over polyp head and around stalk; *D,* snare closed to strangle stalk; *E,* electrocoagulation of stalk; *F,* polyp stalk severed.

easy. However, it is foolish to court disaster, especially if it is suspected that the lesion may be malignant; elective surgery is clearly preferable.

Small Polyps

The majority of 2 to 5 mm sporadic polyps in the colon (as opposed to those in the rectum) prove to be adenomas and should be destroyed or removed.[31-33] Snare polypectomy is possible but small lesions are often difficult to retrieve, even by placing a mucus trap in the suction line and attempting to aspirate the specimen. For this reason the compromise technique of "hot biopsy" has some advantages.[23, 34] A conventional but electrically insulated biopsy forceps is used to grasp the head of the polyp and to pull or tent it toward the center of the lumen (Plate 45-4). Electrocoagulating current is applied and this preferentially heats the narrowed base of the polyp where it is pulled away from the wall, whereas the biopsy is protected within the forceps cups. With hot biopsy only a few seconds are needed to obtain a biopsy and simultaneously destroy the remainder of the polyp. Polyps over 7 to 8 mm cannot be tented up sufficiently with the forceps and these require snare polypectomy. When biopsies are not required, such as when the diagnosis of adenomatous polyposis is already established, small polyps can alternatively be rapidly destroyed with a button electrode, bipolar probe, or laser photocoagulation.

Multiple Polyps

Only 2% of patients have five or more polyps and, even among these, some polyps are small enough for hot biopsy or aspiration after polypectomy. For practical purposes, the colonoscope must be withdrawn to retrieve each polyp that has been removed by snare polypectomy, although a skilled endoscopist can retrieve several at one time with the "long-nose retriever snare" (Plate 45-5) or a basket. Colonoscopic overtube technique (see Chapter 40) also speeds up the retrieval process for multiple polypectomy specimens by shortening the time and lessening the difficulty of reinserting the instrument through the sigmoid colon. The sigmoid colon should be cleared of polyps first to avoid amputation as the overtube is advanced over the insertion tube of the colonoscope. Most endoscopists retrieve single polyps either by

grasping the specimen with the polypectomy snare or by aspirating it onto the tip of the colonoscope. Special polyp grasping forceps are available commercially. Aspiration of the polyp onto the tip of the endoscope often precludes adequate examination of the colon distal to the polypectomy site and necessitates reinsertion of the endoscope to the level of the polyp. In patients such as those with hamartomatous polyposis (Peutz-Jeghers syndrome, juvenile polyposis), in whom the virtual absence of cancer risk makes precise location of particular polyps unimportant, 300 to 400 ml of warm saline solution can be instilled through the accessory channel of the colonoscope with a syringe at a point proximal to the location of the resected polyps. Subsequent to removal of the endoscope, the administration of a suppository or phosphate enema will cause evacuation of the whole polyp load. As many as 100 non-neoplastic or inflammatory polyps have been snared in a single procedure.[35, 36] If 10 or more probable neoplastic polyps are seen, the possibility of adenomatous polyposis makes it important to concentrate on identifying further small polyps in order to estimate more exactly the number present before deciding to snare the larger polyps or to advise surgery.

Chromoscopy (Dye-Spray Technique)

Japanese endoscopists have demonstrated that fine mucosal detail may be rendered more obvious by vital staining or coloration with dyes such as indigo carmine or methylene blue.[37, 38] These chromoscopy techniques are discussed fully in Chapter 10, Part 2. A 25% solution of washable blue fountain-pen ink makes a satisfactory alternative "dye" that can be used to demonstrate otherwise invisible 1 to 3 mm polyps. Representative flat and clean areas of mucosa are chosen, and a washing tube (spray catheter) is used to layer a small amount of the blue solution over the surface. Any polyps present project as pink islands that are easily seen, and biopsies can be obtained (Plate 45-6). Biopsy is essential, since lymphoid follicles and other small mucosal projections may appear similar to small adenomas.

Intramucosal tattooing is a means of marking areas of interest within the colon. A 2 ml submucosal injection of autoclaved black India ink leaves a permanent blue-gray mark visible both internally and on the serosal aspect of the bowel (Plate 45-7). This can be

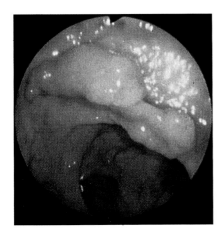

PLATE 45–3. Polyp (tubulovillous adenoma) 3 cm in length is suitable for piecemeal polypectomy.

PLATE 45–4. Ten-second sequence of hot-biopsy destruction and simultaneous biopsy of 5-mm polyp showing elevation to form a pseudopedicle before electrocoagulation.

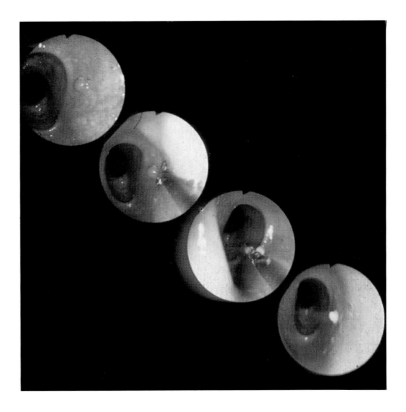

PLATE 45–5. Three 8- to 9-mm polyps retrieved together using long-nosed polyp retriever.

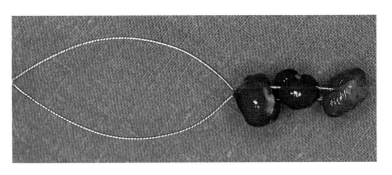

helpful for endoscopic follow-up, for the pathologist, or if necessary for the surgeon if a tattoo marks the site of attempted removal of suspicious or sessile lesions. Polypectomy and retrieval of any specimens should be completed before tattooing, since some ink can reflux during the injection and obscure the field of view in the area being marked.

CONTRAINDICATIONS AND COMPLICATIONS

There are few contraindications to colonoscopy or polypectomy, except after recent myocardial infarction or in a seriously ill patient especially when symptoms suggest impending bowel perforation. Few endoscopists attempt more than careful and limited colonoscopy in a patient obstructed by tumor. Normal bowel preparation is impossible and dangerous in the presence of obstruction. Over-insufflation proximal to the point of obstruction may occur, although this hazard is minimized by the use of readily absorbed carbon dioxide for insufflation.[21] The contraindications and complications of colonoscopy are discussed in Chapter 41.

The risk of postpolypectomy bleeding in reported series is about 2%, whereas the perforation rate associated with polypectomy is about 0.3%.[28, 39] These figures are only slightly higher than those for diagnostic colonoscopy, and represent "worst case" standards, since they derive from the pioneering experience of self-taught colonoscopists. With appropriate technique and equipment, hemorrhage should rarely occur. The risk is highest when polyp stalks are over 1 cm in diameter, this corresponding in most cases to a diameter of 2 cm or more for the head of the polyp.[28] Particular care should be taken before and during snaring of these larger polyps; a coagulation profile is obtained preprocedure in a few centers, blood typing may be done, and in some cases patients are admitted to the hospital overnight after the procedure.

Bleeding, if it occurs, is usually immediate, and if an appropriate length of residual stalk has been left, the snare loop can be quickly replaced on the stalk to strangulate it for 10 to 15 minutes, after which time clotting and thrombosis will usually have occurred (Plate 45–8). If the remaining stalk is too short for this maneuver, or if blood clots obscure the view, the site can be irrigated or injected with a solution of 1:100,000 epinephrine, an intravenous infusion started, and the use of intravenous pitressin considered. Assuming some local electrocoagulation occurred before transection, bleeding will usually stop spontaneously. There is a remote possibility, especially after removal of large polyps, of delayed hemorrhage between 24 hours and 14 days. The risk of both immediate and delayed hemorrhage is minimal if sufficient electrocoagulation precedes polypectomy.

Any risk of perforation following snare polypectomy is greatest during removal of large sessile polyps when there is a danger that a full-thickness portion of bowel wall will be pulled into the snare loop. There are also reports of perforation after removal of small polyps using a snare loop or hot biopsy forceps. These perforations are difficult to explain but are presumably due to point contact of the serosal aspect of the polypectomy site with another structure. In most cases postpolypectomy perforation is localized and the patient can be managed conservatively with rest and antibiotics. If there is any doubt, it is safer to recommend operation. Delayed perforation has also been reported after polypectomy but this is a rare event. More common is the occurrence of lesser degrees of bowel wall damage that result in pain, fever, and leukocytosis without evidence of free intra-abdominal gas. This "postpolypectomy syndrome" is managed conservatively.

ENDOSCOPIC FEATURES AND MANAGEMENT OF NON-NEOPLASTIC POLYPS

A histologic classification of polyps is given in Table 45–1. With the exceptions of the hamartomatous polyposis syndromes, and postinflammatory polyps and bleeding polyps in childhood, most non-neoplastic polyps are coincident findings during investigation for other conditions. Non-neoplastic polyps are frequently covered by normal mucosa and thus often look paler and shinier than neoplastic polyps. They may sometimes be hyperemic, ulcerated, and indistinguishable from neoplastic polyps; therefore representative specimens or biopsies must always be assessed histologically. Even then the distinction between non-neoplastic and neoplastic polyps has been somewhat blurred by the recognition that there can be "mixed" polyps such as those combining metaplastic and adenomatous elements or a focus of dysplastic

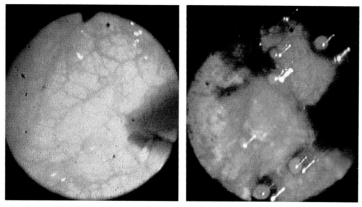

PLATE 45–6. Demonstration of 1- to 2-mm polyps in a patient with adenomatous polyposis, using "dye-spray" technique (1:4 dilution of washable blue ink).

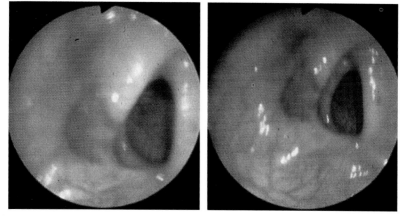

PLATE 45–7. Submucosal tattoo after two years, localizing site of removal of malignant polyp (1 cc sterile black ink injected submucosally).

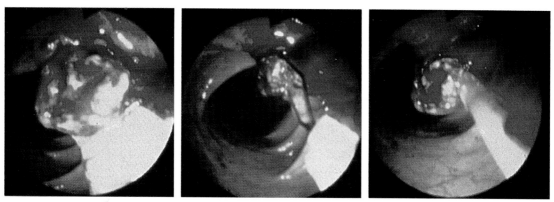

PLATE 45–8. Bleeding polyp stalk grasped and strangulated with snare loop (no further electrocoagulation was required).

TABLE 45–1. **Histologic Classification of Polyps**

Histologic Type (%)	Surgical Series* Percentage with Carcinoma				Colonoscopic Series† Percentage with Carcinoma			
	<1 cm	*1–2 cm*	*>2 cm*	*Total*	*<1 cm*	*1–2 cm*	*>2 cm*	*Total*
Tubular (75)	1	10	35	5	1	3	10	2
Tubulovillous (20)	4	7	46	23	0	4	11	6
Villous (5)	10	10	53	4	0	5	·38	18
	Overall Total 10% with carcinoma				Overall Total 5% with carcinoma			

*Muto et al.[54]
†Gillespie et al.[30]

adenomatous tissue occurring in a hamartomatous polyp.

Hamartomatous Polyps

Hamartomas are localized tumor-like collections of normal tissues arranged in an abnormal and disorganized fashion in an inappropriate site. In the colon, the commonest examples are juvenile and Peutz-Jeghers polyps. Juvenile polyps are also discussed in Chapter 48.

Juvenile polyps are the characteristic polyps of childhood, although they are found sporadically in adulthood. They are sometimes referred to as mucus retention polyps because of cystic inclusions of entrapped mucus that give sections a characteristic "Swiss cheese" appearance (Plate 45–9 and Fig. 45–2). Both the cysts and the crypts of juvenile polyps are lined with essentially normal cells, and the polyp is covered by normal epithelium with mucus-secreting cells. The surface can be ulcerated, and the stroma usually shows marked inflammatory changes. Ulceration or infarction may result in entrapment of tissue and a subsequent bizarre appearance known as "pseudo-invasion."

Endoscopically, a juvenile polyp is usually a smooth-surfaced, shiny lesion 1 to 2 cm in diameter. The stalk is characteristically thin and contains no muscular elements. Because of this juvenile polyps may twist and autoamputate, sometimes with massive hemorrhage; they can also be easily snared with little risk of hemorrhage after electrocoagulation. There may be an increased risk of perforation when juvenile polyps are removed in the thin-walled colon of children; more rapid transection is preferred than that used for polypectomy in adults. Several large polyps may occur in a small child and may be distributed anywhere in the colon, so that examination of the whole bowel is desirable if one polyp is found distally.[40, 41] Follow-up is not normally recommended for isolated juvenile polyps.

Individual juvenile polyps have no malignant potential, but there are families in whom juvenile polyposis (defined as 10 or more juvenile polyps) is associated with a high risk

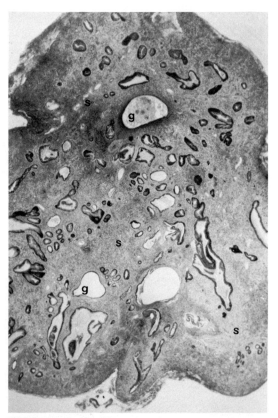

FIGURE 45–2. Juvenile polyp with characteristic abundant stroma (s) within which are widely spaced cystic nondysplastic glands (g). The muscularis mucosae is not involved, a feature believed responsible for the ease with which juvenile polyps undergo auto-amputation (×20).

of cancer.[42] This is probably due to the presence of adenomatous elements in some of the polyps. Patients with multiple juvenile polyps, especially those with a family history of cancer, must therefore undergo either careful colonoscopic follow-up with removal of polyps or prophylactic subtotal colectomy.

Peutz-Jegher polyps of the colon occur in most patients affected by the syndrome of mucocutaneous pigmentation—circum oral, circum anal, palms, soles, and under the nails—with polyposis throughout the gastrointestinal tract from stomach to rectum. Inheritance is mendelian dominant, but sporadic cases of Peutz-Jeghers polyposis occur and isolated Peutz-Jeghers polyps may be found without other features of the syndrome. Colonic polyps are of secondary clinical importance to those in the stomach, duodenum, or small intestine. The colonic polyps appear to have no significant malignant potential, whereas there is a significant risk in the stomach and duodenum. Removal of the jejunal and ileal polyps is mandatory because of the danger of intussusception and catastrophic infarction resulting in the short-bowel syndrome. For this reason the primary investigative procedure for affected patients is the small-bowel x-ray series. This should be repeated at 1½- to 2-year intervals along with surgical removal of any polyps 1 cm or more in diameter as a prophylactic measure. At similar intervals, gastroscopy and colonoscopy allow removal of significant-sized polyps from endoscopically accessible areas[43] (Plate 45–10). During such examinations it is common to see numerous 1 to 3 mm polyps, the majority of which will disappear spontaneously and can therefore be ignored. The tendency to pigmentation and polyp formation in the Peutz-Jeghers syndrome appears to decline progressively after 25 to 30 years of age, by which age three or four laparotomies and numerous endoscopies may have been necessary.

Histologically, Peutz-Jeghers polyps show a characteristic branching framework of muscle fibers derived from the muscularis and spreading between disorganized but otherwise normal mucosal crypts (Fig. 45–3). The entrapped mucous cysts of juvenile polyps are not seen. No dysplasia or neoplastic tissue is present, although "pseudo-invasion" with misplacement of foci of epithelium into the stroma of the polyp head may result after ulceration or local hemorrhage.[44]

Other Mesodermal Polyps

Lipomas occur most commonly in the right colon, sometimes with fatty enlargement of the ileocecal valve but also as single or multiple submucosal rounded elevations 1 to 3 cm in diameter. Pedunculated lipomas are relatively rare. At endoscopy a rounded, shiny lesion that is soft and easily indented by the endoscope tip or the biopsy forceps (pillow sign) is virtually diagnostic of a lipoma[45, 46] (Plate 45–11). Repeated biopsy at the same site will sometimes reveal underlying yellowish fat. Snare polypectomy is rarely indicated once the diagnosis has been made endoscopically, since lipomas are always benign and usually asymptomatic, although intussusception or surface bleeding have been reported. If removal is attempted, electrocoagulation and cutting are difficult to achieve, even with high power, because fat is nonconductive.

Polyps can occasionally be composed of other tissue elements, but the microscopic diagnosis after snare polypectomy usually comes as a surprise because these lesions are covered by normal mucosa. Examples include polypoid hemangiomas, neurofibromas, and leiomyomas.

Endometriosis of the colon usually involves the muscular layers and rarely presents as a submucosal swelling that can be friable or even mimic a carcinoma. Endometriosis is discussed in Chapter 46.

Metaplastic (Hyperplastic) Polyps

During proctoscopy or proctosigmoidoscopy it is common to observe 2 to 5 mm pale or glistening metaplastic (hyperplastic) polyps in the rectum. Essentially these are a normal finding and occur in increasing numbers in old age (Plate 45–12). In the colon only 10% of polyps of this size prove to be metaplastic on biopsy; instead the majority of 2 to 5 mm colonic polyps are adenomas.[31, 47] Larger metaplastic polyps up to 1 cm in diameter are occasionally found, usually as a sessile mound of shiny tissue, but sometimes semipedunculated. Multiple metaplastic polyposis occurs and can be indistinguishable from familial adenomatous polyposis except on biopsy. The differential diagnosis is important, since adenomatous polyposis requires surgery, whereas metaplastic polyposis can be ignored.

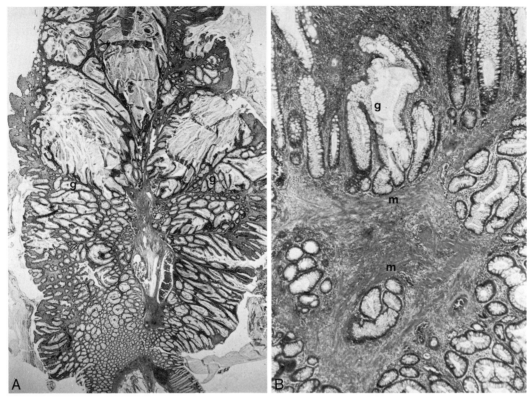

FIGURE 45–3. *A,* Peutz-Jeghers polyp with irregular nondysplastic glands (g) that intermingle with stroma and muscle fibers (m) (×12). *B,* Glands are well seen in a high-power view of *A* (×125).

Histologically, the characteristic features of a metaplastic polyp include elongation of the mucosal crypts with reduced numbers of goblet cells and "saw-toothing" (Fig. 45–4), this last feature being an irregular outline of the epithelial cells.[48] Metaplastic polyps do not exhibit dysplasia and have no malignant potential. The commonly used term "hyperplastic" has been regarded as inappropriate because it suggests abnormal nuclear activity and cellular regeneration. The association of metaplastic polyps with colorectal cancers may be partly due to the increased incidence of metaplastic polyps with age.

Postinflammatory and Inflammatory Polyps

Postinflammatory polyps are most commonly worm-like or thread-like (filiform) tags of essentially normal mucosa that develop after a severe attack of any form of colitis (e.g., ulcerative, Crohn's, amebic, schistosomal or ischemic).[49] Despite their names, they are usually not inflamed, although some may be hyperemic or superficially ulcerated at the tip, and at endoscopy some may have a surface covering of white slough (Plate 45–13). Larger polyps may occur under similar circumstances; these are truly inflammatory, being composed mainly of granulation tissue, and have a misleadingly sinister, irregular appearance despite a benign histology. Occasionally, especially after schistosomal colitis, the exudate and bleeding from numerous larger inflammatory polyps may be sufficient to cause presenting symptoms of anemia and hypoproteinemia. Postinflammatory polyps are sometimes referred to as "pseudopolyps," a term that is technically incorrect. They must not be confused with the plaque-like or polypoid areas of severe epithelial dysplasia that may occur beginning 8 to 10 years after the onset of extensive ulcerative colitis.[50–51] Postinflammatory polyps have less tendency to malignant change than the surrounding mucosa. Therefore screening biopsies should be taken from surrounding mucosa rather than from postinflammatory polyps when searching for dysplasia in association with long-standing ulcerative colitis.

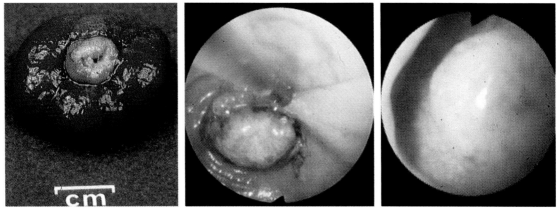

PLATE 45–9.   PLATE 45–10.   PLATE 45–11.

PLATE 45–9. Juvenile polyp (gross specimen).
PLATE 45–10. Peutz-Jeghers polyp showing suggestive pale color.
PLATE 45–11. Lipoma showing rounded contour and shiny normal overlying mucosa.

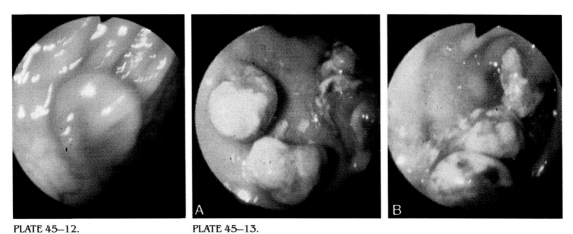

PLATE 45–12.   PLATE 45–13.

PLATE 45–12. Metaplastic polyp showing pale shiny surface and uneven shape.
PLATE 45–13. A & B, Inflammatory polyps showing characteristic surface slough.

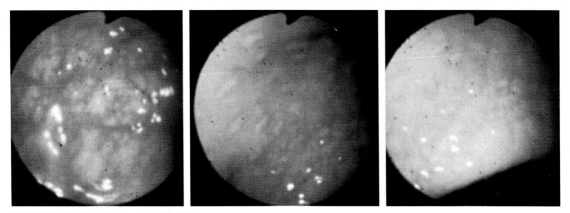

PLATE 45–14. Colonic lymphoid follicles.

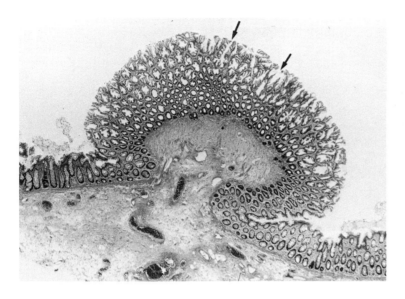

FIGURE 45–4. Metaplastic polyp. Serrated pattern of slightly dilated crypts (*arrows*) is characteristic. They are usually sessile (×25).

Lymphoid Polyps

The intestinal tract is studded with lymphoid tissue. Polyps that arise from this tissue element may present an entire spectrum from isolated polypoid lesions to diffuse lymphoid hyperplasia (Plate 45–14). Nodular lymphoid hyperplasia of the terminal ileum is a normal finding in young persons, and similar 1 to 3 mm nodules may occur in the distal colon of some children[52] (Plate 45–15). This must be considered when screening young members of families with adenomatous polyposis coli. Biopsies are obtained for differentiation. Multiple benign lymphoid polyposis may also occur in the aftermath of an infective process, sometimes associated with an immunoglobulin disturbance. The smallest lesions may be translucent and therefore less obvious on endoscopy than on barium enema, unless the endoscopist carefully inspects the surface using the reflected light-reflex to advantage or the dye-spray technique.

Solitary benign lymphoid polyps, up to about 1 cm in diameter, may occur in the rectum of young adults.[53] They appear as pale, submucosal lesions, the diagnosis being made at histologic examination after snare polypectomy. The single or multifocal tumors of lymphoid tissue are described later.

ENDOSCOPIC FEATURES AND MANAGEMENT OF NEOPLASTIC POLYPS

Adenomas

The commonest neoplastic polyp in the colon and rectum is the adenoma; this is the generic name of polyps having a distinctive abnormal dysplastic epithelium in different architectural arrangements.

The tubular adenoma occurs most frequently; it has a relatively solid head that is often fissured, giving it a lobular appearance. Histologically it has tubules that are characterized by branching and by a neoplastic epithelium that is usually only mildly dysplastic (Fig. 45–5). Tubular adenomas more than 7 to 8 mm in diameter usually have a stalk. At the other end of the architectural spectrum is the villous adenoma, frequently larger, sessile, and having a frond-like structure covered by a dysplastic epithelium that is by comparison more often severely dysplastic. In the architectural spectrum between the common, relatively benign tubular adenoma and the uncommon villous adenoma is the tubulovillous (or villoglandular) adenoma, representing about 20% to 30% of all adenomatous polyps and having an intermediate structure with both branching fronds and tubular elements.

Allocation of a polyp as a particular type of adenoma is a subjective histologic determination. If more than 20% to 25% but less than 75% to 80% of the polyp consists of villous elements, it will be considered tubulovillous, although assessment may vary according to individual opinion and the number of sections taken. Interrelationship of histologic type, size, and malignant tendency of different adenomas is shown in Table 45–1.[30, 35]

The endoscopist can rarely be certain of the histologic type of a small or stalked polyp, except that it is unlikely to be villous. Villous adenomas are usually sessile with an irregular, pale surface (Plate 45–16) that distinguishes them with reasonable certainty from carcinomas, although the possibility of an invasive malignant focus cannot be excluded until all resected tissue has been examined histologically.

The Adenoma-Carcinoma Sequence

It is now generally accepted that, except in ulcerative colitis, most colorectal carcinomas originate from preexisting adenomatous tissue.[54] The dysplastic epithelial surface of an adenoma may appear similar to that of infiltrating carcinoma and behave identically in tissue culture. As a result, severe dysplasia in an adenoma may be referred to as carcinoma in situ or focal carcinoma. This is clinically misleading, since for practical purposes metastasis is never associated with such lesions, there being no lymphatic drainage superficial to the muscularis mucosae. Until the dysplastic cells invade across the muscularis mucosae dividing the epithelial surface from the submucosa the pathologist is not justified in diagnosing carcinoma. As described for hamartomatous polyps, the phenomenon of misplaced epithelium causing the appearance

of "pseudo-invasion" may be confusing, although the misplaced tissue is nondysplastic and not surrounded by the fibrous (desmoplastic) reaction that occurs around carcinomatous tissue.

The relationship between size of an adenoma and risk of malignancy probably represents a statistical relationship between the mass of the polyp and the number of potentially cancerous cells present. Malignancy rarely occurs in tiny adenomas and the overall malignancy rate for adenomas in endoscopic series is about 5%,[30, 55] compared with about 10% for surgical series.[54] The disparity may be due to inclusion in the surgical series of adenomatous polyps removed from cancer patients and also from the pre-endoscopic era policy of delaying operation until polyps showed "suspicious" changes in configuration on follow-up barium enemas.

The existence of an adenoma-carcinoma sequence in the large bowel is supported by much indirect evidence. As well as behaving similarly in tissue culture, adenomas and carcinomas have similar histochemical and chromosomal aberrations. Many early carcinomas have residual adenoma tissue, and the percentage of this benign element decreases in

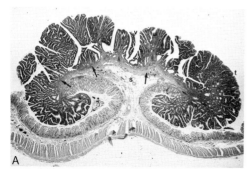
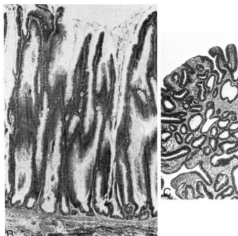
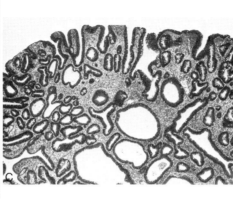
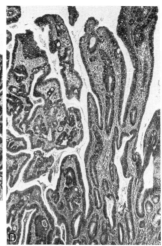

FIGURE 45–5. A, Benign tubulovillous adenoma showing stalk(s), intact even line of muscularis mucosae (arrows), and dysplastic tubular (t) and villous (v) epithelium (×12). A range of adenomatous patterns is seen in B, C, and D: B, villous pattern; C, tubular pattern; D, tubulovillous arrangement (×50).

more advanced carcinomas in which the prior benign tissue of the adenoma is presumed to have been engulfed. The distribution of adenomas and carcinomas in the colon is found in most series to be identical, that is, predominantly in the left colon with a small increased incidence of carcinoma in the cecum that may be related to the increased cecal incidence of sessile villous adenomas. The worldwide geographic incidence of adenomas and carcinomas is also similar, both being rare in Africans and indigenous Japanese and both being more common in Caucasians and "westernized" Japanese such as those living in Hawaii.[56]

Synchronous adenomas are present in many patients with colon cancer; patients with adenomas on the resection specimen have a higher risk of future carcinoma formation.[4, 9, 21] Patients with adenomas have a higher risk of developing colon carcinoma than matched nonpolyp-bearing controls.[57] The risk of both coexistent (synchronous) or subsequent (metachronous) carcinoma increases with increasing numbers of adenomas to an incidence of 100% in patients with adenomatous polyposis.[54] Destruction of adenomas reduces the incidence of cancer in the rectum.[58]

The time required for an adenoma to develop into carcinoma is speculative, although figures have been given for the growth rate of polyps and cancers based on radiologic or clinical observation. Muto et al.[54] suggested an average of 5 years for an adenoma of 1 cm in diameter to develop into a malignancy, although Morson admits (personal communication) that there may be a wide spectrum of behavior as evidenced by the occasional development of carcinoma within one year and the fact that many adenomas do not become malignant within the lifetime of the patient.

The evidence available suggests that environmental, dietary, and genetic factors may be involved in the development of an adenoma. It has been proposed that a recessive gene predisposes to adenoma formation, the actual development of adenomas being triggered in such predisposed persons by environmental factors.[59] Adenoma-bearing subjects according to this theory might be homozygous (pp) for the adenoma-predisposing gene (p), whereas adenomatous polyposis subjects may require only a dominant gene (P) to produce multiple adenomas.[59]

Familial Adenomatous Polyposis

The term "polyposis coli" is now avoided as histologically and anatomically imprecise. To differentiate familial adenomatous polyposis from non-neoplastic forms of polyposis, the presence of adenomas must be proved histologically. Adenomatous polyposis can also involve the small intestine and duodenum. Technically, the definition of adenomatous polyposis requires the presence of 100 adenomas in a surgical specimen, although the number is more often in the thousands (Fig. 45–6). Since many of these may be extremely small or even microscopic, and because of the tendency at endoscopy to underestimate the number of small polyps, demonstration of 25 to 30 adenomas (histologically proved) at colonoscopy is probably sufficient to confirm the diagnosis in a polyposis family member and to consider the possibility in anyone else.

Patients with adenomatous polyposis are usually asymptomatic until development of a carcinoma, which occurs usually between the ages of 20 and 40 years. Great efforts are therefore made to diagnose the condition in an asymptomatic stage by contacting and examining all known blood-relatives of an affected person. The mendelian dominant inheritance of adenomatous polyposis means that about 50% of first-degree relatives should be affected.[59] Fiberoptic sigmoidoscopy is probably the ideal screening examination and should be initiated at about 13 years of age using the dye-spray technique to look for tiny polyps if none are obvious to unaided observation. Total colonoscopy is unnecessary for screening since the distal colon is always involved in affected patients, although the rectum may be relatively spared. Fiberoptic sigmoidoscopy should be repeated every 2 or 3 years until at least age 30, by which time the diagnosis can reasonably be excluded if no polyps have been found. After the diagnosis is confirmed, total colonoscopy is probably justified to check the proximal colon, since polyps are predominately in this segment in some patients, and the presence of numerous or large polyps in the right colon may influence the timing of surgery.

Operation is usually delayed until a socially convenient age (17 to 18 years), since there is no significant risk of carcinoma formation before this. If possible an ileo-anal anasto-

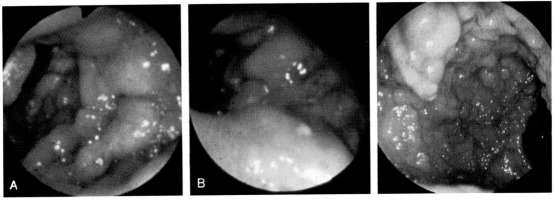

PLATE 45–15.

PLATE 45–16.

PLATE 45–15. *A & B,* Nodular lymphoid hyperplasia of terminal ileum (normal finding).
PLATE 45–16. Encircling sessile villous adenoma showing characteristic pale color.

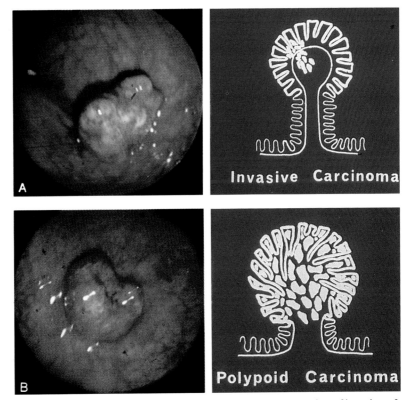

PLATE 45–17. *A,* Malignant adenoma showing irregular outline. *Right,* Diagrammatic representation of invasion of cancer cells below muscularis mucosae. *B,* Polypoid carcinoma on short stalk with ulcerated surface. *Right,* Diagrammatic representation of replacement of entire head of polyp by malignant tissue.

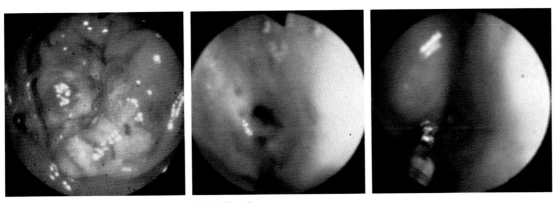

PLATE 45–18.   PLATE 45–19.

PLATE 45–18. Annular carcinoma of colon.
PLATE 45–19. *Left and Right,* Sigmoid colon stricture.

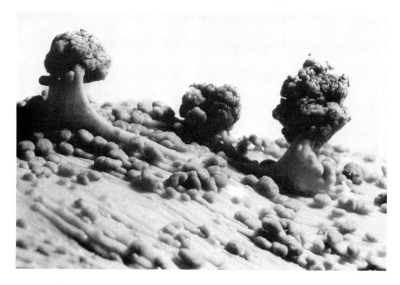

FIGURE 45–6. Detail from surgical specimen of familial adenomatous polyposis. The entire large bowel was carpeted by polyps of varying sizes.

mosis is made, with or without a pouch procedure, to avoid the need for ileostomy. Those patients who refuse surgery and those in whom operation is technically impossible (e.g., extensive intra-abdominal desmoid tumor) can be managed by annual colonoscopy with removal of larger lesions.

Thorough upper gastrointestinal endoscopy will reveal small adenomas in the duodenum of about 80% of older patients with adenomatous polyposis.[60] Gastric polyps may be present in a smaller percentage of patients but are usually hamartomatous and require no therapy. Since duodenal or ampullary (or bile duct) carcinoma occurs occasionally in patients with polyposis, endoscopic surveillance every 2 to 3 years may be justified with snare polypectomy of larger lesions.

Malignant Polyps

A malignant polyp is an adenoma in which malignant cells have spread beneath the muscularis mucosae into the deeper substance of the polyp. In some cases the spread may extend into the stalk of normal tissue, and in some the entire substance of the polyp may be replaced by malignancy. The later circumstance is referred to as a "polypoid carcinoma." Endoscopically and radiologically it is usually impossible to recognize an adenoma containing invasive carcinoma or even a stalked polypoid carcinoma that does not contain any residual adenomatous tissue (Plate 45–17 and Fig. 45–7). Endoscopic signs of malignancy include a thick stalk and an ulcerated or firm polyp head, although soft, rounded polyps on thin stalks may con-

tain cancer, and malignant appearing polyps can prove to be entirely benign. A disproportionately small amount of polyp tissue on a thick stalk may represent the remains of a malignant polyp in which growth of the polyp head had outstripped the blood supply.

After polypectomy, the histologic diagnosis of malignancy in a polyp is most often not expected. If it is certain that the entire lesion has been satisfactorily removed, the principles of subsequent management depend on the pathologist's assessment of the risk of metastasis to local lymph nodes based upon microscopic study of multiple sections of the specimen. Well-differentiated or moderately well-differentiated carcinoma that has not invaded as far as the resection line through the stalk and that does not involve veins or lymphatics is exceedingly unlikely to have spread.[61–63] Although there may be a case for operating in younger patients in whom the mortality of elective colonic resection is low, most endoscopists resist the largely emotional suggestion that even elderly patients should be automatically submitted to the risks of colonic surgery. The relatively high mortality of colonic surgery in elderly patients exceeds the remote chance of finding local tumor extension or involved lymph nodes before the occurrence of distant metastasis. Locally malignant lesions that meet the pathologic criteria can be managed by endoscopic local excision alone. Clinical experience, including several series of patients followed 5 years after polypectomy, supports this conservative policy.[64–68] One dissenting viewpoint appears to be invalid on pathologic grounds.[69] This approach may also be logically applied to

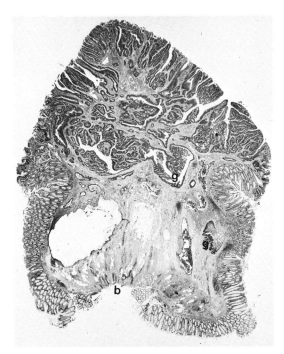

FIGURE 45–7. Malignant polyp in which dysplastic glands have penetrated the muscularis mucosae and invaded the stalk (g). The base of the stalk (b) is free from invasion, a critical feature relevant to management of such polyps (×12).

management of polypoid carcinomas meeting the same criteria.[63]

If malignancy is suspected in a polyp at endoscopy, it is advisable to tattoo the mucosa (vide supra) adjacent to the polypectomy site. If the histologic findings are unexpected, the patient should be re-examined within 2 weeks of the polypectomy before healing obscures the location in order to obtain a biopsy and tattoo the polypectomy site. Thereafter, the site should be examined at 2 and 6 months before proceeding to routine follow-up at 1- to 2-year intervals. Since most malignant polyps occur in the distal colon, a limited colonoscopy to the polypectomy site is sufficient for the first two follow-up examinations.

ADENOCARCINOMA

Endoscopic Diagnosis

The endoscopic diagnosis of adenocarcinoma of the colon rarely presents a problem, since cancers are usually large, reddened, or bleeding with an irregular or ulcerated surface (Plate 45–18). The rarity of 1 to 2 cm flat or ulcerated cancers is evidence against the concept of "de novo" cancer formation in the colon and rectum. For practical purposes intraepithelial carcinoma occurs only in chronic ulcerative colitis (and perhaps granulomatous colitis, although this is debatable).[70] Scirrhous carcinoma of the colon analogous to linitis plastica of the stomach is reported rarely; it is usually metastatic in origin.

A more serious problem for the endoscopist is that invasion may fix or distort the colon so that endoscopic observation is restricted. Strictures in particular can present difficulties since, even if a small-diameter pediatric instrument is available, it may be impossible to maneuver the endoscope tip to obtain satisfactory biopsies (Plate 45–19). Characteristically the margin of invading tumor is covered by a layer of normal mucosa, and endoscopic judgment and dexterity are needed to successfully target biopsies onto a representative area of carcinoma. If standard biopsy forceps are used at least three to four specimens should be obtained, but with a large-channel instrument and large forceps a single, well-placed biopsy may be diagnostic. A snare loop biopsy, when obtainable, provides the pathologist with a larger specimen for histologic assessment. When a stricture is impassable or the forceps will not reach or cannot be directed onto the tumor surface, brushing or washing to obtain a specimen for cytologic evaluation may be diagnostic.[26, 71–73] Even a successful endoscopic biopsy may be too small to show tumor invasion, but it may demonstrate severe epithelial dysplasia and thus differentiate the lesion from an inflammatory mass (e.g., granulation tissue, ischemia, endometrioma, ameboma) and from lymphoma.

Total Colonoscopy in Cancer Patients

The whole colon must be examined in patients with colorectal cancer because of the possibility of other coexistent (synchronous) polyps or cancers.[74] Previously barium enema was the method of choice, but because of significant inaccuracy compared to colonoscopy its use is outdated except where an endoscope cannot be passed through a cancerous segment of the colon.[6, 19, 75] In such cases there may be a place for barium x-ray since barium often passes when endoscopy fails. Sometimes a markedly constricting carcinoma can be passed using a pediatric endoscope or after dilation by endoscopic means including laser photodestruction. When total colonoscopy is performed in patients with adenocarcinoma of the colon, synchronous cancers will be discovered in 3% to 4% of cases and synchronous adenomas will be found in 30% to 40%.[76, 77]

Endoscopic Therapy

Endoscopic therapy has rarely been considered in the management of colon carcinoma because confident assessment of the extent of spread (or resectability) has depended on the operative findings and the histologic findings of the surgical specimen, including the draining lymph nodes. In the future, the availability of increasingly accurate scanning techniques may define patients in whom only palliative measures are justified, since demonstration of distant metastases renders the carcinoma incurable. At present palliative surgical resection is justified clinically to remove the source of offensive rectal discharge and to eliminate the possibility of acute obstruction. There are a number of reports from endoscopic centers on partial endoscopic resection of inoperable colon cancers by electrosurgical means or laser[78]; the long-term results of this approach are unknown at present. Except in elderly patients, in whom operative mortality is clearly relevant, or for patients with rare anaplastic cancers of the colon, the slow-growing nature of most colorectal cancer may permit survival of 5 years or more after palliative surgery. If endoscopy is to become an alternative to palliative surgery the results must be at least comparable, and the endoscopic methods must be demonstrated to be safe and well tolerated by the majority of patients.

Colonoscopy in High-Risk Groups

Colonoscopy may have a role both in preventing cancer and in avoiding unnecessary surgery in groups of patients at high risk for colorectal adenocarcinoma. The cancer-family syndrome, in which cancer develops in first-degree relatives in the 30- to 40-year age group, is a rare but important clinical entity.[79] The anatomic distribution of cancers in such families is less weighted to the distal colon than in the general population, and sporadic polyps (as opposed to polyposis) may be found anywhere in the colon and are presumed antecedents of malignancy. In cancer-family members total colonoscopy is essential, probably at 2- to 3-year intervals, in the expectation either that cancer can be pre-

vented by destroying or snaring polyps or that cancer can be found at an early stage.

Patients in whom both ureters have been implanted into the colon (ureterosigmoidostomy) because of congenital or acquired bladder problems have a risk of colon cancer in the mucosa adjacent to the ureteric stomas that is hundreds of times greater than expected as a chance event.[80–82] It appears that this risk has greatest significance at 10 or more years after surgery. The risk probably remains even if the ureters have been reimplanted into an ileal conduit, unless the stomas and their adjacent colonic mucosa have been removed. The mechanism of carcinogenesis is unexplained, but local bacterial production of nitrosamines from urinary nitrates and nitrites is a plausible hypothesis. Preliminary experience suggests that 2- to 3-year surveillance by fiberoptic sigmoidoscopy will yield a significant number of localized adenomas.[80] Preliminary biopsies must be taken to ensure that any lesion to be snared is indeed neoplastic and not merely an inflammatory enlargement of the stoma. Depending on the surgeon's technique, an ureterosigmoidostomy may appear endoscopically as a small protrusion that is easily mistaken for a polyp (Plate 45–20). Endoscopy can be technically difficult and/or painful in these patients because of surgical fixation of the sigmoid loop; a pediatric instrument with a high degree of flexibility may be the preferred endoscope.

Chronic extensive ulcerative colitis, 8 to 10 years after onset, results in an increased risk of cancer that becomes more than 30 times that of normal individuals by 30 years.[83–85] Multiple cancers may occur in one colon and are often submucosal or underlie a superficial patch or plaque of roughened or irregular mucosa that on biopsy may be dysplastic.[51] The almost invariable association of cancer with overlying or adjacent epithelial dysplasia makes colonoscopy and biopsy at 1- to 2-year intervals mandatory in at-risk patients. Minor mucosal abnormalities are common in longstanding ulcerative colitis, and tumors, especially those in an early stage, are seldom diagnosed radiographically.[86] Dysplasia may be present in mucosa that is entirely flat and featureless at endoscopy. Although pedunculated adenomas may be found sporadically in patients with ulcerative colitis, nonpedunculated adenomas should be assessed with care, since they more likely represent colitis-related dysplasia, for which polypectomy

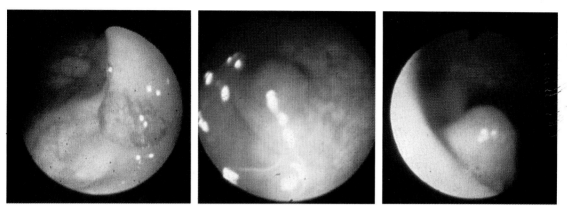

PLATE 45–20. Endoscopic appearance of normal ureteric stomas in sigmoid colon.

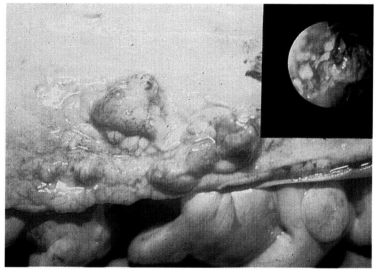

PLATE 45–21. Polypoid dysplasia in ulcerative colitis. Operative specimen with endoscopic view (including dye-spray highlighting nodular adjacent dysplastic mucosa).

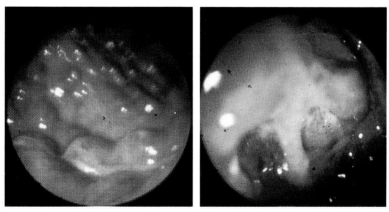

PLATE 45–22. PLATE 45–23.

PLATE 45–22. Multiple lymphomatous nodulesin disseminated lymphomatosis.
PLATE 45–23. Submucosal carcinomatous (ovarian) in sigmoid colon.

alone is not appropriate management. Biopsies taken from mucosa around the base of polypoid dysplasia will usually show abnormal dysplastic epithelium, whereas the mucosa around an adenoma should be histologically normal (Plate 45–21). The problem of adenocarcinoma and dysplasia in association with chronic ulcerative colitis is discussed in Chapter 43.

OTHER MALIGNANT TUMORS

Lymphoma or lymphosarcoma of the colon and rectum may occur as a solitary lesion or as part of a more widespread process. If solitary, the lesion may resemble a broad-based pale polyp at endoscopy, or it can be indistinguishable from carcinoma.[87] It may produce a submucosal or stricturing deformity that is difficult to diagnose, except when abnormal tissue protrudes into the lumen. The presence of multiple 5 to 7 mm polyps with a depressed center is characteristic of the diffuse form of lymphomatous involvement (Plate 45–22); gastroduodenoscopy will often show similar lesions, and this establishes the widespread nature of the process in a given patient. The importance of the histologic diagnosis of lymphoma lies in its responsiveness to chemotherapy or local radiotherapy rather than to surgical treatment. Reduction of the bulk of a localized tumor by piecemeal endoscopic resection may be justified provided that no undue risks are taken.

Kaposi's sarcoma (usually in AIDS patients) shows characteristic blue nodules in the mucosa from which diagnostic biopsies can be obtained.[88] This lesion is discussed in Chapters 42 and 46.

Carcinoid tumors diagnosed colonoscopically are usually localized and nonmetastatic and occur mainly in the rectum as small submucosal tumors; the diagnosis is made histologically. Patients are not subject to the systemic symptoms of the carcinoid syndrome (e.g., flushing) that occur with liver metastases from malignant carcinoids arising in the small intestine.

Melanomas are even rarer lesions occurring in the rectum. Since they are frequently nonpigmented, the diagnosis must be established histologically.

Metastatic carcinoma or carcinoma invading the colon from adjacent organs (e.g., pancreas, uterus, ovary, stomach) may have many endoscopic appearances, and thus diagnosis is difficult. The endoscopic features range from tissue edema or friability that may mimic mild ischemia to strictures or raised submucosal lesions that defy endoscopic diagnosis[89] (Plate 45–23). When the invading tumor reaches the colonic epithelium, it can frequently be differentiated from primary colonic adenocarcinoma histologically, except when the tumor is poorly differentiated.

FOLLOW-UP OF ADENOMA AND CARCINOMA

There is reasonable evidence of a significantly increased risk of both adenoma and carcinoma formation in the years after an adenoma or malignant lesion has been excised from the colon, the risk increasing with age and with the number of neoplastic lesions at the time of initial diagnosis.[90] Of patients who have had one cancer, 5% to 10% will develop another tumor, this occurring at an average interval of 13 years after diagnosis of the first carcinoma.[56] Ten years after an adenoma has been removed, further adenomas (mostly small) are expected in at least 20% to 30% of patients, and carcinomas in 2% to 4%. Furthermore, a redefinition of the exact future risk is required because much of the present evidence is based on inaccurate methods of assessment such as rigid proctosigmoidoscopy and single-contrast barium enema.

At each follow-up examination the whole colon should be examined because many cancers found occur proximal to the sigmoid colon and many of the polyps are proximal to the splenic flexure.[91] Rigid proctosigmoidoscopy alone gives a particularly low yield and should be abandoned as a method of follow-up; at least fiberoptic sigmoidoscopy should be performed if total colonoscopy is not available or technically too difficult to justify its repetition. Total colonoscopy is the preferred procedure, since it allows immediate polypectomy or biopsy and is more accurate than barium enema.[6] When necessary, double-contrast barium enema is acceptable for examination of the proximal colon because colonoscopic assessment is least accurate in this area,[6, 92] but it should be accompanied by fiberoptic sigmoidoscopy to increase the accuracy of assessment in the sigmoid colon. After sigmoid resection or formation of a colostomy, total colonoscopy is particularly easy and is almost always the method of choice for follow-up.

There is a significant risk of missing one or more small polyps during an initial colonoscopy. Therefore, a second total colonoscopy should be performed within one year of the first to establish that the colon has been cleared of all polyps ("clean colon") before initiating surveillance examinations at longer intervals.[93] Ideally these intervals should be determined according to the individual patient's long-term risk, but assessment of this is impossible by currently available data. Based on present evidence, it is probable that the presence of more than one neoplastic lesion at initial evaluation (e.g., two adenomas or one adenoma with a cancer) signifies a higher risk for the subsequent development of neoplastic lesions than that associated with a single adenoma, and that the risk is higher still if more than five adenomas are present initially.[91, 94–96] Also, patients older than 60 years are at higher risk than younger patients, and men are at higher risk than women.[91] Examination every 3 years should therefore be sufficient for younger patients with a single adenoma, and 2-year examinations are probably justified for older patients with more than one lesion. In some patients with numerous adenomas, annual follow-up is justified at least initially.

Whatever the follow-up colonoscopy plan adopted, patients should be warned to undergo endoscopy earlier than scheduled if suspicious symptoms occur, particularly bleeding. The problem of follow-up is essentially one of logistics[93]; too-frequent follow-up of the large numbers of potential patients is always unjustified, since the object is cancer prevention rather than "adenoma hunting."

Editor's note: The management of colorectal polyps that contain invasive malignancy continues to generate considerable discussion. References 97, 98, and 99 are some recent publications pertaining to this topic. There is also growing interest in laser ablation of colorectal polyps, discussed in references 100, 101, and 102. Finally, references 103, 104, and 105 are other recent publications of interest.

References

1. Macrae FA, St John DJB. Relationship between patterns of bleeding and hemoccult sensitivity in patients with colorectal cancers or adenomas. Gastroenterology 1982; 82:891–8.
2. Williams AR, Balasooriya BAW, Day DW. Polyps and cancer of the large bowel: a necroscopy study in Liverpool. Gut 1982; 23:835–42.
3. Eide TJ, Stalsberg H. Polyps of the large intestine in northern Norway. Cancer 1978; 42:2839–48.
4. Roe AM, Jamieson MH, Maclennan I. Colonoscopy preparation with Picolax. J R Coll Surg Edinb 1984; 29:103–4.
5. Marks G, Boggs HW, Castro F, et al. Sigmoidoscopic examinations with rigid and flexible fiberoptic sigmoidoscopes in the surgeon's office. Dis Colon Rectum 1979; 22:162–8.
6. Williams CB, Macrae FA, Bartram CI. A prospective study of diagnostic methods in adenoma follow-up. Endoscopy 1982; 14:74–8.
7. Grobe JL, Kozarek RA, Sanowski RA. Flexible versus rigid sigmoidoscopy: a comparison using an inexpensive 35 cm flexible proctosigmoidoscope. Am J Gastroenterol 1983; 78:569–71.
8. Bohlman TW, Katon RM, Lipshutz GR, et al. Fiberoptic pansigmoidoscopy. An evaluation and comparison with rigid sigmoidoscopy. Gastroenterology 1977; 72:644–9.
9. Winnan G, Berci G, Panish J, et al. Superiority of the flexible to the rigid sigmoidoscope in routine proctosigmoidoscopy. N Engl J Med 1980; 302:1011–2.
10. Winawer SJ, Leidner SD, Boyle C, et al. Comparison of flexible sigmoidoscopy with other diagnostic techniques in the diagnosis of rectocolon neoplasia. Dig Dis Sci 1979; 24:277–81.
11. Zucker GM, Madura MJ, Chmiel JS, et al. The advantages of the 30-cm flexible sigmoidoscope over the 60-cm flexible sigmoidoscope. Gastrointest Endosc 1984; 30:59–64.
12. Schapiro M. Flexible fiberoptic sigmoidoscopy—the long and short of it. Gastrointest Endosc 1984; 30:114–5.
13. Bond JH, Levitt MD. Colonic gas explosion—is a fire extinguisher necessary? Gastroenterology 1979; 77:1349–50.
14. Dodds WJ, Stewart ET, Hogan WJ. Role of colonoscopy and roentgenology in the detection of polypoid colonic lesions. Am J Dig Dis 1977; 22:646–9.
15. Gilbertsen VA, McHugh R, Schumann L, et al. The earlier detection of colorectal cancers: a preliminary report of the results of the occult blood study. Cancer 1980; 45:2899–901.
16. Welin S. Results of the Malmo technique of colon examination. JAMA 1967; 199:369–71.
17. Fork FT, Lindstrom C, Ekelund G. Double contrast examination in carcinoma of the colon and rectum. A prospective clinical series. Acta Radiol (Diag) 1983; 24:177–88.
18. Glerum J, Agenant D, Tytgat GNJ. Value of colonoscopy in the detection of sigmoid malignancy in patients with diverticular disease. Endoscopy 1977; 9:228–30.
19. Farrands PA, Vellacott KD, Amar SS, et al. Flexible fiberoptic sigmoidoscopy and double-contrast barium-enema examination in the identification of adenomas and carcinoma of the colon. Dis Colon Rectum 1983; 26:725–7.
20. Harned RK, Consigny PM, Cooper NB, et al. Barium examination following biopsy of the rectum or colon. Radiology 1982; 145:11–6.
21. Hussein AMJ, Bartram CI, Williams CB. Carbon dioxide insufflation for more comfortable colonoscopy. Gastrointest Endosc 1984; 30:68–70.

22. Williams CB. Colonoscopy in the prevention, detection and treatment of large bowel cancer. In: DeCosse JJ, Sherlock P, eds. Gastrointestinal Cancer. The Hague: Martinus Nijhoff, 1981; 227–54.

23. Cotton PB, Williams CB. Practical Gastrointestinal Endoscopy. Oxford: Blackwell Scientific Publications, 1980.

24. Waye J, Braunfeld S. Surveillance intervals after colonoscopic polypectomy. Endoscopy 1982; 14:79–81.

25. Lennard-Jones JE, Morson BC, Ritchie JK, et al. Cancer in colitis: assessment of the individual risk by clinical and histological criteria. Gastroenterology 1977; 73:1280–9.

26. Williams CB. Diverticular disease and strictures. In: Hunt RA, Waye JD, eds. Colonoscopy. Techniques, clinical practice and colour atlas. London: Chapman & Hall, 1981; 363–81.

27. Dixon AK, Fry IK, Morson BC, et al. Pre-operative computed tomography of carcinoma of the rectum. Br J Radiol 1981; 54:655–9.

28. Macrae FA, Tan KG, Williams CB. Towards safer colonoscopy: a report on the complications of 5000 diagnostic or therapeutic colonoscopies. Gut 1983; 24:376–83.

29. Christie JP. Colonoscopic excision of sessile polyps. Am J Gastroenterol 1976; 66:23–8.

30. Gillespie PE, Chambers TJ, Chan KW, et al. Colonic adenomas—a colonoscopy survey. Gut 1979; 20:240–5.

31. Granqvist S, Gabrielsson N, Sundelin P. Diminutive colonic polyps—clinical significance and management. Endoscopy 1979; 11:36–42.

32. Williams CB, Riddell RH. Colonic polyps and polypectomy. In: Schiller KFR, Salmon PR, eds. Colonoscopic polypectomy. Modern Topics in Gastrointestinal Endoscopy. London: Heinemann Medical Books, 1976; 245–74.

33. Feczko PJ, Bernstein MA, Halpert RD, et al. Small colonic polyps: a reappraisal of their significance. Radiology 1984; 152:301–3.

34. Williams CB. Diathermy-biopsy—a technique for the endoscopic management of small polyps. Endoscopy 1973; 5:215–8.

35. Kropp G. Massenpolypetktomien und Bergungsmodus im Kolon. Dtsch Med Wochenschr 1976; 101:19–20.

36. Hussein AMT, Medany S, Abou el Magd AM, et al. Multiple endoscopic polypectomies for schistosomal polyposis of the colon. Lancet 1983; 1:673–4.

37. Tada M, Katoh S, Kohli Y, Kawai K. On the dye spraying method in colonofiberoscopy. Endoscopy 1976; 8:70–4.

38. Maffioli C, Zeitoun P. Intérêt des colorations en endoscopie digestive. Gastroent Clin Biol 1979; 3:509–14.

39. Frühmorgen P, Demling L. Complications of diagnostic and therapeutic colonoscopy in the Federal Republic of Germany. Results of an enquiry. Endoscopy 1979; 11:146–50.

40. Gleason WA Jr, Goldstein PD, Shatz BA, et al. Colonoscopic removal of juvenile colonic polyps. J Pediatr Surg 1975; 10:519–21.

41. Douglas JR, Campbell CA, Salisbury DM, et al. Colonoscopic polypectomy in children. Br Med J 1981; 281:1386–7.

42. Stemper TJ, Kent TH, Summers RW. Juvenile polyposis and gastrointestinal carcinoma. A study of a kindred. Ann Intern Med 1975; 83:639–46.

43. Williams CB, Goldblatt M, Delaney PV. Top and tail endoscopy and follow-up in Peutz-Jeghers Syndrome. Endoscopy 1982; 14:82–4.

44. Morson BC, Dawson IMP. Gastrointestinal Pathology. Ed 2. Oxford: Blackwell Scientific Publications, 1979; 805.

45. De Beer RA, Shinya H. Colonic lipomas: an endoscopic analysis. Gastrointest Endosc 1975; 22:90–1.

46. Messer J, Waye JD. The diagnosis of colonic lipomas—the naked fat sign. Gastrointest Endosc 1982; 28:186–8.

47. Waye JD, Frankel A, Braunfeld SF. The histopathology of small colon polyps. (Abstr) Gastrointest Endosc 1980; 26:80.

48. Williams GT, Arthur JF, Bussey HJR, et al. Metaplastic polyps and polyposis of the colorectum. Histopathology 1980; 4:155–70.

49. Teague RH, Read AE. Polyposis in ulcerative colitis. Gut 1975; 16:792–5.

50. Lennard-Jones JE, Morson BC, Ritchie JK, et al. Cancer surveillance in ulcerative colitis. Experience over 15 years. Lancet 1983; 2:149–52.

51. Blackstone MO, Riddell RH, Rogers BHG, et al. Dysplasia-associated lesion or mass (DALM) detected by colonoscopy in longstanding ulcerative colitis: an indication for colectomy. Gastroenterology 1981; 80:366–74.

52. Coremans G, Rutgeerts P, Geboes K, et al. The value of ileoscopy with biopsy in the diagnosis of intestinal Crohn's disease. Gastrointest Endosc 1981; 30:167–72.

53. Price AB, Morson BC. Benign lymphoid polyps and inflammatory polyps. In: Morson BC, ed. The Pathogenesis of Colorectal Cancer. London: WB Saunders Co., 1978; 33–42.

54. Muto T, Bussey HJR, Morson BC. The evolution of cancer of the colon and rectum. Cancer 1975; 36:2251–70.

55. Shinya H, Wolff WI. Morphology, anatomic distribution and cancer potential of colonic polyps. An analysis of 7000 polyps endoscopically removed. Ann Surg 1979; 190:679–83.

56. Correa P, Haenszel W. The epidemiology of large-bowel cancer. Adv Cancer Res 1978; 26:1–141.

57. Brahme F, Ekelund GR, Norden JG, et al. Metachronous colorectal polyps; comparison of development of colorectal polyps and carcinomas in persons with or without histories of polyps. Dis Colon Rectum 1974; 17:166–71.

58. Gilbertsen VA, Nelms JM. The prevention of invasive cancer of the rectum. Cancer 1978; 41:1137–9.

59. Bussey HJR, Veale AMO, Morson BC. Genetics of gastrointestinal polyposis. Gastroenterology 1979; 74:1325–30.

60. Tonelli F, De Masi E, Astarita C, et al. Gastric and duodenal polyps associated with familial polyposis coli: personal experience and review of the literature. Ital J Gastroenterol 1981; 13:32–9.

61. Fenoglio CM. Symposium: Colonoscopy in 1977. Polyp-cancer controversy updated. NY State J Med 1978; 78:1889–92.

62. Morson BC, Bussey HJR, Samoorian S. Policy of local excision for early cancer of the colorectum. Gut 1977; 18:1045–50.

63. Morson BC, Whiteway JE, Jones EA, et al. Histopathology and prognosis of malignant colorectal polyps treated by endoscopic polypectomy. Gut 1984; 25:437–44.

64. Wolff WI, Shinya H. Definitive treatment of "malignant" polyps of the colon. Ann Surg 1975; 182:516–25.

65. Rossini FP, Ferrari A, Spandre M, et al. Colonoscopic polypectomy in diagnosis and management of cancerous adenomas: an individual and multicentre experience. Endoscopy 1982; 14:124–7.

66. Shinya H. Follow-up study of the colonoscopic management of colonic polyps with invasive cancer. (Abstr) Gastrointest Endosc 1979; 25:48.

67. Christie JP. Malignant colon polyps—cure by colonoscopy or colectomy? Am J Gastroenterol 1984; 79:543–7.

68. De Cosse JJ. Malignant colorectal polyp. Gut 1984; 25:433–6.

69. Colacchio TA, Forde KA, Scantlebury VP. Endoscopic polypectomy: inadequate treatment for invasive colorectal carcinoma. Ann Surg 1981; 194:704–7.

70. Morson BC, Bussey HJR. Predisposing causes of intestinal cancer. Curr Probl Surg 1970; 1–46.

71. Kline TS, Yum KK. Fiberoptic colonoscopy and cytology. Cancer 1976; 37:2553–6.

72. Winawer SJ, Leinder SD, Hajdu SI, et al. Colonoscopic biopsy and cytology in the diagnosis of colon cancer. Cancer 1978; 42:2849–53.

73. Hunt RH, Teague RH, Swarbrick ET, Williams CB. Colonoscopy in the management of colonic structures. Br Med J 1975; 3:360–1.

74. Unger SW. Colonoscopy: an essential monitoring technique after resection of colorectal cancer. Am J Surg 1983; 145:71–6.

75. von Goumoens E, Nuesch HJ, Kobler E, et al. Wie Sicher ist die Radiologie in der Kolonkarzinomdiagnostic. Schweiz Med Wochenschr 1982; 107:533–4.

76. Langevin JM, Nivatvongs S. The true incidence of synchronous cancer of the large bowel. A prospective study. Am J Surg 1984; 147:330–3.

77. Maxfield RG. Colonoscopy as a routine preoperative procedure for carcinoma of the colon. Am J Surg 1984; 147:477–80.

78. Grossier VW. YAG laser therapy of gastrointestinal tumors. Gastrointest Endosc 1984; 30:311–2.

79. Lynch HT, Harris RE, Organ CH Jr, et al. The surgeon, genetics, and cancer control: the cancer family syndrome. Ann Surg 1977; 185:435–40.

80. Stewart M, Macrae FA, Williams CB. Neoplasia and ureterosigmoidostomy: a colonoscopy survey. Br J Surg 1982; 69:414–6.

81. Thompson PM, Hill JT, Packham DA. Colonic carcinoma at the site of ureterosigmoidostomy: what is the risk? Br J Surg 1979; 66:809.

82. Rossini FP, Ferrari A, Rizello N. Fiberendoscopic evaluation of ureterosigmoidostomies. Endoscopy 1979; 11:249–52.

83. Fuson JA, Farmer RG, Hawk A, et al. Endoscopic surveillance for cancer in chronic ulcerative colitis. Am J Gastroenterol 1980; 73:120–6.

84. Butt JH, Lennard-Jones JE, Ritchie JK. A practical approach to the risk of cancer in inflammatory bowel disease. Med Clin North Am 1980; 64:1203–20.

85. Yardley JH, Bayless TM, Diamond MP. Cancer in ulcerative colitis. Gastroenterology 1979; 76:221–5.

86. Frank PH, Riddell RH, Feczko PJ, et al. Radiological detection of colonic dysplasia (pre-carcinoma) in chronic ulcerative colitis. Gastrointest Radiol 1978; 3:209–19.

87. Greene FL, Livstone EM, McAllister WB Jr, et al. Reticulum cell sarcoma of the large intestine. The role of fiberoptic colonoscopy. Am J Digest Dis 1974; 19:379–84.

88. Tavassolie H, Mir-Madjlessi SH, Sadr-Ameli M-A. The endoscopic demonstration of Kaposi's sarcoma of the colon. Gastrointest Endosc 1983; 29:331–2.

89. Geboes K, De Wolf-Peeters C, Rutgeert P, et al. Submucosal tumors of the colon: experience with twenty-five cases. Dis Colon Rectum 1978; 21:420–5.

90. Morson BC. The evolution of colorectal carcinoma. Clin Radiol 1984; 35:425–31.

91. Macrae FA, Williams CB. Identification of risk factors in follow-up of patients with adenomas. Gut (in press)

92. Laufer I, Smith NCW, Mullens JE. The radiological demonstration of colorectal polyps undetected by endoscopy. Gastroenterology 1976; 70:167–70.

93. Williams CB. The logic and logistics of colon polyp follow-up. In: Glass GBJ, Sherlock P, eds. Progress in Gastroenterology. Vol 4. New York: Grune & Stratton, 1983; 513–25.

94. Kirsner JB, Rider JA, Moeller HC, et al. Polyps of the colon and rectum. Statistical analysis of a long-term follow-up study. Gastroenterology 1960; 39:178–82.

95. Kronborg O, Hage E, Adamsen S, et al. Follow-up after colorectal polypectomy. II. Repeated examinations of the colon every 6 months after removal of sessile adenomas and adenomas with the highest degrees of dysplasia. Scand J Gastroenterol 1983; 18:1095–99.

96. Deyhle P. Results of endoscopic polypectomy in the gastrointestinal tract. Endoscopy 1980; (suppl):35–46.

97. Haggitt RC, Glotzbach RE, Soffer EE, Wruble LD. Prognostic factors in colorectal carcinomas arising in adenomas: implications for lesions removed by endoscopic polypectomy. Gastroenterology 1985; 89:328–36.

98. Cranley JP, Petras RE, Carey WD, et al. When is endoscopic polypectomy adequate therapy for colonic polyps containing invasive carcinoma? Gastroenterology 1986; 91:419–27.

99. Wilcox GM, Anderson PB, Colacchio TA. Early invasive carcinoma in colonic polyps. A review of the literature with emphasis on the assessment of the risk of metastasis. Cancer 1986; 57:160–71.

100. Brunetaud JM, Mosquet L, Houcke M, et al. Villous adenomas of the rectum. Results of endoscopic treatment with argon and Nd:YAG lasers. Gastroenterology 1985; 89:832–7.

101. Mathus-Vliegen EMH, Tytgat GNJ. Nd:YAG laser photocoagulation in colorectal adenoma. Evaluation of its safety, usefulness and efficacy. Gastroenterology 1986; 90:1866–73.

102. Brunetaud JM, Maunoury V, Ducrotte P, et al. Palliative treatment of rectosigmoid carcinoma by laser endoscopic photoablation. Gastroenterology 1987; 92:663–8.

103. Nivatvongs S. Complications in colonoscopic polypectomy. An experience with 1,555 polypectomies. Dis Colon Rectum 1986; 29:825–30.

104. Aldridge MC, Sim AJ. Colonoscopy findings in symptomatic patients without X-ray evidence of colonic neoplasms. Lancet 1986; 2:833–4.

105. Larson GM, Bond SJ, Shallcross C, et al. Colonoscopy after curative resection of colorectal cancer. Arch Surg 1986; 121:535–40.

Chapter 46

MISCELLANEOUS DISORDERS OF THE COLON

BARRY J. LUMB, M.B., F.R.C.P.(C)
RICHARD H. HUNT, M.B., F.R.C.P., F.R.L.P.(C)

A number of miscellaneous conditions are important to the colonoscopist. These may be considered in two broad groups: those that constitute an indication for colonoscopy and those that the colonoscopist may encounter by chance during an examination for a specific but unrelated reason.

CONDITIONS IN WHICH COLONOSCOPY IS INDICATED

Diverticular Disease

Diverticular disease is particularly common in Western countries where it occurs in approximately 10% of patients over age 40 and 35% of patients over age 60.[1] About 10% of patients with diverticular disease will have evidence of hypertrophy of the colonic musculature.[2] Left-sided diverticular disease is the most common (Plate 46–1). This may be silent, or have presenting symptoms of discomfort localized to the left iliac fossa and alteration of bowel habits. These are also the common symptoms of the irritable bowel. Local inflammation can occur and lead to diverticulitis and occasionally perforation with local abscess formation.

Severe disease can present diagnostic problems for both the clinician and the radiologist. In advanced cases, distortion of the sigmoid by circular muscle spasm, fibrosis, and adhesions prevents adequate demonstration of this colonic segment by double contrast barium enema even if the study is of the highest quality possible.[3] In the presence of diverticular disease, carcinoma, a polyp, or inflammatory bowel disease cannot be excluded radiographically. Since diverticular disease and colonic cancer are both more common in the elderly, this association by age provides a rationale for fiberoptic examination in this group of patients. Although laparotomy was heretofore often required for diagnosis because of these problems colonoscopy is now of proved benefit in diverticular disease.[4–6] The results of five reported studies that evaluated colonoscopy in the diagnosis of complicated diverticular disease are listed in Table 46–1.[4, 7–11]

Diverticular disease may result in colonic bleeding that is clinically mild, moderate, or severe. In a review of more than 5000 patients with diverticular disease, Rigg and Ewing[12] reported that 15% had evidence of bleeding. In other reports bleeding was evident in 5% to 41% of patients. More recent studies suggest that minor bleeding is often due to additional associated pathology, whereas massive bleeding, which may occur from the right or left colon,[13] is usually caused by recurrent damage to a diverticulum.[14]

Colonoscopy may be technically difficult and occasionally impossible in patients with severe diverticular disease. Adhesions with fixation of the bowel and luminal distortion seem to be the main reasons for failure to intubate the colon in patients with severe diverticular disease, and success does not seem to be improved by increasing the dosage of sedation or the administration of antispasmodic drugs (Plate 46–2). When the process is long-standing, wide-mouthed diverticula are often present, of which one or more might be falsely interpreted as the lumen. Consequent intubation is potentially hazardous, as it can result in perforation either directly from instrumentation or from excessive air insufflation.[15] At colonoscopy, the well-visualized and perfectly round lumen is unlikely to be the true lumen; rather, the correct channel is usually poorly seen and distorted by irregular mucosal folds and often lies at 90 degrees from the diverticular orifice.[6] Even when intubation of the diseased segment is successful, visualization of the entire mucosal surface may be inadequate because of the associated distortion. Examination of the areas immediately proximal to hypertrophic interhaustral septa may be especially difficult (see Chapter 40 for technique of examination "behind" colonic folds). Therefore, the risk of a false-negative result of colonoscopy is somewhat greater in the presence of severe diverticular disease.[7] Fluoroscopy may be helpful when difficulty with intubation or observation is encountered in relation to diverticular disease.[4, 16]

Acquired Immune Deficiency Syndrome (AIDS) and Sexually Transmitted Diseases

Multiple, simultaneous enteric infections and traumatic anorectal lesions in homosexual men are becoming increasingly recognized.[17, 18] This group of disorders has been collectively referred to as the "Gay Bowel" syndrome.[19, 20] The infectious agents consist of the common venereal agents as well as organisms usually associated with food contamination (Salmonella and Shigella, etc.), tropical illness (Giardia lamblia and Entamoeba histolytica) and parenteral exposure (Hepatitis B and cytomegalovirus [CMV], etc.).[17, 18, 21] The most common presentation is nonspecific proctitis accompanied by one or more of the following complaints: abdominal pain, diarrhea, rectal pain, discharge, and bleeding. The appearance at flexible sigmoidoscopic or colonoscopic examination may be indistinguishable from idiopathic inflammatory bowel disease.[18] The histologic appearance may be non-specific, although some distinguishing characteristics are now being recognized.[18, 21, 22] Diagnosis depends on a high index of suspicion, a detailed history and physical examination, and careful, repeated stool microscopy and culture.

AIDS in previously healthy homosexual men was first described in 1981.[23] By December 1983, over 3000 cases were reported from 42 states in the United States and from 20 other countries.[24] The syndrome has also been recognized in other groups such as those who use illicit intravenous drugs, Haitians, hemophiliacs, female sexual partners of men in high-risk categories, and recipients of blood transfusion from high-risk groups. The underlying immune defect is caused by a viral transmissible agent having an incubation period in excess of one year.[25, 26]

Diagnosis of AIDS requires documentation of an underlying acquired immunodeficiency together with the presence of unusual opportunistic infections (e.g., Pneumocystis carinii) or development of Kaposi's sarcoma or other associated lymphoid malignancy (e.g., Burkitt's lymphoma).[25] In addition, a chronic lymphadenopathy syndrome has been described which may represent a prodrome to AIDS in some patients.[25, 26] Earlier diagnosis and improved supportive measures have led to an apparent decline in mortality (43%); however, Fauci et al.[25] believe that it may eventually approach 100%.

In addition to the wide variety of enteric infestations that occur in homosexual men, there are a few infections unique to patients with AIDS.[25–27] Cryptosporidia are tiny coccidial protozoans that inhabit the microvillus region of intestinal epithelial surfaces. This pathogen has been known to cause an enterocolitic illness in calves and other domestic

TABLE 46–1. **Colonoscopy in Diverticular Disease**

Author	No. Patients	Patients with Carcinoma	Patients with Polyps
Dean and Newell[7]	36	4 (11%)	NSa
Greene et al.[8]	32	7 (22%)	12 (37%)
Hunt et al.[4]	39	6 (15%)	6 (15%)
Sugarbaker et al.[9]	18	4 (22%)	NSa
Boulos et al.[11]	46	3 (14%)	8 (17%)
Total	171	24 (14%)	26 (17%)

NSa = not stated.

animals, and since 1976 several reports have described an acute diarrheal illness in animal workers and immunocompromised patients. In otherwise healthy patients, this is usually a self-limiting illness.[28]

In AIDS and other immunodeficient patients, cryptosporidia may cause a profound watery diarrhea syndrome, the mechanism of which is not currently understood. In contrast to infections in immunologically normal patients, both large and small bowel may be infected.[26, 28–31] Conventional stool examination may be inadequate to detect the organism, and new, more specific techniques are being developed.[28] The laboratory and pathologist should be alerted when this infection is suspected. In particular, biopsy specimens should be very carefully examined for evidence of the protozoan on epithelial surfaces.[29, 31] Electron microscopy may be helpful in some cases.[29, 32] Since colonic involvement has been documented, colonoscopy with multiple biopsies may be diagnostic and is indicated in all cases. The diagnosis of this infection in a patient with AIDS is particularly ominous, since no effective treatment is available and severe morbidity may result.[26, 28–31, 33]

CMV infection is common in the homosexual population, and this virus has been implicated in the pathogenesis of AIDS.[25] Solitary mucosal ulceration caused by CMV has been described in immunocompromised patients such as renal transplant recipients.[34] Knapp et al.[35] reported a case of patchy colonic ulceration in a homosexual man that was initially diagnosed and treated as Crohn's disease; however, subsequent blood, urine, and open lung biopsy cultures were positive for CMV. Careful review of the original histologic specimens from the colon showed the presence of intracellular inclusion bodies characteristic of CMV, and upper gastrointestinal endoscopy revealed similar changes in the gastric and duodenal mucosa.[35] Gertler et al.[36] have also described a homosexual man with disseminated CMV infection involving the esophagus and colon. Flexible sigmoidoscopy showed scattered, yellow-green adherent plaques 2 to 3 mm in diameter surrounded by hyperemic mucosa suggestive of pseudomembranous colitis; however, all cultures and toxin assay for *Clostridium difficile* were negative. At autopsy, multiple, tiny, ulcerating lesions were seen in the cecum and ascending colon, with microscopic changes typical of CMV confined to the ulcerated area.

Kaposi[37] first described patients with "multiple idiopathic sarcoma of skin" in 1872. Prior to the recognition of AIDS, three forms of this condition were known. In North America and Europe it occurs as a localized, nodular tumor on the lower limbs of elderly men, frequently of Ashkenazi Jewish or Mediterranean ancestry. The lesions vary in color from red to blue, are noninvasive, and tend to follow an indolent course with good response to chemotherapy or radiotherapy. In equatorial Africa, a disseminated and invasive form of this disease occurs in young men, usually resulting in a rapidly fatal outcome. Finally, reports of Kaposi's sarcoma occurring in patients with immune deficiency have been described.[26]

Up to December 22, 1983, approximately 34% of AIDS patients reported to the Centers for Disease Control (CDC) in the United States developed Kaposi's sarcoma.[24] Gastrointestinal involvement in cases of Kaposi's sarcoma has been documented in the past; however, in AIDS patients the incidence is much higher and probably exceeds 50% of those with skin lesions.[20, 26, 38–40] In several case reports, the first evidence of Kaposi's sarcoma was found in the stomach, colon, or rectum.[26, 38–40] Oral lesions are highly suggestive of other gastrointestinal lesions.[20]

There is a high incidence of gastrointestinal symptoms in patients with AIDS, and it is difficult to define precisely which features are related to Kaposi's sarcoma. The lesions are frequently asymptomatic; however, overt rectal bleeding, melena, diarrhea, weight loss, abdominal pain, intussusception, obstruction, and perforation have been reported.[25, 26, 38, 39]

There are several diverse descriptions of the colonoscopic appearance of Kaposi's sarcoma.[26, 38, 39, 41–43] One consistent feature is the presence of pigmentation ranging from strawberry red to deep purple. Flat, macular, and polypoid forms have been found that range in size from a few millimeters to several centimeters. The lesions are situated in the submucosa and, although there may be ulceration, superficial biopsy specimens may be negative.[26] Consideration should therefore be given to the use of a larger coagulation biopsy forceps or a polypectomy snare to obtain an adequate specimen.

Gottlieb et al.[26] have recommended complete gastrointestinal investigation of patients with proven or suspected Kaposi's sarcoma, both for pretreatment staging and accurate follow-up. The frequent occurrence of flat lesions suggests that endoscopy is superior to double-contrast radiography for this assessment. During treatment, follow-up by endoscopy has revealed a response to therapy similar to that of cutaneous lesions.

Health care workers should exercise precautions with blood and secretions from patients with AIDS. The CDC have published guidelines for workers who may be exposed to laboratory samples or who are in direct contact with AIDS patients.[44] Endoscopic equipment should be gas-sterilized after use.

Aspects of the "Gay Bowel" syndrome are also discussed in Chapter 42.

Behçet's Syndrome

Behçet's syndrome is a chronic inflammatory disorder of unknown etiology originally described as a triad of aphthous stomatitis, genital ulceration, and ocular inflammation.[45] Subsequently, it has been shown to be a multisystem disorder with articular, vascular, respiratory, cutaneous, neurologic, and gastrointestinal abnormalities.[46, 47] The diagnosis of the syndrome is hampered by the variable clinical manifestations, the frequent delay in their onset, a lack of pathognomonic laboratory features, and a clinical course characterized by exacerbations and remissions.[47] Attempts have been made to define specific diagnostic criteria. Mason and Barnes[48] have identified four major ones: buccal and genital ulceration, eye lesions, and skin lesions. Minor criteria consist of typical involvement of other systems such as non-erosive arthritis, occlusive vascular lesions, meningoencephalitis, and gastrointestinal ulceration. It has been proposed that a minimum of three major criteria or two major and two minor criteria be present to confirm the diagnosis.[48] However, because of the very high incidence of oral ulceration (98%), the diagnosis should probably be provisional if this symptom is absent.[49]

There is a marked variability in the worldwide distribution of Behçet's syndrome. The prevalence is estimated at 0.3 per 100,000 in the United States, 0.6 in Great Britain, and 10 in Japan.[50] Israel and other Middle East countries have an incidence approaching that of Japan.[46] The incidence is increasing in Japan, where it is higher in the northern part of the country.[51] Major morbidity is usually a consequence of neurologic or intestinal involvement or vascular occlusion. In Japan, the syndrome accounts for up to 12% of all acquired causes of blindness before middle age.[47]

Minor gastrointestinal symptoms have been reported in up to 50% of cases. These include abdominal pain, nausea and vomiting, weight loss, malabsorption, constipation, and diarrhea. Significant intestinal involvement is much less common and occurs as a consequence of mucosal ulceration.[47, 48] Lesions have been described throughout the intestinal tract; however, the ileocecal area is most likely to be affected.[46, 48, 50–53]

Major gastrointestinal symptoms and signs also vary. Severe abdominal pain is common, and a symptom complex identical to acute appendicitis has been frequently reported.[51] Bleeding per rectum, with or without associated diarrhea, is also a common presenting symptom.[52] Sudden perforation, which may occur in several locations, may be recurrent, and may occur without warning, is a major source of morbidity and mortality.[51, 54] As a result of this variability in presentation, the preoperative diagnosis in one series was correct in only 22% of 136 patients.[51]

Radiologically the classic description is of a "collar-button"–like ulcer that is well circumscribed and discrete, with even, raised edges.[55] However, there is considerable variability, the appearances ranging from irregular edges to linear ulcers with fissuring.[46, 51–53, 56] The classic radiologic appearance of Crohn's disease or ulcerative colitis has been described in several case reports.[52, 54, 56] The absence of mucosal thickening, luminal narrowing, and preservation of the haustral marking may aid in differentiating Behçet's disease from idiopathic forms of inflammatory bowel disease.[55]

Reports of the colonoscopic appearance of Behçet's colitis typically describe features similar to those barium studies with discrete, well circumscribed ulcers with raised edges and mild surrounding erythema (Plate 46–3); but again, marked variability has been noted.[47, 51, 52, 56] Smith et al.[52] have reported a vesicular lesion that they speculated as representing an early form of an ulcer. Since penetration into the submucosa and muscularis mucosa can occur, care should be taken to avoid overdistention during double contrast barium enema or colonoscopy.[52] Carbon dioxide might be used for luminal distention in this situation, since absorption of any residual gas is much more rapid than air. Biopsies should probably be taken only from the edge of an ulcer as another precaution in avoiding perforation.

Clearly, the presence of colonic ulceration can cause difficulty in differentiating Behçet's colitis from idiopathic ulcerative colitis and Crohn's disease. This is particularly true in those patients with Behçet's syndrome who present with gastrointestinal symptoms or those in whom gastrointestinal symptoms predominate. This is further complicated by the similarity between the extracolonic manifestations of inflammatory bowel disease and the major criteria of Mason and Barnes[48] and others.[47, 52] Predominant involvement of the ileocecal area, with discrete ulcers and normal intervening mucosa, usually suggests the possibility of Crohn's disease as a first consideration. Furthermore, rectovaginal fistula formation has been observed in at least two patients with Behçet's syndrome.[52]

The usual histologic description is of very deep, sharply demarcated ulcers with chronic inflammatory cell infiltrates. Unfortunately, crypt abscess formation and the presence of noncaseating granulomas have also been described in otherwise well-documented cases of Behçet's syndrome, further complicating the differential diagnosis.[52] However, the existence of genital ulceration in 80% of patients,[46] the occurrence of free perforation, and unusual radiologic features should help to correctly diagnose this rare condition.

Pseudomembranous Colitis

Prior to the 1940's pseudomembranous colitis (PMC) was characteristically a catastrophic complication that followed abdominal surgery. With the introduction of antimicrobial agents PMC became more commonly associated with their administration and was thought to arise as a consequence of *Staphylococcus aureus* overgrowth.[57] In 1977, Rifkin et al.[58] reported that the disease was mediated by an enterotoxin that could be neutralized by the *Clostridium sordelli* antitoxin. Shortly afterward two groups of investigators simultaneously isolated *Clostridium difficile* from patients with PMC and demonstrated that this organism could reproduce all the clinical features of the disease and

that it produced an enterotoxin that cross-reacted with the *Clostridium sordelli* antitoxin.[59, 60] Specific techniques to isolate this agent and identify the enterotoxin are now widely available.

The vast majority of patients in whom PMC develops have a history of recent exposure to antibiotics. Although clindamycin was implicated as the most likely antibiotic, it is now clear that the disease can occur following the administration of any antibiotic, aside from vancomycin hydrochloride and the aminoglycosides.[61, 62] There are still occasional cases following surgery in which antibiotics were not used;[57] the disease may also occur spontaneously.[63]

Clostridium difficile has been isolated extensively in the environment of patients with PMC and has also been recovered in the stools and on the hands of hospital staff caring for these patients.[64, 65] This has obvious implications with respect to the pathogenesis of PMC and suggests that the use of enteric precautions for patients suspected of having PMC may be of practical importance.

Clinically, PMC is characterized by diarrhea, abdominal pain, fever, and leukocytosis during antibiotic therapy or as long as 6 weeks after it has been discontinued.[61, 62] The severity of the illness varies. In a prospective study Tedesco et al.[66] showed that typical pseudomembranes were frequently present at sigmoidoscopy in patients who developed only mild diarrhea while taking clindamycin.

The diagnosis of PMC depends on recognition of the appropriate clinical setting, together with endoscopic demonstration of pseudomembranes, positive stool cultures, and toxin assay.[61] Price and Davies[67] have proposed a histologic grading system that has gained popular acceptance.

Endoscopic examination is essential to the diagnosis of PMC. Typically, multiple elevated yellowish–white plaques that vary in size from a few millimeters to complete confluence of the bowel surface are found. The intervening mucosa may be normal or hyperemic and edematous. In areas in which pseudomembranes have not developed, the appearance may be similar to idiopathic inflammatory bowel disease.[61] If classic pseudomembranes are discovered, then appropriate therapy can be instituted before the results of culture or toxin assay are known. The colonoscopic appearance of pseudomembranous colitis is described further in Chapter 42.

In the majority of patients, rigid sigmoidoscopy will be sufficient to establish the diagnosis;[62] however, rectal sparing clearly occurs.[68–72] In 1978, Seppala[69] reported a case of PMC in which sigmoidoscopy showed nonspecific inflammation only. Subsequent colonoscopy, without preparation, demonstrated typical changes of PMC beginning 30 cm from the anus. He recommended that all patients in whom the diagnosis of PMC is strongly suspected have colonoscopy if rigid sigmoidoscopy is not diagnostic. Tedesco[71] also described 6 patients with culture proven *Clostridium difficile* overgrowth but negative sigmoidoscopy. In 5 of these 6 patients colonoscopy revealed typical pseudomembranes scattered throughout the colon. A later, prospective, trial of colonoscopy showed that in 5 of 22 patients the first evidence of pseudomembrane formation appeared more than 25 cm from the anus.[72] Seppala et al[70] also conducted a prospective assessment in 16 patients. They found typical changes at sigmoidoscopy in only 5 patients; 11 of 13 patients who underwent colonoscopy had pseudomembranes beginning at 30 cm from the anus.

Colonoscopy in these patients may be difficult because of the large amounts of mucus and debris that may be present; however, the colonoscope need not be advanced beyond the first clear evidence of pseudomembranes. Because toxic dilation has been described in PMC,[61] overdistention of the colon should be avoided.

Up to 14% of patients may have a relapse following completion of therapy.[73, 74] Bartlett et al.[73] have shown that at colonoscopy done during remission there is complete resolution of the lesions. When patients were re-examined during relapse there was clear evidence of recurrent pseudomembrane formation.

In summary, sigmoidoscopy and stool culture are usually sufficient to confirm the diagnosis of PMC; however, if the diagnosis is strongly suspected despite negative sigmoidoscopy, patients should undergo early colonoscopy.

Endometriosis

Infiltration of the gastrointestinal tract by endometrial tissue should be considered in the differential diagnosis of lower abdominal pain in women of reproductive age. The clinical manifestations arise as a consequence of the normal hormonal response of ectopic endometrial tissue.[75, 76] Estimates of the frequency of endometriosis have been limited by the unknown incidence of asymptomatic disease. The prevalence has been crudely estimated at 10% to 15% of premenopausal women.[77, 78] Williams and Pratt[79] reported a prospective series in which 485 of 968 women undergoing pelvic exploration had evidence of endometriosis. Since these patients were referred for gynecologic consultation, this is certainly an overestimate of the prevalence of the disease in women with a complaint of lower abdominal pain. Earlier studies noted that gastrointestinal structures lying in the pelvic region are more likely to be involved.[78] Williams and Pratt[79] found macroscopic evidence of involvement of the rectosigmoid in 172 patients, the ileum in 9, and the appendix in 17. Clinical evidence of obstruction was found in only 1 patient preoperatively, but 7 patients required bowel resection after the extent of disease became apparent during laparotomy.

The pathogenesis of endometriosis is not understood. Initially, the serosa is involved and under cyclic hormonal influences the islands of the endometrium may differentiate into glandular tissue and enlarge to invade the subserosa and submucosa.[75, 78] Considerable fibrosis and smooth muscle hypertrophy may also occur but mucosal invasion is rare. Rectal bleeding is therefore an uncommon manifestation, and a search for an alternative lesion should be initiated even in patients with known endometriosis.[75] Bleeding secondary to tissue ischemia and ulceration has been described in a patient with intussusception complicating endometriosis.[80]

A temporal change in symptoms and signs during the menstrual cycle is distinctive[75, 79] but not diagnostic, since changes in hormone levels can also influence normal gastrointestinal function, especially motility and thereby produce symptoms.[81] Associated menstrual complaints are also common. All patients suspected of having endometriosis should have a careful pelvic examination; special attention should be focused on the area of the cul de sac, as ectopic tissue is commonly found in this location.[75] In contrast to malignant disease, pain on palpation of infiltrated areas is characteristic.[78]

The radiologic differential diagnosis of a mass involving the distal small bowel or colon includes primary and metastatic carcinoma, lymphoma, inflammatory bowel disease, abscess, and adhesions, in addition to endome-

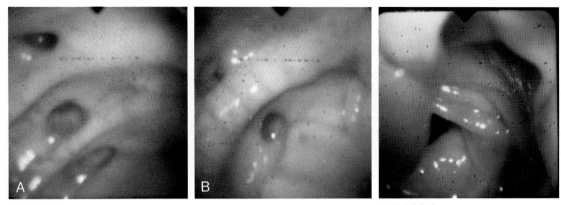

PLATE 46–1.   PLATE 46–2.

PLATE 46–1. *A,* Colonoscopic view of sigmoid diverticula. *B,* Colonoscopic view showing sigmoid diverticula and hypertrophic interhaustral septa. (Courtesy M.V. Sivak, Jr., M.D.)
PLATE 46–2. Severe diverticular disease of sigmoid colon with associated hypertrophy of interhaustral septa, spasm, and deformity. (Courtesy M.V. Sivak, Jr., M.D.)

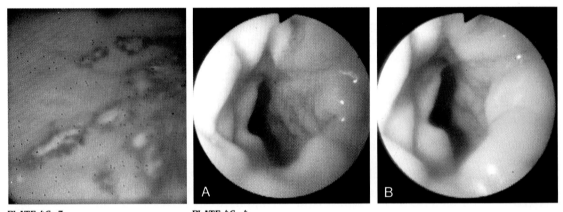

PLATE 46–3.   PLATE 46–4.

PLATE 46–3. Ulcers of Behcet's syndrome at colonoscopy.
PLATE 46–4. *A,* Constriction of distal sigmoid colon in patient with endometriosis. *B,* Submucosal nodules are noted on close inspection, but mucosa is intact. (Courtesy M.V. Sivak, Jr., M.D.)

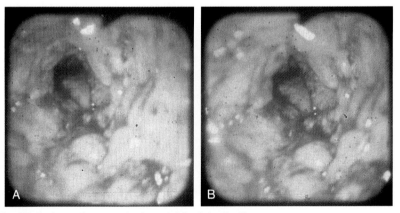

PLATE 46–5. Polyp-like lesions of pneumatosis cystoides intestinalis.

triosis.[82] If the lesion is large, differentiation from primary colonic carcinoma may be difficult.[83, 84] McSwain et al.[85] noted a correct preoperative radiologic diagnosis in only 6 of 11 women who underwent a barium enema. At laparotomy the surgeon's impression of the resected specimen was accurate in only 6 of 14 cases. With smaller lesions, identification of an extraluminal mass is more straightforward.[86, 87] Double-contrast imaging undoubtedly improves diagnostic accuracy.[88]

The role of colonoscopy in endometriosis is not well established. There may be a clear indication for colonoscopy in any patient with symptoms of rectal bleeding, major alteration of bowel habit, lower abdominal pain, or a radiologic diagnosis of an intrinsic or extrinsic mass lesion. At least one group has recommended colonoscopy prior to laparotomy for all patients with endometriosis to rule out significant asymptomatic colon infiltration.[89] An impression of extrinsic compression or occasionally bluish submucosal discoloration may be the only endoscopic abnormality (Plate 46–4). Normal overlying mucosa virtually excludes the possibility of a colonic neoplasm. Biopsy is only rarely diagnostic, since the lesions are submucosal. If the diagnosis is not confirmed after barium contrast studies and colonoscopy, then laparoscopy may clarify the situation.

CONDITIONS THAT MAY BE ENCOUNTERED INCIDENTALLY

Pneumatosis Cystoides Intestinalis

Pneumatosis cystoides intestinalis (PCI) is an unusual condition characterized by the occurrence of multiple, gas-filled cysts in the submucosa and subserosa of the small and large intestine. Occasionally, the stomach, mesentery, and omentum may also be involved.[75]

It has been suggested that the disease be classified into two categories, depending on the presence of other gastrointestinal disease.[90] The primary form occurs in the absence of any other known gastrointestinal disease and has been associated classically with chronic pulmonary disease.[90, 91] Secondary PCI has been associated with complications of endoscopy, including biopsy and polypectomy, but is most commonly associated with pyloroduodenal obstruction.

Although it is clear that both large and small bowel may be involved with these lesions, the frequency of large bowel involvement remains somewhat controversial. In re-

viewing the literature, Koss[91] found only 13 of 213 cases had involvement of the colon alone. A later review by Ecker et al.[90] supported this conclusion. However, more recently several authors have suggested that recognition of colonic involvement is becoming more frequent.[92, 93]

The pathogenesis of PCI has been widely debated; none of the current theories adequately account for both the development and persistence of these cysts.[94, 95] The "mechanical" theory suggests that gas from ruptured pulmonary alveoli may dissect along tissue planes and localize in the intestinal wall. Alternatively, disruption of the intestinal mucosa secondary to obstruction, surgical anastomosis, or instrumentation may allow luminal gas to localize in the intestinal wall. Animal experiments have confirmed that air injected into the mediastinum can dissect through the posterior mediastinum and mesenteric vascular tree to produce a picture similar to PCI.[75] However, this theory does not account for the perpetuation of these cysts, since extraluminal gas in other locations is rapidly reabsorbed.[92] The "biochemical" theory proposes that excess gas produced as a consequence of bacterial metabolism diffuses across the gut wall and is held in equilibrium with blood diffusion. A variety of studies have provided indirect support for this theory. Forgacs et al.[94] have shown that hydrogen may constitute almost half of the gas in these cysts. Hydrogen is produced only as a result of bacterial fermentation, and excess breath hydrogen has been documented in some patients with PCI.[96, 97] Furthermore, improvement in patients with PCI has been documented after administration of metronidazole[98] and other antibiotics that inhibit gut bacteria as well as after the use of elemental diets that decrease the amount of carbohydrate reaching the colonic bacteria.[97] It is most likely that this condition is multifactorial in origin with no single mechanism accounting for all of the clinical features described.

A wide range of symptoms have been associated with PCI but it may also be asymptomatic and, therefore, discovered during radiologic investigation of the abdomen for other reasons.[99] Abdominal pain, diarrhea, constipation, obstruction, intussusception, volvulus, perforation, and the presence of blood, mucus, or pus by rectum are said to be associated with PCI.[75, 90, 91] If the rectum is involved, digital examination may suggest the presence of multiple soft polyps.[90]

Radiologically the diagnosis of PCI is not difficult. Occasionally, pneumoperitoneum may be seen in conjunction with other evidence of this disease. Extraluminal rupture of subserosal cysts is well documented, but the risk of peritoneal contamination is small.[99]

There is increasing use of colonoscopy as the primary mode of investigation in patients with symptoms or signs referable to the colon, and the presence of PCI may not be known prior to this procedure. The colonoscopic appearance may be confused with more common disorders such as multiple colonic polyps, villous adenoma, carcinoma, lymphoma, or submucosal lymphoid hyperplasia.[93] The lesions vary in diameter from a few millimeters to several centimeters, usually protrude into the lumen, and are pale or bluish, with occasional overlying inflammation (Plate 46–5). Their wide base may help to distinguish them from true polyps. Biopsy of the lesions is harmless and often results in deflation of the cyst, sometimes with evidence of gas escaping under pressure.[75, 92, 93]

PCI has been described as a complication of sigmoidoscopy and colonoscopy.[75, 100] Kozarek et al.[101] reported a case of pneumoperitoneum and pneumatosis coli following a difficult colonoscopy without biopsy. At laparotomy the patient had extensive serosal laceration of the colon with no evidence of transmural or mucosal tear. These authors subsequently demonstrated in animal experiments and human cadaveric colons that the air pressure generated by modern light sources was sufficient to cause serosal tears. Although intracolonic pressure during routine colonoscopy may not reach these levels, it is clear that generated pressure may be sufficient to produce serosal tears of the left colon if the colonoscope tip is impacted against the bowel wall. Without prior roentgenography, colonoscopy should not always be considered the cause of PCI when there is evidence of other gastrointestinal disease; PCI has been reported in patients with both sigmoid volvulus and scleroderma, with and without instrumentation.[91, 102–104]

Melanosis Coli and Cathartic Colon

Melanosis coli may be an incidental finding in patients undergoing colonoscopy, especially if there is a history of laxative abuse. The condition was first reported by Cruveilhier in 1829[105] and has been more completely described in the past 50 years.[106, 107] The anthracene group of purgatives is responsible; this includes senna, cascara, rhubarb, and frangula.

The condition occurs most commonly in middle-aged and elderly patients and is thought to be related to fecal stasis as well as to the anthracene cathartics; it may be reversible if the use of the offending agents is discontinued. The presence of melanosis in a patient undergoing investigation for diarrhea strongly suggests laxative abuse.

Endoscopically, the usual healthy pink appearance of the colonic mucosa is replaced by varying degrees of pigmentation (Plate 46–6A). There are usually unpigmented islands of pinkish or yellowish mucosa which give the bowel wall a mottled appearance (Plate 46–6B). Pigmentation may be seen throughout the colon, but it is most prominent in the rectum and cecum. Light microscopy shows the pigment to be lipofuscin in mononuclear cells of the lamina propria and the submucosa. The non-pigmented areas are lymphoid follicles that do not accumulate lipofuscin. Other lesions such as adenomatous polyps or carcinomas are similarly not pigmented.

The anthracene laxatives may also be associated with the "cathartic colon" and, although the changes may be seen anywhere in the colon, the cecum and ascending colon are most commonly affected. The barium enema appearance often mimics that seen in chronic ulcerative colitis with diminished haustral segmentation, smooth-appearing mucosa, and occasionally strictured segments. The latter changes seldom resemble a typical carcinoma; however, colonoscopy may be necessary to exclude malignancy.

Solitary Rectal Ulcer and Non-Specific Ulcer of the Colon

Unusual ulceration in the rectum was first described by Cruveilhier in 1830.[108] The condition of solitary ulcer of the rectum is now well recognized, and the histologic findings are thought to be diagnostic.[109, 110]

The majority of patients are young and healthy. The presenting symptom is fresh, rarely heavy, rectal bleeding, blood being passed with the stool. Mucus is commonly passed after the stool. Pain is unusual but occasionally may be severe and localized in the perineal, left iliac fossa, or sacral areas.

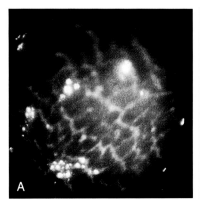

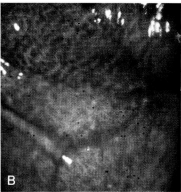

PLATE 46–6. A, Extreme degree of melanosis coli in which mucosa is almost entirely black. (Courtesy M.V. Sivak, Jr., M.D.) B, Mottled appearance of melanosis coli.

The bowel habit has no special characteristics, although irregularity was reported in 26% and regular use of laxatives in a further 18% in the series reported by Madigan and Morson.[109]

It is probable that straining at stool is an important cause of solitary rectal ulcer. It has been suggested that the frequent location of the ulcer on the anterior or anterolateral wall of the rectum indicates incomplete prolapse of the rectal mucosa; this must be excluded in each case.

Diagnosis is important because the appearance may simulate a neoplasm. The lesion often lies across or on the side of a rectal fold and can always be seen with the rigid proctosigmoidoscope about 6 to 10 cm from the anal margin. The ulcer is usually shallow with flat edges that may be irregular, round, or even linear in appearance (Plate 46–7). Biopsies show characteristic features that can confirm the diagnosis.[110] Initially there is replacement of the lamina propria by fibroblasts that are oriented at right angles to the muscularis mucosae, and there are a few associated inflammatory cells. Strands of smooth muscle alongside fibroblasts and thickening of the muscularis mucosae are occasionally found. With progression, these features become more prominent, and marked hypertrophy of the fibers of the muscularis appears. The muscularis fibers become reoriented and point toward the lumen rather than lying parallel to the mucosal surface. The crypts may show branching, distortion, and regeneration.

Treatment is not always necessary, as the condition may be asymptomatic for many years. If symptoms become troublesome, attempts may be made to control them. No local treatment has yet been shown to improve reliably the ulceration although corticosteroid suppositories, increasing dietary bulk with the addition of fiber, and mild tranquilizers may be tried. The patient should be advised to avoid straining at stool. Should these measures fail, surgical intervention should be considered, using either the transanal approach[110] or the transsphincteric approach.[111]

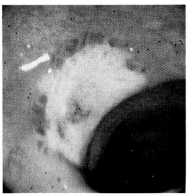

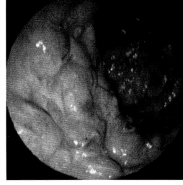

PLATE 46–7. Solitary rectal ulcer on rectal fold.
PLATE 46–8. Colitis cystica profunda.

PLATE 46–7.   PLATE 46–8.

Cecal Ulceration

Discrete cecal ulceration has been reported in an immunosuppressed patient who had evidence of CMV infection.[112] This unusual condition has been most frequently associated with renal transplantation,[34] although these ulcers may also develop in dialysis patients.[113] Gastrointestinal complications of renal transplantation are common and usually associated with a poor prognosis.[114, 115] Undoubtedly this is in part a result of immunosuppressive therapy.

Sutherland et al.[34] reported a series of 12 transplant patients with cecal ulceration. Three patients had coexistent upper gastrointestinal sources of blood loss but had persistent hematochezia after treatment of the proximal lesion. Bleeding was usually acute or subacute and 10 of 12 patients died. Arteriography was diagnostic in 8 patients and colonoscopy in 1. Seven patients had evidence of CMV infection in the ulcer base. Mills et al.[113] reported a series of 5 patients with chronic renal failure and 1 transplant recipient with cecal ulceration. In this series, colonoscopy was diagnostic in 2 cases, although the lesion was overlooked on initial examination in 1 patient. CMV was not found in any of these patients. The 50% mortality in this group emphasizes the poor prognosis for these patients and supports the conclusion of several authors who recommend an aggressive approach to gastrointestinal bleeding in renal transplant and other immunosuppressed individuals.[113–115]

Colitis Cystica Profunda

Colitis cystica profunda (CCP) is a rare, benign disorder of the colon characterized by the presence of multiple, mucus-filled cysts beneath the muscularis mucosa of the bowel wall.[116, 117] Herman and Nabseth[118] reviewed 48 cases reported up to 1973 and classified CCP into localized, segmental, and diffuse forms. The localized form was most common, accounting for 32 cases. In these patients a soft, polypoid mass is usually discovered lying within 12 to 15 cm of the anal verge. Seven patients had segmental involvement, usually in the rectosigmoid area, although localization of the transverse colon has also been described.[119] Six patients had diffuse colonic involvement; this has also been associated with chronic ulcerative colitis.[120]

The clinical features include abdominal pain, tenesmus, and diarrhea with blood or mucus that may result in profound hypoalbuminemia.[121] Proctoscopy in the localized form of CCP will reveal a soft, polypoid mass suggestive of polyp or carcinoma. The distinction between a colonic carcinoma and CCP may be difficult, and there are numerous reports of resection for presumed colon cancer.[116, 117, 120–125]

The radiologic appearance is that of an intraluminal space-occupying lesion. The differential diagnosis, therefore, is extensive and includes adenocarcinoma, lymphoma, benign adenomatous polyps, endometriosis, amebiasis, schistosomiasis, and lymphogranuloma venereum, as well as pseudopolyposis due to ulcerative colitis or Crohn's disease.[126]

The cysts are lined by patches of epithelial cells, and frequently a connection with the colonic lumen can be demonstrated. Localized inflammatory changes and fibrosis of the surrounding tissue are characteristic. Confusion in the histologic interpretation of biopsy and resected specimens between CCP and a colloid-producing carcinoma has been reported.[121, 123, 125]

Endoscopically, the lesions appear as soft, polypoid areas with varying amounts of overlying mucus and inflammation (Plate 46–8). Biopsy by sigmoidoscopy in the localized form, or colonoscopy in the segmental and diffuse forms, should clarify the diagnosis, provided the possibility of CCP is considered.[125, 126]

Editor's note: As a result of the AIDS epidemic, the gastrointestinal endoscopist must be familiar with the manifestations of a relatively large number of infectious and neoplastic disorders of the gastrointestinal tract, colon and rectum that heretofore were considered rare, even esoteric. References 127 and 128 are some recent publications of interest.

References

1. Morson BC, Dawson IMP. Gastrointestinal Pathology. Oxford: Blackwell Scientific, 1979.
2. Parks TG. Post-mortem studies on the colon with special reference to diverticular disease. Proc R Soc Med 1968; 61:932–4.
3. Nicholas GG, Miller WT, Fitts WT, Tondreau RL. Diagnosis of diverticulitis of the colon: role of the barium enema in defining pericolic inflammation. Ann Surg 1972; 176:205–9.
4. Hunt RH, Teague RH, Swarbrick ET, Williams CB. Colonoscopy in the management of colonic strictures. Br Med J 1975; 3:360–1.

5. Hunt RH. Rectal bleeding. Clin Gastroenterol 1978; 7:719–40.
6. Williams CB. Diverticular disease and strictures. In: Hunt RH, Waye JD, eds. Colonoscopy: Techniques, Clinical Practice and Colour Atlas. London: Chapman and Hall, 1981; 363–81.
7. Dean AC, Newell JP. Colonoscopy in the differential diagnosis of carcinoma from diverticulitis of the sigmoid colon. Br J Surg 1973; 60:633–5.
8. Greene FL, Livstone EM, Troncale FJ. Fiberoptic colonoscopy in the management of colonic disease. South Med J 1974; 67:105–10.
9. Sugarbaker PH, Vineyard GC, Lewicki AM, et al. Colonoscopy in the management of diseases of the colon and rectum. Surg Gynecol Obstet 1974; 139:341–9.
10. Hunt RH. The role of colonoscopy in complicated diverticular disease. A review. Acta Chir Belg 1979; 78:349–53.
11. Boulos PB, Karamanolis DG, Salmon PR, Clark CG. Is colonoscopy necessary in diverticular disease? Lancet 1984; 1:95–6.
12. Rigg BM, Ewing MR. Current attitudes on diverticulitis with particular reference to colonic bleeding. Arch Surg 1966; 92:231–2.
13. Casarella WJ, Kanter IE, Seaman WB. Right-sided colonic diverticula as a cause of acute rectal hemorrhage. N Engl J Med 1972; 286:450–3.
14. Meyers MA, Alonso DR, Gray GF, Baer JE. Pathogenesis of bleeding colonic diverticulosis. Gastroenterology 1976; 71:577–83.
15. Williams CB, Lane RH, Sakai V. Colonoscopy: an air pressure hazard. Lancet 1973; 2:729.
16. Hunt RH. Colonoscopy intubation techniques with fluoroscopy. In: Hunt RH, Waye JD, eds. Colonoscopy: Techniques, Clinical Practice, and Colour Atlas. London: Chapman and Hall, 1981; 109–46.
17. Dritz SK. Medical aspects of homosexuality. N Engl J Med 1980; 302:463–4.
18. Baker RW, Peppercorn MA. Gastrointestinal ailments of homosexual men. Medicine 1982; 61:390–405.
19. Heller M. The gay bowel syndrome: a common problem of homosexual patients in the emergency department. Ann Emerg Med 1980; 9:487–93.
20. Saltz RK, Kurtz RC, Lightale CJ, et al. Gastrointestinal involvement in Kaposi's sarcoma. (Abstr) Gastroenterology 1982; 82(Part 2):1168.
21. Quinn TC, Stamm WE, Goodell SE. The polymicrobial origin of intestinal infections in homosexual men. N Engl J Med 1983; 309:576–82.
22. Surawicz CM, Belic L. Rectal biopsy helps to distinguish acute self limited colitis from idiopathic inflammatory bowel disease. Gastroenterology 1984; 86:104–13.
23. Centers for Disease Control. Kaposi's sarcoma and pneumocystitis pneumonia among homosexual men—New York City and California. MMWR 1981; 30:305–8.
24. Centers for Disease Control. Update: acquired immunodeficiency syndrome (AIDS)—United States. MMWR 1984; 32:688–91.
25. Fauci AS (moderator). Acquired immunodeficiency syndrome: Epidemiologic, clinical, immunologic, and therapeutic considerations. Ann Intern Med 1984; 100:92–106.
26. Gottlieb MS (moderator). The acquired immunodeficiency syndrome. Ann Intern Med 1983; 99:208—20.
27. Mildvan D, Mathur U, Enlow RW. Opportunistic infections and immune deficiency in homosexual men. Ann Intern Med 1983; 96(Part 1):700–4.
28. Current WL, Reese NC, Ernst JV, et al. Human cryptosporidiosis in immunocompetent and immunodeficient persons. Studies of an outbreak and experimental transmission. N Engl J Med 1983; 308:1252–7.
29. Chiampi NP, Sundberg RD, Klompus JP, Wilson AJ. Cryptosporidial enteritis and pneumocystis pneumonia in a homosexual man. Hum Pathol 1983; 14:734–7.
30. Soave R, Danner RL, Honig CL. Cryptosporidiosis in homosexual men. Ann Intern Med 1984; 100:504–11.
31. Guarda LA, Stein SA, Cleary KA, Ordonez NG. Human cryptosporidiosis in the acquired immune deficiency syndrome. Arch Pathol Lab Med 1983; 107:562–6.
32. Dobbins WO III, Weinstein WM. Electron microscopy of the intestine and rectum in acquired immunodeficiency syndrome (AIDS). (Abstr) Gastroenterology 1984; 86:1063.
33. Centers for Disease Control. Cryptosporidiosis: assessment of chemotherapy of males with acquired immune deficiency syndrome (AIDS). MMWR 1982; 31:589–92.
34. Sutherland DE, Chan FY, Fourcar E, et al. The bleeding cecal ulcer in transplant patients. Surgery 1979; 86:386–98.
35. Knapp AB, Horst DA, Eliopoulos G. Widespread cytomegalovirus gastroenterocolitis in a patient with acquired immunodeficiency syndrome. Gastroenterology 1983; 85:1399–402.
36. Gertler SL, Pressman J, Price P, et al. Gastrointestinal cytomegalovirus infection in a homosexual man with severe acquired immunodeficiency syndrome. Gastroenterology 1983; 85:1403–6.
37. Kaposi M. Idiopatisches multiples pigment sarkom der Haut. Arch Derm Syphilol 1872; 4:265.
38. Friedman-Kien AE, Laubenstein LJ, Rubinstein P. Disseminated Kaposi's sarcoma in homosexual men. Ann Intern Med 1982; 96(Part 1):693–704.
39. Matthew JS, Gottlieb MS, Lewin KJ, Weinstein WM. Gastrointestinal lesions in homosexual men with acquired cellular immunodeficiency. (Abstr) Gastroenterology 1982; 82(Part 2):1126.
40. Stern JO, Dieterich D, Faust M, et al. Disseminated Kaposi's sarcoma: involvement of the GI tract among a group of homosexual men. (Abstr) Gastroenterology 1982; 82(Part 2):1189.
41. Bianco J, Pratt-Bianco L. Kaposi's sarcoma of the rectum: a case report. Mt Sinai J Med 1983; 50:278–80.
42. Bradin JL Jr. Kaposi's sarcoma of the rectum (Letter). West J Med 1983; 139:109.
43. Tavossolie H, Mir-Madjessi SH, Sadr-Ameli M. The endoscopic demonstration of Kaposi's sarcoma of the colon. Gastrointest Endosc 1983; 29:331–2.
44. Centers for Disease Control. Acquired immune deficiency syndrome (AIDS): Precautions for clinical and laboratory staffs. MMWR 1982; 31:577–80.
45. Behçet H. Ueber rezidivierende apthose, durch ein Virus verursachte geschwure am Mund, am Auge unde an den Genitalien. Dermat Wochenschr 1937; 105:1152–7.
46. Chajek T, Fainaru M. Behçet's disease. Report of 41 cases and a review of the literature. Medicine (Balt) 1975; 54:179–96.
47. Shimizu T, Ehrlich GE, Inaba G, Hayashi K. Beh-

çet's disease. Semin Arthritis Rheum 1979; 8:223–60.

48. Mason RM, Barnes CG. Behçet's syndrome with arthritis. Ann Rheum Dis 1969; 28:95–103.

49. James DG. Behçet's syndrome (editorial). N Engl J Med 1979; 301:431–2.

50. Griffin JW Jr, Harrison HB, Tedesco FJ, Mills LR. Behçet's disease with multiple sites of gastrointestinal involvement. South Med J 1982; 75:1405–8.

51. Kasahara Y, Tanaka S, Nishino M, et al. Intestinal involvement in Behçet's disease: Review of 136 surgical cases in the Japanese literature. Dis Colon Rectum 1981; 24:103–6.

52. Smith GE, Kime LR, Pitcher JL. The colitis of Behçet's disease: A separate entity? Colonoscopic findings and literature review. Am J Dig Dis 1973; 18:987–1000.

53. Baba S, Maruta M, Ando K. Intestinal Behçet's disease: report of five cases. Dis Colon Rectum 1976; 19:428–40.

54. Ketch LL, Buerk CA, Lietchy RD. Surgical implications of Behçet's disease. Arch Surg 1980; 115:759–60.

55. Stanley RJ, Tedesco FJ, Melson GL. The colitis of Behçet's disease: A clinical radiographic correlation. Radiology 1975; 114:603–4.

56. Eng K, Ruoff M, Bystryn J. Behçet's syndrome. An unusual cause of colonic ulceration and perforation. Am J Gastroenterol 1981; 75:57–9.

57. Bartlett JG, Gorbach SL. Pseudomembranous enterocolitis (antibiotic-related colitis). Adv Intern Med 1977; 22:455–76.

58. Rifkin GD, Fekety FR, Silva J Jr, Sack RB. Antibiotic-induced colitis. Implication of a toxin neutralised by Clostridium sordelli antitoxin. Lancet 1977; 2:1103–6.

59. Bartlett JG, Chang TW, Gurwith M, et al. Antibiotic-associated pseudomembranous colitis due to toxin-producing clostridia. N Engl J Med 1978; 298:531–4.

60. George RH, Symonds JM, Dimock R. Identification of Clostridium difficile in patients with pseudomembranous colitis. Br Med J 1978; 1:695.

61. Bartlett JG. The pseudomembranous enterocolitis. In: Sleisenger MH, Fordtran JS, eds. Gastrointestinal Disease. Ed 3. Philadelphia: WB Saunders Company, 1983; 1168–84.

62. Tedesco FJ. Pseudomembranous colitis: Pathogenesis and therapy. Med Clin North Am 1982; 66:655–64.

63. Howard JM, Sullivan SN, Troster M. Spontaneous pseudomembranous colitis. Br Med J 1980; 2:356.

64. Fekety R, Kim K, Brown D, et al. Epidemiology of antibiotic-associated colitis. Isolation of Clostridium difficile from the hospital environment. Am J Med 1981; 70:906–8.

65. Mulligan ME, Rolfe RD, Finegold SM, George WL. Contamination of a hospital environment by Clostridium difficile. Curr Microbiol 1980; 3:173–5.

66. Tedesco FJ, Barton RW, Alpers DH. Clindamycin-associated colitis: A prospective study. Ann Intern Med 1974; 81:429–33.

67. Price AB, Davies DR. Pseudomembranous colitis. J Clin Pathol 1977; 30:1–12.

68. Burbige EJ, Radigan JJ. Antibiotic-associated colitis with normal-appearing rectum. Dis Colon Rectum 1981; 24:198–200.

69. Seppala K. Colonoscopy in the diagnosis of pseudomembranous colitis. (Letter) Br Med J 1978; 2:435.

70. Seppala K, Hjelt L, Sipponen P. Colonoscopy in the diagnosis of antibiotic-associated colitis. A prospective study. Scand J Gastroenterol 1981; 16:465–8.

71. Tedesco FJ. Antibiotic-associated pseudomembranous colitis with negative proctosigmoidoscopy examination. Gastroenterology 1979; 77:295–7.

72. Tedesco FJ, Corless JK, Brownstein RE. Rectal sparing in antibiotic-associated pseudomembranous colitis: a prospective study. Gastroenterology 1982; 83:1259–60.

73. Bartlett JG, Tedesco FJ, Shull S, et al. Symptomatic relapse after oral vancomycin therapy of antibiotic-associated pseudomembranous colitis. Gastroenterology 1980; 78:431–4.

74. Silva J Jr, Batts DH, Fekety R, et al. Treatment of Clostridium difficile colitis and diarrhea with vancomycin. Am J Med 1981; 71:815–22.

75. Earnest DL. Other diseases of the colon and rectum. In: Sleisenger MH, Fordtran JS, eds. Gastrointestinal Disease. Ed. 3. Philadelphia: WB Saunders Company 1983; 1294–323.

76. Meyers WC, Kelvin FM, Jones RS. Diagnosis and surgical treatment of colonic endometriosis. Arch Surg 1979; 114:169–75.

77. Spiro HM. Gastrointestinal Disease. New York: The MacMillan Company, 1983; 755–8.

78. Henriksen E. Endometriosis. Am J Surg 1955; 90:331–7.

79. Williams TJ, Pratt JH. Endometriosis in 1,000 consecutive celiotomies: incidence and management. Am J Obstet Gynecol 1977; 129:245–50.

80. Aronchick CA, Brooks FP, Dyson WL, et al. Ileocecal endometriosis presenting with abdominal pain and gastrointestinal bleeding. Dig Dis Sci 1983; 28:566–72.

81. Wald A, Van Thiel DH, Hoechstetter L. Gastrointestinal transit: the effect of the menstrual cycle. Gastroenterology 1981; 80:1497–1500.

82. Spjut HJ, Perkins DE. Endometriosis of the sigmoid colon and rectum: a roentgenologic and pathologic study. Am J Roentgenol 1959; 82:1070–5.

83. Pillay SP, Hardie JR. Intestinal complications of endometriosis. Br J Surg 1980; 67:677–9.

84. Michowitz M, Hammer B, Lazarovici I, Solowiejczyk M. Endometriosis of the colon. Postgrad Med J 1981; 67:334–7.

85. McSwain B, Linn RJ, Haley RL Jr, Franklin RH. Endometriosis of the colon: report of 14 patients requiring partial colectomy. South Med J 1974; 67:651–8.

86. Kidd R, Freeny PC. Radiographic manifestations of extrinsic processes involving the bowel. Gastrointest Radiol 1982; 7:21–8.

87. Bashist B, Forde KA, McCaffrey RM. Polypoid endometrioma of the rectosigmoid. Gastrointest Radiol 1983; 8:85–8.

88. Gordon RL, Evers K, Kressel HY, et al. Double-contrast enema in pelvic endometriosis. AJR 1982; 138:549–52.

89. Farinon AM, Vadora E. Endometriosis of the colon and rectum: an indication for preoperative colonoscopy. Endoscopy 1980; 12:136–9.

90. Ecker JA, Williams RG, Clay KL. Pneumatosis cystoides intestinalis—bullous emphysema of the intestine. Am J Gastroenterol 1971; 56:125–36.

91. Koss LG. Abdominal gas cysts (pneumatosis cystoides intestinalis hominis). Arch Pathol 1952; 53:523–49.

92. Holt S, Gilmour HM, Buist TAS, et al. High flow oxygen therapy for pneumatosis coli. Gut 1979; 20:493–8.

93. Varano JV, Bonanno CA. Colonoscopic findings in pneumatosis cystoides intestinalis. Am J Gastroenterol 1973; 59:353–60.

94. Forgacs P, Wright PH, Wyatt AP. Treatment of intestinal gas cysts by oxygen breathing. Lancet 1973; 1:579–82.

95. Yale CE. Etiology of pneumatosis cystoides intestinalis. Surg Clin North Am 1975; 55:1297–1302.

96. Gillon J, Tadesse K, Logan RF, et al. Breath hydrogen in pneumatosis cystoides intestinalis. Gut 1979; 20:1008–11.

97. Van Der Linden W, Marsell R. Pneumatosis cystoides coli associated with high H_2 excretion. Scand J Gastroenterol 1979; 14:173–4.

98. Ellis BW. Symptomatic treatment of primary pneumatosis coli with metronidazole. Br Med J 1980; 1:763–4.

99. Rice RP, Thompson WM, Gedgaudas RK. The diagnosis and significance of extraluminal gas in the abdomen. Radiol Clin North Am 1982; 20:819–37.

100. Meyers MA, Ghahremani GG, Clements JL Jr, Goodman K. Pneumatosis intestinalis. Gastrointest Radiol 1977; 2:91–105.

101. Kozarek RA, Earnest DL, Silverstein ME, Smith RG. Air-pressure induced colon injury during diagnostic colonoscopy. Gastroenterology 1980; 78:7–14.

102. Wertkin MG, Wetchler BB, Waye JD, Brown LK. Pneumatosis coli associated with sigmoid volvulus and colonoscopy. Am J Gastroenterol 1976; 65:209–14.

103. Heer M, Altorfer J, Pirovino M, Schmid M. Pneumatosis cystoides coli: A rare complication of colonoscopy. Endoscopy 1983; 15:119–20.

104. Miercort RD, Merrill FG. Pneumatosis and pseudo-obstruction in scleroderma. Radiology 1969; 92:359–62.

105. Cruveilhier J. Cancer avec melanose. In: Bailliere JB, ed. Anatomie Pathologique du Corps Humain. Paris, 1829; 6.

106. Bockus HL, Willard JH, Bank J. Melanosis coli; etiology significance of anthracene laxatives; report of 41 cases. JAMA 1933; 101:1–9.

107. Wittoesch JH, Jackman RJ, McDonald JR. Melanosis coli: General review and study of 887 cases. Dis Colon Rectum 1958; 1:172–80.

108. Cruveilhier J. Ulcere chronique du rectum. In: Bailliere JB, ed. Anatomie Pathologique du Corps Humain, Ed 2. Paris, 1870; 25:4.

109. Madigan MR, Morson BC. Solitary ulcer of the rectum. Gut 1969; 10:871–81.

110. Rutter KRP, Riddell RH. The solitary ulcer syndrome of the rectum. Clin Gastroenterol 1975; 4:505–30.

111. Mason AY. Trans-sphincteric exposure of the rectum. Ann R Coll Surg Engl 1972; 51:320–31.

112. Wolfe BM, Cherry JD. Hemorrhage from cecal ulcers of cytomegalovirus infection: report of a case. Ann Surg 1973; 177:490–4.

113. Mills B, Zuckerman G, Sicard G. Discrete colon ulcers as a cause of lower gastrointestinal bleeding and perforation in end-stage renal disease. Surgery 1981; 89:548–52.

114. Faro RS, Corry RJ. Management of surgical gastrointestinal complications in renal transplant recipients. Arch Surg 1979; 114:310–2.

115. Sawyer OI, Garvin PJ, Codd JE, et al. Colorectal complications of renal allograft transplantation. Arch Surg 1978; 113:84–6.

116. Epstein SE, Ascari WQ, Ablow RC. Colitis cystica profunda. Am J Clin Pathol 1966; 45:186–201.

117. Wayte DM, Helwig EB. Colitis cystica profunda. Am J Clin Pathol 1967; 48:159–69.

118. Herman AH, Nabseth DC. Colitis cystica profunda: localized, segmental, and diffuse. Arch Surg 1973; 106:337–41.

119. Barner JL. Colitis cystica profunda. Radiology 1967; 89:435–7.

120. Castleman B, McNeeley BU. Clinicopathologic conference. Case 3—1972. N Engl J Med 1972; 286:147–53.

121. Castleman B, McNeeley BU. Clinical pathologic conference. Case 41—1966. N Engl J Med 1966; 275:608–14.

122. Howard RJ, Mannax SJ, Eusebio EB. Colitis cystica profunda. Surgery 1971; 69:306–8.

123. Silver H, Stolar J. Distinguishing features of well differentiated mucinous adenocarcinoma of the rectum and colitis cystica profunda. Am J Clin Pathol 1969; 51:493–500.

124. Tedesco FJ, Sumner HW, Kassens WD Jr. Colitis cystica profunda. Am J Gastroenterol 1976; 65:339–43.

125. Clark JF, Muldoon JP. Colitis cystica profunda in an adenoma (adenomatous polyp): report of a case. Dis Colon Rectum 1970; 13:387–9.

126. Goldberg HI, Buchignani J, Rulon DB. RPC of the month from the AFIP. Radiology 1970; 96:447–52.

127. Dworkin B, Wormser GP, Rosenthal WS, et al. Gastrointestinal manifestations of the acquired immunodeficiency syndrome: a review of 22 cases. Am J Gastroenterol 1985; 80:774–8.

128. Friedman SL, Wright TL, Altman DF. Gastrointestinal Kaposi's sarcoma in patients with acquired immunodeficiency syndrome. Endoscopic and autopsy findings. Gastroenterology 1985; 89:102–8.

Chapter 47

ANOSCOPY

DAVID G. JAGELMAN, M.S., F.R.C.S., F.A.C.S.

The examination of the anal canal and lower rectum is termed anoscopy. This procedure is complemented by visual examination and palpation of the perianal skin, digital palpation of the anal canal, and proctosigmoidoscopy. Even before considering this a detailed history is essential with particular reference to bowel function, rectal bleeding, anal pain or discomfort, and prolapse. The history will often help to define the etiology of the anal symptoms. Additional studies such as double contrast radiologic examination of the large bowel, fiberoptic sigmoidoscopy, or colonoscopy may be indicated as supplementary investigations.

ANORECTAL SYMPTOMS

Rectal bleeding is the most frequent symptom requiring anorectal examination. Whether the blood is bright red or dark, of small or large volume, with or without mucus, after defecation or without defecation are important features in the history. Bleeding caused by hemorrhoids is mostly bright red and usually follows defecation; if associated with pain a fissure in ano should be considered. Dark red rectal bleeding is usually due to causes other than hemorrhoids and requires a more extensive colonic examination. Ulcerative proctitis causes rectal bleeding often mixed with mucus and is often confused with hemorrhoidal bleeding or diarrhea. Close questioning, however, will determine that the blood and mucus are often passed alone, and the patient will have one or less solid bowel movements daily even to the point of constipation. Blood mixed with bowel movement suggests a higher rectal or colonic lesion. A history of clots and dark rectal bleeding may indicate rupture of perianal hematoma and will often be preceded by increasing anal pain and perianal swelling.

Rectal pain or discomfort is another frequent symptom requiring anorectal examination. The pain may be so severe and the associated anal spasm so marked that urgent examination under anesthesia should be recommended. In this situation an acute anal fissure should be suspected or a perianal or, more specifically, an intersphincteric abscess may be implicated. It is inappropriate to pursue anoscopic or proctoscopic examination with this degree of pain without the benefit of anesthesia. Less acute fissures, perianal hematoma, perianal abscess, and anal carcinoma can and will have anal pain as a presenting symptom. Anal discomfort of intra-anal distribution can be caused by descending perineum syndrome and internal rectal procidentia, prolapsing internal hemorrhoids as well as proctalgia fugax. External perianal discomfort such as itching and irritation can be caused by brim irritation, poor hygiene, skin infections, or nondescript pruritus ani.

A history of a perianal lump with or without pain may indicate perianal hematoma or so-called thrombosed external hemorrhoid, hypertrophied anal papilla, prolapsing internal hemorrhoid, external skin tag, or perianal skin tumor.

EXAMINATION

The anus and rectum can be examined either in the lateral position or in the knee-chest position. Personal preference and experience with both methods suggest that the knee-chest position is more satisfactory. A special examination table with tilt and leveling features further enhances the examination.

Most patients are embarrassed and apprehensive about anorectal examination and

960

their anxiety should be considered at all times. They should be comfortable in the examining position and during the procedure the examiner should explain what is being done. Above all, the aim should be the avoidance of pain. Preparation for the examination is not required prior to the office visit and can easily be accomplished with a small disposable, flexible tip enema. Adequate toilet facilities should be close by.

The examination itself is composed of three elements: inspection, palpation, and anoscopy.

Inspection

Visual inspection of the perianal area with the patient comfortable in the knee-chest position is carried out first. This often requires gentle traction on the buttocks. Good illumination is necessary, preferably from a high-intensity overhead lamp.

The perianal skin should be examined for a variety of different disorders. Skin tags as a result of a remote thrombosed external hemorrhoid or the classic edematous tags seen in Crohn's disease as part of the perianal Crohn's complex are characteristic (Plates 47–1 and 47–2). Posterior or anterior skin tags or so-called sentinal tags are typical features of a chronic fissure in ano (Plate 47–3). Ulcerated lesions, either traumatic from irritation or tumor, or the ulcerated chronic lesions of Crohn's disease can be extensive (Plates 47–4 through 47–7). Pilonidal sinuses or cysts will be evident (Plate 47–8). The presenting features of squamous cell carcinoma (Plate 47–9), Paget's disease or Bowen's disease may include discolored areas with or without some superficial ulceration or induration. Skin fibromas, perianal warts (Plates 47–10 and 47–11), and in some patients, small sebaceous cysts may be seen around the anus. Draining abscesses (Plate 47–12) or fistulas (Plate 47–13) can be easily identified. Patients with a prolapsing internal hemorrhoid will often demonstrate heaped up or lax skin in the primary hemorrhoid positions. Some other common disorders are shown in Plates 47–14, 47–15, and 47–16.

Gentle eversion of the anus with the fingers close to the anus on the perianal skin will almost always demonstrate a fissure in ano, prolapse of internal hemorrhoids (Plates 47–17 and 47–18), and hypertrophied anal papillae. External fistulous openings may also be seen with or without a small bead of pus exiting (Plate 47–19). Intra-anal warts may also be seen as well as lower rectal adenomatous polyps (Plate 47–20).

Perianal rashes as a result of pruritus ani (Plate 47–21) and various skin infections or excessive use of perianal creams and subsequent allergic reactions may be seen. Skin scrapings, ultraviolet light examination, or skin biopsy may be necessary to determine the cause of such rashes.

Palpation and Digital Examination

The perianal area should be palpated to determine the texture of any perianal lesions. Induration is usually indicative of perianal abscess or fistula. The course of a fistulous tract can usually be determined by following the induration from the draining external opening.

Digital examination of the anus and distal rectum using a soft, thin, well-lubricated glove should follow thorough visual inspection and perianal palpation. At the conclusion of each digital examination the examining finger should be checked for blood or pus.

The internal digital examination is useful in detecting not only anal pathology but also other pelvic disorders. Pelvic abscesses can be felt through the rectal wall as a tender boggy mass. The cervix can be palpated easily in women and must not be confused with a rectal tumor. Masses in the rectovaginal pouch such as ovarian tumor, endometriosis, or more commonly an enlarged uterus with fibroids are detectable. Prostatic enlargement, the presence of hard nodules, or obliteration of the prostatic groove should be sought in men. The seminal vesicles are also palpable. In patients with carcinoma of the lower third of the rectum, enlarged retrorectal lymph nodes can be felt. Rarely, other extrarectal tumors such as chordoma and teratoma have been detected. It is a good practice to consider carefully the possibility that any one of these lesions may be present before concentrating on lower rectal and anal pathology.

Internal induration in conjunction with abscess or fistula disease may indicate upward extension of the septic focus in the submucosal, intersphincteric, or ischiorectal fossa planes. Indeed, internal fistulous openings can often be felt, usually in the posterior midline at the level of the dentate line. At times pus can be seen on the examining finger.

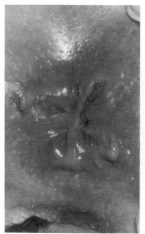 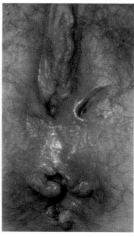 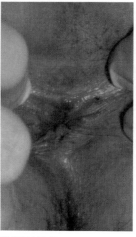 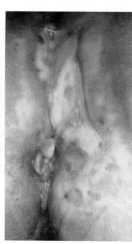

PLATE 47–1.   PLATE 47–2.   PLATE 47–3.   PLATE 47–4.

PLATE 47–1. Fissures and edematous sentinel tags in Crohn's disease.
PLATE 47–2. Crohn's perineum with fissures, fistulas, and edematous tags.
PLATE 47–3. Chronic posterior fissure in ano.
PLATE 47–4. Severe irradiation injury to the perianal skin.

The texture of the lower rectal mucosa can also be determined by digital examination. For example, the mucosa will feel somewhat granular in ulcerative colitis. Alterations from the normal smooth texture can be detected in other inflammatory diseases; if there is mucosal hemorrhage, blood is frequently noted on the examining finger.

Rectal carcinomas as far as 10.0 cm from the anal verge can usually be palpated. Even some sigmoid lesions can be felt through the upper rectum if the sigmoid loop has arched over and become adherent to the upper rectum. Distal rectal carcinomas can be palpated, and mobility, the presence or absence of central ulceration, depth of invasion, and an estimate of size should be determined. Other palpable lesions in the lower rectum and anal canal include rectal polyps, warts, and anal papillae; their size and location should be documented. The posterior lower third of the rectum should be carefully examined by finger palpation, since this is a potentially blind area at endoscopic examination because

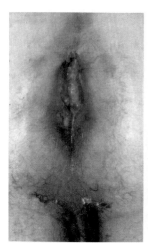 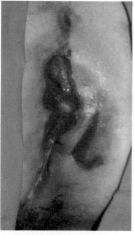 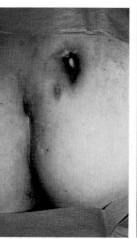 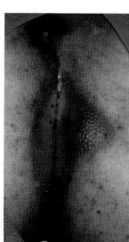

PLATE 47–5.   PLATE 47–6.   PLATE 47–7.   PLATE 47–8.

PLATE 47–5. Perianal Crohn's disease with destruction of overlying skin.
PLATE 47–6. Perianal and perivaginal cutaneous Crohn's disease.
PLATE 47–7. Colonic Crohn's disease with fistula appearing adjacent to sacrum.
PLATE 47–8. Pilonidal sinus with abscess and central midline pits.

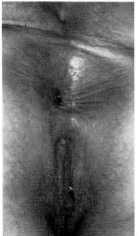
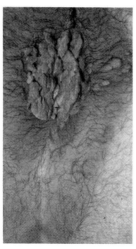
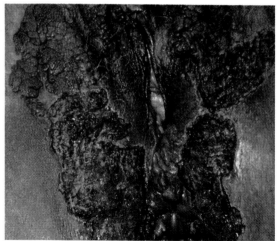

PLATE 47–9.   PLATE 47–10.   PLATE 47–11.

PLATE 47–9. Small squamous cell carcinoma of anal canal.
PLATE 47–10. Anal condylomata.
PLATE 47–11. Perianal and perivaginal condylomata during laser treatment.

of the normal angle formed by the luminal axes of the anus and rectum and because this area may receive only cursory observation if the anoscope or proctoscope is withdrawn quickly.

Anal sphincter function can also be evaluated during digital examination by asking the patient to actively contract the anal sphincter. The anorectal sphincter is anatomically deficient anteriorly, more so in women. Because anal sphincter tone is lost during anesthesia, it is important to document normal or deficient tone preoperatively. A decrease in tone may be detected in the elderly patient with a lax sphincter. In those patients incontinent after fistulotomy or other forms of anal trauma, decreased tone and a defect in the anorectal sphincter ring will be evident; this simple evaluation is useful to the surgeon when attempts at sphincter repair are to be made.

Much information can be gained from a digital examination although the examiner's finger is too often inserted and withdrawn without regard to the wide range of important observations that are possible. For the inexperienced examiner a checklist of important points as outlined is useful. A disciplined

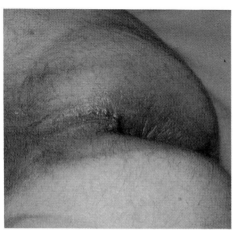
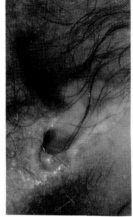
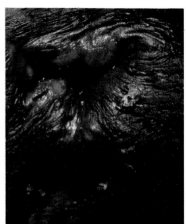

PLATE 47–12.   PLATE 47–13.   PLATE 47–14.

PLATE 47–12. Large ischiorectal abscess.
PLATE 47–13. Chronic fistula in ano.
PLATE 47–14. Anal herpes with severe discrete ulcers.

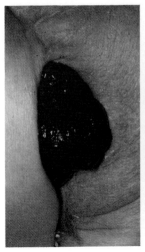 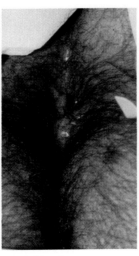 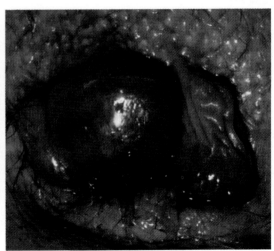

PLATE 47–15.   PLATE 47–16.   PLATE 47–17.

PLATE 47–15. Complete rectal procidentia.
PLATE 47–16. Thrombosed perianal hematoma.
PLATE 47–17. Thrombosed prolapsed internal hemorrhoid.

mental review of the list as the examination proceeds insures that maximum information will be obtained and reduces the possibility that vital clinical information will be lost.

Anal Endoscopy (Anoscopy)

Anoscopy is complemented by inspection and palpation and by other more extensive examinations such as fiberoptic sigmoidoscopy, colonoscopy, and radiologic double contrast examination of the large bowel. As well as being a diagnostic procedure it is also useful in treatment of internal hemorrhoids by sclerotherapy or elastic band ligation.

The choice of anoscope is according to personal preference. The normal range of diameter is 2 to 3 cm and the length is from 5 to 8 cm. There are a number of different designs; some have straight ends, others are open in one quadrant and allow the lower rectum and anal canal to bulge into the lumen of the instrument upon removal of its introducer. Some instruments have built-in

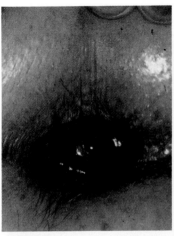  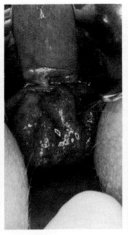 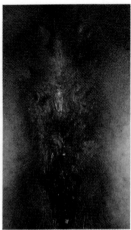

PLATE 47–18.   PLATE 47–19.   PLATE 47–20.   PLATE 47–21.

PLATE 47–18. Thrombosed gangrenous prolapsed internal hemorrhoids.
PLATE 47–19. Perianal abscess partially draining.
PLATE 47–20. Prolapsing rectal villous adenoma.
PLATE 47–21. Severe pruritus ani.

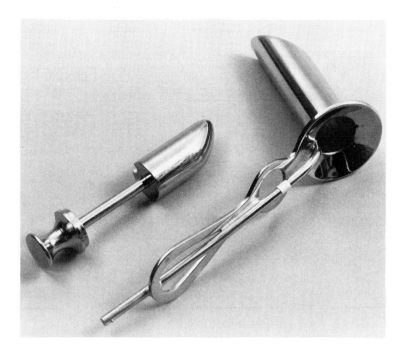

FIGURE 47–1. Anoscope with built-in fiberoptic light system and beveled slit feature.

fiberoptic lighting that facilitates the examination (Fig. 47–1).

The anoscope should be well lubricated. If insertion causes pain the examination should be terminated. The patient's comfort is extremely important and an on-going explanation of what is being done and what sensations to expect will help to allay the anxiety of the patient and enlists a greater degree of cooperation.

The method of insertion involves gentle forward pressure with some rotation followed by posterior angulation of the tip to compensate for the normal anorectal angle. When the instrument is fully inserted the introducer is removed. If an instrument has a slit, rotation of the anoscope to visualize the full circumference of the anal canal may be necessary. If rotation is required, it may be necessary to insert the introducer again to facilitate this rotation.

Anoscopy has a special advantage in the diagnosis of internal hemorrhoids and their treatment by injection or elastic band ligation. Examination of the lower rectum and anal canal is enhanced by asking the patient to bear down gently. This is of further aid in the diagnosis and treatment of prolapsing or enlarged hemorrhoids by causing them to bulge into the lumen of the instrument.

Anoscopy also permits visual examination of the lower rectal mucosa. This is particularly helpful in patients with proctitis; swabs can be taken for bacteriologic study when gonococcal proctitis is suspected. In ulcerative proctitis swabbing the mucosa with a cotton swab will precipitate contact bleeding, and a smear of the rectal mucosa on a glass slide to determine if leukocytes are present may be helpful in the differential diagnosis of early or mild cases. Anoscopy is also a useful examination for fissures and internal fistulous openings.

CONCLUSION

Inspection and palpation of the perianal and intra-anal tissues and the use of anoscopy are essential in the appropriate and thorough evaluation of anorectal symptoms. These procedures should be completed systematically in combination with proctosigmoidoscopic examination. Failure to do so may result in a missed diagnosis; this is further compounded by the inherent limitations of a rigid proctosigmoidoscopy and fiberoptic examinations of the large bowel and rectum in the examination of the most distal aspect of the rectum and anal canal.

Chapter 48

COLONOSCOPY IN THE PEDIATRIC PATIENT

ROBERT WYLLIE, M.D.

Colonoscopy has become an established procedure for the diagnosis, evaluation, and treatment of large bowel diseases in pediatric patients, the number of procedures performed having increased dramatically during the past 10 years. The utilization and importance of colonoscopy will continue to increase as instruments specifically designed for pediatric patients come into routine use; advances in therapeutic endoscopy are expected to further enhance the usefulness of the procedure. There are differences between pediatric and adult patients, however, that not only influence the approach to the patient but also therapeutic decisions when abnormalities are suspected or identified.

PROCEDURE FOR COLONOSCOPY

Bowel Preparation

Most pediatric colonoscopists recommend a liquid diet for 48 hours prior to the procedure. In a child with diarrhea, this is usually the only preparation necessary for a successful examination. In other patients, magnesium citrate, approximately 1 oz per year of age, to a maximum of 10 oz, is given the day before the procedure, followed by saline enemas the night before and the morning of the procedure. If further preparation is needed, bisacodyl (Dulcolax tablets or suppositories) or senna syrup (Senokot X-prep) may be helpful.

The lavage method of colon preparation in which relatively large quantities of electrolyte solutions are taken orally has been well accepted by adult patients.[1] The experience with this method has not been as favorable in pediatric patients. Young children and even adolescents often object to the taste and volume of liquid that must be consumed for an adequate preparation.

Endoscopy Unit and Personnel

The physical qualities of the endoscopy unit have an important bearing on the pediatric patient's reaction to the procedure. Some portion of the unit should be designed and furnished in a manner appropriate to the age and interests of young patients. It is extremely helpful if the pediatric patient can recognize a "familiar face" throughout the procedure. Especially important is a description of the procedure prior to arrival in the endoscopy unit. A pediatric endoscopy nurse can often fill this role. During the procedure it is frequently necessary to have a second assistant who attends to technical matters such as the medication, equipment, record keeping, and collecting specimens. The first assistant devotes his or her time to holding, monitoring, and reassuring the patient, functions that in the case of infants and children will take the entire attention of one person. These concepts are the same for upper gastrointestinal endoscopy and are discussed further in Chapter 13.

Medication

With pediatric patients, the goal of premedication is not only sedation and the least discomfort but also amnesia for the procedure. A decade ago many endoscopists relied on general anesthesia for these purposes. This has some disadvantages, and although the morbidity and mortality are not prohibitive, most pediatric endoscopists now perform colonoscopy with intravenous sedation. Usually a combination of meperidine (1 to 2

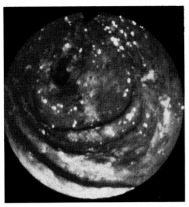

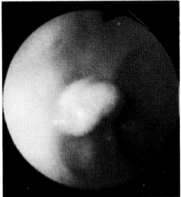

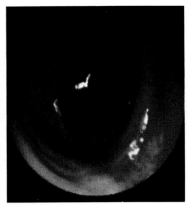

PLATE 48—1.
PLATE 48—2.
PLATE 48—3.

PLATE 48—1. Colitis associated with Henoch-Schönlein purpura in 5-year-old boy.
PLATE 48—2. Simple juvenile polyp.
PLATE 48—3. Lymphangioma in 3-year-old girl with hematochezia.

as esophageal varices must also be considered. The role of colonoscopy in these conditions depends on the clinical setting, but it is frequently of assistance in diagnosis.

Colon Polyps

Colonic polyps are a common cause of moderate rectal bleeding in childhood (Plate 48–2). Almost all polyps in the pediatric age group are hamartomas without significant malignant potential. Referred to as juvenile, retention, or inflammatory, these polyps are uncommon during the first year of life but gradually increase in frequency and reach a peak between 5 and 6 years of age. They again become uncommon after the early teenage years.

Juvenile polyps can occur anywhere in the colon; 8% are within the distal 20 cm of the bowel.[11] They are associated with painless, bright red rectal bleeding that is often inter-

mittent. Although not usually associated with significant hemorrhage, Hassal et al.[2] described bleeding sufficient to cause anemia in 10 of 26 patients with juvenile polyps. Most juvenile polyps autoamputate and may be mistaken for clots in the stool. Occasionally they prolapse from the rectum or act as a lead point in an intussusception.

At endoscopic examination, most have a relatively large, smooth head on a thin stalk, a configuration that probably explains their propensity for autoamputation. The surface at the tip of the head is often hemorrhagic with evidence of secondary inflammation. Necrosis may be caused by interruption of the blood supply to the polyp when the pedicle is twisted. Because of autoamputation, a stalk will occasionally be seen without the head of the polyp. At least 20% of patients have multiple polyps, the true frequency being unknown since evaluation has

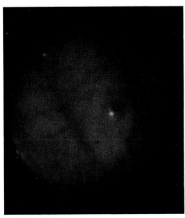

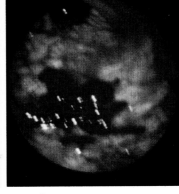

PLATE 48—4. Arteriovenous malformation in 6-year-old boy with hematochezia.
PLATE 48—5. Arteriovenous malformation in 15-year-old girl with intermittent hematochezia and anemia.

PLATE 48—4.
PLATE 48—5.

often been terminated following identification of an initial lesion. Recurrence rates are biased by the same limited evaluation; the reported frequency is approximately 25%.

Isolated adenomas have been reported in the pediatric age group, but are uncommon.[12] A single case has been described of a mixed type of polyp with both juvenile and adenomatous elements. Macroscopically, these lesions are indistinguishable from hamartomatous polyps and cannot be identified by their gross appearance at colonoscopy.

Juvenile polyposis coli must be considered in patients with multiple polyps. These are grossly and microscopically indistinguishable from simple juvenile polyps. They may occur anywhere in the gastrointestinal tract, but are most common in and often limited to the colon.[13] Many members of the patient's pedigree may have the disorder, although in the majority of cases reported, only a single affected family member has been identified. The main symptoms are anemia, hypoproteinemia, malnutrition, and growth retardation.[14] Associated anomalies occur in about 20% of the patients, including cardiac defects, intestinal malrotation, enlarged and unusually shaped heads, and Meckel's diverticulum.[14]

The malignant potential in juvenile polyposis has yet to be resolved. Theoretically, it should be at least equal to the malignant potential of the tissues from which these polyps arise. The mucosa of the large intestine is prone to neoplastic growth so that the development of adenomas and carcinomas would not be unexpected in juvenile polyps. The majority of polyps in juvenile polyposis have the same histologic characteristics as isolated juvenile polyps, although areas of atypia with mild to moderate dysplasia have been identified. The percentages of patients with adenomatous changes are approximately the same, whether polyps are single or multiple in juvenile polyposis. Intestinal carcinoma has been reported in patients and family members;[15] the frequency is increased if multiple family members are affected.[14]

An association between juvenile polyposis and adenomatous polyposis coli has been suggested based on the occurrence of the two diseases within the same family. The hypothesis put forth by Habr-Gama et al.[3] is that hamartomas and adenomas represent the same genetic pattern with different phenotypic expression. Like familial (adenomatous) polyposis coli, juvenile polyposis should be considered a possible marker of potential neoplastic change in the patient and his family.

Single polyps in pediatric patients should be resected and examined histologically. Complete colonoscopy must be performed to look for additional polyps that may cause anemia or be a marker for a more serious potential problem. If no other polyps are identified, further follow-up is probably not required. In patients with multiple polyps, all or at least a number of specimens should be submitted for histologic analysis. This group of patients should probably undergo periodic examination in anticipation of the development of juvenile polyposis and possible malignant changes. If an adenoma is identified, follow-up colonoscopy, as in adult patients, is essential.

Meckel's Diverticulum

Meckel's diverticulum may also be a cause of painless rectal bleeding in pediatric patients. This structure represents a persistence of the omphalomesenteric duct. The persistence of the duct itself is not associated with bleeding and is usually asymptomatic. In the adult, Meckel's diverticulum is usually attached to the antimesenteric border of the ileum within 100 cm of the ileocecal valve. Its frequency in autopsy series is 0.3% to 3.0%.[16, 17] Bleeding, the most frequent complication, can occur when the diverticulum is lined by ectopic gastric mucosa. The bleeding arises from ulceration of the ileal tissue adjacent to the ectopic stomach mucosa, most often during the first 2 years of life. Although colonoscopy will not usually identify the source of hemorrhage, it will localize it to the small bowel so that the appropriate radionuclide studies can be performed.

Vascular Lesions

Vascular lesions in children are rare but have been reported as a cause of intermittent rectal bleeding.[18-22] Hemorrhage is the most common presenting symptom. Other clinical features include abdominal pain with intussusception and signs of obstruction. The lesions can be divided into two general varieties: large cavernous hemangiomas (Plate 48–3) and small networks of "capillaries" or telangiectasias (Plate 48–4). Approximately half the patients also have cutaneous hemangiomas. Electrocoagulation has been successful in treating smaller vascular lesions in two of our pediatric patients. Both patients presented with chronic intermittent hematochezia with mild anemia (Plate 48–5).

Many syndromes have been associated with vascular lesions of the gastrointestinal tract including "blue-rubber-bleb" nevus disease, Osler-Weber-Rendu syndrome, CRST syndrome (calcinosis cutis, Raynaud's phenomenon, sclerodactyly, and telangiectasia), dyschondroplasia (Maffucci's syndrome), and diffuse neonatal hemangiomatosis.

"Blue-rubber-bleb" nevus disease is characterized by cavernous hemangiomas on the upper limbs, trunk, and in the gastrointestinal tract. Familial transmission as well as sporadic cases have been reported.[23]

The CRST syndrome has rarely been associated with gastrointestinal hemorrhage. The Osler-Weber-Rendu syndrome is probably the best known of the hereditary telangiectasias, its classic features being recurrent hemorrhage from telangiectatic lesions in the nasopharynx and gastrointestinal tract. The lesions are also found on the skin, characteristically on the palms of the hands and nail beds. Intestinal telangiectasia has also been associated with pseudoxanthoma elasticum and Turner's syndrome.[24, 25]

Lymphonodular Hyperplasia

Lymphonodular hyperplasia or a "lymphoid follicular pattern" of the colon is a postulated cause of painless rectal bleeding.[26, 27] It has been associated with a variety of other pathologic conditions including immunodeficiency states and Hirschsprung's disease.[28–31] The mechanism of bleeding is thought to be thinning of the mucosa overlying the lymphatic tissue with trauma from the passage of fecal material or an endoscope leading to ulceration and hematochezia. However, in a prospective study of 48 patients no correlation could be found between the presence or absence of the nodules and any symptom complex.[32] In the children tested, no immunologic abnormality was found.

Lymphatic tissue nodules can be found throughout the gastrointestinal tract. They are particularly prominent in children, in whom they are found in 15% to 50% of air contrast barium enemas. The nodules are most conspicuous in children under 5 years of age.[33] At colonoscopy, smooth-surfaced, 1 to 2 mm yellowish-white nodules are noted and are most prominent in the rectum, sigmoid, and descending colon. Larger nodules

may have a central umbilication. The etiology of lymphoid hyperplasia is unknown, but it is thought to be a nonspecific response to antigenic stimulation, most often infection. The response is self-limited and does not require any specific therapy. Colonoscopy is indicated when there is difficulty in differentiating this benign condition from multiple polyps. This question may also arise in reference to the small intestine; endoscopic examination and biopsy of the terminal ileum during a colonoscopy may clarify abnormalities noted on small bowel x-rays.

Inflammatory Bowel Disease

Ulcerative Colitis

Ulcerative colitis has an incidence of 2.8 to 7.2 per 100,000 population[34] with a prevalence rate from 4.1 to 79.9 cases per 100,000.[35] Presenting symptoms develop in 30% to 40% of patients before 21 years of age.[36] The most common symptom is diarrhea, followed by rectal bleeding and abdominal pain, fatigue, weight loss, nausea and vomiting, and fever (Table 48–2).[37] Approximately half the pediatric and adolescent patients will have an insidious onset with low-grade fever accompanied by mild diarrhea.

Early endoscopic findings include hyperemia, edema, and loss of the normal vascular pattern; those of more progressive disease are granularity and friability with shallow, small ulcerations and erosions. Later changes include deeper ulcerations with pseudopolyp formation, shortening of the bowel with loss of interhaustral septae and mucosal bridging.[38] Direct examination with biopsy of the colonic mucosa is essential for diagnosis, as

TABLE 48–2. **Presenting Features in Ulcerative Colitis**

Finding	Adults (N = 465)	Children (N = 125)
Diarrhea	44%	53%
Rectal bleeding	39%	20%
Weight loss		10%
Abdominal pain	1%	5%
Arthritis		4%
Growth failure		2%

N = Number of patients studied.
Adapted from: Grand RJ, Homer DR. Inflammatory bowel disease in childhood and adolescence. Pediat Clin North Am 1975; 22:835–50.

TABLE 48–3. **Ulcerative Colitis and Carcinoma of Colon in 9 Pediatric Patients**

Age at Initial Diagnosis of Ulcerative Colitis (Years)	Duration of Disease Before Diagnosis of Cancer (Years)
4	12
8	11
8	15
11	15
11	15
12	16
16	11
18.5	22
19.5	14

From: Farmer RG, Michener WM, Mortimer EA. Long term prognosis of ulcerative colitis with onset in childhood or adolescence. J Clin Gastroenterol 1979; 1:301–5.

TABLE 48–4. **Initial Clinical Features in Crohn's Disease**

Finding	Patients (N = 175)	No. with Findings at Diagnosis Adults (N = 140)	Children (N = 66)
Abdominal pain	52%	85%	79%
Diarrhea	25%	62%	84%
Weight loss	2%	50%	40%
Fever		41%	72%
Rectal bleeding	6%	13%	30%
Arthritis	3%		20%
Mass	2%		10%

N = Number of patients studied.
Adapted from: Grand RJ, Kelts DG: Inflammatory bowel disease. Curr Probl Pediatr 1980; 10:1–40.

well as the assessment of the extent of disease and the progress of therapy.

Onset of ulcerative colitis in childhood is not associated with any greater risk for the development of carcinoma than is associated with onset during later years. Cancer surveillance is begun after 7 years since dysplastic changes have been infrequently encountered before 8 to 10 years' duration of disease.[39] In our long-term follow-up of 336 pediatric patients, carcinoma developed in 9 (Table 48–3). Colonoscopic surveillance for carcinoma and precancerous changes (dysplasia) is patterned after the approach to follow-up of adult patients (see Chapter 43). Multiple biopsies should be obtained sequentially from the cecum to the rectum with special attention to suspicious areas such as raised or irregular mucosal surfaces. If the endoscopic and histologic evaluation of the colon is unremarkable except for the presence of chronic ulcerative colitis, the evaluation is currently being repeated at an interval of 1 to 2 years. If dysplasia is found, follow-up at shorter intervals is required.

Crohn's Disease

The onset of Crohn's disease in the pediatric age group is often subtle with long delays between the onset of symptoms and diagnosis. The most common initial symptoms are diarrhea, abdominal pain, and fever (Table 48–4); these occur in more than 70% of patients. Weight loss is noted in approximately 40%, bleeding in 30%; 20% of the patients have arthritis as an initial manifes-

tation. An inflammatory mass is palpable in 10%.[36]

Pediatric patients with Crohn's disease can be divided into three prognostic groups according to the location of the disease.[42] Those with isolated small bowel disease tend to develop intestinal obstruction, perianal disease, and fistulae (Table 48–5). Occasionally, growth retardation may be the only manifestation of the disease. Arthritis, pyoderma,

TABLE 48–5. **Clinical Features of Crohn's Disease: Small Intestine Pattern**

Clinical Feature	Patients (%)*
Perianal disease	40 (26)
Internal fistulae	27 (18)
Intestinal obstruction	47 (31)
Growth retardation	10 (6)
Arthritis	11 (7)
Pyoderma	1
Erythema nodosum	4 (3)
Iritis or uveitis	0
Liver disease	0
Toxic megacolon	5 (4)
Died	2
Lost to follow-up	0

*Total number of patients = 151.
Follow-up greater than 5 years = 94 (62%); mean follow-up = 7.2 years.
Definitions: Perianal disease—any perianal fistula or abscess; internal fistula—enteroenteric, to another organ or space or enterocutaneous; growth retardation—less than 3rd percentile on growth curve; liver disease—any evidence for hepatobiliary disease; toxic megacolon—acute illness with dilation of colon to more than 7 cm diameter (plain x-ray film of abdomen).
From: Farmer RG, Michener WM. Prognosis of Crohn's disease with onset in childhood or adolescence. Dig Dis Sci 1979; 24:752–7.

TABLE 48–6. **Clinical Features of Crohn's Disease: Colon Pattern**

Clinical Feature	Patients (%)*
Perianal disease	31 (19)
Internal fistulae	25 (15)
Intestinal obstruction	31 (19)
Growth retardation	13 (8)
Arthritis	16 (10)
Pyoderma	2
Erythema nodosum	5 (4)
Iritis or uveitis	1
Liver disease	4 (3)
Toxic megacolon	19 (12)
Died	8 (5)
Lost to follow-up	6 (4)

*Total number of patients = 162.
Follow-up greater than 5 years = 107 (66%); mean follow-up = 7.6 years.
Definitions: Same as Table 48–5.
From: Farmer RG, Michener WM. Prognosis of Crohn's disease with onset in childhood or adolescence. Dig Dis Sci 1979; 24:752–7.

TABLE 48–7. **Clinical Features of Crohn's Disease: Ileocolic Pattern**

Clinical Feature	Patients (%)*
Perianal disease	64 (36)
Internal fistulae	34 (19)
Intestinal obstruction	45 (26)
Growth retardation	13 (7)
Arthritis	12 (7)
Pyoderma	1
Erythema nodosum	4 (2)
Iritis or uveitis	0
Liver disease	1
Toxic megacolon	7 (4)
Died	2 (1)
Lost to follow-up	3 (1)

*Total number of patients = 175.
Follow-up greater than 5 years = 115 (68%); mean follow-up = 7.4 years.
Definitions: Same as Table 48–5.
From: Farmer RG, Michener WM. Prognosis of Crohn's disease with onset in childhood or adolescence. Dig Dis Sci 1979; 24:752–7.

erythema nodosum, liver disease, iritis, and uveitis are uncommon. Toxic megacolon occurs in about 5% of these patients. Children with isolated colonic disease also have perianal inflammation, fistulae, and tend to develop intestinal obstruction (Table 48–6). Arthritis, growth retardation, and toxic megacolon each occurs in about 10% of patients; liver disease develops in 5% and erythema nodosum, iritis, uveitis, and pyoderma occur infrequently. In combined ileal and colonic Crohn's disease, perianal inflammation occurs in one third of patients, intestinal obstruction in one fourth, and fistulae in almost 20% (Table 48–7). The frequencies for growth retardation, cutaneous, ophthalmic and hepatic problems are similar to those in children with isolated large bowel disease.

Crohn's disease is usually diagnosed by barium contrast radiography and/or endoscopy. Colonoscopy during the early stages of the disease usually reveals aphthous ulcers with segments of erythema and edema separated by normal mucosa. As the disease progresses, serpiginous ulcerations with undermined edges and a "cobblestone" appearance may develop. Rectal suction biopsies provide larger, less distorted specimens than those obtained with endoscopic forceps. In some series, suction specimens have increased diagnostic yield by 50%.[43] In patients with isolated small bowel disease, intubation of the terminal ileum at colonoscopy may aid in distinguishing benign conditions from Crohn's ileitis.

The incidence of carcinoma in Crohn's disease appears to be greater than that of the normal population, but the risk is not of the magnitude associated with ulcerative colitis. Since the risk has not been precisely defined, patients are not routinely screened for dysplastic mucosal changes.

References

1. Thomas G, Brozinsky S, Isenberg JI. Patient acceptance and effectiveness of a balanced lavage solution (Golytely) versus the standard preparation for colonoscopy. Gastroenterology 1982; 82:435–7.
2. Hassall E, Barclay GN, Ament ME. Colonoscopy in childhood. Pediatrics 1984; 73:594-9.
3. Habr-Gama A, Alves PRA, Gama-Rodriques JJ, et al. Pediatric colonoscopy. Dis Colon Rectum 1979; 22:530–5.
4. Williams CB, Laage NJ, Campbell CA, et al. Total colonoscopy in children. Arch Dis Child 1982; 57:49–53.
5. Byrne WJ, Evler AR, Campbell M, Eisenach K. Bacteremia in children following upper gastrointestinal endoscopy or colonoscopy. J Pediatr Gastroenterol Nutr 1982; 1:551–3.
6. Gans SL, Ament M, Cristie DL. Pediatric endoscopy with flexible fiberscopes. J Pediatr Surg 1975; 10:375–80.
7. Holgersen LO, Mossberg SM, Miller RE. Colonoscopy for rectal bleeding in childhood. J Pediatr Surg 1978; 13:83–5.
8. Vincent M, Smith LE. Management of perforation due to colonoscopy. Dis Colon Rectum 1983; 26: 61–3.
9. Livstone EM, Cohen GM, Troncale FJ, et al. Diastatic serosal lacerations: an unrecognized complication of colonoscopy. Gastroenterology 1974; 67: 1245–7.
10. Hillemeier C. Rectal bleeding in childhood. Pediatrics in Review 1983; 5:35–41.

11. Roth SI, Helwig EB. Juvenile polyps of the colon and rectum. Cancer 1963; 16:468–79.

12. Louw JH. Polypoid lesions of the large bowel in children with particular reference to benign lymphoid polyposis. J Pediatr Surg 1968; 3:195–209.

13. Veale AMO, McColl I, Bussen HJR, et al. Juvenile polyposis coli. J Med Genet 1966; 3:5–16.

14. Bussey HJ, Veale AMO, Morson BC. Genetics of gastrointestinal polyposis. Gastroenterology 1978; 74:1325–30.

15. Stemper TJ, Kent TH, Summers RW. Juvenile polyposis and gastrointestinal carcinoma: a study of a kindred. Ann Intern Med 1975; 83:639–46.

16. Johns TNP, Wheeler JR, Johns FS. Meckel's diverticulum disease: a study of 154 cases. Ann Surg 1959; 150:241–56.

17. Soltero MJ, Bill AH. The natural history of Meckel's diverticulum and its relation to incidental removal. Am J Surg 1976; 132:168–73.

18. Fisher SE, Harrison M, Adkins JC. Colonoscopic diagnosis of vascular anomalies in children. Clin Pediatr 1979; 18:299–303.

19. Rodesch P, Cadranel S, Peeters JP, et al. Colonic endoscopy in children. Acta Paediatr Belg 1976; 29:181–4.

20. Skovgaard S, Sorensen FH. Bleeding hemangioma of the colon diagnosed by colonoscopy. J Pediatr Surg 1976; 11:83–4.

21. Soehendra N. Colonoscopy in children. Proctology 1979; 1:8.

22. Abrahamson J, Shandling B. Intestinal hemangiomata in childhood and a syndrome for diagnosis: a collective review. J Pediatr Surg 1973; 8:487–95.

23. Morris SJ, Kaplan SR, Ballan K, et al. Blue-rubber-bleb nevus syndrome. JAMA 1978; 239:1887.

24. Haddad HM, Wilkins L. Congenital anomalies associated with gonadal aplasia: review of 55 cases. Pediatrics 1959; 23:885–902.

25. Goodman RM, Smith EW, Paton D, et al. Pseudoxanthoma elasticum: a clinical and histopathological study. Medicine 1963; 42:297–334.

26. Capitanio MA, Kirkpatrick JA. Lymphoid hyperplasia of the colon in children. Radiology 1970; 94:323–7.

27. Kaplan B, Benson J, Rothstein F, et al. Lymphonodular hyperplasia of the colon as a pathologic finding in children with lower gastrointestinal bleeding. J Pediatr Gastroenterol Nutr 1984; 3:704.

28. Knutsen AP, Merten DF, Buckley RH. Colonic nodular lymphoid hyperplasia in a child with antibody deficiency and near normal immunoglobins. J Pediatr 1981; 98:420–3.

29. Wolfson JJ, Goldstein G, Krivit W, et al. Lymphoid hyperplasia of the large intestine associated with dysgammaglobulinemia. Am J Roentgenol 1970; 108:610–4.

30. Ament ME, Ochs HD, David SD. Structure and function of the gastrointestinal tract in primary immunodeficiency syndromes: a study of 39 patients. Medicine 1973; 52:227–48.

31. Shannon R, Vickers TH. Multiple colonic polyposis in Hirschsprung's disease. Aust NZ J K Surg 1967; 37:108–13.

32. Riddlesberger MM Jr, Lebenthal E. Nodular colonic mucosa of childhood: normal or pathologic? Gastroenterology 1980; 79:265–70.

33. Theander G, Tragardh B. Lymphoid hyperplasia of the colon in childhood. Acta Radiol (Diagn) 1976; 17:631–48.

34. Garland CF, Lilienfeld AM, Mendeloff AI, et al. Incidence rates of ulcerative colitis and Crohn's disease in fifteen areas in the United States. Gastroenterology 1981; 81:1115–24.

35. Monk M, Mendeloff AI, Siegel CI, et al. An epidemiological study of ulcerative colitis and regional enteritis among adults in Baltimore. I. Hospital incidence and prevalence 1960 to 1963. Gastroenterology 1967; 53:198–210.

36. Grand RJ, Homer DR. Inflammatory bowel disease in childhood and adolescence. Pediat Clin North Am 1975; 22:835–50.

37. Michener WM. Ulcerative colitis in children. Pediatr Clin North Am 1967; 14:159–73.

38. Waye JD. The role of colonoscopy in the differential diagnosis of inflammatory bowel disease. Gastrointest Endosc 1977; 23:150–4.

39. Lennard-Jones JE, Morson BC, Ritchie JK, Williams CB. Cancer surveillance in ulcerative colitis. Experience over 15 years. Lancet 1983; 2:149–52.

40. Farmer RG, Michener WM, Mortimer EA. Long term prognosis of ulcerative colitis with onset in childhood or adolescence. J Clin Gastroenterol 1979; 1:301–5.

41. Grand RJ, Kelts DG. Inflammatory bowel disease. Curr Probl Pediatr 1980; 10:1–40.

42. Farmer RG, Michener WM. Prognosis of Crohn's disease with onset in childhood or adolescence. Dig Dis Sci 1979; 24:752–7.

43. Hill RB, Kent TH, Hansen RN. Clinical usefulness of rectal biopsy in Crohn's disease. Gastroenterology 1979; 77(4 Pt 2): 938–44.

Chapter 49

FLEXIBLE SIGMOIDOSCOPY

JAMES W. MANIER, M.D.

The flexible sigmoidoscope has been a controversial instrument in the United States since its introduction in 1976. With the passing of time its place in the practice of medicine is gradually becoming better defined. It is now apparent that its use should not be limited to endoscopists alone. Although it has been shown that the fiberoptic instrument is better tolerated than the rigid sigmoidoscope[1-4] and that more lesions are discovered because of the greater depth of insertion,[1, 2, 5-8] major questions remain such as training of nonendoscopists in the procedure, its safety in the hands of the nonendoscopists, cost effectiveness, and the best length of the instrument.

INSTRUMENTATION

A large number of flexible sigmoidoscopes are offered by several manufacturers. For the most part these are fiberoptic instruments based on the principles outlined in Chapter 2. However, an electronic-type instrument built around a charge couple device is also available (Welch Allyn) (see Chapter 10, Part 6). Because of the electronic endoscope, the term flexible sigmoidoscope is used to encompass all available instrument types.

Characteristics of Flexible Sigmoidoscopes

In addition to basic differences in the method of image transmission, there are other major and minor differences between various flexible sigmoidoscope models. The length of the insertion tube is the one major difference. Flexible sigmoidoscopes can be broadly classified into 35-cm and 60-cm lengths, although there are slight variations from these norms from one manufacturer's

model to another. Some flexible sigmoidoscopes are built for electrosurgical procedures such as polypectomy (Figs. 49–1 and 49–2). There are slight differences in the degree of tip deflection, accessory channel diameter, depth of focus, and angle of the field of view. Some instruments are equipped for photography. Some have automatic air insufflation and water irrigation mechanisms similar to those found with most colonoscopes. Others employ a hand-operated bulb for air insufflation and/or an attached syringe for irrigation. The external suction connection is on the umbilical section of the endoscope in some cases and on the control section of the instrument in others. Some operators find that the latter allows easier cleaning of the suction line should it become obstructed by fecal debris. The suction line connection is on the control section of most newer model flexible sigmoidoscopes. Some of the characteristics of flexible sigmoidoscopes commercially available in the United States are given in Tables 49–1 and 49–2 (Figs. 49–1 to 49–7). There are also a variety of light sources for use with flexible sigmoidoscopes; these also have varying characteristics and capabilities but will not be discussed here.

Cost

The cost of equipment for flexible sigmoidoscopy can be a major consideration. For the individual office practice of a nonendoscopist physician, price may be a significant factor. Price may also be a consideration for the medical center in which a number of instruments and light sources may be required for screening sigmoidoscopy programs for large numbers of patients. Generally, the cost of the equipment increases in proportion to capability, except that there are only minor differences in price with respect to the length

Text continued on page 980

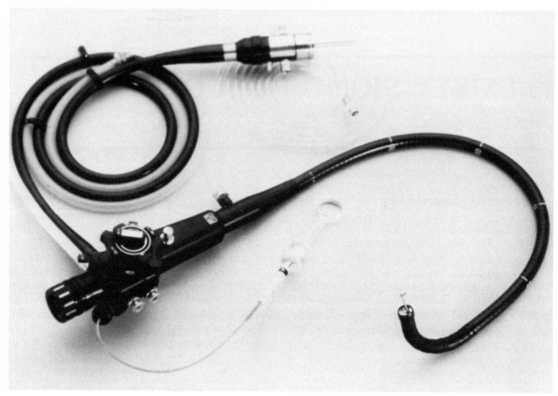

FIGURE 49–1. Olympus CF-ITS2 fiberoptic sigmoidoscope.

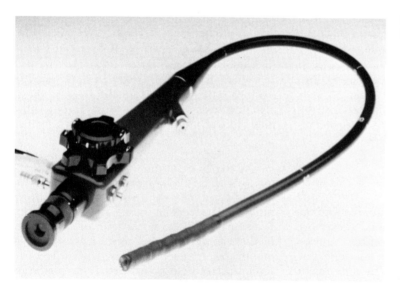

FIGURE 49–2. Olympus OSF fiberoptic sigmoidoscope.

TABLE 49–1. **Specifications of 60-cm Flexible Sigmoidoscopes**

Specification	Manufacturer								
	Olympus	Olympus	Fujinon	Fujinon	Pentax	Reichert	American ACMI	American ACMI	Welch Allyn
Model	OSF-60	CPF-P10-S	SIG-E2	SIG-PC	FS-34A	SC-5	T915	TX915	80055
Length (cm)	60	63	72.5	65	62	65	61	62	60
Diameter (mm)	12.2	12.2	13	13	11.5	13.6	13	13.2	13.5
Tip deflection									
(degrees up/down)	180	180	180	180	180	180	180	180	180
(degrees left/right)	160	160	160	160	160	160	165	165	160
Field of view (degrees)	100	120	105	105	95	100	75	—	90
Depth of focus (mm)	3–100	5–100	2–120	4–120	3–100	10–70	5–80	—	3–100
Diameter accessory channel (mm)	3.2	3.2	3.7	3.7	3.7	3.2	3.3	3.3	3.0
Suction	External	External	Internal	External	External	External	External	External	External
Air insufflation	Automatic	Automatic	Automatic	Automatic	Automatic	Automatic	Automatic	Automatic	Automatic
Irrigation	Manual	Can be automatic	Automatic	Manual	Automatic	Manual	Manual	Automatic	Manual
Immersible	No	Yes	No	No	No	No	No	No	No
Cost, 1984 dollars (approx.)	2900	5400	4200	2700	3250	2275	3275	4550	7560 w/TV monitor and processor
(with light source)	(3250)		(4500)	(2900)	(3500)	(2650)			

TABLE 49–2. **Specifications of 35-cm Flexible Sigmoidoscopes**

Specification	Manufacturer			
	Olympus	Fujinon	Reichert	Reichert
Model	OSF-35	PRO-PC	FPS-3	SC-35
Length (cm)	35	35	35	35
Diameter (mm)	12.2	13	13.2	13.4
Tip deflection				
(degrees up/down)	180	180	175	170
(degrees left/right)	160	160	—	140
Field of view (degrees)	100	105	75	90
Depth of focus (mm)	3–100	4–120	10–70	10–70
Diameter accessory channel (mm)	3.2	3.7	2.6	2.6
Suction	External	External	External	External
Air insufflation	Automatic	Automatic	Manual	Automatic
Irrigation	Manual	Manual	Manual	Manual
Immersible	No	No	No	No
Cost, 1984 dollars (approx.)	2700	2500	1200	1775
(with light source)	(3050)	(2700)	(1475)	(2150)

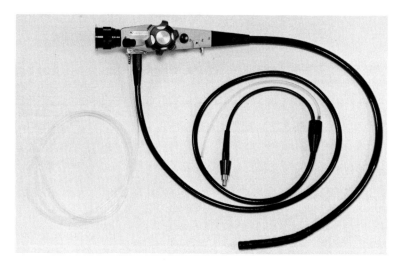

FIGURE 49–3. Reichert (A. O. Scientific) SC4B fiberoptic sigmoidoscope.

FIGURE 49–4. Reichert (A. O. Scientific) FPS-3 fiberoptic sigmoidoscope.

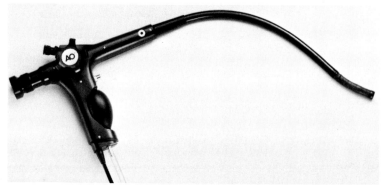

FIGURE 49–5. A.C.M.I. TX-915 fiberoptic sigmoidoscope.

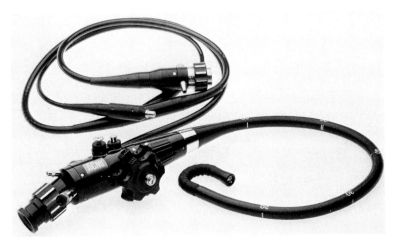

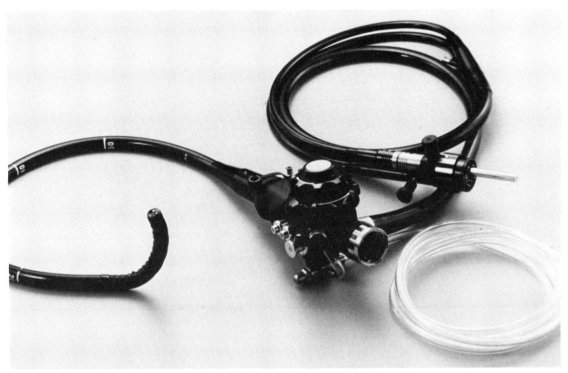

FIGURE 49–6. Pentax SIG-E2 fiberoptic sigmoidoscope.

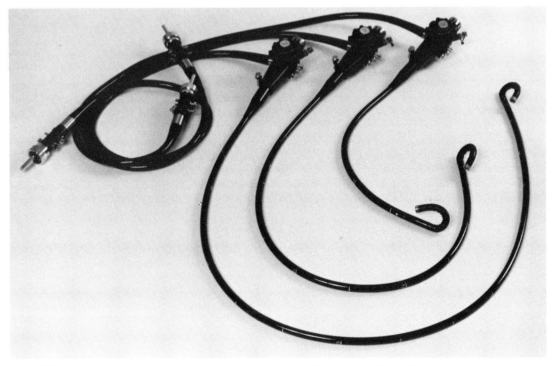

FIGURE 49–7. Fujinon 65-cm fiberoptic sigmoidoscope, 147-cm and 183-cm fiberoptic colonoscopes.

of the insertion tube. The cost of a 35-cm length instrument is usually only a few hundred dollars less than that of a 60-cm length instrument made by the same manufacturer. However, increased capability of the instrument in other respects increases its costs. Some options such as the ability to take photographs may be a necessity in a teaching center but an expensive luxury in an office practice. Four-way tip deflection markedly increases cost, but this is a necessity, especially in 60-cm length instruments. An accessory channel is also required for all sigmoidoscopes. Although extensive patient preparation is not necessary for flexible sigmoidoscopy, fecal material and enema fluid may nevertheless be present at examination, and since the accessory channel is also the suction channel, a larger-diameter channel is advantageous. This also allows the use of a larger forceps for biopsy. It has been shown that biopsy specimen size is greater with larger forceps and that these larger pieces of tissue may be obtained with no increased risk of bleeding or perforation.[9]

One often overlooked factor in the purchase decision is the availability, quality, and promptness of manufacturer's service for repair of malfunctioning equipment. In this author's opinion, good service is the single most important criterion in the decision to purchase a flexible sigmoidoscope, light source, and acccessories from any manufacturer.

INSERTION TUBE LENGTH

The ideal length for the flexible sigmoidoscope is still debated (see section on 35-cm instruments). In the greatest measure this must be determined on an individual basis and must be influenced by the experience and competence of the physician(s) who will use the equipment. Insertion tube diameter does not seem to influence acceptance of the procedure by patients or ease of insertion except for attempts to pass the instrument through a stricture. The importance of differences in instrument characteristics, especially length, is not entirely clear at present.

35-cm Flexible Sigmoidoscope

The 35-cm length flexible sigmoidoscope has been introduced because of concerns about cost and the safety of the 60-cm sigmoidoscope in the hands of nonendoscopists.

Hocutt et al.[10] trained family practice residents in the use of a 35-cm fiberoptic instrument. Training included attendance at one or two 1-hour conferences, perusal of a seven-page instruction booklet, and supervision by a preceptor during examinations. One resident averaged 28.5 cm insertion depth after 18 examinations and another averaged 29.7 cm after 40 procedures. The overall average for participants in the program after 102 endoscopies was 27.7 cm. The average time of examination was 13.4 minutes. There were no complications. The fiberoptic procedure was preferred by 94% of 36 patients who had been examined previously with a rigid proctosigmoidoscope.

Schapiro et al.[11] trained three gastrointestinal assistants, skilled in assisting at colonoscopy, with a prototype 35-cm fiberoptic sigmoidoscope with four-way tip deflection. Average examination time was 5 minutes. Average length of insertion was 24 cm. X-ray films showed that this insertion depth rarely included the entire sigmoid colon. Fourteen percent of the patients had significant pathologic findings. Immediately after each of the trainees' examinations, the supervising gastroenterologist repeated the procedure with a 60-cm fiberoptic sigmoidoscope. Analysis of the findings from this second examination disclosed that the trainees had overlooked less than 1% of the lesions found by the supervising physician within the range of the 35-cm endoscope. The missed lesions were all diminutive polyps. The second examination by an experienced gastroenterologist also resulted in a 16% increase in the yield of significant lesions because of greater depth of insertion with the 60-cm length instrument. Ninety-four percent of the patients preferred the examination with the 35-cm endoscope in comparison with their previous sigmoidoscopy experience with a rigid instrument. Seventy-six percent preferred the 35-cm flexible instrument examination to that with the 60-cm length instrument.

Winawer et al.[12] have reported the results of 200 examinations performed by a primary care physician with prior but limited experience with rigid sigmoidoscopy. The trainee observed a number of colonoscopies and 60-cm fiberoptic sigmoidoscopic examinations, and then briefly received "hands-on" instruction from an endoscopist using a colon model and a 35-cm endoscope. He then examined several patients under the supervision of the endoscopist. During the first 50 procedures by the trainee, insertion time was less than 8 minutes in 24%, less than 10 minutes in 58%, and less than 12 minutes in 72%. During the next 150 procedures 94% of examinations took less than 8 minutes and 97% less than 10 minutes. Comparison of the trainee's results with a random sample of 400 patients undergoing rigid sigmoidoscopy at the same clinic revealed that use of the 35-cm endoscope doubled the average insertion depth (16 to 30 cm) and provided a sensitive examination of the distal 30 to 35 cm of rectosigmoid.

We have found in our studies at the Lovelace Medical Center that our internists required only one third more time for introduction of the 60-cm fiberscope beyond an insertion depth of 30 cm.

Grobe et al.[13] compared 35-cm fibersigmoidoscopy to rigid proctosigmoidoscopy in 71 consecutive patients. Average examination time was 3.6 minutes for the rigid and 4.2 minutes for the fiberoptic examination. Mean insertion length was 21 cm with the rigid instrument and 29.5 cm with the flexible one. Discomfort was quantitated by patients according to a discomfort index (0 = none, 1 = mild to moderate, 2 = severe). During the rigid examination 29.6% of patients experienced no discomfort versus 69.0% during flexible examination. Severe discomfort was noted by 19.7% during the rigid examination compared with 5.6% during the fiberoptic procedure. Significant pathologic findings were discovered in 8 patients during examination with the rigid instrument; the flexible sigmoidoscope revealed important findings in 13 patients. One rectal carcinoma and seven polyps were detected by both procedures. Another nine polyps were discovered only by use of the 35-cm flexible instrument.

Logically, the diagnostic yield should be greater with the 60-cm length sigmoidoscope than that obtained with the 35-cm instrument. Marks et al.,[5] for example, found that one half of the 400 polyps they identified with the 60-cm endoscope were beyond the 30-cm level. Direct comparisons between 60-cm and 35-cm flexible sigmoidoscopes have been reported[14-16] (Table 49–3).

Zucker et al.[14] found no clear advantage of one instrument length over the other. In their study of 96 patients who underwent both examinations there was no significant difference in the number of polyps found with either instrument. The authors found that it was not possible to utilize the full length of the 60-cm fiberoptic sigmoidoscope in 38 cases because of stool in the colon; the average depth of insertion of the 60-cm instrument was only 44 cm. The time required for the 35-cm examination was significantly less than for the 60-cm procedure. Patient discomfort was less with the shorter instrument.

Dubow et al.[15] examined 258 asymptomatic patients aged 45 and older in a random fashion with both 35-cm and 60-cm instruments. Full insertion of the 60-cm instrument was achieved in 78.8% of cases versus 98.5% with the 35-cm endoscope. Mean insertion depth was 55.9 cm versus 34.9 cm. The 35-cm examination required significantly less time than the 60-cm procedure and was preferred by the majority of patients. Forty-nine of 50 known polyps were found with the 60-cm endoscope and 38 with the 35-cm fiberscope. However, in 80% of the patients with polyps, at least one polyp was found during the 35-cm procedure. The authors regarded 35-cm flexible sigmoidoscopy as fulfilling many of the criteria of a screening procedure.

TABLE 49–3. **Comparison of Studies of 60-cm and 35-cm Flexible Sigmoidoscopy**

Results	60-cm			35-cm		
	Zucker et al.[14]	*Dubow et al.*[15]	*Sarles et al.*[16]	*Zucker et al.*[14]	*Dubow et al.*[15]	*Sarles et al.*[16]
No. examinations	96	258	100	96	258	100
Insertion depth (mean, cm)	44	56	60	28	35	34
Examination time (mean, min)	9.8	5.7	9.6	6.4	2.5	4.2
No. cancers found	6	—	2	6	—	2
No. polyps found	25	49	24	21	38	18

In the study by Sarles et al.,[16] the yield of pathologic findings for the 35-cm examination did not differ significantly from that for the 60-cm procedure. Patients noted less discomfort with the 35-cm instrument. The results obtained with the 60-cm sigmoidoscope by an operator experienced in colonoscopy are undoubtedly better than those of a physician who undertakes the same examination without prior endoscopic experience. The mobility of the sigmoid colon on its mesentery is one of the main technical problems in colonoscopy. The competent colonoscopist has learned either to maintain the sigmoid loop in a relatively straight configuration or to manipulate the sigmoid loop to advantage. As a result, the real depth of insertion of the flexible sigmoidoscope for the experienced endoscopist will in most cases be greater than that achieved by the inexperienced examiner. In many cases the colonoscopist will pass the 60-cm instrument well into the descending colon.

Depth of Insertion

The depth of insertion of a flexible sigmoidoscope does not accurately indicate the actual length of the colon examined. Lehman et al.[17] assessed the anatomic extent of fiberoptic sigmoidoscopy by placing a metal clip on the colonic mucosa at the point of deepest insertion. The location of the clip was then determined during barium enema. Examinations were performed by house staff under the supervision of an experienced endoscopist who completed the examination when the trainee was unable to do so. There was no prolonged effort to straighten the sigmoid colon. The 60-cm instrument was inserted to the maximum possible depth in 58 patients. Study of the position of the clips indicated that at least 75% of the sigmoid colon was examined in all these cases, and that in 81% the area viewed included the sigmoid–descending colon junction. At least one half of the descending colon was seen in 34%, and in 7% the instrument tip reached a point proximal to the splenic flexure. In 15 patients in this study the 60-cm instrument was only inserted to a depth of 30 to 35 cm. The position of the clips in these patients disclosed that at least 50% of the sigmoid colon was examined in 60%, and that at least 75% was examined in 33%. Although the 35-cm instrument was inserted to the splenic flexure in 6%, the entire sigmoid was viewed in only 13% of the examinations. The authors attrib-

uted these results in part to the wide range in length and differences in tortuosity of the sigmoid in any group of patients. In general, the anatomic extent of the examination decreased in proportion to the depth of insertion of the sigmoidoscope.

In a similar study by Ott et al.,[18] in which the anatomic extent of the fiberoptic sigmoidoscopy procedure was evaluated radiographically, full insertion of the 60-cm instrument (accomplished in 74%) made possible the examination of the entire sigmoid colon in 45% of patients. The authors attributed failure to examine the entire sigmoid to poor colon preparation, patient intolerance, previous pelvic surgery, and redundancy of the sigmoid. In this study, however, a plain x-ray film was used to assess the location of the tip of the instrument at maximum insertion. In the study by Lehman et al.[17] it was shown that this technique overestimated or underestimated the extent of visualization in 27% of the cases.

Instrument Choice

At present it is difficult or impossible to make recommendations concerning the "best" flexible sigmoidoscope for nonendoscopists. Each insertion tube length has certain advantages and disadvantages. The cost of either length instrument is approximately the same. With respect to the frequency of instrument breakdown, one manufacturer found this to be 25% higher for their 60-cm instrument than for their 35-cm model (personal communication, American Optical Company, 1983). For those with little experience in endoscopic procedures, it is easier to learn to perform 35-cm flexible sigmoidoscopy safely and with the greatest possible patient comfort. However, the yield for flexible sigmoidoscopy in the hands of an experienced examiner will usually be greater with a 60-cm instrument.

TRAINING

The level of training necessary to achieve a reasonable level of competence in flexible sigmoidoscopy and how this should be carried out are still debatable issues. There is general agreement that some training is necessary. Most endoscopists who teach the procedure believe short 2- to 3-day courses with some work in plastic models is not a satisfactory approach, although it may be a means of introducing students to the principles of fiberoptic endoscopy.

Johnson et al.[19] introduced the 60-cm flexible fiberscope as a screening tool into their family practice residency program in 1980. Five faculty members were trained in the procedure by a gastroenterologist faculty member. Residents were instructed in the mechanics, limitations, and cleaning procedures of the sigmoidoscope. A 1-hour teaching session on fiberoptic sigmoidoscopy was then presented during the first month of the academic year to all residents in the program. Faculty members experienced in fiberoptic sigmoidoscopy were present during all family practice clinics, as was the endoscope and its teaching attachment. After the first 100 procedures (approximately 20% by faculty) the instrument was introduced to an average depth of 49 cm. Fifteen polyps, three cancers, one case of ulcerative colitis, and two cases of Crohn's disease were found. In this teaching environment each resident performed between 25 and 50 examinations. After almost 3 years, over 400 examinations had been done with no complications.

We have trained 10 general internists in 60-cm fiberoptic sigmoidoscopy at the Lovelace Medical Center. The physicians became comfortable with the procedure after performing 8 to 10 examinations. On an average, competence was obtained after 20 examinations. Average time of examination was 10 minutes with no complications occurring during the period of training. Patient pain and discomfort seemed to be related to the technique and ability of the individual examiner rather than to the level of experience.

McCray[20] trained five physicians experienced in rigid sigmoidoscopy in fiberoptic sigmoidoscopy. Four of the five became competent after performing an average of 50 examinations. The only complication during the training period was impaction of the instrument in a patient's rectum, the endoscope being removed by the instructor without injury to patient or endoscope.

Schapiro et al.[21] offered training with a 35-cm fiberoptic sigmoidoscope to active staff physicians of two community hospitals utilizing their own patients. Seventy-five percent of physicians who were offered the program enrolled; 85% of this group attended an introductory session but only 10% completed the program. When subsequently asked why they did not continue the course, physicians noted concern about using their own patients, personal time constraints, and worry about cost benefits of fiberoptic sigmoidos-

copy. Schapiro et al.[21] found that seven training sessions seemed adequate to train most physicians. An additional five examinations with a 60-cm fiberscope led to proficiency with this instrument. Endoscopic pathology was easily identified by the trainee physicians, and no complications occurred during the study.

It seems likely that much of the future training of physicians in flexible sigmoidoscopy will be given in residency programs. For those physicians who are already in practice, proper training will have to be on a preceptorial basis with experienced endoscopists.

INDICATIONS AND CONTRAINDICATIONS

Indications

Endoscopists disagree on the indications for flexible sigmoidoscopy (Table 49–4). Certainly the present list is incomplete as new uses are regularly reported. Most endoscopists agree that the procedure is excellent for routine polyp-cancer surveillance at 2- to 5-year intervals in asymptomatic patients over age 45.[1, 5, 6, 22, 24–26] It is the preferred instrument for evaluation of the distal colon prior to a barium enema, since the sigmoid colon is less well examined radiographically owing to its anatomic configuration.[5, 22] It can be introduced more easily in the patient with a physical disability such as a stroke than the rigid sigmoidoscope when the examination is performed in the left lateral decubitus position.[22] In patients with rectal complaints such as tenesmus or pruritus, it should be the first diagnostic modality after the history and physical examination.[22, 24] It can be of assistance in delineating the nature of indeterminate or uncertain findings on barium enema in the rectum or distal sigmoid colon and can be used as an initial procedure in evaluating the genesis of an acute colitis.[22, 25] It can determine the basis of a mass found in association with sigmoid diverticular disease and may help in evaluating functional lower bowel complaints.[22, 24, 25] It is suggested in some reports that reproduction of a patient's symptoms during the examination is a useful diagnostic finding,[24] although this is debatable.

Indications that are somewhat more controversial include the following. It has been used for sigmoid volvulus decompression. However, subsequent elective sigmoid resec-

TABLE 49–4. **Indications for Fiberoptic Sigmoidoscopy***

	Manier[22]	Marks et al.[5]	Vellacott and Hardcastle[6]	Holt and Wherry[23]	Bohlman et al.[1]
No. patients	304	1012	350	116	120
Screening	56.9	20.1	15.3	9.5	30.8
Symptom resolution	28.1	31.4	29.6	44.8	54.2
Polyp surveillance	1.3	19.5	36.6	28.4	
Cancer follow-up	4.2	13.0	18.5	6.1	11.7
X-ray confirmation	1.3	7.3		5.2	
Preoperative clearance		0.5			
Anatomosis inspection		1.3			
IBD monitoring	8.2	1.3		3.4	3.3
Rigid scope failure		1.7		2.6	
Other indications		3.9			

*Except for the number of patients in each series, data are given as percentage of examinations.
Modified from: Manier JW. The role of flexible sigmoidoscopy in the practice of a gastroenterologist. Gastrointest Endosc 1983; 29:122–3.

tion is preferred since a volvulus will otherwise recur in approximately 50% of patients.[25] The instrument has been used for follow-up after resection of sigmoid carcinoma to inspect the anastomosis for local recurrence and for surveillance of the rectal segment for recurrence and removal of polyps in patients with familial polyposis who have undergone ileal rectostomy.[22, 24]

Flexible fiberoptic sigmoidoscopy does not substitute for colonoscopic surveillance for polyp recurrence after colonoscopic polypectomy and for dysplasia in inflammatory bowel disease or in follow-up after surgery for colon cancer.[22, 26] Colonoscopy is also the only acceptable endoscopic method for the direct observation of unexplained radiographic abnormalities proximal to the sigmoid colon, for the determination of the proximal extent of ulcerative colitis, and for the evaluation of Crohn's colitis.[22, 26]

It is imperative that the limitations imposed by the length of the flexible sigmoidoscope, the need for adequate training, and the cost-benefit effectiveness of flexible sigmoidoscopy be kept firmly in mind by physicians who undertake the procedure. It should also be remembered that fiberoptic sigmoidoscopy is only one part of the evaluation of colonic symptoms and/or lesions, and that other modalities such as barium enema, colonoscopy, and fecal occult blood testing have important places.[7, 27, 28]

It is probable that the major use of the flexible sigmoidoscope will be in the office practice of medicine in ambulatory patients undergoing routine surveillance examinations for colonic polyps and cancer. It is with respect to this indication that the procedure has its greatest potential to impact favorably on a major health care problem in countries with a high incidence of colonic neoplasia. In the United States, current recommendations for screening of patients with no known risk factors include an annual digital rectal examination after age 40, an annual stool guaiac determination after age 50, and sigmoidoscopy every 3 to 5 years after age 50 provided two initial sigmoidoscopies one year apart are negative.

Contraindications

There are relatively few absolute contraindications to flexible sigmoidoscopy; common sense dictates that the procedure should not be performed in patients with suspected bowel perforation, acute peritonitis, acute fulminant colitis or toxic megacolon, large aneurysms, acute diverticulitis, and paralytic ileus. There are also some relative contraindications such as severe cardiac or respiratory disease, late stages of pregnancy, severe coagulation disorders, pelvic adhesions, and suspected ischemic bowel necrosis.

PREPARATION

Since routine surveillance will likely constitute the major indication for flexible sigmoidoscopy in terms of numbers of patients examined, the preparation for the examination must be simple, easily and rapidly administered, and effective in cleaning the distal 60 to 70 cm of the large bowel.

In general, three types of preparation have been recommended: a single phosphosoda enema immediately prior to the examination,[1, 3, 6, 23, 29] two enemas before the study,[2, 5, 8] or a laxative given somewhat in advance plus an enema prior to the examination.[30] A review of studies concerned with various methods of preparation supports the view that a single enema is as effective as two enemas and perhaps more effective (Table 49–5). This may be because the second enema washes down fecal debris from more proximal areas of the colon. However, what is most impressive is that a high degree of success is obtained with all types of preparation.

It is important in my experience that the enema be given with the patient in the left lateral decubitus position and with instructions to retain the enema until the urge to defecate becomes well established. Placing a cot in the restroom near the toilet reduces anxiety over premature defecation on the floor and improves patient compliance. We studied the preparation procedure in 49 consecutive patients prepared with a single enema. The mean time for preparation was 4 minutes with a range of 2 to 10 minutes. If the initial preparation is found to be inadequate upon introduction of the endoscope, it is a simple procedure to return the patient to the restroom and repeat the preparation.

TECHNIQUE OF FLEXIBLE SIGMOIDOSCOPY

One of the advantages of flexible sigmoidoscopy is that the procedure can be carried out with the patient lying in the lateral decubitus position, a distinctly more comfortable position than the knee-chest or the tilt table positions commonly used in rigid sigmoidoscopy. Although the rigid examination can also be performed with the patient in a lateral decubitus position, this is more difficult for the examiner even when the patient is placed at the edge of the examining table. Frequently the rigid instrument must be placed at an upward angle relative to the position of the examiner. Since this position is uncomfortable for the endoscopist, it frequently compromises the success of the procedure. Flexible sigmoidoscopy can also be performed with the patient kneeling across the standard tilt table, although it is rarely necessary to tilt the patient's head down more than a few degrees, if at all. Sedation is seldom, if ever, necessary for flexible sigmoidoscopy.

Digital rectal examination and anoscopy (see Chapter 47) are important aspects of the procedure. It is often difficult to adequately visualize the anal canal using a flexible sigmoidoscope. The rectal ampulla, especially the posterior aspect, is also a blind area unless a retroflexion maneuver is performed in the rectum.

The procedure is begun with a rectal examination performed by the examiner with a well-lubricated, gloved index finger. This must be done gently, pushing the ball of the tip of the finger obliquely through the anal orifice in its wider anterior-posterior axis. The rectal examination allows the exclusion of a low-lying obstruction such as a tumor that would interfere with subsequent passage of the endoscope, and it also lubricates the anal canal.[10, 31]

After the rectal examination a well-lubricated anoscope is passed into the anal canal and the canal is thoroughly inspected[24, 31] (see Chapter 47).

After the anoscope is removed, the lubri-

TABLE 49–5. **Preparation for Fiberoptic Sigmoidoscopy**

Method	Results		No. Patients	Author(s)
	*Adequate**	*Inadequate**		
Single enema	90.0	10.0	120	Bohlman et al.[1]
	98.0	2.0	468	Crespi et al.[29]
	97.4	2.6	116	Holt and Wherry[23]
	93.3	6.7	306	Manier[22]
	95.4	4.6	350	Vellacott and Hardcastle[6]
Two enemas	49.0	21.3	516	Leicester et al.[2]
	96.8	3.2	1012	Marks et al.[5]
	80.0	20.0	342	Winnan et al.[8]
Enema plus laxative	82	18	175	Record et al.[30]

*Percentage of patients examined.

cated flexible sigmoidoscope is inserted into the rectum obliquely, so as to take advantage of the longer anterior-posterior dimension of the anal sphincter, and then advanced further into the rectum. The endoscope must be advanced several centimeters before attempting to deflect the tip. Premature attempts at deflection accomplish nothing until the entire bending section of the instrument is in the rectum.

The initial endoscopic view may reveal only a "red-out" because the instrument tip is against the mucosa. In this situation the instrument should be slowly withdrawn until the lumen comes into view. Only then should the instrument be advanced.

The technique of flexible sigmoidoscopy is similar to that for the early stages of the colonoscopy procedure (see Chapter 40). The instrument is advanced using tip deflection, torque, and alternating insertion and withdrawal. The use of air insufflation must be kept to a minimum because overdistention of the colon accentuates its acute angles and bends, which makes advancement of the instrument more difficult. Acute tip angulation may limit advancement of the instrument because the angulated portion of the insertion tube becomes the forward point rather than the instrument tip. Some of the force exerted to advance the endoscope is thus diverted to the adjacent bowel wall instead of in the direction of the lumen. This usually causes the patient some discomfort and is a potential source of damage to the bowel wall if the endoscopist does not understand what is happening.

The importance of attempting to keep some portion of the bowel lumen in view at all times cannot be overstated. Certain endoscopic clues help to determine the direction of the lumen. Generally this involves observation of the shadows and highlights (reflections) produced by the endoscope light as it illuminates the mucosal surface. Looking for an arc of mucosa against a shadowed background is helpful. The lumen will be behind the mucosal arc. If the colon is deflated or in spasm, the lumen will be found at the center of converging folds. Shadows also may help find the lumen. Reflection of the endoscope light may result in an arc-shaped pattern of highlights; generally the lumen will be in a direction opposite the inner aspect of the curve of the arc. If one side of the circular image is brighter than the other, the lumen will usually be found by

directing the instrument tip away from the bright area.

Modern instruments with wide-angle fields of view make it possible to locate the lumen of the bowel in most situations. In the past, instrument capabilities necessitated the use of a maneuver known as "slide-by," because of limited tip deflection and a relatively narrow angle of view. In this maneuver the general direction of the lumen is determined using the type of observation suggested above, and then the instrument is gently advanced in this direction even though the lumen, at least at the outset of the maneuver, is not visualized. If the technique is properly performed, the mucosa is observed to "slide" past the tip of the endoscope, hence the terms "slide-by" and "slide-maneuver." This maneuver should be rarely necessary with current flexible sigmoidoscopes. However, in some situations, severe diverticulosis for example, it may be difficult to keep the lumen in view at all times. If a slide-maneuver is unavoidable, the tip should not be flexed too acutely. The instrument should be advanced slowly and advancement should be discontinued if the vascular pattern of the bowel blanches or a total red-out occurs. These observations indicate that the instrument tip is imbedded in the mucosa and that considerable and possibly hazardous force is being exerted. Withdrawal of the endoscope will often straighten out the colon, allowing advancement subsequently, a maneuver preferable to slide-by.

Three techniques for insertion of the fiberoptic sigmoidoscope have been described.[32] These are intubation by elongation, looping, and accordionization.

Intubation by elongation is accomplished by pushing the insertion tube forward while keeping the lumen in view. This technique is successful if the sigmoid is relatively short and straight. Unfortunately, in other, more tortuous colons, it will only stretch the sigmoid on its mesentery; advancement will be prevented as acute angulation in the sigmoid develops.

Intubation by looping is most effective in redundant sigmoid colons.[32] Here, advantage is taken of the increased mobility of the colon by inserting the endoscope and simultaneously applying counterclockwise torque. This displaces the colon toward the abdominal wall, and eventually the tip of the instrument reaches the more distal bowel in a gentle curve that prevents formation of an acute angle at the sigmoid–descending colon junction, thus allowing advancement into the more proximal bowel. Tip deflection must be kept at a minimum for this maneuver so that the instrument follows the gentle curve of the bowel wall produced by application of counterclockwise torque to the insertion tube.

The third technique, accordionization, unlike the first two, attempts to pull the colon down over the insertion tube as opposed to simply pushing the instrument upward into the bowel.[32] This is accomplished by an engineering principle called dithering, in which the scope is rapidly advanced a short distance into the bowel while clockwise torque is applied. The push advances the instrument and the clockwise torque straightens the sigmoid curve. The endoscope is then slowly withdrawn the same distance it was advanced while counterclockwise torque is applied. This results in plication of the colon onto the instrument in an accordion-like fashion. The maneuver is repeated in a rhythmic fashion at a rate of about one cycle per second. While performing this technique, it is important to avoid overdistention of the colon and to keep tip deflection to a minimum and directed toward the angle of the lumen rather than around bends and into it. Never advance immediately into the lumen when it comes into view but rather continue to dither torque in order to accordionize as much bowel onto the insertion tube as possible. The technique of accordionization is particularly helpful in sigmoid colons composed of multiple small tight loops.

During insertion, the major effort is to advance the instrument as far as possible without producing undue discomfort for the patient. Lesions are sought predominantly during withdrawal of the endoscope.

The rectal ampulla is a blind area if the endoscope is simply withdrawn from the rectum to the anal canal. Therefore, a retroflexion maneuver should be part of every examination to seek out lesions just beyond the anal sphincter. With newer flexible sigmoidoscopes this is usually easily accomplished by upward deflection and gentle advancement of the instrument, beginning in the distal rectum, until the insertion tube is seen entering the rectum through the anus.[26] We studied this technique in over 200 cases and were able to accomplish the maneuver in 95% of attempts without damage to the endoscope or injury to the patient. It must be emphasized that this maneuver allows visualization of the distal rectum but not the anorectal sphincter area, which can only be visualized with the anoscope.

CLEANING THE FLEXIBLE SIGMOIDOSCOPE

The methods required for cleaning flexible sigmoidoscopes are similar to those for other gastrointestinal endoscopes.[33] Our effective yet simple method is as follows.

The instrument should be left attached to the light source and suction outlet. The insertion tube is submerged in warm tap water containing a detergent and scrubbed using a small gauze pad until all debris is removed. The suction (accessory) and air-water channel valves and the distal hood are removed, and these areas of the instrument are cleaned with tap water containing detergent using a cotton-tipped applicator or a toothbrush. Warm, soapy water is then drawn through the suction channel followed by a thorough scrubbing of the channel with a cleaning brush supplied by the manufacturer. Finally, the suction channel and insertion tube of the scope are rinsed in clear water. Some flexible sigmoidoscopes can be totally immersed in water, but the control section of others is not water-tight and will be damaged if it becomes wet.

To disinfect the instrument, 50 ml of alkaline glutaraldehyde is drawn into the suction (accessory) channel of the instrument and left in place while the insertion tube is placed in a large container of glutaraldehyde and left there for 5 minutes.[34] Gloves must be worn during cleaning with glutaraldehyde to protect hands against caustic injury. After disinfection the accessory-suction channel and insertion tube are rinsed thoroughly in clear water.

The control surface and handle of the instrument are then cleaned using a sponge soaked in 70% alcohol. The umbilical cord is wiped with gauze pads soaked in glutaraldehyde that is then removed by wiping with gauze pads soaked in water. The entire sigmoidoscope is then dried and the suction air channel cleared of residual liquid by continued suction of air through the channel. If the instrument will not be used in a short period of time for another examination, it should be hung in a closet with the insertion tube and umbilical cord hanging down.

In a personal study undertaken several years ago, I found that this type of cleaning required 2 to 10 minutes, with an average time of 5 minutes.

RESULTS OF FLEXIBLE SIGMOIDOSCOPY

Experienced endoscopists have shown that the level of discomfort experienced by most patients is at least no greater than and in many cases less than that associated with rigid proctosigmoidoscopy.[1-4] The time required for insertion of the flexible sigmoidoscope is about twice that necessary for rigid proctosigmoidoscopy.

The nature and incidence of pathologic findings at flexible sigmoidoscopy depend upon the initial indications for the procedure. More lesions will be reported from series of symptomatic patients than in those for whom the primary objective is surveillance of asymptomatic population groups. The reason for surveillance (e.g., previous polyp or colonic cancer, positive family history of cancer, and evaluation of patients over age 45) will also affect the frequency and nature of positive findings (see Table 49–4). The yield of lesions is three to four times that found on rigid sigmoidoscopy.

McCallum et al.[35] reported the results of flexible sigmoidoscopy in 1015 patients with a variety of symptoms. The mean depth of insertion was 49 cm. Eighty-five neoplastic lesions were discovered in 78 patients (7.7%), the majority of which were proximal to the 20-cm level of insertion. Peak yield occurred in patients in their seventh decade; no cancers were found in patients less than 40 years of age.

There are relatively few reports of the use of flexible sigmoidoscopy in asymptomatic patients according to the guidelines for screening.[36-39] Ibrahim et al.[36] performed 60-cm flexible sigmoidoscopy in 409 wood and metal worker employees of an automobile company because an increase in mortality from colon cancer had been noted among wood worker employees. Some patients were under 50 years of age, and no information was obtained regarding risk factors such as a history of colon adenomas. The average depth of insertion of the sigmoidoscope was 55 cm, and the average time required for each procedure was 10 minutes. The prevalence of polyps was 10.76%, only one of which contained an in situ carcinoma. The majority of polyps were found in patients 50 years of age and older. In the study by

Wherry,[37] 417 asymptomatic patients with an average age of 52 years underwent screening with flexible sigmoidoscopy with a 60-cm instrument. Seventy-three polyps were found in 52 patients. One half of the polyps were proximal to 25 cm and one-third were over 1.0 cm in diameter.

Rosevelt and Frankl[38] reported on colorectal cancer screening by a nurse practitioner using a 60-cm fiberoptic instrument in 825 patients. The majority of patients were asymptomatic (75 had a history of rectal bleeding) and underwent the procedure as part of a routine health evaluation. Polyps, 79% of which were proximal to 25 cm, were found in 72 patients. The yield of positive findings was greatest (10.6%) for patients aged 50 and older.

Yarborough and Waisbren[39] reported their findings in 483 asymptomatic patients. Ninety-four polyps were found in 86 of 435 patients aged 50 and older. Eighteen of these polyps contained carcinoma; one adenocarcinoma was discovered in this age group. A solitary polyp was found in each of 8 patients from a group of 48 patients under 50 years old.

Polyps are an important finding because of the known malignant potential of adenomatous polyps. It must be remembered that only 60% of polyps are found in the sigmoid and descending colon.[40] The presence of an adenomatous polyp signifies that the entire colonic mucosa is at increased risk of neoplasia; multiplicity of colon polyps is a frequent finding. Therefore, it must be emphasized that if a polyp is found on flexible sigmoidoscopy, a subsequent colonoscopy must be performed to search for additional polyps that may be present in the more proximal colon not examined by the flexible sigmoidoscope.

COMPLICATIONS

When evidence of acute diverticulitis or ischemic colitis is discovered, I believe that further introduction of the endoscope serves little purpose and increases the risk of instrument-induced bowel perforation through an area weakened by the disease process.[41, 42] Acute ulcerative colitis also should be a contraindication for further introduction of the instrument because of the risk of precipitating a toxic megacolon or perforating a disease-damaged colon.[43] If the instrument cannot be easily and quickly introduced through a circumferential carcinoma, it should be withdrawn using as little air insufflation as possible, since a marked increase in air pressure above a partially obstructed colon that does not allow escape of air distally can blow out the cecum.

Perforation of the colon during flexible sigmoidoscopy is a very uncommon occurrence. Marks et al.[5] encountered one perforation in 1,012 cases (0.1%). There were no perforations in the report of 5000 procedures by Traul et al.[44] In many reported series there were no complications.[1, 6, 8, 13, 17, 35, 39, 45]

Although there are no case reports of endocarditis following colonoscopy, two cases of enterococcal endocarditis have been reported following flexible sigmoidoscopy.[46, 47] Flexible sigmoidoscopy–associated bacteremia has been shown to be a rare occurrence.[48, 49] Currently, antibiotic prophylaxis is not recommended for patients with valvular heart disease who are to undergo flexible sigmoidoscopy without biopsy.[50] However, in certain clinical situations in which the consequences of bacteremia may be catastrophic (for example, patients with prosthetic heart valves, artificial joints, arteriovenous shunts for hemodialysis, and severe neutropenia), a strong argument can be made for antibiotic prophylaxis.

COST-BENEFIT EFFECTIVENESS OF FLEXIBLE SIGMOIDOSCOPY

There is no question that the rigid sigmoidoscope is less expensive to purchase than the flexible sigmoidoscope and that its life expectancy is limited only by its nonmetal parts. The flexible sigmoidoscope is far more sophisticated mechanically and optically. Maintenance and repair costs can be expected to be greater with the more complex instrument. Over the years, it has been my experience that fiberoptic instruments have become more rugged. Perhaps greater skill on the part of endoscopists has also reduced the demands made of the instrument.

Some years ago I evaluated the performance of an early-model fiberoptic sigmoidoscope. This instrument was in daily use by nine gastroenterologists and several medical residents. During 1387 procedures the instrument had to be returned to the manufacturer five times for repairs at a cost of $4496. During this time the instrument generated

gross revenues at $50 per procedure of $69,350. Experience with newer instruments suggests an even better record. Our current fiberoptic sigmoidoscope has needed no repairs in over 2 years of daily use by two gastroenterologists, seven fellows in Gastroenterology, and general internists.

The impact of widespread use of flexible sigmoidoscopy on health care in the United States is a very important issue. The question of what to charge for the procedure is a professional and economic issue that is beyond the scope of this chapter. However, the technical and professional charges for flexible sigmoidoscopy probably add up to a greater overall cost to the health-care consumer than that for rigid proctosigmoidoscopy. To what degree this is justified by somewhat greater overhead cost in terms of equipment and time devoted to the procedure, by greater patient comfort and acceptance, and by the increased yield due to the more extensive examination is a professional ethical issue that engenders some controversy. Any screening test to be considered ideal should have certain attributes. It should be simple and quick, convenient for the patient as well as painless, safe, sensitive and specific, and inexpensive. If, as I have stated, the main value of flexible sigmoidoscopy will be the screening of patients for colorectal neoplasia, it must fulfill as many of these attributes as well as possible. At a time in the United States when health care costs are prominent national issues addressed by diverse groups with legitimate interests in these problems, an expensive test will likely be rejected as a screening test. Given the magnitude of the problem of colonic cancer, this is a point worth pondering.

There is no doubt that colorectal neoplasia is a significant problem in many developed countries including the United States. Statistics indicate that the mortality of colon cancer (the major significant lesion sought on sigmoidoscopy) is approximately 60% in the United States.[51]

The direct costs of treating patients with incurable disease and the indirect cost to society with the loss of productive individuals are surely great. I estimated a direct cost of $25,000 to $30,000 (1985 dollars) for treatment of a patient with non-resectable colonic carcinoma. Aside from the issue of cost, the suffering of patients with incurable colon carcinoma must also be considered.

Dutton,[52] reporting in 1978, concluded

that in his unit the cost for detection of a curable neoplastic lesion was $7000 (based on a $20 fee for rigid sigmoidoscopy and an incidence rate for such lesions of 0.2%). Based on data in the literature, two to four times as many lesions will be found with flexible sigmoidoscopy than with rigid proctosigmoidoscopy. In 1982 Johnson et al.[53] reported an identical cost of $7000 per curable lesion detected by the flexible sigmoidoscope using a detection rate of 1.4% in their unit and a fee of $140.

Despite the difficulties in dealing with colorectal neoplasia, our knowledge of its pathogenesis is greater than that for most other cancers. There is considerable evidence that the precursor lesion has been identified in the adenomatous polyp, and the means to interrupt the polyp-cancer sequence are at hand (see Chapter 45).

Gilbertsen's[54] work showed that rigid sigmoidoscopy with polypectomy led to a decrease in the incidence of rectal cancer from an expected 70 to 80 cases to 12 cases. Although comparable data are not available for flexible sigmoidoscopy, it is logical to assume that an even greater benefit would occur. Furthermore, a study such as Gilbertsen's, which was reported in 1974, might have less satisfactory results if performed today because of the statistically demonstrated shift in the distribution of colorectal cancers from distal to proximal.[55-58]

Editor's note: The superiority of flexible sigmoidoscopy in comparison to rigid sigmoidoscopy in screening for colorectal neoplasia is well established. However, certain aspects of flexible sigmoidoscopy remain controversial. Issues include the instrument length most appropriate for physicians without formal training in endoscopy, the level of training that such physicians require, the cost-benefit ratio of the procedure, selection of patients, patient compliance, and the required frequency of the examination. References 59 to 62 are recent publications that address some of the issues. References 63 to 65 are other recent publications relevant to this chapter.

References

1. Bohlman TW, Katon RW, Lipshutz, et al. Fiberoptic pansigmoidoscopy: an evaluation and comparison with rigid sigmoidoscopy. Gastroenterology 1977; 72:644–9.
2. Leicester RJ, Pollett WG, Hawley PR, Nicholls RJ. Flexible fiberoptic sigmoidoscopy as an outpatient procedure. Lancet 1982; 1:34–5.
3. Manier JW. Fiberoptic pansigmoidoscopy: an evaluation of its use in office practice. Gastrointest Endosc 1978; 24:119–20.
4. O'Connor JJ. Flexible fiberoptic sigmoidoscopy. A study of 746 cases. Am J Proctol Colon Rectal Surg 1981; 32:8–9.
5. Marks G, Boggs HW, Castro AF, et al. Sigmoidoscopic examinations with rigid and flexible fiberoptic sigmoidoscopes in the surgeon's office. Dis Colon Rectum 1979; 22:162–8.
6. Vellacott KD, Hardcastle JD. An evaluation of flexible fiberoptic sigmoidoscopy. Br Med J 1981; 283:1583–6.
7. Winawer SJ, Leidner SD, Boyle C, Kurtz RC. Comparison of flexible sigmoidoscopy with other diagnostic techniques in the diagnosis of rectocolon neoplasia. Dig Dis Sci 1979; 24:277–81.
8. Winnan G, Berci G, Panish J, et al. Superiority of the flexible to the rigid sigmoidoscope in routine proctosigmoidoscopy. N Engl J Med 1980; 302:1011–2.
9. Manier JW. Comparison of biopsies obtained with two sizes of biopsy forceps by two techniques. (Abstr) Gastrointest Endosc 1982; 28:139.
10. Hocutt JE Jr, Jaffe R, Owens GM, Walters DT. Flexible fiberoptic sigmoidoscopy. AFP 1982; 26:133–41.
11. Schapiro M, Gillman L, Kerlin J, Mann S. Flexible sigmoidoscopy by the GI assistant in the community hospital. Gastrointest Endosc (Abstr) 1981; 27:138.
12. Winawer SJ, Cummins R, Baldwin MP, Ptak A. A new flexible sigmoidoscope for the generalist. Gastrointest Endosc 1982; 28:233–6.
13. Grobe JL, Kozarek RA, Sanowski RA. Flexible versus rigid sigmoidoscopy: A comparison using an inexpensive 35-cm flexible proctosigmoidoscope. Am J Gastroenterol 1983; 78:569–71.
14. Zucker GM, Madura MJ, Chmiel JS, Olinger EJ. The advantages of the 30-cm flexible sigmoidoscope over the 60-cm flexible sigmoidoscope. Gastrointest Endosc 1984; 30:59–64.
15. Dubow RA, Katon RM, Benner KG, et al. Short (35 cm) versus long (60 cm) flexible sigmoidoscopy: a comparison of findings and tolerance in asymptomatic patients screened for colorectal neoplasia. Gastrointest Endosc 1985; 31:305–8.
16. Sarles HE, Haynes WC, Sanowski RA, et al. The long and short of flexible sigmoidoscopy: Does it matter? (Abstr) Gastrointest Endosc 1984; 30:145.
17. Lehman GA, Buchner DM, Lappas JC. Anatomical extent of fiberoptic sigmoidoscopy. Gastroenterology 1983; 84:803–8.
18. Ott DJ, Wu WC, Gelfand DW. Extent of colonic visualization with the fiberoptic sigmoidoscope. J Clin Gastroenterol 1982; 4:337–41.
19. Johnson RA, Quam M, Rodney WM. Flexible sigmoidoscopy. J Fam Pract 1982; 14:757, 62–3 passim.
20. McCray RS. A fiberoptic sigmoidoscopy training program for cancer screening physicians. (Abstr) Gastrointest Endosc 1981; 27:137.
21. Schapiro M, Auslander MO, Getzig SJ, Klasky I. Flexible fiberoptic sigmoidoscopy training of nonendoscopic physicians in the community hospital. (Abstr) Gastrointest Endosc 1983; 29:186.
22. Manier JW. The role of flexible sigmoidoscopy in the practice of a gastroenterologist. Gastrointest Endosc 1983; 29:122–3.
23. Holt RW, Wherry DC. Flexible fiberoptic sigmoid-

oscopy in a surgeon's office. Am J Surg 1980; 139:708–10.

24. Morrissey KP. Flexible fiberoptic sigmoidoscopy in the practice of a surgeon. Gastrointest Endosc 1983; 29:124–5.

25. Previti FW, et al. Detorsion of sigmoid volvulus by flexible fiberoptic sigmoidoscopy. J Med Sci 1981; 78:288–9.

26. Hogan WJ. Flexible sigmoidoscopy versus colonoscopy—when to use which instrument. Gastrointest Endosc 1983; 29:126–8.

27. Winawer SJ, Andrews M, Flehinger B, et al. Progress report on controlled trial of fecal occult blood testing for the detection of colorectal neoplasia. Cancer 1980; 45:2959–64.

28. Gilbertsen VA, McHugh R, Schuman L, Williams SE. The earlier detection of colorectal cancers: a preliminary report of the results of the occult blood study. Cancer 1980; 45:2899–901.

29. Crespi M, Casale V, Grassi A. Flexible sigmoidoscopy: a potential advance in cancer control. Gastrointest Endosc 1978; 24:291–4.

30. Record CO, Bramble MG, Lishman AH, Sandle GI. Flexible sigmoidoscopy in outpatients with suspected colonic disease. Br Med J 1981; 283:1291–2.

31. Manier JW. Some questions and answers concerning flexible sigmoidoscopy. (Abstr) Gastrointest Endosc 1978; 24:205.

32. Coller JA. Technique of flexible fiberoptic sigmoidoscopy. Surg Clin North Am 1980; 60:465–79.

33. Geenen JE, Pfeifer M, Simonsen L. Cleaning and disinfection of endoscopic equipment. Gastrointest Endosc 1978; 24:185–6.

34. Washington JA II, et al. Endoscopes: disinfection or sterilization? Hospital Infection Control 1978; 5:34–64.

35. McCallum RW, Meyer CT, Marignani P, et al. Flexible sigmoidoscopy: diagnostic yield in 1015 patients. Am J Gastroenterol 1984; 79:433–7.

36. Ibrahim MAH, Batra SK, Schuman BM, Viola FV III. Fiberoptic sigmoidoscopy in screening pattern makers for colon cancer at their work place. Am J Gastroenterol 1984; 79:262–4.

37. Wherry DC. Screening for colorectal neoplasia in asymptomatic patients using flexible fiberoptic sigmoidoscopy. Dis Colon Rectum 1981; 24:521–2.

38. Roosevelt J, Frankl H. Colorectal cancer screening by nurse practitioner using 60-cm flexible fiberoptic sigmoidoscope. Dig Dis Sci 1984; 29:161–3.

39. Yarborough GW, Waisbren BA Sr. The benefits of systematic fiberoptic flexible sigmoidoscopy. Arch Intern Med 1985; 145:95–6.

40. Tedesco FJ, Waye JD, Avella JR, Villalobos MM. Diagnostic implications of the spatial distribution of colonic mass lesions (polyps and cancers). A prospective colonoscopic study. Gastrointest Endosc 1980; 26:95–7.

41. Forde KA, Lebwahl O, Wolff M, Voorhees AB. The endoscopic corner. Am J Gastroenterol 1979; 72:182–5.

42. Forde KA. Colonoscopy in complicated diverticular disease. Gastrointest Endosc 1977; 23:192–3.

43. Waye JD. Endoscopy in inflammatory bowel disease. Clin Gastroenterol 1980; 9:279–80.

44. Traul DG, Davis CB, Pollock JC, Scudamore HH. Flexible fiberoptic sigmoidoscopy—The Monroe Clinic experience. A prospective study of 5000 examinations. Dis Colon Rectum 1983; 26:161–6.

45. Hilsabeck JR. Experience with routine office sigmoidoscopy using the 60-cm flexible colonoscope in

private practice. Dis Colon Rectum 1983; 26:314–8.

46. Rodriguez W, Levine JS. Enterococcal endocarditis following flexible sigmoidoscopy. West J Med 1984; 140:951–3.

47. Rigilano J, Mahapatra R, Barnhill J, Gutierrez J. Enterococcal endocarditis following sigmoidoscopy and mitral valve prolapse. Arch Intern Med 1984; 144:850–1.

48. Goldman GD, Miller SA, Furman DS, et al. Does bacteremia occur during flexible sigmoidoscopy? Am J Gastroenterol 1985; 80:621–3.

49. Kumar S, Abcarian H, Prasad L, Lakshmanan S. Bacteremia associated with lower gastrointestinal endoscopy: Fact or fiction? II. Proctosigmoidoscopy. Dis Colon Rectum 1983; 26:22–4.

50. Shulman ST, Amren DP, Bisno AL, et al. Prevention of bacterial endocarditis. A statement for health professionals by the committee on rheumatic fever and infective endocarditis of the council on cardiovascular disease in the young. Circulation 1984; 70:1123A–7A.

51. Cancer statistics 1983. 1983; CA 30:23–38.

52. Dutton JJ. Sigmoidoscopy as a periodic screening test. J Fam Pract 1978; 7:1041–6.

53. Johnson RA, Quam M, Rodney WM. Flexible sigmoidoscopy. J Fam Pract 1982; 14:757–70.

54. Gilbertsen VA. Proctosigmoidoscopy and polypectomy in reducing the incidence of rectal cancer. Cancer 1974; 34:936–9.

55. Snyder DN, Heston JF, Beigs W, Flannery JT. Changes in site distribution of colorectal carcinoma in Connecticut, 1940–1973. Dig Dis 1977; 22:791–7.

56. Rhodes JB, Holmes FF, Clark GM. Changing distribution of primary cancers in the large bowel. JAMA 1977; 238:1641–3.

57. Beart RW, Melton LJ III, Maruta M, et al. Trends in right and left-sided colon cancer. Dis Colon Rectum 1983; 26:393–8.

58. Mamazza J, Gordon PH. The changing distribution of large intestinal cancer. Dis Colon Rectum 1982; 25:558–62.

59. Lehman GA, Hawes R, Roth B, Hast J. A study of optimal length of flexible fiberoptic sigmoidoscopes for initial endoscopic training. Dis Colon Rectum 1986; 29:878–81.

60. Sarles HE Jr, Sanowski RA, Haynes WC, Bellapravalu S. The long and short of flexible sigmoidoscopy: does it matter? Am J Gastroenterol 1986; 81:369–71.

61. Hawes R, Lehman GA, Hast J, et al. Training resident physicians in fiberoptic sigmoidoscopy. How many supervised examinations are required to achieve competence? Am J Med 1986; 80:465–70.

62. Bowman MA, Wherry DC. Training for flexible sigmoidoscopy. Gastrointest Endosc 1985; 31:309–12.

63. Wanebo HJ, Fang WL, Mills AS, Zfass AM. Colorectal cancer. A blueprint for disease control through screening by primary care physicians. Arch Surg 1986; 121:1347–52.

64. Bat L, Pines A, Ron E, et al. A community-based program of colorectal screening in an asymptomatic population: evaluation of screening tests and compliance. Am J Gastroenterol 1986; 81:647–51.

65. Rozen P, Fireman Z, Figer A, Ron E. Colorectal tumor screening in women with a past history of breast, uterine, or ovarian malignancies. Cancer 1986; 57:1235–9.

Section V

LAPAROSCOPY

Chapter 50

TECHNIQUE OF LAPAROSCOPY

H. JUERGEN NORD, M.D.

HISTORY OF LAPAROSCOPY

Laparoscopy was first introduced as a gastrointestinal endoscopic procedure on September 23, 1901, when Georg Kelling,[1, 2] in Hamburg, Germany, presented his concept of "The Inspection of the Esophagus and Stomach with Flexible Instruments." He recognized the utility of a pneumoperitoneum and explored this new technique mainly in dogs but also in two patients. Hans Christian Jacobaeus[3] was the first to report on the practicality and clinical significance of this procedure and also originated the term "laparoscopy." Heinz Kalk[4] improved laparoscopic equipment and technique and developed laparoscopy as a valuable diagnostic procedure in diseases of the liver.

Initially, telescopes had 90-degree side-viewing optics of the type used in cystoscopes. The 50-degree foroblique optic is now the most frequently used instrument. The English physicist Harold Hopkins[5, 6] introduced computer-designed glassrod optics in the 1960's. Image brightness was further improved with the development of computer-designed conventional lenses with special types of glass and lens coatings that have an antiglare effect.

Extracorporal light sources with fiberoptic light transmission supplanted the use of intracorporal incandescent bulbs. These cold light sources with halogen and xenon-arc lamps provided maximal illumination of the abdominal cavity without the risk of burns to the intestine because of the heat generated by the older Edison bulbs. Until the 1940's, reports on laparoscopy and early atlases were illustrated in black and white or water color drawings. In the 1930's Norbert Henning[7] adapted a single lens reflex (SLR) camera for endoscopic photography, first for gastroscopy and later for laparoscopy. Other developments followed: black and white and color photographs, an electronic intracorporal flash resulting in endophotographs of optimal organ illumination and unsurpassed brilliance, and direct color television transmission of laparoscopic images.

Accessory procedures have been developed that complement visual observation. Ruddock,[8] the father of laparoscopy in the United States, introduced forceps liver biopsy followed by electrocoagulation. Other ancillary procedures such as direct cholecystography and cholangiography and splenoportography have also been developed.

EQUIPMENT

Equipment for exploratory laparoscopy is less complicated than modern flexible fiberoptic endoscopes. The basic design principles have not appreciably changed in years. A routine abdominal exploration can be performed with a minimum of equipment. The entire laparoscopy set is less expensive than a standard intestinal fiberoptic endoscope, and if properly cared for will last for years.

Equipment for Pneumoperitoneum

For a successful laparoscopy it is essential to establish and maintain a workspace for the telescope by means of a pneumoperitoneum. This requires a needle, connecting tube, and an insufflator. Any needle that can penetrate the anterior abdominal wall is adequate, but the Veres needle is preferred by most examiners. This needle has an established, satisfactory performance record for over 40 years (Fig. 50–1). It consists of an inner blunt needle with lateral porthole for the exit of insufflated gas, and an outer spring-loaded

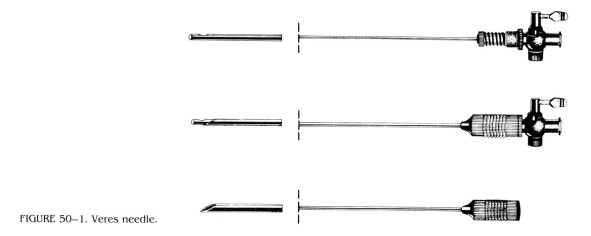

FIGURE 50–1. Veres needle.

needle with a sharp beveled edge. The blunt inner needle protrudes beyond the outer sharp needle in the resting position. During insertion the inner blunt needle is pushed back by the resistance of the abdominal wall, allowing the sharp outer needle to cut into and penetrate the layers of the abdominal wall. When the needle has completely perforated the abdominal wall, the blunt inner needle will be protruded by its spring and thus prevent injury to the underlying viscera. The hub of the needle is then connected by a Luer fitting and plastic tube to the insufflator.

During earlier periods, room air was insufflated by a syringe, three-way stopcock, and a micropore air filter. Although some examiners still prefer air and have used it safely during many procedures, an automatic insufflator for nitrous oxide or carbon dioxide is generally preferred today. Yokes for both gases are available for adaptation of insufflators. These units have a self-contained 10-liter internal tank that must be filled from an external gas cylinder. This provides for controlled insufflation and prevents accidental abdominal overdistention from a high-volume, high-pressure external gas source. The insufflator is equipped with several gauges that allow easy monitoring of various aspects of the pneumatic system. These are: a visual gas flow indicator, an intra-abdominal pressure gauge that indicates the dangerous high-pressure range (>30 mm Hg), an internal tank gauge that shows the volume of gas insufflated (1 to 10 liters), and a gas reservoir pressure gauge (Fig. 50–2). The most important of these is the intra-abdominal pressure gauge.

Observation of the intra-abdominal pressure allows the operator also to monitor the position of the needle within the abdomen and avoid injury to the viscera and accidental omental insufflation. If the port of the Veres needle becomes occluded, for example by burying of the needle in the omentum, and gas flow is interrupted, the resultant and sometimes abrupt increase in pressure will be shown by this gauge and the needle can be changed to a more appropriate position.

A typical insufflator such as the one shown (Fig. 50–2) has switches for several purposes. One of these is an on-off switch; in the off position the gas flow is completely shut down. There is a switch to fill the internal tank, and there is also a manual-automatic switch. In the "automatic" position the insufflator automatically replaces gas lost during endoscopy. Different manufacturers provide units that combine the insufflator, light source, and electrosurgical units on special carts. This type of laparoscopic insufflator greatly contributes to the overall safety of laparoscopy.

The choice of gas, carbon dioxide or nitrous oxide, depends on the type of laparoscopy planned. Carbon dioxide is preferred for gynecologic laparoscopy, which is frequently performed under general anesthesia and may involve electrosurgery. In the peritoneal cavity, carbon dioxide combines with water to form carbonic acid, which may irritate the peritoneum and cause pain and discomfort during the procedure.[9] Carbon dioxide is more rapidly absorbed than room air or nitrous oxide and does not support combustion. Accidental intravascular injection of small amounts appears to have no side effects or complications. However, hypercarbia and

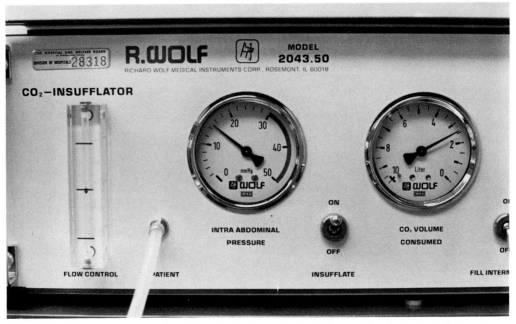

FIGURE 50–2. Nitrous oxide/carbon dioxide insufflator (partial view). The gas flow indicator has risen to second line of flow gauge indicating adequate flow of gas. Intra-abdominal pressure is 14 mm Hg. Two and one half liters of gas have been insufflated.

cardiac arrhythmias have been reported with carbon dioxide.[10, 11]

For diagnostic laparoscopy under local anesthesia and without the use of electrosurgery, nitrous oxide is the gas of choice. The patient's pain perception is much less than with carbon dioxide, and nitrous oxide is more rapidly absorbed from the abdominal cavity than room air, although at a lesser rate than that of carbon dioxide.

Experienced examiners have used electrosurgery safely in the presence of nitrous oxide, but there is at least a theoretic possibility of explosion. Nitrous oxide will support combustion in mixtures with hydrogen and methane, gases that may diffuse from the intestine into the peritoneal cavity. Actual concentrations of these gases within the abdominal cavity have not been measured. However, electrosurgery is seldom necessary during diagnostic laparoscopy. In the rare case when electrocoagulation is contemplated, it is advisable to use carbon dioxide until the question of the safety of nitrous oxide during electrocoagulation is resolved.

Laparoscopes and Light Sources

Laparoscopes of high optical quality, minimal glare, and maximal illumination using glass fiber light transmission are available from various manufacturers in different types and diameters from 5 to 10 mm. The essential components are a metal tube with ocular (proximal end), optical lenses, and objective (distal end). However, several major developments have improved the basic instrument. In the late 1950's and 1960's glass fibers were incorporated as light-transmitting bundles. This enabled the use of high-intensity cold light projectors for optimal illumination. This also eliminated the need for an intracorporal incandescent bulb and thereby an element of "dead length" from the instrument. In 1967 electronically configured glass rod lenses were introduced. Within the telescope, air spaces between the rods acted as lenses and resulted in improved image resolution, brightness and contrast, performance gains that would have otherwise required an increase in telescope diameter.[5] This development provided a stimulus for other instrument manufacturers to improve their conventional optics through use of computer-designed multiple glass lens systems with up to 20 glass/air interspaces, multiple coatings, and special optical glasses to reduce glare and further improve image brightness.

From a functional standpoint, there are two types of laparoscope: diagnostic (double

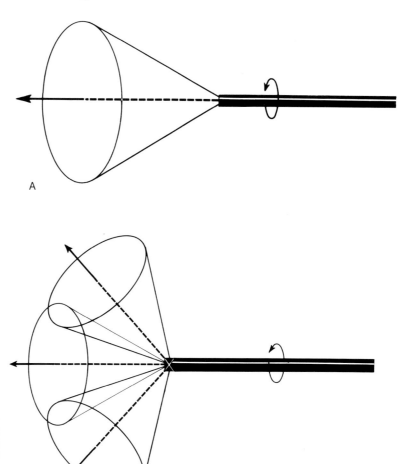

FIGURE 50–3. A, Forward-viewing (0-degree) telescope with 65-degree field of view. Axial rotation does not change image size. B, Side-viewing (50-degree) telescope. Axial rotation provides panoramic view.

puncture), and operative (single puncture) with built-in channel for accessory instruments. Their field of view of 65 degrees qualifies them as wide-angle telescopes but is narrow enough to avoid significant peripheral image distortion. The viewing angle indicates the degree of deflection of the axis of the visual field from the long axis of the instrument. Thus, a 0-degree optic would be a forward-viewing, and a 90-degree optic side-viewing with the visual field oriented perpendicular to the instrument axis. Optics with viewing angles of 0, 10, 20, 50, 70, 80, and 90 degrees are available and even a retrograde optic of 120 degrees is offered.

Only three optics are clinically important: the forward optic (0 degrees), which is popular with beginners because it is easier to orient, the foroblique optic (50 degrees), which is more suitable for abdominal exploration, especially of the liver with its convex surface, and the operative optic with a 10-degree viewing angle. The semiside-viewing

or 50-degree foroblique-viewing telescope is the preferred instrument and is superior to forward-viewing telescopes (Fig. 50–3 and Plate 50–1). With the use of axial rotation along with insertion and withdrawal of the telescope a complete panoramic view may be obtained and upper and under organ surfaces can be observed. Operative laparoscopes are forward-viewing with a slight (10-degree) deviation of the optical beam because of the integral instrument channel. Laparoscopes are designed to work at close distances. Lent's optics provide a true 1:1 image at a distance of 3 cm from an object, magnification at closer distances, and diminution at distances greater than 3 cm.

Light-transmitting cables are usually glass fiberoptic bundles. They are generally of lesser optical quality than viewing optical fibers since the fiber bundles are nonaligned and therefore afflicted with significant light loss. Furthermore, at any coupling, for example, the light source to the fiberoptic bun-

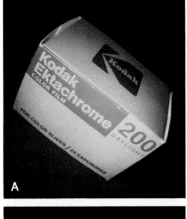
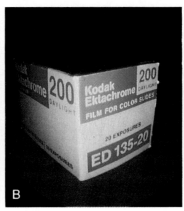
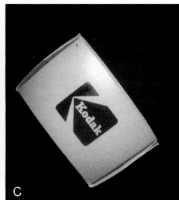
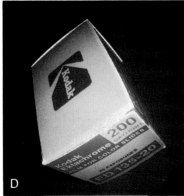

PLATE 50–1. *A-D,* Superiority of 50-degree telescope is demonstrated in photographing different views of film box by simply rotating telescope on its longitudinal axis.

dle cable, or cable to telescope, there is an additional loss of light of at least 15% to 20%. For television, motion picture photography, or high-quality still photography, telescopes with continuous integral light-transmitting bundles rather than connections are preferred. Cables can also be fitted with various adaptors that permit use of various conventional light sources.

Standard light sources are usually equipped with halogen lamps (150 watts), reflecting mirrors, and condensor lenses that focus the light beam on the end of the light-transmitting bundle. For television or still or ci-

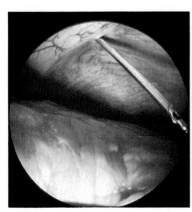
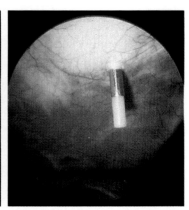

PLATE 50–2. PLATE 50–3. PLATE 50–4.

PLATE 50–2. Veres cannula freely positioned in abdominal cavity.
PLATE 50–3. Laparoscopic view of preperitoneal anesthetic block for second puncture site.
PLATE 50–4. Accessory trocar sleeve properly positioned in right upper quadrant.

nephotography or when the light is split by using a teaching attachment for a second observer, high-intensity light sources that have xenon lamps of up to 1000 watts are preferred.

Equipment for Endophotography

Most manufacturers now offer light sources with electronic vacuum tubes for flash photography. Standard light sources are unsatisfactory for still photography because their light output is inadequate. An SLR camera such as the Olympus OM-1 model is available in most endoscopy suites. Since the camera will only be used in the manual mode regardless of whether or not the light source has manual or automatic settings for photography, a camera with an automatic mode (e.g., Olympus OM-2) is not necessary. A camera with exchangeable focusing screens (see technique of laparoscopic photography) is required. Polaroid cameras with special lenses for 1 or 4 images per photographic print are also available. The focal length of the camera lens determines the size of the image on the film. The longer the focal length, the larger the size of the image. Larger images require more light. When purchasing photographic equipment and a camera lens with longer focal length, be certain that the available light is adequate. The standard 50 mm focal length lens frequently used by amateur photographers gives too small a picture (13 mm diameter). A commercial 100 mm lens provides an image of adequate size (24 mm diameter), and its cost is affordable. Several manufacturers provide quickmount adaptors that couple lenses to telescopes.

Some manufacturers provide a device with lens, adaptor for the telescope, and built-in light meter in one unit (e.g., Olympus SM-EFR OM-adaptor, 110 mm focal length) for use with their special automatic light sources. In such a system a synchronizing cord coordinates the action of the shutter with the electronic flash of the light source. Any telescope of adequate diameter (10 mm) to allow sufficient light transmission may be used. Preferably the light-transmitting bundle should be an integral part of the telescope.

A wide variety of films are available for still photography. The film must be matched with the light source. Newer light sources with a color temperature in the daylight range require daylight type film. In most instances a high-speed daylight film with an ASA rating of 200 or 400 is best (e.g., Kodak Ektachrome). Lower-speed films render a photograph with less grain, but are usually unacceptable because the available light is insufficient. Experience with the newer high-speed ASA 1000 films is limited at present.

The choice between color slides or prints is an individual one. Slides have greater brightness and are well suited to teaching conferences and lectures. Prints can be attached to the endoscopy report as part of the permanent record. This is also possible with Polaroid prints (Polaroid film type 779) that provide an image in 90 seconds. These are usually of lesser quality than photographs provided by the previous techniques but are adequate to complement the written report and for use by other consultants.

Accessory Equipment

Telescopes at room temperature will fog immediately when introduced into the 37°C environment of the abdominal cavity unless they are prewarmed to body temperature. An electric telescope heater with four autoclavable tubular inserts is available (Fig. 50–4). The same results can be achieved less expensively by wrapping an electric heating pad around previously sterilized telescopes that have been covered by a sterile towel.

Various accessory instruments are available for use through the instrument channel of the operative laparoscope (single puncture technique) or via a second puncture accessory trocar. A trocar sleeve with insulated shaft and automatic valve to prevent loss of the pneumoperitoneum plus a trocar are needed for the second puncture technique. The preferred trocar has a 3 mm diameter and a conical atraumatic point rather than a pyramidal one. This device permits rapid exchange of accessories and is telescope-independent and therefore allows for greater maneuverability of accessory instruments. In general, the 3 mm diameter accessory instruments inserted through this trochar are easier to use than bulky 5 mm accessories. Of all the available accessories, the tactile probe marked at 1-cm intervals is the most important. We use it routinely for exploration, palpation of various organs, elevation of right and left hepatic lobes, freeing organs of overlying omentum, and measuring lesions, so that it greatly complements the visual examination.

Various biopsy needles are available for

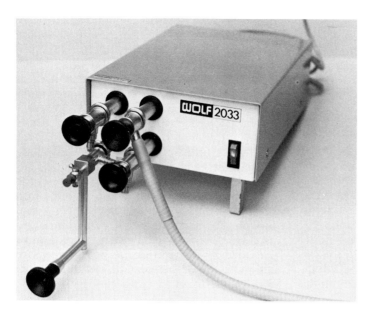

FIGURE 50–4. Electric telescope heater with autoclavable tubular inserts shown with two standard laparoscopes, operating laparoscope, and telescope with integral light-transmitting bundle.

laparoscopic liver biopsy. In general we prefer the 30 cm long, 2 mm wide Franklin-Silverman biopsy cannula (outer cannula with inner slit cannula). This provides adequate tissue cylinders even when the liver is cirrhotic. The most distal parts of the needle are not hollow and prevent the specimen from sliding out. The Silverman-Boeker needle is identical except that the ends are open. Menghini needles of 1.4 and 1.8 mm diameter with internal specimen-trapping metal insert and ejector are also available. To avoid damage to the delicate tips of these needles when passing them through the trocar sleeve and opening the flap valve, an insertion sleeve with rubber sealing cap should first be introduced to hold the valve open. Spleen and biliary puncture cannulas complete the set, also known as the "Freiburg" biopsy set.[12]

The "Tru-cut" biopsy needle that is used for direct percutaneous puncture gives equally good specimens. The longer, 15 cm version should be used because of the height of the intra-abdominal gas cupula. Recently a modified Tru-cut needle long enough to fit through the second puncture sleeve and thus avoid an additional skin puncture has become commercially available. It is spring-loaded, works fast and reliably, and avoids the frequent "dry" biopsies of beginners.

A Menghini needle set (1.4 and 1.8 mm diameter needle) for a direct percutaneous

approach including a trocar sleeve (2.3 mm) for rapid change of needles is also available.

Biopsies of focal lesions are best obtained using a forceps with lancet-shaped jaws (Robbers forceps) or a double spoon forceps. A grasping forceps for retrieval of a dropped biopsy specimen or foreign body, a retractable cytology brush, ascites drainage tube, button electrode and "skinny" needle for aspiration cytology are less often needed but should be available. If a single puncture operative laparoscope is used, a different, longer set of accessories is required. When accessories are to be used with the operative telescope, a set of rubber sealing caps of various sizes is needed to prevent escape of intra-abdominal gas. These are placed over the insertion port of the telescope; accessories are then passed through the rubber seal and into the telescope channel.

Additional items of standard equipment are necessary for the skin incision and closure. To avoid crowding all equipment on one tray, which also makes proper sterilization difficult, all necessary equipment should be assembled on three instrument trays for adequate steam autoclaving and gas sterilization.[13] The first of these should contain all the equipment for local anesthesia, skin incision and closure, and dressing, as listed in Table 50–1 (Fig. 50–5). The second tray contains laparoscopes and a second puncture set as listed in Table 50–2 (Fig. 50–6). The

TABLE 50–1. **Equipment for Local Anesthesia, Skin Incision and Closure, and Dressing (Tray 1)**

2 10-cc Glass syringes, Luerlock
3 Needles (25″ × ⅝″, 4″ × 1½″, 4″ × 3½″)
Metal cup with 30 ml 1% lidocaine
Metal cup with 30 ml 0.9% NaCl solution
2 Knife handles with #11, #15 blades
6 Small towel clips
2 Curved mosquito forceps
2 Straight mosquito forceps
1 Needle holder
Suture (4–0, 2–0 silk, cutting needle)
1 Adson tissue forceps
1 Dressing forceps
1 Suture scissors
8 Sponges
3 Band-Aids, Steri-Strip
6 Linen towels

third contains needles, biopsy forceps, and other less frequently used instruments listed in Table 50–3 (Fig. 50–7).

CARE OF EQUIPMENT

All instruments should be thoroughly cleaned with a soft brush, mild soap, and warm water. All distal objective lenses, ocular windows, and all fiber-end surfaces on light cables and telescopes must be cleaned individually with alcohol-soaked cotton swabs. Metal instruments should *never* be used for cleaning, since they may damage telescopes and accessory equipment. Stopcocks, valves, and forceps mechanisms should be lubricated with a special instrument oil. All light-transmission cables should be handled with extreme care, since mishandling breaks individual optical fibers and reduces light-transmitting capacity. To avoid irreversible damage, they should never be submerged in water, pulled, kinked, or stretched.

Our gastroenterology assistants clean all equipment in the endoscopy suite and pack and seal the individual trays before they are sent to Central Supply for sterilization. Therefore, no personnel unfamiliar with the special characteristics of the equipment will handle it; this is not guaranteed if telescopes and accessories are sent to the operating room cleaning area. Repairs have been minimal, and after more than a decade of regular use the equipment is in optimal optical and technical condition.

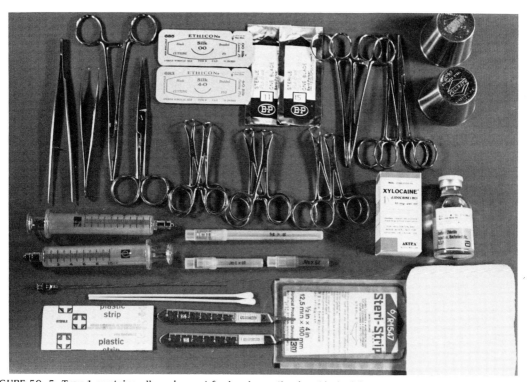

FIGURE 50–5. Tray 1 contains all equipment for local anesthesia, skin incision, closure, and dressing (see text).

TABLE 50–2. **Laparoscopes and Second Puncture Set (Tray 2)**

Veres needle
Laparoscopes
   0-degree forward optic
   50-degree foroblique optic
   10-degree optic operating (Jacobs-Palmer)
Light-transmitting cables
Tubular inserts for telescope preheater
Laparoscope trocar sleeve with trocar
Second puncture trocar sleeve with trocar
Tactile (palpating-measuring) probe
Set of assorted rubber sealing caps

Sterilization

Cold Sterilization (Disinfection)

A 2% solution of active glutaraldehyde (Cidex) is suitable for all telescopes and accessories. Within a short period it destroys most microorganisms including *Mycobacterium tuberculosis* and viruses. It does not affect rubber, plastics, and lens cements. Disinfection is achieved after 10 minutes of soaking. Several patients can be examined in one morning, using one set of telescopes and trocar, which can be cleaned and sterilized by this method between cases.

Gas Sterilization

Gas sterilization is also suitable for all telescopes and accessories. Ethylene oxide is recommended. The temperature should not exceed 60° C (140° F), and the gas pressure should be between 6 and 7 pounds and not exceed 8 pounds. Because of the toxicity of ethylene oxide, airing of the trays for a number of hours is necessary, usually overnight.

Steam Autoclaving

Before telescopes are considered for steam autoclaving the manufacturer's instructions should be checked carefully. Even under ideal conditions heat and pressure during a steam autoclave cycle will reduce the life span of any optical system. It is therefore recommended that all telescopes be gas-sterilized or cold soaked to ensure maximum life expectancy, unless otherwise required. In general, the maximum sterilization cycle must not exceed 10 minutes at 134°C (272° F) at 2.2 atmospheric pressure.[14, 15] Accessories can usually be steam autoclaved. Insulated and non-insulated equipment should be separated into two groups before being placed on trays.

Special Precautions

There are some important "don'ts" in caring for equipment. Instruments containing a lens system or electric bulb should never be boiled. Solvents (except alcohol or acetone) should never be used to clean the instruments. Never sterilize instruments in carbolic

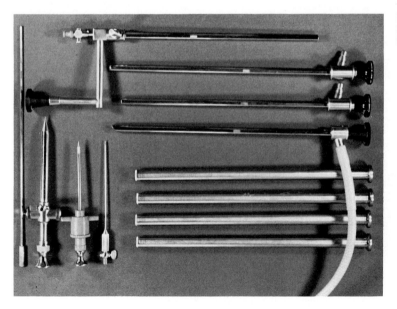

FIGURE 50–6. Tray 2 contains laparoscopes and second puncture set (see text).

TABLE 50–3. **Needles, Biopsy Forceps, and Other Less Frequently Used Instruments (Tray 3)**

"Freiburg" biopsy set
Biopsy forceps with lancet-shaped jaws (Robbers forceps)
Biopsy forceps (double spoon)
Grasping forceps
Tru-cut biopsy needle
Cytology brush
Button electrode for coagulation
Ascites drainage tube

acid, and do not steam autoclave standard fiber illuminated telescopes. Instruments should not be immersed in any solution beyond the time recommended by the manufacturer of the solution. Bichloride of mercury or other corrosive solutions can never be used as germicides. Do not use clamps or forceps when handling instruments or pick up or handle several instruments in a bunch. Telescopes should not be grasped at the distal end; grasp them at the eyepiece end. Instruments or cables should not be piled one on top of another because the weight of heavy instruments can cause fiber breakage.

ROOM SETUP

Laparoscopy requires a room of at least 150 square feet with access to all four sides of the endoscopy table. There should be adequate storage space for supplies and sufficient counter space to set up trays and accessories for the procedure.

Sterile instruments and techniques are required for laparoscopy, but the procedure need not be performed in an aseptic operating room.[14, 16] Scheduling a laparoscopy procedure in a busy operating room may be difficult because operating room regulations may require the presence of an anesthesiologist and/or other personnel. The operating room staff is usually unfamiliar with the special aspects of gastrointestinal laparoscopy, and operating and recovery room services are expensive. There is no published evidence to indicate an increase in the frequency of infectious complications for laparoscopy performed in an endoscopy room.[17]

Sinks for the preoperative scrub and cleanup after the procedure are needed in the endoscopy suite. A rheostat switch for dimming ceiling lights facilitates endoscopic observation, and an operating-room type light with spotlight is helpful for the local anes-

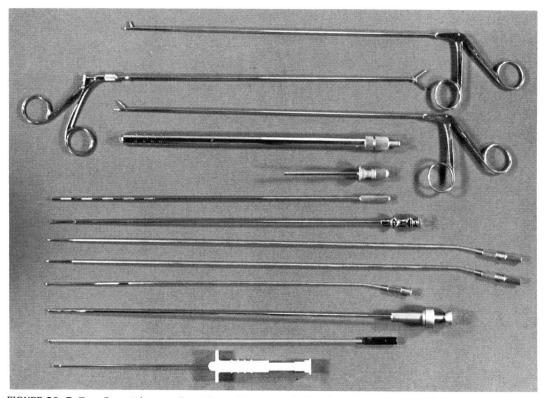

FIGURE 50–7. Tray 3 contains needles, biopsy forceps and other less frequently used instruments (see text).

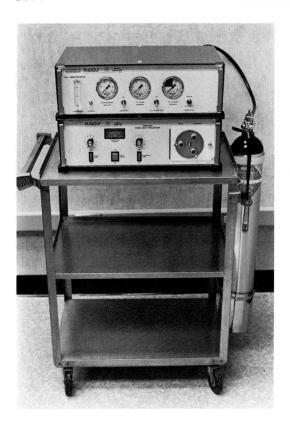

FIGURE 50–8. Insufflator, light source, and gas tank are assembled on movable cart for positioning at endoscopy table.

thesia, skin incision, Veres needle and trocar insertion, and skin closure aspects of the procedure. Air conditioning is helpful since gowns are worn and the patient is draped with large sheets.

A movable cart may be readily adapted to hold insufflator, light source, separate light source for photography, and gas cylinder (Fig. 50–8). It should be positioned so that it does not impair the tilting maneuvers of the endoscopy table. The operator must be able to view the insufflator during introduction of the pneumoperitoneum. Tray 1 (Table 50–1) containing equipment for local anesthesia and skin incision and closure should be placed on a Mayo stand to the operator's left within easy reach. As the equipment is being set out before the procedure the following should be added to this tray: Veres needle, trocar, tactile probe, Freiburg biopsy set, Robbers forceps, and rubber sealing caps. The standard laparoscopy procedure including biopsy can be carried out by one examiner with one circulating assistant/nurse to monitor the patient and operate the table, insufflator, and light sources.

One small item on the counter setup has been helpful. Should the telescope tip touch any viscera such as omentum or become submerged in ascitic fluid, photography usually becomes impossible because the optics cannot be properly wiped or cleaned, and photos will be blurred. A small, sterilized electric coffee pot that contains sterile water heated to boiling can be used to clean the optics. The telescope tip is briefly dipped into the water. Then, wiping the objective with clean gauze removes any oily film and assures clear photographs.

An endoscopy table that can be tilted in all directions allows for complete abdominal exploration. Lateral tilting is mandatory. Pillows propped under the patient as a method of tilting are a poor substitute. If available, an operating room table serves this function. However, the "Maquet" endoscopy table is best for laparoscopy (Fig. 50–9A). It is a floor-mounted, fixed-column table with electric motor–operated hydraulics. The table top is rotatable 360 degrees and can be adjusted horizontally and vertically so that the examination may be performed in a comfortable

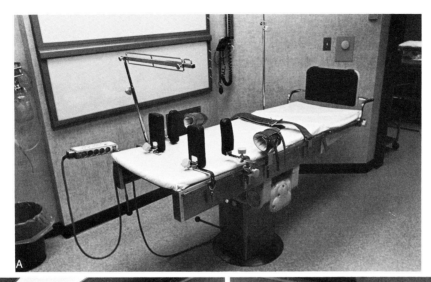

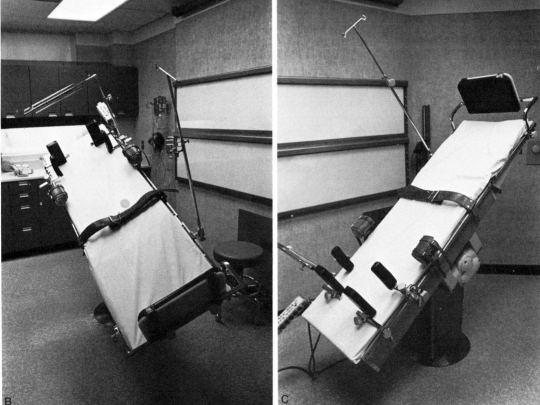

FIGURE 50–9. *A*, Maquet endoscopy table with various attachments (Model 1531.90; U.S. Importer, Siemens Corp.). *B*, Right lateral and head-up tilting of Maquet table. Position 4 for examination of left upper quadrant and spleen. *C*, Thirty-degree Trendelenburg position. Position 7 for examination of lower abdomen and pelvis.

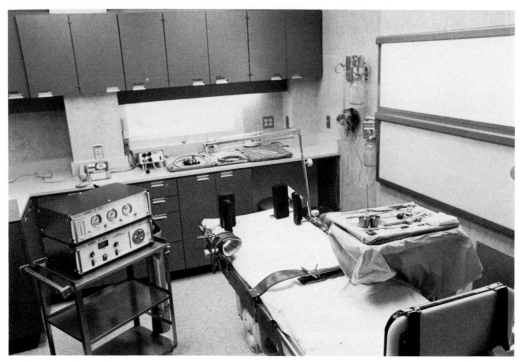

FIGURE 50–10. Complete room setup.

sitting position. Various attachments such as shoulder and lateral supporting braces, foot rest, and straps prevent the patient from sliding when the table is in an extreme position. Wristlets prevent the patient from inadvertently touching the sterile operative field. The table may be tilted 45 degrees laterally to either side and inclined 30 degrees head up and head down (Trendelenburg) (Fig. 50–9B and C).

The complete pre-endoscopy room setup is shown in Figure 50–10.

ENDOSCOPIC TECHNIQUE

Preoperative Evaluation, Patient Education, and Preparation

The patient scheduled for laparoscopy should be admitted to the hospital no later than the day before the procedure. Usually a complete history and physical examination have been performed and the proper indication has been selected (see Chapter 51).

Attention should be given to several points of special importance in the patient's evaluation. A history of prior surgery and the presence of abdominal scars have a bearing on site selection. Although an uncomplicated abdominal hysterectomy or appendectomy is not a contraindication and presents no in-

creased risk, a history of appendiceal perforation followed by diffuse peritonitis and a high probability of diffuse intra-abdominal adhesions is a contraindication. Inflammatory bowel disease, especially Crohn's disease of the small intestine, may present significant problems during introduction of pneumoperitoneum. Extensive upper abdominal surgery may prevent inspection of the area of interest due to adhesions.

Proper assessment of the patient's bleeding and clotting status is of utmost importance. A normal prothrombin time and platelet count are not safeguards against bleeding. More important than wide-ranging laboratory assessment is a detailed history of any bleeding tendency in the patient or his or her family. If this arouses any suspicion, additional clotting factors should be determined in addition to the routine studies of complete blood count, platelet count, prothrombin time, and partial thromboplastin time. Even though the liver bleeding time does not appear to correlate with routine clotting studies,[18] any abnormality in these parameters should not be ignored. Because the bleeding site can be inspected for adequate clot formation, and it is possible to compress and coagulate the bleeding point if necessary, laparoscopy can be performed when the prothrombin time is 4 seconds over control and the platelet count is as low as 50,000 cu mm.

The necessity for the procedure, the technique, potential benefit, and possible complications should be discussed with the patient on the day before the procedure; questions should be encouraged and answered frankly. It is frequently helpful if other family members are present. Patient education film cassettes or pamphlets can also be helpful.[19] The extent to which complications should be discussed is a matter of judgment in the individual case. Some patients are inquisitive, whereas others do not wish to be given any details. In this latter case, a separate discussion with a family member should take place. A well-informed patient who fully understands what to expect usually requires minimal sedation, and the procedure is uneventful. The operative permit may be attended to at the conclusion of the patient interview and instruction session. Generally, the permit must be witnessed by someone who is not a member of the team responsible for the patient's medical care.

The patient's abdomen is thoroughly examined by the operator on the day before the procedure unless this was done during the initial evaluation. The examination is repeated on the day of the procedure immediately prior to the abdominal scrub. Special attention should be focused on palpable organs and masses, scars, evidence of ascites, signs of portal hypertension, and abdominal wall vascular markings, in relation to the ways in which these findings will influence entry site, intra-abdominal inspection, and selection of biopsy sites.

Several parts of the laparoscopy procedure should be practiced with the patient during the physical examination of the abdomen. The cooperation of the patient is important, especially the elevation of the anterior abdominal wall and tensing of the muscles during insertion of the pneumoperitoneum needle and trocar. The patient will usually try to accomplish this by arching the back. This is incorrect. It projects the spine and large vessels anteriorly and may present a risk during insertion of sharp instruments. To achieve a maximal distance between viscera and anterior parietal peritoneum, the patient's back should be pressed flat against the mattress. The patient can be taught to perform the correct maneuver by sliding one hand under the back and placing the other on the anterior abdominal wall. The patient is then asked to perform the Valsalva maneuver and elevate the anterior abdominal wall against one of the examiner's hands while simultaneously pushing his or her back firmly against the examiner's other hand.

Shaving the abdomen is necessary only if there is extensive hair growth. The patient should be told that under no circumstances should the pubic hair be shaved. Otherwise, an uninformed prep team will often shave the entire abdomen despite specific instructions to spare the pubic area; shaving this area is part of the standard preparation for abdominal surgery. Large inguinal or umbilical hernias should be taped firmly to prevent bulging herniation and associated patient discomfort during the pneumoperitoneum. A hiatal hernia is no longer considered a contraindication.[20] Also, routine enemas are not necessary. If a patient has a history of constipation and abdominal examination reveals a stool-filled colon or the abdominal film reveals significant fecal material in the large intestine that might interfere with the examination, one to two enemas the night before might be helpful. Laxatives should be avoided because they may cause abdominal cramps and diarrhea during the laparoscopy.

The patient should be instructed to empty his or her urinary bladder before coming to the endoscopy suite. A full bladder can present a risk during needle and trocar insertion and causes discomfort. If an intravenous line is running, the flow rates should be adjusted to "keep open"; otherwise, rapid infusion of fluid during a prolonged examination may result in bladder filling and discomfort to the patient.

A minimal number of preoperative laboratory tests are necessary, mainly relating to the clotting status. However, it would be unusual in today's practice if the patient did not have a prior chest x-ray and chemistry profile, or in cases of suspected liver disease one or more noninvasive imaging procedures. The results of such tests should be carefully reviewed beforehand.

Attention to all the points mentioned may make the difference between a smooth and successful examination and a difficult and painful one for patient and physician alike.

Premedication

The operator must decide which of the patient's medications may be stopped safely prior to the procedure and which drugs, antihypertensives for example, will be continued. For exploratory laparoscopy, general anesthesia is unnecessary and undesirable because the cooperation of the patient is needed during the procedure and the risk of general anesthesia equals that of laparoscopy. The patient should be fasting for at least 8 hours prior to the procedure. A sedative taken the evening before the examination is helpful if the patient is especially apprehensive. The type of premedication and dosage depends on the patient's general condition, associated illnesses, and operator preference. We prefer meperidine (Demerol), 50 to 100 mg intramuscularly, 30 minutes prior to the procedure combined with 0.6 mg atropine sulfate intramuscularly. At the examination table the degree of sedation is further titrated to the proper level with 5 to 10 mg diazepam (Valium) intravenously. An intravenous access line in the right forearm is helpful if additional sedation is required, as might occur during a prolonged procedure. Patients occasionally complain of shoulder pain caused by elevation of the diaphragm due to the pneumoperitoneum. Additional analgesic administration will usually alleviate this discomfort.

Asepsis and Preparation of the Abdomen

As mentioned, laparoscopy requires sterile technique and aseptic instruments, especially those parts of the instruments that enter the abdominal cavity. We consider the black eyepiece (ocular) of the telescope and teaching attachment nonsterile since these touch the examiner's eyelashes and orbita. Cameras cannot be sterilized. Endophotography is usually done prior to biopsy, and thus results in a break in sterile technique. However, a simple change of gloves after photodocumentation is sufficient to maintain proper sterile technique.

The only exposure to scrub procedures, asepsis, and proper surgical gowning for many gastroenterologists occurs during medical school clerkship, since most no longer serve rotating internships. For this reason, these procedures should be reviewed with operating room personnel. Examiners are usually fully gowned and gloved, including cap and face mask. However, European laparoscopists do not wear caps and masks routinely, and they have the same low or nonexistent infection rates as their American colleagues.

The patient's abdomen is scrubbed with Betadine solution or PhisoHex from nipple line to pubic hair line, starting from the umbilicus with ever widening circles until the entire area is covered; this process is repeated twice. Special attention should be given to cleansing the umbilicus with cotton tip applicators. A laparotomy sheet with slit is draped over the patient and attached to the anesthesia screen to block the patient's view into the operative field.

Site Selection

Proper site selection for pneumoperitoneum and telescope is one of the most important aspects of safe and successful laparoscopy. In selecting a site, the main purpose of the examination must be considered. For example, if a lesion is suspected high in the dome of the right hepatic lobe, the site might be moved somewhat cranially, although not so far as to prevent negotiation around the falciform ligament. If the pelvis is the primary area of interest, an infraumbilical incision in the linea alba may be more appropriate. The usual trocar entry site for exploratory laparoscopy in an abdomen without previous surgery or other extenuating circumstance is 3 to 5 cm or two finger breadths to the left and cranial to the umbilicus (Fig. 50–11). This places the incision at the medial aspect of the rectus abdominis

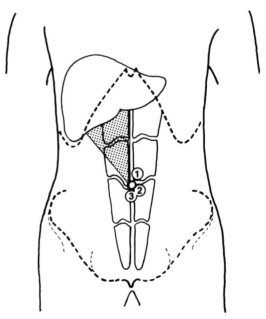

FIGURE 50–11. Entry site for telescope trocar in "medical" laparoscopy. Preferred site is 1; 2 and 3 are alternative sites. Shaded area should be avoided, since this is region of widely variable falciform and round ligaments.

muscle in a relatively avascular area. A more lateral approach may risk laceration of the epigastric vessels and bleeding. For gynecologic laparoscopy the entry is usually in the inferior umbilical fold. In women concerned about the small scar in the left upper abdomen after medical laparoscopy, the umbilicus is an appropriate site provided the patient does not have portal hypertension, which results in the presence of collateral vessels in this area.

When there is a mass in the left upper aspect of the abdomen or organ enlargement, an enlarged left hepatic lobe or splenomegaly, for example, a site directly to the left of the umbilicus or infraumbilical in the linea alba is appropriate (Fig. 50–11). The shaded area indicated in Figure 50–11 should be avoided, since the falciform and round ligaments are in this position; these may contain vessels of significant diameter in cases of portal hypertension. Furthermore, the gallbladder, because of its variable position, may be inadvertently punctured by instruments inserted into this area. The trocar site should

be at least 5 cm from the edge of any organ or mass and 3 to 5 cm from any scar.

Surgical scars also have a bearing on site selection (Fig. 50–12). A veil of adhesions will usually be attached to the undersurface of any abdominal scar; viscera may also be attached to the anterior abdominal wall in the region of a scar. The location and length of a scar does not always correspond to the extent of intra-abdominal adhesions. Lower abdominal scars after uncomplicated surgery, e.g., appendectomy or gynecologic operations, generally present no problems and the classic entry site may be used (Fig. 50–12D). With an upper abdominal midline scar an intra-abdominal site usually permits examination of the regions on both sides of the scar-associated intra-abdominal adhesions. If the prime area of interest is more to the right, site 2 should be used; if it is to the left, site 3 is preferable (Fig. 50–12A). The most commonly encountered scar in the upper abdomen is probably that resulting from a cholecystectomy. The adhesions associated with this may make the inspection of the

FIGURE 50–12. A–D, Common abdominal scars with standard entry site for trocar 1 and alternatives 2 and 3.

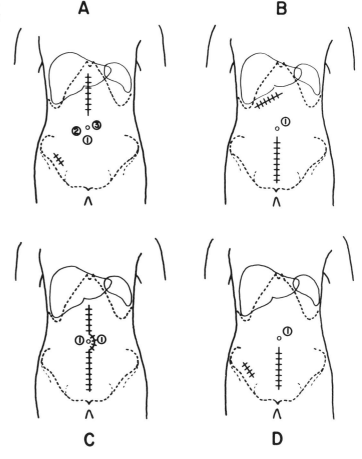

right lobe of the liver impossible; the patient should be advised of this before the procedure. In this situation, a good view of the left lobe is possible using the standard entry site (Fig. 50–12*B*). If the problem under investigation is diffuse liver disease, a biopsy obtained from the left lobe may be satisfactory. In many cases of postcholecystectomy adhesions, portions of the right lobe may still be visualized, and one may be able to negotiate the telescope through an opening in the adhesions. With an extensive midline scar, the operator must decide if entry on the left or right is preferable. This will mainly depend on the prime indication for laparoscopy. If a site to the right of the scar is chosen, the variable position of the gallbladder, which may even reach into the lower abdomen, should be kept in mind. A cholecystogram or ultrasonography may be indicated to determine the exact location (Fig. 50–12*C*). The beginner should limit himself initially to examinations of the nonoperated abdomen and attempt cases with abdominal scars only after having had experience with simpler examinations.

Pneumoperitoneum

The operator stands at the left side of the patient, with the instrument tray within easy reach to his left. The second examiner, if available, assists from the opposite side. Most examiners now prefer insertion of Veres cannula and telescope trocar at the same site. This technique avoids a second puncture of skin and peritoneum that is required when using the classic technique in which the insertion point is between the middle and outer third of the Richter-Monroe line connecting the umbilicus with the left iliac crest.

After the appropriate site has been chosen (Figs. 50–11 and 50–13) the local anesthetic is injected. A significant sensation of pain occurs only at the skin and peritoneum. Twenty to forty milliliters of 1% lidocaine (with or without epinephrine) are infiltrated in an area 1 cm in transverse and 2 cm in longitudinal dimension. Using a 25-gauge needle the anesthetic is initially injected intracutaneously, creating an "orange peel" effect (Fig. 50–14). Then the deeper layers are infiltrated using a 21-gauge, 1.5-inch needle. A sharp, somatic pain sensation indicates that the needle tip reached the peritoneum. A good preperitoneal block of 10 ml or more of anesthetic will assure an easier and pain-free examination. Multiple skin punctures should be avoided. The patient should be informed of each successive step in the procedure and the sensations to expect.

A skin incision 10 mm in length is made with one smooth stroke using a number 15 scalpel blade (Fig. 50–15). The length should

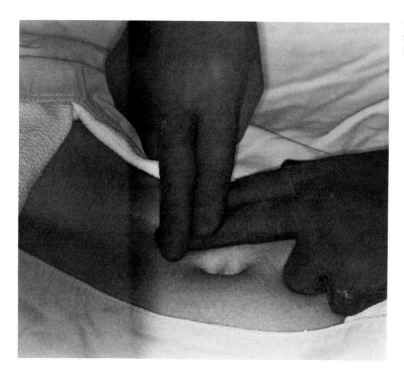

FIGURE 50–13. Classic entry site two-finger breadths above and to left of umbilicus.

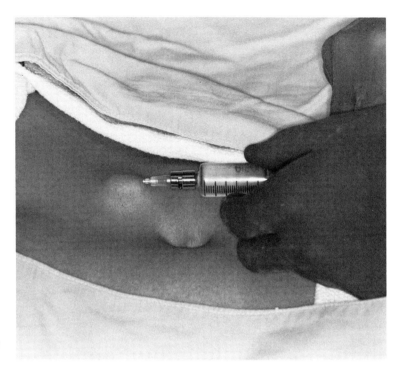

FIGURE 50–14. Intracutaneous injection of anesthetic.

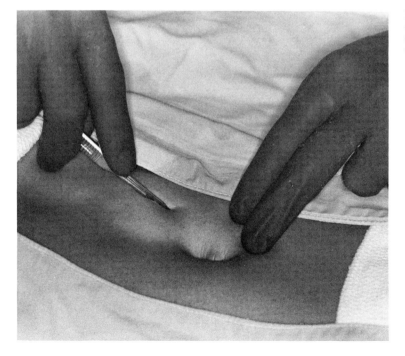

FIGURE 50–15. Skin incision should not exceed width of trocar. A scalpel with #15 blade is used.

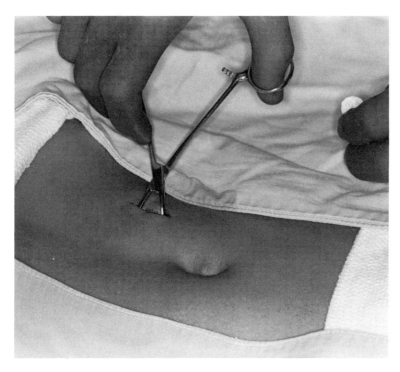

FIGURE 50–16. Dissection of subcutaneous tissue using mosquito forceps.

not exceed the diameter of the trocar sleeve. A large incision is unnecessary and undesirable. The subcutaneous tissue, if substantial, is bluntly dissected using a curved mosquito forceps (Fig. 50–16). This should never be done with a knife. Small bleeding vessels are usually compressed, and bleeding is arrested by the trocar sleeve. Ligation is not required.

In patients with portal hypertension the incision site is always selected between cutaneous vessels, and only the skin is carefully incised; other instrumentation is kept to an absolute minimum. Abdominal wall venous bleeding can be massive and may be fatal in this setting. In young athletic patients with little subcutaneous fat tissue the firm anterior

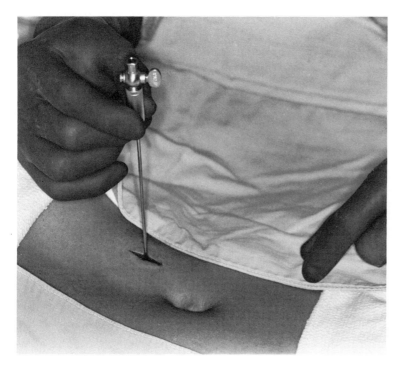

FIGURE 50–17. Insertion of Veres cannula. Stopcock should be in open position. Needle should be held at its hub so that the spring mechanism is not blocked.

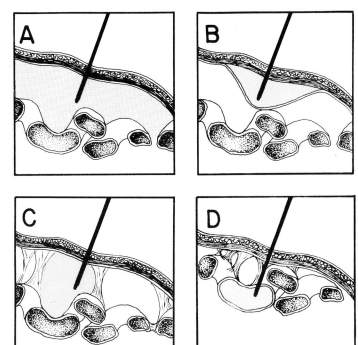

FIGURE 50–18. Various positions of Veres cannula within abdomen. *A*, Normal position. *B*, Preperitoneal insufflation. *C*, Insufflation of chamber caused by adhesions resulting in asymmetric insufflation. *D*, Position of needle in viscus adherent to anterior abdominal wall because of adhesions.

rectus fascia may be weakened using a scalpel but only under direct vision.

Before the Veres needle is inserted, the patient is asked to perform a Valsalva maneuver, tensing the abdominal wall and avoiding arching the back. The Veres needle is then inserted through the wound perpendicular to the abdominal surface (Fig. 50–17). Two distinct "pops" should be felt as the needle penetrates the anterior fascia and posterior rectus fascia with peritoneum. Negative aspiration assures that the needle lies freely in the abdominal cavity (Plate 50–2 and Fig. 50–18*A*) and has not punctured any viscus or vessel. A few milliliters of saline should be injected through the Veres cannula; flow through the cannula should be free and unobstructed. The fluid meniscus on the top of the cannula should disappear rapidly after the syringe is disconnected. These steps assure that the cannula is properly positioned before gas is insufflated.

The gas tubing is then connected and the switches on the nitrous oxide insufflator are set to "insufflate" and "manual." Under normal conditions free flow is shown by the gas flow indicator, usually at a rate of 1 liter/min given the normal flow resistance of the Veres needle of less than 8 mm Hg. Hepatic dullness to percussion should disappear rapidly; the entire abdomen should be percussed periodically during insufflation to check for the tympany that indicates a generalized pneumoperitoneum.

Occasionally the Veres needle may penetrate the posterior fascia but not the peritoneum (Fig. 50–18*B*). At this point insufflation will result in dissection and preperitoneal insufflation. This usually precludes laparoscopy for 24 hours. Adhesions may form a chamber within the abdomen. If the needle has been inserted into such a space, asymmetric abdominal distention and discomfort will result (Fig. 50–18*C*). Should the needle lie within a hollow viscus marked discomfort and absence of a free pneumoperitoneum occur (Fig. 50–18*D*). This is usually recognizable when the intra-abdominal pressure gauge indicates increased pressure. If the position of the needle in the abdominal cavity is in doubt a cross table lateral x-ray may be helpful. In cases of ascites, it may be necessary to drain 1½ to 2 liters of fluid to allow space for the pneumoperitoneum. Drainage of this amount is usually well tolerated by a cirrhotic patient. In exudative ascites due to tumor or infection, a greater volume of fluid may be removed, but it is not necessary to drain all the ascitic fluid for successful laparoscopy.

The volume of gas required for an adequate pneumoperitoneum varies widely. The safe. However, in a multiparous woman or an individual with a soft abdomen and weaker abdominal wall muscles, a greater height may be required.

Trocar Insertion

The Veres needle is withdrawn and the patient is again asked to perform the maneuver to tighten the abdominal wall. The assistant may support the flanks of a patient with ascites or flaccid abdominal walls. The trocar with its sleeve is inserted using controlled downward force and a twisting, rotatory motion (Fig. 50–21). Insertion may require significant pressure. We prefer the conical rather than the pyramidal trocar because it is less traumatic, only splitting rather than cutting the layers of the abdominal wall. Once the "two pops" are felt and the resistance of the abdominal wall is overcome, the inserting force is immediately arrested and the trocar is withdrawn into its sleeve. A hissing sound of escaping gas from the opened lateral stopcock indicates that the trocar sleeve is properly positioned. After the trocar is removed from the sleeve, the sleeve may be inserted further with ease using gentle forward force

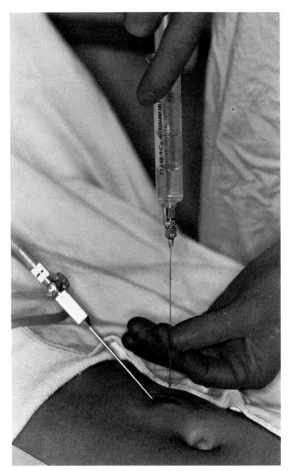

FIGURE 50–19. Estimation of height of gas cupula using a thin ("skinny") needle.

proper tightness of the abdominal wall is more important than the absolute volume of gas insufflated. The required volume ranges from 1500 to 7000 ml with an average of 3000 ml of nitrous oxide.[17]

The height of the gas cupula can be estimated using a thin needle (22 gauge × 15 cm). The needle with attached syringe containing 2 to 3 ml of saline is inserted into the abdomen next to the Veres needle. Continuous slow aspiration and observation of the gas bubbles in the fluid as the needle is advanced allows accurate estimation of the depth of the pneumoperitoneum and "working space" for trocar insertion (Fig. 50–19). By tilting the needle and rotating it so that its tip describes a circle one can also test for adhesions under the site for insertion of the trocar (Fig. 50–20). In an appropriately insufflated peritoneal cavity with firm abdominal wall, a cupula at least 8 cm high is usually

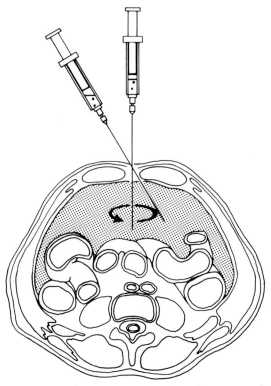

FIGURE 50–20. Estimation of depth of pneumoperitoneum and testing for adhesions under site for trocar insertion.

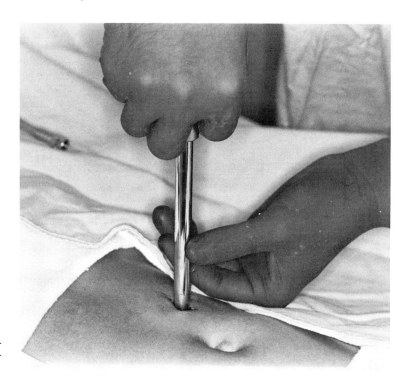

FIGURE 50–21. Insertion of trocar using controlled force and rotating motion.

and slight left-right axial rotation (Fig. 50–22A). With complete removal of the trocar, the trumpet valve of the trocar sleeve closes automatically to prevent further escape of gas. Occasionally the trocar tip but not the sleeve will have entered the abdomen (Fig. 50–22B), at which point the trocar should not be withdrawn; it should be withdrawn only after the sleeve has fully penetrated the abdominal wall (Fig. 50–22C and D).

The gas tubing is reconnected and the insufflator switches are set on "insufflate" and "automatic." The intra-abdominal pressure gauge should indicate slight fluctuations in intra-abdominal pressure with respiration. The proximal trocar sleeve is cleaned of any blood and secretions with cotton-tipped ap-

plicators so that the distal telescope objectives are kept clean when passing through the trocar sleeve (Fig. 50–23).

The side-viewing 50-degree telescope is preferred for abdominal exploration. By rotating the telescope around its axis and advancing and retracting it through the trocar sleeve, a complete panoramic view of the abdominal cavity and its organs is achieved. Forward optics cannot provide this complete visual field or the degree of inspection of inferior and superior surfaces of the liver achieved with the 50-degree foroblique telescope and axial rotation. With prograde optics the dome of the liver can only be seen tangentially; the 50-degree optics provide an en face view.

FIGURE 50–22. Stepwise trocar insertion. A, Trocar tip just tents peritoneum. B, Tip but not yet the sleeve has entered abdomen. Trocar should not be withdrawn. C, Once sleeve has fully penetrated abdominal wall, inner trocar is removed. D, Trocar sleeve is further advanced with ease using rotating motion.

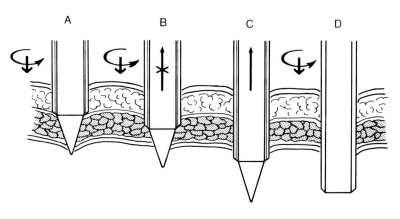

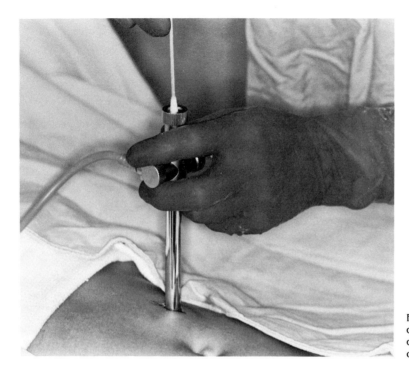

FIGURE 50–23. Trocar sleeve is cleaned with cotton-tipped applicators to assure clean telescope objectives.

Second Puncture Technique

Some examiners prefer passing the palpating probe and biopsy instruments through the instrument channel of the Jacobs-Palmer operating laparoscope, using a single puncture technique (Fig. 50–24). Since the telescope must follow each motion of the probe, biopsy needle or forceps, the maneuverability and view are somewhat restricted.

We prefer and recommend the double puncture technique (Fig. 50–25). It brings the accessory instruments directly to the point where they are needed by means of the small 4 mm accessory trocar and sleeve. This technique has the advantage of greater telescope-independent maneuverability in the use of accessory devices.

If, after an initial exploratory survey, it is thought necessary to use an accessory, the

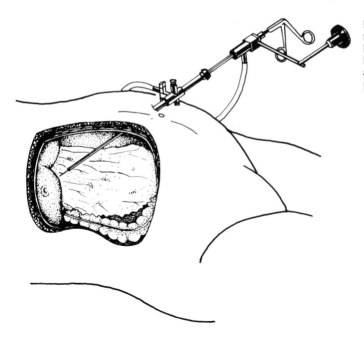

FIGURE 50–24. Single puncture technique using Jacobs-Palmer operating laparoscope. Robbers forceps is inserted into integral instrument channel in an attempt to obtain biopsy of focal neoplastic lesion in right hepatic lobe.

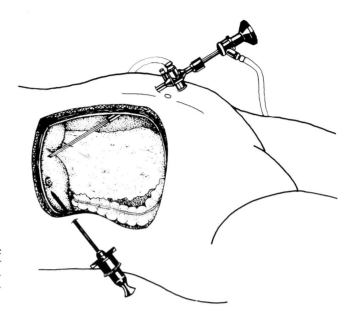

FIGURE 50–25. Second (double) puncture technique. Accessory trocar in right anterior axillary line allows greater mobility of accessory instruments. Their movement is telescope independent.

accessory trocar site is selected. Generally this will be a point along the right anterior axillary line in most cases subcostally, although the last intercostal space is acceptable when the liver is small or shrunken. To place the second trocar at a higher point along this line entails a risk of a pneumothorax and restricts mobility especially toward the left upper abdomen. In selecting a site one should be certain that instruments can be easily maneuvered past the inferior edge of the falciform ligament to reach the left hepatic lobe and left upper quadrant. Transillumination of the abdominal wall using telescope-transmitted light allows selection of an avascular area for the incision in patients with portal hypertension. The operator may indent the abdominal wall at the selected site with a finger so that the corresponding spot on the peritoneal side can be viewed laparoscopically (Fig. 50–26). The selected site can then be related to the position of the intra-

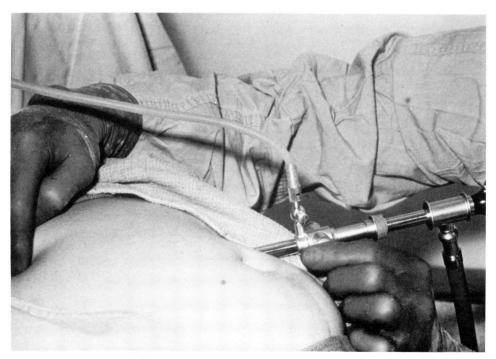

FIGURE 50–26. Site selection for accessory trocar.

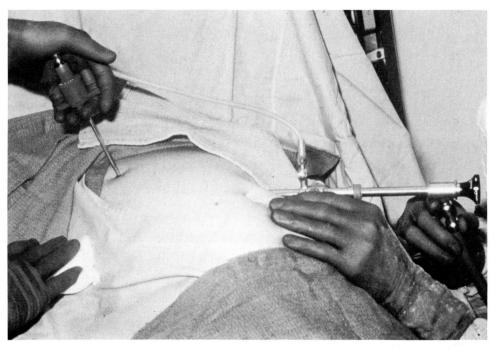

FIGURE 50–27. Insertion of accessory trocar with endoscopic monitoring.

abdominal organs and structures. Minor adjustments can then be made so that the placement of the second puncture site is optimal. The skin is infiltrated over an area of 1 sq cm in a manner similar to that described for the Veres needle. The needle is easily identified through the laparoscope as it tents and penetrates the wall; observation allows minor adjustments in placing the needle so that adequate preperitoneal injection of the anesthetic is assured (Plate 50–3). A small 4 mm stab wound using a number 11 blade is made, nicking only the skin. Trocar insertion is monitored from the peritoneal side, adjusting the direction of the trocar to avoid injury to underlying structures (Fig. 50–27). After the trocar sleeve has fully penetrated (Plate 50–4), various instruments may be inserted as needed. When instruments are withdrawn an automatic valve prevents escape of gas.

The entire second puncture procedure adds only 3 to 5 minutes to the total examining time, and the overall exploratory capability is greatly enhanced. Suturing is not required, and a small, additional adhesive strip is the only visible sign after the procedure. As a rule the small stab wound leaves no visible scar.

Technique of Abdominal Exploration

A competent laparoscopist must be able to identify correctly the various normal and abnormal structures in the abdominal cavity and therefore must be first a student of normal anatomy. Review of an atlas or textbook of anatomy is advisable, and study of the available excellent atlases and textbooks of laparoscopy greatly enhances understanding of anatomy.[12, 21–23] Thorough knowledge avoids such errors as referring to the appendix fibrosa of the hepato-phrenic ligament (Plate 50–5) or the phrenicocolic ligament (Plate 50–6), an important early site of portal-systemic collaterals, as adhesions. Riedel's or quadrate lobes will be correctly identified and the Anomaly of Zahn[24] over the dome of the right lobe of the liver will not be overlooked. The competent laparoscopist finds no challenge in naming the various folds on the inferior abdominal wall. The vas deferens crossing the inguinal fold will never be overlooked (Plate 50–7) nor mistaken for a fibrous band or nerve. Attention should also be directed to the female pelvis (see Chapter 57); the gynecologist is also well advised to turn the laparoscope cephalad to scan upper abdomen, liver, and spleen.

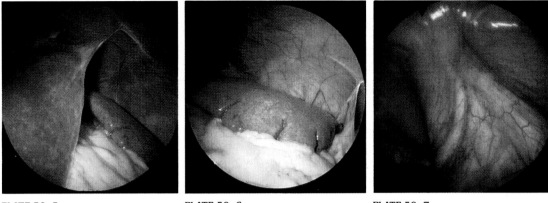

PLATE 50—5.   PLATE 50—6.   PLATE 50—7.

PLATE 50—5. Left upper quadrant. Lateral aspect of left liver lobe with appendix fibrosa of hepatophremic ligament. This sail-like structure is widely variable and frequently confused with adhesions. Spleen with medial crenated margin is seen in back.

PLATE 50—6. Left upper quadrant. Normal spleen is characterized by its crenated medial margin. This organ is frequently covered by omentum. Structure at inferior pole of spleen is not an adhesion but the phrenicocolic ligament. In portal hypertension portal systemic collaterals develop earliest in this structure. It is therefore important to identify correctly this ligament if early portal hypertension is suspected.

PLATE 50—7. Right lower quadrant, anterior abdominal wall. External iliac vessels form a fold with bluish vein in its lateral margin; the artery lies medial to it. White cord crossing this fold is vas deferens, readily identified in male patients.

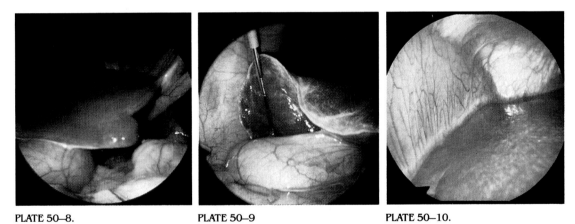

PLATE 50—8.   PLATE 50—9   PLATE 50—10.

PLATE 50—8. Normal right upper quadrant. Normal right hepatic lobe with smooth surface and sharp edge is seen. Gallbladder with characteristic Robin's-egg blue and vascular markings lies in foreground. Falciform ligament with round ligament in its free anterior aspect separate right and left liver lobes. Portions of stomach in foreground and diaphragmatic dome in background are also visible.

PLATE 50—9. Lateral aspect of right liver lobe. Exploration of undersurface of right lobe using the probe is demonstrated. Hepatic surface is normal with some increased capsule thickening, especially in the edge. "Draping" effect of liver as it hangs over probe is characteristic of its soft consistency and is absent in a fibrotic or cirrhotic organ. Normal gallbladder with its widely variable position reaches far to right. Portions of parietal peritoneum of lateral abdominal wall with normal vascular markings are also seen.

PLATE 50—10. Normal falciform ligament. This view with portions of left hepatic lobe in foreground shows normal falciform ligament that is seen from its left side. Delicate sail-like structure and fine reticular network of vessels are evident. Central tendon of diaphragm is seen in top center.

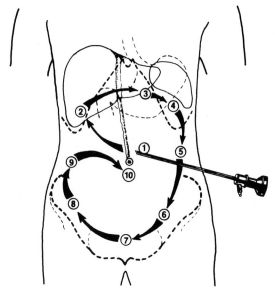

FIGURE 50—28. Technique of abdominal exploration using a standard sequence of steps and positions (see text).

To avoid errors of omission, a complete abdominal exploration should be carried out in a standardized sequence of steps and standard table positions (Fig. 50—28) as suggested in the following paragraphs. The various positions described reemphasize the importance of an endoscopy table, such as the Maquet table, that can be tilted in all directions. It may be necessary to modify the sequence according to the individual patient and/or the preference of the physician. The patient remains supine in all the following positions and the examination table is tilted.

First Position

The patient is horizontal, the examiner at the patient's left side, and the telescope is directed toward the mid-right upper quadrant. The abdominal viscera (omentum, small bowel) directly below the Veres needle and trocar insertion site should be inspected first to exclude any possible injury. Next the falciform and round ligaments are identified as general landmarks. This position gives an overall view of the abdominal cavity including inferior portions of the right and left hepatic lobes, anterior portion of the stomach, and omentum, as well as any adhesions or abnormalities of the large and small bowel, peritoneum and ascites.

Second Position (Right Upper Abdomen) (Plates 50—8 and 50—9)

The patient is positioned 30 degrees head up—feet down with his or her right shoulder

elevated 45 degrees. The laparoscopist is on the patient's left side, directing the telescope toward the right upper quadrant. The structures and organs visualized in this position include the right hepatic lobe, gallbladder, falciform and round ligaments, right dome of the diaphragm, and duodenum. This is also the standard position for guided liver biopsy.

Third Position (Upper Mid-Abdomen) (Plate 50—10)

The patient is in a 30-degree head up—feet down position. The examiner remains on the left side and the telescope is directed toward the upper mid-abdomen. In this position the left hepatic lobe with corresponding diaphragm, falciform ligament, round ligament, and anterior wall of stomach are visualized. Early changes of portal hypertension are well appreciated in this position with the sail-like extension of the falciform ligament.

Fourth Position (Left Upper Quadrant) (Fig. 50—9B; Plates 50—5 and 50—6)

The patient's position is 30 degrees head up—feet down with 45-degree elevation of the left shoulder. The examiner is now at the patient's right side directing the telescope toward the left upper quadrant. The organs and structures to be visualized include the left hepatic lobe with hepatophrenic ligament, left dome of the diaphragm (right ventricular pulsations should be noted), spleen and splenophrenic ligament, phrenicocolic ligament, anterior wall and greater curvature of stomach.

Fifth Position (Left Lumbar Region)

The patient is horizontal except that the left side of the table is tilted upward 30 degrees. The examiner is on the patient's right and the telescope is directed toward the left flank. The descending colon, small intestine, and omentum should be visualized.

Sixth Position (Left Lower Quadrant) (Plate 50—11)

The patient is in a 30-degree head down—feet up position with the left side of the table tilted upward 30 degrees. The examiner remains at the patient's right side directing the telescope toward the left lower quadrant. This allows observation of the descending and sigmoid colon, omentum, small bowel, and in men the inguinal rings (medial, lateral) and vas deferens.

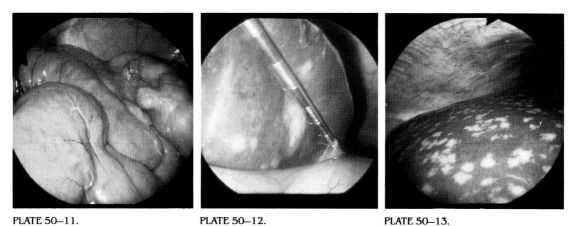

PLATE 50–11.   PLATE 50–12.   PLATE 50–13.

PLATE 50–11. Left lower quadrant. Foreground shows some loops of small bowel with omentum. Some white lymphatics on small bowel surface are evident. Sigmoid colon with wide-mouth diverticulum lies in background.
PLATE 50–12. Proper elevation of left hepatic lobe in patient with metastatic adenocarcinoma originating from pancreas.
PLATE 50–13. Sarcoidosis of liver, right hepatic lobe.

Seventh Position (Pelvis) (Fig. 50–9C)

The table is tilted so that the patient is in a 30-degree head down–feet up position with shoulders parallel to the floor. The examiner now changes to the patient's left side and directs the laparoscopic view into the lower mid-abdomen and pelvis. In this position the urinary bladder, sigmoid colon, small bowel, and omentum are visualized. In addition, in women the uterus, fallopian tubes, and ovaries are observed.

Eighth Position (Right Lower Quadrant)

In this position the patient is in a 30-degree head down–feet up position with the table tilted 30 degrees upward on the right side. The examiner directs the telescope toward the right lower quadrant working from the patient's left side. The ascending colon with appendix, small bowel, terminal ileum, and omentum can be visualized; in men the right inguinal rings and vas deferens can also be seen.

Ninth Position (Right Flank Region)

The patient is horizontal except that the right side of the table is tilted upward 30 degrees. The examiner is on the left and directs the view toward the right flank. Organs and structures to be visualized include the ascending colon, small intestine, omentum, and peritoneum.

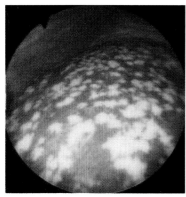

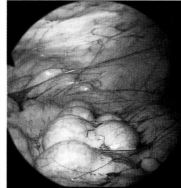

PLATE 50–14. Polaroid photograph of same lesion shown in Plate 50–13.
PLATE 50–15. Mid-abdomen, transverse colon viewed from left side. Haustra and a central tenia of transverse colon are evident. There is a significant amount of preperitoneal fat on anterior abdominal wall.

PLATE 50–14.   PLATE 50–15.

Tenth Position (Periumbilical Region)

The patient is horizontal and the examiner is at the left; the telescope is directed straight downward toward the center of the abdomen. The omentum, small intestine, and peritoneum should be visualized.

At this point the exploration is complete. The abdominal cavity is scanned in a panoramic fashion for a last time, biopsy sites are re-inspected to assure complete hemostasis, and the telescope is withdrawn.

Special Considerations

Palpating Probe

The range of abdominal exploration is greatly enhanced by routine use of the palpating probe. This allows inspection of the undersurface of the right and left hepatic lobes (Plates 50–9 and 50–12), especially in cases of suspected metastatic disease. Actual palpation with the probe also gives a good appreciation of tissue consistency. The firmness of tumor lesions or a cirrhotic liver can be appreciated without difficulty. The proper way of lifting the liver is shown in Plate 50–12. Sliding the probe under the organ parallel to its edge rather than perpendicular to it allows lifting of a broader region with less discomfort.

If the tip of the probe is slid over the normal liver surface a light line will appear as blood is pressed out of the tissue. Normal liver color reappears in 1 or 2 seconds. When there is fatty infiltration the probe describes a yellow line. The technique has been called "xanthography–yellow writing" and is helpful when a fatty liver is suspected.

The appendix can be identified in 75% of all cases in position 8 using a probe.[25] A suction probe can be especially helpful, allowing lifting of the appendix and inspection of all sides from base to tip.

Inspection of the Pancreas

Inspection of parts of the pancreas was first reported in 1972 by Meyer-Burg[26] using a supragastric approach. Other techniques using an infragastric route and observation of the head of the pancreas in the duodenal C loop have been described (see Chapter 52).[27, 28]

Since the pancreas is a retroperitoneal structure it is not primarily accessible by laparoscopy. In slender patients, portions of the pancreas may be seen through a fat-free omentum; these have a characteristic yellow color but lack the usual glitter of fat. The body and tail may be viewed by elevating the patient's head and left shoulder (position 3 or 4). The stomach and omentum will slide caudad freeing the region under the left hepatic lobe. A 50-degree foroblique viewing telescope is then brought under the left liver lobe elevating it with a view onto the minor omentum and lesser sac. With scissors or Robbers forceps, an incision is made into the omentum whereupon the pancreas can be directly observed through the incision. When the telescope is inserted into the lesser sac, larger portions of the gland may be inspected.

Tissue may be obtained using a thin ("skinny") needle for aspiration cytology or Robbers forceps and Menghini (1.2 mm) and Tru-cut needles for biopsy. The diagnostic yield is high and because complications such as pancreatitis or fistula formation are infrequent, laparoscopic pancreatic biopsy is a remarkably safe procedure.[29] Since the depth of biopsy is difficult to control with Menghini and Tru-cut needles, forceps biopsy or aspiration for cytology is recommended. The thin needle with its extreme flexibility is difficult to direct once it has penetrated the abdominal wall. A simple solution to this problem is to insert an 18-gauge needle first into the abdominal wall. This can then be used as a perfect trocar sleeve for the thin needle, making it easy to direct the needle tip to an area for aspiration cytology.

Flexible Laparoscopy

A flexible, small-caliber fiberoptic endoscope has been adapted for laparoscopy; the feasibility of this technique has been demonstrated.[30] With the superiority of present telescope optics and the 50-degree viewing angle we see no advantage in a fiberoptic flexible instrument over the standard classic technique.

Biopsy Techniques

Direct Vision Liver Biopsy

Exploratory laparoscopy, especially in the evaluation of diseases of the liver, would be incomplete without direct vision biopsy as originated by Kalk et al.[31] Three types of needles are available: the 1.4 and 1.8 mm Menghini, the Vim-Silverman, and the Tru-cut, as well as a forceps for focal lesions (see Accessory Equipment).

In general the right lobe of the liver is preferred for biopsy. Biopsy of the more variable shape and thickness of the left lobe may entail some increased risk, but a biopsy can be safely obtained from this lobe when the right lobe is inaccessible because of adhesions or when multiple liver biopsies are indicated, e.g., lymphoma staging. Before biopsy, the undersurface of the left lobe should be inspected to insure that its thickness at the biopsy site is adequate. The preferred sites for direct vision biopsy are shown in Figure 50–29. The liver edge, the region over the gallbladder, and the area of the porta hepatis should be avoided for obvious reasons. The biopsy needle should enter the liver at an angle 30 degrees from the surface of the organ to avoid deeper regions and vessels with the risk of increased bleeding.

The Menghini technique, the preferred method for percutaneous liver biopsy, is used widely and requires no special explanation.[32] After the needle (usually the 1.8 mm diameter needle) has been inserted into the accessory trocar, a site is chosen that appears safe and that can be inspected without difficulty at all times. While the operator advances the needle tip 0.5 to 1 cm into the liver parenchyma at a 30-degree angle, the assistant creates a vacuum by withdrawing the plunger of the attached syringe. The needle is then thrust 2 cm into the liver and withdrawn while the patient holds his or her breath. The specimen is ejected with a special plunger after the internal trapping probe has been

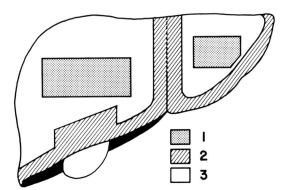

FIGURE 50–29. Sites for direct vision liver biopsy. (1) Optimal site. (2) This site should be avoided because of thinness of liver edge as well as underlying structures such as gallbladder, large vessels, and bile ducts. (3) Alternative site depending on special circumstances.

removed. Bleeding is minimal and ceases rapidly.

The biopsy site can be easily compressed with the palpating probe, another advantage of the 30-degree angle approach (Fig. 50–30). Clot formation is evident after several minutes. In some cases of cirrhosis with portal hypertension, a fountain of blood may emerge from the biopsy site when a branch of the portal system is punctured. Even in these cases, persistent compression of the biopsy site will usually suffice to control bleeding. In the unusual situation in which these conservative measures fail, coagulation with a suction electrode will control bleeding. Some examiners use coagulation routinely after each biopsy,[33] but we found no need of this in more than 15 years.

FIGURE 50–30. Control of post–liver biopsy bleeding with compression of biopsy port with probe.

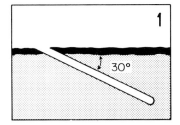

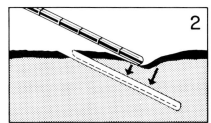

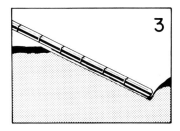

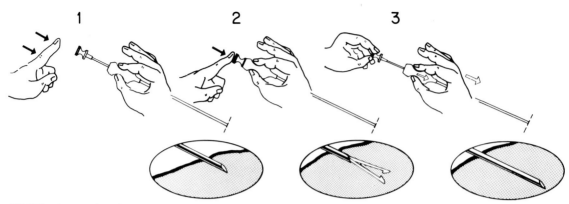

FIGURE 50–31. Vim-Silverman liver biopsy technique. Note three steps of holding outer cannula steady while advancing inner split needle into liver, cutting and trapping liver cylinder. By holding inner needle steady, the outer cannula is advanced over it and finally the entire apparatus is withdrawn.

One disadvantage of the Menghini technique is that the specimen is frequently fragmented in cases of fibrosis or cirrhosis. A particulate specimen has been taken as indirect evidence of cirrhosis, since this occurs in 11% of such cases compared with only 2% of normal or noncirrhotic livers.[34] If the second puncture technique with an accessory trocar is not used, the biopsy may be obtained through the operating laparoscope or by a direct percutaneous approach. A special shorter set of instruments is available for the direct vision percutaneous technique.

We prefer the Vim-Silverman technique (Fig. 50–31) because it gives a larger, unfragmented specimen and has the same low incidence of bleeding complications. Beginners sometimes have difficulty with the three steps and fail to obtain a specimen. However, the principle is simple and once understood should present no problems. Before biopsy the inner split needle is retracted into the outer sheath. With the entire apparatus in

this position, the operator advances the needle 0.5 to 1 cm into the parenchyma, again using the 30-degree angle approach (Step 1). The actual biopsy then takes place. While the assistant holds the outer cannula firmly in place with his left hand the inner needle is rapidly advanced with the right index finger until its hub reaches the hub of the outer cannula with a pop (Step 2). The inner needle is then held steady, and the outer cannula is advanced over the inner needle with a twisting that cuts and traps the specimen (Step 3). Finally, the entire apparatus is withdrawn and disassembled, and the specimen is removed.

The Tru-cut technique employs the same principle and is in its three steps identical to the above-described Vim-Silverman technique (Fig. 50–32). It is reliable and cuts a 2-cm specimen that is then trapped in its chamber. In the past a direct percutaneous approach using a longer 15-cm version of the needle was necessary. However, a modi-

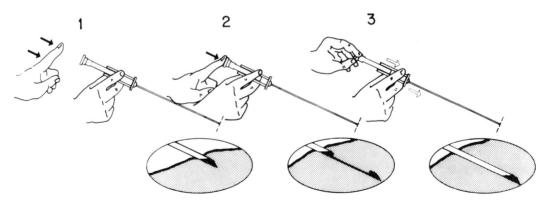

FIGURE 50–32. Tru-cut biopsy technique using same basic three steps as with Vim-Silverman technique.

fied type with spring mechanism has become available (Wolf Instrument Co.) that can be used directly through the accessory trocar. This makes an additional skin puncture unnecessary, and its spring release mechanism avoids some of the difficulties encountered by beginners.

Occasionally, a biopsy specimen cylinder may be lost on the liver surface. It is possible to recover the specimen in such a case using a grasping forceps, although this usually causes some crush artifact in the specimen. It is simpler in most cases to obtain a new biopsy.

Biopsies can be obtained of focal liver lesions such as tumor with any of the above techniques, but a lancet-shaped forceps (Robbers) appears best suited.[35] The periphery of a focal lesion is the preferred site rather than its center since biopsies of the latter usually yield only necrotic tissue. The lesions may be of various sizes. Smaller ones are preferred for biopsy since this avoids the larger vessels in larger metastases that may give rise to increased bleeding. The fixed portion of the double lancet-shaped forceps is fully inserted into the tumor edge, the hinged movable part is closed over it, and the forceps is then withdrawn (Fig. 50–33). Some crush artifact is usual with any forceps biopsy specimen.

Biopsy specimens are transferred into a 10% formaldehyde solution for fixation and further processing in the pathology department. For tissue culture, a small portion of the biopsy is placed in a sterile container prior to fixation. Quantitative analysis for iron or copper requires special considerations for needles and containers. Suspected hepatic porphyria may be confirmed immediately by exposing the specimen to ultraviolet light. The unfixed biopsy cylinder will exhibit red fluorescence if the patient has this disease.

If biopsy appears to be too dangerous, material for cytology can be obtained by aspiration with a thin ("skinny") needle. A retractable cytology brush for liver or peritoneal lesions is highly effective and extremely safe. In one series of 100 consecutive cases, the diagnostic yield was 94% for tumors involving the liver and 100% for those of the peritoneum.[36]

Peritoneal Biopsy

Peritoneal biopsies may be obtained with any of the various forceps available for this purpose. Depending on the tissue consistency, a cupped or cutting instrument can be used. The peritoneum is very pain sensitive. Pulling on the visceral peritoneum may cause dull visceral pain and a vasovagal response. For biopsy of the parietal peritoneum some form of local anesthesia is advisable. This is best accomplished from the peritoneal side using any fine needle such as the biliary puncture cannula via the accessory trocar. Percutaneous anesthesia involves additional pain as the needle penetrates the skin.

Biopsy of Other Organs

The need for biopsy of the spleen is much less than that for liver biopsy. A 1.2 or 1.4 mm Menghini needle or a thin ("skinny") needle for aspiration cytology is used. Increased bleeding is a definite risk after needle biopsy. However, conservative measures appear to be sufficient for control of bleeding without resorting to electrocoagulation.[17] "Skinny" needles are used for aspiration cytology of lymph nodes.

Splenoportography, Cholecystocholangiography, Transhepatic Cholangiography, and Ultrasonography

These combined laparoscopic-radiographic procedures require x-ray capability in the endoscopy suite. To perform laparos-

FIGURE 50–33. Biopsy of focal liver lesion using Robbers forceps.

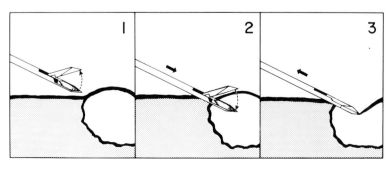

copy in the radiology department is extremely cumbersome and in many instances impractical.

Percutaneous and laparoscopic splenoportography have largely been replaced by direct visceral arteriography and evaluation of the venous phase of angiographic studies. Although laparoscopic splenoportography provides excellent radiographs and appears safe in experienced hands,[37–39] it receives little use in present day practice.

Cholecystocholangiography and transhepatic cholangiography are also largely of historical importance.[40, 41] These studies have been replaced by the technically simpler methods of percutaneous transhepatic cholangiography (PTC) and ERCP.

There have been some preliminary attempts at laparoscopic sonography, especially for evaluation of the pancreas and retroperitoneal masses. It is too soon to say if the method has clinical significance when compared with transcutaneous ultrasonography.

Therapeutic Laparoscopy

Therapeutic laparoscopy is mainly concerned with gynecologic indications (see Chapter 57). In the rare case of prolonged bleeding after liver biopsy that cannot be controlled by conservative measures, a few bursts of coagulating current through the suction-coagulating probe will usually control the bleeding.[33]

Although adhesions are frequently encountered, they are only rarely the cause of abdominal pain. To prove that adhesions are the true cause, the exact area of pain localization should first be marked by injecting methylene blue. If adhesions are found at laparoscopy in the regions of peritoneum so marked, tugging and pulling them with a probe should predictably reproduce the pain: only then is there a clear indication for adhesiolysis. Various insulated forceps and scissors are available for this purpose. In avascular adhesions the task is easy and without risk. But if vessels are present, the gastroenterologist will probably consult a surgeon with experience in laparoscopy. In a patient with portal hypertension, adhesions should be left alone because they are the sites of portal-systemic collateral vessels.

The most common type of intervention is removal of a foreign body from the abdominal cavity, usually an intrauterine device that has perforated the uterus or a catheter tip sheared off during paracentesis. Extraction with a grasping forceps through the accessory trocar is usually not difficult.[42–44] Exact localization of a radiopaque foreign body with biplane radiographics prior to laparoscopy is mandatory.

Completion of Procedure and Postoperative Care

After the telescope has been removed the accessory trocar is withdrawn. The pneumoperitoneum is deflated by activating the trumpet valve of the main trocar which is then also withdrawn. Small amounts of gas that remain in the abdominal cavity are absorbed in a few days. Gloves should be changed prior to skin closure.

The incision is closed using 1 to 2 sutures (4–0 silk with cutting needle), skin clips or Steri-Strips. The latter can also be used for the stab wound of the accessory trocar (Fig. 50–34). Incision and puncture sites are then covered with adhesive tape. In case of ascites, the skin should only be loosely approximated. This allows drainage of ascites but this generally ceases in a few days. Tight skin closure facilitates dissection of ascites into abdominal wall, scrotum, or vulva. Sutures should be removed in 5 to 7 days. Patients may take showers as long as the incision is protected by tape; tub baths are permissible after the sutures have been removed.

Twenty-four hours of bedrest with close monitoring of vital signs is only necessary if a liver biopsy has been performed. In other cases the patient may get up earlier depending on overall condition and degree of sedation. The most common postoperative complaint is shoulder pain secondary to diaphragmatic irritation. The pain is usually controlled by an analgesic.

The laparoscopic findings should again be discussed with the patient in the afternoon following the procedure, since postoperative sedation may preclude a clear understanding of the significance of the findings at an earlier time.

Laparoscopic Photography

Laparoscopic photography is more difficult than other gastrointestinal photodocumentation. Distances in the abdominal cavity are greater, and the dark color of the liver ab-

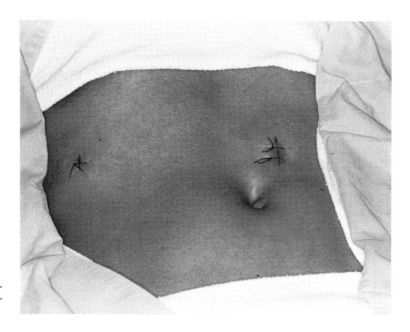

FIGURE 50–34. Skin closure using 4–0 silk. Skin clips or Steri-Strips can also be used.

sorbs more light. General principles of endoscopic photography are discussed in Chapter 4.

The basic equipment for laparoscopic photography has been described in an earlier section. If the camera is used for other types of endophotography, the regular focusing screen must be exchanged for a microprism of the clear-field type with hair-line for easy focusing (e.g., Olympus focusing screen No. 1–12). The camera design should allow for rapid exchange of screens (e.g., Olympus OM-series). Since the diameter of the telescope is smaller than the diameter of the standard camera lens, only the central portion of the lens is used. Expensive lenses with special correction for peripheral distortion are therefore not necessary. To assure that all the light transmitted through the telescope reaches the film, the lens aperture should be fully opened by selecting the lowest F-stop on the lens aperture ring, e.g., F-stop 2.8 for 100 mm lens. The synchronization selector should be set on "X" and the time exposure at 1/15 sec (in some cases 1/30 sec, 1/60 sec). This assures that the shutter is in the open position for the duration of the electronic flash discharge (1/500 to 1/2000 sec).[13] Because of these extremely short exposure times it is not necessary for the patient to hold his or her breath. The cardiac pulsations of the right ventricle readily observed at the left diaphragmatic dome and transmitted aortic pulsations or intestinal peristalsis usually do not result in image distortion.

The special focusing screen allows proper focusing of the image, especially for close-up shots of surface detail. Since the operator is usually concerned with other aspects of laparoscopy and comfort of the patient, it is difficult and cumbersome to worry about flash intensity, focusing, F-stops, etc. It is therefore more convenient to use a fixed focus. For Wolf telescopes with 100 mm commercial lens and 1 dopter quickmount adaptor, a focus setting of 1.5 m (5 ft) will usually assure sharp images except for very close-up photos. The Olympus adaptor (SM-EFR) is also easily focused.

The intensity of the flash is either automatically regulated by the light source or selected manually (see special manufacturer's instructions). If a camera has a built-in automatic light meter this should be switched to manual or turned off. For routine photography it is easiest to rely on the flash intensity automatically selected by the light source. Experts prefer the manual mode with "bracketing" of various shots for optimal object illumination. Differing degrees of light absorption between a dark liver surface and a brilliant, shiny peritoneum or omentum present a problem for the automatic light meter within the adaptor or light source. Usually a compromise is reached, but over- or under-exposed photos might result depending on the reading of the light sensor. When the light intensity in the same view varies greatly from one surface to another the telescope can be rotated to "recompose" the picture so that it will have one predominant color or brightness.

Some investigators have attempted to resolve the difficulties of proper illumination by introducing a quartz rod into the abdomen through a separate trocar. The rod is attached to an external flash globe. Its discharge is synchronized with the camera shutter.[33, 45] However, this requires an additional skin puncture. Newer light sources with large telescopes and integral light-transmitting bundles usually provide adequate illumination.

Polaroid systems provide instant photodocumentation. A print of reasonable quality is available in 90 seconds and can be attached to the patient's chart as an objective record for review by referring physician and consultants. Since Polaroid films are of slow speed there is not enough light for the image to fill the entire frame, which is a waste of film. Some cameras allow rotation of the camera body to expose 4 or 6 images on a single print. Polaroid film gives a lesser quality photograph than color negative or positive film, but it nevertheless serves the purpose of complementing the operative report. Two photographs are shown (Plates 50–13 and 50–14) of the liver of a 30-year old woman with sarcoidosis involving the liver to demonstrate the difference between transparency and Polaroid photography.

Photography is best carried out after abdominal exploration is complete and before biopsies are taken. Blood from the biopsy site will obscure surface details and absorbs light. Since cameras cannot be sterilized, obtaining photographs entails a break in sterile technique. The trocar entry site should be protected by wrapping an additional sterile towel around the telescope which also covers the operative field. After photodocumentation, which adds about 5 minutes to the examination, gloves should be changed.

Laparoscopic photography has reached a state of perfection such that the examiner not primarily interested in photography is able to obtain usable pictures. Each procedure should be documented on film as a permanent, objective record.

Normal Abdomen

Some photographic examples of normal laparoscopic findings have been presented. The color plates are reproductions of transparencies and have therefore lost some of the color brilliance and brightness of the originals (Plates 50–5 through 50–11 and Plate 50–15).

References

1. Kelling G. Über die Besichtigung der Speiseröhre und des Magens mit biegsamen Instrumenten. Presentation at the 73, Versammlung dtsch. Naturf. Hamburg Ärzte, 1901.
2. Kelling G. Uber die Besichtigung der Speiseröhre und des Magens mit biegsamen Instrumenten. Verhandl Ges dtsch Naturf Ärzte 1902; 73:117.
3. Jacobaeus HC. Über die Möglichkeit, die Zystoskopie bei Untersuchung seröser Höhlungen anzuwenden. Münch Med Wochenschr 1910; 57:2090.
4. Kalk H. Erfahrungen mit der Laparoskopie (Zugleich mit Beschreibung eines neuen Instrumentes). Z Klin Med 1929; 111:303–48.
5. Hopkins HH. Optical principles of the endoscope. In: Berci G, ed. Endoscopy. Ed 2. New York: Appleton-Century-Crofts, 1976:3–26.
6. Hopkins HH. Physics of the fiberoptic endoscope. In: Berci G, ed. Endoscopy. Ed 2. New York: Appleton-Century-Crofts, 1976; 27–63.
7. Henning N, Keilhack H. Farben-photography der Magenhöhle. Dtsch Med Wochenschr 1938; 54:1328.
8. Ruddock JC. Peritoneoscopy. West J Surg 1934; 42:392–405.
9. Sharp JR, Pierson WP, Brady CE III. Comparison of CO_2 and N_2O induced discomfort during peritoneoscopy under local anesthesia. Gastroenterology 1982; 82:453–6.
10. El-Minawi WF, Wahbi O, El-Bagouri IS, et al. Physiologic changes during CO_2 and N_2 pneumoperitoneum in diagnostic laparoscopy. A comparative study. J Reprod Med 1981; 26:338–46.
11. Scott DB, Julian DG. Observations on cardiac arrhythmias during laparoscopy. Br Med J 1972; 1:411–3.
12. Beck K. Color Atlas of Laparoscopy. Ed 2. Philadelphia: WB Saunders, 1984; 508.
13. Nord HJ, Boyce HW Jr. Manual of Laparoscopic Technique. R. Wolf Med Instr Corp, Chicago, III, Second Printing, 1983.
14. Loffer PD. Disinfection versus sterilization of gynecologic laparoscopy equipment. The experience of the Phoenix Surgicenter. J Reprod Med 1980; 25:263–6.
15. Guidelines for preparation of laparoscopic instrumentation. AORN J 1980; 32:65–6, 70, 74.
16. Guidelines for establishment of gastrointestinal endoscopy areas. Guidelines for clinical application. Am Soc Gastrointest Endosc, 1983.
17. Meyer-Burg J, Henning H. Laparoskope. In: Ottenjahn R, Classen M, eds. Gastroenterologische Endoskopie. Stuttgart: Enke, 1979; 243–307.
18. Ewe K. Bleeding after liver biopsy does not correlate with indices of peripheral coagulation. Dig Dis Sci 1981; 26:388–93.

19. Some answers to questions about gastrointestinal laparoscopy. Patient education pamphlet. Am Soc Gastrointest Endosc, 1982.
20. Henning H, Merkel W, Look D. Laparoskopie bei Hiatus hernia? Z Gastroenterol 1969; 7:83.
21. Berci G, ed. Endoscopy. Ed 2. New York: Appleton-Century-Crofts, 1976; 805.
22. Bruguera M, Borda JM, Rodes J. Atlas of Laparoscopy and Biopsy of the Liver. Philadelphia: WB Saunders, 1979; 215.
23. Dagnini G. Clinical Laparoscopy. Padua: Piccin Med Books, 1980.
24. Boyce HW Jr, Nord HJ. The hepatic "nodule." Gastrointest Endosc 1981; 27:104–5.
25. Lindner H, Henning H, Zienau HL, et al. Die Appendix vermiformis im laparoskopischen Bild. In: Lindner H, ed. Fortschritte der gastroenterologischen Endoskopie. Vol. 8. Baden-Baden: G. Witzstrock, 1977; 9–11.
26. Meyer-Burg J. The inspection, palpation, and biopsy of the pancreas by peritoneoscopy. Endoscopy 1972; 4:99.
27. Strauch M, Lux G, Ottenjahn R. Infragastric pancreoscopy. Endoscopy 1973; 5:30.
28. Look D, Henning H, Lüders CJ. Darstellung und Biopsie des Pancreaskopfes bei der Laparoskopie. Z Gastroenterol 1972; 10:209–14.
29. Ishida H. Peritoneoscopy and pancreas biopsy in the diagnosis of pancreatic diseases. Gastrointest Endosc 1983; 29:211–8.
30. Sanowski RA, Kozarek RA, Partyka EK. Evaluation of a flexible endoscope for laparoscopy. Am J Gastroenterol 1981; 76:416–9.
31. Kalk H, Brühl W, Sieke E. Die gezielte Leberpunktion. Dtsch Med Wochenschr 1943; 69:693.
32. Menghini G. One-second needle biopsy of the liver. Gastroenterology 1958; 35:190–9.
33. Jensen DM, Berci G. Laparoscopy: Advances in biopsy and recording techniques. Gastrointest Endosc 1981; 27:15–5.
34. Lindner H. Percutaneous liver biopsy with the Menghini needle. Experiences with over 1000 cases. Med Welt 1962; 43:2265–78.
35. Robbers H, Hess H. Ein neues Gerät zur gezielten Leberpunktion. Dtsch Med Wochenschr 1951; 76:248.
36. Lightdale CJ, Hajdu SI, Luisi CB. Cytology of the liver, spleen, and peritoneum obtained by sheathed brush during laparoscopy. Am J Gastroenterol 1980; 74:21–4.
37. Wannagat L. Die laparoskopische Splenoportographie. Klin Wochenschr 1955; 33:750–8.
38. Wannagat L. Die Splenoportographie. Leber Magen Darm 1973; 3:3–10.
39. Rösch J. Splenoportographie. In: Schinz HR, ed. Ergebnisse der Medizinischen Strahlenforschung, Vol. I. Stuttgart: Thieme, 1964.
40. Wannagat L. Laparoskopische Cholezystographie und transhepatische Cholangiographie. In: Demling L, ed. Klinische Gastroenterologie. Stuttgart: Thieme, 1973.
41. Rosenbaum FJ. Die laparoskopische Cholangiographie. Klin Wochenschr 1955; 33:39–41.
42. Whitmore RJ, Lehman GA. Laparoscopic removal of intraperitoneal catheter. Gastrointest Endosc 1979; 25:75–6.
43. Lemay JL, Dupas JL, Capron JP, Robine D. Laparoscopic removal of the distal catheter of ventriculoperitoneal shunt (Ames valve). Gastrointest Endosc 1979; 25:162–3.
44. Valle RF. Laparoscopic removal of translocated retroperitoneal IUDs. Gastrointest Endosc 1981; 27:28–30.
45. Berci G, Hasler G, Helmuth JF. Permanent Film Records. In: Berci G, ed. Endoscopy. Ed 2. New York: Appleton-Century-Crofts, 1976; 242–70.

Chapter 51

INDICATIONS, CONTRAINDICATIONS, AND COMPLICATIONS OF LAPAROSCOPY

CHARLES J. LIGHTDALE, M.D.

Through a keyhole opening, laparoscopy exposes the peritoneal cavity and its contents in a clear, bright view that is stunning in its clarity. Laparoscopic photographs can be spectacular. Perhaps most astonishing is the common experience of quietly conversing with the lightly sedated patient while inspecting the viscera.

INDICATIONS

Indications for laparoscopy derive from the intra-abdominal organs that can be brought into view. The liver, seen remarkably well, is the main attraction for the gastroenterologist (Table 51–1). The need to examine large areas of parietal and visceral peritoneum and evaluation to determine the cause of ascites are also major indications. The omentum and the serosal surfaces of the stomach, small bowel, colon, and appendix may be seen, but indications for inspection of these areas are less common. Posterior organs and surfaces are not completely seen, and consequently the indications to perform laparoscopy for evaluation of these areas are few, although portions of the spleen are routinely seen, and parts of the pancreas may sometimes be visualized (see Chapter 52). Examination of the internal female pelvic organs is a major indication for laparoscopy. Therapeutic or operative maneuvers may be performed, usually under general anesthesia. For the most part, this is the province of the gynecologist or surgeon (see Chapter 57). However, systematic exploration of the ab-

TABLE 51–1. **Indications for Laparoscopy**

1. **Liver Disease**
    Focal lesions, benign and malignant
    Diffuse disease, cirrhosis
2. **Staging for Cancer Treatment**
    Liver and peritoneal metastases
        Hodgkin's disease, lymphomas
        Primary hepatocellular carcinoma
        Miscellaneous preoperative
3. **Peritoneal Disease**
    Ascites of unknown etiology
    Metastatic and primary cancer
    Tuberculosis, other infections
    Adhesions
    Endometriosis
    Portal hypertension
    Fever of unknown etiology
    Pain of unknown etiology (acute, chronic)
    Abdominal trauma
    Mass of uncertain nature
    Foreign body removal
4. **Pelvic Disease**
5. **Disease of the Spleen**
6. **Pancreatic Disease**

dominal cavity at laparoscopy, including the pelvis, is advocated as good medical practice.[1-7]

Liver Disease

Laparoscopy provides a superb view of the liver (Plate 51–1). More than two-thirds of

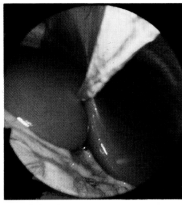 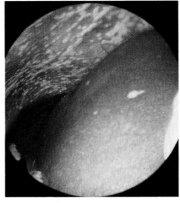 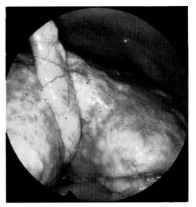

PLATE 51–1.   PLATE 51–2.   PLATE 51–3.

PLATE 51–1. 1. Laparoscopic view of normal right upper quadrant. Liver surface is smooth and mahogany brown. In foreground liver is seen resting on yellow omentum; round ligament is seen and in background is smooth, shiny parietal peritoneum.

PLATE 51–2. 1 to 3 mm tiny liver metastases from primary breast cancer, and multiple flat white metastatic nodules on parietal peritoneum. CT of abdomen showed no abnormalities. Liver and peritoneal forceps biopsies confirmed diagnosis pathologically.

PLATE 51–3. Diffusely infiltrating hepatocellular carcinoma in cirrhotic liver. Whitish tissue is clearly neoplastic with areas of prominent neovascularity. Site for needle biopsy was chosen to avoid large surface vessels, and biopsy was accomplished with minimal bleeding.

PLATE 51–4. Tiny 2-4 mm nodules in liver of patient with Hodgkin's disease. At initial presentation, small scattered lesions such as these are often the only disease present in liver. Blind biopsies are likely to miss such lesions. Accurate biopsies can be obtained at laparoscopy.

PLATE 51–5. Hodgkin's disease on splenic surface. These tiny nodules resemble liver lesions seen at initial staging for treatment (see Plate 51–4). More often than not, Hodgkin's disease is not evident on splenic surface, and diagnostic yield of splenic biopsy is low compared to pathologic analysis after splenectomy.

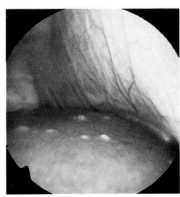 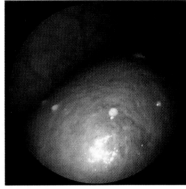

PLATE 51–4.   PLATE 51–5.

PLATE 51–6. Intensely green, cholestatic liver with tense, distended (Courvoisier) gallbladder due to common duct obstruction from pancreatic cancer.

PLATE 51–7. In this patient with cirrhosis, ascites was thought to be due to portal hypertension that is evident from increased vascularity seen on parietal peritoneum. In foreground, however, there is large tumor metastasis on falciform ligament due to metastatic retroperitoneal sarcoma. There were multiple metastases to peritoneum and omentum. A dark pool of ascites is in background.

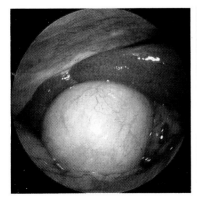 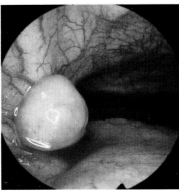

PLATE 51–6.   PLATE 51–7.

the hepatic surface may be seen depending on technique, body habitus of the patient, and pathology. Color, consistency, and contour of the liver are rapidly documented. Structures as small as 1 mm in size may be observed without difficulty.[1, 5, 6]

Malignant Liver Disease

Since the liver may be examined in such fine detail, laparoscopy is particularly useful for the diagnosis of diseases that produce focal defects in the liver. Diagnosis of malignant liver disease as a major indication for laparoscopy is discussed in Chapter 52. Based on autopsy and surgical studies, it has been established that metastatic liver disease will be evident on the liver surface in about 90% of cases.[8, 9] Even small, early, metastatic foci may be detected on the surface, and direct vision biopsy is highly accurate. Intraparenchymal, subsurface liver lesions may cause a bulge in the hepatic contour, and deep needle biopsies in these areas can be diagnostic. The diagnostic accuracy of laparoscopy in malignant liver disease ranges from 70% to 90%.[10–16] The diagnosis is highly specific, since false-positive biopsy specimens are rare. The sensitivity rate was 92% in a report from Memorial Sloan-Kettering Cancer Center in which technetium-99m scans were used to guide deep biopsies if no surface lesions were evident.[16]

After a careful medical history and physical examination, standard biochemical blood tests of liver function are the most commonly used second step in screening for malignant liver disease. In the study from Memorial, these tests had a reasonably high sensitivity of 86%, but a low specificity of 49% because of the large number of false-positive results.[16]

Laparoscopy in Relation to Other Methods of Diagnosis

Liver Imaging

Tests that provide an image of the liver are generally ordered in an effort to increase specificity in the diagnosis of malignant liver disease. Radionuclide liver scans were most commonly ordered, but these are rapidly being replaced by computed tomography (CT) and ultrasonography.[16] These tests, by detecting bile duct dilation, have revolutionized the management of jaundiced patients.[17] These tests are also useful in differentiating focal from diffuse liver disease, and in this context their sensitivity and specificity are superior to radionuclide scans. Ultrasonography is less expensive than CT, but the

results are more operator-dependent, more difficult to interpret, and more often nondiagnostic. Ultrasonography detects focal lesions in the liver as small as 2 cm, whereas the newest rapid-scan CT machines may detect lesions in the 1 to 2 cm range. The vascularity of focal lesions is best assessed by CT with intravenous contrast.[18–20]

In general, CT is the most accurate test in determining the number, location, size, and density of focal lesions in the liver. The value of magnetic resonance imaging (MRI) in focal and diffuse liver disease is not yet determined but initial results are promising.[21] In most cases, histologic confirmation is required because false-positive and false-negative results occur with all imaging modalities[22] although there are notable exceptions. In hemangioma of the liver, ultrasonography and CT with contrast can be diagnostic, and biopsy can be avoided.[17, 19] Polycystic disease is another example. For the most part, however, specific histologic results cannot be predicted on the basis of imaging studies, and a liver biopsy must be obtained.

Percutaneous Liver Biopsy

Percutaneous aspiration biopsy of the liver using the Menghini method, although relatively safe and inexpensive, is inaccurate for the diagnosis of malignant liver disease.[10, 23, 24] Results of studies have shown an overall yield of 40% to 49% for this so-called "blind" biopsy method. A second biopsy with aspiration cytology may increase the yield by as much as 20%; nevertheless this may still be inadequate.[25, 26] In advanced malignant disease with extensive replacement of normal liver, the likelihood of obtaining a positive biopsy result is about 70%. In early disease with a normal scan and slightly abnormal biochemical tests of liver function, the probability of the needle's striking cancerous tissue is low, perhaps 30% or less.

Laparoscopy has been consistently more accurate in diagnosing malignant liver disease than the standard percutaneous method described by Menghini. Jori and Peschle[10] performed a "blind" percutaneous biopsy immediately before laparoscopy in 48 patients. In metastatic disease, the "blind" biopsy specimen was positive in only 31%; that obtained at laparoscopy was positive in 87.5%. In primary liver cancer 70% of cases were documented by the initial biopsy, and 95% at laparoscopy. In the Memorial Hospital study of 60 patients found to have malignant liver disease at laparoscopy, the "blind" biopsy result within 2 weeks prior to laparoscopy was negative in 23 patients.[16]

Scan-Directed Biopsy

It has been known for some time that aiming a needle at an area of the liver that is abnormal on radionuclide scans will increase the diagnostic yield of percutaneous biopsy.[26] The problem with this, particularly with needles inserted subcostally, is the risk of puncturing major vessels, bile ducts, gallbladder, or adjacent viscera. Cysts, possibly echinococcal, cannot be differentiated from other radionuclide scan defects. In recent years, it has been shown that these risks can be decreased using ultrasonography or CT to guide the biopsy needle. Accuracy with modern scanners ranges from 65% to 90%.[27–30]

Since biopsies directed by ultrasonography or CT have a significantly higher yield, they are replacing "blind" biopsy for the diagnosis of malignant liver disease. Ultimately, laparoscopy must be compared to these procedures with regard to accuracy, morbidity, and expense. Such comparisons must be made in well-matched patients. Any series that includes a high percentage of patients with massive metastatic disease will have a high accuracy rate whatever the technique.

Laparoscopy has several advantages over scan-guided aspiration biopsy in the diagnosis of malignant liver disease. Laparoscopy can detect surface lesions only a few millimeters in diameter that are beyond the resolving power of the most modern CT scanners. Biopsy can be directed to small areas with pinpoint precision. Small peritoneal lesions, usually not detectable on any scanning modality, may similarly be documented by laparoscopy (Plate 51–2). Scan-directed aspiration needles usually have small diameters (0.6–0.9 mm) for safety, and cytology specimens or at best small tissue fragments are obtained. These are not always sufficient for morphologic analysis or special staining procedures. Laparoscopic biopsies using larger needles or forceps almost always provide adequate tissue for a specific diagnosis. Biopsy of vascular areas can be avoided at laparoscopy, and post-biopsy bleeding can be controlled under direct vision.[2]

Laparoscopy has some limitations in the diagnosis of malignant liver disease. It is technically impossible to see certain regions of the liver including the extreme superior, right lateral, and posterior areas. Neoplastic disease localized to these areas is likely to be overlooked. Adhesions or retained ascites may conceal an area of the liver containing malignant disease. Finally, small malignant foci located deeply within the liver parenchyma may be overlooked if they do not cause a bulge in the surface contour.[16]

Differentiation from Focal Benign Disease

Accurate diagnosis in malignant liver disease is crucial for proper therapy and prognostic guidance. Differentiation of benign from malignant lesions is also critical. Laparoscopy assessment and directed biopsy are highly effective in diagnosing a variety of infectious, granulomatous, fibrous, and vascular abnormalities that may affect the liver and mimic malignancy.[1, 4, 5] Conditions such as amebiasis, schistosomiasis, sarcoidosis, and tuberculosis are diagnosed at laparoscopy, as are cysts, hematomas, infarcts, and scars. Lesions such as these may be confused clinically with neoplastic disease, particularly in patients with a history of malignancy. Normal anatomic variations in liver contour can produce apparent focal defects on radionuclide scans, as can diffuse liver diseases such as hepatitis, fatty liver, and cirrhosis.[16] Ultrasonography and CT offer clarification in many of these situations, especially by defining dilated bile ducts.[17] However, a negative scan-directed biopsy leaves open the possibility that a focal lesion was overlooked. In many cases nothing less than a tissue diagnosis will suffice. Laparoscopy is ideally suited to this purpose.

There are also instances where laparoscopy without biopsy is useful for visual confirmation of a diagnosis. For example, hemangioma may be accurately diagnosed by CT, MRI, red cell scan, or angiography but, in some cases, hemangiomas mimic neoplastic liver disease. At laparoscopy, hemangiomas usually can be distinguished from metastases, photographic documentation can be performed, and a dangerous biopsy avoided.

Diagnostic tests, particularly imaging modalities, must be ordered selectively to avoid unnecessary expense and morbidity. Laparoscopy is a well-tolerated, accurate, and usually definitive method of diagnosing focal liver disease, benign and malignant. The ability to detect and obtain biopsies of small lesions makes the procedure particularly useful in the diagnosis of early malignant disease and in staging.

Staging of Malignancy

Prospective evaluation of patients for the extent of spread of malignant disease, usually before primary treatment, is termed staging. Advances in both medical and surgical oncology have resulted in situations where treatment will be drastically altered depending on involvement of liver or peritoneum. For example, wide surgical excision with en bloc lymph node dissection is considered to offer the best chance for prolonged survival in many primary cancers. Yet, if malignancy has spread to the liver or peritoneum, radical surgery would be excessive. Patients with cancers from such primary sites as lung, breast, pancreas, and rectum have been spared radical surgery when liver metastases have been documented at laparoscopy.[31–35]

In some of these patients, abnormal levels of liver enzymes in the blood suggest the correct diagnosis, but this is not always the case.[16] Early lesions may be too small to be evident by the usual imaging methods, and even in the case of a positive scan, the accurate diagnosis of liver metastases is often so crucial in planning surgical treatment that histologic documentation is mandatory. Ultrasonography and CT may be used to guide biopsies in staging, but the advantages of laparoscopy, to reiterate, are that very small lesions less than 1.0 cm may be detected and biopsies obtained when standard imaging techniques give false-negative results. In addition, direct control of bleeding from biopsy sites is possible, and the peritoneum may be evaluated.

Elevated biochemical tests of liver function may not be indicative of liver metastases. These are nonspecific and abnormal in many liver diseases. For example, some primary malignancies such as head and neck and esophageal cancers are associated with heavy alcohol consumption. Radionuclide scans may be difficult to interpret or falsely interpreted as positive for metastases in alcoholic liver disease. Ultrasonography and CT may clarify the situation in some cases, but the true diagnosis may often require laparoscopic inspection and pathologic analysis of an adequate biopsy specimen.[36–39]

Resection of localized liver metastases, mostly of colonic origin, has been reported in several recent series to result in 5-year survival in about 20% of cases.[40–42] The carcinoembryonic antigen (CEA) test has been used for follow-up of patients after resection of primary colon cancer, and a positive test has been taken as a guide for "second-look" surgery.[43] Laparoscopy has been employed with elevated CEA levels to document unre-

sectable liver metastases and avoid repeat laparotomy.

Primary Liver Cancer

There has been considerable advancement in the surgical technique for partial resection of the liver during the past 10 years. Improvements have resulted in better control of bleeding, and better postoperative drainage has reduced the incidence of infection. Although there is recent interest in resecting localized metastatic disease, the benefit of excising resectable primary hepatocellular carcinoma is more established.[40, 44]

Resection is much more likely to lead to prolonged survival if there is a single, localized focus of hepatocellular carcinoma.[41] Laparoscopy can be used preoperatively for evaluation of the extent of the disease. Peritoneal and diaphragmatic metastases and malignant ascites are commonly encountered and easily confirmed at laparoscopy. Documentation of such metastatic spread at laparoscopy means that laparotomy for resection would be futile and should not be performed. Multiple areas of disease in both liver lobes also indicate unresectability, and may be documented by laparoscopy and guided biopsy.[45]

Hepatocellular carcinoma developing in cirrhotic patients is often diffuse or multifocal at presentation (Plate 51–3). Severe cirrhosis often precludes major hepatic resection in any case. Differentiation of regenerating nodules from tumor foci may be difficult, but is more certain under direct laparoscopic inspection with guided biopsy than on scans. Small areas of peritoneal metastases and small volumes of malignant ascites are also best detected by laparoscopy.[46]

Whereas most metastatic cancers to the liver are relatively nonvascular, primary hepatocellular carcinoma is often characterized by an extensive vascular network (Plate 51–3). The risk of post-biopsy bleeding from a hepatocellular carcinoma is, therefore, greater. In addition, hepatocellular carcinoma superimposed on chronic liver disease may develop in many patients, and blood clotting may be compromised.[45, 46] At laparoscopy, a biopsy site away from large surface vessels can be selected, and any post-biopsy bleeding can be controlled under direct vision.[2] Directed aspiration biopsy using other imaging techniques does not have these advantages. Multiple needle passes are often made to insure representative sampling of the tumor area, and the material obtained is cytologic in nature and may be difficult to interpret. Atypical hepatocytes from cirrhotic nodules may be difficult to differentiate from well-differentiated cancer cells in a small aspiration specimen.

Lymphoma

In Hodgkin's disease, advances made in medical rather than in surgical therapy make liver involvement a key issue in planning treatment. With involvement of the liver, chemotherapy is almost always indicated rather than radiation therapy alone.[47, 48]

The spread of Hodgkin's disease has been codified in the widely used Ann Arbor staging system.[48, 49] Stage I is involvement of a single lymph node area; Stage II, two or three lymph node areas; Stage III, lymph nodes on both sides of the diaphragm, with splenic involvement being Stage IIIns; Stage IV is extralymphatic involvement, with involvement of the liver being Stage IVh. Laparotomy studies have shown that Hodgkin's disease almost always moves through these stages in a regular progression after arising in one lymph node area, so that hepatic Hodgkin's disease without splenic involvement is a rarity.

At the time of initial presentation, Hodgkin's disease metastases in the liver are usually too small to be detectable on liver scans (Plate 51–4).[1, 50] CT scans of the abdomen have been useful in staging retroperitoneal lymph node involvement, but have added little to staging of liver involvement.[48] False-negative clinical staging of the liver remains high, about 20% on average, and false-positives are in the same range. The high false-positivity is attributed to the effects of extrahepatic Hodgkin's disease. Cholestasis, inflammatory infiltrates, and granulomas can occur in the liver in the absence of hepatic involvement with Hodgkin's disease, leading to abnormal blood tests and equivocal CT scans, results that are often misleading. It is partly for this reason that staging laparotomy was found useful in Hodgkin's disease. Percutaneous "blind" liver biopsy was ineffective when measured against the laparotomy standard, missing more than half the cases of hepatic Hodgkin's disease.[51, 52]

DeVita et al.,[53] at the National Cancer Institute, used percutaneous biopsy and laparoscopy to evaluate the liver in 25 patients with positive abdominal lymphangiograms and splenomegaly, and documented liver disease in 28%. A matched control group undergoing full laparotomy had an equal percentage of hepatic Hodgkin's disease.

Based on these results they advised against percutaneous biopsy prior to laparoscopy to avoid added hospitalization and expense. In early Hodgkin's disease, laparoscopic biopsy has tripled the diagnostic yield of "blind" needle biopsy.[50]

The results of laparoscopy measured against the laparotomy standard have been determined by two groups of investigators by performing laparoscopy before surgery in patients scheduled to undergo staging laparotomy. Cornell University Medical College investigators documented hepatic Hodgkin's disease in 4 of 34 patients at laparoscopy.[54] Chemotherapy was instituted in these 4 patients without laparotomy. The remaining 30 patients underwent staging laparotomy, and 1 was found to have hepatic Hodgkin's disease. Of 121 patients at the National Tumor Institute in Milan, 7 were found to have Hodgkin's disease in the liver at laparoscopy.[55] Of the remaining patients, 2 additional cases of hepatic Hodgkin's disease were confirmed at laparotomy. A positive staging examination is usually more definitive than a negative, but in staging the liver in Hodgkin's disease, laparoscopy approaches the laparotomy standard.

When to use laparoscopy in staging the liver for Hodgkin's disease will vary between oncologists and institutions, depending in part on treatment protocols.[48] For example, in some centers patients with Stage III disease are treated with extended field radiation alone, whereas patients with Stage IV disease receive chemotherapy; the discovery of Stage IVh disease, hepatic metastases, thus becomes crucial.

Laparoscopy is useful in Hodgkin's disease primarily to stage the liver. It is usually not helpful in diagnosing involvement of deep retroperitoneal lymph nodes unless they are grossly enlarged.[53–55] Splenic involvement may be observed, but whereas splenic biopsy is considered safe by some laparoscopists, the diagnostic yield of a splenic needle biopsy is low compared to examination of the total spleen after splenectomy (Plate 51–5).[5, 55]

The absence (A) or presence (B) of systemic symptoms (weight loss, night sweats, fever) may be important in planning treatment.[48] Some oncologists treat Stage IIA with radiation and IIB with chemotherapy. Symptomatic patients are more likely to have hepatic metastases.

There is a tendency to use chemotherapy for earlier stages of Hodgkin's disease than in the past, even when all disease appears to be confined to the lymphatic system. In addition, local radiation is sometimes given. Splenectomy is not performed routinely. However, many oncologists wish to use laparoscopy to stage the liver as accurately as possible, short of major surgery, as a guide to prognosis and the choice of chemotherapy regimen.

Laparoscopy also increases diagnostic accuracy in non-Hodgkin's lymphoma metastatic to the liver, more than doubling the yield of percutaneous biopsy.[56–59] The Ann Arbor staging system for Hodgkin's disease is also applied to the non-Hodgkin's lymphomas, but the latter are often multifocal at diagnosis. Furthermore, non-Hodgkin's lymphomas do not follow a regular progression through stages as does Hodgkin's disease, and histologic study plays a more important role in deciding on treatment. However, it is still frequently useful to document the presence of liver metastases before treatment is started.[60]

In both Hodgkin's disease and non-Hodgkin's lymphoma, laparoscopy has been used as a repeat procedure to evaluate the effect of treatment on previously confirmed liver metastases. Decisions regarding continued treatment can be difficult; effectively treated areas may be residual fibrous scars that create misleading defects for the various imaging techniques. The nature of these areas can be clarified by laparoscopic observation and guided biopsy.[61]

Diffuse Liver Disease

Morphologic confirmation is usually not necessary in acute diffuse liver disease such as acute viral or toxic hepatitis. In difficult diagnostic situations percutaneous needle biopsy is generally sufficient for diagnosis.[62] In the setting of chronic hepatitis, however, there may be an uneven distribution of morphologic abnormalities that can lead to sampling errors when assessment is based on "blind" biopsy technique.[63, 64] Laparoscopy affords the opportunity to obtain biopsies from different areas of the liver, concentrating on those that appear most abnormal.[65]

The laparoscopic appearance of the liver may also add to or clarify the histologic analysis of the biopsy specimen.[3] For example, it is usually not difficult to detect areas of fatty metamorphosis characterized by pale, yellow infiltration. Expert laparoscopists have described surface changes typical of chronic

active hepatitis, marked by arteriolar proliferation and varying fibrous bands[1, 5, 66] (see Chapter 53). Primary biliary cirrhosis has been distinguished by multiple, slightly raised red patches, and fine fibrosis.[67]

Cirrhosis

Laparoscopy has been most useful in chronic liver disease in determining the presence of cirrhosis (see Chapter 54). This applies to cirrhosis that develops from alcoholism or chronic hepatitis. Percutaneous needle biopsy has been used widely to diagnose cirrhosis, but false-negative results are a significant problem. In a review of English and German literature by Nord,[68] the average false-negative rate was 20%. Laparoscopy, with visual and histologic diagnosis combined, decreased false-negativity to 9%. A prospective, randomized trial of "blind" biopsy versus laparoscopy showed a false-negative rate of 20% for biopsy alone, and 6% for laparoscopy and biopsy.[69] Percutaneous biopsy is a simpler, less expensive method; laparoscopy is more accurate.

The importance of establishing the diagnosis of cirrhosis in a particular patient must be considered in choosing percutaneous "blind" biopsy or laparoscopy. There are advantages to laparoscopy in addition to greater accuracy. The differentiation between cirrhosis and hepatic neoplasm is a frequent problem. In patients referred for laparoscopy at Memorial Sloan-Kettering Cancer Center with suspected liver neoplasm, cirrhosis was the most common benign diagnosis.[16] Various imaging techniques and percutaneous biopsies often do not confirm cirrhosis or eliminate the possibility of neoplastic disease. Laparoscopy is very effective in this setting.

Clinical deterioration in a patient with known cirrhosis raises the possibility of hepatocellular carcinoma in addition to worsening of the cirrhotic process. Serum alpha-fetoprotein elevation strongly suggests the former diagnosis, but a high level is not always present, and histologic confirmation is desirable.[44] At laparoscopy, areas of primary hepatocellular carcinoma usually can be differentiated from regenerating nodules, and directed biopsies clarify the pathologic process when there is uncertainty about any area (see Chapters 52 and 53).[45, 46]

Jaundice

Observation of the liver and gallbladder at laparoscopy will usually point to the basic abnormality in patients with jaundice.[5, 70] Gallstones can be detected visually and by palpation of the gallbladder; chronic cholecystitis or gallbladder cancer can usually be diagnosed. In obstructive jaundice, the liver has a mottled green color; there may be a distended "Courvoisier" gallbladder (Plate 51–6). In intrahepatic cholestasis and hepatic duct carcinoma, the gallbladder is collapsed.

The etiology of jaundice is usually confirmed by ultrasonography, CT, endoscopic retrograde cholangiopancreatography (ERCP) or thin needle percutaneous cholangiography. Laparoscopic cholangiography has been performed successfully in several centers but this approach has become unnecessary in most instances.[1, 5] In obstructive jaundice that appears to be caused by malignant disease, laparoscopy may be a means to obtain a tissue diagnosis of liver or peritoneal metastases. Laparotomy can thus be deferred in selected patients, and the obstruction treated by endoscopic or percutaneous drains or biliary endoprostheses.[39] Laparoscopy has a major advantage over percutaneous CT or ultrasonographically directed needle biopsies in obstructive jaundice. At laparoscopy, small biopsy specimens and cytologic brushings can be taken with great accuracy directly from surface tumor nodules, and the risk of puncturing a dilated bile duct is decreased.[71]

Pancreas

The pancreas, situated deeply in the upper retroperitoneum, was considered inaccessible at laparoscopy. However, in 1972 German laparoscopists developed methods to visualize parts of the pancreas by using a supragastric approach.[72] Subsequently, techniques with an infragastric approach were described.[73] A limiting factor was interference by omental fat. More recently, a method was described from Japan in which an omentotomy was used to circumvent this problem.[74] These techniques may represent an improvement in the diagnosis of acute and chronic pancreatitis in some difficult diagnostic cases when clinical tests and imaging methods have not been definitive (see Chapter 52).[75]

Pancreatic cancer may sometimes be diagnosed by directed biopsy at laparoscopy.[72–75] Thin-needle aspiration of the pancreas under CT or ultrasonographic guidance is currently in widespread use.[27] None of these methods is likely to be diagnostic for early pancreatic cancer or have an impact on survival. Laparoscopy, however, is advantageous in the diagnosis of small liver and peritoneal metastases from pancreatic cancer that may not be evident by other imaging methods and may thus make laparotomy unnecessary.[39]

Spleen

The spleen is largely a posterior organ, although the splenic tip is usually seen in normal subjects. Congestive splenomegaly due to portal hypertension, as well as that associated with infiltrative diseases, is usually evident, although the appearance of the splenic surface is often not diagnostic. Gross tumor nodules are sometimes evident on the surface, and direct biopsies as well as cytologic brushing specimens may be obtained at laparoscopy[76] (Plate 51–5). Splenic biopsy has a higher risk of excessive bleeding than liver biopsy, and most laparoscopists do not routinely obtain biopsies of the spleen. Some European laparoscopists, however, believe that a biopsy of the spleen can be safely performed.[5] In a report from the National Tumor Institute in Milan, 121 splenic biopsies were performed at laparoscopy during staging for Hodgkin's disease with no complications.[55] The diagnostic yield was only 35%, however, compared with that for analysis of the entire spleen after splenectomy. Tumor nodules are usually small and scattered beneath the surface.[1, 47] Splenic biopsy is not considered worthwhile on a routine basis in Hodgkin's disease because of the low diagnostic yield.

Peritoneum

The falciform and round ligaments are major points of orientation within the anterior peritoneal space created by the pneumoperitoneum. The phrenicocolic and left lateral triangular ligaments are also usually identified at laparoscopy.[3] Intra-abdominal adhesions can be easily detected. These are usually the result of prior surgery, but may be related to other inflammatory conditions. Adhesions to the gallbladder usually accompany cholecystitis. Multiple, fine ("violin string") adhesions around the liver suggest chlamydial or gonococcal perihepatitis (Fitzhugh-Curtis syndrome).[5] However, adhesions around the liver can be due to any previous inflammatory condition. In some cases, an adhesion points to a neoplastic lesion beneath the liver capsule.[38] Adhesions in the lower quadrants may be suggestive of pelvic inflammatory disease or chronic appendiceal disease.[77]

Increased vascularity in the peritoneum, due to portal hypertension, may be detected at laparoscopy.[5] If the umbilical vein is patent, it may be markedly enlarged, almost pencil-thick, and bulging. The falciform ligament will usually show an increase in the size and number of blood vessels, and areas around adhesions in particular may also be marked by localized prominent vascularity. Portal hypertension is usually due to cirrhosis, and congested lymph vessels and lymphatic cysts may be evident on the liver surface[1] (see Chapter 54).

Ascites of uncertain origin is a major indication for laparoscopy[5] (see Chapter 55). Paracentesis, usually performed initially, is often not diagnostic. Large areas of parietal peritoneum can be inspected at laparoscopy. Tuberculous peritonitis with chronic ascites may be diagnosed by directed forceps biopsy of peritoneal granulomas.[78] The diagnosis of primary mesothelioma can be confirmed, as well as metastatic malignant disease to the peritoneum and omentum (Plate 51–7).[79]

Ovarian carcinoma is the most common source of peritoneal metastases. In one study, 77% of patients were found at laparoscopy to have metastases to the peritoneum and diaphragm 1 month after primary surgery.[80] Laparoscopy has also been used for post-treatment follow-up in ovarian carcinoma.[81–83] Colon, pancreas, breast, and lung cancer are other primary malignancies that metastasize commonly to the peritoneum.[31, 84] Forceps biopsies of peritoneal metastases can be performed safely and easily at laparoscopy.[39]

Miscellaneous Indications

Intra-abdominal lymph nodes are mainly located posteriorly and retroperitoneally. Large nodes containing metastatic disease can often be exposed and biopsies obtained at laparoscopy.[85] However, smaller lymph glands are usually inaccessible, and laparoscopy has not proved useful in staging the abdominal nodes in conditions such as Hodgkin's disease.[53–55]

The nature of most abdominal masses may be determined by CT and ultrasonography. Management often requires a laparotomy although this is not always the case. In some instances, laparoscopy is useful in establishing the nature and location of the mass preoperatively along with a tissue diagnosis.

Fever of unknown origin may also resist all attempts at noninvasive diagnosis, in which case liver biopsy or laparotomy is often recommended. Laparoscopy can successfully resolve this clinical problem; it has been particularly effective in diagnosing lymphoreticular malignancies and granulomatous diseases as the cause of fever.[86, 87]

Laparoscopy has been useful in chronic abdominal pain syndromes when the cause remains obscure despite thorough evaluation.[88, 89] Endometriosis and adhesions have been implicated most often as causes of pain in such cases (see Chapter 57). Laparoscopic lysis of adhesions and electrocoagulation of endometrial implants have been accomplished and have been successful therapeutically in some cases.[90, 91] Laparoscopy has been used by surgical teams in the emergency setting of abdominal trauma to determine the extent of injury and need for surgery[92–95] (see Chapter 56). The procedure has also been helpful in instances of unclear acute abdominal pain and possible appendicitis in patients at high risk for complications associated with general anesthesia and exploratory laparotomy.[96, 97] Laparoscopic appendectomy has been reported.[98] Liver abscesses may be drained with laparoscopic guidance, but this may usually be accomplished under CT or ultrasonographic guidance.[99, 100] Abdominal foreign bodies, such as cut-off catheters or intrauterine devices that have perforated into the abdomen, have been successfully removed at laparoscopy.[101–103]

CONTRAINDICATIONS

Acute or unstable cardiopulmonary conditions are considered absolute contraindications to laparoscopy (Table 51–2). However, there is a continuum of relative risk in more chronic disorders that depends on the patient's degree of cardiovascular and/or pulmonary compensation. A relative contraindication must be balanced against the need for diagnosis and the risks of the alternative methods of diagnosis, the option usually being general anesthesia and laparotomy.[104] For example, elderly patients with chronic cardiopulmonary disorders are often at increased risk for general anesthesia, but with gentle technique, reassurance, and minimal sedation they tolerate laparoscopy under local anesthesia very well.

Peritoneal adhesions as a contraindication to laparoscopy must also be considered in relation to the necessity of establishing a diagnosis. Adhesions can also be considered a spectrum of technical problems and relative risk; depending on their cause, they may contraindicate laparoscopy to a greater or lesser degree. A history of generalized peritonitis is usually an absolute contraindication to laparoscopy because of the likelihood of multiple, dense internal adhesions that could lead to bleeding or bowel perforation on insertion of the trocar, or prevent adequate exploration. Prior abdominal surgery also produces adhesions, but here the risks are relative. The adhesions are likely to be more localized and can be avoided in many cases.[105] In weighing the decision to perform a laparoscopy, the relative risk increases with the number of prior operations and the extent of the surgery. Most adhesions are located directly under the surgical scar.[3] For laparoscopy of the liver, prior surgical procedures in the lower abdomen such as appendectomy, hysterectomy, or sigmoid colectomy usually do not cause adhesions that limit examination. Uncomplicated cholecystectomy usually leaves adhesions that obscure the right lobe of the liver but not the left. Procedures involving more extensive dissection, subtotal gastrectomy or right hemicolectomy for example, can produce massive adhesions in the right upper quadrant. The laparoscopic approach to the patient with adhesions is discussed in Chapter 50.

Infection involving the abdominal wall such that sterile insertion of the laparoscope is impossible is a contraindication to laparoscopy. A more commonly encountered and usually absolute contraindication is intestinal obstruction with dilated bowel loops in which there is a significant risk of injury to the bowel during insertion of the pneumoperitoneum needle or main trocar.

Abdominal hernias may incarcerate during insufflation of the pneumoperitoneum, but this is rare; hernias therefore are only a relative contraindication to laparoscopy.[106] Laparoscopy is technically more difficult in obese patients but usually can be safely accomplished except in the most morbid states. However, patients must be able to lie supine for about 20 minutes, and uncooperative patients should not be examined laparoscopically under local anesthesia.

Coagulation disorders that cannot be corrected usually contraindicate laparoscopy. Mild abnormalities, however, may be acceptable when there is a strong indication to perform the procedure. Increased bleeding does not correlate directly with mild coagulation defects.[107] A thin laparoscope can be used to minimize abdominal wall bleeding; biopsy specimens should be small and supplemented by thin-needle aspiration or brush cytology; post-biopsy bleeding can be controlled with pressure, direct application of hemostatic agents, or electrocautery.[2, 71]

Tense ascites prevents laparoscopy, and large amounts of ascitic fluid may obscure observation. A rapid paracentesis may be performed in patients with an exudative ascites that has a high concentration of protein, as ascitic fluid re-accumulation is likely to be slow. Paracentesis may be performed just before laparoscopic exploration. In tense transudative ascites, however, as in cirrhosis with portal hypertension, it is dangerous to remove large volumes of the ascitic fluid rapidly.[108] Careful diuresis and paracentesis over several days may be needed, with replacement and monitoring of intravascular volume to avoid precipitation of renal insufficiency.[109]

COMPLICATIONS

As an invasive procedure, diagnostic laparoscopy under local anesthesia is remarkably safe. This is especially impressive considering that frequently the only adequate alternative is exploratory laparotomy, which has a much higher morbidity and cost.[110, 111]

Untoward laparoscopy sequelae are most conveniently divided for the purpose of discussion into mild and severe complications and mortality. The description of mild complications (e.g., transient pain or pneumoomentum) varies widely in the literature. Severe complications are documented with greater accuracy and are readily identified by required surgical management or prolonging hospitalization. Complications for each phase of the procedure may also be analyzed separately as being related to induction of the pneumoperitoneum, trocar insertion, and biopsy.

In assessing the overall complication rate of laparoscopy, several factors must be considered. An important variable is the skill and experience of the operator.[112] In some series the results of a single individual or group are reported, in others the combined results of large surveys. Most surveys indicate

TABLE 51–2. **Contraindications to Laparoscopy**

Absolute
1. Unstable cardiopulmonary states
2. Uncorrectable or severe coagulopathy
3. History of generalized peritonitis
4. Bowel obstruction
5. Abdominal wall infection
6. Uncooperative patient (for local anesthesia)

Relative
1. Chronic cardiopulmonary disorders
2. Correctable or minimal coagulopathy
3. Prior abdominal surgery
4. Abdominal hernias
5. Obesity
6. Tense ascites (transudate from portal hypertension)

that errors and complications of laparoscopy are more common in early experience. With regard to gynecologic laparoscopy, Mintz[112] reported a mortality of 0.03% in 53,100 procedures performed by beginners, and a mortality of 0.005% in 40,409 procedures by experienced laparoscopists. It is clear that the complication rate is higher for beginners. This also seems to hold true for those who perform the procedure infrequently.[106, 112, 113]

An overview of laparoscopic complications can be obtained from several large surveys (Table 51–3). As reviewed by Vilardell and Marti-Vicente,[7] in several individual series of more than 2,000 diagnostic laparoscopies there was no mortality. As a rough guide, however, based on large surveys (Table 51–3), it seems that minor complications occurred in about 1 of 100 procedures, severe complications in about 1 of 500, and death in about 1 of every 2000 procedures.

In a classic report from Germany in 1966, Brühl[114] accumulated retrospective results of

63,845 laparoscopies from 67 investigators. The overall complication rate was 2.5%, of which 1.9% were mild and 0.6% were severe, with a mortality of 0.029%. In 1968 Vilardell et al.[108] reported another important but smaller survey of 1455 laparoscopies from the School of Gastroenterology in Barcelona. The overall complication rate was 1.2%, of which 0.6% were severe with a mortality of 0.13%. In a survey of 21,387 laparoscopies performed between 1972 and 1974, Look[115] reported a complication rate of 1.57%, with severe complications in 0.173% and a mortality of 0.014%. In the 1974 American Society for Gastrointestinal Endoscopy Survey, 93 investigators reported results of 4404 laparoscopies.[116] The overall complication rate was 0.7%, with a mortality of 0.02%. Incorporating these data with other results from Europe and Japan, Henning and Look[106] reviewed 94,382 diagnostic laparoscopies performed between 1968 and 1977.[106, 115–119] The overall complication rate was 0.87% and the mortality 0.064%. In another survey of 46,364 laparoscopies from 17 groups, a serious complication occurred in 0.149% with a 0.054% mortality. This included 10,157 procedures performed by the group at Fohrenkamp in the Federal Republic of Germany from 1967 to 1981; there were only 3 serious complications (0.029%) and 1 death (0.009%).[106]

Some of the complications reported in earlier series include errors that would be unlikely at present. For example, in the report of Vilardell et al.[108] of 1455 laparoscopies there were 3 cirrhotic patients in whom hepatic coma developed after rapid withdrawal of ascitic fluid, 1 of whom died. In Brühl's[114] large survey, there were 8 fatal cases of bile peritonitis following liver biopsy in patients with extrahepatic cholestasis.

Compilations of surveys provide approximations of the average complication rate, but the degree of risk can vary in individual cases. The presence or absence of a relative contraindication and the basic condition of the patient are important factors. For example, seriously ill patients, such as those with advanced malignancy or those with severe malnutrition, are at increased risk.

Complications associated with various stages of laparoscopy are listed (Table 51–4). The most common complications are associated with improper placement of the pneumoperitoneum needle. Subcutaneous emphysema and pneumo-omentum occur most

TABLE 51–3. **Laparoscopy Complication Rate**

Reference	No. Cases	Total (%)	Serious (%)	Mortality (%)
Bruhl[114]	63,845	2.5	0.60	0.029
Vilardell et al.[108]	1455	1.2	0.6	0.13
Look[115]	21,387	1.57	0.17	0.014
Henning, Look[106]	46,364		0.149	0.054
Silvis et al.[116]	4404	0.7		0.02
Paologgi, Debray[117]	34,597	0.5		0.09
Wittman et al.[118]	2322	0.3		0.04
Takemoto et al.[119]	31,672	0.87		0.076
Average		1.09	0.38	0.05

TABLE 51–4. **Complications of Laparoscopy Based on 46,364 Cases from 17 Reports Reviewed by Henning and Look**[106]

	Complication	**Incidence (%)**
1. Associated with pneumoperitoneum	Pneumomentum	0.72
	Subcutaneous emphysema	0.26
	Vasovagal hypotension	0.14
	Abdominal wall bleeding	0.09
	Omental bleeding	0.09
	GI tract perforation	0.06
	Mediastinal emphysema	0.03
	Liver, spleen injury	0.02
	Pneumothorax	0.01
	Arrhythmia	0.01
	Myocardial infarction or arrest	Rare
	Air embolus	Rare
	Herniation	Rare
	Aortic or retroperitoneal injury	Rare
	Ovarian cyst perforation	Rare
2. Associated with laparoscope insertion	Abdominal wall bleeding	0.21
	Liver, spleen injury	0.02
	GI tract perforation	0.02
	Omental injury	0.01
	Tear of adhesion	0.01
	Bleeding from intra-abdominal artery	Rare
	Gallbladder perforation	Rare
	Cyst perforation	Rare
3. Associated with liver biopsy	Bleeding	0.20
	Bile peritonitis	0.04
	Perforation of viscus	Rare
4. Post-laparoscopy	Prolonged pain	0.04
	Hernia at insertion site	0.01
	Infection	Rare
	Fever	Rare
	Hepatic coma	Rare

frequently although in general these are not serious. Mediastinal emphysema, pneumothorax, and air embolus are rare. Abdominal wall bleeding and laceration or perforation of major blood vessels, organs, or bowel occur rarely during placement of either the pneumoperitoneum needle or the main trocar.

Biopsy accounts for the highest percentage of serious complications associated with diagnostic laparoscopy. This usually involves bleeding from liver biopsy sites. Other operative maneuvers, with electrocautery, as are carried out during gynecologic or therapeutic laparoscopy, will have an additional low risk of bleeding or burns.[2, 120]

Pain during the procedure may be related to the pneumoperitoneum. Carbon dioxide causes more discomfort than nitrous oxide or air. It may also cause hypercarbia and arrhythmias and is not recommended despite its greater blood solubility.[121, 122] Pain may also be related to traction on the peritoneum during laparoscopic exploration. Pain for

more than 1 or 2 hours after the procedure is unusual and may represent a complication such as hepatic subcapsular hematoma after liver biopsy.[106]

Infection is a rare complication of laparoscopy and performance of the procedure in an endoscopy suite rather than an operating room does not increase this risk.[108] Incisional hernia and malignant implantation at the laparoscopic insertion site have been reported but are rare.[123]

Complications during laparoscopy can be avoided by careful training that emphasizes a systematic approach, attention to detail, and continuous review.[124] The rational understanding of each phase of the procedure and of the maneuvers taken to avoid accidents should be stressed. Close supervision of beginners is essential. With attention to proper laparoscopic technique and appropriate selection of patients according to indications and contraindications, risks are low and benefits high.

References

1. Beck K. Color Atlas of Laparoscopy. Philadelphia: WB Saunders, 1984.
2. Berci G. Laparoscopy in General Surgery. In: Berci G, ed. Endoscopy. Ed 2. New York: Appleton-Century-Crofts, 1976; 302–400.
3. Boyce HW Jr. Laparoscopy. In: Schiff L, Schiff ER, eds. Diseases of the Liver. Ed 5. Philadelphia: JB Lippincott, 1982; 333–48.
4. Bruguera M, Borda JM, Rodes J. Atlas of Laparoscopy and Biopsy of the Liver. Philadelphia: WB Saunders, 1979.
5. Dagnini G. Clinical Laparoscopy. Padua: Piccin Medical Books, 1980.
6. Lightdale CJ. Diagnostic laparoscopy in gastroenterologic practice. In: Jerzy Glass GB, Sherlock P, eds. Progress in Gastroenterology, Vol. 4. New York: Grune & Stratton, 1983; 461–75.
7. Vilardell F, Marti-Vicente A. Peritoneoscopy (laparoscopy). In: Bockus HL, ed. Gastroenterology, Vol. 4. Philadelphia: WB Saunders, 1976; 65–82.
8. Hogg L Jr, Pack GT. Diagnostic accuracy of hepatic metastases at laparotomy. Arch Surg 1956; 72:251–2.
9. Ozarda A, Pickren J. The topographic distribution of liver metastases: Its relation to surgical and isotope diagnosis. J Nucl Med 1962; 3:149–52.
10. Jori GP, Peschle C. Combined peritoneoscopy and liver biopsy in the diagnosis of hepatic neoplasm. Gastroenterology 1972; 63:1016–9.
11. Kuster G, Biel F. Accuracy of laparoscopic diagnosis. Am J Med 1966; 42:388–93.
12. Sauer R, Fahrlander H, Fridrich R. Comparison of the accuracy of liver scans and peritoneoscopy in benign and malignant primary and metastatic tumors of the liver. 222 confirmed cases examined by both methods simultaneously. Scand J Gastroenterol 1973; 8:389–94.
13. Van Waes L, D'Haveloose J, Demeuienaere L. Diagnostic accuracy of laparoscopy in the detection of liver metastases. A prospective study. (Abstr) Gastroenterology 1978; 74:1107–12.
14. Whitcomb FF Jr, Gibb SP, Boyce HW Jr. Peritoneoscopy for the diagnosis of left lobe lesions of the liver. Arch Intern Med 1978; 138:126–7.
15. Riemann JF: Peritoneoscopy in the diagnosis of liver metastases. In: Weiss L, Gilbert HA, eds. Liver Metastasis. Boston: Hall Medical Pub, 1982; 244–54.
16. Lightdale CJ, Winawer SJ, Kurtz RC, Knapper WH. Laparoscopic diagnosis of suspected liver neoplasms. Value of prior liver scans. Dig Dis Sci 1979; 24:588–93.
17. Lightdale CJ. Screening for diffuse and focal liver disease: A gastroenterologist's viewpoint. J Clin Ultrasound 1984; 12:93–4.
18. Snow JH Jr, Goldstein HM, Wallace S. Comparison of scintigraphy, sonography and computed tomography in the evaluation of hepatic neoplasms. AJR 1979; 132:915–8.
19. Berland LL, Lawson TL, Foley WD, et al. Comparison of pre- and postcontrast CT in hepatic imaging in the detection of metastatic disease. AJR 1982; 138:853–8.
20. Smith TJ, Kemeny MM, Sugarbaker PH, et al. A prospective study of hepatic imaging in the detection of metastatic disease. Ann Surg 1982; 195:486–91.
21. Smith FW, Mallard D Jr, Reid A, Hutchinson JM. Nuclear magnetic resonance tomographic imaging in liver disease. Lancet 1981; 1:963–6.
22. Mansi G, Savarino V, Picciotto A, et al. Comparison between laparoscopy, ultrasonography, and computed tomography in widespread and localized liver disease. Gastrointest Endosc 1982; 28:83–5.
23. Menghini G. One-second needle biopsy of the liver. Gastroenterology 1958; 35:190–9.
24. Conn HO, Yesner R. A re-evaluation of needle biopsy in the diagnosis of metastatic cancer of the liver. Ann Intern Med 1963; 59:53–61.
25. Grossman E, Goldstein MJ, Koss LG, et al. Cytological examination as an adjunct to liver biopsy in the diagnosis of hepatic metastases. Gastroenterology 1972; 62:56–60.
26. Conn HO. Percutaneous versus peritoneoscopic liver biopsy. Gastroenterology 1972; 63:1074–5.
27. Ferrucci JT Jr, Wittenberg J, Mueller PR, et al. Diagnosis of abdominal malignancy by radiologic fine-needle aspiration biopsy. AJR 1980; 134:323–30.
28. Schwerk WB, Schmitz-Moormann P. Ultrasonically guided fine-needle biopsies in neoplastic liver disease: cytohistologic diagnoses and echo pattern of lesions. Cancer 1981; 48:1469–77.
29. Zornoza J, Wallace S, Ordonex N, Lukman J. Fine-needle aspiration biopsy of the liver. AJR 1980; 134:331–4.
30. Nosher JL, Plafker J. Fine needle aspiration of the liver with ultrasound guidance. Radiology 1980; 136:177–80.
31. Lightdale CJ, Knapper WH, Winawer SJ. Laparoscopy at a cancer center. Clin Bull 1976; 6:8–14.
32. Maltz C, Lightdale CJ. The Zollinger-Ellison syndrome: A new approach. Clin Bull 1979; 9:165–7.
33. Margolis R, Hansen HH, Muggia FM, Kannouwa S. Diagnosis of liver metastases in bronchogenic carcinoma. A comparative study of liver scans, function tests, and peritoneoscopy with liver biopsy in 111 patients. Cancer 1974; 34:1825–9.
34. Pirogov AI, Wagner RI, Matytsin AN. The potentialities and prospects for surgical methods of diagnosis of cancer of the lung. J Surg Oncol 1980; 13:99–105.
35. DeSouza L, Shinde S. The value of laparoscopic liver examination in the management of breast cancer. J Surg Oncol 1980; 14:97–103.
36. Bruguera M, Bordas JM, Mas P, Rodes J. A comparison of the accuracy of peritoneoscopy and liver biopsy in the diagnosis of cirrhosis. Gut 1974; 15:799–800.
37. Harbin WP, Robert NJ, Ferrucci JT. Diagnosis of cirrhosis based on regional changes in hepatic morphology. Radiology 1980; 135:273–83.
38. Lightdale CJ. Laparoscopic diagnosis of malignant liver disease. NY State J Med 1981; 81:45–7.
39. Lightdale CJ. Clinical applications of laparoscopy in patients with malignant neoplasms. Gastrointest Endosc 1982; 28:99–102.
40. Fortner JG, Maclean BJ, Kim DK, et al. The seventies evolution in liver surgery for cancer. Cancer 1981; 47:2162–6.
41. Foster JH, Berman MM. Solid liver tumors. Major Probl Clin Surg 1977; 22:1–342.
42. Lightdale CJ, Sherlock P. Management of metastatic liver disease. In: Popper H, Schaffner F, eds. Progress in Liver Diseases. Vol. 8. New York, Grune & Stratton, 1982; 649–62.

43. Attiyeh FF, Stearns MW Jr. Second-look laparotomy based on CEA elevations in colorectal cancer. Cancer 1981; 47:2119–25.
44. Maltz C, Lightdale CJ, Winawer SJ. Hepatocellular carcinoma. New directions in etiology. Am. J Gastroenterol 1980; 74:361–5.
45. Vilardell F. The value of laparoscopy in the diagnosis of primary cancer of the liver. Endoscopy 1977; 9:20–2.
46. Lightdale CJ. Laparoscopy and biopsy in malignant liver disease. Cancer 1982; 50:2672–5.
47. Aisenberg AC. The staging and treatment of Hodgkin's disease. N Engl J Med 1978; 299:1228–32.
48. Rosenberg SA. Hodgkin's disease. In: Holland J, Frei E III, eds. Cancer Medicine. Ed 2. Philadelphia: Lea & Febiger, 1982; 1478–1502.
49. Carbone PP, Kaplan HS, Musshoff K, et al. Report of the Committee on Hodgkin's Disease Staging Classification. Cancer Res 1971; 31:1860–1.
50. Bagley CM Jr, Thomas LB, Johnson RE, et al. Diagnosis of liver involvement by lymphoma: results in 96 consecutive peritoneoscopies. Cancer 1973; 31:840–7.
51. Glatstein E, Guernsey JM, Rosenberg SA, Kaplan HS. The value of laparotomy and splenectomy in the staging of Hodgkin's disease. Cancer 1969; 24:709–18.
52. Givler RL, Brunk SF, Hass CA, et al. Problems of interpretation of liver biopsy in Hodgkin's disease. Cancer 1971; 28:1335–42.
53. DeVita VT Jr, Bagley CM Jr, Goodell B, et al. Peritoneoscopy in the staging of Hodgkin's disease. Cancer Res 1971; 31:1746–50.
54. Coleman M, Lightdale CJ, Vinciguerra VP, et al. Peritoneoscopy in Hodgkin's disease. Confirmation of results by laparotomy. JAMA 1976; 236:2634–6.
55. Beretta G, Spinelli P, Rilke F, et al. Sequential laparoscopy and laparotomy combined with bone marrow biopsy in staging Hodgkin's disease. Cancer Treat Rep 1976; 60:1231–7.
56. Huberman MS, Bunn PA Jr, Matthews MJ, et al. Hepatic involvement in the cutaneous T-cell lymphomas: Results of percutaneous biopsy and peritoneoscopy. Cancer 1980; 45:1683–8.
57. Chabner BA, Johnson RE, Young RC, et al. Sequential nonsurgical and surgical staging of non-Hodgkin's lymphoma Ann Intern Med 1976; 85:149–54.
58. Castellani R, Bonadonna G, Spinelli P, et al. Sequential pathologic staging of untreated non-Hodgkin's lymphomas by laparoscopy and laparotomy combined with marrow biopsy. Cancer 1977; 40:2322–8.
59. Bonadonna G, Castellani R, Narduzzi C, et al. Pathological staging in adult previously untreated non-Hodgkin's lymphomas. Recent Results Cancer Res 1978; 65:41–50.
60. DeVita VT Jr, Fisher RI, Johnson RE, Berard CW. Non-Hodgkin's lymphomas. In: Holland JF, Frei E III, eds. Cancer in Medicine. Ed 2. Philadelphia: Lea & Febiger, 1982; 1502–37.
61. Anderson T, Bender RA, Rosenoff SH, et al. Peritoneoscopy: a technique to evaluate therapeutic efficacy in non-Hodgkin's lymphoma patients. Cancer Treat Rep 1977; 61:1017–22.
62. Sherlock S. Chronic hepatitis. Diseases of the Liver and Biliary System. Ed 6. Oxford: Blackwell, 1981; 270–94.
63. Soloway RD, Baggenstoss AH, Schoenfield LJ, et al. Observer error and sampling variability tested in evaluation of hepatitis and cirrhosis by liver biopsy. Am J Dig Dis 1971; 16:1082–6.
64. Abdi W, Millan JC, Mezey E. Sampling variability on percutaneous liver biopsy. Arch Intern Med 1979; 139:667–9.
65. Lindner H. Why laparoscopy? Gastrointest Endosc 1973; 19:176–9.
66. Heit HA, Johnson LF, Rabin L. Liver surface characteristics as observed during laparoscopy correlated with biopsy findings. Gastrointest Endosc 1978; 24:288–90.
67. Minami Y, Seki K, Nishikawa M, et al. Laparoscopic findings of the liver in the diagnosis of primary biliary cirrhosis: "reddish patch," a laparoscopic feature in the asymptomatic stage. Endoscopy 1982; 14:203–8.
68. Nord HJ. Biopsy diagnosis of cirrhosis: Blind percutaneous versus guided direct vision techniques—A review. Gastrointest Endosc 1982; 28:102–4.
69. Pagliari L, Rinaldi F, Craxi A, et al. Percutaneous blind biopsy versus laparoscopy with guided biopsy in diagnosis of cirrhosis. A prospective randomized trial. Dig Dis Sci 1983; 28:39–43.
70. Irving AD, Cuschieri A. Laparoscopic assessment of the jaundiced patient: a review of 53 patients. Br J Surg 1978; 65:678–80.
71. Lightdale CJ, Hajdu SI. Brush cytology of the liver and peritoneum at laparoscopy. Gastrointest Endosc 1978; 24:169–71.
72. Meyer-Burg J, Ziegler U, Palme G. Zur supragastralen Pankreaskopie Ergebnisse aus 125 Laparoskopien. Dtsch Med Wochenschr 1972; 97:1969–71.
73. Cuschieri A, Hall A, Clark J. Value of laparoscopy in the diagnosis and management of pancreatic carcinoma. Gut 1978; 19:672–7.
74. Ishida H. Peritoneoscopy and pancreas biopsy in the diagnosis of pancreatic diseases. Gastrointest Endosc 1983; 29:211–8.
75. Look D, Henning H. Laparoscopic inspection and biopsy of the pancreas. In: Fruhmorgen P, Classen M, eds. Endoscopy and Biopsy in Gastroenterology. Berlin, Heidelberg, New York: Springer-Verlag, 1980; 198.
76. Lightdale CJ, Hajdu SI, Luisi CB. Cytology of the liver, spleen, and peritoneum obtained by sheathed brush during laparoscopy. Am J Gastroenterol 1980; 74:21–4.
77. Steptoe PC. Laparoscopy: diagnostic and therapeutic uses. Proc R Soc Med 1969; 62:439–41.
78. Wolfe JH, Behn AR, Jackson BT. Tuberculous peritonitis and role of diagnostic laparoscopy. Lancet 1979; 1:852–3.
79. McCallum RW, Maceri DR, Jensen D, Berci G. Laparoscopic diagnosis of peritoneal mesothelioma. Report of a case and review of the diagnostic approach. Dig Dis Sci 1979; 24:170–4.
80. Rosenoff SH, Young RC, Anderson T, et al. Peritoneoscopy: A valuable staging tool in ovarian carcinoma. Ann Intern Med 1975; 83:37–41.
81. Smith WG, Day TG Jr, Smith JP. The use of laparoscopy to determine the results of chemotherapy for ovarian cancer. J Reprod Med 1977; 18:257–60.
82. Piver MS, Lele SB, Barlow JJ, Gamarra M. Second-look laparoscopy prior to proposed second-look laparotomy. Obstet Gynecol 1980; 55:571–3.

83. Mangioni C, Bolis G, Incalci MD, et al. Laparoscopy and peritoneal cytology as markers in the follow-up of ovarian epithelial tumors. Recent Results Cancer Res 1978; 68:146–51.

84. van der Spuy S, Levin W, Smith BJ, et al. Peritoneoscopy in the management of breast cancer. S Afr Med J 1978; 54:402–3.

85. Meyer-Burg J, Ziegler U. The intra-abdominal inspection and biopsy of lymph nodes during peritoneoscopy. Endoscopy 1978; 10:41–3.

86. Solis-Herruzo JA, Munoz-Yagiii T, Ruizdelgado C. Laparoscopic findings in polyarteritis nodosa. Endoscopy 1981; 13:9–13.

87. Trujillo NP. Peritoneoscopy and guided biopsy in the diagnosis of intra-abdominal disease. Gastroenterology 1976; 71:1083–5.

88. Kierse M, Vandervellen R. Laparoscopy in chronic pelvic pain. Endoscopy 1973; 5:27–30.

89. Lundberg WI, Wall JE, Mathers JE, Laparoscopy in evaluation of pelvic pain. Obstet Gynecol 1973; 42:872–6.

90. Yuzpe AA. Operative laparoscopy. J Reprod Med 1974; 13:27–32.

91. Cohen MR. Laparoscopy and the management of endometriosis. J Reprod Med 1979; 23:81–4.

92. Sherwood R, Berci G, Austin E, Morgenstern L. Minilaparoscopy for blunt abdominal trauma. Arch Surg 1980; 115:672–3.

93. McSwain NE Jr. Visual examination for blunt abdominal trauma. JACEP 1977; 6:56–7.

94. Cortesi N, Zambarda E, Manenti A, et al. Laparoscopy in routine and emergency surgery: Experience with 1,720 cases. Am J Surg 1979; 137:647–9.

95. Sugal E, Gyr K, Fahrlander H. Peritoneoscopy in abdominal emergencies—a valuable tool. Endoscopy 1982; 14:97–9.

96. Leape LL, Ramenofsky ML. Laparoscopy for questionable appendicitis: Can it reduce the negative appendectomy rate? Ann Surg 1980; 191:410–3.

97. Anderson JL, Bridgewater F. Laparoscopy in the diagnosis of acute lower abdominal pain. Aust NZ J Surg 1981; 51:462–4.

98. de Kok HJ. A new technique for resecting the non-inflamed non-adhesive appendix through a mini-laparotomy with the aid of the laparoscope. Arch Chir Nederl 1977; 29:195–8.

99. Staples DC, Dale JA. Peritoneoscopically guided needle aspiration of amebic liver abscess. Gastrointest Endosc 1980; 26:21–2.

100. Iwamura K. Therapeutic utilization of laparoscopy in liver abscess cases. Tokai J Exp Clin Med 1981; 6:275–84.

101. Osborne JL, Bennett MJ. Removal of intraabdominal intrauterine contraceptive devices. Br J Obstet Gynecol 1978; 85:868–71.

102. Lemay J, Dupas J, Capron J, Robine D. Laparoscopic removal of the distal catheter of ventriculoperitoneal shunt (Amer valve). Gastrointest Endosc 1979; 25:162–3.

103. Whitmore RJ, Lehman GA. Laparoscopic removal of intraperitoneal catheter. Gastrointest Endosc 1979; 25:75–6.

104. Friedman IH, Wolff WI. Laparoscopy: a safer method for liver biopsy in the high risk patient. Am J Gastroenterol 1977; 67:319–23.

105. Marti-Vicente A, Villalona RJ, Rodríquez J, Alcala FM. Peritoneoscopy examination following abdominal operations. Gastrointest Endosc 1979; 25:144–5.

106. Henning H, Look D. Laparoskopie Atlas und Lehrbuch. Stuttgart: Thieme, 1985.

107. Ewe K. Bleeding after liver biopsy does not correlate with indices of peripheral coagulation. Dig Dis Sci 1981; 26:388–93.

108. Vilardell F, Seres I, Marti-Vicente A. Complications of peritoneoscopy: a survey of 1,455 examinations. Gastrointest Endosc 1968; 14:178–80.

109. Reynolds TB, Cowan RE. Peritoneoscopy. In: Wright R, Alberti K, Karran S, Millward-Sadler GH, eds. Liver and Biliary Disease. Philadelphia: WB Saunders, 1979; 543–56.

110. Meeker WR Jr, Richardson JD, West WO, et al. Critical evaluation of laparotomy and splenectomy in Hodgkin's disease. Arch Surg 1972; 105:222–9.

111. Brogadir S, Coleman M, Vinciguerra VP, et al. Morbidity of staging laparotomy in Hodgkin's disease. Clin Res 1975; 23:336A.

112. Mintz M. Risks and prophylaxis in laparoscopy. A survey of 100,000 cases. J Reprod Med 1977; 18:269–72.

113. O'Kieffe DA, Boyce HW Jr. Peritoneoscopy: Has this procedure come of age? Med Ann DC 1972; 41:437–40.

114. Brühl W. Zwischenfalle und Komplikationen bei der Laparoskopie und gezielten Leberpunktion. Ergebuis einer Umfrage. Dtsch Med Wochenshr 1966; 51:2297–9.

115. Look D. Riskien der Laparoskopischen untersuchung. In: Lindner H, ed. Laparoskopie und Leberbiopsie. Baden-Baden: Verlag G Witzstrock, 1975; 41–3.

116. Silvis SE, Nebel O, Rogers G, et al. Endoscopic complications. Results of the 1974 American Society for Gastrointestinal Endoscopy Survey. JAMA 1976; 235:928–30.

117. Paolaggi J, Debray C. Accidents de la laparoscopie. Enquete nationale. Ann Gastroenterol Hepatol 1976; 12:335–9.

118. Wittman I, Bodo M, Lendvai I. Komplikationen bei der gastroenterologischen Endoskopie. Akt Gastrologie 1979; 8:379–87.

119. Takemoto T, Okita K, Fukumoto Y, et al. Complications of laparoscopy in Japan. Gastroenterol Jpn 1980; 15:140–3.

120. Taylor PJ. Gynecologic laparoscopy. Obstet Gynecol Ann 1979; 8:333–67.

121. Sharp JR, Pierson WP, Brady CE III. Comparison of CO_2 and N_2O-induced discomfort during peritoneoscopy under local anesthesia. Gastroenterology 1982; 82:453–6.

122. Minoli G, Gerruzzi V, Spinzi GC, et al. The influence of carbon dioxide and nitrous oxide on pain during laparoscopy: A double-blind, controlled trial. Gastrointest Endosc 1982; 28:173–5.

123. Döbrönte Z, Wittmann T, Karácsony G. Rapid development of malignant metastases in the abdominal wall after laparoscopy. Endoscopy 1978; 10:127–30.

124. Soderstrom RM, Butler JC. A critical evaluation of complications in laparoscopy. J Reprod Med 1973; 10:245–8.

Chapter 52

LAPAROSCOPY OF ABDOMINAL TUMORS

FRANCISCO VILARDELL, M.D., D.Sc.
ARMANDO MARTI-VICENTE, M.D.

Laparoscopy has been a diagnostic procedure in Europe since the turn of the century, although its use in the United States has been more recent.[1-3] There remains a wide difference of opinion concerning the indications for the procedure, which are perhaps now more limited because of the advent of new imaging techniques. In general, laparoscopy should be performed when abdominal malignancy is suspected, other methods of investigation have not resolved the question, and laparotomy should be avoided. In our experience, laparoscopy is unrivaled for the detection of early metastatic involvement of the peritoneum and the diaphragm, as well as in the diagnosis of gallbladder cancer. The procedure is useful for the diagnosis of primary and secondary tumors of the liver. Laparoscopy has a definite place in the staging of lymphomas and in the management of gynecologic tumors. Several detailed reviews assessing the role of laparoscopy have been published.[4-9]

TECHNIQUE

The technique of laparoscopy and the use of laparoscopic equipment are discussed elsewhere (see Chapter 50).

Most authors, including ourselves, use local anesthesia for gastroenterologic laparoscopy. In some instances in which discomfort is expected or with uncooperative patients, short-acting intravenous anesthesia has been employed without an undue increase in morbidity.[10, 11]

Equipment

Of the various instruments offered by manufacturers, we prefer the Wolff telescope with an 11-mm trocar (Richard Wolff GmbH, Knittlingen, West Germany) and the Jacobs-Palmer operating laparoscope. The latter instrument is particularly useful when adhesions make visualization of a needle biopsy site difficult.[12] For biopsy we prefer a long Spinelli needle (Biocut). Instruments designed for close-up photography and inspection are of limited use in tumor diagnosis.[13] Photography with a Polaroid camera is a rapid method for documentation of visual findings.[14] Laparoscopy has been performed with a fiberscope; prototype flexible laparoscopes are available (Olympus), although the overall utility of this type of instrument is not yet established.[15] A double telescope technique improves liver visualization.[16] Ultrasound laparoscopy, a new technique under investigation in a number of centers, may be an important advance since it offers the prospect of demonstrating very small tumors within the liver that are not visualized by the standard method of observation.[17-19]

Cytologic Sampling During Laparoscopy

We make extensive use of a cytologic technique in which the surface of suspicious lesions of the liver, spleen, peritoneum, or ovaries is abraded using brushes similar to those employed with standard fiberscopes.[20] A brush is introduced either through a second abdominal incision that is also used for biopsy or via the operating channel of the Jacobs-Palmer laparoscope (Plate 52–1). After brushing, cells may also be aspirated for cytologic study from a lesion with a fine (0.8-mm) needle. The yields for abrasive and aspiration cytology have been similar, brush cytology being preferred when the liver surface is clearly involved by tumor, and aspiration when lesions are seen below the capsule of the liver.

We performed cytologic studies in 600 patients with suspected intra-abdominal cancer. In 387 cases of pathologically confirmed malignancy, cytologic findings were positive in 325 (84.0%), suspicious for cancer in 25 (6.5%), and negative in 37 (9.5%). Of 143 patients in whom laparoscopy was reported to be negative, cytologic study gave a suspicious result in only one instance. Of 70 additional patients in whom the laparoscopic findings were consistent with malignancy, but in whom biopsy specimens were negative, cytologic study added 17 (25%) positive diagnoses. A false-positive result has not occurred thus far in our experience. Other investigators also report excellent results for cytologic sampling in conjunction with laparoscopy.[21] However, false-positive diagnoses have been reported in instances of liver disease in which "reactive" hepatocytes may be present.[22]

Direct Cholangiography During Laparoscopy

Cholangiography by direct puncture of the liver parenchyma with a Chiba needle under laparoscopic guidance has been advocated when obstructive jaundice is suspected.[23] However, this method has not gained widespread acceptance.

RISKS OF LAPAROSCOPY

The complications of laparoscopy are discussed elsewhere (see Chapter 51). With respect to malignancy, most complications arise when biopsy of necrotic or vascular tumors is attempted.[24–28] Cytologic sampling (see below) is a more suitable and safer method of diagnosis of these types of lesions. Splenic biopsy has been performed with minimal risk, particularly for the staging of lymphoma. In one series comprising 1243 biopsies of the spleen, there was only one severe accident (uncontrollable hemorrhage) that

had to be resolved by splenectomy.[29] Malignant seeding of the needle track following biopsy of some carcinomas has been reported.[30] The rapid development of metastases in the abdominal wall after laparoscopy has also been observed.[31]

Adhesions from previous operations, which are frequently encountered in the laparoscopic assessment of patients suspected of having recurrent malignancy, do not contraindicate laparoscopy. Scars from previous laparotomies usually do not prevent a satisfactory examination.[32–36] Of 3000 laparoscopies in our institution, 836 (28%) were performed on patients with laparotomy scars.[34] In 571 of these cases (68%), the entire liver surface was well visualized, whereas in 235 instances (28%), only one of the two liver lobes could be inspected, either partially or in its entirety. The examination could not be performed in 28 patients. Minor complications occurred in 7 patients. In particular, scars located on the abdominal wall below the umbilicus did not prevent adequate examination of the liver surface.

MALIGNANT LIVER TUMORS

Metastatic Carcinoma of the Liver

Endoscopic Aspects

Metastatic liver disease is perhaps the most common indication for laparoscopy. Although the general diagnosis of metastatic liver involvement is not difficult, no metastatic tumor has features that are pathognomonic of a specific diagnosis, except perhaps cases of metastatic melanoma. Diagnoses of malignancy can also be incorrect, even by experienced laparoscopists. Unfortunately, as in all visual diagnostic procedures, the opinion of the laparoscopist may be influenced by prior knowledge of the clinical circumstances and condition of the patient. Biopsy and/or cytologic studies are thus essential to substantiate the endoscopic impression.

Four general types of metastatic liver involvement may be recognized at laparoscopy: nodular, massive, locally invading, and infiltrative.

Nodular. A nodular pattern is the most common type of liver involvement, about 90% of metastases being of this type (Plates 52–2 and 52–3).[5]

One or several nodules are seen on the surface of the liver. These are usually whitish-gray or yellowish with a surrounding red-

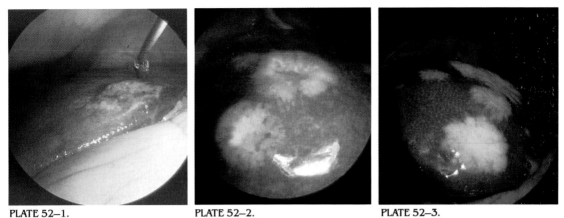

PLATE 52–1.   PLATE 52–2.   PLATE 52–3.

PLATE 52–1. Cytology brush abrading the surface of liver metastasis.

PLATE 52–2. Typical metastatic nodules from carcinoma of the colon in the right lobe of the liver. Rounded contour and central umbilication are readily apparent.

PLATE 52–3. Liver metastases from pancreatic cancer on a deep green liver surface secondary to complete biliary obstruction.

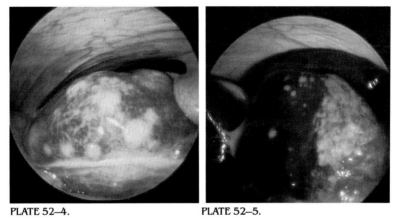

PLATE 52–4.   PLATE 52–5.

PLATE 52–4. Massive type of liver metastases. Left lobe of the liver is occupied by a multicentric tumor mass.

PLATE 52–5. Metastatic melanoma. Inferior surface of left lobe of the liver is invaded by a large tumor mass consisting of black nodules.

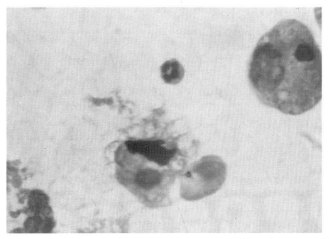

PLATE 52–6. Cytologic specimen from a case of metastatic melanoma. One malignant-looking cell has large melanin deposits in its cytoplasm (Papanicolaou stain, x 400).

dish halo that is caused by increased vascularity. Anomalous vessels are characteristic of most metastatic tumors. The vessels are irregular in size, shape, diameter, and course, with aberrant branching patterns. Metastatic nodules are usually found to be hard when palpated with a probe. As a result of central necrosis, the center of the nodule is often depressed, an appearance that is given various descriptive terms such as "umbilicated," "moon crater," and "volcano." A central depression is much less common in nonepithelial tumors and hepatocellular carcinoma. Nodules may be of various sizes, solitary or confluent.

The gross morphology of a metastatic nodule may be of some assistance in determining the source of the primary tumor. Small miliary nodules are often seen in prostate and breast carcinomas, whereas large confluent nodules are generally secondary to carcinoma of the gastrointestinal tract. Polypoid nodules are frequently seen with metastases from hypernephroma and carcinoid tumors. Metastases from epidermoid malignancies such as bronchial and esophageal neoplasms are usually not umbilicated.[5]

Liver parenchyma not involved by metastatic nodules may be normal in appearance or, when there is massive involvement, it may appear congested, dark red, or violaceous.

Massive. The massive type of metastatic disease to the liver is a rarer form. A white-yellow tissue involves one lobe of the liver and occasionally the entire liver surface, which is stone-hard and has a veined, streaked, marble-like appearance. Abnormal vessels and isolated nodules may also be present (Plate 52–4).

Locally Invading. A whitish-gray or yellow plaque of hard tissue infiltrates the liver adjacent to the gallbladder and the hilum of the liver in a radiating fashion in the locally invading type of metastatic involvement. The limits between the involved and the normal parenchyma are indistinct. The abnormal tissue is hard and surrounded by abnormal, interrupted vessels.

Infiltrating. True infiltrating secondary tumors are very rare.[5] The liver is enlarged but its color and shape are normal. Sometimes only the presence of abnormal vessels or ecchymotic spots on the surface of the liver and/or a hard consistency on palpation suggest a diagnosis of malignancy. Enlargement of the caudate lobe may be noted, especially when the Budd-Chiari syndrome occurs, as a result of hepatic vein compression by a tumor mass.[37]

Differential Diagnosis

Although the diagnostic accuracy of laparoscopy is high in metastatic liver disease, errors in diagnosis may occur. Benign lesions such as liver adenomas, calcified hemangiomas and cysts, and fibrin deposits on the liver surface may be mistaken for metastatic tumors[4, 5, 7] even at laparotomy.[38] Small abscesses and solitary tuberculomas of the liver may mimic a secondary neoplasm.[39] Hydatid cysts of the liver, with their whitish discoloration and increased vascularity, may be confused with carcinoma. In our series, 8 of 34 such cases, and 12 of 26 cases in another series of liver hydatid cysts, were diagnosed as malignancies.[9]

Diagnostic Accuracy

More than two-thirds of the liver surface can be readily inspected by the laparoscopist. Good views are usually obtained of the left lobe of the liver, an area in which blind biopsy is hazardous.[40, 41] However, the extreme superior, right lateral, and posterior areas are not visible.[2–4, 7] Nevertheless, autopsy studies clearly demonstrate that in about 90% of cases metastases on the liver surface will be visible by laparoscopy.[42] In addition, solitary superficial metastases that may be difficult to detect by imaging techniques occur in about 8% of cases.[43]

Laparoscopy may be used to guide the decision for or against cancer surgery. Patients with cancers from such primary sites as the lung, breast, stomach, and colon may be spared radical surgery when early metastatic involvement is discovered. In uncontrolled series the accuracy of the procedure in determining the presence of metastases approached 90%.[44–49] In one of the few prospective studies, 15 of 47 (32%) consecutive patients with resectable abdominal tumors, verified at surgery within 1 to 5 days, were found to harbor liver metastases.[50] Liver metastases were suspected on the basis of clinical findings and biochemical tests in only 4 of the 15 patients who were found to have metastatic liver involvement at laparoscopy. Surgical exploration revealed liver metastases in 3 of the 32 patients with negative findings at laparoscopy. The overall accuracy of laparoscopy in this series was 94%.

Laparoscopy is particularly useful for staging carcinoma, for example, lung or esophageal carcinoma, in patients who also consume excessive amounts of alcohol.[8] In such patients it may be difficult to determine the cause of abnormal liver function tests.

Laparoscopy is of great value in staging cancer in those instances in which surgical treatment does not involve laparotomy, as in cancer of the breast and of the lung. In as many as 8.5% of patients with primary breast tumors considered to be localized, laparoscopy showed liver metastases of less than 1 cm in diameter.[51, 52] Liver metastases were found by laparoscopy in one series in 7% of patients with lung cancer without apparent liver involvement.[4] Others have reported similar results.[53, 54] Mulshine et al[55] studied 157 consecutive patients with small cell lung cancer with a variety of procedures, including computed tomography (CT) and radionuclide liver scan, to detect liver metastases prior to therapy. Metastases were found in 26% of patients. Laparoscopy was the most sensitive method and was found to be especially useful after percutaneous biopsy; this approach increased detection of hepatic metastases in 9 additional cases.

Laparoscopy detected liver metastases in about 5% of patients with cancer of the upper two-thirds of the esophagus and in 25% of those with cancer of the lower third.[4] Shandall and Johnson[56] found that laparoscopy obviated the need for laparotomy in many cases of esophageal carcinoma, although these authors found the procedure to be of less value in gastric carcinoma. However, in a series of 126 patients with nonstenosing gastric carcinoma, preoperative laparoscopy indicated liver metastases in 52 cases; laparotomy was thus avoided in these cases.[57]

The accuracy of laparoscopic biopsy is as high as 90% in most series.[58, 59] A sensitivity of 94% and a specificity of 95% have been reported.[60] The greater the experience of the operator, the better the results, as shown by the comparison of results of consecutive series from the same institution.[59] The likelihood of a positive tissue diagnosis of carcinoma by biopsy does not seem to improve if more than one biopsy is obtained from each liver lobe when the liver surface is apparently normal.[59] However, liver scans may provide information on the probable location of metastases. Even if no surface lesions are seen, the scan can be used to guide insertion of the biopsy needle. A sensitivity of 92% has been achieved with this technique.[61]

In our experience comprising 457 patients with carcinoma, liver biopsies were positive in 387 (84.6%). An increased yield (8.0%)

may be expected if cytologic techniques are used simultaneously.[20]

Melanoma

Metastases from melanoma are readily diagnosed because of bluish-black discoloration. Central necrosis is present in some instances, and then the dark pigment is more obvious at the bottom of the crater.[7] Sometimes many dark, slightly protruding nodules are seen on a congested and irregular liver surface.[4] Metastases occasionally appear as slightly elevated plaques resembling shale[4] (Plates 52–5 and 52–6). The laparoscopic picture of metastatic melanoma may be atypical, such as a mixture of pale and dark nodules. With a truly infiltrating tumor the liver surface acquires a grayish tint without losing its smoothness. In these instances, melanoma may be difficult to differentiate endoscopically from lipofuscin deposits (see Chapter 53).[4] Involved abdominal lymph nodes can sometimes be detected because of their shiny blue-black discoloration, which contrasts with the yellow background of peritoneal fat.[4]

About 6% of melanomas metastasize silently into the liver.[4] Laparoscopic staging of melanoma was performed by Bleiberg et al,[62] and the liver was found to be invaded in 23% of patients in whom only local or regional evidence of melanoma was apparent.

Hepatocellular Carcinoma

Laparoscopy has been highly effective in the biopsy-proved diagnosis of hepatocellular carcinoma.[58, 63, 64] Cytologic study can be an important adjunct to biopsy, since in many highly vascularized tumors biopsy may be contraindicated. The presence of concomitant cirrhosis is readily documented by laparoscopy.

Endoscopic Aspects

Hepatocellular carcinoma can usually be differentiated from surrounding cirrhotic nodules by its color, friability, and irregularity.[65] Several endoscopic types may be encountered.[63]

Solitary Nodule. The solitary nodule of hepatocellular carcinoma appears as a single, irregular nodule or mass, whitish or darker, violaceous, congested, and often multicolored. Most of the time the nodule is stone hard (Plate 52–7).

Multiple Nodules. In the multinodular type

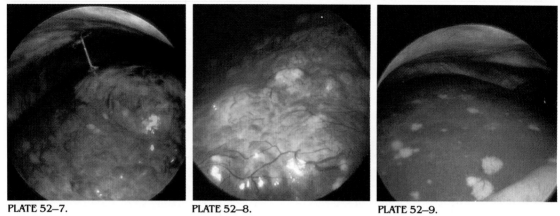

PLATE 52–7.   PLATE 52–8.   PLATE 52–9.

PLATE 52–7. Hepatocellular carcinoma. Large irregular tumor mass featuring large, tortuous, abnormal vessels on a background cirrhotic liver.
PLATE 52–8. Cirrhotic liver with white and yellowish prominent nodules. Biopsy and cytology confirmed the presence of multinodular hepatocellular carcinoma.
PLATE 52–9. Cholangiocarcinoma. Surface of the left liver lobe is invaded by a number of flat, rounded nodules, without central depression. Biopsy confirmation.

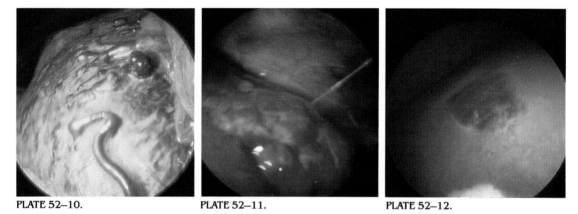

PLATE 52–10.   PLATE 52–11.   PLATE 52–12.

PLATE 52–10. Angiosarcoma. Large tumor mass with fibrin deposits featuring very large tortuous vessels and an angiomatous soft module.
PLATE 52–11. Polylobulated white-pinkish mass, well circumscribed and hard on palpation. The background liver surface is normal. This is a benign adenoma in a patient taking oral contraceptives.
PLATE 52–12. Flat, irregular, bright red plaque typical of a hemangioma on an otherwise normal liver surface.

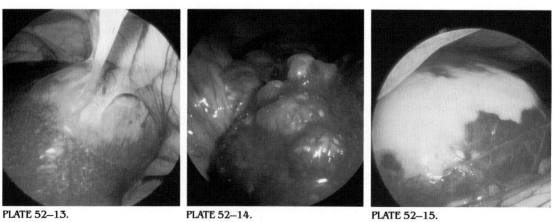

PLATE 52–13.   PLATE 52–14.   PLATE 52–15.

PLATE 52–13. Primary cyst of the liver with whitish-blue surface. Adhesions are seen between the cyst and the falciform ligament. The visible liver parenchyma is normal. Appearance may be confused with that of a hydatid cyst.
PLATE 52–14. Polycystic liver disease. Several bluish and white cysts are seen implanted on a congested liver parenchyma.
PLATE 52–15. Hydatid cyst of the liver occupying the entire left lobe of the liver, featuring a white membrane devoid of vessels. The remaining liver parenchyma appears flattened and congested.

of hepatocellular carcinoma the liver surface is studded with nodules that are irregular in shape, variable in size, sometimes surrounding a larger mass, usually very hard, and encircled by large abnormal vessels. The nodules are white, yellowish-gray, dark red, violaceous, or brown-green when bile is produced by the tumor cells. This polychromatic appearance is distinctive and makes diagnosis relatively easy. In general, nodules of hepatocellular carcinoma do not show the central necrosis that is typical of metastases, although the absence of this feature is not specific.[66] In our experience, both lobes of the liver are more often involved in hepatocellular carcinoma when there is no associated cirrhosis.

Cirrhotic Type. The cirrhotic type is the most common appearance of hepatocellular carcinoma. Laparoscopy demonstrates the presence of cirrhosis and, in a few instances, there is nothing present to suggest primary carcinoma. Most often, however, large, irregular, white-yellow or reddish nodules that have abnormal vascularization (Plate 52–8) and greater firmness to palpation suggest the diagnosis and are the proper sites for biopsy. The finding of whitish areas of hard tissue separating typical-appearing cirrhotic nodules should also alert the endoscopist to the presence of carcinoma. Furthermore, the detection of hemorrhagic ascites can be an indication of hepatocellular carcinoma.[8]

Carcinoma in Association with Hemochromatosis. Primary hepatocellular carcinoma occurs rarely in association with hemochromatosis. It can be diagnosed by the presence of polychromatic or whitish nodules on a typical brown liver.[4]

Biopsy

Some authors recommend that biopsy not be performed when the laparoscopic diagnosis of hepatocellular carcinoma is obvious because of the danger of hemorrhage,[63, 67] although most endoscopists usually attempt to obtain a biopsy. Puncture of the selected biopsy site first with a fine needle has been recommended.[4] If significant bleeding ensues, there should be no further attempt to obtain tissue. We first use the cytologic techniques of brushing and fine needle aspiration and then obtain a biopsy if the initial cytologic sampling suggests that it is safe to do so. Laparoscopic biopsy provides tissue in almost all cases.[68–71]

Diagnostic Accuracy

The Spanish Society of Gastrointestinal Endoscopy surveyed 190 cases of primary liver cancer; laparoscopic biopsies were positive in 154 (81%), the accuracy being greater in patients without cirrhosis.[64] Our experience with primary liver tumors comprises 193 cases. In 179 (92.7%) the diagnosis of malignancy was confirmed by laparoscopy. The areas of liver not involved by tumor were otherwise normal in only 34 cases. Cirrhosis was diagnosed in 118 cases and chronic liver disease in 41 (unpublished data). Erroneous diagnoses in these cases of primary cancer included hydatid cyst of the liver, retroperitoneal tumors, and metastatic malignancy.

Staging

Laparoscopy may play a role in staging hepatocellular carcinoma, particularly when only one lobe of the liver seems to be involved. Laparotomy can be avoided if anterior wall metastases, peritoneal seeding, involvement of both lobes, and other intra-abdominal metastases are discovered.[72, 73]

Cholangiocarcinoma

Cholangiocarcinoma is more uncommon than hepatocellular carcinoma, the relative incidence among primary liver cancers ranging from 5% to 30% at autopsy.[74] These tumors cannot be distinguished endoscopically from metastatic implants of cancers of the larger bile ducts. Malignant nodules are whitish-yellow, often with a central depression similar to that which occurs with the more common metastatic tumors (Plate 52–9). The surface of the liver is often dark green owing to bile stasis as a result of invasion of the bile ducts by tumor. Histologically cholangiocarcinoma greatly resembles tumors of the extrahepatic bile ducts or gallbladder or tumors of pancreatic origin. Spread toward the gallbladder bed may occur, the laparoscopic picture then being indistinguishable from that of gallbladder carcinoma with local involvement of the liver.[74]

We studied 19 cases of proved cholangiocarcinoma from 1964 to 1983. These comprised 9.8% of all primary liver tumors encountered during this period. In no case was the diagnosis confirmed by the endoscopist, but a biopsy compatible with cholangiocarcinoma was obtained in all cases. Absolute confirmation, however, could be obtained only at autopsy. Cytologic examination has an important role in the diagnosis of cholangiocarcinoma since bile stasis may increase the likelihood of bile leakage and peritonitis after biopsy.[9] Cytologic sampling gave a positive result in 7 of our last 9 cases.

Angiosarcoma

Although it is the most common malignant mesenchymal neoplasm of the liver, angiosarcoma (malignant hemangioendothelioma) is a rare tumor. An association with polyvinyl chloride has prompted the follow-up of workers from chemical plants in which this substance is used, and liver damage, including hepatic fibrosis and portal hypertension, has been shown by laparoscopy.[75] Other cases have been associated with Thorotrast injections.

Laparoscopic findings include fibrosis, large nodules, white plaques of fibrin deposition, and increased vascularity.[7] In our experience, we have found only one case of angiosarcoma. The liver was greatly enlarged, the main feature being large multilobulated nodules measuring several centimeters in diameter. Some nodules were dark red, others brownish. Very large, tortuous, abnormal vessels surrounded the nodules. The lesions were relatively soft on palpation (Plate 52–10).

Leiomyosarcoma

Hepatic leiomyosarcoma is an extremely rare tumor. A single large mass or multiple nodules in a greatly enlarged liver may be the presenting features of this lesion. A primary hepatic leiomyosarcoma was diagnosed at laparoscopy in a 69-year-old man with a 2-year history of hepatomegaly and abdominal swelling. Endoscopy revealed multiple nodules on the entire surface of the liver. A specific diagnosis was made by laparoscopic biopsy. The patient did not undergo laparotomy.[76]

BENIGN LIVER TUMORS

With the exception of angiomas, benign liver tumors are uncommon conditions that are usually found incidentally during laparoscopy.

Adenomas

Reports of adenomas of the liver prior to the introduction of oral contraceptives are rare.[77] Adenomas are sharply demarcated and often appear encapsulated, which accounts for their relative hardness on palpation.[5] Their usual appearance is a well-defined, yellowish-white, sometimes multilobulated bulge above the liver surface. Adenomas may be very vascular despite their pale color, and therefore not conspicuous. They are usually solitary, although multiple tumors have been observed[78] (Plate 52–11).

Hemangiomas

Hemangiomas are the most common of all benign tumors of the liver. They were found in 8 of 1000 laparoscopies in one series,[5] 12.5% of them in patients with cirrhosis.

Small angiomas appear as bluish or violaceous nodules or flat rounded areas beneath Glisson's capsule. They are well circumscribed and their surface is usually smooth, although it may be irregular, multinodular, or berry-like (Plate 52–12). Their structure is cavernous.[79] Larger hemangiomas present as rounded masses, which may be pedunculated, but are usually embedded in the liver parenchyma.[5] They have an undulating surface with furrows that are the consequence of fibrous partitions that divide the tumor into compartments. Hemangiomas are soft on palpation, unless thrombosis, calcification, or extensive fibrosis has occurred. Even large hemangiomas are demarcated from the surrounding parenchyma, although their contour may be irregular or scalloped. Large, "old" hemangiomas may have a thick capsule that may modify their color from blue or cyanotic to gray.[7] They may be of uneven consistency, with hard areas due to calcifications or thrombosis alternating with soft spots. The lack of abnormal vessels on their surface differentiates hemangiomas from hepatocellular carcinoma. Rarely, a regenerating nodule in cirrhosis may be very vascular and mimic an angioma.[4]

Peliosis Hepatis

Small reddish-purple areas are occasionally found on the surface of the liver, appearing as multiple round or triangular flat spots measuring as large as 2.0 mm in diameter.[80] This laparoscopic picture is produced most often by peliosis hepatis (see Chapter 53). Biopsy specimens may show the typical blood-filled cavities that are usually not lined by endothelium.[77] Peliosis hepatis is not as rare as previously thought, having been found in 20 of 3035 laparoscopies in one series.[81]

CYSTS OF THE LIVER

Nonparasitic Cysts

Solitary cysts of the liver are as a rule unexpected laparoscopic findings, since nowadays liver cysts are diagnosed by imaging techniques without the help of laparoscopy. Small cysts are dark blue, well-circumscribed, smooth, and rounded spots, a few millimeters in diameter. Larger cysts are sky-blue instead of violaceous or black. They are often dome-shaped, but occasionally may protrude like a ball or be pedunculated.[5] Their walls are thin without vessels. Adhesions are rare. On palpation they are soft and elastic and the liquid contents are often perceived because of the transparency of the wall (Plates 52–13 and 52–14).

Hydatid Cysts

At laparoscopy, hydatid cysts appear as spheres, domes, or rounded plaques arising from the liver parenchyma or the liver edge. Their walls are smooth and whitish, sometimes resembling mother-of-pearl or cartilage. Their margins are usually well delineated. The cysts are surrounded by vessels that follow a linear course with normal branching patterns, and the large, irregular, abnormally branching vessels seen in malignant tumors are absent. Adhesions are present in more than 50% of cases.[5] Sometimes a severe inflammatory reaction with adhesions around the cyst may produce a confusing picture, especially when the calcified walls of the cyst result in a very hard consistency to palpation. In such cases differentiation from tumors may be difficult. Multilocular cysts may also give rise to an unusually knobby configuration, which may be mistaken for spreading malignancy. In fact, primary liver cancer is sometimes confused with hydatid cysts laparoscopically (Plate 52–15).

Laparoscopy is not very accurate in the diagnosis of hydatid cysts. In one series of 41 patients, endoscopy was diagnostic in 66.8% of cases, and in 24.6% of cases cysts were not visible because of adhesions or their intrahepatic location.[82] A positive diagnosis was made by laparoscopy in 26 of 34 of our cases, but there were both false-positive and false-negative interpretations, and the lesion could not always be differentiated from primary hepatocellular carcinoma.[83]

CARCINOMA OF THE GALLBLADDER

Carcinoma of the gallbladder is an infrequent malignancy; most of the time it is a papillary or scirrhous adenocarcinoma, although squamous types are recognized.[84] The tumor may rise from the fundus or the neck of the gallbladder; rapid spread to local lymph nodes and the adjacent liver parenchyma often causes obstructive jaundice. Widespread dissemination often includes the duodenum and causes symptoms resembling duodenal stenosis. About 50% of cases are associated with obstructive jaundice, and in these there is little indication for laparoscopic examination. In the remainder, laparoscopy can be useful, particularly if atypical signs of cholecystitis are present.[85]

Endoscopic Aspects

Unfortunately many tumors are large when discovered and have already invaded the hilum of the liver. Liver metastases may be detected in about 40% of cases[85–87] (Plate 52–16).

Small carcinomas can be recognized if a circumscribed thickening of the gallbladder wall appearing as a plaque surrounded by confluent abnormal vessels is discovered.[7] Larger, more extensive tumors produce a rigid, distended gallbladder, the wall of which is usually thickened, opaque white or bluish, with hard and soft zones on its surface and congested, tortuous vessels. In some instances the gallbladder may be small, hard, and infiltrated by a white tissue that is also invading the neighboring liver.

Differentiation from chronic calculous cholecystitis may be extremely difficult in some cases, since stones inside the gallbladder may be also hard on palpation, much like the localized thickening and firmness of carcinoma.[5] Other signs of malignancy include hydrops of the gallbladder with confluent adhesions on the superior surface of the liver, liver metastases in the neighborhood of the gallbladder bed, and an irregular, firm omental mass enveloping the gallbladder with numerous tortuous vessels. The gallbladder surface may be hidden by adhesions, and only the hardness of a suspicious area may alert the endoscopist to the presence of malignancy.

Carcinoma of the gallbladder fundus usually results in extensive liver metastases by lymphatic spread, whereas carcinoma of the

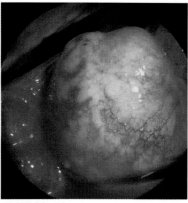

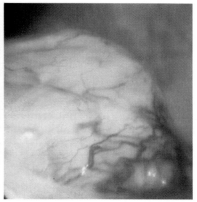

PLATE 52–16.   PLATE 52–17.

PLATE 52–16. Gallbladder carcinoma. On an enlarged gallbladder with an irregularly thickened wall, there is large whitish plaque encircled by large numbers of abnormally tortuous vessels. Cytologic confirmation.
PLATE 52–17. Carcinoma of the pancreas. Large tumor mass protruding in the center of the abdominal cavity emerging below the stomach. The stone-hard tumor is covered by many irregular vessels.

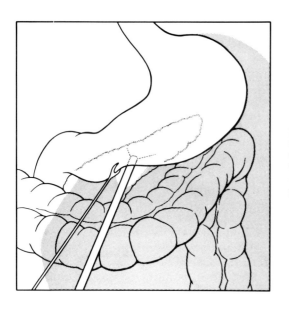

PLATE 52–18. Examination of lesser sac according to Cuschieri et al.[97] The laparoscope has been passed through an aperture created in the greater omentum close to the stomach, which is raised by the tactile probe. (From Cuschieri[97] A. et al. GUT 1978; 19:672–677. By permission.)

PLATE 52–19. Supragastric bursoscopy according to Ishida. The lesser omentum is incised with a forceps, then the laparoscope is advanced into the lesser peritoneal sac through the incision to permit direct inspection of the body and tail of the pancreas. (From Ishida H. Gastrointest Endosc 1983; 29:211–218. By permission.)

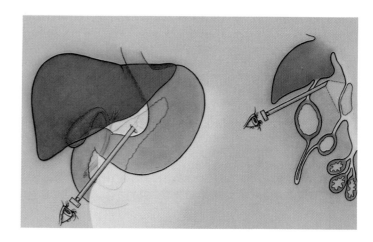

body and neck may sometimes result in local invasion of the gallbladder bed almost without any visible abnormalities of the gallbladder wall.[4] Secondary hydrops due to carcinoma is not rare, the neoplasm in these cases remaining occult except for the enlarged gallbladder. The diagnosis may then be impossible to confirm, unless the hilum region is invaded with a resultant enlarged, green liver.

Diagnostic Accuracy

In one series of 24 cases, a mass with tortuous vessels covered by omentum was found in 8 cases and liver metastases near the gallbladder in 7 cases; in the remaining patients, either a solitary nodular gallbladder or a neoplastic lesion invading the gallbladder bed was identified. In only 3 cases was a single metastatic nodule seen on the liver surface. A tissue diagnosis was obtained in 15 of 23 patients. Metastatic lesions were visible in 39% of cases.[87] Dagnini et al[88] reported laparoscopic findings in 98 patients with carcinoma of the gallbladder. In 30 patients there were hard, white plaques on the gallbladder wall. Local metastases were present in 89 patients. Histologic confirmation was obtained by biopsy in 90% of patients; this required a biopsy from the gallbladder in only 3 patients. In another series of 33 cases, metastases were present in 14; the diagnosis was unmistakable in 10, probable in 9. Evidence of biliary obstruction was detected in 26 cases.[86] In one series, cytologic examination of bile aspirated by puncture of the gallbladder gave a positive diagnosis in 10 of 12 cases.[89] In our experience with laparoscopic cytology, a positive result was obtained in 29 of 37 patients (79%) with gallbladder carcinoma.

The wall thickness of the gallbladder can be measured accurately by experienced observers using ultrasonography.[90] However, inflammatory disease can also produce thickening of the wall,[91] so that further experience will be necessary to determine whether ultrasonography can replace laparoscopy in the diagnosis of gallbladder cancer. The diagnosis of carcinoma was correct in 8 of 12 patients in one series, but other conditions were falsely diagnosed as carcinoma in a number of cases.[92] A diagnosis of carcinoma was made in 88% of 18 proved cases in another series.[93] Comparative studies of laparoscopy and ultrasonography in the diagnosis of gallbladder carcinoma are lacking, but it is probable that in advanced cases with metastases the accuracy of both techniques will be similar.

CARCINOMA OF THE PANCREAS

Laparoscopic inspection of the pancreas is hindered by its retroperitoneal situation. However, in 1972, Meyer-Burg[94] described a method that allowed at least partial visualization of the pancreas. Since that report, a variety of maneuvers have been perfected for this purpose.[95–98] Without these special methods, only very large tumors of the pancreas can be detected at laparoscopy (Plate 52–17).

Technical Aspects

Meyer-Burg employed the supragastric route. This consisted essentially of placing the patient on his or her right side with the head end of the table elevated 30 degrees. With the patient in this position it is possible to slide the laparoscope under the left lobe of the liver. The pancreas can then be inspected through the transparent lesser omentum (provided there is no fat deposition) and appears as a yellowish-pink mass. In a later report, Meyer-Burg et al[99] stated that visualization of the pancreatic body was possible with this method in about 60% of patients. Inspection of the head of the pancreas through the duodenal loop is feasible.[95]

So-called infragastric pancreoscopy has been described as another method for inspection of the pancreas.[96] This technique consists of visualizing the pancreas by means of a laparoscope introduced from the left side, while a grasping forceps inserted via a 5-mm trocar in a second puncture site draws the gastrocolic ligament downward. Through another small trocar a hole is made in the gastrocolic ligament through which the laparoscope is passed into the lesser peritoneal sac. This method permits inspection of a considerable part of the body of the pancreas.

Another infragastric route has been described by Cuschieri et al.[97] The greater curvature of the stomach is lifted with the tip of the palpating probe, and the transparent lesser omentum close to the greater curvature is identified. A "window" is perforated with the tip of the probe and the laparoscope advanced through the hole. Insufflation with carbon dioxide will distend the lesser sac, allowing inspection of the body and part of the tail of the pancreas. Cytologic aspiration with a thin needle may then be performed.

The presence of fat in the omentum, which limits visibility, is the main limiting factor in all laparoscopic techniques for visualization of the pancreas (Plate 52–18).

The supragastric approach to the pancreas described by Ishida[98] is probably the most perfected technique. After inspection of the head of the pancreas, the head end of the procedure table is raised about 30 degrees, and the lesser omentum under the left lobe of the liver is exposed as much as possible. The left hepatic lobe is then lifted with the tip of the laparoscope. If no fat deposits are present, the body of the pancreas can be visualized through the transparent omentum. A forceps is then inserted from the left upper part of the abdomen, and the lesser omentum is cut to allow introduction of the laparoscope into the lesser sac. Biopsies may then be obtained, as well as specimens by needle aspiration for cytologic examination (Plate 52–19).

Results

Meyer-Burg et al[99] reported visualization of the body of the pancreas in 85 of 125 cases. Twenty pancreatic carcinomas were diagnosed. Cytologic aspirates were positive in 13 of 17 cases (76%); biopsies were positive in 6 of 13 cases. Metastases were present in 14 cases. Cuschieri et al[97] reported successful inspection of the pancreas in 6 of 10 instances. Ishida[98] reported experience with 71 tumors of the pancreas: of 38 cases of carcinoma of the pancreatic head, 12 (32%) were diagnosed by laparoscopy. Diagnostic accuracy was greater in cancer of the body and tail, with successful diagnosis in 28 of 33 examinations (85%). A false-positive diagnosis of cancer was made with respect to the head of the pancreas in 1 of 13 cases (7.7%) and with respect to the tail in 4 of 32 cases (12.5%). Liver metastases were present in 11% of patients with carcinoma of the head of the pancreas and in 50% of those with tumors of the body or tail. Peritoneal spread was found in 24% of patients with cancer of the head and in 61% of those with cancer of the body or tail. Overall, a positive result was obtained in 70% by cytologic study of fine needle aspirates of the pancreas. Cytologic results were better with cancer of the body and tail (81.8%) than with tumors in the head

of the gland (57.5%). A biopsy was obtained from the pancreas in 44 of the 71 reported cases. This yielded a positive tissue diagnosis in 50% of cancers arising in the head and in 84.6% of cancers of the body and tail regions. By combining the results of cytodiagnosis and biopsy, a positive diagnosis of carcinoma was obtained in 74.1% of cancers of the head and 87.5% of those of the body or tail of the pancreas. Although there were no fatalities in the study of Ishida,[98] complications occurred in 7 cases (3.3%), including acute pancreatitis, spillage of necrotic tissue into the peritoneal cavity, hemorrhage, and leakage of pancreatic juice.

Laparoscopic visualization with biopsy and/or needle aspiration of the pancreas requires considerable expertise and experience. The fact that carcinoma of the head of the pancreas is usually not visualized, although it is the most common location of the tumor, is an important drawback. Ishida's technique seems to be accurate for the diagnosis of carcinoma of the body and tail; however, since these lesions are so rarely resectable at any stage, the information obtained may have little practical value. In addition, fine needle aspiration for cytodiagnosis may also be performed using other less invasive imaging techniques. In some patients, however, laparoscopy may have some usefulness in avoiding laparotomy if liver or peritoneal metastases are demonstrated.

Warshaw et al[100] performed laparoscopy in 40 patients with proved and potentially treatable pancreatic cancer. Laparoscopy was obtained prior to laparotomy in these patients in whom other studies had failed to reveal metastases. In 14 cases laparoscopy disclosed 1- to 2-mm metastatic nodules involving the liver, parietal peritoneum, and/or omentum. In all 14 patients the therapeutic plan was altered based on these findings. Unsuspected metastases that were not found at laparoscopy were discovered at surgery in an additional 3 patients. These false-negative laparoscopic examinations were attributed to incomplete examination of the liver in 2 cases and to a centrally located hepatic lesion in the remaining case.

LYMPHOMA

Although laparotomy is the procedure of choice for staging of Hodgkin's disease in most centers,[101–103] laparoscopy may be used to avoid surgical intervention, since the morbidity of laparotomy with splenectomy in lymphoma may be significant.[104] In fact, laparoscopy has been used extensively in several institutions for the staging of lymphomas.[105–107]

The Ann Arbor staging system for Hodgkin's disease is widely accepted; the disease is classified in four stages: (1) stage I: disease of a single lymph node or nodal area; (2) stage II: involvement of two or three contiguous lymph node areas; (3) stage III: lymph nodes involved on both sides of the diaphragm (stage IIIns denotes splenic involvement); and (4) stage IV: extralymphatic spread (stage IVh indicates liver metastases). Hodgkin's disease is known to advance through these stages as a regular progression. Although treatment protocols vary, there is general agreement that stage IV is always an indication for chemotherapy rather than radiation therapy alone. Thus a staging laparotomy can be avoided if liver invasion can be proved by laparoscopic biopsy.

Biopsy Techniques

At least one biopsy should be taken from each liver lobe at laparoscopy. Some authors recommend an average of three needle biopsies and, if possible, at least one biopsy of the spleen. Wedge liver biopsies can also be taken from suspicious areas. The group from the National Cancer Institute[106] suggests taking six liver biopsies. The following protocol is recommended by Dagnini[4]:

1. When both liver and spleen appear to be normal, four liver biopsies (two from each lobe) should be taken together with two biopsies away from the hilum of the spleen. Although splenic rupture during laparoscopy has been reported,[108] biopsy of the spleen does not seem to increase the morbidity of laparoscopy unduly.

2. When a focal lesion on the liver surface is suspected, a biopsy should be obtained from the suspicious area in addition to the other biopsies noted above.

3. If gross involvement of the spleen is detected, a biopsy of the lesion should be obtained along with the four liver biopsies noted above.

4. Areas of gross liver involvement should be sampled by either needle or forceps biopsy, and needle biopsies should also be obtained from adjacent normal parenchyma. Biopsy of the spleen is unnecessary in this instance, since by definition the spleen is always involved when metastatic Hodgkin's disease of the liver is present.

Endoscopic Aspects

The early stage of liver involvement by Hodgkin's disease may be manifested by very tiny whitish or yellowish macules spread over an otherwise normal liver surface. The appearance resembles that of fatty deposition.[5] More advanced lesions result in larger, whitish, flat areas of discoloration with irregular, fuzzy margins.[4] Miliary lesions, indistinguishable from those of miliary tuberculosis, may be observed. These are small whitish nodules with well-circumscribed edges that are scattered in large numbers over the liver surface. In other areas of the liver parenchyma, white "smudges" of the type already described are seen. Large masses and confluent nodules resembling metastatic carcinoma but without central depression and necrosis are the rule in advanced cases. Umbilicated nodules are quite rare in lymphoma.[4, 106] Only when there is extensive spread of the malignancy throughout the abdomen can lymph nodes be visualized. Meyer-Burg and Ziegler[109] succeeded in obtaining biopsies of abdominal lymph nodes in these instances, but this procedure is probably of little practical value (Plate 52–20).

The laparoscopic findings in Hodgkin's and non-Hodgkin's lymphomas are very similar, and a differential diagnosis cannot be made endoscopically (Plate 52–21).

Diagnostic Accuracy

An accuracy of 80% to 93% may be expected in the diagnosis of lymphoma by laparoscopic examination when compared with diagnosis by laparotomy.[107, 110, 111] The accuracy of laparoscopy in the diagnosis of stage IV non-Hodgkin's lymphoma is stated to be somewhat greater.[112] Among the advantages of laparoscopy over laparotomy are its lesser morbidity, the avoidance of severe infections (e.g., by varicella-zoster), and the possibility of starting chemotherapy without delay after surgery.[8, 113]

One study included 105 patients in whom blind liver biopsy did not reveal the presence of lymphoma.[114] Laparoscopy with multiple liver biopsies performed in 91 of these patients disclosed liver involvement in 26 cases (29%). In another series of 127 patients with Hodgkin's disease, 15% had liver involve-

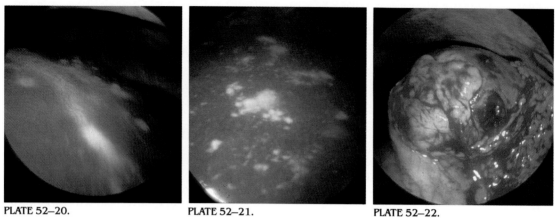

PLATE 52—20.   PLATE 52—21.   PLATE 52—22.

PLATE 52—20. Hodgkin's disease of the liver. Small flat or slightly protruding nodules are seen alongside an enlarged lymphatic vessel.

PLATE 52—21. Non-Hodgkin's lymphoma of the liver. White and yellow soft plaques and nodules of various sizes and shapes are seen on the surface of the liver. Differentiation from Hodgkin's disease is impossible.

PLATE 52—22. A large, hard, yellowish irregular mass with abnormal vascularization is implanted on the inferior aspect of the spleen. Biopsy confirmed a diagnosis of metastatic rhabdomyosarcoma.

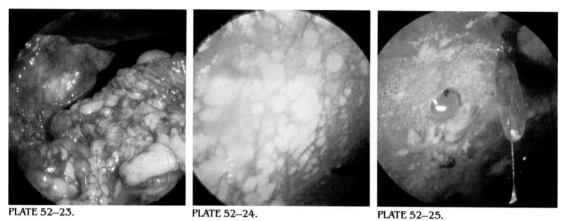

PLATE 52—23.   PLATE 52—24.   PLATE 52—25.

PLATE 52—23. Disseminated peritoneal metastases on the entire omentum, featuring hemorrhagic areas. In the deep background the liver edge is visualized with metastatic implants on it.

PLATE 52—24. The falciform ligament is studded with whitish soft plaques and nodules, soft and friable on palpation. Biopsy confirmed the presence of peritoneal mesothelioma.

PLATE 52—25. Pseudomyxoma peritonei. Mucoid, sticky, gelatinous nodules on a "dirty" looking parietal peritoneum, secondary to an ovarian tumor.

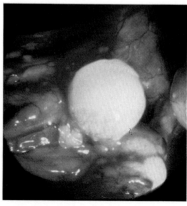

PLATE 52—26. Multiple hydatid cysts in the peritoneal cavity. Cysts of various sizes are disseminated on the parietal peritoneum. A large cyst, devoid of vessels, soft and translucent, is apparent in the center of the picture.

ment diagnosed by laparoscopy; laparotomy showed liver lesions in 18% of 33 patients with a negative laparoscopic examination.[106] Another group found liver involvement in 6% of patients and splenic infiltration in an additional 10% of 80 patients with negative laparoscopic findings.[115] Laparoscopy may also be useful in the diagnosis of T-cell lymphomas; in one series, liver involvement was diagnosed in three patients by blind biopsy, whereas laparoscopy increased the yield to seven.[112]

Our personal experience comprises 236 lymphomas (147 Hodgkin's disease and 89 non-Hodgkin's lymphomas). Laparotomy detected liver lesions in nine cases with negative laparoscopic findings (18% of cases). Laparotomy was avoided as a result of laparoscopy in 64 patients (27.1%). Among the complications encountered, there were three instances of intraperitoneal hemorrhage of little importance and one case of parietal hematoma.

Laparoscopy may be used repeatedly to evaluate the results of treatment in patients with previously documented lymphomatous liver metastases.[116] Effectively treated areas in the liver may leave residual fibrous scars that may cause difficulties in interpretation of various imaging procedures.[8] The nature of these scars can be clarified by laparoscopy.[117] A brownish discoloration of localized areas of disease of the liver surface may be found in some cases after chemotherapy.

PERITONEAL TUMORS

Laparoscopy is probably the most useful single procedure in the diagnosis of peritoneal cancer, especially when early serosal or diaphragmatic involvement is suspected. Laparoscopy is extremely helpful in the differential diagnosis of exudative or chylous ascites (see Chapter 55), since it allows biopsy and/or cytologic study of any suspicious lesion (Plate 52–22). It will provide confirmation of a diagnosis of malignancy when the primary site is unknown. Laparoscopy is of value in the preoperative staging of tumors and can be used in assessing the results of chemotherapy, especially in tumors of gynecologic origin.[118] Peritoneal involvement by tumors is also discussed in Chapter 55.

Endoscopic Aspects

Carcinoma

Malignant involvement of the peritoneum usually has the appearance of white or pinkish nodules or plaques scattered on the visceral and parietal peritoneum. Metastases often appear waxy and may have increased vascularization consisting of abnormal tortuous vessels (Plate 52–23). The peritoneum is usually opaque and granular with disseminated petechiae. When large growths are present, differentiation from tuberculous peritonitis may be difficult, especially if the nodules are soft, friable, or fungating. Although vascular congestion is more often a feature of inflammatory than malignant conditions, malignant nodules are frequently surrounded by a vascular halo, whereas tuberculous nodules may arise on an entirely normal background. Abundant fibrin deposition and adhesions are more often features of tuberculosis.[4] Hemorrhagic ascites is often conspicuous in carcinomatous invasion, but it is not a truly distinctive feature, and errors in interpretation are common unless biopsies are obtained. The presence of pale, semisolid, translucent material is typical of pseudomyxoma peritonei.[119] The great majority of peritoneal metastases are secondary to carcinomas; however, lymphoid tumors may also invade the peritoneum. Intestinal lymphomas invade the serosal surface of the bowel in about 20% of cases,[120] and peritoneal involvement has been reported in about one-third of non-Hodgkin's lymphomas.[121]

Mesothelioma

Mesothelioma is a rare variety of cancer that involves the peritoneum in about 25% of cases (see also Chapter 55).[122] The endoscopic picture may vary from that of numerous whitish, miliary deposits in the parietal peritoneum[123] to large, glistening nodules with associated plaques resembling icing on a cake.[124] The peritoneum usually has no signs of inflammation. In the few reported cases, the diagnosis was made by forceps biopsy that showed the typical appearance of mesothelioma.[123, 124] Multiple biopsies are necessary, since the pathologist may encounter difficulty in differentiating this lesion from metastatic adenocarcinoma.[124] In any patient with clinical symptoms consistent with mesothelioma, a small portion of a biopsy specimen should be placed in glutaraldehyde for electron microscopy, since this method of diagnosis may be decisive.[122]

We have seen three patients with peritoneal mesothelioma, and in none of them was the diagnosis suspected endoscopically. In one case the entire parietal peritoneum was studded with irregularly distributed, whitish, flat nodules and plaques. Palpation elicited bleeding, and most tumor masses were soft and friable. Several biopsies were taken, and the pathologic findings were compatible with papillary mesothelioma. After appropriate chemotherapy, a repeated laparoscopy showed that most nodules and plaques had disappeared (Plate 52–24).

Pseudomyxoma Peritonei

In pseudomyxoma peritonei the abdominal cavity is filled with sponge-like milky or yellowish masses, some of them adhering to the peritoneal surface. The size of the lesions varies from that of a peppercorn to that of a cherry; they usually cover the whole peritoneal surface. Biopsies disclose large mucoid areas surrounded by a fibrous connective tissue framework that includes inflammatory cells. Obviously malignant areas may also be seen.[119] Pseudomyxoma peritonei is of ovarian origin 50% of the time, and the primary tumor can often be detected by laparoscopy.[125] In 25% of instances, the tumor is appendiceal in origin.[125] To the best of our knowledge, the latter diagnosis has not been made by laparoscopy (Plate 52–25).

Diagnostic Accuracy

There is little factual information reported on the accuracy of laparoscopy in the diagnosis of peritoneal tumors. Although in some instances inflammatory conditions may be mistaken for carcinomatous involvement, usually biopsy will make a correct diagnosis. Laparoscopy demonstrated widespread malignancy in 52 cases and peritoneal infiltration in 76 instances in a series of 922 patients with cancer in whom this examination was performed to assess the extent of the disease.[126] In another study, diaphragmatic involvement was demonstrated in 77% of 30 patients with ovarian carcinoma.[118] Laparoscopy has been used extensively in the follow-up of treated patients with gynecologic malignancies.[116, 127] Serosal involvement and peritoneal metastases were present in 22% of 130 patients with gastric cancer and in 12% of 160 patients with intestinal tumors studied by Dagnini.[4]

The accuracy of cytologic examination of peritoneal malignancies in our laboratory is about 85%. With both biopsy and cytology, very few cases of peritoneal involvement by tumors will be overlooked.

Hydatid Cysts of the Peritoneum

If laparoscopy is performed soon after rupture of a hydatid cyst in the abdominal cavity, the only significant finding is congestion of the peritoneal surface and ascites; microscopically, large amounts of eosinophils are present in the peritoneal exudate.[5] When endoscopy is performed months or years later, the typical whitish, gray, or blue spherical masses of various sizes are seen emerging from the peritoneal fat and the intestinal loops. They are elastic and soft to palpation. The lesions are usually well vascularized, but no abnormal vessels are seen. This is a rare finding, but to the experienced laparoscopist it should not be difficult to distinguish this picture from that of peritoneal malignancy (Plate 52–26).

LAPAROSCOPY IN CANCER DIAGNOSIS

Laparoscopy is an excellent technique for the evaluation of focal hepatic abnormalities, the diagnosis of cirrhosis, and the detection of early peritoneal involvement by malignant disease. Despite the availability of excellent instruments and biopsy methods for at least 30 years, the use of laparoscopy in English-speaking countries has increased only in the past decade. This is probably more the result of interest on the part of gynecologists than of gastroenterologists. Unfortunately, there is a lack of properly designed studies that allow an accurate perspective of laparoscopy in comparison with new scanning and imaging techniques.

Laparoscopy and Isotopic Scanning Methods

The isotopic liver scan has been reported to have an accuracy of up to 84% and false-positive rates ranging from 17% to 37% in the detection of liver metastases.[128] The high false-positive diagnostic rate is the main drawback of isotopic scans. However, this is not a problem for laparoscopy. In one study the accuracy of liver scanning and laparoscopy was evaluated in 222 cases, of which 123 were liver tumors.[129] The sensitivity of the liver scan was 79% with a false-positive rate of 18%. The sensitivity of laparoscopy was also 80%, but there were no false-positive diagnoses. In a similar study the sensitivity of laparoscopy was 92% and the specificity 100%.[61] Comparative figures have been reported by others[50]: sensitivity for laparoscopy was 91% and specificity 100%; false-positive liver scans varied between 18% and 50%. Laparoscopy is more accurate than scintigraphy in the diagnosis of primary liver cancer.[130]

The combination of laparoscopy and liver scanning provides an accurate diagnosis of hepatic malignancy.[131] Previous knowledge of the site of metastases based on liver scanning may enhance the yield of laparoscopic biopsy when tumor implants are not evident on the liver surface.[61]

Laparoscopy and Ultrasonography

There are very few reports comparing the efficacy of ultrasonography (US) with laparoscopy in the detection of liver tumors. In one study, hepatic metastases were correctly diagnosed by US in 92% of patients later checked by laparoscopy. US was considered normal in only 2% of patients later proved to have metastases by laparoscopy.[132] US does not have the high rate of false-positive diagnosis associated with isotopic scanning, although the sensitivities are similar.[133, 134]

Laparoscopy and Computed Tomography

The diagnostic accuracy of computed tomography (CT) and US was compared with that of laparoscopy in one study.[135] US disclosed lesions in the liver of 39 of 47 patients with neoplasms (83%), but the findings were pathognomonic in only 63.8% of cases. CT revealed hepatic abnormalities in 21 of 24 cases (87.5%) and highly suspicious or definite changes in 17 (70.8%). In all these patients, metastatic disease was found by laparoscopy. Both US and CT did not diagnose diffuse liver disease or early cirrhotic changes in many cases. Radionuclide scans provide similar findings.[136-138] In one of the few prospective studies available comparing CT and laparoscopy, both techniques gave the same information in 20 of 30 patients; CT provided significant data undetected by laparoscopy in 8 patients, and laparoscopy discovered small peritoneal implants missed by CT in 2 cases.[139] In another study of 73 patients with malignant disease, liver metastases were diagnosed by CT in 16 cases and by laparoscopy in 14, but peritoneal involvement was diagnosed again by laparoscopy in 3 patients with normal CT scans.[140] Response to che-

motherapy was documented in 4 cases only by laparoscopy.

Conclusions

Laparoscopy should be compared with modern scan techniques in terms of accuracy, morbidity, and cost-effectiveness in a large series of well-matched patients, a difficult undertaking. Any series that includes a high percentage of patients with widely disseminated malignant disease will show high accuracy rates, whatever the technique.[141] Laparoscopy can detect minute lesions of the liver surface as well as small peritoneal lesions that are beyond the resolving power of scanning methods. Benign tumors of the liver are more easily identified by laparoscopy than by scanning methods. There is evidence that metastases to the left lobe of the liver are better recognized by laparoscopy than by CT or US.[140] However, both US and CT are superior to laparoscopy for detecting malignant biliary obstruction, a common occurrence in abdominal cancer. Thin needle biopsy, as employed with scanning procedures, may not always be diagnostic because of the small size of the tissue fragments retrieved, the insufficiency of cytology samples, or the incidence of false-positive interpretations.[142] Laparoscopy will usually allow a standard type of biopsy while avoiding highly vascularized areas and also will usually allow the complementary brushing technique for collection of cytologic specimens. Moreover, bleeding after laparoscopic biopsy can often be controlled. Laparoscopy will avoid unnecessary laparotomies when properly performed after imaging techniques have failed to provide a definite diagnosis of liver metastases. Laparoscopy should probably be the procedure of choice when early peritoneal involvement is suspected.

References

1. Ruddock JC. Peritoneoscopy: a critical review. Surg Clin North Am 1957; 37:1249–60.
2. Reynolds TB, Cowan RE. Peritoneoscopy. In: Wright R, Alberti KG, Karran S, Millward-Sadler GH, eds. Liver and Biliary Disease. Philadelphia: WB Saunders Co, 1979; 543–56.
3. Boyce HW Jr. Laparoscopy. In: Schiff L, Schiff ER, eds. Diseases of the Liver. Ed. 5. Philadelphia: JB Lippincott, 1982; 333–48.
4. Dagnini G. Clinical Laparoscopy. Padua: Piccin Medical Books, 1980.
5. Solis Herruzo JA. Diagnostico Diferencial Laparoscopico. Madrid: Ed. Paz Montalvo, 1975.

6. Bruguera M, Bordas JM, Rodes J. Atlas of Laparoscopy and Biopsy of the Liver. Philadelphia: WB Saunders Co, 1979; 215.

7. Beck WK. Color Atlas of Laparoscopy. Ed. 2. Philadelphia: WB Saunders Co, 1984.

8. Lightdale C. Diagnostic laparoscopy in gastroenterologic practice. In: Glass GBJ, Sherlock P, eds. Progress in Gastroenterology, Vol. IV. New York: Grune and Stratton, 1983; 461–76.

9. Vilardell F, Marti-Vicente A. Peritoneoscopy (laparoscopy). In: Bockus HL, ed. Gastroenterology, Vol. IV. Ed. 3. Philadelphia: WB Saunders Co, 1976; 65–82.

10. Michel H, Raynaud A. Advantages of laparoscopy under general anesthesia. Acta Endoscop 1981; 11:97–9.

11. Bleiberg H, Rozencweig M, Mathieu M, et al. The use of peritoneoscopy in the detection of liver metastases. Cancer 1978; 41:863–7.

12. Jacobs E. A new operating photographic peritoneoscope. Gastrointest Endosc 1971; 18:33–4.

13. Leuschner U, Reetberg H, Leinweber W, Nildgrube HY. Uber den Wert der Lupenoptik nach Lent fur die Laparoskopie. Z Gastroenterol 1977; 15:715–21.

14. Schroder G. Praxisgerechte laparoskopische Fotodokumentation mit der Polaroid Kamera. Leber Magen Darm 1978; 8:118–9.

15. Sanowski RA, Kozarek RA. Laparoscopy using a flexible endoscope. Acta Endoscop 1982; 12:61–4.

16. Sugarbaker PH. Optimizing peritoneoscopic visualization of the liver utilizing a double telescope technique. Surg Gynecol Obstet 1981; 152:655–7.

17. Ohta Y, Fujiwara K, Sato Y, et al. New ultrasonic laparoscope for diagnosis of intra-abdominal diseases. Gastrointest Endosc 1983; 29:289–93.

18. Frank K, Bliesze H, Bonhof JA, et al. Laparoscopic sonography: a new approach to intraabdominal disease. JCU 1985; 13:60–5.

19. Fukuda M, Mima S, Tanabe T, et al. Endoscopic sonography of the liver—diagnostic application of the echolaparoscope to localize intrahepatic lesions. Scand J Gastroenterol [Suppl] 1984; 102:24–38.

20. Marti-Vicente A, Cabre-Fiol V, Enriquez J, et al. Laparoscopic cytology in the diagnosis of abdominal tumors. Scand J Gastroenterol 17 (Suppl 78) 1982; 183.

21. Lightdale CJ, Hajdu SI, Luisi CB. Cytology of the liver, spleen and peritoneum obtained by sheathed brush during laparoscopy. Am J Gastroenterol 1980; 74:21–4.

22. Carney CN. Cytology and liver biopsy. Gastroenterology 1980; 78:190.

23. Cortesi N, Canossi GC, Zambarda E. Laparoscopic cholangiography in the diagnosis of cholestasis: experience with 103 cases. Gastrointest Radiol 1978; 3:185–90.

24. Takemoto T, Okita K, Fukumoto Y. Complications of laparoscopy in Japan. Gastroenterol Jpn 1980; 15:140–3.

25. Henning H. Laparoscopy. In: Beker S, ed. Diagnostic Procedures in the Evaluation of Hepatic Diseases. New York: Alan R. Liss Inc. 1983; 469–88.

26. Manenti A, Manenti F, Villa E, et al. Complications in laparoscopy: a survey of 6563 cases. Acta Endoscop 1980; 10:373–9.

27. Vilardell F, Seres I, Marti-Vicente A. Complications of peritoneoscopy. A survey of 1455 examinations. Gastrointest Endosc 1968; 14:178–80.

28. Manenti A, Ferrari A, Gibertini G Jr, et al. Laparoscopic liver biopsy—a survey of 3000 cases. Acta Endoscop 1983; 13:21–4.

29. Dagnini G, Caldironi MW, Marin G, et al. Laparoscopic splenic biopsy. Endoscopy 1984; 16:55–8.

30. Sakurai M, Okamura J, Seki K, Kuroda C. Needle tract implantation of hepatocellular carcinoma after percutaneous liver biopsy. Am J Surg Pathol 1983; 7:191–5.

31. Dobronte Z, Wittman NT, Karacsony G. Rapid development of malignant metastases in abdominal wall after laparoscopy. Endoscopy 1978; 10:127–30.

32. Smith VM, Cuevas AP. Peritoneoscopy and abdominal adhesions: intentional perforation to improve visibility. Gastrointest Endosc 1969; 15:142–4.

33. Pleissner I, Berndt H, Gutz HJ. Laparoscopy following abdominal operations. Endoscopy 1978; 10:187–91.

34. Marti-Vicente A, Villalona Rodriguez J, Martinez Alcala F. Peritoneoscopy examination following abdominal operations. Gastrointest Endosc 1979; 25:144–5.

35. Terruzzi V, Introzzi GL, Minoli G, et al. Abdominal adhesion and laparoscopy in liver diseases. Acta Endoscop 1981; 6:397–403.

36. Serour GI, Kandil O, Askalani H, et al. Laparoscopy on patients with previous lower abdominal surgery: a new technique. Int J Gynaecol Obstet 1982; 20:357–62.

37. Craxi A, Gatto G, Maringhini A, et al. Laparoscopy in Budd-Chiari syndrome. Ital J Gastroenterol 1982; 14:21–3.

38. Fletcher MS, Everett WG, Hunter JO, et al. Benign liver nodules presenting as apparent hepatic metastases: a report of 5 cases. Br J Surg 1980; 67:403–5.

39. Bhargava DK, Verma K, Malaviya AN. Solitary tuberculoma of liver: laparoscopic, histologic, and cytologic diagnosis. Gastrointest Endosc 1983; 29:329–30.

40. Whitcomb FF Jr, Gibbs SP, Boyce HW Jr. Peritoneoscopy for the diagnosis of left lobe lesions of the liver. Arch Intern Med 1978; 138:126–7.

41. Lehmann EE. Laparoscopy. In: Zakim D, Boyer TD, eds. Hepatology. A Textbook of Liver Disease. Philadelphia: WB Saunders Co, 1982; 126–7.

42. Foster JH, Berman MM. Solid Liver Tumors. Philadelphia: WB Saunders Co, 1977.

43. Schulz W, Hort W. The distribution of metastases in the liver. Virchows Archiv A 1981; 394:89–96.

44. Rosenoff SH, Young RC, Anderson T, et al. Peritoneoscopy: a valuable staging tool in ovarian carcinoma. Ann Intern Med 1975; 83:37–41.

45. Gaisford WD. Peritoneoscopy: a valuable technic for surgeons. Am J Surg 1975; 130:671–7.

46. Robinson HB, Smith GW. Applications for laparoscopy in general surgery. Surg Gynecol Obstet 1976; 143:829–34.

47. Friedmann IH, Grossman MB, Wolff WI. The value of laparoscopy in general surgical problems. Surg Gynecol Obstet 1977; 144:906–8.

48. Saleh JW. Peritoneoscopy: an alternative approach to unresolved intra-abdominal disease. Am J Gastroenterol 1978; 69:641–5.

49. Lewis A, Archer TJ. Laparoscopy in general surgery. Br J Surg 1981; 68:778–80.

50. Van Waes L, D'Haveloose J, Demeulenaere L. Diagnostic accuracy of laparoscopy in the detection of liver metastases. A prospective study. (Abstr) Gastroenterology 1978; 74:1107.

51. De Souza LJ, Shinde SR. The value of laparoscopic

liver examination in the management of breast cancer. J Surg Oncol 1980; 14:97–103.

52. Van der Spuy S, Levin W, Smit BJ, et al. Peritoneoscopy in the management of breast cancer. S Afr Med J 1978; 54:402–3.

53. Margolis R, Hansen H, Muggia F, et al. Diagnosis of liver metastases in bronchogenic carcinoma. A comparative study of liver scans, function tests, and peritoneoscopy with liver biopsy in 111 patients. Cancer 1974; 34:1825.

54. Pirogov AI, Wagner RI, Matytsin AN. The potentialities and prospects for surgical methods of diagnosis of cancer of the lung. J Surg Oncol 1980; 13:99–105.

55. Mulshine JL, Makuch RW, Johnston-Early A, et al. Diagnosis and significance of liver metastases in small cell carcinoma of the lung. J Clin Oncol 1984; 2:733–41.

56. Shandall A, Johnson C. Laparoscopy or scanning in oesophageal and gastric carcinoma? Br J Surg 1985; 72:449–51.

57. Geisenhainer G. Die Bedeutung der explorativen Laparoskopie fur die praoperative Diagnostik des Magenkarzinoms. Z Aerztl Fortbild (Jena) 1979; 73:558–62.

58. Jori GP, Peschle C. Combined peritoneoscopy and liver biopsy in the diagnosis of hepatic neoplasm. Gastroenterology 1972; 63:1016–9.

59. Bleiberg H, Rozencweig M, Longeval E, et al. Peritoneoscopy as a diagnostic supplement to liver function tests and liver scan in patients with carcinoma. Surg Gynecol Obstet 1977; 145:821–5.

60. Angehrn FG, Schmid P, Pescia R, et al. Lebermetastasen: diagnosticher Wert von Bluttests, Szintigraphie und Laparoskopie. Dtsch Med Wochenschr 1976; 101:1047–55.

61. Lightdale CJ, Winawer SJ, Kurtz RC, Knapper WH. Laparoscopic diagnosis of suspected liver neoplasms. Value of prior liver scans. Dig Dis Sci 1979; 24:588–93.

62. Bleiberg H, La Meir E, Lejeune F. Laparoscopy in the diagnosis of liver metastases in 80 cases of malignant melanoma. Endoscopy 1980; 12: 215–8.

63. Debray C, Paolaggi JA, Mugnier B, Barret C. La laparoscopie dans les cancers primitifs du foie (a propos de 50 operations). Nouv Presse Med 1973; 2:2659–62.

64. Vilardell F. The value of laparoscopy in the diagnosis of primary cancer of the liver. Endoscopy 1977; 9:20–2.

65. Reynolds TB. Diagnostic methods for hepatocellular carcinoma. In: Okuda K, Peters RL, eds. Hepatocellular Carcinoma. New York: John Wiley, 1976; 437–48.

66. Jacobs E. La laparoscopie dans le diagnostic du cancer primitif du foie. Arch Fr Mal App Dig 1972; 61:407–15.

67. Leuschner M, Leuschner U, Hubner K, et al. Blind liver biopsy or guided biopsy? A prospective study. Acta Endosc 1982; 12:23–5.

68. Frey P, Schmid M, Knoblauch M. Die Klinik des Leberkarzinoms. Dtsch Med Wochenschr 1975; 100:1625–9.

69. Trujillo NP. Peritoneoscopy and guided biopsy in the diagnosis of intra-abdominal disease. Gastroenterology 1976; 71:1083.

70. Alvarez SZ, Carpio R. Endoscopic diagnosis of primary cancer of the liver. Ann Acad Med Singapore 1980; 9:219–21.

71. Alpert E. Primary tumors of the liver: etiologic and diagnostic features. Viewpoints Dig Dis 1982; 14:9–12.

72. Balasegaram M. Current concepts in the management of primary liver-cell carcinoma. Clin Oncol 1975; 1:111–20.

73. Conn HO. Nuclide scanning, ultrasonography and liver biopsy in the diagnosis of hepatic tumors: a comparative evaluation of the available techniques. Clin Gastroenterol 1976; 5:665–80.

74. Mori W, Nagasako K. Cholangiocarcinoma and related lesions. In: Okuda K, Peters RL, eds. Hepatocellular Carcinoma. New York: John Wiley, 1976; 227–46.

75. Marsteller HJ. Klinische und laparoskopische Aspekte der Leberschaden bei Chemiearbeitern in der Vinylchlorid Polymerisation. Leber Magen Darm 1975; 5:196–202.

76. O'Leary MR, Hill RB, Levine RA. Peritoneoscopic diagnosis of primary leiomyosarcoma of liver. Hum Pathol 1982; 13:76–8.

77. Edmonson HA. Benign epithelial tumors and tumor-like lesions of the liver. In: Okuda K, Peters RL, eds. Hepatocellular Carcinoma. New York: John Wiley, 1976; 309–30.

78. Friedman IH, Wolff WI. Laparoscopy: a valuable adjunct to the general surgeon's armamentarium. Am J Surg 1978; 135:160–3.

79. Ishak KG, Rabin L. Benign tumors of the liver. Med Clin North Am 1975; 59:995–1013.

80. Ito T. Peritoneoscopy of peliosis hepatis. Endoscopy 1982; 14:14–8.

81. Solis-Herruzo JA, Colina F, Munoz-Yague MT, et al. Reddish-purple areas on the liver surface: the laparoscopic picture of peliosis hepatis. Endoscopy 1983; 15:96–100.

82. Carrasquer J, Carrasco D, Garrido G, et al. Utilidad de la laparoscopia en el diagnostico de la hidatidosis hepatica. Rev Esp Enferm Apar Dig 1976; 47:317–28.

83. Vilardell F. Echinococcus (hydatid) cysts of the liver. In: Bockus HL, ed. Gastroenterology, Vol. III. Ed. 3. Philadelphia: WB Saunders Co, 1976; 570–5.

84. Gazet JC. Primary carcinoma of the gallbladder. In: Gazet JC, ed. Carcinomas of the Liver, Biliary Tract, and Pancreas. London: Edward Arnold, 1983; 82–103.

85. Debray C, Hardouin JP, Paolaggi JA, et al. Les cancers primitifs de la vesicule biliaire. Donnees cliniques et evolutives a propos de 52 observations. Arch Mal Appar Dig 1965; 54:5–24.

86. De Dios J, Vega JF, Hita Perez J, et al. Valor de la laparoscopia en el diagnostico del cancer de vesicula biliar. Estudio de 34 cases. Rev Esp Enferm Apar Dig 1973; 41:867–74.

87. Bhargava DK, Sarin S, Verma K, Kapur BM. Laparoscopy in carcinoma of the gallbladder. Gastrointest Endosc 1983; 29:21–2.

88. Dagnini G, Marin G, Patella M, Zotti S. Laparoscopy in the diagnosis of primary carcinoma of the gallbladder. A study of 98 cases. Gastrointest Endosc 1984; 30:289–91.

89. Kimura R, Wakui K, Ishioka K, et al. Significance of peritoneoscopic examination, direct cholangiography, and cytological examination of aspirated bile in the diagnosis of biliary and pancreatic malignancies. Tohoku J Exp Med (Suppl) 1976; 118:145–8.

90. Phillips G, Pochaczevsky R, Goodman J, Kumari S. Ultrasound patterns of metastatic tumors in the gallbladder. J Clin Ultrasound 1982; 10:379–83.

91. Allibone GW, Fagan CJ, Porter SC. Sonographic features of carcinoma of the gallbladder. Gastrointest Radiol 1981; 6:169–73.

92. Suramo I, Paivansalo M, Myllyla V, et al. Ultrasonography of carcinoma of the gallbladder. Fortschr Roentgen Nukl 1983; 139:680–3.

93. Dalla Palma L, Rizzatto G, Pozzi-Mucelli RS, Bazzacchi M. Grey-scale ultrasonography in the evaluation of carcinoma of the gall bladder. Br J Radiol 1980; 53:662–7.

94. Meyer-Burg J. The inspection, palpation, and biopsy of the pancreas. Endoscopy 1972; 4:99–101.

95. Look D, Henning H, Luders CJ. Darstellung und Biopsie des Pankreaskopfes bei der Laparoskopie. Z Gastroenterol 1972; 10:209–14.

96. Strauch M, Lux G, Ottenjann R. Infragastric pancreoscopy. Endoscopy 1973; 5:30–2.

97. Cuschieri A, Hall AW, Clark J. Value of laparoscopy in the diagnosis and management of pancreatic carcinoma. Gut 1978; 19:672–7.

98. Ishida H. Peritoneoscopy and pancreas biopsy in the diagnosis of pancreatic diseases. Gastrointest Endosc 1983; 29:211–8.

99. Meyer-Burg J, Ziegler U, Kirstaedter HJ, Palmer G. Peritoneoscopy in carcinoma of the pancreas. Report of 20 cases. Endoscopy 1973; 5:86–90.

100. Warshaw AL, Tepper JE, Shipley WU. Laparoscopy in the staging and planning of therapy for pancreatic cancer. Am J Surg 1986; 151:76–80.

101. Urlaub BJ, Mack E. Evaluation and complications of 107 staging laparotomies for Hodgkin's disease. Ann Surg 1979; 190:45–7.

102. O'Holleran TP, Mastio GJ. An evaluation of the staging laparotomy in Hodgkin's disease. Arch Surg 1980; 115:694–5.

103. Sterchi JM, Myers RT. Staging laparotomy in Hodgkin's disease. Ann Surg 1980; 191:570–5.

104. Brogadir S, Fialk MA, Coleman M, et al. Morbidity of staging laparotomy in Hodgkin's disease. Am J Med 1978; 64:429–33.

105. De Vita VT Jr, Bagley CM Jr, Goodell B, et al. Peritoneoscopy in the staging of Hodgkin's disease. Cancer Res 1971; 31:1746–50.

106. Bagley CM Jr, Thomas LB, Johnson RE, et al. Diagnosis of liver involvement by lymphoma: results in 96 consecutive peritoneoscopies. Cancer 1973; 31:840–7.

107. Beretta G, Spinelli P, Rilke F, et al. Sequential laparoscopy and laparotomy combined with bone marrow biopsy in staging Hodgkin's disease. Cancer Treat Rep 1976; 60:1231.

108. Dancygier H, Jacob RA. Splenic rupture during laparoscopy. (Letter) Gastrointest Endosc 1983; 29:63.

109. Meyer-Burg J, Ziegler U. The intra-abdominal inspection and biopsy of lymph nodes during peritoneoscopy. Endoscopy 1978; 10:41–3.

110. Coleman M, Lightdale CJ, Vinciguerra VP, et al. Peritoneoscopy in Hodgkin disease. Confirmation of results by laparotomy. JAMA 1979; 236:2634.

111. Hoeffken K, Schmidt CG. Laparoskopie bei Morbus Hodgkin. Dtsch Med Wochenschr 1976; 101:814–8.

112. Huberman MS, Bunn PA Jr, Matthews MJ, et al. Hepatic involvement in the cutaneous T-cell lymphomas. Results of percutaneous biopsy and peritoneoscopy. Cancer 1980; 45:1683–8.

113. Veronesi U, Spinelli P, Bonadonna G, et al. Laparoscopy and laparotomy in staging Hodgkin's and non-Hodgkin's lymphoma. Am J Roentgenol 1976; 127:501–3.

114. Chabner BA, Johnson RE, Young RC, et al. Sequential nonsurgical and surgical staging in non-Hodgkin's lymphoma. Ann Intern Med 1976; 85:149–54.

115. Castellani R, Bonadonna G, Spinelli P, et al. Sequential pathologic staging of untreated non-Hodgkin's lymphomas by laparoscopy and laparotomy combined with bone-marrow biopsy. Cancer 1977; 40:2322–8.

116. Dagnini G. Considerations about laparoscopic follow-up of the abdominal localizations of malignant tumors undergoing therapy. Acta Endoscop 1982; 12:91–3.

117. Anderson T, Bender RA, Rosenoff SH, et al. Peritoneoscopy: a technique to evaluate therapeutic efficacy in non-Hodgkin's lymphoma patients. Cancer Treat Rep 1977; 61:1017–22.

118. Rosenoff SH, Young RC, Anderson T, et al. Peritoneoscopy: a valuable staging tool in ovarian carcinoma. Ann Intern Med 1975; 83:37–41.

119. Benvestito V, Boscia F, Moschetta R, et al. Laparoscopic diagnosis of pseudomyxoma peritonei. In: Marcozzi G, Crespi M, eds. Advances of Gastrointestinal Endoscopy. Proceedings of the 2nd World Congress of Gastrointestinal Endoscopy. Padua: Piccin Medical Books, 1972; 407–11.

120. Walsh DB, Williams G. Surgical biopsy studies of omental and peritoneal nodules. Br J Surg 1971; 58:428–33.

121. Ehrlich AN, Stalder G, Geller W, Sherlock P. Gastrointestinal manifestations of malignant lymphoma. Gastroenterology 1968; 54:1115–21.

122. Antman KH. Current concepts: malignant mesothelioma. N Engl J Med 1980; 303:200–2.

123. Salky BA. Laparoscopic diagnosis of peritoneal mesothelioma. (Letter) Gastrointest Endosc 1983; 29:65–6.

124. McCallum RW, Maceri DR, Jensen D, Berci G. Laparoscopic diagnosis of peritoneal mesothelioma. Report of a case and review of the diagnostic approach. Dig Dis Sci 1979; 24:170–4.

125. Fernandez RN, Daly JM. Pseudomyxoma peritonei. Arch Surg 1980; 115:409–14.

126. Cortesi N, Zambarda E, Manenti A, et al. Laparoscopy in routine and emergency surgery. Experience with 1720 cases. Am J Surg 1979; 137:647–9.

127. Lacey CG, Morrow CP, Disaia PJ, Lucas WE. Laparoscopy in the evaluation of gynecologic cancer. Obstet Gynecol 1978; 52:708–12.

128. Boyd WP Jr. Relative accuracy of laparoscopy and liver scanning techniques. Gastrointest Endosc 1982; 28:104–6.

129. Sauer R, Fahrlander H, Fridrich R. Comparison of the accuracy of liver scans and peritoneoscopy in benign and malignant primary and metastatic tumours of the liver. Scand J Gastroenterol 1973; 389–94.

130. Horica CA, Pescia R, Akovbiantz A, et al. Diagnose von Lebermetastasen und primarem Hepatome mit Szintigraphie. Laparoskopie und Laparotomie. Schweiz Med Wochenschr 1975; 105:1708–11.

131. Blackwell JN, Dean ACB, MacLeod IB, et al. Laparoscopy and radioisotope imaging in the investigation of suspected liver disease. Dig Dis Sci 1981; 26:507–12.

132. Erckenbrecht J, Waltenberg M, Sonnenberg A, et

al. Ist die sonographisce Diagnose der Leberzirrhose und Metastasenleber zuverlassig? Dtsch Med
Wochenschr 1981; 106:894–7.
133. Lammer J, Beaufort F, Tolly E, Hackl A. Lebermetastasen: Sonographie oder Szintigraphie? Wie-
ner Med Wochenschr 1983; 133:433–6.
134. Bondestam S, Lahde S, Annala R, et al. Scintigraphy and sonography in the investigation of liver
metastases. Diagn Imaging 1980; 49:339–42.
135. Mansi C, Savarino V, Picciotto A, et al. Comparison
between laparoscopy, ultrasonography, and computed tomography in widespread and localized
liver diseases. Gastrointest Endosc 1982; 28:83–5.
136. Temple DF, Parthasarathy KL, Bakshi SP, Mittel-
man AE. A comparison of isotopic and computerized tomographic scanning in the diagnosis of
metastasis to the liver in patients with adenocarcinoma of the colon and rectum. Surg Gynecol
Obstet 1983; 156:205–8.
137. Mulder GL, Butzelaar RM, van der Schoot JB, et
al. Computerized tomography and radionuclide
scan in surgical patients—A comparative prospective study in detecting liver metastases. Neth J Surg
1981; 33:66–74.
138. Alderson PO, Adams DF, McNeil BJ, et al. Computed tomography, ultrasound, and scintigraphy
of the liver in patients with colon or breast carcinoma: a prospective comparison. Radiology 1983;
149:225–30.
139. Barth RA, Jeffrey RB Jr, Moss AA, Liberman MS.
A comparison study of computed tomography and
laparoscopy in the staging of abdominal neoplasms.
Dig Dis Sci 1981; 26:253–6.
140. Bleiberg H, Osteaux M, Peetrons PH. Laparoscopic
evaluation of computed tomography (CT) and ultrasonography (US) in liver and abdominal tumor
dissemination. Acta Endoscop 1982; 12:51–60.
141. Lightdale CJ. Laparoscopy and biopsy in malignant
liver disease. Cancer 1982; 50:2672–5.
142. Schwerk WB, Durr HK, Schmitz-Moormann P.
Ultrasound guided fine-needle biopsies in pancreatic and hepatic neoplasms. Gastrointest Radiol
1983; 8:219–225.

Chapter 53

HEPATOMEGALY AND INFLAMMATORY DISEASE OF THE LIVER AND GALLBLADDER

PROFESSOR DR. MED. HARALD HENNING

Great credit belongs to Kalk for clarifying the morphogenesis of liver cirrhosis and defining the link between acute viral hepatitis and hepatic cirrhosis. His systematic laparoscopic examinations resulted in an understanding of the macroscopic morphology of chronic hepatitis as well as the correlation between visible and histologic findings.[1-4] Kalk's work focused attention on the benefits of direct observation of the liver and resulted in the widespread use of laparoscopy in Germany in the diagnosis of liver disease.

Over the years the relative necessity, merits, and justification of targeted versus blind percutaneous liver biopsy have been discussed. This debate will, no doubt, continue. In our experience, the combination of laparoscopic inspection of the liver and histologic evaluation of a selective liver biopsy has, without any doubt, the highest degree of diagnostic reliability. In addition, laparoscopy affords information on the early stages of development of portal hypertension and disturbances in lymph drainage up to and including the formation of ascites, information that cannot be obtained by microscopic evaluation of a cylinder of liver tissue obtained by blind percutaneous liver puncture as a sole diagnostic procedure.

Present-day non-invasive techniques such as ultrasonography, computed tomography (CT), and scintigraphy, and also invasive procedures such as endoscopic retrograde cho-

langiopancreatography (ERCP) and percutaneous transhepatic cholangiography (PTC), are capable of providing decisive information when there is clinical and biochemical evidence of obstruction to the flow of bile. The indications for laparoscopy in this instance are limited. Laparoscopy may occasionally be of assistance in clarifying the nature, location, or spread of a cholestatic process or when there is doubt as to whether a lesion is malignant and a directed biopsy might provide an answer.

The interpretation of findings at laparoscopy usually occasions little difficulty, provided the examining physician is thoroughly familiar with the normal anatomic features. However, it is much more difficult to evaluate changes in the surface details of the liver for the purpose of differential diagnosis. Constant observation and comparison of findings are essential for this purpose, and in this respect the experience afforded by an adequate number of regularly performed examinations is indispensable. As with many types of endoscopy, experience refines the ability to observe. In our opinion, the minimum number of examinations required to achieve satisfactory expertise is five per week.

As in all other endoscopic procedures, complete mastery of technique is a prerequisite for acquiring experience in laparoscopy. This skill is acquired only from constant practice. Practice and experience form the basis for the interpretation of subtle findings that in many cases will have serious consequences for the patient.

DIFFUSE ALTERATIONS OF THE LIVER

The technical improvements in laparoscopic optical systems introduced since 1970 make it possible to detect details in the surface features of the liver that formerly were not seen. Some of the features that should be noted are inclusions (fat, pigments, circumscribed areas of discoloration), the nature and number of arterial and venous blood vessels, lymphatics, and the configuration and extent of fibrosis, scars, or cirrhotic transformation.

Acute Hepatitis

Acute viral hepatitis is almost never an indication for laparoscopy. In the few cases in which a laparoscopic exploration is performed for differential diagnosis, the liver is found to be moderately enlarged, very red, or, as a result of hyperbilirubinemia, pale brown, with a smooth surface and rounded edges (Plate 53–1). The architecture of the liver lobules cannot be distinguished. Small arteries or veins are rarely seen. However, an increase in lymph vessels can frequently be observed, particularly with close inspection. This finding indicates increased lymph flow.

Cholestatic acute viral hepatitis is a less common form of the disease that is often problematic with respect to differential diagnosis and has an uncertain pathogenesis. Laparoscopy in this disease discloses a smooth liver surface with the whole liver covered by a uniform distribution of green spots.

In all cases of acute viral hepatitis, the spleen is enlarged, presenting a congested appearance with rounding of the caudal pole and crenate margin. The spleen is usually very red.

The liver may return to normal after recovery from acute viral hepatitis. Apparently, in most cases, however, there is a persistent accentuation of the hexagonal lobular architecture by delicate interlobular fibrosis (Plate 53–2).

Partial dystrophy of the liver, superficial flat scarring, or the so-called potato liver may develop after severe viral hepatitis[3] (Plates 53–3 and 53–4). Such morphologic changes are, however, not associated with any disorder of liver function, nor is progression of these processes to be expected. Although such changes can occasionally be impressive, they must not be misinterpreted as an indication of severe liver disease or macronodular cirrhosis. Even after the most severe form of viral hepatitis, there may be no scars.

Some patients with apparent viral hepatitis may have a protracted clinical course over many years. Biochemically, the process remains moderately active, and histologic changes are compatible with chronic persistent hepatitis or a mildly active chronic aggressive hepatitis. We have followed such patients laparoscopically for more than 10 years. Laparoscopy reveals the picture of acute viral hepatitis with no signs of any scarring or cirrhotic transformation. Our observations suggest that these conditions are typical "precursors" of the non-A, non-B viral infection.

Chronic Hepatitis Due to Viral Infection

Chronic Persistent Hepatitis

In chronic persistent hepatitis the surface of the liver is usually smooth and reddish brown to brick red. Arterial and venous vessels are not visible, but lymph vessels are clearly increased, although not congested to any marked degree (Plate 53–5). Occasionally, interlobular fibrosis may be present, which, on close-up inspection, gives the liver surface an irregular appearance. All things considered, the laparoscopic appearance in chronic persistent hepatitis is similar or identical to that of healing acute viral hepatitis or protracted inflammation; splenic congestion is not marked.

Chronic Active (Aggressive) Hepatitis

In contrast to acute viral hepatitis and chronic persistent hepatitis, the surface of the liver in chronic aggressive hepatitis is no longer mirror smooth, but has an irregular "wavy" appearance (Plate 53–6). The irregularity of the surface is due to muddy yellow indentations in the parenchyma that are manifestations of circumscribed dystrophy, flat scars, fibrotic processes, and incipient regenerative nodules. The color of the organ varies within wide limits from salmon pink to pale muddy hues that can give the liver a variegated appearance.[5]

Blood vessels are seen mainly as long, bright red arteries, while only a few short, dichotomously branched, bluish veins are

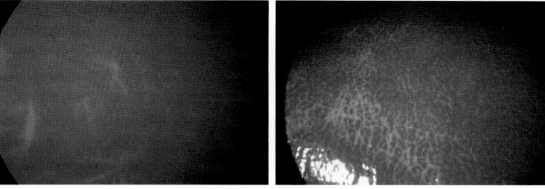

PLATE 53—1.   PLATE 53—2.

PLATE 53—1. Acute hepatitis: red, smooth liver surface. The normal hexagonal structure of the liver lobules is not visible.
PLATE 53—2. Healed acute hepatitis: Normal colored, smooth liver surface. Significant interlobular fibrosis demarcates the shape of the liver lobules.

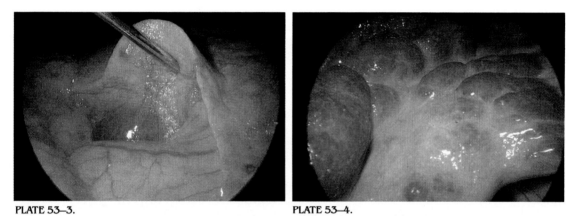

PLATE 53—3.   PLATE 53—4.

PLATE 53—3. Postdystrophic scar: Flat connective tissue at the margin of the left liver lobe.
PLATE 53—4. Postdystrophic scar: Large areas of liver regenerations representing the so-called potato liver.

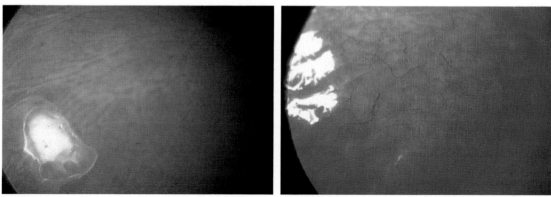

PLATE 53—5.   PLATE 53—6.

PLATE 53—5. Chronic persistent hepatitis: Smooth liver surface with an increased number of lymphatic vessels, representing an increase of lymph flow.
PLATE 53—6. Chronic aggressive hepatitis: Breakup of the light reflex demonstrates the irregularity of the liver surface. Corkscrew-like arterial vessels have developed.

noted. Somewhat congested lymph vessels are occasionally found; these indicate increased lymph production.

Red patches that are circumscribed but not sharply delimited or petechia-like hemorrhages can be found in highly inflammatory cases[6] (Plate 53–7). Under magnification, these are identifiable, in part, as tufts of arterial vessels resembling spider nevi.[5]

The fibrosis in chronic active hepatitis differs fundamentally from that of healed acute viral hepatitis. In the latter, the fibrotic changes are oriented to the structure of the hexagonal lobules, i.e., the fibrosis is periportal. In chronic aggressive hepatitis, the fibrotic changes consist of bands or cords of varying widths that form round rather than hexagonal patterns; they demarcate areas of regenerative parenchymal proliferation that vary in diameter and elevation above the surface; these may be the forerunners of cirrhotic nodules (Plate 53–8).

The laparoscopic appearance of chronic aggressive hepatitis becomes more typical the more marked the inflammatory activity and the more advanced the cirrhotic transformations.

Cirrhosis

With progression of the process of hepatic fibrosis, dome-shaped regenerative nodules become more predominant. In the active inflammatory stage, the "ensheathing" cords of connective tissue tend to be yellowish-white and are not sharply delimited. Newly sprouting blood vessels and congested lymph vessels accompany cirrhotic transformation. Some of the lymph vessels may have bead-like dilations in which the valves of the vessel are visible (Plate 53–9). Active inflammation is also indicated by the red patches and the petechial changes described above.

There is a synchronous increase in the size of the spleen with the development of cirrhosis; its color can vary widely between reddish brown and dove-blue.

Alcoholic Liver Injury

More or less prominent orange and yellow discolorations on the surface of the liver are the laparoscopic correlates of fatty infiltration (Plate 53–10), depending on the extent of the fatty infiltration. The underlying color of the liver and the nature of its capsule also influence the appearance. The intensity of the discolorations also differs from one area to another. When fatty infiltration is markedly zonal, an accentuation of the lobular structure becomes visible on the surface of the liver, which then has an appearance reminiscent of the markings of a leopard.[7] If fatty infiltration is more diffuse and confluent, the structures are blurred. It is not possible to correlate the laparoscopic appearance and the histologic distribution pattern of fatty infiltration reliably.

With increasing storage of fat, the liver becomes larger, and the anterior margin becomes blunted or rounded, the right lobe usually being more markedly affected than the left. If fatty infiltration is not accompanied by inflammation, the surface of the organ remains smooth.

In contrast to uncomplicated hepatic steatosis, "fatty liver hepatitis," a result of chronic liver damage due to alcohol, leads to irregularities of the liver surface that are caused by loss and replacement of parenchymal cells (necrobiosis), circumscribed postdystrophic scars, and reactive fibrosis.[8] The extent of fatty infiltration plays only a secondary role in this process, although the fat content may be discrete if alcohol consumption has stopped abruptly. In this process the manifestations of inflammatory activity are similar to those of chronic aggressive hepatitis: patchy red discoloration of the liver surface that is more or less extensive and an increase of venous capsule vessels that usually display dichotomous branching (Plate 53–11). In severe cases of alcoholic hepatitis, green dots as a consequence of intrahepatic cholestasis can also be found. If excessive alcohol consumption has persisted over a long period, the liver acquires a darker brown color with the onset of cirrhosis.

Complete recovery of the liver occurs within about 3 weeks if abstinence from alcohol begins at the stage of fatty infiltration. However, a fine-mesh reticular fibrosis will remain as a consequence of the necrobiotic processes.

Immoderate consumption of alcohol for at least 5 years leads, via necrobiotic processes, to a progressive cirrhotic transformation of the liver that typically results in a considerably enlarged micronodular organ (Plate 53–12).[9] The transformation can be so finely nodular that the surface of the liver appears smooth on cursory inspection. However, this micronodular cirrhosis is not always found. Sometimes in advanced stages it is only pos-

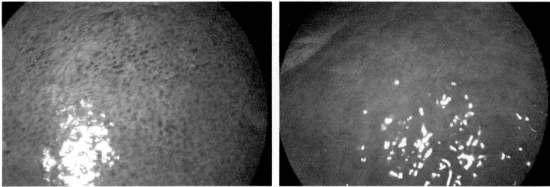

PLATE 53–7.　　　　　　　　　　　　PLATE 53–8.

PLATE 53–7. Chronic agressive hepatitis: Irregular liver surface. Red spots on the liver surface represent a high degree of inflammatory activity.
PLATE 53–8. Chronic aggressive hepatitis: Very early stages of the cirrhotic transformation are indicated by flat, elevated nodules.

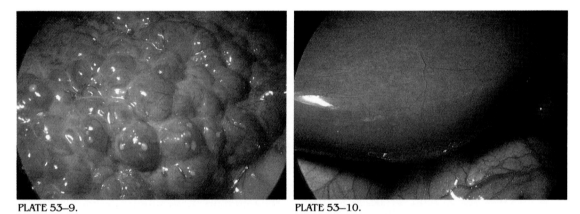

PLATE 53–9.　　　　　　　　　　　　PLATE 53–10.

PLATE 53–9. Postnecrotic liver cirrhosis: Complete cirrhotic transformation of mixed macronodular and micronodular types. On the top of the nodules a few white lymph cysts are visible.
PLATE 53–10. Fatty liver infiltration: The margin of the right lobe is rounded, and there is yellowish demarcation of the liver lobules.

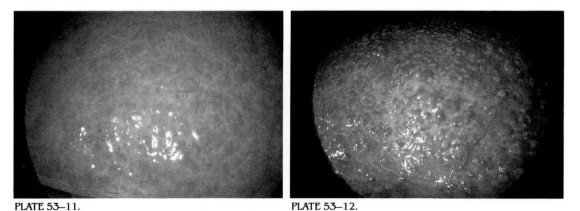

PLATE 53–11.　　　　　　　　　　　　PLATE 53–12.

PLATE 53–11. Chronic alcoholic hepatitis: The liver surface is irregular and there is fatty infiltration, multiple small venous vessels, and developing micronodular transformation.
PLATE 53–12. Alcohol-toxic liver cirrhosis: Complete micronodular transformation of the liver with diffusely distributed white lymph cysts.

sible to recognize islands of parenchyma "embedded" in large "plates" of connective tissue. Furthermore, cirrhosis caused by alcohol may also result in medium-sized to large nodules. When abstinence is practiced and the liver recovers its regenerative power, large regenerative nodules can develop.[10] Complications of liver cirrhosis such as portal hypertension, ascites, and metabolic decompensation are no different in alcoholic cirrhosis than in cirrhosis due to other causes. Results of an 18-year Scandinavian study indicate that development of hepatocellular carcinoma must be expected in 13% of patients with alcoholic cirrhosis (quoted by Thaler[11]).

Toxic Liver Injury

Laparoscopic differentiation of drug-related toxic hepatitis from chronic aggressive hepatitis is often difficult, especially since the appearance of the liver varies considerably, depending on the duration of ingestion and the dosage of an injurious drug. Thus, the liver surface may have normal smoothness, or it may have post-necrotic scars or cirrhotic transformation. In our experience, typical findings include both a yellowish-white thickening of the periportal areas from which cotton wool–like "fingers" project into the liver lobules and a dirty reddish-brown to grayish-brown color of the organ. The color can vary widely, depending on the extent of current inflammation, the development of fibrotic or cirrhotic processes, and the presence of associated cholestasis. Even in advanced processes, the vascular tufts so characteristic of chronic aggressive hepatitis are absent.[12] Cholestasis is the predominant finding in cases of injury due to methyltestosterone or chlorpromazine.

Administration of the radiologic contrast material Thorotrast results in a particularly marked hepatic fibrosis.[13] Although the use of this agent was discontinued in the 1940's, there may still be individual patients with Thorotrast-induced liver injury. Thorotrast also induces the development of cholangiocarcinoma, hemangiosarcoma, and hepatocellular carcinoma.[14, 15] Vinyl chloride–induced disease in industrial workers results in marked liver fibrosis, which can lead to portal hypertension with splenomegaly. As with Thorotrast, multicentric hemangiosarcomas have also been observed as a result of exposure to vinyl chloride.

Nonspecific Reactive Hepatitis

Nonspecific reactive hepatitis morphologically is very similar to chronic persistent hepatitis. It occurs primarily with extrahepatic intra-abdominal disorders such as enteritis, colitis, or ulcer disease and can be seen in association with common viral infections. This underscores the importance of histologic evaluation in such cases.

There are few reports of laparoscopic observations in primary sclerosing cholangitis, a rare condition that is occasionally associated with chronic ulcerative colitis or Crohn's disease. Beck[16] mentioned the condition in connection with a case of primary stenosing bile duct sclerosis with marked cholestasis and isolated occlusion of the right hepatic duct. Lindner et al.[17] considered stellate vascular tufts to be characteristic changes in the surface of the liver.

Cholestatic Syndrome

The surface of the liver exhibits normal smoothness in newly developed cases of diffuse cholestasis in which all segments of the liver are uniformly affected by a greenish-yellowish discoloration (Plate 53–13). In such cases, laparoscopy cannot differentiate between intrahepatic and extrahepatic causes of cholestasis. However, with high degrees of obstruction, inspection of the gallbladder is useful (see below).

Intrahepatic and extrahepatic forms of cholestasis can be differentiated by inspection of the liver when cholestasis has been present for longer periods, since each form has typical laparoscopic findings. The liver surface remains mirror smooth in intrahepatic cholestasis even when the condition has been present for a number of weeks (Plate 53–13). In contrast, surface irregularities quickly develop when cholestasis is due to extrahepatic causes. Initially this appears as a fine granulation followed later by fibrotic changes in the capsule. If occlusion of the bile ducts persists, a situation always associated with intermittent cholangitis, the laparoscopic appearance can become highly variegated; the color and texture result from a mixture of cholestasis, inflammation, lymph vessel congestion, connective tissue proliferation, dystrophic processes, and the formation of scattered abscesses throughout the liver. This situation can progress within a period of several weeks to produce fully developed secondary biliary cirrhosis.

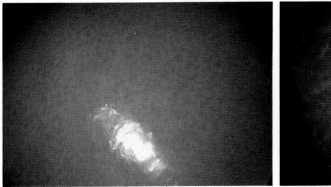 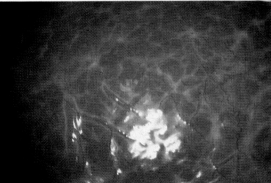

PLATE 53–13.   PLATE 53–14.

PLATE 53–13. Intrahepatic cholestatis: Early Ajmalin liver injury. There is a muddy greenish-yellowish discoloration of the liver, the surface is smooth, and green spots demarcate the liver lobules.

PLATE 53–14. Dubin-Johnson syndrome: So-called black liver disease. Bluish-brown discoloration is present in all areas.

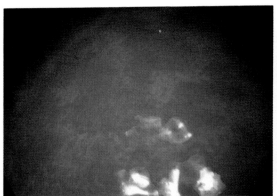 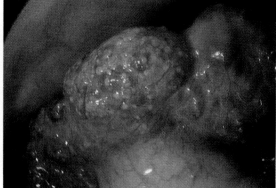

PLATE 53–15.   PLATE 53–16.

PLATE 53–15. Primary biliary cirrhosis (chronic nonsuppurative destructive cholangitis): This is an early stage of the disease in which typical "geographical" surface markings are noted on the liver surface.

PLATE 53–16. Primary biliary cirrhosis: Late stage of the disease with complete micronodular cirrhosis and extensive cholestasis.

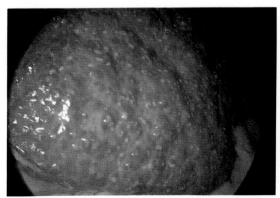 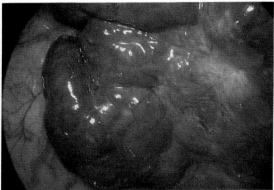

PLATE 53–17.   PLATE 53–18.

PLATE 53–17. Hemochromatosis: Micronodular cirrhosis with dark-brown coloration. Many white lymph cysts are visible.

PLATE 53–18. Wilson's disease: Postnecrotic scarred liver and macronodular regenerations in a 16-year-old young man.

The laparoscopic appearance of the gallbladder is highly significant in the differential diagnosis of the cholestatic syndrome. With distal obstruction of the common bile duct, the gallbladder is typically distended to a marked or extreme degree; it displays a delicate, thin-walled appearance, usually with no increase in the presence of injected vessels. Palpation of a gallbladder with this appearance using a probe scarcely produces any indentation; rather, the organ moves in toto as if it were solid.[18] This finding, known clinically as Courvoisier's sign, is seen particularly in carcinoma of the head of the pancreas. In intrahepatic cholestasis, a poorly filled, flaccid gallbladder with apparently thickened walls is seen.

Pigmentation

Lipofuscin

The presence of lipofuscin in the liver appears laparoscopically as if all sections of the liver were uniformly "sprinkled" with livid blue color. This results in a dot pattern oriented to the structure of the lobules that augments the normal lobular pattern, this finding being visible on closer inspection of the surface. Color is the decisive differential diagnostic feature vis-a-vis discrete cholestasis of recent onset. Knowledge of the appearance of lipofuscin deposition is thus a matter of practical importance for the laparoscopist.

Porphyria

The laparoscopic appearance of chronic hepatic porphyria is characterized by gray patches on the surface of the liver in 70% of cases.[19-21] Under ultraviolet light, which can be introduced into the abdominal cavity during laparoscopy, these gray areas are induced to emit a red fluorescence.[22]

Examination of a core of liver tissue under ultraviolet light (wavelength 366 nm) immediately after the biopsy is obtained is a reliable method of diagnosing chronic hepatic porphyria. A homogeneous red fluorescence is regularly found if porphyria cutanea tarda is present; the red fluorescence is reticular or punctiform in latent forms of porphyria.

Dubin-Johnson Syndrome

Extreme discoloration of the liver as a result of deposition of a slate-gray to bluish-gray pigment is found in the syndrome described by Dubin and Johnson[23] in 1954 as "chronic idiopathic jaundice." The laparoscopic appearance of this rare autosomal recessive disorder is extremely impressive and fully merits the description of "black liver disease" (Plate 53-14).[24]

Malaria

Pigment deposition in the liver after malaria is difficult to distinguish macroscopically from the Dubin-Johnson syndrome. Iwata et al.[25] found this pigmentation in 5 of 15 patients subjected to laparoscopy; the pigment was demonstrated histologically in 14 of the same patients.

Primary Biliary Cirrhosis (Chronic Nonsuppurative Destructive Cholangitis)

After Schmid[26] expressed the opinion that laparoscopy was merely capable of evaluating cirrhotic transformation of the liver, Lindner et al.[17, 27] systematically observed 38 patients with primary biliary cirrhosis (35 women, 3 men). These authors were able to correlate laparoscopic aspects of this disease with the various stages described by Scheuer.[28] They were thus able to demonstrate the development of this condition laparoscopically. In addition to the findings described by Lindner et al.[17, 27] and by Beck,[16] Minami et al.[29] observed irregular reddish areas that varied in diameter from 0.5 cm to 3 cm on the surface of the liver in cases of asymptomatic primary biliary cirrhosis. This observation is in agreement with our experience that these "geographical" surface markings are virtually pathognomonic for stage I of primary biliary cirrhosis, since we have never observed this finding in any other liver disease (Plate 53-15). A marking that resembles a leopard skin in the lighter-colored areas is noteworthy and has been reported by Lindner et al.[17] and by Beck.[16] Occasionally, this latter pattern will be almost indistinguishable from that of confluent fatty infiltration.

Connective tissue proliferation is manifested by a very finely granular structuring of the liver surface. This may obscure the true extent of cirrhotic transformation; histologic examination of biopsy specimens may reveal that this has already taken place. However, palpation of the surface of the liver with a probe to determine its consistency may provide an indication of cirrhosis (Plate 53-16).

Various stages in the development of primary biliary cirrhosis can be found at the same time "side by side" in different sections of the liver. This characteristic is extremely difficult to detect by means of percutaneous liver biopsy alone. Also, the early phases of development of primary biliary cirrhosis are frequently difficult to distinguish histologically from chronic aggressive hepatitis. For these reasons, we believe that laparoscopy with guided biopsy (including, when necessary, additional biopsies from areas of differing appearance) makes the diagnosis of primary biliary cirrhosis more reliable and also improves staging.

Hemochromatosis

The liver parenchyma becomes progressively darker brown in hemochromatosis owing to the storage of iron. The laparoscopic appearance of the surface of the liver corresponds with this, unless fibrosis of the capsule, with its resulting grayish-white coloration, masks the brown color (Plate 53–17). Fischer[30] found the typical dark brown liver in about half of his 51 cases.

Fibrosis becomes more marked the longer hemochromatosis remains untreated. Initially this is net-like; later there is septate fibrosis that can progress to a fully developed cirrhosis, usually of the finely nodular type, that may be accompanied by splenomegaly, portal hypertension, and ascites. Among his observations Fischer[30] also described the presence of a macronodular liver with and without scars. Hemochromatosis is one of the diseases that has a predisposition for the development of hepatocellular carcinoma (see Chapter 52).

Wilson's Disease

Laparoscopically, Wilson's disease does not usually present as typical liver cirrhosis, but rather as a post-necrotic scarred organ with macronodular regeneration, often with broad cicatricial fields (Plate 53–18). In the early stages, marked connective tissue proliferation and scars may even be absent, although changes similar to those in chronic aggressive hepatitis are present. Sternlieb and Scheinberg[31] thus urged that in cases of "idiopathic chronic hepatitis," even in patients up to 30 years of age, Wilson's disease be considered in the differential diagnosis. Thaler[11] emphasized that the detection of a fatty liver in early childhood in the absence of any alimentary cause should always raise the suspicion of Wilson's disease.

FOCAL LESIONS OF THE LIVER

Non-Parasitic Cystic Liver

Subcapsular hepatic cysts "come in all sizes";[32] the largest in our experience had a diameter of about 7 cm. The wall of the cyst is usually cloudy or opaque, white or pale blue in color, but occasionally also greenish, suggesting the presence of bile (Plate 53–19). A subcapsular solitary cyst is usually an incidental finding. We have not drained such a cyst by puncture during laparoscopy. Spontaneous rupture is very rare.[33]

Within the framework of the rare polycystic disease not only cystic kidneys but also a cystic liver can develop, the latter representing a virtually complete cystic transformation of the liver (Potter's syndrome). The laparoscopic appearance of polycystic liver disease is highly impressive, since typical liver parenchyma is barely visible.[34] The different-sized hepatic cysts have no uniform coloration, since their contents are apparently mixed sometimes with blood, sometimes with bile.

Hemangioma

Hemangiomas, as with subcapsular cysts, are usually fortuitous laparoscopic findings. Small, superficial hemangiomas in particular will escape detection by other imaging methods such as ultrasonography. At laparoscopy, they attract attention because of their purple color; they are usually multilocular and raised only slightly above the level of the liver capsule (Plate 53–20).[35]

We have observed only one really large cavernous hemangioma, which was in a 50-year-old woman. It projected from below the margin of the left lobe of the liver along with several bluish-red nodules that were about 5 cm in diameter. During more than 15 years this lesion has not resulted in any clinical symptoms.

Hepatic Peliosis

Laparoscopically, the presenting symptoms of peliosis hepatis are livid reddish, rounded, triangular, or stellate patches within the plane of the capsule of the liver (Plate 53–21).[36] The patches may occasionally become confluent, forming a net-like configuration. They may vary in size from 0.5 to 2.0 mm (see Chapter 52). We first observed such patches of extravasated blood in patients with

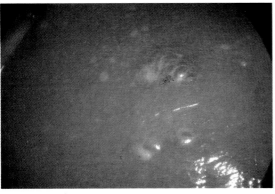
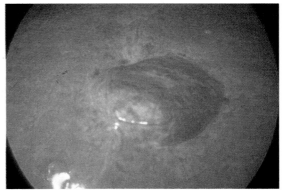

PLATE 53–19.   PLATE 53–20.

PLATE 53–19. Multiple subcapsular benign hepatic cysts.
PLATE 53–20. Benign hemangioma on the surface of the right lobe of the liver, 2 cm in diameter.

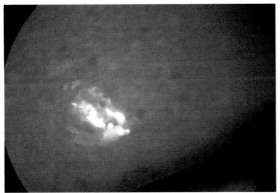
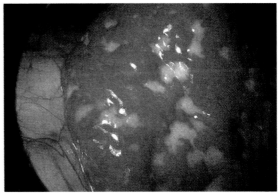

PLATE 53–21.   PLATE 53–22.

PLATE 53–21. Peliosis hepatis: Multiple livid reddish patches are noted within the plane of the left liver capsule.
PLATE 53–22. Cholangiofibromatosis: Diffuse "infiltration" of the liver by benign cholangiofibromas, so-called cholangio-dysplastic pseudocirrhosis.

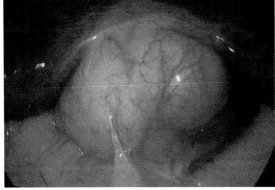
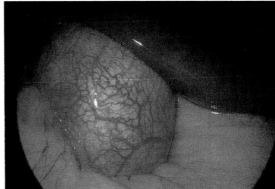

PLATE 53–23.   PLATE 53–24.

PLATE 53–23. Adenomyomatosis of the gallbladder: Bulging of the gallbladder wall similar to a diverticulum, but, in fact, representing hyperplasia of the Rokitansky-Aschoff sinus.
PLATE 53–24. Cholecystitis: The stage of inflammatory vascular reaction.

alcoholic liver damage; pigmentations resembled the marks of an indelible pencil.

The number and distribution of peliotic patches on the surface of the liver vary markedly from case to case. They may be disseminated over both lobes, occur as a solitary lesion, or appear as scattered foci. However, the large numbers of circumscribed areas that are occasionally observed are without any apparent specific cause. Hepatic peliosis is generally an incidental laparoscopic finding of no pathologic significance even though spontaneous abdominal hemorrhage resulting in death has been known to occur.[37]

Liver Abscess

Non-parasitic liver abscesses are rarely mentioned in the literature on laparoscopy. At most, multiple small cholangitic abscesses are reported.[19, 38] These, uncharacteristically, are yellowish-white elevations on the surface of the liver. In contrast to tuberculous nodules, these small abscesses that may be associated with biliary obstruction have no surrounding vascular reaction.

Focal Nodular Hyperplasia

Laparoscopically, these benign lesions are readily recognizable by their pale pink to orange-red color and slight elevation above the capsule of the liver. They vary in size from a few millimeters to more than 5 cm in diameter. The echogenicity of the liver in focal nodular hyperplasia is very similar to that of normal parenchyma, making this condition difficult to detect by ultrasonography. Therefore, laparoscopy becomes of considerable importance in diagnosis. Furthermore, laparoscopy is important in assessing the size of the nodules, including increases that may be a criterion for surgical intervention.[39] Nodular disorders of the liver are also discussed in Chapter 55.

Cholangiofibroma

Cholangiofibromas present at laparoscopy as white or yellowish-white, round to oval patches 2 to 10 mm in diameter. Most are not elevated above the normal plane of the capsule. Approximately 5% of these lesions have a flat, prominent cystic-nodular appearance.[40] Diffuse "infiltration" of the liver by cholangiofibromas is known as cholangio-dys-plastic pseudocirrhosis (Plate 53–22). Cholangiofibromas can be differentiated from other circumscribed lesions only by obtaining a forceps biopsy. The absence of splenic involvement in cholangioma is a differential point vis-a-vis sarcoidosis.

Sarcoidosis

Ursin et al.[41] have collected the laparoscopic findings in 50 patients with sarcoidosis (23 men, 27 women). These authors found changes in the liver surface in 82% of patients with histologically confirmed hepatic sarcoidosis. In 31 of the 50 patients the changes could be characterized as two to five scattered, rarely grouped, round to oval nodules with diameters of 0.5 to 2.0 mm. Most of these nodules were within the plane of the capsule or only slightly raised, were sharply demarcated from the liver parenchyma, and occasionally had delicate extensions into the parenchyma ("pseudopodia"). In a few cases there was a disseminated "scattering" of foci on both lobes of the liver that varied in size up to pinhead diameter. Ten patients had coarsely nodular plaque or tumor-like grayish-white infiltrates. In part, these lesions formed well-demarcated, irregularly shaped plaques or prominent hemispherical conglomerates. Apparently these larger lesions were comprised of confluent smaller lesions. In 10 of these patients, corresponding lesions were also detected in the spleen; in one case, the liver was macroscopically unremarkable. Sarcoid involvement of the parietal and visceral peritoneal surfaces is discussed in Chapter 55.

PARASITIC LIVER DISEASE

Echinococcosis

The first reports of laparoscopic findings in echinococcosis in the 1960's are descriptions of *Echinococcus cysticus* infection reported from Spain, a country where echinococcosis is common (see Chapter 52).[42, 43] In a number of cases interpretation of the cystic findings was difficult, since the wall of the cyst was irregularly thickened and, in part, bore nodules. Also, pericystic vascular reactions, such as are seen with metastatic tumors, were sometimes visible. Palpation of the lesion with a probe proved useful for differentiation of this condition from a tumor; in the latter case the lesion was hard, and in the former the soft cystic quality was demonstrated. Extensive and well-developed adhesions were frequently present in the area of an echinococcal cyst. In rare cases there will be involvement of the spleen.[44]

Although only infestations with *E. cysticus* are observed in Spain, the percentage of cases of *Echinococcus alveolaris* infestation is high in other endemic areas. Between 1956 and 1969, 351 cases of echinococcosis were reported in Switzerland; 35% were due to *E. alveolaris*.[45] Mörl[46] described the tumor-like configuration of *E. alveolaris* with an accumulation of numerous small white to gray-colored cysts that reached the size of a hazelnut. In this disorder, the risk of biopsy is low, so that histologic differentiation from malignant lesions is possible.

Amebic Abscess

An amebic abscess is not a collection of pus; it represents an area of cytolytic necrosis of liver tissue in which amebas are not detectable. Occasionally, an amebic abscess is found to be the cause of fever of unknown origin.[47] Therapeutic aspiration of the contents of the cyst via selective puncture has been performed.[48, 49] There is no characteristic macroscopic appearance; the correct diagnosis can be made only by reference to an appropriate clinical setting. Usually, numerous adhesions to the anterior wall of the abdomen are found in the region of the lesion.[50]

Schistosomiasis

The laparoscopic finding in the early stages of chronic schistosomiasis is a marked septate fibrosis of the liver. Parasite eggs can frequently be detected in the biopsy specimens. Lent[6] described characteristic small white nodules in the capsule of the liver, which probably represent egg tubercles. We have found similar nodules, which are rather hard, in the region of the mesentery of the appendix.

An increase in the number and size of blood vessels in the falciform ligament develops with advancing fibrosis as an expression of incipient portal hypertension; ascites soon follows. Laparoscopically, advanced stages of schistosomiasis present the fully developed picture of a medium-sized to coarsely nodular cirrhosis with the marked vascularity of portal hypertension and with ascites.[51–53]

Visceral Larva Migrans

Llanio and Sotto[54] described the laparoscopic picture of visceral larva migrans based on 20 examinations performed in Cuba. It is of interest that 15 procedures were performed in adults. In all cases there were typical whitish-yellow, raised, straight or arched cords 2 to 5 cm in length on the surface of the liver, together with whitish-yellow circumscribed patches having a diameter of only a few millimeters. Follow-up laparoscopy after successful treatment revealed fibrotic transformation of the larval tracts.

Pentastomum Denticulatum

The laparoscopic presentation of the larva of the tongue worm *Linguatula serrata* is an approximately pea-sized fibrotic area beneath the capsule of the liver; the lesion may also calcify after death of the larva.[55, 56] Infestation with this worm and involvement of the liver are harmless for humans. From the standpoint of differential diagnosis, the pentastomum denticulatum nodule can be distinguished from other circumscribed forms of fibrosis only by obtaining a biopsy. Histologically, a calcified structure surrounded by a tough fibrotic capsule is found.

DISORDERS OF THE GALLBLADDER

Anatomic Features

The normal gallbladder is a bluish-gray, opaque, hemispheric structure, the fundus of which projects more or less beyond the right margin of the liver. Blood vessels—an artery with concomitant veins—are usually found in its wall. These often have a "three-lane" appearance.[57] Occasionally, a number of lymph vessels of a delicate gray tone may be observed.

Typically, there is an incisure of the liver margin in the region of the gallbladder. This varies in size, and it may be acute-angled, arched, or rectangular in configuration.[58] To the best of our knowledge, this incisure has no anatomic name, although it is situated at the beginning of the Rex-Cantli-Serege line that separates the embryologic right and left lobes of the liver. We have given it the name "incisura vesicae felleae hepatis."

Adenomyomatosis

Formerly, we misinterpreted bulges in the gallbladder wall as diverticula[58]; we now are

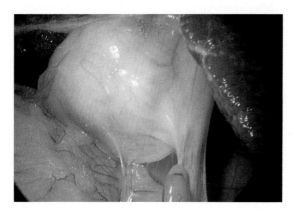

PLATE 53–25. Shrunken gallbladder: Postcholecystitis adhesions. The irregular shape of the thickened gallbladder wall is caused by multiple gallstones.

able to identify these structures as adenomyomatosis—hyperplasia of the Rokitansky-Aschoff sinus (Plate 53–23).[59] Knowledge of adenomyomatosis, which we detected in 17 of 1821 patients undergoing laparoscopy, is important in the differential diagnosis vis-a-vis carcinoma of the gallbladder. Oral cholecystography and ultrasonography are frequently unreliable in the recognition of adenomyomatosis.

Inflammatory Changes

Inflammatory changes of the wall of the gallbladder are impressive and easily detected. Hara et al.[60] have suggested the following classification: Type 0, normal; Type I, edema and congestion; Type II, blood vessel changes in the gallbladder wall (Plate 53–24); Type III, turbidity and wall changes; Type IV, pericholecystic adhesions; Type V, shrunken gallbladder (Plate 53–25).

Laparoscopy is not indicated in acute cholecystitis except perhaps occasionally in the differential diagnosis of the acute abdomen. In contrast, we believe laparoscopy has a role in establishing the presence of chronic cholecystitis, and thus the need for cholecystectomy, in patients with cholelithiasis.

References

1. Kalk H. Fortschritte der Laparoskopie. Dtsch med Wochenschr 1942; 68:677–81.
2. Kalk H. Die chronischen Verlaufsformen der Hepatitis epidemica Beziehung zu ihren anatomischen Grundlagen. Dtsch med Wochenschr 1947; 72:308–13.
3. Kalk H. Uber die Leberzirrhose nach Hepatitis epidemica. Arztl Wochenschr 1948; 3:161–5.
4. Kalk H, Brühl W, Sieke W: Die gezielte Leberpunktion. Dtsch med Wochenschr 1943; 69:693.
5. Look D. Laparoskopische Aspekte der "chronischen Hepatitis." In: Lindner H, ed. Fortschritte der gastroenterologischen Endoskopie. Baden-Baden, Brussels, Koln: Witzstrock, 1976:73–7.
6. Lent H. Kriterien und Bedeutung laparoskopischer Aktivitats-beurteilung entzundlicher Lebererkrankungen. In: Lindner H, ed. Laparoskopie und Leberbiopsie. Baden-Baden, Brussels, Koln: Witzstrock, 1975:104–14.
7. Müller K. Laparoskopische Aspekte der Fettleber. Leber Magen Darm 1971; 1:111–6.
8. Thaler H. Die Fettleber und ihre pathogenetische Beziehung zur Leberzirrhose. Virchows Arch (Pathol Anat) 1962; 335:180–210.
9. Boyce HW Jr. Peritoneoscopy views of alcoholic cirrhosis and portal hypertension. Hosp Med 1971; 7:60–5.
10. Bordas JM, Bru C, Bruguera M, Rodes J. Aspecto seudotumoral del higado en la hepatitis alcoholica aguda. Rev Esp Enferm Apar Digest 1980; 57(Suppl 3):77–80.
11. Thaler H. Leberkrankheiten: Histopathologie, Pathophysiologie, Klinik. Berlin, Heidelberg, New York: Springer Verlag, 1982.
12. Look D, Henning H, Lindner H. Laparoskopische Befunde bei medikamententoxischen Lebererkrankungen. In: Lindner H, ed. Fortschritte der gastroenterologischen Endoskopie. Baden-Baden, Brussels, Koln: G. Witzstrock, 1977:21–3.
13. Frenger W, Heinkel K. Zum laparoskopischen Bild der Thorotrastleber. Med Bildd Roche 1962; 2:18–21.
14. Thiel H, Schott D, Schejbal V, Hörster HG. Panmyelopathie und metastasierendes Hämangioendotheliom der Leber nach Thorotrastapplikation. Med Klin 1979; 74:1451–5.
15. Yamada S, Hosoda S, Tateno H, et al. Survey of Thorotrast-associated liver cancer in Japan. J Natl Cancer Inst 1983; 70:31–5.
16. Beck K, ed. Farbatlas der Laparoskopie. Stuttgart, New York: F. K. Schattauer, 1980.
17. Lindner H, Dammermann R, Kloppel G. The laparoscopic staging of primary biliary cirrhosis. Endoscopy 1977; 9:68–73.
18. Henning H. Der Beitrag der Laparoskopie zur Differentialdiagnose biliarer Erkrankungen. In: Lindner H, ed. Laparoskopie und Leberbiopsie, Baden-Baden, Brussels, Koln: Gerhard Witzstrock, 1975: 151–4.
19. Beck K, ed. Farbatlas der Laparoskopie. Stuttgart, New York: F. K. Schattauer, 1968.
20. Henning H, Look D, v. Bruan H, Luders CJ. Die Laparoskopie-heute. Indikation und morphologischer Befund. Internist prax 1971; 11:385–99.

21. Solis-Herruzo JA. Cuadro laparoscopico de la porfiria cutanea tarda (Estudio de 23 casos). Gaceta Med Bilbao 1973; 24:197–200.
22. Look D, Henning H. Chronische hepatische Porphyrien. Diagnostik 1974; 7:496–8.
23. Dubin IN, Johnson FB. Chronic idiopathic jaundice with unidentified pigment in liver cells; new clinico-pathologic entity with report of 12 cases. Medicine 1954; 33:155–97.
24. Edwards RH. Inheritance of the Dubin-Johnson-Sprinz syndrome. Gastroenterology 1975; 68:734–49.
25. Iwata K, Tanabe K, Maruto H, et al. Liver in patients with malaria. Acta Hepato Jap 1982; 23:909–14.
26. Schmid M. Das laparoskopische Bild der primaren biliaren Zirrhose. Z Gastroenterol 1974; 12:48.
27. Lindner H, Dammermann R, Kloppel G. Zur laparoskopischen Studieneinteilung der primarbiliaren zirrhose. In: Lindner H, ed. Fortschritte der gastroenterologischen Endoskopie, Bd. 7, S. 78. Baden-Baden, Brussels, Koln: G. Witzstrock, 1976: 78–83.
28. Scheuer PJ. Primary biliary cirrhosis. Proc R Soc Med 1967; 60:1257–60.
29. Minami Y, Seki K, Nishikawa M, et al. Laparoscopic findings of the liver in the diagnosis of primary biliary cirrhosis: "Reddish patch," a laparoscopic feature in the asymptomatic stage. Endoscopy 1982; 14:203–8.
30. Fischer R. Klinik und Therapie der idiopathischen Hamochromatose. Erfahrungen bei 51 eigenen Fallen. Leber Magen Darm 1976; 6:316–29.
31. Sternlieb I, Scheinberg IH. Chronic hepatitis as a first manifestation of Wilson's disease. Ann Intern Med 1972; 76:59–64.
32. Banche M, Ferrari A, Roatta L. Il ruolo della laparoscopia nella diagnosi delle formazioni cistiche del fegato. Minerva Gastroenterol 1975; 21:45–8.
33. Nymark J. Ruptur nicht nonparasitaere levercyster. Ugeskr Laeg 1979; 141:1580–1.
34. Niemetz D, Sokol A, Meister L. Polycystic disease of the liver. Report of two cases diagnosed by peritoneoscopy. Ann Intern Med 1949; 31:319–24.
35. Eckardt V, Beck K. Benigne Hamangiome der Leber. Leber Magen Darm 1974; 4:337–42.
36. Schonlank FW. Ein Fall von Peliosis hepatis. Virchows Arch Pathol Anat 1916; 222:358–64.
37. Bagheri SA, Boyer JL. Peliosis hepatitis associated with androgenic anabolic steroid therapy. A severe form of hepatic injury. Ann Intern Med 1974; 81:610–8.
38. Muller B, Plantier M. Small abscess of the liver detected by peritoneoscopy during biliary lithiasis. Arch Mal Appar Dig 1961; 50:972–5.
39. Tung LC, Haring R, Gortz G, Jautzke G. Gutartige Lebertumoren—Die fokale nodulare Hyperplasie. Der Kassenarzt 1982; 22:3322–30.
40. Henning H, Friedrich K, Lüders CJ. Laparoskopischer Aspekt und klinische Relevanz von Cholangiofibromen. Z Gastroenterol 1982; 20:744–51.
41. Ursin E, Spech HJ, Liehr H. Laparoskopie und Lebersarkoidose. Med Klin 1974; 69:681–6.
42. Hernandez Guido C, Miranda Baiocchi R. Valor de la laparoscopia para el diagnostico de la hidatidosis hepatica y su diferenciacion de otros procesos tumorales. Rev Esp Enfern Apar Dig 1963; 22:94–7.
43. Seres L, Marti A. Valor de la laparoscopia en el diagnostico del quiste hidatidico del higado. Rev Esp Enferm Apar Dig 1967; 38:84–9.
44. Mörl M, Herrmann HJ. Parasitosen der Leber. Dtsch Arztebl 1979; 76:1619–26.
45. Drolshammer F, Wiesmann E, Eckert J. Echinokokkose beim Menschen in der Schweiz 1956–1969. Schweiz med Wochenschr 1973; 103:1337–41.
46. Mörl M. Lebertumoren—Laparoskopische Aspekte. Fortschr Med 1976; 94:1876–8.
47. Farid Z, Trabolski B, Kilpatrick ME, et al. Amoebic liver abscess presenting as fever of unknown origin (FUO). Serology, isotope scanning and metronidazole therapy in diagnosis and treatment. J Trop Med Hyg 1982; 85:255–8.
48. Salky B, Finkel S. Laparoscopic drainage of amebic liver abscess. Gastrointest Endosc 1985; 31:30–2.
49. Staples DC, Dale JA. Peritoneoscopically guided needle aspiration of amebic liver abscess. Gastrointest Endosc 1980; 26:21–2.
50. Arguello M, Cortes E, Ahumada JJ. Amibiasis colica y hepatica, medios de diagnostico, tratamiento y evolucion. Rev Fac Med (Bogota) 1972; 28:237–61.
51. Iwamura K. Hepatic involvement of schistosomiasis japonica. Tokai J Exper Clin Med 1977; 2:143–50.
52. dos Passos Galvao Filho. La Laparoscopia En La Cirrhosis Hepatica Por S. Mansoni. IV World Congress of Digestive Endoscopy. Abstracts. Madrid, June 1–3, 1978.
53. Abd El-Rahman N, Gawad G, Manialawi M. Schistosomiasis of GI tract: Evaluation by fiberscopy and laparoscopy. First Cairo International. Teaching Conference in Gastrointestinal Endoscopy. Cairo, January 20–22, 1979.
54. Llanio R, Sotto A. Larva migrans visceralis. Diagnostic par laparoscopie. Sem Hop Paris 1972; 48:1223–5.
55. Pickert H, Muller K. Geschwulste der Leber im laparoskopischen Bild. Med Mitt 1969; 30:9–16.
56. Solis-Herruzo JA. Atlas de Diagnostico Diferencial Laparoscopico. Madrid: Editorial Paz Montalvo, 1975.
57. Otto K. Das venose Gefabsystem der Gallenblase. Fortschr Med 1971; 89:437–40.
58. Pickert H, Müller K, Henning H. Anomalien und Normvarianten der Gallenblase und Leber im laparoskopischen Bild. Med Mitt (Schering) 1967; 28:7–13.
59. Look D, Kloppel G. Die Adenomyomatose der Gallenblase. In: Henning H, ed. Fortschritte der gastroenterologischen Endoskopie. Baden-Baden, Brussels, Koln, New York: G. Witzstrock, 1979.
60. Hara TS, Sakaue T, Shinoda R, et al. Laparoscopic observations on gallbladder surface. (II) (Correlation between cholecystographic findings and laparoscopic types on gallbladder.) Proceedings of the 14th Autumnal Meeting, Niigata, Japan, 1972.

Chapter 54

LAPAROSCOPY IN CIRRHOSIS AND PORTAL HYPERTENSION

GIORGIO DAGNINI, M.D.

CIRRHOSIS OF THE LIVER

Cirrhosis of the liver is a frequent and serious disease characterized by such evident and specific morphologic changes that an accurate diagnosis is possible by inspection alone. Therefore, laparoscopy is the most suitable procedure for identification of cirrhosis in living patients. Furthermore, laparoscopic examination of the liver with modern instruments can reveal even the subtlest alterations, a circumstance in which a diagnosis may nevertheless be confirmed by direct visualization and multiple guided biopsies. The information thus gained can be useful in classifying the type of cirrhosis, in formulating a possible etiology and pathogenesis, and in estimating the prognosis. Laparoscopy may also reveal associated pathology.

In addition to its diagnostic value, laparoscopy has contributed much to the knowledge of cirrhosis and its complex natural history. This is the result of systematic observations of the various phases of the evolution of the disease. Over 50 years ago Kalk used laparoscopy to demonstrate the transformation of chronic hepatitis into cirrhosis. This phenomenon seems obvious today, but at that time it was obscure.

Laparoscopic Findings in Cirrhosis

Surface Nodulation

The primary and specific laparoscopic finding in cirrhosis is the presence of regenerative nodules on the hepatic surface.

The parenchymal nodules of cirrhosis vary in size, shape, and character. They may be as small as a grain of millet or a peppercorn (Plate 54–1). Medium nodules are the size of a pea, and large ones range from walnut size to 7 cm or more in diameter. The small and medium-sized nodules are usually regular in shape, uniform in size, round, numerous, and close together. Larger nodules are more often irregular in shape, vary in size, and thus give the surface a coarse, irregular appearance.

Small and medium-sized nodules are surrounded by thin septa of light gray fibrous tissue. Larger nodules may also be separated by thin and sometimes incomplete septa. However, much more frequently they are isolated by wide, deep furrows of pale, retracted fibrous tissue. These areas of scarring are often deeply depressed with a white background; they may be linear, simple or branched, polygonal or stellate (Plate 54–2). Post-necrotic scarring may be extensive and appears as vast, flat areas bordering nodular zones. At times, the process may result in a smooth white fibrous layer that can involve most of a lobe.

Regenerative nodules may be markedly elevated (Plate 54–1) ("semispherical nodular type")[1] or barely raised above the surface, although clearly evident.

Sometimes the regenerative nodules are not very pronounced and therefore are barely perceptible to the laparoscopist. It may be difficult to determine whether the surface is really nodular. Furthermore, the surface may appear nodular when there is a marked increase in hepatic connective tissue, although the normal lobular architecture remains. Thus, the laparoscopic diagnosis of cirrhosis can be demanding: if there are nodules, the diagnosis is cirrhosis; if not, the diagnosis is only hepatic sclerosis, which can be the end result of diverse pathologic processes.[2] In such circumstances, a specific diagnosis can be made only by obtaining a biopsy.

Careful examination of the surface with incident light can be useful in determining whether nodules are present. Nodules, even if not very elevated, reflect the light as numerous small luminous points (Plate 54–3). If, instead, the surface is rough but not nodular, the light is irregularly dispersed.

In some cases, histologic findings demonstrate cirrhosis despite the presence of a smooth liver surface at laparoscopy. There are forms without nodules, e.g., the so-called smooth or glabrous cirrhosis (Plate 54–4). Although these are difficult to diagnose macroscopically, careful examination will sometimes reveal rare, isolated, slightly raised nodules. Close-up examination, which magnifies the image, can reveal surface changes of an underlying cirrhosis. The lobular pattern is not visible even with the frequently associated fatty infiltration that usually accentuates the lobular design. In its place are flat, round, hazy, red-brown areas that stand out against the pale yellow background (Plate 54–5). Even though not protuberant, these areas represent regenerative nodules; we propose calling these "flat cirrhotic lesions."

The color of the nodules varies. In common cirrhosis they are pink, pale or dark gray, or red or red-brown. With cholestasis the apex of the nodules is dark green. Certain conditions are characterized by different and distinct colors that suggest particular types of cirrhosis. With intense steatosis the nodules are yellowish, with accumulation of hemosiderin or lipofuscin they are rust-brown, and with copper accumulation they are brown with blue overtones.

Other Findings

Changes in Form and Volume

The shape of the liver is generally not altered in cirrhosis. The greatest changes in configuration occur in macronodular cirrhosis in which one or both hepatic lobes may consist of a few regenerative nodules, varying in size and shape and divided by deep grooves or by extensive areas of retracted scar tissue. In such cases the liver is grossly deformed and sometimes termed "potato liver" or polylobar liver (Plate 54–6).

A cirrhotic liver may be normal, increased, or decreased in size. Laparoscopy permits an evaluation of the dimensions of the two lobes in relation to specific reference points and to the thickness of the lobe itself. It therefore gives a fairly accurate idea of liver volume.

A clinical impression of hepatomegaly can be confirmed by comparing the position of the liver margin with the subcostal border. The position of the latter is determined by exerting external pressure with a hand placed under the costal margin while observing the resultant indentation of the abdominal wall laparoscopically.

The most common laparoscopic method of estimating size consists of studying the relation between the anterior margin (sometimes termed the liver edge) and the hepatic insertion of the round ligament. In a liver of normal size, the insertion corresponds to the hepatic margin. If the liver is enlarged, the anterior margin extends beyond or inferior to the insertion of the ligament, and if decreased in size, the margin appears to be behind, i.e., superior to the ligament.

The thickness of the two lobes in the anterior-posterior dimension is also important in judging the size of the organ (Plate 54–7). In some cases a large increase in thickness is associated with only a slight extension in the inferior direction. Although the round ligament is on almost the same line as the anterior margin, the liver must still be considered enlarged. In contrast, the margin may extend beyond the round ligament, but the liver cannot be considered enlarged since the lobes are thin.

Increases or decreases in size may involve both lobes equally or may be asymmetric, with volume changes in only one lobe or enlargement of one lobe and diminution of the other.

Changes in Consistency

The consistency of a cirrhotic liver is usually increased because of the presence of fibrous tissue. The degree of firmness varies with the stage of the cirrhosis. In fully developed forms the liver is hard. The firmer consistency is evident even with simple inspection because the two lobes no longer rest upon or conform to the underlying organs, but instead appear rigid and abnormally elevated, often exposing the posterior surface to laparoscopic observation. This is particularly apparent on the left where the lobe, which is normally molded to the gastric surface, is elevated and only barely touches the underlying stomach (Plate 54–8).

The firmness and rigidity of the liver can be appreciated by palpation with a probe at laparoscopy. When the liver edge is raised by

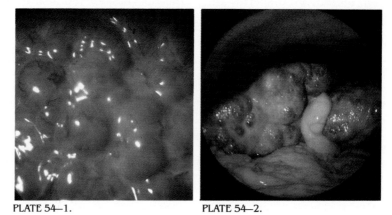

PLATE 54—1.   PLATE 54—2.

PLATE 54—1. Medionodular cirrhosis. Elevated nodules with a regular shape and thin septa.
PLATE 54—2. Macronodular cirrhosis. Extensive scarring, and the partially filled gallbladder has a thickened wall.

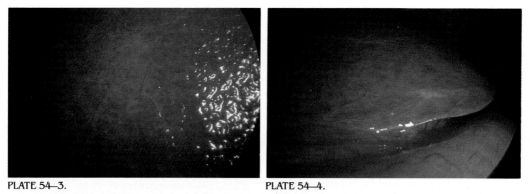

PLATE 54—3.   PLATE 54—4.

PLATE 54—3. Micronodular cirrhosis. Small, barely protruding nodules are visible only by the reflected light.
PLATE 54—4. Glabrous cirrhosis. Flat cirrhotic lesions without evidence of nodules in the left lobe. The margin of the lobe is thin, and the consistency of the liver is increased.

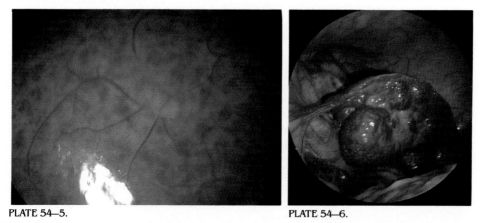

PLATE 54—5.   PLATE 54—6.

PLATE 54—5. "Histologic cirrhosis." The surface of the liver is smooth, and there is no distortion of the reflected light. The normal lobular design has been destroyed and replaced by round spots (flat cirrhotic lesions). The biopsy result was cirrhosis.
PLATE 54—6. Macronodular cirrhosis. The left lobe is atrophic with large, coarse nodules and extensive scars ("potato liver").

a probe, the lobe remains rigid and does not deform as lifting pressure is applied with the probe. Resistance encountered as a biopsy needle is introduced into the parenchyma provides the experienced endoscopist with another method for assessment of the degree of firmness.

A hard liver is a consistent and characteristic finding in cirrhosis. Sometimes, however, even in the presence of a clear-cut surface nodulation, the changes in consistency are modest. Such a finding is more likely in the early stages of cirrhosis with limited fibrosis.

Changes in Liver Edge

Changes occur in the liver margin or edge in cirrhosis. The hepatic border may be thin, as in the normal liver; more often, however, it is narrow or sharp, especially when the lobe is small and regular in shape (Plate 54–4). Sometimes the margin is bordered in its entirety by a narrow, continuous white ribbon of fibrosis that glistens (Plate 54–9). This is a common finding that can also be observed in other disorders, principally chronic hepatitis. The margin may also appear notched or scalloped, with indentations and protrusions of varying dimensions (Plate 54–10). It can be more or less thickened and rounded, which usually occurs when the entire lobe is enlarged (Plate 54–7). The outline of the edge may then be regular or grossly irregular and may be bordered by the aforementioned fibrous band.

Other Surface Changes

If the liver capsule is normal and therefore transparent, all characteristics of the parenchyma are visible. In cirrhosis, however, the capsule is sometimes thickened and opaque owing to prior inflammation. Capsular thickening may be diffuse or localized and varies in degree. Examination of the parenchyma may therefore be limited to varying degrees (Plate 54–11). Sometimes even the nodules are hidden. In general, the capsule is less altered on the inferior surface, where the liver parenchyma is more visible.

Color. The color of the liver must be evaluated with care because color is a subjective finding that varies with the intensity and quality of the illumination and with the distance between the laparoscope and the surface of the organ: it appears lighter close up, darker from afar. Therefore, the variations in color in cirrhosis can be significant.

The liver may be a normal reddish-brown, but more often it is a paler gray-brown or pink-gray because of the presence of fibrous tissue. Many different nuances of color are created by combinations of various colors, the regenerative nodules, and the surrounding pale gray connective tissue. This variegated pattern is the most common appearance.

Certain color changes may have a particular significance. Bright red indicates acute or subacute inflammation, an active phase in the cirrhotic process (Plate 54–12). Yellow is typical of associated steatosis, an entity that determines color variations from pale to bright yellow (Plate 54–13). Rust brown, particularly of the nodules, corresponds to hemosiderin deposits (Plate 54–14), and blue-brown indicates copper accumulation. Gray-blue spots, which are more or less extensive and diffuse, indicate the presence of abnormal amounts of porphyrin. A green liver, whether diffusely colored or stippled, is evidently caused by cholestasis (Plate 54–15). These findings and their precise significance will be discussed.

Capsular Vessels. The liver surface may be diffusely or partially a bright red of varying intensity. High magnification reveals that this is due to an increased number of small capsular vessels of increased caliber as well as capillaries that form an often thick and hazy network (Plate 54–16). This is the characteristic appearance of "active" congestion. An analogous alteration is the change that occurs in small veins in passive congestion in which the vessels appear turgid and thickened, dark red, and well-defined.

Lymphatic vessels may seem more numerous, enlarged, turgid, and often branched in cirrhosis. They are semi-transparent and shining (Plate 54–17). These changes may be isolated or associated with other changes in the superficial vasculature and may indicate either inflammation or stasis-congestion.

Lymphatic Microcysts. Small, whitish, glassy formations, similar to the head of a pin and containing liquid, are often found on the surface of a cirrhotic liver. Frequently numerous, they are found primarily near the hepatic margins. These are the so-called lymphatic microcysts (Plates 54–14, 54–18). They resemble tubercular nodules, and careful examination is required for this differentiation. Lymphatic microcysts are not visible at autopsy and are, therefore, a laparoscopic finding only. They form as a result of parenchymal induration that blocks normal lymph drainage. Microcysts are found in other forms of hepatic sclerosis, although they are

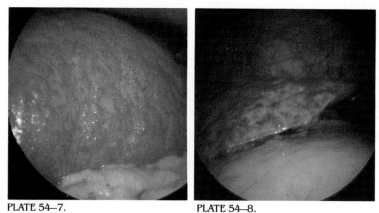

PLATE 54—7.   PLATE 54—8.

PLATE 54—7. Hypertrophic micronodular cirrhosis. There is a marked increase in thickness of the left lobe with rounded margins. Fine nodules are present.
PLATE 54—8. Atrophic mixed cirrhosis. The thin left lobe is evidently rigid, as it no longer rests on the underlying stomach.

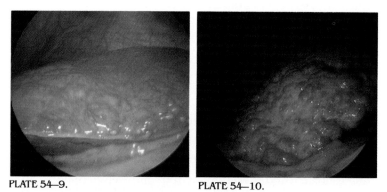

PLATE 54—9.   PLATE 54—10.

PLATE 54—9. Mixed cirrhosis. Nodules are clearly elevated. Margin is bordered by a thin white fibrous band.
PLATE 54—10. Mixed cirrhosis. The irregular margin of the left lobe is composed of nodules.

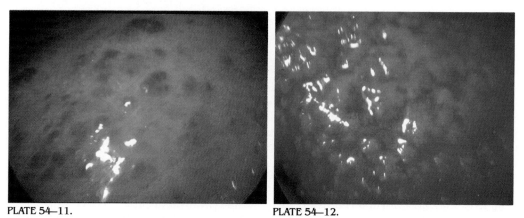

PLATE 54—11.   PLATE 54—12.

PLATE 54—11. Chronic diffuse perihepatitis. Extreme right lobe capsular thickening. Only small areas of parenchyma can be visualized.
PLATE 54—12. Micromedionodular cirrhosis. There is a remarkable degree of active congestion in this view of the right lobe.

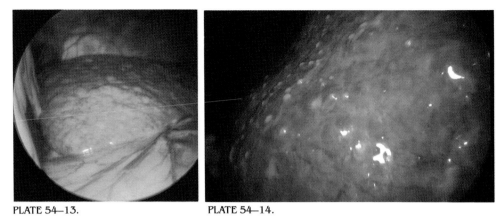

PLATE 54–13.   PLATE 54–14.

PLATE 54–13. Fatty micromedionodular cirrhosis. The left lobe is bright yellow.
PLATE 54–14. Hypertrophic micronodular cirrhosis. Rusty brown overtones indicate secondary hemochromatosis of the right lobe. Numerous lymphatic microcysts are present.

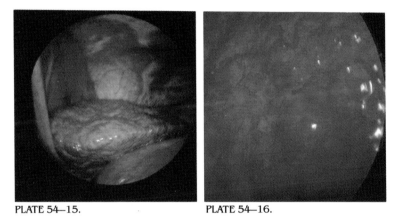

PLATE 54–15.   PLATE 54–16.

PLATE 54–15. Micromedionodular cirrhosis. The green left lobe indicates diffuse and marked cholestasis. Congestion and inflammation of the gastric serosa are seen in the foreground, and there is intense congestion of the diaphragmatic parietal peritoneum, which is covered with extensive fibrinous whitish plaques. This patient had associated spontaneous bacterial peritonitis.
PLATE 54–16. Micromedionodular cirrhosis. Small capsular vessels are developed to a marked degree on the right lobe.

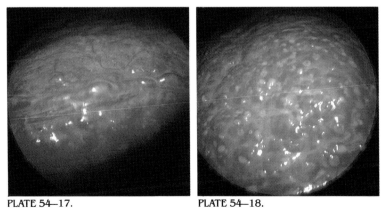

PLATE 54–17.   PLATE 54–18.

PLATE 54–17. Hypertrophic micromedionodular cirrhosis. The margin of the left lobe is thickened and lymphatic vessels are distended. There is stasis in the small veins.
PLATE 54–18. Micromedionodular cirrhosis. Lymphatic microcysts are numerous in the left lobe.

---

fairly indicative of cirrhosis and can be used as supporting evidence of the diagnosis when other evidence is less than certain.

Gallbladder Changes

In hepatic cirrhosis, as in other chronic hepatic diseases, gallbladder changes are a common, although inconsistent, finding. The gallbladder may be normal greenish-blue with a thin wall, or the wall may be thickened, whitish (Plate 54–2), and edematous. Owing to dysfunctional emptying, the gallbladder may be dilated, but there is never the extremely tense wall found with distal obstruction of the biliary system (see Chapter 52). Although tense, the wall is easily indented with the palpating probe. In some cases the organ is small with a thickened wall. Alterations of the parietal vasculature of the gallbladder may be observed: either a diffuse reddening due to active congestion or enlargement and turgor of the small veins as a result of venous stasis.

Signs of Portal Hypertension

The earliest signs of portal hypertension in the form of collateral circulations in the small peritoneal vessels can be revealed by laparoscopy. These require a careful search with shifting of the patient to appropriate decubitus positions that reveal the sectors of the abdominal wall where portacaval anastomoses exist that permit formation of collateral channels.

The earliest findings are collateral small vessels that are seen only by laparoscopy. Other techniques, such as arteriography and sonography, visualize only larger caliber vessels that, when dilated, are a later manifestation of portal hypertension. The earliest evidence of collateral circulation occurs in the various sectors of the accessory portal system, the phrenocolic ligament, and the system of Retzius. Collateral vessels can also be found on adhesions between the visceral and parietal peritoneum. These findings are most useful in supporting a diagnosis of cirrhosis when the diagnosis is otherwise uncertain.

Ascites

Laparoscopy reveals even small amounts of ascites that are not clinically apparent in cirrhosis, another useful finding that supports the diagnosis. Ultrasonography also demonstrates small amounts of fluid in the abdomen, and this has decreased the importance of laparoscopy in this respect. Laparoscopy not only demonstrates the presence of ascites, but permits the aspiration of samples of the fluid even when the most minimal volume is present. This greatly enhances diagnosis by allowing complete characterization of the ascites (see Chapter 55).

Etiology of Cirrhosis

The etiology of cirrhosis is usually determined by combined epidemiologic, clinical, and histologic investigations.[3] We believe that laparoscopy is also indispensable, since this is the only method of defining the macroscopic character of the lesions and following their evolution during the course of the disease.

Cirrhosis is the end stage of many different hepatic disorders. At this final stage several alterations can lose their specificity. The morphology may also be profoundly changed by diverse associated or superimposed cirrhogenic factors, as frequently occurs with alcoholism and viral hepatitis. However, some laparoscopic findings remain that may suggest an etiology. The list of possible etiologic factors in cirrhosis proposed by Anthony et al.[3] will be used as a point of reference (Table 54–1).

Venous outflow obstruction (veno-occlusive disease, Budd-Chiari syndrome) and prolonged severe cardiac stasis produce progressive hepatic alterations known as cardiac cirrhosis. This form does not, however, have the characteristics of a true cirrhosis. Rather,

TABLE 54–1. **Etiologic Factors in Cirrhosis**

A. Cirrhosis with established etiologic associations:
  1. Viral hepatitis
  2. Alcoholism
  3. Metabolic disorders (e.g., hemochromatosis, Wilson's disease, alpha$_1$-antitrypsin deficiency, type IV glycogenosis, galactosemia)
  4. Biliary disease (intrahepatic and extrahepatic)
  5. Venous outflow obstruction (veno-occlusive disease, Budd-Chiari syndrome)
  6. Toxins and therapeutic drugs (e.g., certain pyrrolizidine alkaloids with allyl side chains, methotrexate, oxyphenisatin, alpha-methyldopa)
  7. Intestinal bypass operations for obesity
  8. Other (e.g., sarcoidoses)

B. Debatable etiologic factors:
  1. Autoimmunity
  2. Mycotoxins
  3. Schistosomiasis
  4. Malnutrition
  5. Others

C. Cirrhosis of unknown etiology:
  1. With well-defined pattern—Indian childhood cirrhosis
  2. Without well-defined pattern—"cryptogenic" cirrhosis

Adapted from Anthony et al.[3]

there are features of hepatic fibrosis: the liver is enlarged, the capsule is often thickened (Plate 54–19), and the surface, which is wine red, is rough or granular but lacks true regenerative nodules (Plate 54–20). In our opinion, venous stasis alone will not cause cirrhosis unless associated with other etiologic factors.

A causal relationship between cirrhosis and toxins and therapeutic drugs has not been demonstrated. We have studied many patients when they are undergoing polychemotherapy, at the end of such therapy, and after lapses of months and years, and have observed hepatic disease and hepatic sclerosis, often severe, with extensive scarring and prominent parenchymal atrophy. But we have never positively identified regenerative nodules in these patients and have therefore never found an example of cirrhosis.

Experience with laparoscopy in patients who have undergone intestinal bypass surgery is extremely limited.

We have occasionally observed a granulomatous hepatitis in sarcoidosis, in which the liver is indurated with a surface that is grossly altered by numerous and deep scars. However, this appearance differs from true cirrhosis, which, according to our own experience and that of others,[4, 5] is not found in sarcoidosis. Evidence of portal hypertension can nevertheless be found in these forms.[5]

With regard to debatable etiologic factors as a category of Anthony et al.,[3] there are no specific laparoscopic findings for these factors. Malnutrition has been recognized as a cause of cirrhosis. Some of the characteristics of these conditions can be considered along with alcoholism. Cirrhosis of unknown etiology, very common in our experience, clearly cannot present characteristic laparoscopic findings.

The established associations between etiologic factors and cirrhosis include alcoholism, viral hepatitis, metabolic disorders, and biliary disease.

Alcoholism

Alcoholic cirrhosis is generally characterized by a regular, dense nodulation with small and medium-sized elements. The nodules are homogeneously distributed and separated by thin septa. This is the appearance of a micronodular or septal cirrhosis (Plates 54–1, 54–3).

Steatosis is a common, perhaps obligatory, finding in cirrhosis, which gives the liver a yellow tone. Alcoholic cirrhosis is sometimes indifferently referred to as micronodular, septal, or fatty. However, fatty accumulation is not extensive enough in all cases to justify the use of this last term. True fatty cirrhosis is characterized by a large, rigid liver with small, regular nodules. The organ is overtly yellow, often with pink or bright yellow-orange spots and variegations that result from a combination of yellow nodules and the cinnabar red background produced by inflammatory necrosis (Plate 54–21). Fatty cirrhosis is characteristic of alcoholic cirrhosis, and this appearance is the most specific finding for this disorder.

The laparoscopic finding of cirrhosis without nodules is also suggestive of alcoholic cirrhosis. These smooth or glabrous forms, which often have an important component of steatosis (Plate 54–5), are almost always a result of alcoholism, and in such cases an alcoholic etiology is highly probable.

Another finding that suggests alcoholism as the cause of cirrhosis is iron accumulation, which appears as a rust brown overtone (Plate 54–14). This secondary accumulation of iron in association with cirrhosis must not be confused with that of the primary hemochromatosis, which has different characteristics and a different significance (see below).

Viral Hepatitis

Cirrhosis as a result of viral hepatitis is more often macronodular or "post-necrotic," a form that is easily recognized by direct observation. There are large or enormous nodules and extensive scarring that corresponds to the cirrhotic evolution of a massive hepatitis with extensive necrosis (Plates 54–2, 54–6). In pure forms of viral induced post-necrotic cirrhosis, steatosis is absent.

The laparoscopic findings described above for alcohol-related and viral-related cirrhosis are the typical, perhaps theoretic, appearances. It cannot be said, however, as some have affirmed, that the "small and medium nodule" or "septal" forms are synonymous with nutritional/alcoholic cirrhosis or that the macronodular appearance must necessarily be the result of a viral hepatitis with necrosis. Apart from the etiologic associations, micronodular forms can, in fact, be observed in cases with a viral etiology, and macronodular forms may be produced by alcoholism alone. An etiologic diagnosis is particularly difficult when regular small and medium-sized nodules surrounded by narrow septa are associated with vast, irregular, and retracted scars and large nodules that have a clearly post-necrotic aspect (Plate 54–22). The systematic use of laparoscopy documents the occurrence of innumerable transitional forms of cirrhosis. This phenomenon can be explained by repetitive episodes of extensive necrosis against a background of micronodular cirrhosis, which are due to recurrent alcoholic injury or superimposed episodes of hepatitis that result in extensive, profound scars. These macroscopic findings of a "mixed" cirrhosis do not permit conclusions as to the original etiology of the disorder.

Metabolic Disorders

Some metabolic disorders cause forms of cirrhosis that have particular macroscopic characteristics that permit accurate diagnosis at laparoscopy. Most importantly, the cirrhosis of Wilson's disease and hemochromatosis can be identified. However, other varieties in this category of disorders do not have distinguishing macroscopic characteristics, although one distinctive form of cirrhosis not included in the list of Anthony et al.[3] is that which can develop in "porphyria cutanea tarda."

Hemochromatosis. As noted, alcoholic cirrhosis may be accompanied by hemosiderin deposition in hepatocytes. This presents as a classic cirrhosis, i.e., an atrophic or mildly hypertrophic liver generally with small and medium-sized nodules and a characteristic rust brown color. Depending on the amount of iron and the existence of associated phenomena such as steatosis, inflammatory reactions, or connective tissue proliferation, the color may vary toward yellow, red, or gray.

The hepatic pathology caused by a primary disorder in iron metabolism has substantially different laparoscopic features. There is always an enormous hepatomegaly with a substantial increase in the thickness of the liver. The surface is uniformly granular or rough and brown with rust overtones (Plate 54–23). Sometimes a grayish connective tissue in a web-like pattern can be seen but without much tendency to retraction.

Another differential point revealed only by laparoscopy is the finding of portal hypertension. In secondary iron deposition the disease is a true cirrhosis, and therefore collateral circulations are often found in the various possible sites. With primary hemochromatosis, even when severe or in the late stages, the finding of portal hypertension is exceptional.

Wilson's Disease. In the early stages of the cirrhosis of Wilson's disease typical lesions will be present that are easily recognized at laparoscopy. However, this disease evolves over a long period and findings will change with the duration. At first the liver is enlarged with a smooth, reddish surface that is covered with numerous spots 5 to 10 mm in diameter that are dark bluish and either flat or slightly raised. In the later stages these lesions, which are uniformly distributed, become nodular and retain the dark coloration at their apices. The connective tissue component of the disease is not well developed, as is evident from the brown-red color of the liver and from the barely increased firmness in the consistency of the parenchyma (Plate 54–24).

Porphyria Cutanea Tarda. Chronic hepatic disease is almost always present in porphyria cutanea tarda. A true cirrhosis occurs in about 30%, and this can be diagnosed laparoscopically.[6] The appearance is that of a micronodular cirrhosis that is distinguished by the gray-blue color of the nodules, particularly of their central raised areas. Macroscopically, the appearance resembles Wilson's disease, but the differential diagnosis is easy because of the red fluorescence of the hepatic tissue under ultraviolet light in porphyria. This will be revealed by illumination with a Wood's lamp.

Biliary Disease

Cirrhosis secondary to biliary disease can have macroscopic characteristics that suggest an etiology. The principal finding, related to cholestasis, is the coloration, which varies from gray to dark green depending on the degree of stasis.

When presented with such an appearance, the differential diagnosis includes the following: (1) A common cirrhosis in which the cholestasis is not etiologic but secondary to associated pathology such as an acute hepatitis (either viral or alcoholic), hepatic failure, or mechanical obstruction; (2) a secondary biliary cirrhosis or pure cholestatic cirrhosis caused by prolonged extrahepatic obstruction, e.g., by calculi or biliary stricture; (3) a cholangitic cirrhosis as a consequence of a chronic inflammatory process of the intrahepatic biliary tree; and (4) primary biliary cirrhosis. It may be difficult to distinguish the exact cause, and the differential points can be subtle. In some cases laparoscopy reveals useful, at times decisive, information. In other cases it is less advantageous or may not be beneficial.

Common cirrhosis with superimposed cholestasis can be diagnosed when the typical

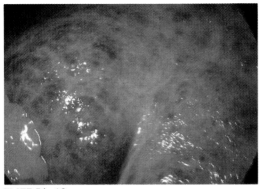

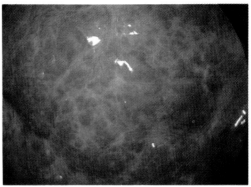

PLATE 54—19.

PLATE 54—20.

PLATE 54—19. "Cardiac cirrhosis." Capsular thickening and fibrosis are present.
PLATE 54—20. "Cardiac cirrhosis." There is venous stasis, and the surface of the liver is rough and fibrotic although without real regenerative nodules.

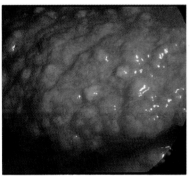

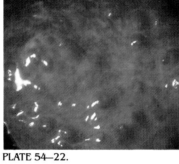

PLATE 54—21. Hypertrophic alcoholic fatty cirrhosis. Yellow nodules are seen.
PLATE 54—22. Mixed cirrhosis. Detailed view of nodules of various dimensions as well as large areas of scar tissue.

PLATE 54—21.

PLATE 54—22.

PLATE 54—23. Primary hemochromatosis. There is marked hepatomegaly. The left lobe is increased in thickness with rounded margins and a rough surface. Note brown coloration.
PLATE 54—24. Cirrhosis in Wilson's disease.

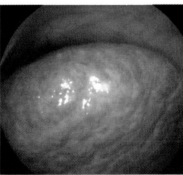

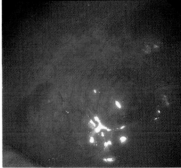

PLATE 54—23.

PLATE 54—24.

and characteristic findings of cirrhosis are present and the nodules are "tattooed" with green. However, when there is a regular nodularity and a diffuse and intense green color, it is difficult to distinguish cirrhosis with superimposed cholestasis from a primary cholestatic cirrhosis. Other signs, direct or indirect, may confirm the existence of obstruction, e.g., evidence of a primary carcinoma of the gallbladder; an enlarged, tense gallbladder as a sign of distal bile duct obstruction; an empty, collapsed gallbladder as evidence of proximal biliary obstruction; or hepatic or peritoneal metastases.

Cholangitic biliary cirrhosis results from an inflammatory process of the intrahepatic biliary ducts. At laparoscopy the color of the liver varies from brown to green, but it often has a gray hue because of capsular thickening. The capsular changes may take the form of wide bands or deep, retracted, and congested strips, sometimes with associated adhesions (Plate 54–25). These findings are the result of repeated and protracted inflammation of the superficial bile canaliculi and the surrounding hepatic tissue with scar tissue repair of the necrotic areas. Eventually alterations of the gallbladder also occur, including chronic inflammation, retraction, thickening of the wall, congestion, and adhesions between the gallbladder and neighboring structures.

The appearance of the liver in primary biliary cirrhosis varies with the stage of the disease, although there are no specific characteristics that permit laparoscopic diagnosis. The liver may be enlarged and hard, with alterations that resemble congestive changes. Or the surface may be almost unchanged, showing only the disappearance of the lobular design. There may be nodules that are barely visible or obvious. The stippled green color of cholestasis can also be present (Plate 54–26). In general, laparoscopy, insofar as macroscopic findings are concerned, does not contribute to the diagnosis.

Laparoscopic Liver Biopsy

The histologic confirmation of alterations in the hepatic architecture characterized by parenchymal destruction, fibrosis, and regenerative nodules is the basis for the morphologic diagnosis of cirrhosis. It has long been recognized that in series of patients the results of transcutaneous biopsy (the more frequently used procedure) differ significantly from those of laparoscopic biopsy.

Transcutaneous Biopsy

In 1973 Lindner[7] claimed that "percutaneous biopsy alone carries an unacceptably high risk of diagnostic error." This conclusion was based on his vast experience, a review of the literature,[8–10] and the results of a questionnaire sent to all German-speaking hepatologists in 1971. In a total of 33,372 cases, there was an incomplete or mistaken diagnosis in 15% to 50% in relation to cirrhosis, the highest error rate being found in the macronodular forms.

There are two reasons for discrepancies between the results of laparoscopic and percutaneous biopsies. The sample obtained with the biopsy needle may be small and often fragmented and precludes adequate study of the hepatic architecture.[11, 12] The needle may penetrate uninvolved areas or regenerative nodules (Plate 54–27), so that the microscopic appearance of the sample is normal (false negative). Or an area of trivial capsular fibrosis, the result of an insignificant local process, may be sampled with the needle, in which case the microscopic appearance may give the false impression of cirrhosis (false positive). Anthony et al.[3] have observed that "the needle of Menghini tends to aspirate soft liver parenchyma preferentially, leaving the tougher connective tissue behind." This is a particular problem when nodules are large. The histologic diagnosis of cirrhosis based on blind transcutaneous biopsy is therefore unreliable to a certain degree.

Pagliaro et al.[13] randomized 126 patients with a clinical diagnosis of chronic diffuse liver disease to either percutaneous liver biopsy (64 patients) or laparoscopy with guided biopsy (62 patients). The presence of cirrhosis was either recognized or eliminated in 82% of patients in the percutaneous biopsy group. The presence or absence of cirrhosis was correctly recognized by guided laparoscopic biopsy in all cases. The difference in these results was statistically significant. The inaccurate events in the percutaneous biopsy group were mostly false-negative results.

Nord[12] compared the accuracy of blind percutaneous biopsy with that of guided laparoscopic biopsy in a review of the literature. He pointed out that the number of studies available for review was small and many had shortcomings. Newer types of cutting biopsy needles were not used in any of the studies reviewed. The mean false-negative rate with the blind percutaneous biopsy was 24%; the mean false-negative rate for guided laparoscopic biopsy was virtually the same at 25% (range 7% to 51%). The false-negative rate for laparoscopic diagnosis averaged 9% (range 4% to 18%), but when laparoscopic diagnosis was combined with histologic evaluation of biopsies, the accuracy was greater than that for blind biopsy alone.

Laparoscopic Biopsy

New Techniques

The complications of liver biopsy include hemorrhage and bile leakage. Hemorrhage can be stopped at laparoscopy with various maneuvers, including compression with the palpation probe, instillation of coagulants, .

and diathermy electrocoagulation. Biopsy accidents are nevertheless dangerous. Bile leakage that cannot be arrested with these methods may occur (laparoscopic complications are discussed in Chapter 51). The complication rate in our series is similar to that reported elsewhere.[14-16] Until December 1981 we obtained biopsies of the liver on 8321 occasions in a total of 8828 laparoscopy procedures. There were 9 serious episodes of hemorrhage (0.11%) that resulted in the deaths of 2 patients and serious bile leakage in 2 patients (0.02%) with 1 death.[17]

In order to deal with laparoscopic accidents without resorting to surgery we have developed a simple instrument, the "bioplug," that permits the introduction of a compressed fibrin plug into the biopsy hole through the laparoscope (Plate 54–28). This plug is capable of immediately blocking both bleeding and bile leaks. In our more recent experience with 3347 biopsy procedures we have had no further complications.[18, 19] Undoubtedly, techniques such as this reduce the risk of guided laparoscopic liver biopsy, probably to a level that is less than the complication rate for blind percutaneous biopsy.

The development of cutting biopsy instruments is an interesting technical advance, especially in relation to cirrhosis. With this type of needle, which has almost completely replaced the aspiration type, a regular and integral sample (a 2 to 3 cm cylinder) can almost always be obtained, even when the parenchyma is very hard, as in cirrhosis.[20] This method provides the best possible specimen for histologic evaluation (see Chapter 50 for a discussion of biopsy techniques).

We have compared the results of biopsies obtained with a Menghini needle during laparoscopy in 224 cases of chronic hepatic disease with the results in 311 cases in which biopsies were obtained with a cutting needle.[21] In the Menghini needle group 14% of the samples were inadequate and did not permit a diagnosis, whereas in the cutting needle group the percentage of inadequate specimens decreased to 4%.

Multiple Biopsies

During laparoscopy, multiple specimens can be taken from any area of the right and left hepatic lobes without increasing patient discomfort. More abundant pathologic material from different areas of the liver makes histologic diagnosis more precise than is possible with a single sample. The advantages of multiple biopsies are evident and well recognized by those who regularly perform lap-

aroscopies.[1, 11, 12] The value of multiple specimens without laparoscopy has also been recognized.[22, 23] However, the ease with which two, three, or more biopsies can be obtained during laparoscopy in exactly the points chosen, including the left lobe, as well as a more random sampling of the liver when necessary, makes this method preferable to the less precise method of several passes with a needle through the same percutaneous puncture site.

Guided Biopsies

Precise selection of tissue samples is the principal advantage of guided laparoscopic biopsy. Its greatest importance is in relation to focal processes. However, even with diffuse hepatic disease it is important to select the most representative area for the biopsy. One of the major difficulties with blind biopsies is that the sample may come from a part of the liver in which the process is less well developed or the changes are insignificant. Even those diseases that are customarily considered diffuse, especially chronic hepatic disease and cirrhosis, are not evenly developed throughout the entire liver. Although small biopsy specimens will generally be representative of certain diffuse processes, such as fatty metamorphosis and acute hepatitis, sampling errors are more likely to occur in less diffuse diseases in which changes are patchy, such as chronic hepatitis and cirrhosis.[12] Laparoscopic observation has demonstrated that definitive cirrhotic nodules may be present in only one lobe or a part of a lobe, whereas alterations that are consistent with a diagnosis of chronic hepatic disease but not fibrosis are present in other zones (Plate 54–29).

For the reasons outlined above, the most reliable histologic diagnosis is achieved by obtaining specimens with a cutting biopsy needle at laparoscopy, taking samples from the most representative areas as well as multiple samples from different zones when necessary.

Indications for Laparoscopic Biopsy

Laparoscopic biopsy is indicated to establish or confirm a diagnosis, to determine the activity of a disease process, and to obtain information pertaining to the etiology of the disease.

Biopsy Diagnosis of Cirrhosis

There are inherent errors and uncertainties when the diagnosis of cirrhosis is based solely on laparoscopic evidence. This is particularly true when it is difficult to determine

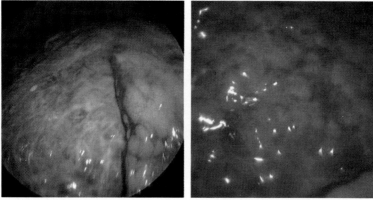

PLATE 54–25.   PLATE 54–26.

PLATE 54–25. Cholangitic secondary biliary cirrhosis. The right lobe is green, and there are clearly visible nodules and linear scars with signs of active inflammation. The omentum is partially adherent to the liver.
PLATE 54–26. Primary biliary cirrhosis. Cirrhosis is fully developed with evident nodules and congestion.

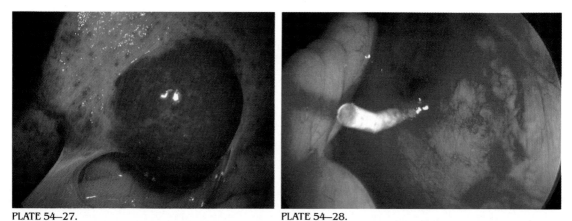

PLATE 54–27.   PLATE 54–28.

PLATE 54–27. Vast areas of scarring and large regenerative nodules are present on the hepatic surface. Biopsy results will vary with the sample chosen.
PLATE 54–28. Mononodular primary liver cancer. This tumor is highly vascularized. A "bioplug" has been introduced into the site to arrest bleeding.

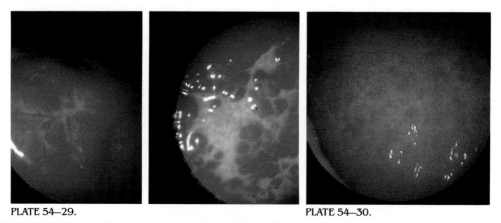

PLATE 54–29.   PLATE 54–30.

PLATE 54–29. Cirrhosis with limited nodules. The left lobe (left) has a smooth, congested surface with retracted scars. Biopsy showed chronic active hepatitis. The right lobe (right) shows areas of scarring and regenerative nodules. The biopsy specimen revealed cirrhosis.
PLATE 54–30. Laparoscopic findings do not permit a macroscopic differentiation between hepatitis and cirrhosis.

whether the surface is smooth or nodular, and made even more difficult if nodules are scarce or absent. The pathologist may also be faced with uncertainties and dubious situations, and the diagnosis based on histologic findings may be at odds with the laparoscopic assessment. However, combining the results of macroscopic evaluation and histologic examination provides the most certain diagnosis.[8, 13, 24–26] Macroscopic and histologic findings must be complementary,[24] but complete agreement between the two parameters is found in only 49% to 89% of cases. The differences probably relate to subjective judgment[27] but also to the precision of diagnostic criteria, both microscopic and laparoscopic, and the degree of morphologic evidence produced by the evolving cirrhosis.

Ideally, there will be complete agreement between histologic and laparoscopic findings, in which case the diagnosis is certain. When the conclusions drawn from each method of assessment differ, however, which should be considered most indicative of the state of the liver? Based on our experience,[21] several scenarios are possible when laparoscopy is performed in cases of chronic hepatic disease to determine whether cirrhosis is present.

1. The concordance between biopsy results and laparoscopy diagnosis will be high in cases in which diffuse nodules are evident. The laparoscopy diagnosis will be cirrhosis, and the biopsy will reveal at least one regenerative nodule surrounded by fibrous tissue and will confirm the diagnosis in 80% of cases (Fig. 54–1).

2. When laparoscopy discloses definite nodules, but with localization of the findings of cirrhosis to one lobe or part of a lobe, the biopsy from this area will reveal cirrhosis in more than 80% of cases (Fig. 54–1).

3. When the liver surface is smooth and regular or slightly irregular (rough, scarred) in limited areas or there is evidence of steatosis, cirrhosis cannot be diagnosed by observation alone. Histologic results confirm the absence of cirrhosis in 62% of such cases, render an "uncertain" (altered structure without evidence of nodules) result in 27%, and indicate cirrhosis in the remaining 11% (Fig. 54–1).

4. When the liver surface is diffusely irregular (grooved, undulating, rough) or when nodules are not clearly evident, the laparoscopic diagnosis is hepatic sclerosis, "doubtful" or "uncertain" (Plate 54–30). The biopsy results will be consistent with these uncertain findings in 45% of cases, will demonstrate cirrhosis in 35%, and will not demonstrate any evidence of cirrhosis in the remaining 20% (Fig. 54–1).

In summary, the importance of the biopsy result in the diagnosis of cirrhosis must be considered with respect to the general principle that, when faced with two opposing results, the positive finding (cirrhosis) should be given precedence and the negative finding discounted. The importance of biopsy is therefore inversely proportional to the significance of laparoscopic findings and vice versa. The concordance between the laparoscopy and the biopsy findings in cases in which

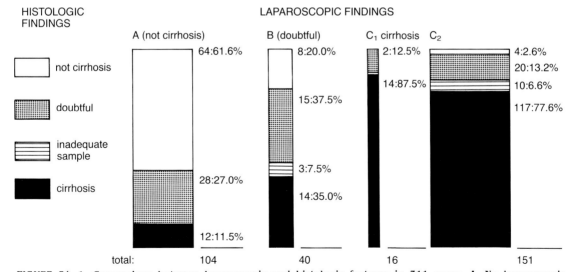

FIGURE 54–1. Comparison between laparoscopic and histologic features in 311 cases. A, No laparoscopic evidence of cirrhosis; B, laparoscopic findings reveal "doubtful" or "uncertain" cirrhosis; C₁, cirrhosis in a limited area of the liver; C₂, generalized "diffuse" cirrhosis.

nodules are evident at laparoscopy practically eliminates the value of histologic examination.[1, 21, 28] If the biopsy fails to disclose cirrhosis, the possibility of a false-negative result must be considered. Therefore, when the macroscopic diagnosis of cirrhosis is certain, biopsy may be superfluous, and when coagulation parameters are markedly abnormal, biopsy can and should be avoided. Conversely, histologic findings must be considered definitive when cirrhosis is demonstrated in a liver that at laparoscopy appears to be free of cirrhosis with a smooth surface or with indefinite nodules. In the latter case multiple biopsies should always be obtained in diverse parts of the organ.

Evaluation of Disease Activity

The activity of cirrhosis is judged histologically by the extent and severity of necrosis and the consequent inflammatory reaction (round cell infiltration of the portal spaces, areas of fibrosis, etc.). Histologic assessment of activity, although interesting, does not have absolute value. Often this does not correspond to the clinical and laboratory evaluation of disease activity. This is explained by the fact that the activity of the disease may vary from area to area and one small sample is not necessarily representative.[29] The biopsy may also reveal changes due to secondary phenomena in the course of cirrhosis, e.g., infection, ischemic necrosis, and biliary obstruction.

Etiologic Diagnosis

It would be inappropriate to attempt a complete discussion of the causes of cirrhosis. However, some of the essential facts will be presented in relation to what has been said about macroscopic findings. Histologic study is important for confirmation of laparoscopic findings that are considered indicative of a pathologic process. It may specify the type of lesion and define severity and/or extent. Histologic study may also add information over and above that obtained by macroscopic examination that substantiates the diagnosis or suggests an etiology when laparoscopy fails to indicate a cause.

Supporting evidence for a laparoscopic diagnosis of alcoholic cirrhosis includes the micronodular pattern, steatosis, and, in later stages, hemosiderosis. More characteristic of alcoholic liver disease are features of alcoholic hepatitis, including swelling of hepatocytes, focal infiltration, and Mallory's hyalin. The last is not always present nor specific for an alcohol-induced process.

The diagnosis of post-hepatitis cirrhosis is facilitated by demonstration of hepatitis B surface antigen with immunofluorescence and immunoperoxidases, although the antigen is not invariably present. Other significant findings are ground-glass hepatocytes and intense inflammatory activity.

The laparoscopic features of primary hemochromatosis are confirmed by histologic findings: an increase in portal fibrosis and the formation of septa with hemosiderin accumulation in hepatocytes and phagocytes. The parenchyma is almost unaltered, and there is a low level of inflammatory activity. The particular histologic feature of Wilson's disease is the demonstration of copper accumulation in the nodules.

In primary biliary cirrhosis there are no characteristic laparoscopic features so that the diagnosis depends on biopsy. The lesion, which changes during the course of the disease, involves the portal spaces. The bile ducts are hyperplastic or necrotic and are surrounded by a dense infiltration of lymphocytes, plasma cells, eosinophils, and granuloma-type epithelioid cells. Later, in the frankly cirrhotic stage, the space is replaced by connective tissue, the bile ducts disappear, and new perilobular ducts are formed (Hering's ducts). The histologic picture is practically pathognomonic but difficult to recognize with one small needle biopsy. Although observations made at laparoscopy are not particularly useful for diagnosis, the procedure does permit more extensive sampling of the liver vis-à-vis multiple biopsies.

Histologic findings do not add important information to the laparoscopic diagnosis of secondary biliary cirrhosis. In general, other methods of establishing the presence and cause of biliary obstruction are preferred. For these reasons, and especially because of the risk of bile leakage, biopsy is usually not advisable when laparoscopic findings clearly indicate secondary biliary cirrhosis.

Laparoscopic Classification of Cirrhosis

The cirrhoses have been classified with reference to pathogenesis, morphologic findings, and eponyms.[30–32] The liver undergoes many progressive morphologic alterations in the long, complex evolution of cirrhosis from the earliest stages to the death of the patient. The morphologic categories of cirrhosis do not represent specific diseases, but rather

TABLE 54–2. **Laparoscopic Classification of Liver Cirrhosis**

Based on nodularity
 Size of the nodules
  Micro- and medionodular cirrhosis
  Macronodular cirrhosis
  Mixed cirrhosis
 Extent of nodule formation
  Diffuse nodulation
  Limited nodulation
 No evidence of nodules
  With other laparoscopic signs of cirrhosis:
   "Glabrous" cirrhosis
  Without other laparoscopic signs of cirrhosis:
   "Histologic" cirrhosis

Based on liver size
 Hypertrophic cirrhosis
 Atrophic cirrhosis
 Atrophic-hypertrophic cirrhosis

Based on possible etiology
 Alcoholic cirrhosis
 Post-hepatic cirrhosis
 Metabolic disorders
  Hemochromatosis
   Primary
   Secondary
  Wilson's disease
  Porphyria cutanea tarda
 Biliary disease
  Primary biliary cirrhosis
  Secondary biliary cirrhosis
   Cholestatic
   Cholangiolitic

different stages and forms of a single process.[3, 31] Our system, based on laparoscopic findings, resembles a postmortem classification, the main elements being nodularity, the size of the liver, and suggested etiology (Table 54–2).

Nodularity

The following features should be assessed regarding the nodularity of the liver in cirrhosis (Table 54–2): (1) absence of nodules, (2) extent of nodule formation (from scattered to diffuse), and (3) nodule size. These will be considered in reverse order.

Size

The classification of cirrhosis as micronodular and macronodular is almost universally accepted. In the micronodular form the nodules are small, less than 3 mm in diameter (Plates 54–3, 54–7). The term micronodular is preferred to all other synonyms, including septal, portal, mononodular, and Laennec's cirrhosis. The nodules of macronodular cirrhosis are more than 3 mm in diameter. They also have an irregular shape with septa and large areas of connective tissue (Plates 54–2,

54–6). The term macronodular should be used in preference to post-necrotic and irregular. The less well-established term of medionodular indicates nodules from 3 mm to 6 mm in diameter.[33] Aside from nodule size, the appearance of the medionodular form resembles that of micronodular cirrhosis. Large and small nodules may be present in about the same proportions, in which case the appearance may be classified as mixed. Large, irregular, deep scars are frequently present in the mixed form and are usually indicative of previous massive necrosis (Plates 54–9, 54–10, 54–22). The morphologic classification of cirrhosis according to nodule size must be based on gross observation because the macronodular and mixed forms cannot be recognized with certainty by needle biopsy alone.

There have been attempts to correlate the morphologic classification according to nodule size with prognosis. Harihara et al.[33] reported a 5-year survival rate of 70% for the micronodular forms, 14% for macronodular, and 42% in the mixed form. None of the patients with macronodular cirrhosis was alive after 10 years.

Extent of Nodule Formation

Conceptually, cirrhosis of the liver is a diffuse process that involves the entire organ. In many cases, however, this is not entirely true. Anthony et al.[3] stated that focal abnormalities, e.g., focal nodular hyperplasia, do not constitute cirrhosis. However, they added also that the nodules of cirrhosis do not develop simultaneously in all parts of the liver and that it would be extremely difficult to determine the exact time of onset of cirrhosis even if the virtual impossibility of continuous observation could be disregarded. Thus, the differentiation between precirrhotic lesions and frank cirrhosis is almost always imprecise. However, Scheuer[29] has written that "An impression may be gained that cirrhosis is at an early stage of development on the one hand, or fully developed on the other." Nevertheless, the diagnosis of the earliest stages of cirrhosis remains problematic, especially when based on the results of blind biopsy without the aid of macroscopic findings.

In about 10% of all cases of cirrhosis in our experience there are simultaneous and substantial differences in the laparoscopic findings between the two lobes of the liver. On the right, for example, the appearance may be that of simple chronic hepatitis; on

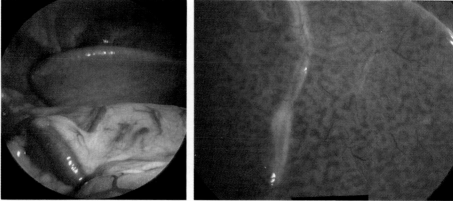

PLATE 54—31.   PLATE 54—32.

PLATE 54—31. Atrophic glabrous cirrhosis. There is no evidence of nodules on the left lobe although the consistency of the lobe was increased. The swollen mesenteric vein in the foreground indicates portal hypertension.
PLATE 54—32. Hepatic steatosis. The hepatic surface is smooth with an accentuated but regular lobular design. Biopsy demonstrated severe steatosis.

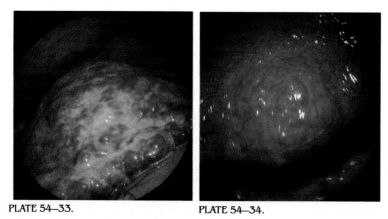

PLATE 54—33.   PLATE 54—34.

PLATE 54—33. Mononodular primary liver cancer with cirrhosis. A large mass occupies most of the right lobe.
PLATE 54—34. Micronodular cirrhosis. An elevated parenchymal nodule is seen. This could be primary liver cancer or hyperplasia. Biopsy revealed hyperplasia.

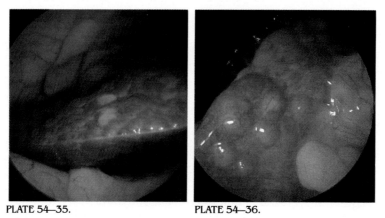

PLATE 54—35.   PLATE 54—36.

PLATE 54—35. Multinodular primary liver cancer with cirrhosis. Two barely elevated whitish tumor nodules are seen.
PLATE 54—36. Diffuse infiltrative primary liver cancer with cirrhosis. Some pale cirrhotic nodules with neoplastic infiltration are present.

the left cirrhotic nodulation may be evident (Plate 54–29). Biopsies confirmed the differences: specimens from the smooth right lobe revealing a chronic hepatitis or dubious changes of cirrhosis; those from the left lobe showing definite cirrhosis. Cirrhosis is not necessarily a uniform process, at least in its early stages.

These findings suggest the existence of another form of cirrhosis that could be termed "limited nodulation" in addition to the more common and classic "diffuse form" of nodulation. The former may represent one stage in the evolution of the disease. These "incomplete" cirrhoses might correspond to an early stage in the development of cirrhosis. Although the natural history and further evolution of limited and incomplete nodulation are not established, the identification of these forms could have a substantial prognostic significance if indeed these findings represent a true early stage of a disorder destined to evolve into cirrhosis. The value of laparoscopy in determining prognosis in such a circumstance should be obvious. Even when limited nodulation is present, the results of guided laparoscopic biopsies correlate with the laparoscopic findings (Plate 54–1).

No Evidence of Nodules

As emphasized above, in some cases cirrhosis can be found histologically, even though the surface of the liver is smooth at laparoscopy. The frequency of this occurrence ranges from a minimum of 0.5%[34] to a maximum of 5% to 10%.[28] In our classification scheme the forms of cirrhosis without visible nodules at laparoscopy should be further distinguished into two different types.

There may be other laparoscopic findings that suggest cirrhosis in some cases without nodules or with rare or poorly defined nodules. These findings include a firm consistency of the parenchyma to palpation, changes in the margin as described above, decreased volume, lymphatic microcysts, evidence of early portal hypertension, and small amounts of ascites. With experience, it is possible to diagnose cirrhosis by laparoscopy in such cases. This is the so-called smooth or "glabrous" form of cirrhosis (Plate 54–31).

In other cases of cirrhosis in which the surface is completely smooth and sometimes even shiny, the evidence of cirrhosis at laparoscopy may be very subtle. A loss of the normal lobular pattern on the surface may be found along with flat parenchymal spots

that are frequently associated with steatosis ("flat cirrhotic lesions") (Plate 54–5). The only other findings are an increase in volume and a firm consistency, elements that do not alone justify a diagnosis of cirrhosis. This appearance is very different from massive steatosis (Plate 54–32). Using strict criteria, cirrhosis cannot be diagnosed with these findings, and biopsies, preferably multiple, are necessary to establish that cirrhosis is present. We propose the classification of "histologic cirrhosis" in such cases, which constitute about 10% of cases in which the hepatic surface is smooth. The etiology of the cirrhosis in these cases is almost always alcoholic.

Liver Size

The cirrhotic liver may be termed hypertrophic, atrophic, or normotrophic with reference to changes in size. There is no general agreement that the distinction between atrophic (Plates 54–6, 54–31) and hypertrophic (Plates 54–7, 54–14, 54–17) cirrhosis is important. For example, the atrophic cirrhotic liver has been regarded as simply one possible outcome in the usual evolution of cirrhosis and a finding that has no significance. It is also believed that an estimate of the total volume of existing functional parenchyma is essential. Caroli et al.[35] confirmed the prognostic importance of a quantitative assessment of functioning liver tissue. In this view, the amount of hepatic tissue present is proportional to the size of the liver, and for this reason it is important to specify size in cirrhosis as normal, hypertrophic, or atrophic.

The trophic changes may be diffuse or one lobe may be atrophic, whereas the other lobe is normal or hypertrophic. Caroli et al.[35] classified these forms as "atrophic-hypertrophic."

Some authors have proposed a relationship between volume changes and prognosis. For example, Harihara et al.[33] reported a 5-year survival rate of 71% with right lobe hypertrophy and 30% with right lobe atrophy. The 10-year survival rates were 53% and 12%, respectively.

Etiology

It is possible to formulate a classification of cirrhosis based on etiology. However, this is not a true laparoscopic classification and requires the integration of macroscopic and histologic findings.

Cirrhosis and Primary Liver Cancer

The close relationship between cirrhosis and primary liver cancer is evident in clinical experience and autopsy studies.[36-41] There is also evidence of an increase in the frequency of this association[42, 43] Although liver tumors are discussed elsewhere (see Chapter 52), certain aspects that relate directly to cirrhosis will be considered here.

Frequency in Laparoscopic Experience

Primary liver tumors are found in 1% to 1.6% of all laparoscopies performed, depending on the population studied. From 66% to 95% are associated with cirrhosis.[34, 44-46] Carcinomas develop in about 7% of all cases of cirrhosis.[34] The most common type of primary liver cancer found with cirrhosis is hepatocarcinoma, which makes up about 93% of the total.

In a total of 10,000 laparoscopies, we have found 232 cases (2.3%) of primary cancer.[47, 48] Cirrhosis was present in 146 (63%) of these cases, and absent in 86 (37%). Primary liver carcinoma was the diagnosis in about 2772 cases of cirrhosis we observed from 1968 to 1982. The increasing incidence of these tumors cited in autopsy studies[38] is confirmed by laparoscopy.[44, 46] In our experience, carcinoma was encountered in 3.5% of all cases of cirrhosis in the 5-year period between 1968 and 1972. From 1973 to 1977 the incidence of primary liver carcinoma in cirrhotic patients was 6%. To some extent this may be attributed to improved diagnostic techniques, although there also appears to be a real increase in the incidence of primary liver carcinoma.

Unlike primary liver cancer unassociated with cirrhosis, the tumor when associated with cirrhosis is more common in men (about five times more common in our experience) and in the elderly. In the 40- to 45-year-old age group we have observed carcinoma in less than 2% of patients with cirrhosis. This increases to 10% between ages 55 and 60 with further increases being encountered beyond this age range.

We have not found a correlation between carcinoma and type of cirrhosis (micronodular or macronodular).

There is an established relationship between primary liver cancer and the hepatitis B virus.[41, 49, 50] For example, the results of a prospective multi-centered study conducted in Italy demonstrated a significant correlation with serologic hepatitis B virus markers, but not with alcohol abuse.[51]

Laparoscopic Findings and Diagnosis

Primary liver tumors assume one of the following macroscopic forms: (1) solitary nodule, (2) multiple nodules, and (3) diffuse infiltration. Primary hepatic carcinoma is also discussed in Chapter 52, but some laparoscopic features will be presented here along with an outline of relevant diagnostic problems.[36, 44-46, 52-56]

Solitary Nodule

A small or medium-sized node may be observed, or a solitary massive tumor may involve one lobe entirely with consequent enlargement and deformity. Diagnosis is not difficult when the tumor is superficial and is a hard, whitish-pink, yellowish, or variegated nodule (Plate 54–33), often with a marked vascular component (Plate 54–28). However, a small mononodular tumor can be a problem, since it may be easily confused with a hyperplastic nodule (Plate 54–34). A centrally located tumor can be especially problematic, since the lobe may be enlarged and/or deformed although the tumor is not visible. Surface changes such as venous congestion with accentuation of the lobular design and circumscribed, yellowish areas of steatosis are indirect evidence of its presence.

Multiple Nodules

The liver is covered with many raised nodules, varying from pea to walnut sizes in this form. The nodules are usually white and resemble lard (Plate 54–35), a characteristic appearance that makes diagnosis easy. Nevertheless, differentiating multinodular hepatocellular carcinoma from multiple metastatic nodules of another primary source can be difficult. Cholangiocarcinoma may have the morphologic features of metastases: raised nodes or flat plaques with central umbilication. However, the chance of an error in cases of cirrhosis is reduced by the fact that hepatic metastases in association with cirrhosis are rare (the ratio of primary to secondary cancer is 9 to 1 in our experience). Cholangiocarcinoma, the most likely metastatic lesion to cause such uncertainty in differential diagnosis, is rare in cirrhosis. Biopsy specimens usually provide a definitive diagnosis.

Diffuse Infiltration

This form of primary liver carcinoma is only found with cirrhosis. There is a more or less extensive infiltration of the parenchyma without evidence of well defined nodules.

The appearance varies. In some cases the liver is nodular, with small or medium-sized nodules, but some of these will be unlike regenerative nodules; they are hard and bright pinkish-white, sometimes with yellowish overtones. Although the form of the cirrhotic nodules is conserved, the elements are partially or completely replaced by neoplastic tissue (Plate 54–36). In other cases there is only a fine whitish network that may be thickened in places forming small, flat, white plaques. This appearance may be difficult to differentiate from insignificant capsular thickening. Only a biopsy specimen will confirm or eliminate a suspicion of cancer, but neoplastic infiltration must be suspected if a specimen is to be obtained from the proper place (Plate 54–37).

The Biopsy

A biopsy is the only method of obtaining an accurate and conclusive diagnosis, especially when macroscopic findings are subtle or uncertain (Plates 54–34, 54–38). There is usually not much risk in obtaining a biopsy. A large mass should be palpated with a probe first to determine whether it is soft and cystic as a result of liquefaction necrosis; puncture is dangerous in this circumstance. When the tumor is vascular, larger caliber vessels must be avoided as the biopsy is obtained. The risk of bleeding is reduced when a fibrin plug is inserted into the puncture tract (vide supra).

When a biopsy is obtained from clearly evident large nodules, the histologic results are reliable. The central portion of the nodule should be avoided, since this is frequently necrotic and neoplastic cells may be unrecognizable. Rather, the sample should be taken from the periphery of the lesion near the non-neoplastic hepatic parenchyma. When lesions are small, uncharacteristic, and/or deep to the surface, it may be difficult to select a proper biopsy site. Then the surface must be examined carefully with a high magnification laparoscope to locate suspicious areas and palpated with a probe to identify areas of increased firmness. Areas with a smooth surface that appears almost normal but lacks a lobular design should be considered with circumspection (Plate 54–39).

A biopsy should be taken from every suspicious point and inspected directly, preferably with a magnifying glass. If the specimen is whitish or variegated brown-red, it probably contains neoplastic tissue. Biopsies from the aforementioned normally colored, smooth areas will often have whitish tissue only in the portion from the deeper level of the liver.

Indications for Laparoscopy in Cirrhosis

The usual indications for laparoscopy in cirrhosis are confirmation of the diagnosis, determination of the type of cirrhosis, and investigation of portal hypertension. The second of these was discussed above.

Confirmation of the Diagnosis

It is useful to distinguish cases of cirrhosis with a complete and typical clinical pattern from those in which the picture is incomplete or atypical.

Complete and Typical Clinical Manifestations

When there are typical manifestations of frank cirrhosis, diagnosis is seemingly easy and laparoscopy superfluous. Nevertheless, when patients with a conclusive clinical diagnosis are studied by laparoscopy, a consistent rate of incorrect diagnoses will be found.

We performed laparoscopy for diagnostic confirmation in a series of 1079 patients who were thought to have cirrhosis on the basis of clinical and laboratory evidence. Cirrhosis was confirmed in 1015 patients. Of the others, 40 had chronic hepatic disease without cirrhosis, 6 had hepatocarcinoma, and 12 had various disorders of the liver, peritoneum, and other abdominal organs. In 6 patients the liver was apparently normal. This is not to suggest that laparoscopy must be performed in all cases in which cirrhosis is diagnosed on clinical and laboratory evidence, but when morphologic studies are considered necessary for precise diagnosis, laparoscopy is the most reliable and decisive means of obtaining the necessary information.

Laparoscopy is always indicated when the diagnosis of cirrhosis is uncertain: either the clinical manifestations and results of other methods of investigation do not permit a conclusive diagnosis, or the clinical findings are atypical and possibly attributable to other pathologic conditions.

Partial or Atypical Findings

Symptoms and Physical Findings. The classic clinical features of cirrhosis are so frequently absent that partially developed clinical manifestations are usual. Therefore, this cannot be considered atypical.

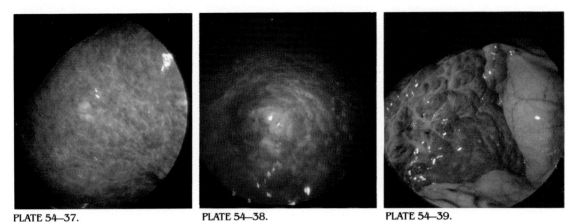

PLATE 54—37.   PLATE 54—38.   PLATE 54—39.

PLATE 54—37. Diffuse infiltrative primary liver cancer with cirrhosis. There is a thin white network and small flat plaques.
PLATE 54—38. Micronodular cirrhosis. An elevated parenchymal nodule could be a primary liver cancer. Biopsy revealed metastases from esophageal carcinoma.
PLATE 54—39. Mixed cirrhosis. An elevated area without nodules is present on the inferior surface of the right lobe. A guided biopsy demonstrated primary liver cancer.

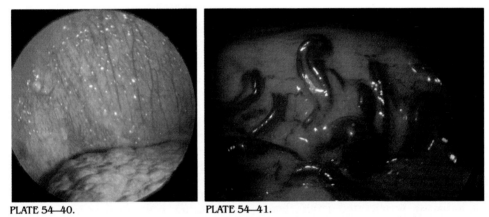

PLATE 54—40.   PLATE 54—41.

PLATE 54—40. Mixed cirrhosis. The falciform ligament in the background of this view of the left liver lobe appears congested, with numerous small granules that reflect the light. This finding was due to superimposed peritoneal miliary tuberculosis.
PLATE 54—41. Marked enlargement of the veins of the greater curvature of the stomach.

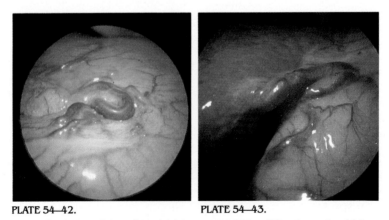

PLATE 54—42.   PLATE 54—43.

PLATE 54—42. Collateral circulation of the veins of the lesser curvature of the stomach, which are raised and distended.
PLATE 54—43. Markedly enlarged paraumbilical vein originates from the anterior and medial margin of the right lobe and enters the fat at the base of the round ligament.

The principal and most important atypical symptoms, which can be found in the same patient in various combinations, are abdominal pain, fever, jaundice, hepatomegaly, and variations in the characteristics of ascitic fluid that are not typical of cirrhosis (see Chapter 55). Clinical manifestations such as these may lead to other noninvasive examinations that in many patients reveal other associated disease(s). We have studied 139 patients with atypical presentations.[32] At laparoscopy 50% were found to have a simple cirrhosis; 50% had other associated or superimposed pathology. The results of this study are given in Table 54–3.

Abdominal pain, an unusual symptom in cirrhosis, and/or pain on palpation of the liver, an uncommon finding in uncomplicated cirrhosis, should lead to a suspicion of neoplasm. Pain may be episodic or continuous, the latter being more common when a neoplasm is the cause. Abdominal pain in conjunction with a clinical picture of cirrhosis is a strong indication for laparoscopy. Of 28 patients who underwent laparoscopy because of pain in a clinical setting of cirrhosis, 16 were found to have hepatocarcinoma (Table 54–3).

A prolonged fever with marked temperature elevation is not consistent with a diagnosis of simple cirrhosis. Associated inflammation of the gallbladder or peritoneum or a hepatic tumor was found in 50% of such cases (Table 54–3).

Jaundice associated with cirrhosis is usually mild and varies in intensity over the course of the disease, being more prominent during periods of hepatic insufficiency. This is supportive evidence of cirrhosis. However, deep, prolonged, and nonfluctuating jaundice that resembles cholestatic jaundice is atypical and requires further investigation. Laparoscopy may demonstrate simple cirrhosis with cholestasis, as was the case in 18 of 25 such patients in our series, although in 3 patients this type of jaundice was due to a primary or metastatic hepatic tumor (Table 54–3).

When the liver is enlarged, particularly to a marked degree with an irregular shape and hard consistency, further investigation is indicated, including laparoscopy. Cirrhosis alone, especially that due to alcoholism, may have these features, as was found in 39 of 63 patients with atypical hepatomegaly. However, in 15 of these patients laparoscopy revealed hepatocarcinoma (Table 54–3).

TABLE 54–3. **Laparoscopic Diagnosis of Liver Cirrhosis with Atypical Clinical Symptoms; 139 Cases**

Atypical Symptom or Finding	No.	Laparoscopic Diagnosis	
		Simple Cirrhosis	*Cirrhosis Complicated by*
Pain	12	5	Hepatocarcinoma (6)
			Chronic cholecystitis (1)
Pain/jaundice	3	2	Chronic cholecystitis (1)
Pain/fever	4	—	Hepatocarcinoma (3)
			Gallbladder hydrops (1)
Pain/atypical ascites	4	—	Hepatocarcinoma (2)
			Subacute nonspecific peritonitis (1)
			Peritoneal tuberculosis (1)
Pain/hepatomegaly	5	—	Hepatocarcinoma (5)
Fever	9	5	Chronic cholecystitis (2)
			Hepatocarcinoma (1)
			Gallbladder hydrops (1)
Fever/jaundice	1	1	—
Fever/atypical ascites	3	2	Peritoneal tuberculosis (1)
Fever/hepatomegaly	1	1	—
Jaundice	12	3	Hepatocarcinoma (2)
			Cholangitis (4)
			Extrahepatic cholestasis (2)
			Chronic cholecystitis (1)
Jaundice/atypical ascites	2	2	—
Hepatomegaly	26	18	Hepatocarcinoma (8)
Hepatomegaly/atypical ascites	7	5	Hepatocarcinoma (2)
Atypical ascites	50	30	Subacute nonspecific peritonitis (8)
			Hepatocarcinoma (7)
			Peritoneal tuberculosis (2)
			Peritoneal carcinomatosis (1)
			Perihepatitis (2)
Total	139	74	(65)

Laboratory Findings. Variations in the characteristics of ascitic fluid in cirrhosis are discussed in Chapter 55. The typical ascites associated with cirrhosis is transudative. However, variations are common. Laparoscopy is often indicated when analysis of the fluid produces an atypical result. In about 70% of such cases in our experience, however, laparoscopy still reveals only uncomplicated cirrhosis. But even when cirrhosis is confirmed, laparoscopy may reveal the presence of an associated disorder, most often neoplastic or inflammatory. Negative laparoscopic findings, except for cirrhosis, do not necessarily eliminate another cause of ascites. For example, "spontaneous bacterial peritonitis," now recognized as a relatively common complication of cirrhosis,[57-59] is not a laparoscopic diagnosis. Peritoneal tuberculosis is a rare but important complication of cirrhosis that is fatal if unrecognized and untreated (Plate 54–40).[60]

Laboratory results may sometimes increase a diagnostic dilemma even when cirrhosis is suspected clinically. Biochemical parameters of liver function may be only slightly abnormal or even normal in cirrhosis. Conversely, there may be clearly abnormal laboratory findings, but these may not be entirely characteristic of cirrhosis. Marked elevations of certain serum enzyme levels, such as alkaline phosphatase and transpeptidases, are not typical, and elevations of the erythrocyte sedimentation rate and increased alpha-globulin levels suggest an associated inflammatory process. The presence of alpha-fetoprotein, especially in high titers, suggests malignant degeneration. Laparoscopy is indicated when clinical evidence suggests cirrhosis and the results of laboratory tests are not in agreement or suggest that some disorder may be present other than, or in addition to, cirrhosis.

Other Diagnostic Procedures. Radionuclide liver scans, computed tomography (CT), and ultrasonography of the liver may yield results that are inconsistent with simple cirrhosis. The merits of these studies in cirrhosis are beyond the scope of this chapter. However, diagnosis is most accurate when based on macroscopic and histologic findings. This does not negate the value of these studies, but when faced with atypical or inconclusive results, laparoscopy is frequently diagnostic.

PORTAL HYPERTENSION

Evidence of portal hypertension may be found by physical examination (splenomegaly, cutaneous collateral circulation, etc.), esophagoscopy (varices), abdominal ultrasonography and CT (dilated veins), and angiography (venous phase abnormalities), and by a variety of other invasive and noninvasive methods. Each provides a somewhat different perspective of this clinical problem. Laparoscopy, although not indicated for diagnosis, can also be used to advantage in studying portal hypertension vis-à-vis observation of the veins of the portal system from within the abdomen.[25, 61, 62]

Laparoscopic Findings

The principal laparoscopic findings in portal hypertension involve the abdominal venous collateral circulation and the spleen.

Abdominal Collateral Circulations

Collateral circulations may be found by laparoscopy in areas where portal-systemic anastomoses can develop. Specifically, these are: (1) omental and gastric veins, (2) paraumbilical veins, (3) umbilical veins, and (4) small peritoneal veins.

Omental and Gastric Veins

Normally, vessels in the greater omentum are barely visible. In portal hypertension, however, the omentum may appear grooved by tortuous, entwined veins of varying diameter. Although these vessels may be large and distended, they are usually bright red. This color indicates active blood flow and contrasts with the dark color of equally distended veins in which flow is stagnant as a result of local obstruction caused, for example, by tumors.

Dilation and turgor of the veins of the greater curvature of the stomach may be found in portal hypertension (Plate 54–41). However, this is a less reliable sign of elevated portal pressure because these findings also occur occasionally without pathologic findings.

The veins of the lesser gastric curvature can also be visualized at laparoscopy (Plate 54–42). These may exhibit changes that are isolated or accompany vascular alterations on the greater curvature. This finding is important because it indicates hypertension in the left and right gastric veins and, almost always, the presence of gastroesophageal varices.

Paraumbilical Veins

Another valuable laparoscopic sign of portal hypertension is distention and turgor of the paraumbilical veins. These are accessory portal veins that originate from the abdominal wall at the umbilicus and follow the falciform ligament near or directly behind the round ligament to the liver. Usually, blood from this region is carried to the left branch of the portal vein through the right and left paraumbilical veins. When the portal system is obstructed below the entry of the paraumbilical veins, these veins are not affected. When the obstruction is upstream from their point of entry, the direction of flow in the paraumbilical veins is reversed, and a collateral circulation is formed that empties into the vena cava through anastomoses with the superior and inferior epigastric veins and the internal thoracic and subcutaneous abdominal veins.

At laparoscopy the veins appear distended. They originate directly from the hepatic parenchyma at the anterior and medial margins of the right lobe and follow the falciform ligament to the umbilical region (Plate 54–43). Usually, only one vein is affected. Occasionally, enlarged paraumbilical veins arise from both lobes and then join to form a single trunk. These collateral circulations are definite evidence of portal hypertension due to intrahepatic obstruction.

Recanalization of the Umbilical Vein

Recanalization of the umbilical vein results in the so-called Cruveilhier-Baumgarten syndrome. A distinction is made between this and Cruveilhier-Baumgarten anomaly (or disease), in which there is congenital patency of the umbilical vein, usually in the absence of liver disease. The term Cruveilhier-Baumgarten syndrome refers to recanalization of the umbilical vein in association with liver disease and portal hypertension. Large, tortuous vessels of the abdominal wall are the prominent clinical features of the syndrome. Auscultation of the abdominal wall frequently discloses a continuous bruit.

At laparoscopy the round ligament resembles a large, distended, and tortuous blue vein with a U-shaped curve (Plate 54–44). The umbilical vein may sometimes reach monstrous dimensions. As a laparoscopic

finding, recanalization of the umbilical vein is an unequivocal sign of portal hypertension.

Small Peritoneal Veins

The small peritoneal veins undergo characteristic changes in portal hypertension that can be visualized at laparoscopy. These vessels are too small to be studied by any other imaging technique, including arteriography. The importance of laparoscopy in portal hypertension is based on the ability to observe the distribution and alterations of these small vessels. Structures and areas where small vessel collateral circulation may be observed are: the falciform ligament and diaphragm, gallbladder system, veins of Retzius, phrenocolic ligament, and adhesions.

The peritoneal vessels are normally thin and form a loose, barely visible network. Portal hypertension results in changes in these small vessels on both the parietal and the visceral surfaces. Raised, tortuous, dilated vessels are visible on the serosa of the intestinal loops, where they form a dense vascular network (Plate 54–45). The most marked changes involve the parietal peritoneum, where the vessels are increased in number and diameter, distended with blood, and raised. There are numerous anastomoses, and actual vascular plexuses are sometimes observed. It is important to differentiate these changes of passive congestion, where the vessels appear distinct and well demarcated against the peritoneum, which retains its normal color, from those of active congestion, where the vessel borders are hazy and the peritoneum is reddened.

Falciform Ligament and Diaphragm. Alteration of the small vessels of the falciform ligament in portal hypertension is due to formation of a collateral circulation in the accessory portal veins of the diaphragm that results in a dense vascular network (Plate 54–46). An accentuated venous pattern on the falciform ligament is often found in normal subjects; this may be particularly visible against the thin membrane of the ligament. This finding can be considered significant only when the passive congestion is conspicuous and extends to the peritoneal vessels of the upper abdominal wall, which indicates communication with the systemic circulation.

Gallbladder System. Small vessel collateral circulation involving the gallbladder is due to increased pressure in the cystic accessory por-

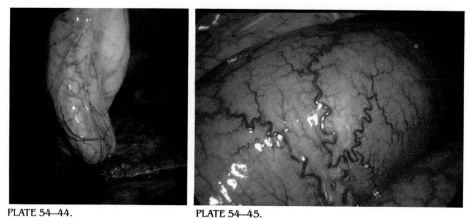

PLATE 54—44.   PLATE 54—45.

PLATE 54—44. Dilated and tortuous umbilical vein in hepatic cirrhosis.
PLATE 54—45. Small veins on the serosa of the small intestine. Collateral circulation from portal hypertension.

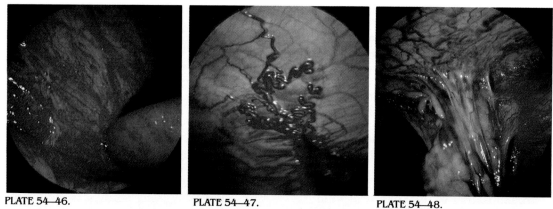

PLATE 54—46.   PLATE 54—47.   PLATE 54—48.

PLATE 54—46. Micronodular cirrhosis. There is enormous development of the veins of the falciform ligament. The anteromedial margin of the liver is in the right foreground.
PLATE 54—47. Small distended veins on the parietal peritoneum above the insertion of the phrenocolic ligament.
PLATE 54—48. Numerous enlarged and turgid veins on a postsurgical adhesion and on the superior abdominal wall at the point of attachment of the adhesion.

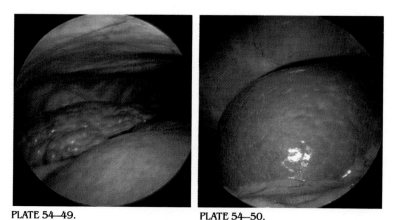

PLATE 54—49.   PLATE 54—50.

PLATE 54—49. Greatly enlarged spleen in the foreground elevates the left lobe of the liver. The appearance of the liver is consistent with an atrophic mixed cirrhosis.
PLATE 54—50. Fibrous or fibrocongestive splenomegaly in hepatic cirrhosis.

tal veins that results in retrograde flow into the vena cava. The veins on the visible portions of the gallbladder will be congested. This is an infrequent finding but is highly indicative of portal hypertension.

Veins of Retzius. Parallel vertical veins with frequent anastomoses can be found in the lateral recesses of the abdominal cavity along the line of junction of the visceral and parietal peritoneum. These vessels represent the collateral circulation between veins of the intestinal wall (portal vein tributaries) and the parietal veins (tributaries of the vena cava) through the system of Retzius. At laparoscopy these vessels are hidden by the intestines, but they can be seen if a careful search is made, placing the patient in right and left lateral decubitus positions to facilitate observation of the lateral recesses.

Phrenocolic Ligament. The most lateral part of the greater omentum is attached to the abdominal wall directly beneath the spleen, in contact with its inferior border, forming the phrenocolic ligament. This is best observed with the patient in the right lateral decubitus position. Normally the ligament stretches between the upper wall and the abdominal viscera and contains varying amounts of fat and a few blood vessels. In portal hypertension, numerous dilated veins of variable caliber originate from the visceral veins of the abdomen and run through the ligament to end on the upper wall near its insertion (Plate 54–47).

Adhesions. Any surgical or post-inflammatory adhesion extending between the visceral and parietal intra-abdominal surfaces may have a rich venous network. This is a typical sign of portal hypertension, the adhesion serving as a bridge across which portal blood can, under the influence of the increased portal pressure, drain into the systemic circulation (Plate 54–48).

Splenic Changes

If the spleen is of normal size, it is difficult to observe at laparoscopy when the patient is supine. The patient must be placed in particular positions, which requires an electrically controlled laparoscopy table that is capable of extreme inclinations (see Chapter 50). (Our table is built to our specifications by Malvestio, Padova, Italy).

The patient is placed in the maximum reverse Trendelenburg position and then tilted to a right lateral decubitus position. This maneuver exposes the grooved medial margin of the spleen as well as its anterior and inferior surfaces; the superior border, the posterior surface, and the lateral margin remain hidden. Usually the spleen can be adequately explored in about 70% to 80% of cases, more frequently if it is enlarged. In some cases, however, the spleen will not be seen despite use of extreme changes in patient position. It may lie too deeply within the abdomen, or it may be covered with a large amount of adherent omental fat that cannot be displaced with a probe. The spleen can be hidden behind post-surgical or inflammatory adhesions or behind a dilated splenic flexure of the colon.

The technical aspects of laparoscopic observation of the spleen are less of a problem than interpretation of findings. Laparoscopic observation is limited to an external examination, which is less informative than gross pathologic study of the cut surface. The splenic capsule is fibrous, not particularly transparent, and often thickened by perisplenic inflammation, and so the underlying parenchyma is often hidden.

The only laparoscopic finding of any significance with respect to the spleen in cirrhosis is splenomegaly (Plate 54–49), although laparoscopy is not necessary to establish the presence of this abnormality. Minor degrees of splenomegaly may not be appreciated at laparoscopy. Besides a general increase in volume, the inferior border of the spleen may extend below the costal margin. The enlarged spleen also displaces the phrenocolic ligament in a lateral-inferior direction. The color of the spleen varies from deep wine-red to pale gray-red. The surface may be smooth and tense or rough and irregular and covered by a retracted fibrous network (Plate 54–50). The consistency may be normal or variably increased.

This description corresponds to so-called fibrous or fibrocongestive splenomegaly, which may reflect a primary pathologic disorder of the spleen or changes secondary to cirrhosis. In some cases laparoscopy can differentiate primary from secondary splenic enlargement. However, there are no specific morphologic alterations that permit a certain diagnosis. Venous portacaval anastomoses on the adjacent parietal peritoneum and in the phrenocolic ligament are consistent with splenomegaly secondary to portal hypertension. However, marked splenomegaly may occur in portal hypertension without any changes in intra-abdominal vessels, in which case it is usually not possible to differentiate primary from secondary splenic enlargement. No correlation has been demonstrated between the degree of splenomegaly revealed at laparoscopy and wedged hepatic vein pressure.[63]

Utility of Laparoscopy in Portal Hypertension

Laparoscopy can add unique and important information to the clinical evaluation of portal hypertension. We believe that this technique is essential for a complete evaluation of portal hypertension for two reasons: (1) Laparoscopic exploration of the liver is reliable and accurate in the investigation of liver disease, especially in problematic cases. (2) Laparoscopy is the only technique with which small vessel collateral circulations can be studied.

Study of the Liver

Laparoscopic study of the liver, the key organ in portal hypertension, will usually indicate whether the cause of portal hypertension is intrahepatic, prehepatic, or posthepatic. Most cases are intrahepatic, i.e., due to cirrhosis. Although this diagnosis is generally not difficult, cirrhosis may also present with isolated manifestations of portal hypertension, such as gastrointestinal hemorrhage or ascites or as radiologic or endoscopic evidence of esophageal varices. Diagnosis of the cause of portal hypertension is then more difficult, although precise evaluation of the liver by laparoscopy will generally resolve this problem. This may reveal otherwise asymptomatic and unsuspected cirrhosis or some other hepatic disease. When the liver is macroscopically and microscopically normal, portal hypertension is almost certainly prehepatic. Laparoscopy also supplies topographic information on the intra-abdominal collateral circulation. A particularly significant finding is the presence of collateral circulations only in the left hypochondrium. This occurs with isolated thrombosis of the splenic vein. When laparoscopy of the liver reveals severe signs of chronic venous congestion, posthepatic portal hypertension (Budd-Chiari syndrome, and other causes) must be considered.[7]

Small Peritoneal Vessels

Laparoscopic study of the small peritoneal vessels will reveal the first signs of portal hypertension and permit identification of different "types" of collateral circulation.

Early Signs of Portal Hypertension. The earliest and subtlest changes of portal hypertension occur in the smallest caliber vessels; these are visible at laparoscopy. Collateral circulations tend to form first in the falciform ligament, phrenocolic ligament, paracolic gutters, and within adhesions. As a result of the ability to observe these areas, laparoscopy is the most sensitive technique for recognition of the presence of portal hypertension, even when of moderate degree and in an early stage.

Types of Collateral Circulation. Although the importance of the large vessel collateral circulations (those revealed by esophagogastroscopy, ultrasonography, and CT) is obvious, the less well-recognized collateral circulations that utilize the small peritoneal vessels have equal relevance because of the profusion of these channels. When details of the small vessel circulation provided by laparoscopy are used together with information from other sources on the status of large vessel collateral circulations, an accurate representation of the entire collateral circulation for a given patient can be constructed.

The total collateral circulation in the individual case is made up of a mixture of component venous channels. This may include all available collateral channels or a lesser number.[62] The reason or reasons for this are obscure. With the help of laparoscopy three types of collateral circulations can be found in cirrhosis, each with a different clinical picture.

Type 1 is characterized laparoscopically by extensive involvement of the smaller abdominal vessels; the gastric veins are spared, and varices will not be present at esophagogastroscopy. Type 2 is the opposite of type 1. The peritoneum is normal, and the collateral circulation is exclusively via the gastric veins (right, left, and short). Gastroesophageal varices are a significant finding at gastroscopy and arteriography. In type 3 all or most available channels, including small peritoneal vessels and larger veins, are utilized in the total collateral circulation. The effect of the portal hypertension is evenly distributed throughout the intra-abdominal venous system, and the clinical picture is characterized by ascites and gastrointestinal bleeding, although the latter occurs less frequently and later in the course of the disease.[64]

We used this classification in 311 cases of cirrhosis. Type 1 occurred in 119 cases (38.4%), type 2 in 50 cases (16%), and type 3 in 142 cases (45.6%). There were no instances of variceal hemorrhage in those patients classified as type 1; ascites was present in 51 patients (42.9%) in this group. In those patients classified as having type 2 portal hypertension there were 3 patients (1.5%) with ascites; bleeding occurred in 34 patients (68%) and there was a strong tendency for bleeding to develop at an early stage of the disease. For those patients with a type 3 collateral circulation, ascites was present in 67 (47%) and bleeding in 41 (29%).

This classification, based on laparoscopy for defining small vessel collaterals as well as other methods such as esophagogastroscopy for identification of large vessel collaterals, is useful in predicting the probability of variceal bleeding. It appears that the risk of bleeding is highest in patients with type 2 collateral circulation, less common in those with type 3, and decidedly uncommon in patients with type 1 circulation. This laparoscopic-endoscopic method of classification can be used to advantage in conjunction with Inokuchi endoscopic criteria for predicting hemorrhage from gastroesophageal varices.[65, 66]

References

1. Fukumoto Y, Okita K, Kodama T, et al. Peritoneoscopic findings and liver function in chronic liver disease. Endoscopy 1980; 12:68–75.
2. Antia FP, Kalro RH, Desai HG. Peritoneoscopy: a diagnostic aid for separation of hepatic cirrhosis and non-cirrhotic portal fibrosis. Indian J Med Sci 1978; 32:95–8.
3. Anthony PP, Ishak KG, Nayak NC, et al. The morphology of cirrhosis: definition, nomenclature, and classification. Bull WHO 1977; 55:521–40.
4. Ursin E, Spech HJ, Liehr H. Laparoskope und Lebersarkoidose. Med Klin 1974; 69:681–6.
5. Le Verger JC, Gosselin M, Lauhois B, et al. Sarcoidose el hipertension portale. Presentation de 2 cas et revue de la litterature. Gastroenterol Clin Biol 1977; 1:661–9.
6. Beck K, Dischler W, Oehlert W. Farbatlas der laparoskopie. Stuttgart: F. K. Schattauer Verlag, 1980; 499.
7. Lindner H. Laparoscopy in hepatic vein thrombosis (Budd-Chiari syndrome). Endoscopy 1973; 5:104–6.
8. Gros von H. Laparoscopie oder perkutane Leberbiopsie? Munch Med Wochenschr 1973; 115:492–4.
9. Vido I, Wildhirt L. Korrelation des laparoskopischer und histologischen Befundes bei chronischer Hepatitis und Leberzirrhose. Dtsch Med Wochenschr 1969; 94:1633–7.
10. Vido I, Winckler K. Diagnose der Leberzirrhose anhand laparoskipischer und histologischer Befunde. Med Klin 1972; 67:400–2.
11. Belaiche J, Compain P, Chaput JC, et al. Comparaison entre l'efficacité de la laparoscopie et de la ponction-biopsie dirigée a l'aiguille de Menghini dans le diagnostic de cirrhose du foie. Sem Hop Paris 1976; 12:751–6.
12. Nord HJ. Biopsy diagnosis of cirrhosis: blind percutaneous versus guided direct vision techniques. A review. Gastrointest Endosc 1982; 28:102–4.
13. Pagliaro L, Rinaldi F, Craxi A, et al. Percutaneous blind biopsy versus laparoscopy with guided biopsy in diagnosis of cirrhosis. A prospective, randomized trial. Dig Dis Sci 1983; 28:39–43.
14. Dibray CH, Paolaggi JA. Accidents de la laparoscopie. Ann Med Interne 1976; 127:689–92.
15. Henning G, Look D, Paradisi Barrios CI. Laparoscopy. Its possibilities and limits. Acta Endoscop 1978; 8:329–44.
16. Manenti A, Manenti F, Villa E, et al. Complications in laparoscopy: a survey of 6563 cases. Acta Endoscop 1980; 10:373–9.
17. Dagnini G, Bergamo S, Caldironi MW, et al. Incidenti della laparoscopia: rapporto su 7870 casi. Giorn Ital Gastroent End Dig 1980; 3:9–14.
18. Dagnini G, Caldironi MW, Marin G, et al. Tamponamento per via laparoscopica con spugna di fibrina negli incidenti di biopsia d'organo. Giorn Ital End Dig 1981; 4:339–44.
19. Dagnini G, Caldironi MW, Marin C, et al. Fibrin sponge plugging of bioptic hemorrhages during laparoscopy. Gastrointest Endosc 1985; 1:35–6.
20. Holund B, Poulsen H, Schlichelng P. Reproducibility of liver biopsy diagnosis in relation to the size of the specimen. Scand J Gastroenterol 1980; 15:329–35.
21. Zotti S, Papaleo E, Marin G, et al. Laparoscopy and liver biopsy in the morphological diagnosis of cirrhosis: concordance and diagnostic validity. Ital J Gastroenterol 1981; 13:14–7.
22. Abdi W, Millan JC, Mezey E. Sampling variability on percutaneous liver biopsy. Arch Intern Med 1979; 139:667–9.
23. Czaja AI, Wolf AM, Baggenstoss AH. Clinical assessment of cirrhosis in severe chronic active liver disease. Mayo Clin Proc 1980; 55:360–4.
24. Lindner H. Why laparoscopy? Acta Gastroenterol Belg 1973; 36:595–602.
25. Herrerias Gutierrez JM, Perez Mijaris R. La laparoscopia en el diagnostico de la hipertension portal. Rev Esp Enferm Apar Dig 1974; 44:767–74.
26. Heit HA, Johnson LF, Rabin L. Liver surface characteristics as observed during laparoscopy correlated with biopsy findings. Gastrointest Endosc 1978; 24:288–90.
27. Orlandi F. Observer error in morphological diagnosis of chronic active hepatitis and cirrhosis. Ital J Gastroenterol 1979; 11:5–8.
28. Capelle PH, Conte-Marti Mme. Interet de l'examen histologique du foie par ponction-biopsie quand la laparoscopie montre un foie paraissant peu altere. Sem Hop Paris 1971; 47:172–6.
29. Scheuer PJ. Liver biopsy in the diagnosis of cirrhosis. Gut 1970; 11:275–8.
30. Galambos JT. Classification of cirrhosis. Am J Gastroenterol 1975; 64:437–51.
31. Popper H. Pathological aspects of cirrhosis. A review. Am J Pathol 1977; 87:228–64.
32. Dagnini C, Bergamo S, Caldironi MW, et al. Validità e limiti delle prove diagnostiche in epatologia. Laparoscopia ed epatobiopsie. Attualità in diagnostica e terapia delle vie biliari. Rome: II Pensiero Scientifico Editore, 1980.
33. Harihara S, Monna T, Yamamoto S. The prognostic value of peritoneoscopic findings in patients with liver cirrhosis. Gastroenterol Jpn 1980; 15, 4:379–84.

34. Solis-Herruzo JA. Atlas de Diagnostico Diferencial Laparoscopico. Madrid: Montalvo, 1975; 163–5.
35. Caroli J, Ribet A, Parae A. Précis des maladies du foie, du pancreas et des voies biliaires. Paris: Masson, 1975.
36. Caroli J, Marcus N, Grynglat A, et al. Le cancer primitif du foie sur cirrhose. Rev Med Chir Mal Foie 1970; 45:292–8.
37. Gislon J, Barge J, Feldmann C. L'étude comparative des cirrhoses avec ou sans cancer primitif du foie. Arch Br Mal App Dig 1976; 65:369–78.
38. Peters RL, Afroudakis AP, Tatter D. The changing incidence of association of hepatitis B with hepatocellular carcinoma in California. Am J Clin Pathol 1977; 68:1–7.
39. Burnett RA, Patrick RS, Spilg WG, et al. Hepatocellular carcinoma and hepatic cirrhosis in the West of Scotland: a 25-year necroscopy review. J Clin Pathol 1978; 31:108–10.
40. Norredam K. Primary carcinoma of the liver. Acta Path Microbiol Scand 1979; 87:227–36.
41. Omata M, Ashcavai M, Leiw CT, Peters RL. Hepatocellular carcinoma in the U.S.A.: etiologic considerations. Gastroenterology 1979; 76:279–87.
42. Aoki K. Cancer of the liver, international mortality trends. World Health Stat Q 1978; 31:28–50.
43. Saracci R, Repetto F. Time trends of primary liver cancer: indication of increased incidence in selected cancer registry populations. JNCI 1980; 65:241–7.
44. Safrany L. Die laparoskopische Diagnose des primaren Leberkarzinomas. Endoscopy 1970; 4:213–7.
45. Etienne JP, Chaput JC, Feydy P, et al. La laparoscopie dans le cancer primitif du foie de l'adulte. Ann Gastroenterol Hepatol 1973; 9:49–56.
46. Vilardell L. The value of laparoscopy in the diagnosis of primary cancer of the liver. Endoscopy 1977; 9:20–3.
47. Caldironi MW, Milanesi P, Zotti S, et al. Laparoscopic findings of primary liver cancer in adults. Scand J Gastroenterol 1982; 17(Suppl 78):733.
48. Caldironi MW, Zotti S, Milanesi P, et al. Primary liver cancer in adults: epidemiologic considerations derived from laparoscopic experience. Scand J Gastroenterol 1982; 17(Suppl 78):103.
49. Maupas PH, Melnick JL, eds. Hepatitis B virus and primary hepatocellular carcinoma. Progress in Medical Virology. Vol 27. New York: S. Karger, 1981.
50. Shafritz AD, Kew CM. Identification of integrated hepatitis B virus DNA sequences in human hepatocellular carcinoma. Hepatology 1981; 1:1–8.
51. Pagliaro L. Carcinoma primitivo del fegato: fattori di rischio. Ie Fegato 1982; 28:17–29.
52. Jacobs MI. La laparoscopie dans le diagnostic du cancer primitif du foie. Arch Er Mal App Digest 1972; 61:407–16.
53. Paolaggi JA, Mugnier B, Barret C, et al. La laparoscopie dans le diagnostic des cancers primitifs du foie. A prospos de 50 observations. Acta Gastroenterol Belg 1973; 36:609–25.
54. Anguilar Reina J, Reina Campos E, Truullo Rodriguez L, et al. Posibilidades de la laparoscopia con optica convencional y de aumento en el diagnostico del cancer hepatico primitivo. Rev Esp Enferm Apar Dig 1977; 49:203–13.
55. Herrerias Gutierrez JM, Jimenez Salnz M, Garrido Peralta M. Aspectos actuales del cancer primitivo de higado (III). Algunos aspectos diagnosticos. Rev Esp Enferm Apar Dig 1977; 49:665–74.
56. Herrerias JM, Vilasco A, Manilla A, et al. Aspectos actuales del cancer primitivo de higado en el adulto (IV). Anatomia patologica. Rev Esp Enferm Apar Dig 1977; 49:789–800.
57. Conn HO. Spontaneous bacterial peritonitis. Gastroenterology 1976; 70:455–7.
58. Kammerer J, Talib M, Dupeyron C, et al. Peritonites bacteriennes spontanées du cirrhotique. Gastroenterol Clin Biol 1979; 3:709–18.
59. Carrer MLE, Poupon RY, Ballet F, et al. Les infections du liquide d'ascite chez le cirrhotique: étude clinique et biologique de 36 episodes observes au cours d'une année. Gastroenterol Clin Biol 1980; 4:640–5.
60. Dagnini G, Zotti S, Caldironi MW, et al. La diagnosi di tubercolosi peritoneale in associazione alla cirrosi epatica. Minerva Dietol Gastroenterol 1978; 24:107–10.
61. Pozo Camaron A, Rodriguez Cortis J, Pajares Carcia JM. Le laparoscopia en el diagnostico de la hipertension portal. Estudio comparativo con la esplenoportografia. Rev Esp Enferm Apar Dig 1974; 44:775–84.
62. Dagnini G. L'importanza della laparoscopia nello studio dell'ipertensione portale. Minerva Med 1975; 66:432–42.
63. Zuin R, Gatta A, Merkel C, et al. Evaluation of peritoneoscopic and oesophagoscopic findings as indexes of portal hypertension in patients with liver cirrhosis. Ital J Gastroenterol 1982; 14:214–9.
64. Herrerias JM, Osorio M, Moreno M, et al. Correlaciones entre el diagnostico histopatologico de cirrosis y la nodulacion y dureza del higado observados en la laparoscopia. Rev Esp Enferm Apar Dig 1974; 42:149–54.
65. Japanese Research Society for Portal Hypertension. The general rules for recording endoscopic findings on esophageal varices. Jpn J Surg 1980; 10:84–7.
66. Beppu K, Inokuchi K, Koyanagi H, et al. Prediction of variceal hemorrhage by esophageal endoscopy. Gastrointest Endosc 1981; 27:213–8.

Chapter 55

LAPAROSCOPY IN ASCITES AND PERITONEAL DISEASES

WILLIAM P. BOYD, JR., M.D.

Disorders of the peritoneum are commonly associated with ascites, and so ascites will be the primary topic of this chapter. The pathogenesis of ascites secondary to peritoneal disease is uncomplicated compared with the complexity of ascites formation in chronic liver disease. Nevertheless, the clinical presentations of these two large groups of disorders may be remarkably similar. When specific diagnosis cannot be determined from an adequate history, physical examination, noninvasive laboratory studies, and diagnostic paracentesis, exploratory laparoscopy under local anesthesia becomes the best method of evaluation.

ASCITES

General Considerations

The initial evaluation of a patient with ascites includes a thorough history to elicit clues to the etiology. Symptoms of acute or chronic liver disease are often nonspecific, and nonspecific malaise and fatigue may actually suggest a disorder of the liver. Other elements in the history that are suggestive of hepatic disease include alcohol abuse, use of potentially hepatotoxic substances (primarily prescribed drugs) and prior blood transfusions. Standard liver enzyme determinations are usually required to establish the liver as the target of injury. The history must also be complete with respect to other organ systems, primarily the cardiovascular (right heart failure), pancreatic (chronic or acute disease), renal (nephrotic syndrome), and pulmonary (tuberculosis).

Stigmata of chronic liver disease noted on physical examination suggest a hepatic basis for ascites. This could prove to be an incorrect assumption. Paracentesis is still necessary to evaluate for concomitant disorders that are common in patients with chronic liver disease, such as tuberculosis or bacterial peritonitis. In addition to the stigmata of chronic liver disease (e.g., spider angiomata, palmar erythema, hepatomegaly), physical examination must also probe for findings suggestive of other associated diseases such as right heart failure.

Regardless of physical and laboratory findings that suggest a cause of ascites, the majority of patients should undergo a diagnostic paracentesis to exclude a complicating infection and/or to classify the ascites as consistent or inconsistent with the presumed underlying cause. In the case of abdominal infection, paracentesis is reasonably accurate.

Infection

Spontaneous bacterial peritonitis may occur in any patient with ascites. A prompt diagnosis at an early stage of this serious illness may be confirmed by analysis of the characteristics of the ascitic fluid. Bar-Meir et al.[1] found that a white cell count of more than 500 per cu mm of ascitic fluid accurately differentiated infected from noninfected fluid in over 90% of cases. However, patients taking diuretic drugs may also have elevations in their ascitic white counts of over 500.[2] The differential of the white cell count is of assistance in that the finding of more than 250 polymorphonuclear cells suggests spontaneous bacterial peritonitis.[1] Nevertheless, false positive interpretations may occur. It has been suggested that measuring the pH of the ascitic fluid will obviate this difficulty.

In one study the pH of the ascitic fluid from 6 patients with spontaneous bacterial peritonitis ranged from 7.12 to 7.31 compared with a range of 7.42 to 7.50 in 50 patients with sterile ascites.[3]

Tuberculous peritonitis, although less common than spontaneous bacterial peritonitis, is not a rare disease and should be considered in several clinical scenarios: (a) ascites of recent onset; (b) ascites in patients with unexplained fever or chest x-ray film evidence of tuberculosis; and (c) exudative ascites with a preponderance of lymphocytes. The ascites of tuberculous peritonitis is generally found to be exudative with a protein content greater than 3 g,[1] to have a white cell count greater than 250 cells per cu mm,[2, 3] and to contain a preponderance of lymphocytes (usually 90% or more).[2, 3] Of related interest in the evaluation of ascites is the observation that there is a relatively high (18%) incidence of pleuropulmonary tuberculosis when a left pleural effusion is associated with chronic liver disease and ascites.[4] These patients did not have tuberculous peritonitis.

Differential Diagnosis

As noted, ascitic fluid is also sampled to ascertain its characteristics in relation to the clinical impression. If the patient has cirrhosis clinically and the fluid is transudative and without evidence of infection, then it may be decided to discontinue further evaluation for the cause of the ascites. If the ascites is exudative, further evaluation is generally advisable, usually including laparoscopy. Two exceptions to this are pancreatic ascites, which can be diagnosed by the extreme amylase elevation in the fluid,[5] and chylous ascites with its high lipid concentration and microscopic fat droplets.[6] These disorders generally require different diagnostic approaches. Chylous ascites may be seen in otherwise uncomplicated cirrhosis[7] as well as in constrictive pericarditis.[8] The major causes of exudative ascites are tuberculosis, bacterial infection, neoplasm, pancreatitis with pseudocyst formation, nephrosis, myxedema, and the Budd-Chiari syndrome. Unfortunately, these disorders may also present with transudative ascites, albeit some quite rarely (tuberculous, for example). As should be apparent, laparoscopy can and must play an important role in the evaluation of ascites, particularly if it is exudative.

LAPAROSCOPY IN ASCITES
Technique

Although the technical aspects of the laparoscopy procedure are much the same whether or not ascites is present (see Chapter 50), several points merit discussion. These include: the timing of the procedure, the quantity of fluid to be removed, postprocedure leakage of ascitic fluid, and infection.

The optimal timing of laparoscopy in the patient with ascites can be problematic. In transudative ascites, vascular compromise as a result of the rapid loss of ascitic fluid is a cause for concern. If a patient is responding to diuresis, it is advisable to wait several weeks until much of the fluid is gone. If this is impossible or the patient has exudative ascites, laparoscopy may be performed with several precautions. An intravenous line should be started to replace fluid loss if necessary with either normal saline or plasma or both. Fluids should be replaced if substantial quantities of fluid are lost and/or there is evidence of vascular compromise such as hypotension. The pulse may be an invalid indicator of cardiovascular status when atropine is given prior to the procedure.

The Veres needle is an excellent paracentesis needle so that the ascitic fluid can be removed just prior to air insufflation. The amount of fluid to remove is a matter of judgment.

Some laparoscopists recommend complete drainage of the abdomen so that there will be no fluid covering the viscera during the examination. I prefer to remove enough fluid to allow laparoscopy, but not more than 2 to 3 liters so that there is not much risk of vascular compromise. This usually permits satisfactory observation of all pertinent structures, although tilting of the procedure table is required for a complete examination (Plate 55–1A and B). With this method the volume of gas required for an adequate pneumoperitoneum will be decreased since the ascitic fluid will "layer out" posteriorly.

After the procedure is completed, it is recommended that the primary site be sutured somewhat more loosely than normal to allow some leakage of fluid. If the wound is closed tightly, the fluid may find another route of escape and significant scrotal or labial edema may occur. Leaking ascites may be a postprocedure problem that can prolong hospital stay but will rarely be of substantial medical significance.

Infection of ascitic fluid after laparoscopy has not been a problem, although it should be considered if unexplained fever, leukocytosis, or encephalopathy occur.

General Results

Laparoscopy is an efficacious procedure in the diagnosis of the cause of ascites. The overall accuracy in two reports was 97% and 80.5%.[9, 10] The number of possible disorders that may be responsible for ascites is large, so that laparoscopy becomes an interesting exercise in differential diagnosis that challenges the powers of observation and deduction of the endoscopist. Villa et al.[11] reported 223 cases of ascites examined laparoscopically and noted the following distribution of diagnoses: cirrhosis, 113 (51%); metastatic carcinoma, 54 (24%); tuberculous peritonitis, 27 (12%); congestive heart failure, 14 (6%); pancreatitis, 5 (2%); cystic disease, 4 (2%); septic peritonitis, 1; vascular conditions, 2; myxedema, 1; and lymphomas, 2.

Laparoscopic Diagnosis

Uncommon Hepatic Disorders

Although laparoscopy of liver disease is extensively discussed elsewhere (see Chapters 52–54), ascites may occur in several uncommon hepatic conditions as the only manifestation of liver disease. Cirrhosis may also behave in this manner.

Partial Nodular Transformation

Partial nodular transformation of the liver is a rare disorder that may produce ascites.[12] This condition is best appreciated by gross inspection of the liver since it consists of nodule formation in part of the liver, most prominently the perihilar area. A biopsy specimen from any portion of the liver may be unimpressive since fibrosis is not part of the pathogenesis of this disorder; rather, it is the result of an abnormal pattern of liver cell growth. Portal hypertension in this condition may result from primary portal vein thrombosis or intrahepatic portal vein thrombosis.[13] In one case reported, nodular transformation of the caudate lobe of the liver resulted in compression of the extrahepatic portal vein.[14] In light of the reluctance of ascites to form in isolated portal vein thrombosis, one wonders if more subtle changes are present at the small portal vein radicles within the liver or at the level of the space of Disse.

Nodular Regenerative Hyperplasia

Partial nodular transformation should not be confused with nodular regenerative hyperplasia, in which there is nodule formation in the parenchyma and presumably an increase in intrahepatic pressure. This lesion can be appreciated microscopically in an adequate sample of the liver, although it may not be demonstrable in a small needle biopsy specimen. Generally, the two disorders are distinct on gross inspection, partial nodular transformation being perihilar with large nodules, and nodular regenerative hyperplasia being diffuse throughout the liver with very small nodules. However, a case with overlapping features of both disorders has been reported.[15]

Formerly, nodular regenerative hyperplasia had been primarily associated with Felty's syndrome. However, many unrelated chronic diseases have been associated with the disorder more recently. Wanless et al.[16] reported 9 cases of various disorders, mostly hematologic (e.g., myeloma, rheumatoid arthritis, myeloid metaplasia), and suggested that the lesion was due to portal vein thrombotic occlusions with secondary liver cell atrophy and regeneration. Nodular regenerative hyperplasia can mimic micronodular cirrhosis at laparoscopy with a homogeneous distribution of small nodules over the hepatic surface. Biopsy and correlation with the clinical history generally categorize the disorder correctly.

Radiation Liver Injury

Radiation liver injury is an uncommon lesion that may cause ascites. A report of a patient who had tense, transudative ascites is illustrative.[17] At laparoscopy the liver surface was reddish-purple and irregular, and a biopsy revealed sinusoidal congestion and dilation. Radiation hepatitis is known to produce a veno-occlusive–like injury pattern that is almost always transient.[18] This lesion is not dissimilar to the Budd-Chiari syndrome, a lesion that should be familiar to all laparoscopists, in light of the frequency with which this examination is performed in patients with predisposing causes such as cancer and heart disease. The lesion of Budd-Chiari is generally described as a bluish discoloration of the liver surface against a light brown background.[19] Veno-occlusive disease is seen in other clinical settings, such as after chemotherapy for acute leukemia.[20]

Cardiac Disease

The liver may transmit "en passant" elevated pressure from the level of the heart

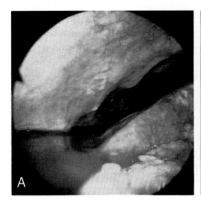
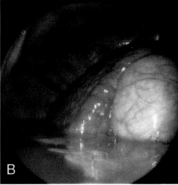

PLATE 55–1. *A,* Right upper quadrant view demonstrates residual ascites. Close inspection reveals nodularity of the peritoneum due to tuberculosis. *B,* Partial removal of ascitic fluid. View of right upper quadrant demonstrates cirrhotic liver.

PLATE 55–2. Parietal peritoneum in mesothelioma. The peritoneum is more diffusely erythematous and irregular than seen in other lesions.
PLATE 55–3. Multiple nodules in the mesentery of a patient with peritoneal mesothelioma. (Photography courtesy of Dr. J. Cunningham.)

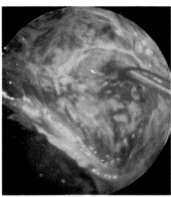

PLATE 55–2.   PLATE 55–3.

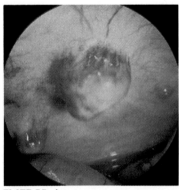
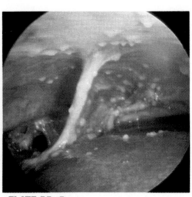

PLATE 55–4. Varying size nodules of adenocarcinoma on parietal peritoneum.
PLATE 55–5. Multiple small nodules of metastatic adenocarcinoma scattered over peritoneum and liver.

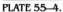

PLATE 55–4.   PLATE 55–5.

and cause portal hypertension sufficient to produce ascites and/or esophageal varices. Although clinically significant portal hypertension primarily occurs in constrictive pericarditis or severe tricuspid regurgitation, it may occur in any state that causes elevation of right-sided pressures and hepatic venous stasis. This can be appreciated by the finding of esophageal varices in 6.7% of patients with congestive heart failure in an autopsy study.[21]

The laparoscopic appearance is an enlarged bluish to bluish-red liver that is often largely covered by a whitish "icing" material, the latter being a nonspecific perihepatitis reaction.

Nonhepatic, Nonperitoneal Disorders

There are several nonhepatic, nonperitoneal causes of ascites. One of the most important is pancreatic ascites. As discussed, this diagnosis is made by paracentesis when the ascites is found to have an amylase level substantially higher than that in the serum. Laparoscopy is said to be indicated in pancreatic ascites for the detection of pancreatic swelling that may indicate pseudocyst formation and changes of pancreatitis such as local hyperemia and fatty necrosis.[22] In my view, laparoscopy is unnecessary. Other imaging techniques such as computed tomography (CT) and/or endoscopic retrograde cholangiopancreatography (ERCP) are more likely to be revealing (see Chapter 38). Pancreatic ascites is almost always a complication of chronic pancreatitis, although it may also occur as a result of pancreatic trauma.

Nephrogenous ascites is a rather refractory form that occurs in patients with renal failure who are undergoing hemodialysis. The ascitic fluid tends to be exudative (protein >3 g), although transudates have been reported. The occurrence of nephrogenous ascites does not depend on prior peritoneal dialysis, occurring in some patients who have only been on maintenance hemodialysis.[23] Laparoscopy must be performed to rule out peritoneal or subtle liver disease. There are no specific laparoscopic findings, and the diagnosis is one of exclusion.

Two rare causes of exudative ascites merit comment. There is a case report of ascites in a patient with plasmacytomas throughout the peritoneal cavity, representing recurrence of a previously resected intestinal plasmacytoma.[24] The ascitic fluid was chylous and contained 10 abnormal plasma cells per milliliter. The other case is one of exudative ascites in a patient with scleroderma in whom laparoscopy failed to reveal any liver or peritoneal abnormality.[25]

Laparoscopy has been used in preoperative evaluation and postoperative follow-up of patients with ovarian carcinoma (see Chapter 57). In addition to the overall peritoneal surface, the diaphragm deserves particular attention when evaluating patients with ovarian carcinoma since the presence of metastases in this area may be overlooked.[26] Laparoscopy as a second-look evaluation after surgery for ovarian cancer has been shown to be of value in a study that demonstrated prolonged survival in patients clinically free of disease who had a negative laparoscopy after completing their treatment protocol.[27]

An unusual case of a patient with ascites on the basis of intrauterine device–related pelvic inflammatory disease has been reported.[28]

Malignant Diseases

Disruption of the integrity of the peritoneal membrane is manifested by weeping of fluid into the peritoneal cavity whether the insult is malignant, infectious, or inflammatory. The most common of these causes is malignancy.

Mesothelioma

The single primary malignancy of the peritoneum is mesothelioma. This tumor is known to be due to exposure to the environmental carcinogen asbestos. Patients may manifest either pleural or peritoneal primary mesothelioma or both. The ratio of pleural to peritoneal involvement is 2.7:1.[29] The most common presenting symptoms are abdominal pain and weight loss. Approximately 90% of patients with peritoneal mesothelioma have ascites.[30] Cytologic examination of the exudative ascitic fluid is rarely definitive, thus making direct biopsy a requirement for diagnosis. Moertel[30, 31] has stated that laparotomy or autopsy is necessary to establish the diagnosis. However, there are numerous reports of diagnosis by laparoscopic exploration and biopsy.[32–34]

At laparoscopy the peritoneum is studded with 1 to 2 mm whitish miliary nodules and occasionally larger nodules. Commonly there is significant inflammation of the peritoneal surface, which has a striking erythematous and irregular appearance (Plate 55–2). Irregular nodules may be noted in the mesentery (Plate 55–3). Biopsy specimens should be examined by both light and electron microscopy to ensure correct identification of the tumor.

Metastatic Carcinoma

Metastatic carcinoma is one of the commonest of the various groups of peritoneal diseases to cause ascites. Metastatic disease to the peritoneum is usually adenocarcinoma with lesser contributions from lymphoma, carcinoid, myeloma, and other malignancies. Adenocarcinoma involving the peritoneum presents as abdominal distention often accompanied by pain and weight loss. As noted, cytologic examination of the ascites may or may not be helpful.

At laparoscopy the lesion appears as multiple nodules of varying size scattered over both the parietal and visceral peritoneum. However, there is considerable variability in the appearance of the metastatic lesions, the spectrum ranging from small "miliary" nodules to large bulky nodules to virtually flat whitish lesions (Plates 55–4 to 55–7). Again,

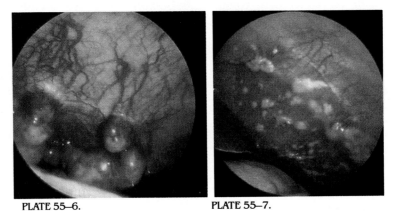

PLATE 55—6.   PLATE 55—7.

PLATE 55—6. Large, multiple nodules on peritoneum in patient with carcinoma at base of tongue.
PLATE 55—7. Whitish nodules, some nearly flat, on peritoneum in patient with adenocarcinoma of pancreas.

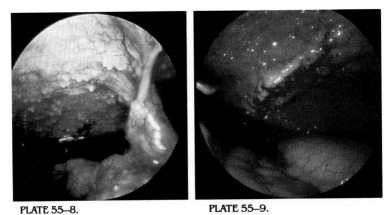

PLATE 55—8.   PLATE 55—9.

PLATE 55—8. Typical small nodules of tuberculous peritonitis. (Photograph courtesy of Dr. Harrison Parker, Milwaukee, WI.)
PLATE 55—9. Site of biopsy of several coalesced tuberculous nodules.

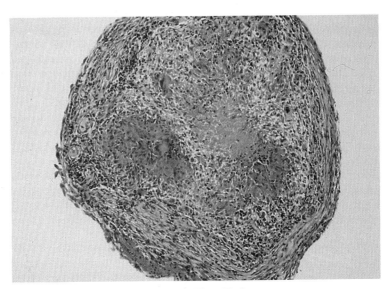

PLATE 55—10. Microscopy of biopsy from lesion seen in Plate 55—9.

biopsy is required for specific diagnosis and to exclude lesions with a similar appearance such as tuberculous peritonitis. The importance of laparoscopy is underscored, in my experience, by the failure of CT to detect metastatic peritoneal lesions.

The major role of laparoscopy in lymphomas is that of a staging procedure (see Chapter 52). Lymphomas, primarily non-Hodgkins, occasionally cause peritoneal disease that leads to ascites. Ehrlich et al.[35] reported 61 of 323 patients as having serosal and omental involvement, some of whom had ascites. Lewin et al.[36] noted that of an original group of 117 patients, 44 progressed to more advanced disease, and that 4 patients (9%) with progressive disease had peritoneal involvement.

Chronic lymphocytic leukemia has on occasion produced ascites. The fluid is generally a transudate with an increased cell count. Cytologic analysis may demonstrate atypical lymphocytes suggestive that the ascites is related to the primary disease.[37] However, the actual pathogenesis is unclear; in some instances ascites may be due to portal hypertension secondary to hepatic infiltration by tumor cells.

Myeloid metaplasia and multiple myeloma may alter peritoneal integrity and produce ascites. Myeloid metaplasia is a recognized cause of exudative ascites that is generally assumed to be secondary to portal hypertension. Gorshein and Brauer,[38] however, found actual implantation of metastatic myeloid tissue on the peritoneum. They surmised occult leakage from the spleen, although clear evidence for this was lacking. Peritoneal implants have been noted to cause ascites in multiple myeloma.[39] The paracentesis in this instance revealed a protein content of 2.5 g and many plasma cells. The myeloma was of IgA paraprotein type, as has been the case in most reported cases of myeloma ascites.

Pseudomyxoma Peritonei

Pseudomyxoma peritonei is a curious disorder in which pale, translucent, jelly-like globules or nodules are found in the peritoneal cavity either free-floating, attached to peritoneal surfaces, or both, as is most usual. Pseudomyxoma peritonei is a descriptive term applied in both benign and malignant disease. The largest subset of patients with pseudomyxoma peritonei have underlying cystadenocarcinoma of the ovary. In a review of 38 patients the origin was ovarian in 45%; the appendix in 29%; and of indeterminate origin in 26%.[40] Higa et al.[41] submit that true

generalized disease is in the main due to either ovarian or appendiceal cystadenocarcinoma and that use of the term should therefore be restricted accordingly. Nevertheless, the term is used when the syndrome is caused by benign disease. As an example, there is a relatively recent report of a mucocele of the appendix producing the full syndrome.[42]

The diagnosis is suggested radiographically by characteristic curvilinear calcifications on a plain abdominal film, although this is a rare finding.[43] Typically, cytologic study of the paracentesis reveals no malignant cells because of their scarcity even when the underlying cause is malignancy. Gelatinous material that suggests the diagnosis may be found in the fluid. Nevertheless, in most instances laparoscopy is required for definitive diagnosis. The characteristic laparoscopic appearance is that of multiple, globular nodules scattered over the peritoneal surfaces and floating free in straw-colored ascites.[44,45]

Infectious Diseases

Spontaneous bacterial peritonitis, previously mentioned, will not be discussed since it is an infection of previously existing ascites. Laparoscopy plays no role in detection or the confirmation that it is spontaneous, as by eliminating primary causes such as bowel perforation.

Tuberculous Ascites

The major infectious cause of ascites is tuberculosis. The pathogenesis of peritoneal tuberculosis is unclear but presumed to be reactivation of prior disease. Many of the patients have no other evidence of tuberculosis, specifically no evidence of pulmonary tuberculosis. Some patients have underlying, perhaps predisposing conditions, such as hepatic disease, particularly alcoholic liver disease.

The presenting symptoms are abdominal distention, fever, and weight loss. The disease is insidious in that most patients have had symptoms for more than 3 months at diagnosis. The cardinal indication of the disease, for both patient and physician, is abdominal distention due to ascites. As noted, the fluid is usually exudative. In one series, 89% of cases had fluid protein values over 3 g,[1] but 11% of the patients had transudative ascites. Most patients will have elevated ascitic fluid cell counts (>300) with a preponderance of lymphocytes (approximately 90%).[2] In addition, low ascitic glucose concentrations have been described.[46] Definitive diagnosis re-

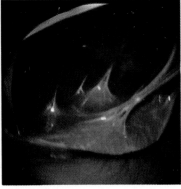 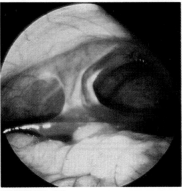 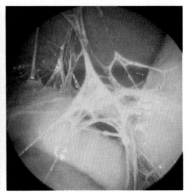

PLATE 55–11.　　　　　　　PLATE 55–12.　　　　　　　PLATE 55–13.

PLATE 55–11. String-like adhesions in patient with recent gonococcal infection.
PLATE 55–12. Perihepatic adhesions in patient with amebic abscess.
PLATE 55–13. Peritoneal dialysis patient with adhesions. (Photograph courtesy Dr. John Cunningham, Charleston, S.C.)

quires demonstration of the acid-fast organism in the fluid or a biopsy with compatible histology. It is very rare to find *Mycobacterium tuberculosis* on examination of the ascitic fluid. Culture of the fluid will yield the organism in nearly one half of cases, but this may require up to 6 weeks; a negative result does not eliminate the possibility of tuberculous peritonitis. Therefore, biopsy is necessary.

Blind peritoneal biopsy has been successful in the diagnosis of tuberculous peritonitis; however, for several reasons laparoscopy is preferred. The bias is that guided biopsy has a higher yield than blind biopsy. However, the primary reasons for laparoscopy are increased safety and wider diagnostic capability. Patients who have underlying liver disease may have portal hypertension, in which case the risk of bleeding may be increased for blind biopsy. Laparoscopy affords visual inspection, not only to insure that the biopsy properly samples the lesion, but also to assess the status of the liver and other intra-abdominal structures.

Laparoscopy reveals multiple, uniform, white miliary nodules generally less than 5 mm in size studding the parietal and visceral peritoneal surfaces. In most instances the peritoneum appears virtually covered with miliary nodules (Plate 55–8); however, at times there are larger coalesced lesions (Plate 55–9). Biopsy specimens of these lesions reveal typical caseation necrosis (Plate 55–10). In addition, adhesions may be present throughout the abdomen. Rarely, there may be tuberculosis of the liver with cheesy, white nonumbilicated nodules on the liver surface.

Ascites occurred in only 9% of cases in a large series of patients with hepatobiliary tuberculosis.[47] Of note, biliary obstruction from tuberculous lymph node involvement was found in 35% of the 130 cases in this series. Biopsy specimens from suspected tuberculous lesions should be cultured in addition to the standard histologic evaluation. Chronic cases may present as "dry" tuberculous peritonitis (without ascites) in which the laparoscopic manifestations are a thickened, dull peritoneal surface and multiple adhesions. In the absence of the typical nodules, biopsy specimens must be taken from nonspecifically abnormal areas of the peritoneum. If the microscopic findings are also nonspecific, the etiology is more likely to be prior pelvic infection, cholecystitis, pancreatitis, or one of the other infectious causes of peritonitis such as *coccidioides*.[1]

Coccidioides immitis Peritonitis

Coccidioides immitis was first reported as a cause of peritonitis by John Ruddock,[48] a pioneer in American laparoscopy. A more recent report of 7 cases of *C. immitis* peritonitis includes 2 cases diagnosed by laparoscopy and biopsy.[49] The laparoscopic findings are similar to those of tuberculous peritonitis, the main feature being multiple small nodules. The diagnosis is made by finding a granuloma containing spherules of *C. immitis* in a biopsy specimen.

Other Infectious Causes of Peritonitis

Other very rare infectious causes of peritonitis (ascites) include strongyloidiasis,[50] amebiasis,[51] acariasis,[52] and schistosomiasis.[53] In the case of *Strongyloides*, it is not surprising that invasive microscopic filariform larvae can on occasion penetrate the gut and become established in the abdominal cavity. Amebic peritonitis is primarily the result of bowel perforation or rupture of a hepatic abscess, although it also appears that *Entamoeba histolytica* is able to penetrate the bowel wall.[51] *Ascaris lumbricoides* as a cause of peritonitis, however, is enigmatic. How this large worm reaches the peritoneal cavity without leaving any evidence of its exit from the gut is unknown. In a case of schistosomiasis the peritoneum was found to be studded with gray-yellow nodules varying from several millimeters to several centimeters in size.[53] The biopsy specimen from this lesion revealed *schistosoma mansoni*.[53]

Any of the aforementioned infections may closely mimic peritoneal carcinomatous metastasis.

Inflammatory Diseases

Noninfectious diseases may mimic metastatic carcinoma. Sarcoidosis is well known for its ability to mimic metastatic carcinoma of the liver, even to the point of producing umbilicated lesions. This disorder also has a lesser known ability to "metastasize" to the peritoneum and mimic carcinomatous peritonitis.[54] Laparoscopically, small white nodules are noted on the peritoneum. The diagnosis is based on a compatible biopsy in a clinical setting of sarcoidosis.

Other benign diseases that can involve the peritoneum include Crohn's disease, Whipple's disease, and eosinophilic gastroenteritis.

Crohn's disease may produce white miliary nodules over the visceral and parietal peritoneum as well as in the mesentery.[55]

Whipple's disease may present as exudative ascites. Isenberg et al.[56] reported the case of a man with weight loss, low-grade fever, and increasing abdominal girth. The ascites was exudative and had an elevated cell count that was 60% polymorphonuclear leukocytes. At laparoscopy, multiple 1 to 2 mm pale yellow nodules were scattered over the peritoneum. Biopsy specimens revealed the characteristic macrophages of Whipple's disease containing periodic acid–Schiff-positive diastase-resistant material. In addition to the nodules described by Isenberg et al.,[56] Henning (personal communication) has observed lymphangiectasias in the visceral peritoneum on the small bowel, a finding also seen in intestinal lymphangiectasia and rarely in normal persons.

Eosinophilic gastroenteritis is more likely to be diagnosed by intestinal biopsy; however, ascites may develop if there is transmural involvement of the gastrointestinal tract. McNabb et al.[57] reported a case of peritonitis in which there was an exudative ascites with a protein content of 4.2 g and a cell count of 7488 with 92% eosinophils.

MISCELLANEOUS NONASCITIC PERITONEAL CONDITIONS

Perihepatitis

The finding of adhesions between the liver and the peritoneum is nonspecific and may be the result of prior surgery or intra-abdominal infection of many types. However, in the particular case of string-like adhesions, as opposed to heavy veil-like adhesive bands, the cause may be perihepatitis due to one of several agents.

The classic perihepatitis syndrome is the Fitz-Hugh-Curtis syndrome described originally as acute gonococcal peritonitis of the right upper quadrant in women.[58, 59] In the typical case, the patient has presenting symptoms of right upper quadrant pain that is very similar to that of acute cholecystitis and a vaginal discharge that is positive for gonococcus. Treatment with an appropriate antibiotic leads to a dramatic clinical recovery, generally within 2 days.

Laparoscopy is useful in the Fitz-Hugh-Curtis syndrome when symptoms are atypical and cervical smears are nondiagnostic. The typical finding is "violin-string"–like adhesions between the anterior surface of the liver and the peritoneum (Plate 55–11). Evidence of fallopian tube involvement may also be noted, reflecting the pelvic inflammatory disease. This syndrome has been reported secondary to *Chlamydia trachomatis*[60] as well as coxsackie-B infection.[61] Hepatic abscess is another lesion that commonly produces adhesions (Plate 55–12).

Adhesions of any cause may produce abdominal pain. However, many patients have adhesions without abdominal pain. Laparoscopy may play a role in establishing a relationship between intra-abdominal adhesions and pain; manipulation of an adhesion may reproduce the patient's symptoms.

Patients undergoing peritoneal dialysis may develop peritonitis, which may require investigation to elucidate the cause. Laparoscopy is particularly difficult in these patients because of their propensity to develop adhesions. Cunningham and Tucker[62] have reported the use of the Tenckhoff catheter to establish the pneumoperitoneum and subsequent air-contrast radiography to allow safe entry of the laparoscope. With this technique, an adequate examination was carried out in 3 patients. A spider-like array of adhesions was found (Plate 55–13) in one of these patients who had a nonspecific inflammatory peritoneal reaction with eosinophils predominant in the biopsy specimen (aptly named eosinophilic peritonitis by the authors).[62]

Lipomas and Cysts

Benign lesions of the peritoneum may be noted during diagnostic laparoscopy. Lipomas of the peritoneum are incidental findings. These only require recognition and any form of intervention should be avoided. Of greater concern is the rare finding of peritoneal cysts. Primary peritoneal cysts may be solitary or multiple, may or may not be fixed to the mesentery, and may produce abdominal pain.[62] Their pathogenesis is unclear, although trauma has been suggested.[63]

References

1. Bar-Meir S, Lerner E, Conn HO. Analysis of ascitic fluid in cirrhosis. Dig Dis Sci 1979; 24:136–44.
2. Hoefs JC. Increase in ascites white blood cell and protein concentrations during diuresis in patients with chronic liver disease. Hepatology 1981; 1: 249–54.
3. Gitlin N, Stauffer JL, Silvestri RC. The pH of ascitic fluid in the diagnosis of spontaneous bacterial peritonitis in alcoholic cirrhosis. Hepatology 1982; 2:408–11.
4. Mirouze D, Juttner HU, Reynolds TB. Left pleural effusion in patients with chronic liver disease and ascites. Dig Dis Sci 1981; 26:984–8.
5. Donowitz M, Kerstein MD, Spiro HM. Pancreatic ascites. Medicine 1974; 53:183–95.
6. Press OW, Press NO, Kaufman SD. Evaluation and management of chylous ascites. Ann Intern Med 1982; 96:358–64.
7. Dagnini G: Cirrhosis of the liver. In: Dagnini G. Clinical Laparoscopy. Padua, Italy: Piccin Medical Books, 1982; 157–80.
8. Marshall JB, Pola L. Chylous ascites secondary to constrictive pericarditis. A discussion of pathophysiologic mechanisms. Dig Dis Sci 1982; 27:84–7.
9. Hall TJ, Donaldson DR, Brennan TG. The value of laparoscopy under local anesthesia in 250 medical and surgical patients. Br J Surg 1980; 67:751–3.
10. Coupland GAE, Townend DM, Martin CJ. Peritoneoscopy—use in assessment of intra-abdominal malignancy. Surgery 1981; 89:645–9.
11. Villa F, de Guzman S, Steigmann F. Peritoneoscopic findings in ascites. Gastrointest Endosc 1968; 14: 48–51.
12. Sherlock S, Feldman CA, Moran B, Scheur PJ. Partial nodular transformation of the liver with portal hypertension. Am J Med 1966; 40:195–203.
13. Boyer JL, Hales MR, Klatskin G. Idiopathic portal hypertension due to occlusion of intrahepatic portal veins by organized thrombi. A study based on postmortem vinylite-injection corrosion and dissection of the intrahepatic vasculature in 4 cases. Medicine 1980; 53:77–91.
14. Fletcher MS, Wight DGD. Partial nodular transformation of the caudate lobe of the liver presenting with ascites. Postgrad Med J 1980; 56:276–9.
15. Shedlofsky S, Koehler RE, DeSchryver-Kecskemeti K, Alpers DH. Noncirrhotic nodular transformation of the liver with portal hypertension: clinical angiographic and pathological correlation. Gastroenterology 1980; 79:938–43.
16. Wanless IR, Godwin TA, Allen F, Feder A. Nodular regenerative hyperplasia of the liver in hematologic disorders: A possible response to obliterative portal venography. Medicine 1980; 59:367–79.
17. Schwartz H, Tenge JR, Parker HW. Laparoscopic diagnosis of low dose radiation-induced hepatitis. Am J Gastroenterol 1978; 70:167–70.
18. Reed GB Jr, Cox AJ Jr. The human liver after radiation injury. A form of veno-occlusive disease. Am J Pathol 1966; 48:597–711.
19. Lindner H. Laparoscopy in hepatic vein thrombosis. Endoscopy 1973; 5:104–6.
20. Griner PF, Elbadawi A, Packman CH. Veno-occlusive disease of the liver after chemotherapy of acute leukemia. Report of two cases. Ann Intern Med 1976; 85:578–82.
21. Luna A, Meister HP, Szanto PB. Esophageal varices in the absence of cirrhosis. Am J Clin Pathol 1968; 49:710–7.
22. Dagnini G. Ascites. Incidence and characteristics in congestive heart failure and neoplasm of the liver. In: Dagnini G. Clinical Laparoscopy. Padua, Italy: Piccin Medical Books, 1982; 18–9.
23. Bichler T, Dudley DA. Nephrogenous ascites. Am J Gastroenterol 1982; 77:73–4.
24. Higby DJ, Ohnuma T. Plasmacytoma cell ascites. NY State J Med 1975; 75:1074–6.
25. Quagliata F, Sebes J, Pinstein ML, Schmidt LW. Long bone erosions and ascites in progressive systemic sclerosis (scleroderma). J Rheumatol 1982; 9:641–4.
26. Bagley CM, Young RC, Schein PS, deVita VT. Ovarian cancer metastatic to the diaphragm—frequently undiagnosed at laparotomy. Am J Obstet Gynecol 1973; 116:397–400.
27. Berek JS, Griffiths CT, Leventhal JM. Laparoscopy for second-look evaluation in ovarian cancer. Obstet Gynecol 1981; 58:192–8.
28. Wilson RO, Sueldo CE. Exudative ascites produced by pelvic inflammatory disease. Obstet Gynecol 1983; 61:54s–5s.
29. Antman KH. Clinical presentation and natural history of benign and malignant mesothelioma. Sem Oncol 1981; 8:313–20.
30. Moertel CG. Peritoneal mesothelioma. Gastroenterology 1972; 63:346–50.
31. Moertel CG. The peritoneum. In: Holland JF, Frei E, eds. Cancer Medicine. Philadelphia: Lea & Febiger, 1982:1836–66.
32. Eslami B, Lutcher CL. Antemortem diagnosis in two cases of malignant peritoneal mesothelioma. Am J Med Sci 1974; 267:117–21.
33. McCallum RW, Maceri DR, Jensen D, Berci G. Laparoscopic diagnosis of peritoneal mesothelioma.

A report of a case and review of the diagnostic approach. Dig Dis Sci 1979; 24:170–4.

34. Salky BA. Laparoscopic diagnosis of peritoneal mesothelioma. Gastrointest Endosc 1983; 29:65–6.

35. Ehrlich AN, Stalder G, Geller W, Sherlock P. Gastrointestinal manifestations of malignant lymphoma. Gastroenterology 1968; 54:1115–21.

36. Lewin KJ, Ranchod M, Dorfman RF. Lymphomas of the gastrointestinal tract. A study of 117 cases presenting with gastrointestinal disease. Cancer 1978; 42:693–707.

37. May JT, Costanzi JJ. Ascites in chronic leukemia. Oncology 1982; 39:55–8.

38. Gorshein D, Brauer MJ. Ascites in myeloid metaplasia due to ectopic peritoneal implantation. Cancer 1969; 23:1408–12.

39. Koeffler HP, Clinem J. Multiple myeloma presenting as ascites. West J Med 1977; 127:248–50.

40. Fernandez RN, Daly JM. Pseudomyxoma peritonei. Arch Surg 1980; 115:409–14.

41. Higa E, Rosai J, Pizzimbono CA, Wise L. Mucosal hyperplasia, mycinous cystadenoma and mucinous cystadenocarcinoma of the appendix. Cancer 1973; 32:1525–41.

42. Pozo A, Pajares J. Peritoneoscopic appearance of pseudomyxoma peritonei. Endoscopy 1975; 7: 176–9.

43. Douds HN, Pitt MJ. Calcified rims: characteristic but uncommon radiologic finding in pseudomyxoma peritonei. Gastrointest Radiol 1980; 5: 263–6.

44. Novetsky GJ, Berlin L, Epstein AJ, Miller SH. Pseudomyxoma peritonei. J Comput Assist Tomogr 1982; 6:398–9.

45. Chui CJ. Pseudomyxoma peritonei diagnosed by peritoneoscopy. Aust N Z J Surg 1975; 45:277–9.

46. Brown JD, Dac An N. Tuberculous peritonitis. Am J Gastroenterol 1976; 66:277–82.

47. Alvarez SZ, Carpio R. Hepatobiliary tuberculosis. Dig Dis Sci 1983; 28:193–200.

48. Ruddock JC, Hope RB. Coccidioidal peritonitis: Diagnosis by peritoneoscopy. JAMA 1939; 113: 2054–5.

49. Saw EC, Shields SJ, Comer TP, Huntington RW. Granulomatous peritonitis due to *coccidioides immitis*. Arch Surg 1974; 108:369–71.

50. Lintermans JP. Fatal peritonitis: An unusual complication of strongyloides stercoralis infestation. Clin Pediatr 1975; 14:974–5.

51. Kapoor OP, Nathwani BV, Joshi VR: Amoebic peritonitis: A study of 73 cases. J Trop Med Hyg 1972; 75:11–5.

52. Reddy CR, Venkateswar RD, Sarma EN, Swamy GM. Granulomatous peritonitis due to ascaris lumbricoides and its ova. J Trop Med Hyg 1975; 78: 146–9.

53. Blumberg H, Srinivasan K, Parnes I. Peritoneal schistosomiasis simulating carcinoma. NY State J Med 1966; 66:758–61.

54. Wong M, Rosen SW. Ascites in sarcoidosis due to peritoneal involvement. Ann Intern Med 1962; 57:277–80.

55. Daum F, Boley SJ, Cohen MI. Miliary Crohn's disease. Gastroenterology 1974; 67:527–30.

56. Isenberg JI, Gilbert SB, Pitcher JL. Ascites with peritoneal involvement in Whipple's disease. Gastroenterology 1971; 60:305–10.

57. McNabb PC, Fleming CR, Higgins JA, Davis GL. Transmural eosinophilic gastroenteritis with ascites. Mayo Clin Proc 1979; 54:119–22.

58. Curtis AH. A cause of adhesions in the right upper quadrant. JAMA 1930; 94:1221–2.

59. Fitz-Hugh T Jr. Acute gonococci peritonitis of the right upper quadrant in women. JAMA 1934; 102:2094–6.

60. Wood JJ, Bolton JP, Cannon SR, et al. Biliary-type pain as a manifestation of genital tract infection: The Curtis-Fitz-Hugh syndrome. Br J Surg 1982; 69:251–3.

61. Friedrich VK, Henning H. Laparoskopisches bild der perihepatitis nach akater Coxsackie-virus erkrankung (Morbus disease). Z Gastroenterol 1982; 20:448–51.

62. Cunningham JT, Tucker CT. Peritoneoscopy in chronic peritoneal dialysis: Use in evaluation and management of complications. Gastrointest Endosc 1983; 29:47–50.

63. Watts HG. Peritoneal cysts. Aust NZ J Surg 1968; 37:374–7.

Chapter 56

EMERGENCY LAPAROSCOPY

GEORGE BERCI, M.D.

The introduction of abdominal lavage by Root et al.[1] expedited the recognition of patients with intra-abdominal bleeding. As years passed, it was found that surgical exploration was not required in every case of hemoperitoneum, and that the incidence of unnecessary diagnostic laparotomy in cases of blunt abdominal trauma is about 20%. In one fifth of these patients no visceral injury or significant bleeding site was found and, therefore, no further intervention was necessary. Even the introduction of computed tomography (CT), a complex and expensive diagnostic study, has not eliminated unnecessary laparotomies.[2] Unnecessary surgery represents a significant burden and expense for patients with respect to increased morbidity and extended hospitalization.

The concept of laparoscopic examination of the intra-abdominal organs on an emergency basis is not new.[3, 4] However, early reports advocated the use of standard laparoscopes and accessory equipment. These instruments are highly satisfactory for elective procedures, but they are not suitable for emergency laparoscopy. We developed a miniature laparoscope that has a diameter almost identical to that of a lavage catheter.[5] This instrument is easier, faster, and safer to introduce than the larger standard instrument. With this laparoscope emergency laparoscopy can be performed with the patient on a bed or stretcher in the emergency room, an intensive care unit, or even a hospital room. The procedure is performed with the patient under local anesthesia and intravenous sedation. The patient's condition must be monitored continuously throughout the examination.[6]

We reported our results with emergency laparoscopy in 1980 and again in 1983.[5, 6]

INDICATIONS

The indications for emergency laparoscopy include the following: (1) mental obtundation, (2) history or evidence of blunt abdominal trauma or abdominal stab wound(s), (3) unexplained hypotension, and (4) equivocal signs of an intra-abdominal emergency on physical examination.

At initial evaluation the physical signs and other evidence of acute intra-abdominal conditions of an emergency nature may be lacking in a patient who is obtunded for any reason, including head trauma, alcoholism, and drug ingestion. Multiple injuries are often present in patients who suffer trauma. Acute alcohol intoxication and drug ingestion may also be associated with blunt abdominal trauma. Physical signs of intra-abdominal hemorrhage or significant organ damage may not be evident at the initial evaluation of a patient who has sustained abdominal trauma. Hypotension can have many possible causes. When thorough evaluation does not suggest an etiology, intra-abdominal hemorrhage and other acute events must be included in the differential diagnosis. Depending on clinical circumstances, the usual signs of intra-abdominal hemorrhage or perforation may be absent, especially during the early phase of the patient's course. Therefore, there are many clinical situations in which a rapid and accurate diagnosis that includes a proper assessment of treatment priorities can influence the eventual outcome for patients who have sustained severe trauma.

In my opinion, peritoneal lavage in cases of trauma is an overly sensitive examination. Furthermore, what constitutes a clearly positive test is controversial.[6] There is, in fact, considerable overlap between positive and negative results, so that interpretation frequently remains in doubt in the difficult clinical situations for which the test is intended.

TECHNIQUE

A complete laparoscopy instrument set should be prepared on a mobile cart. However, the standard telescope set and trocar should be replaced with the special instruments for emergency laparoscopy (Fig. 56–1). Our set-up includes the following: (1) a 4 mm (outer diameter) telescope (30-degree forward-oblique view with fiberoptic illumination) sometimes referred to as a minilaparoscope (Karl Storz Endoscopy of America, Inc.); (2) pneumoperitoneum needle with spring-loaded blunt stylette; (3) accessory trocar with valve and stylette (4 mm outer diameter); (4) 5 mm trocar with rotating valve; and (5) palpation (suction-coagulation) probe with trumpet valve and electrical contact for connection to an electrosurgical generator. The last of these, the suction-coagulation-palpation probe is one of the most important accessories. It acts as the "extended finger" of the endoscopist. It provides interrupted suction for evacuation of fluid or blood and can be used to obtain fluid specimens for laboratory evaluation.

The technique of emergency laparoscopy is in most respects similar to that of routine diagnostic laparoscopy (see Chapter 50). However, there are always slight variations in technique. For emergency laparoscopy I prefer the following approach.

The usual site for insertion of the pneumoperitoneum (Veres) needle is immediately below the umbilicus in the midline. It may be necessary to select another site, however, if previous abdominal scars are present. After suitable local anesthesia has been administered, a stab wound skin incision is made with a blade (No. 11) to allow introduction of the spring-loaded pneumoperitoneum needle. Aspiration should be performed immediately after the needle has entered the peritoneal cavity to be certain that the needle did not enter a blood vessel or the lumen of an intestine. The needle is then attached to an insufflation device by means of which nitrous oxide is to be delivered into the peritoneal cavity at a rate of 1.0 to 1.2 liters per minute. When the pneumoperitoneum is sufficient for laparoscopy, the needle is removed, the stab incision is enlarged, and the 5 mm trocar is introduced through the incision into the peritoneal cavity. Since the trocar is small, it is only necessary to lengthen the stab wound incision by a few millimeters. The prewarmed 4 mm minilaparoscope is then advanced through the trocar. Further technical details of this procedure have been described in previous reports.[5, 6]

Examination of the abdomen should be systematic, including all quadrants, pelvis, and the suprahepatic spaces. The accessory 4 mm trocar may be introduced in a second puncture site. This should be prepared as above with a local anesthetic and requires a stab wound. The suction-coagulation-palpation probe is then introduced through the trocar for the purposes of palpation, retraction, and manipulation of intra-abdominal organs and structures as well as suction and coagulation. The second puncture with introduction of the trocar and probe should be performed under direct vision, i.e., the site

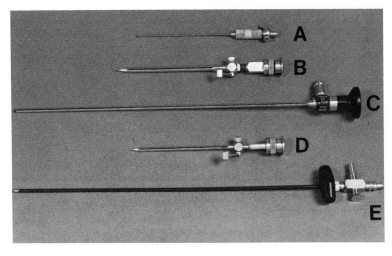

FIGURE 56–1. Instruments for emergency laparoscopy. A, Pneumoperitoneum needle; B, 5 mm examining trocar; C, 30 degree forward oblique view telescope (4 mm); D, accessory trocar with valve and stylette (4 mm); E, suction-coagulation-palpation probe. (Manufacturer: K. Storz Endoscopy of America, Inc.)

chosen for introduction of these accessories should be observed laparoscopically from within the abdomen. Selection of the site depends to some degree on what the laparoscopist wishes to manipulate. Generally, the second puncture site is placed laterally in the right or left upper quadrant.

When the examination is complete, the abdomen is desufflated (via the trocar), all instruments are removed, and the stab wounds closed with one or two metallic clips. Antibiotics are administered only if there is some specific indication for their use. Emergency laparoscopy usually requires no more than 15 to 20 minutes.

LAPAROSCOPIC FINDINGS

Hemoperitoneum

One of the major observations to be made during laparoscopy is the presence or absence of blood within the peritoneal cavity. In this respect the location and quantity of blood are important.

The mode of distribution of blood within the abdomen can provide clues to the location of the bleeding site. For example, blood will be confined to the pelvic area in the case of pelvic fractures. Pelvic fracture is also a common cause of false positive results with peritoneal lavage.

Quantitative assessment of the volume of blood present in the abdomen is difficult, but an impression can be gained with some experience. A useful method for assessing the amount of blood present is to divide hemoperitoneum into minimal, moderate, and severe categories.

The refinement and accuracy of the observations made by emergency laparoscopy provide a far greater latitude in the decision-making process in hemoperitoneum, a distinct advantage in comparison with peritoneal lavage alone.

Minimal Hemoperitoneum

With minimal hemoperitoneum a small amount of blood will be seen in the lateral peritoneal gutter or streaks of blood will be seen between intestinal loops. If there is no increase in this small volume of blood during the procedure, and if the search for a bleeding site has been unrevealing, then the patient can usually be treated conservatively and observed. If the bleeding site is found, the bleeding may amount to a minimal ooze

or it may have stopped completely. In our experience, a bleeding site is found in only 50% of patients classified as having a minimal hemoperitoneum. Extremely small volumes of blood in the peritoneal cavity, as in the case of minimal hemoperitoneum, are nevertheless sufficient to produce a positive result by peritoneal lavage.

Moderate Hemoperitoneum

If 10 to 20 ml of blood can be found in one of the lateral gutters, the patient is considered to have moderate hemoperitoneum. In such cases the second trocar should be introduced immediately as described above. The suction-coagulation-palpation probe should be introduced and the hemoperitoneum evacuated. A thorough and systematic search is then initiated, making use of the suction cannula as a palpation-manipulation probe.

If organ injury with bleeding is discovered (liver laceration, for example), the site of injury should be observed carefully. If the bleeding is brisk, surgical intervention is indicated. If the bleeding site is not found after 5 to 10 minutes of diligent searching and the gutters refill with blood to the previous level, the bleeding vessel is probably not within the range of observation, and surgical intervention should be considered. If a small laceration that is oozing a small amount of blood or one that already shows evidence of cessation of bleeding is found, or if blood clots are seen in the vicinity of the laceration but no active bleeding, then patients with such injuries can be managed by observation alone. The suction-coagulation-palpation probe may be used to aspirate blood from an oozing lesion to better assess the rate of blood loss; in selected cases coagulation may also be applied. If injuries are found that require immediate operation, precise localization of the injury facilitates selection of the optimal incision.

Severe Hemoperitoneum

If aspiration with the pneumoperitoneum needle clearly results in blood in the syringe on two or three attempts, or if this does not result in aspiration of blood but laparoscopic observation displays intestinal loops floating in, or surrounded by a pool of blood, then the indication for immediate operation is obvious. Blood in the lateral gutters to a depth of two or more finger breadths should also be classified as severe hemoperitoneum.

Organ Perforations

In cases of perforation of one of the hollow intra-abdominal organs, yellowish fluid will be seen in gutters. This can be aspirated and sent for laboratory analysis such as amylase and bile content, pH, and bacterial culture. However, this finding, in general, is consistent with perforation and represents an indication for surgery.

If several hours have elapsed between the trauma and the examination, the actual injury may not be seen. However, it may be suspected because of indirect findings such as a conglomerate of omentum in one particular area, or a small aggregation of edematous, hyperemic intestinal loops. The palpation probe can be of help by moving such loops or omentum.

Perforation of the retroperitoneal segment of the duodenum or pancreatic injuries will escape detection at laparoscopy. Fortunately, these lesions are rare and other diagnostic measures will help to clarify this clinical picture.

Splenic Injury

Splenic injury is characterized by accumulation of blood in the left gutter. A spleen that is normal in size is seldom seen in the left upper quadrant because it is usually covered by omentum. The omentum covering the spleen is elevated by a pool of blood or a blood clot. Frequently, the elevated omentum will have a bluish color.

Splenic injury can have serious consequences and is often an indication for splenectomy. However, conservation of the spleen is also desirable and can be accomplished in suitable and selected cases.[7] In some cases of splenic trauma the laparoscopic appearance may be that of a minimal hemoperitoneum with blood present in the area of the spleen but without a significant bulge or bluish color of the omentum lying over the spleen. This assessment requires judgment and experience. However, if the injury is found to be minimal at laparoscopy, and the patient's vital signs are stable, conservative management with very careful observation can be initiated even if the spleen scan denotes splenic injury.

Liver Injury

Deceleration injuries are frequently characterized by lacerations on the anterior surface or dome of the liver lobe and in the vicinity of the round or falciform ligament. These areas are easily observed at laparoscopy. The undersurface of the liver can also be inspected with the aid of the palpation probe by gently lifting up segments of the right lobe and the entire left lobe. If a laceration is found, the telescope is advanced and the area is observed closely under magnification for a few minutes. In the case of a small, oozing laceration, compression or coagulation may be employed. However, if at the end of the observation period bleeding persists, then laparotomy must be considered.

Penetrating Injury

Laparoscopy is not performed for gunshot wounds of the abdomen. However, wounds produced by slow penetration and stab wounds in which it is uncertain whether the peritoneal cavity was entered are not a contraindication to laparoscopy. In one review of 89 stab wounds of the abdomen it was found that an unnecessary surgical exploration was performed in one third of the patients.[8]

When laparoscopy may be of assistance in determining the presence or extent of intra-abdominal injury as a result of a stab wound, our approach is as follows: The skin is temporarily closed to provide a seal for the pneumoperitoneum. Laparoscopic observation in the region of the presumed penetration is highly accurate with respect to excluding or confirming that the parietal peritoneum has been penetrated. If inspection of the parietal surface indicates that the abdomen was entered, the area underlying the penetration site should be inspected with the aid of the palpation probe. Loops of bowel should be lifted and pushed gently aside to look for signs of bleeding, serosal injury, leakage of fluid, and other signs of perforation or hemorrhage.

RESULTS

Our results in 129 patients examined by emergency laparoscopy are summarized. The outcome of the procedure can be classified as follows: (1) negative findings, no surgery; (2) positive findings, no surgery; and (3) positive findings followed by surgical exploration.

Negative Laparoscopy (No Operation)

There were 72 cases (55.8%) in this category. No hemoperitoneum or other abnormalities were discovered, and none of these patients subsequently required exploratory laparotomy.

Positive Laparoscopy (No Operation)

Minimal or moderate hemoperitoneum was found in 33 cases (25.5%). However, there was no identifiable injury, or only minimal lacerations were seen in these patients. These patients were therefore observed in an intensive care unit.

Only one patient required laparotomy subsequent to this decision. This 35-year-old, semi-comatose man was admitted with a compression skull fracture after a motor vehicle accident. Laparoscopy revealed minimal hemoperitoneum in the left (lower) gutter without other abnormalities. The patient's condition improved and oral feeding was begun on the third postadmission day. Abdominal pain in the left lower quadrant, with fever and leukocytosis, developed in two days. On the eighth postadmission day an exploratory operation was performed. A sealed perforation of the sigmoid colon near the rectosigmoid junction was found.

Positive Laparoscopy (Operation)

Severe hemoperitoneum was present at emergency laparoscopy in 24 patients (18.6%), all of whom underwent surgery. The source of bleeding or organ perforation was found endoscopically and confirmed at surgery in all but one patient. In the latter case 700 ml of blood were evacuated at operation but no source of bleeding was found. The 24 cases included 3 liver lacerations, 11 splenic injuries (in 6 patients the spleen was saved with splenorrhaphy), 4 organ perforations, and 6 arterial bleeders.

Complications

In one patient, a minimal amount of hemoperitoneum was interpreted as being caused by injury to the omentum during insertion of the trocar. Fresh coagulum was seen in the area. Observation only was required.

DISCUSSION

Emergency laparoscopy is extremely helpful in avoiding unnecessary abdominal explorations in cases of hemoperitoneum where peritoneal lavage reveals intra-abdominal bleeding. Most of our patients who sustained multiple injuries and were at high surgical risk were elderly. Abdominal surgery in these patients would have significantly increased postoperative morbidity, and therefore it was important to avoid any unnecessary operations. The technique of emergency laparoscopy is not difficult. It provides a safe, fast, and accurate method of diagnosis in cases where the presence and/or extent of intra-abdominal injury is uncertain or unknown. In our experience, the use of emergency laparoscopy has avoided surgery in a significant number of patients. Unfortunately, traumatic injury is a common occurrence that results in significant loss of life and morbidity. A complete and accurate evaluation is of great importance in such cases, and in this respect emergency laparoscopy can have a significant role.

References

1. Root HD, Hauser CW, McKinley CR, et al. Diagnostic peritoneal lavage. Surgery 1965; 57:633–7.
2. Federle MP, Crass RA, Jeffrey RB, Trunkey DD. Computed tomography in blunt abdominal trauma. Arch Surg 1982; 117:645–50.
3. Gazzaniga AB, Stanton WW, Bartlett RH. Laparoscopy in the diagnosis of blunt and penetrating injuries to the abdomen. Am J Surg 1976; 131:315–8.
4. Carnevale N, Baron N, Delany HM. Peritoneoscopy as an aid in the diagnosis of abdominal trauma: a preliminary report. J Trauma 1977; 17:634–41.
5. Sherwood R, Berci G, Austin E, Morgenstern L. Minilaparoscopy for blunt abdominal trauma. Arch Surg 1980; 115:672–3.
6. Berci G, Dunkelman D, Michel SL, et al. Emergency minilaparoscopy in abdominal trauma. An update. Am J Surg 1983; 146:261–5.
7. Morgenstern L, Shapiro SJ. Techniques of splenic conservation. Arch Surg 1979; 114:449–54.
8. Donaldson LA, Findlay IG, Smith A. A retrospective review of 89 stab wounds to the abdomen and chest. Br J Surg 1981; 68:793–6.

Chapter 57

GYNECOLOGIC LAPAROSCOPY FOR THE GASTROENTEROLOGIST

A. ALBERT YUZPE, M.D.

Gynecologists began to perform laparoscopy a decade and a half ago, and since that time this procedure has become the second most frequently performed gynecologic surgical procedure, surpassed only by dilation and curettage. During this short span of time, laparoscopy has evolved from a simple diagnostic procedure, with minimal capabilities, to a sophisticated diagnostic and operative technique in which biopsies may be obtained and tissues and organs manipulated, transected, electrocoagulated, drained, suspended, or mechanically occluded. In short, gynecologic laparoscopy has a wide range of diagnostic and operative applications. For the gynecologist, the laparoscope has become a window to the pelvis and abdomen.

Most gynecologic laparoscopies, diagnostic as well as therapeutic, are performed under general anesthesia, in contrast to gastrointestinal laparoscopy, which is usually performed with local anesthesia (see Chapter 50). Tubal sterilization, accounting for about 60% of all gynecologic laparoscopies, is performed for the most part under general anesthesia, although the use of local anesthesia is increasing. Despite widespread preference for general anesthesia, laparoscopy remains predominantly an out-patient procedure, hospitalization being required only for patients with unrelated but potentially complicating illnesses or those who reside at a great distance.

There is an interesting contrast between patients undergoing laparoscopy for a gynecologic indication and those in whom the indication relates to the gastrointestinal tract or liver. Patients in the former group are rarely seriously ill and undergo the procedure for one or more of the indications listed in Table 57–1. The gastroenterologist's patient frequently has an acute or chronic hepatic disorder, often with some degree of hepatic decompensation and/or portal hypertension.

Since the laparoscope provides a view of the whole abdominal cavity, both gynecologist and gastroenterologist must consider the entire abdomen and pelvis and visualize each organ to the maximum reasonable extent at each procedure.

Unfortunately, gynecologists tend to focus their attention at laparoscopy on the pelvis and often do not turn the laparoscope to visualize the upper abdominal contents. The laparoscopic view of the upper abdomen is compromised to some degree by technique,

TABLE 57–1. **Indications for Gynecologic Laparoscopy**

Diagnostic	
Infertility	Abdominal trauma
Pelvic pain and/or mass	Habitual abortion
Acute	Cryptic malignancy
Chronic	Peritoneal fluid
Suspected ectopic pregnancy	collection
Suspected endometriosis	Endocrine disorders
Assessment of possible	Genetic disorders
candidates for tuboplasty	Menstrual dysfunction
"Second look" procedures	Ascites
Anatomic anomalies	
Amenorrhea—primary or	
secondary	
Therapeutic	
Tubal sterilization	Ovarian cyst aspiration
Lysis of adhesions	Retrieval of oocytes
Fulguration of endometriosis	Uterine suspension
Removal of foreign bodies	Biopsy

since gynecologic laparoscopy is performed with the patient in the Trendelenburg position. However, in most cases, the appendix, liver, gallbladder, lower border of the stomach, falciform ligament, and diaphragm are easily seen. The spleen is rarely, if ever, visualized in the usual gynecologic laparoscopy position. Presumably, many gastroenterologists are of the same opinion, vis-à-vis the pelvic organs, as the gynecologist.

The purpose of this chapter is to familiarize those whose use of laparoscopy is directed to the gastrointestinal tract and liver with the more common disorders of the pelvic organs of women so as to dispel any reluctance to visualize these structures, even though their evaluation is not of primary interest. A treatise on gynecologic laparoscopy cannot be presented here, but there are standard texts that can be used as reference sources.[1, 2] Pelvic findings of a gynecologic nature are often discovered when laparoscopy is performed to determine the cause of pelvic pain. The very same abnormalities may also be encountered as incidental findings when laparoscopy is performed for some other indication. Therefore, a familiarity with the appearance of the normal female pelvis, its variants, and the more prevalent pathologic conditions is essential to the gastroenterologist-laparoscopist.

TECHNIQUE

Unless contraindicated, all gynecologic laparoscopies are performed with the aid of a uterine manipulator in order to mobilize the uterus, fallopian tubes, and ovaries. This permits complete visualization of all structural surfaces. Few, if any, gastroenterologic laparoscopists avail themselves of such instruments, and therefore complete inspection of the female pelvis may be less than adequate. At the same time, partial visualization is preferable to none.

Whenever possible, the systematic approach to evaluation of the female pelvis should include evaluation of the anterior cul-de-sac, round ligaments, uterus, fallopian tubes, ovaries and their suspensory ligaments, uterosacral ligaments, broad ligaments, and posterior cul-de-sac. A blunt-tipped manipulating probe is of great value in mobilizing pelvic structures, whether or not a uterine manipulator is used.

Gynecologic findings that the gastroenterologist will most likely encounter at laparoscopy are listed in Table 57–2.

TABLE 57–2. **Common Gynecologic Abnormalities Likely to Be Encountered at Laparoscopy**

Endometriosis
Other gynecologic causes of pelvic
  pain
        Pelvic inflammatory disease (PID)
        Adhesions
Pelvic masses
        Ovarian cyst
        Solid ovarian tumor
        Uterine fibroids
Genital anomalies
Foreign bodies
        Perforated intrauterine device
        Splints, stents, drains

PELVIC DISORDERS

Endometriosis

Widespread use of laparoscopy has demonstrated that endometriosis is much more common than expected in the general population. Once considered a disease of older white women of higher socioeconomic status who had delayed childbearing, it is now known to be an "equal opportunity" disease that is fairly common in adolescents with otherwise unexplained pelvic pain, in multiparous patients, and in black women.

The laparoscopic findings of endometriosis vary, and the extent of the disease at laparoscopy does not necessarily correlate with the degree of pelvic pain. Endometriosis may be asymptomatic, yet there may be extensive involvement of the pelvic structures. The extent may also be minimal although the patient's symptoms are incapacitating. Any of the findings of endometriosis may be discovered at the time of laparoscopy, either incidentally or during the investigation for pelvic and/or abdominal pain.

It is important not only to recognize endometriosis but also to stage it. The staging method established by the American Fertility Society is of considerable assistance in evaluating treatment modalities. Photographs of the findings should also be obtained so that accurate comparisons can be made when and if a subsequent "second look" laparoscopy is performed to evaluate the response to therapy. This type of evaluation is extremely important because fertility may be affected in women with endometriosis regardless of the extent of the disease.

The gastroenterologist will be the primary endoscopist when vague pelvic-abdominal pain is caused by endometriosis in the adolescent with no associated menstrual symptoms or in the patient with gastrointestinal symptoms, primarily rectal, as the sole manifestation of the disease. When the presenting symptoms are dysmenorrhea, dyspareunia, or infertility, the gynecologist usually confirms the diagnosis.

The laparoscopic features of endometriosis vary (Plates 57–1 to 57–11). Scattered "mulberry or gunpowder" lesions may be seen on any of the smooth surfaces of the pelvis, but primarily in the anterior (Plate 57–1) and more commonly in the posterior cul-de-sac (Plate 57–2). Superficial implants on the serosa of the fallopian tubes (Plate 57–3), uterus, supporting ligaments (especially uterosacral ligaments) (Plate 57–4), and on the surface of the ovaries (Plate 57–5) are also extremely common. The serosa of the bowel may be affected. When endometriosis is suspected, laparoscopy should be performed during the immediate premenstrual or early menstrual phase of the reproductive cycle so that bleeding lesions may be seen (Plate 57–6); in many cases, evidence of retrograde menstruation is also seen (retrograde menstruation remains the most widely accepted theory of the pathogenesis of this condition). With increasing involvement, distortion of the fallopian tubes, adherence of the ovaries to the pouch of Douglas, posterior leaf of the broad ligament, and lateral pelvic walls (Plate 57–7), and ovarian enlargement with ovarian endometrioma (chocolate cysts) may be seen (Plate 57–8).

Rectal involvement with advancement and adherence of the rectum to the posterior surface of the uterus is frequently seen, with resultant obliteration or at least partial obliteration of the cul-de-sac (Plate 57–9). Often the rectum is elevated (advanced) above the level of the cervical-fundal junction with chocolate cysts in both ovaries that extend toward the midline, the so-called "kissing ovaries" appearance. With extensive disease the pelvic structures may have a "frozen pelvis" appearance with the uterus in fixed retroversion or densely adherent to the rectum and ovaries, which, in turn, are immobile and fill the cul-de-sac. Fallopian tubes, generally not occluded at the fimbria, may be clearly visible and appear healthy, although immobilized by extensive adhesions.

Obvious stigmata of endometriosis may not be present in some cases. However, certain findings may nevertheless suggest the presence of the disease. These subtle abnormalities include hemosiderin staining of the anterior and/or posterior cul-de-sac (Plate 57–10), and peritoneal defects (Plate 57–11), the latter primarily involving the posterior leaf of the broad ligament and posterior cul-de-sac. Such defects have been referred to as the "Allan-Masters syndrome" and in the past have been linked to trauma during pregnancy, labor, and delivery. However, it appears that they are extremely common in endometriosis. Endometrial implants are often present on the inner surfaces of the margins of the defects. Inserting a manipulating probe into the defect with elevation of the margin will often demonstrate the presence of a typical "gunpowder" lesion.

When either suggestive or pathognomonic findings of endometriosis are present, the gastroenterologist should carefully document the extent and severity of the disorder in written and photographic forms. The best method is the staging classification of the American Fertility Society. Specific staging forms, available from this society, should be used for this purpose.

Management of minimal endometriosis, i.e., endometrial implants, is by electrocoagulation or by carbon dioxide laser vaporization. This is acceptable if performed with proper instruments and a high frequency, low voltage, low output electrosurgical generator in the case of electrocoagulation, and with assurance that there is no risk of injury to surrounding structures. If the lesions are adjacent to or overlie the ureter on the lateral pelvic sidewall or are in close proximity to other vital structures electrosurgery is contraindicated.

Whether the gastroenterologist should proceed beyond staging to laparoscopic treatment of minimal disease is problematic. There are many factors to consider, including community and hospital standards of practice and the wishes of the patient as determined prior to the procedure. The type of anesthesia employed for the procedure is relevant; local anesthesia is unsuitable. It is unwise for those without training and experience in electrocoagulation of endometrial implants to undertake laparoscopic treatment of minimal endometriosis, especially when the operator also lacks thorough knowledge of pelvic anatomy as well as experience in the manipulation of the pelvic structures. When there is extensive disease and/or disease implants near vital structures, the patient should always be referred to a gynecologist for further management.

At times, lesions may be suggestive but not

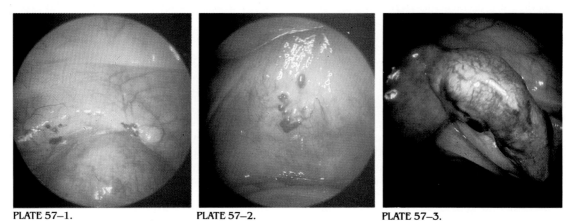

PLATE 57—1.   PLATE 57—2.   PLATE 57—3.

PLATE 57—1. "Mulberry" or "gunpowder" lesions of endometriosis on the vesico-uterine peritoneal fold (anterior cul-de-sac).
PLATE 57—2. Superficial endometriosis implants (mulberry or gunpowder lesions) in the posterior cul-de-sac.
PLATE 57—3. Endometriosis involving the serosa and endosalpinx of the isthmic portion of the fallopian tube. The tube is thickened and occluded in the affected area.

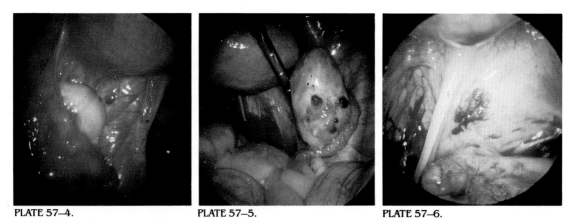

PLATE 57—4.   PLATE 57—5.   PLATE 57—6.

PLATE 57—4. Typical endometriosis implants and scarring of the uterosacral ligament.
PLATE 57—5. Endometriosis implants on the surface of the ovary. The ovary is not enlarged.
PLATE 57—6. Superficial endometriosis implants actively bleeding in the immediate premenstrual or early menstrual phase of the cycle.

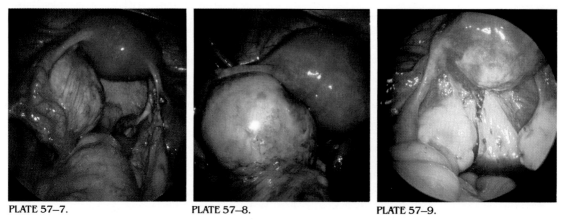

PLATE 57—7.   PLATE 57—8.   PLATE 57—9.

PLATE 57—7. Dense adherence of the ovary to the pelvic side wall, preventing mobilization and visualization of the undersurface of the ovary.
PLATE 57—8. Ovarian endometrioma.
PLATE 57—9. Endometriosis of the cul-de-sac causing advancement of the rectum onto the posterior surface of the uterus. The cul-de-sac is partially obliterated by this rectal involvement, and the ovaries are generally found adherent in the cul-de-sac on either side of the rectal advancement.

diagnostic of endometriosis so that a biopsy becomes necessary for diagnosis. A specimen can be obtained safely when the lesions are not close to vital structures such as the ureters, bladder, or bowel. Shallow biopsies obtained with any of several types of biopsy forceps will provide the gynecologist who will subsequently treat the patient with a pathologic diagnosis. If the biopsy site bleeds, electrocoagulation can be used for hemostasis, but generally bleeding stops rapidly and no treatment is required. However, if electrocoagulation is necessary, the same principles as noted above for any electrocoagulation procedure in the pelvis should be applied, i.e., the use of high frequency electrosurgical generators with low voltage and low power output. Bipolar coagulation instruments should be used if possible.

The appendix and the other areas of the gastrointestinal tract should be examined, since involvement of these regions is common in endometriosis.

A clinical emergency may occasionally arise as a result of rupture of a large ovarian endometrioma. The gastroenterologist may be involved when laparoscopy is performed for diagnosis. Evidence of a ruptured endometrioma is an indication for immediate laparotomy. However, endometriosis rarely results in this type of acute abdominal emergency that requires the participation of a gastroenterologist in diagnostic laparoscopy.

Acute Pelvic Pain

The investigation of pelvic pain that is potentially of gynecologic origin is one of the most frequent reasons that a gastroenterologist becomes involved in laparoscopy; a gynecologist may not be available or the provisional diagnosis may be gastrointestinal in nature. The differential diagnosis of pelvic pain includes a great number of disorders such as acute inflammatory bowel disease, acute appendicitis, acute salpingo-oophoritis, and ectopic gestation. Two important and relatively common disorders are ectopic gestation and pelvic inflammatory disease.

Ectopic Gestation

An ectopic gestation, particularly when unruptured, should be recognizable. Varying amounts of dark red unclotted blood may be seen in the cul-de-sac along with a segmental fusiform distention of the fallopian tube. Examples of isthmic and ampullary unrup-

tured ectopic pregnancies are shown in Plates 57–12 and 57–13.

Acute Pelvic Inflammatory Disease

Acute pelvic inflammatory disease (PID) is often difficult to diagnose or distinguish clinically from ectopic gestation or acute appendicitis. Generally, although not consistently, the findings of acute PID are bilateral. Cervical movement, especially toward the affected adnexa, tends to produce more severe pain in the ectopic gestation than in acute PID, but this is by no means diagnostic. An acutely inflamed appendix, especially if pelvic in location or perforated, may cause a secondary salpingo-oophoritis or salpingitis, with pelvic abscess formation, and may be indistinguishable clinically from acute salpingitis. Investigative methods such as ultrasonography and other laboratory studies are valuable in this clinical problem, although the solution lies with direct laparoscopic visualization of the area in question. Examples of acute and chronic PID are shown in Plates 57–14 and 57–15. As with endometriosis, photographic documentation of the extent of the disease is extremely valuable for the gynecologist, who must subsequently select an appropriate form of primary therapy, and for follow-up of the patient, which may include the management of fertility problems.

Acutely inflamed areas should not be manipulated, especially where pus may be present, to avoid disruption of a walled-off abscess. Pooling of pus or turbid fluid will often be seen in the cul-de-sac in acute pelvic inflammatory processes. Whether pus or turbid fluid, the contents of the cul-de-sac should be aspirated with a suction cannula and cultured for aerobic and anaerobic organisms. Then the pelvis should be thoroughly irrigated with normal saline. If possible, a tissue specimen should be obtained by direct scraping. This is especially helpful when culturing for *Chlamydia*, a frequent cause of acute PID, which usually cannot be cultured unless the specimen contains tissue or cells as opposed to fluid alone. Brushes may be inserted through a second or accessory puncture at laparoscopy to obtain cell samples by "brushing" various tissues. The instillation of antibiotics directly into the peritoneal cavity, in our experience, has not proved to be more advantageous than immediate postoperative treatment with systemic antibiotic therapy.

Laparoscopic manipulation should be kept to a minimum and further surgical intervention should not be undertaken in cases of

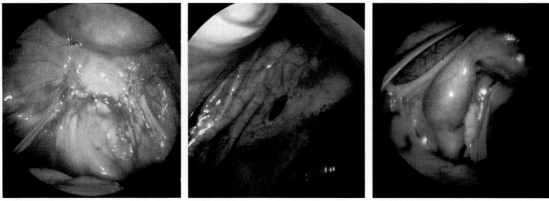

PLATE 57–10.   PLATE 57–11.   PLATE 57–12.

PLATE 57–10. Hemosiderin staining of the cul-de-sac, with scarring in the uterosacral ligaments, but no visible typical mulberry or gunpowder lesions.

PLATE 57–11. Allen-Masters syndrome – a defect generally found in the posterior leaf of the broad ligament or cul-de-sac and frequently seen in association with endometriosis. Superficial implants may be seen on the undersurface of the inner aspect of the peritoneal defect, or as in this case, around the margin of the defect.

PLATE 57–12. Unruptured isthmic estopic pregnancy, with typical bluish discoloration of the fallopian tube.

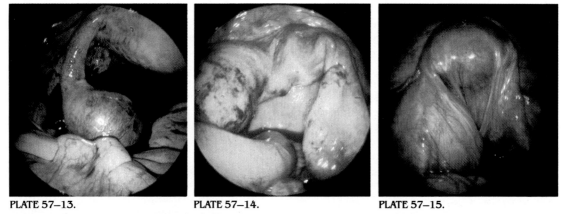

PLATE 57–13.   PLATE 57–14.   PLATE 57–15.

PLATE 57–13. Ampullary unruptured ectopic pregnancy, with accumulation of blood in the cul-de-sac.

PLATE 57–14. Acute pelvic inflammatory disease, with a left tubo-ovarian mass. Note the marked edema and pallor of the pelvic organs. In other instances the pelvic structures may appear to be engorged and very dark red; they may be covered with fibrinous exudate.

PLATE 57–15. Chronic pelvic inflammatory disease with left retro-ovarian mass, peritubal and parovarian adhesions, and obliteration of the cul-de-sac by filmy adhesion.

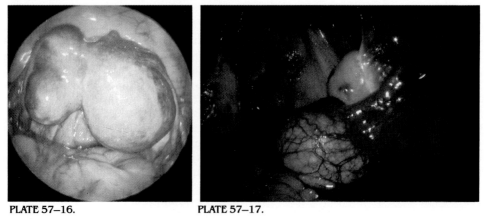

PLATE 57–16.   PLATE 57–17.

PLATE 57–16. Multiple uterine fibroids.

PLATE 57–17. Large parovarian cyst. Note that it is entirely separate from the ovary and should not be confused with an ovarian cyst.

acute PID. In the case of chronic disease, the adhesions are generally so extensive that lysis alone is usually of no value and therefore should be avoided. Bleeding is a complication of laparoscopic lysis of adhesions, and the lack of demonstrable value of lysis makes this form of treatment unwarranted.

Pelvic Masses

The incidental discovery of a pelvic mass at laparoscopy for a nongynecologic indication is relatively common because the pelvic examination is frequently omitted by physicians, other than gynecologists, or performed in a cursory or inexpert fashion during physical examination. When a pelvic mass is discovered, there are important decisions to be made with respect to the nature of the lesion, vis-à-vis benign versus malignant, and whether immediate or future surgical intervention is indicated. As a general rule, the inexperienced individual should not attempt needle aspiration of an ovarian lesion. Whenever possible, an experienced gynecologist should come to the endoscopy room to study such lesions and to plan or perform definitive therapy.

Uterine Fibroids

Uterine fibroids are a frequent finding; they are virtually never malignant (Plate 57–16). A single subserosal or intramural lesion may be present; when multiple, uterine fibroids may totally distort the uterine architecture. Other than documentation of their size and extent, photographically and by written description, no other action is required.

Ovarian and Parovarian Masses

An ovarian mass presents a different, more difficult problem than the uterine fibroid. If the mass is cystic, the decision to aspirate its contents is problematic. Aspiration of a cyst that proves to be malignant may result in leakage of fluid from the ovary and dissemination of malignant cells. This possibility is of constant concern to gynecologists. Some recommend that ovarian cysts never be aspirated, whereas others suggest selective aspiration provided the cyst is (1) smooth, with no external papillary excrescences; (2) less than 5 cm in diameter; (3) freely mobile; and (4) "benign" in appearance as best as can be discerned.

Aspiration using a small-bore needle (22-gauge spinal needle) inserted transabdominally under direct vision may be performed with little risk of leakage if the entire lesion is aspirated. Specimens require pathologic, cytologic, and bacteriologic evaluation. Some gynecologists have suggested that subsequent fenestration of the cyst wall can be considered definitive therapy. However, the majority of gynecologists recommend avoidance of such procedures.

Ovarian endometriomas (Plate 57–8) have a fairly typical appearance and are generally associated with other stigmata of endometriosis. Aspiration should not be performed, since disease at this stage requires further surgical management by laparotomy regardless of whether the lesion is aspirated.

Cysts of mesonephric remnants located in the mesosalpinx, the "parovarian" area, are frequently seen and are often large (Plate 57–17). These cystic structures are separate from the ovary; the fallopian tube is often draped or stretched over the lesion. Depending on its size, the cyst may require definitive surgery or may be managed by aspiration (Plate 57–18), as described for small, benign, cystic ovarian lesions. The fluid should be evaluated cytologically. In such cases the structure is easily collapsed and will often not recur. When these cystic lesions are located near the distal end of the fallopian tube, they may produce prolonged traction on the tube, causing elongation of its pedicle followed by torsion of the entire adnexa (Plate 57–19). Immediate surgery then becomes necessary, and if treatment is delayed, there may be loss of the adnexa due to gangrene.

Benign cystic teratoma (dermoid cyst) is a common finding. The ovary appears smooth, often with a yellowish discoloration seen through the capsule. Needle puncture of such a lesion should not be performed, since leakage of the sebaceous contents may result in profound peritoneal irritation. The abnormality that most closely resembles a dermoid cyst is the ovarian endometrioma. In the latter, other findings of endometriosis may be present and assist in distinguishing these two lesions. However, this may not be the case, and if there is doubt, the lesion should not be punctured. If a dermoid cyst is punctured inadvertently, the puncture site will usually seal if a small-bore needle was used. However, fluid that leaks from the puncture site should be aspirated and the pelvic cavity should be irrigated. Dermoid cysts and endometriomas are frequently bilateral (10% to 15%), and therefore this is not a distinguishing feature.

Assessment of solid ovarian lesions is more

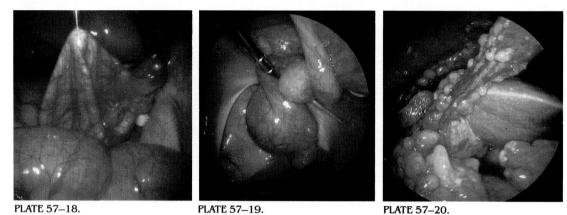

PLATE 57–18. PLATE 57–19. PLATE 57–20.

PLATE 57–18. Management of a parovarian cyst by needle aspiration.
PLATE 57–19. Spontaneous torsion of the fallopian tube. The tube is twisted on itself at least three times.
PLATE 57–20. Carcinoma of the ovary involving the falciform ligament and omentum.

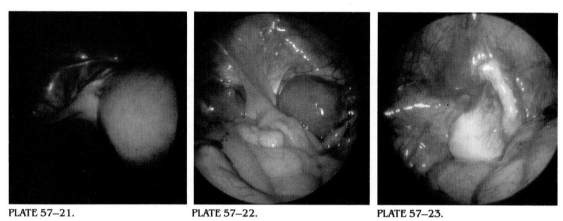

PLATE 57–21. PLATE 57–22. PLATE 57–23.

PLATE 57–21. Unicornuate uterus.
PLATE 57–22. Complete duplication of the genital tract, including two uteri separated by a fold of vesico-uterine peritoneum (uterus didelphys). There is also duplication of the cervix and a septate vagina.
PLATE 57–23. Rokitansky-Küster-Hauser syndrome. A rudimentary uterus is located on each pelvic sidewall, with no midline uterus formed. The fallopian tube and ovary are normal. The patient is endocrinologically normal with the only phenotypic stigma being vaginal agenesis.

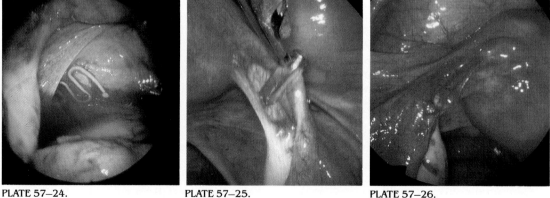

PLATE 57–24. PLATE 57–25. PLATE 57–26.

PLATE 57–24. A Lippes loop intrauterine contraceptive device lying free in the cul-de-sac.
PLATE 57–25. A tubal occlusive device (Filschie clip) for female sterilization. In time, the clip is often covered with a thin layer of peritoneum.
PLATE 57–26. Tubal occlusive Silastic ring (Falope ring) for female sterilization. This device has been in place for several months and is already covered with a peritoneal film. The fallopian tube has separated, with the proximal and distal stumps visible on either side of the ring.

difficult than that of cystic lesions. Benign and malignant ovarian disease may present as a solid ovarian tumor. In general, benign solid ovarian lesions are smooth and uniform. Ovarian fibromas are frequently white, firm excrescences on the surface of the ovary and do not grossly distort its architecture. As with cystic lesions, if the operator is uncertain as to the diagnosis, a gynecologist should be consulted at the time whenever possible. If this is impossible and the lesion appears to be unilateral and benign, a biopsy of the ovary may be taken, preferably with a Palmer biopsy drill forceps, although various types of punch biopsy forceps are also available.

Ovarian carcinoma is insidious. The presenting symptom may be only vague abdominal distention or anorexia. In such cases, endoscopy may disclose a significant volume of ascites. Observation is greatly facilitated by aspirating ascitic fluid prior to laparoscopy (insufflating carbon dioxide into ascitic fluid produces a "bubbling effect" similar to that which occurs when water is added to washing soap). If ascites is present, ovarian carcinoma is generally extensive with metastatic involvement of the entire pelvis and omentum and frequently the falciform ligament and even the liver (Plate 57–20).

Total removal or at least debulking of the tumor has importance in ovarian carcinoma in relation to survival rates and response to further therapy. Therefore, operability should be carefully assessed at laparoscopy, and a gynecologist should be consulted for this purpose, if at all possible at the time of the endoscopic procedure. Usually, biopsy specimens from multiple sites can be easily obtained, and electrocoagulation is not necessary. Aspiration of intra-abdominal fluid, even intraperitoneal washing with saline, for cytologic study is possible when early malignant disease is suspected but no gross lesions are present for biopsy. Occasionally, a very early lesion that proves to be malignant on biopsy will be an incidental finding on the surface of an ovary. In such cases, the survival rate is extremely high when the lesion is treated vigorously.

Genital Anomalies

Malformations of the uterus are common and should be recognized by the endoscopist, although no other management is necessary. The most frequently encountered abnormalities are failure of development of part of the uterus (unicornuate uterus) (Plate 57–21) and duplication of the genital tract (double uterus) (Plate 57–22). Midline uterine fusion defects are also seen (Plate 57–23); these are generally diagnosed early in life, since they are associated with primary amenorrhea and vaginal agenesis. Secondary sexual characteristics develop normally in all of these conditions, since ovarian function is unaffected. Ovarian anomalies are usually diagnosed early in life because of their endocrine manifestations with or without associated somatic abnormalities.

Foreign Bodies

The most frequently encountered foreign body of gynecologic origin in the pelvis is an intrauterine device (IUD) that has perforated the uterus. The device, if "nonmedicated, noncopper-containing," is generally seen lying free in the cul-de-sac (Plate 57–24). These devices rarely, if ever, cause symptoms or problems, especially if they are of the open configuration (Lippes loop). Closed configuration varieties (Bernberg bow) may result in bowel obstruction, but such devices are rarely used today. If a nonmedicated device is lying free in the cul-de-sac, it can be easily removed through the channel (3 or 5 mm) of an operating laparoscope or through a second puncture trocar using a grasping forceps.

Copper-containing IUDs cause considerable tissue reaction when they enter the peritoneal cavity and are generally involved in extensive adhesions with only the string of the device being visible. Firm traction, using a grasping forceps, on the string of such a device usually results in release of the IUD to the point where it can be removed laparoscopically. In some cases, adhesions around or attached to the device must be cut using a hook scissors to free it for removal, but this is rare.

Polyethylene tubal stents used for bridging anastomoses at the time of tubal surgery may be found in the pelvis. These usually cause no symptoms or problems. When discovered, they are usually lying free in the peritoneal cavity and are easily removed with a grasping forceps.

Tubal clips that have been used for sterilization may be encountered; it is only necessary to recognize and note the presence of these devices. The types most frequently employed for female sterilization are the Hulka,

Bleier and Filshie clips (Plate 57–25). The other type of mechanical occlusive sterilization device is the Silastic band or Falope ring (Plate 57–26). These foreign bodies are generally covered with a peritoneal overgrowth after they have been in place for some time, and thus they may not be clearly visible. Since mechanical occlusive devices for female sterilization are used extensively, their appear-

ance should be familiar to all who perform laparoscopy.

References

1. Phillips JM, ed. Laparoscopy. The American Association of Gynecologic Laparoscopists, Department of Publications, 1977.
2. Phillips JM, ed. Endoscopy in Gynecology. The American Association of Gynecologic Laparoscopists, Department of Publications, 1978.

INDEX

Note: Numbers in *italics* refer to illustrations; numbers followed by (t) indicate tables.